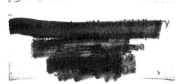

D1476365

Vascular
Anesthesia

Second Edition

Vascular Anesthesia

Edited by

Joel A. Kaplan, MD

Executive Vice President
Chancellor, Health Sciences Center
Professor of Anesthesiology
University of Louisville
Louisville, Kentucky

Associate Editors

Carol L. Lake, MD, MBA, MPH

Professor and Chair
Department of Anesthesiology and Perioperative Medicine
School of Medicine
University of Louisville
Louisville, Kentucky

Michael J. Murray, MD, PhD

Professor and Chair
Department of Anesthesiology
Mayo Clinic
Jacksonville, Florida

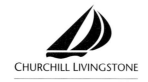

CHURCHILL LIVINGSTONE

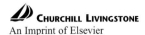
An Imprint of Elsevier

The Curtis Center
170 S Independence Mall W 300E
Philadelphia, Pennsylvania 19106

VASCULAR ANESTHESIA   ISBN 0-443-06620-5
Copyright © 2004, Elsevier, Inc. All rights reserved.

NOTICE

Anesthesiology is an ever-changing field. Standard safety precautions must be followed, but as new
research and clinical experience broaden our knowledge, changes in treatment and drug therapy
may become necessary or appropriate. Readers are advised to check the most current product information
provided by the manufacturer of each drug to be administered to verify the recommended dose, the method
and duration of administration, and contraindications. It is the responsibility of the treating physician,
relying on experience and knowledge of the patient, to determine dosages and the best treatment for each
individual patient. Neither the publisher nor the editor assumes any liability for any injury and/or damage
to persons or property arising from this publication.

Previous edition copyrighted 1991.

International Standard Book Number 0-443-06620-5

Vice President Global Surgery: Richard H. Lampert
Acquisitions Editor: Natasha Andjelkovic
Publishing Services Manager: Tina Rebane
Project Manager: Norm Stellander

Printed in the United States of America

Last digit is the print number: 9   8   7   6   5   4   3   2   1

To our families and loved ones for their support and understanding,

and

To the pioneers of vascular surgery and anesthesia.
They led the way for our students, who will continue the journey.

Joel A. Kaplan, MD
Carol L. Lake, MD, MBA, MPH
Michael J. Murray, MD, PhD

CONTRIBUTORS

Shihab U. Ahmed, MB, BS, MPH
Instructor, Department of Anesthesia,
Harvard Medical School;
Medical Director, Pain Clinic,
Department of Anesthesia and Critical Care,
Massachusetts General Hospital,
Boston, Massachusetts

Riva R. Akerman, MD
Clinical Instructor of Anesthesiology,
Department of Anesthesiology,
Columbia University,
New York, New York

Dimitri Arnaudov, MD
Assistant Professor in Clinical Anesthesiology,
Keck School of Medicine of the University of
Southern California;
Attending Anesthesiologist, University Hospital of the
University of Southern California,
Norris Cancer Center, and Los Angeles County and
University of Southern California Medical Center,
Los Angeles, California

Brian A. Aronson, MD
Assistant Professor of Radiology and
Chief, Vascular and Interventional Radiology,
University of Louisville Hospital,
Louisville, Kentucky

Perry Bechtle, DO
Department of Anesthesiology, Mayo Clinic,
Jacksonville, Florida

Maxim Benbassat, MD
Assistant Professor, Department of Anesthesiology,
Keck School of Medicine of the
University of Southern California;
Attending Anesthesiologist, Los Angeles County Medical
Center, Norris Cancer Institute, Doheny Eye Institute, and
University Hospital of the University of Southern California,
Los Angeles, California

Arnold J. Berry, MD, MPH
Professor of Anesthesiology, Emory University School of
Medicine; Anesthesiologist, Emory University Hospital,
Atlanta, Georgia

Kathleen H. Chaimberg, MD
Assistant Professor, Department of Anesthesiology and
Critical Care, Dartmouth Medical School, Hanover;
Attending Anesthesiologist and Director, Vascular
Anesthesia, Dartmouth Hitchcock Medical Center,
Lebanon, New Hampshire

Claudia Crawford, MD
Department of Anesthesiology, Mayo Clinic,
Jacksonville, Florida

Kevin C. Dennehy, MB, BCh, FFARCSI
Assistant Professor, Harvard Medical School, Boston;
Staff Anesthesiologist, North Shore Medical Center,
Salem, Massachusetts

Christine A. Doyle, MD
Staff Physician, O'Connor Hospital,
San Jose, California

Peter F. Dunn, MD
Instructor, Department of Anesthesia,
Harvard Medical School;
Clinical Director,
Department of Anesthesia and Critical Care,
Massachusetts General Hospital, Boston, Massachusetts

Marcel E. Durieux, MD, PhD
Professor of Anesthesiology,
University of Virginia, Charlottesville, Virginia;
Professor of Anesthesiology,
University of Maastricht,
Maastricht, The Netherlands

Lee A. Fleisher, MD
Professor and Chair,
Department of Anesthesiology,
University of Pennsylvania School of Medicine,
Philadelphia, Pennsylvania

Gligor Gucev, MD, MS
Assistant Professor, Keck School of Medicine
of the University of Southern California;
Anesthesiologist, Los Angeles County and University of
Southern California Medical Center and
Norris Cancer Institute,
Los Angeles, California

Yoogoo Kang, MD
Professor of Anesthesiology, Thomas Jefferson University;
Director, Hepatic Transplantation Anesthesiology,
Thomas Jefferson University Hospital,
Philadelphia, Pennsylvania

Mathai Kurien, MD
Instructor, Anesthesiology, Thomas Jefferson University;
Staff Anesthesiologist, Thomas Jefferson University Hospital,
Philadelphia, Pennsylvania

Christine Lallos, MD
Assistant Professor,
Department of Anesthesiology and Critical Care,
Emory University School of Medicine, Atlanta, Georgia

Catherine K. Lineberger, MD
Associate Professor of Anesthesiology,
Duke University Medical School;
Residency Program Director,
Department of Anesthesiology, Duke University Health System,
Durham, North Carolina

Philip D. Lumb, MB, BS, FCCM
Professor and Chairman, Department of Anesthesiology,
Keck School of Medicine of the
University of Southern California;
Attending Anesthesiologist, University Hospital of the
University of Southern California, Norris Cancer Center, and
Los Angeles County and University of Southern California
Medical Center, Los Angeles, California

Berend Mets, MB, ChB, PhD
Eric A. Walker Professor and Chair, Department of
Anesthesiology, Penn State College of Medicine, and
Penn State Milton S. Hershey Medical Center,
Hershey, Pennsylvania

Alexander Mittnacht, MD
Instructor, Anesthesiology, Mt. Sinai School of Medicine;
Assistant Attending Anesthesiologist, Mt. Sinai Medical
Center, New York, New York

Monica Myers Mordecai, MD
Instructor, Anesthesiology, Mayo Clinic College of
Medicine, Rochester, Minnesota;
Consultant, Department of Anesthesiology, Mayo Clinic,
Jacksonville, Florida

Michael J. Murray, MD, PhD
Professor, Mayo Medical School,
Rochester, Minnesota; Consultant and Chair,
Department of Anesthesiology, Mayo Clinic,
Jacksonville, Florida

Christopher J. O'Connor, MD
Associate Professor of Anesthesiology,
Rush-Presbyterian-St. Luke's Medical Center,
Rush Medical College, Chicago, Illinois

Ronald G. Pearl, MD, PhD
Professor and Chair, Department of Anesthesia,
Stanford University, Stanford, California

Imre Redai, MD
Assistant Professor of Anesthesiology,
Department of Anesthesiology,
Columbia University, New York, New York

David L. Reich, MD
Professor of Anesthesiology, Mt. Sinai School of Medicine;
Attending Anesthesiologist,
Vice-Chair for Academic Affairs, and
Co-Director of Cardiothoracic Anesthesia,
Mt. Sinai Medical Center, New York, New York

Paul Roekaerts, MD, PhD
Director of ICU, Department of Anesthesiology,
University Hospital, Maastricht, The Netherlands

Timothy S. J. Shine, MD
Assistant Professor,
Mayo Medical School, Rochester, Minnesota;
Consultant, Mayo Clinic, Jacksonville, Florida

Robert N. Sladen, MBCHB, MRCP (UK), FRCPC
Professor and Vice-Chair, Department of Anesthesiology,
College of Physicians and Surgeons of Columbia
University;
Director, Cardiothoracic and Surgical Intensive Care Units,
Columbia Presbyterian Hospital,
New York, New York

Mark Stafford Smith, MD, CM, FRCPC
Associate Professor and Director of Duke Cardiothoracic
Anesthesia and Critical Care Fellowship,
Department of Anesthesia,
Duke University Medical Center,
Durham, North Carolina

Danja Strümper, MD
Department of Anesthesiology
University of Münster Medical School,
Münster, Germany

Madhav Swaminathan, MBBS, MD
Assistant Clinical Professor of Anesthesiology,
Duke University Medical Center,
Durham, North Carolina

Christopher A. Troianos, MD
Chair and Program Director,
Department of Anesthesiology
Mercy Hospital of Pittsburgh,
Pittsburgh, Pennsylvania

Kenneth J. Tuman, MD
The Max Sadove Professor of Anesthesiology,
Rush Medical College;
Vice-Chair, Department of Anesthesiology,
Rush-Presbyterian-St. Luke's Medical Center,
Chicago, Illinois

Gail A. Van Norman, MD
Clinical Associate Professor, Department of Anesthesiology,
and Affiliate Associate Professor,
Department of Medical History and Ethics,
University of Washington, Seattle;
Staff Anesthesiologist, St. Joseph Medical Center,
Tacoma, Washington

Colleen Walker, DO
Resident, Department of Anesthesiology,
Mercy Hospital of Pittsburgh,
Pittsburgh, Pennsylvania

Mark P. Yeager, MD
Professor of Anesthesiology and Medicine,
Dartmouth Medical School, Hanover;
Dartmouth-Hitchcock Medical Center,
Lebanon, New Hampshire

PREFACE TO THE FIRST EDITION

THIS book was written to improve anesthesia care for all patients undergoing vascular surgery. Patients with cardiac disease undergoing vascular surgical procedures have benefitted from many of the innovations developed during cardiac surgery (eg, V_5 electrocardiographic lead), but still are often treated as second class citizens in many medical centers. Cardiac anesthesia and thoracic anesthesia are well-recognized fields; in these surgical procedures, anesthesia is usually managed by dedicated subspecialists who spend a large percentage of their time in these areas. Vascular anesthesia has been slower to develop its own identity, but clearly it has arrived. There are now dedicated subspecialists, clinical rotations by residents in the field, fellowship programs, exciting new procedures such as liver transplantation, increasing research, numerous textbooks, and the *Journal of Cardiothoracic and Vascular Anesthesia* that all recognize the field.

The content of this book ranges from preoperative management of the vascular surgical patient or the patient with cardiac disease undergoing major noncardiac surgery, through a selection of the anesthetic, monitoring, and cardiovascular support needed, to postoperative care of the patient in the intensive care unit. The book is organized into four parts, consisting of twenty-three chapters and hundreds of illustrations. The four major areas covered are (1) preoperative assessment and management; (2) cardiovascular physiology and pharmacology; (3) specific anesthetic considerations; and (4) postoperative management. The emphasis throughout is on using the most advanced monitoring techniques to determine the proper therapeutic interventions. All aspects of patient care are presented in the belief that preoperative and postoperative management of the patient are as important as intraoperative management.

The material in *Vascular Anesthesia* was written by the acknowledged experts in each specific area. It is the most authoritative and timely collection of material in the field. It is not a book that reflects one institutions's preference, or a "how to" management style, but instead is intended to provide the scientific foundation in each area as well as the clinical basis for practice. All the chapters have been coordinated in an effort to avoid unnecessary duplication and conflicting opinions, as much as possible, in such a diverse field as vascular anesthesia. Whenever possible, material has been integrated from other fields of anesthesiology, cardiology, cardiovascular pharmacol-ogy, vascular surgery, and critical care medicine to present a complete clinical picture. *Vascular Anesthesia* should serve as the definitive text in the field for anesthesia residents, vascular anesthesia fellows and attendings, cardiologists, vascular surgeons, intensivists, and others interested in the management of the patient for vascular surgery.

In conjunction with my other texts, *Cardiac Anesthesia* and *Thoracic Anesthesia, Vascular Anesthesia* now completes the triad and covers the full range of activities of the modern cardiovascular and thoracic anesthesiologist. Hopefully, it will futher contribute to the widespread application of the techniques and procedures that have been learned in the cardiac surgical operating rooms, which should increasingly be applied to the cardiac patient undergoing noncardiac surgery. This is a larger group of patients than those undergoing cardiac surgery, who are often sicker and will not have their underlying cardiac disease corrected by the operative procedure. In addition, they frequently are not as well evaluated preoperatively, monitored as well intraoperatively, or cared for in as intensive a manner in the postoperative period. Thus, this group continues to have a higher morbidity and mortality than cardiac surgical patients. Clearly, it is the field where we should put our greatest effort to improve patient care.

I gratefully acknowledge the contributions made by the authors of the individual chapters. They are the experts who have helped the field of vascular anesthesia to become established at the major medical centers and are the teachers of our young colleagues practicing anesthesiology around the world. This book would not have been possible without their hard work and expertise.

My sincere appreciation also goes to my secretaries, Joanie Esbri-Cullen and Margorie Fraticelli, whose long hours helped make this text a reality. In addition, thanks are in order for the staff of the contributing authors who sent us the original manuscripts from their institutions. My gratitude also goes to Toni Tracy, President of Churchill Livingstone Inc., for her support with this project, and David Terry for his hard work in putting together all the pieces of the book.

Finally, thanks again to Norma, with whom I just celebrated twenty-five years of dotting the I's and crossing the T's.

Joel A. Kaplan, MD

PREFACE TO THE SECOND EDITION

THE second edition of *Vascular Anesthesia* was written for the purpose of continuing to improve the perioperative management of patients undergoing noncardiac vascular surgery. Since the publication of the first edition in 1991, vascular surgery and the subspecialty of vascular anesthesia have continued to grow at a rapid pace. They have evolved from their empirical clinical roots focused on peripheral vascular surgery and amputation to today's evidence-based practices leading to multiple clinical choices, including advanced medical therapies, as well as minimally invasive and invasive surgical procedures. To maintain its place as the standard reference textbook in the field, this edition has been completely revised, expanded, and updated.

The material in this book was written by the acknowledged international authorities in each specific area related to vascular anesthesia. The authors come from leading academic departments of anesthesiology, critical care medicine, surgery, and radiology. This edition has added two associate editors: Carol L. Lake, MD, MBA, MPH, and Michael J. Murray, MD, PhD. They also serve as associate editors of the *Journal of Cardiothoracic and Vascular Anesthesia* along with the editor, Joel A. Kaplan, MD. They add particular areas of expertise in major vascular surgery, care of the cardiac patient, clinical monitoring, and postoperative management of noncardiac surgical patients with severe vascular disease.

The second edition of *Vascular Anesthesia* is the most comprehensive and up-to-date collection of material in the field. The multi-authored text provides authoritative information on a broad and comprehensive scale that is not possible in a single-authored book or one that describes the practices at a single medical institution. Each chapter aims to provide the scientific foundation from the literature in the area, as well as the clinical basis for practice. All of the chapters have been coordinated to minimize unnecessary duplication and conflicting opinions. Where possible, material has been integrated from the fields of anesthesiology, cardiology, vascular surgery, critical care medicine, and the basic sciences of anatomy, physiology, pharmacology, genetics, and molecular biology to present a complete clinical picture. Thus, the book should continue to serve as the definitive text in the field for anesthesia residents, vascular surgery and transplantation fellows and attendings, vascular surgeons, cardiologists, and others interested in the management of patients for noncardiac vascular surgery or patients with extensive vascular disease for any type of noncardiac surgery.

The content of this book ranges from the preoperative assessment of the vascular surgery patient, through the anesthetic and intraoperative management, to the postoperative care. Special emphasis has been placed throughout the book on three areas: (1) lowering cardiac risk by following the American College of Cardiology/American Heart Association Guidelines for Perioperative Cardiovascular Evaluation published in 2002; (2) reducing the extent of surgery by selecting radiologic vascular interventional procedures or minimally invasive surgery when appropriate; and (3) minimizing the stress of a surgical procedure by providing excellent perioperative pain control.

The book is organized into four parts consisting of 20 chapters with numerous tables and illustrations. The four major areas covered are (1) cardiovascular anatomy, physiology, and pharmacology; (2) preoperative assessment and management; (3) specific perioperative considerations; and (4) postoperative management. Throughout, cardiovascular physiology and pathophysiology are incorporated into the discussions of patient management during different vascular surgical procedures. The latest techniques and equipment utilized in newer forms of treatment such as vascular stenting, endovascular repairs, and thoracic epidural anesthesia are covered. All aspects of patient care are presented in the belief that preoperative and postoperative care is as important as intraoperative management.

In the first edition, Dr. Kaplan stated in the Preface that the text "... will contribute to the widespread application of the techniques and procedures that have been learned in the cardiac surgical operating room, which should increasingly be applied to the cardiac patient undergoing noncardiac surgery." This is certainly true today as well. In 1991, transesophageal echocardiography (TEE) was rarely being used outside of cardiac surgery, whereas today it is routinely used in many hospitals for patients with severe vascular disease. TEE with color-flow Doppler has even become the diagnostic procedure of choice for some types of thoracoabdominal aneurysms or aortic dissections. Another example of our rapid progress involves the pharmacologic management of patients with severe coronary artery disease (CAD) and/or congestive heart failure (CHF). These patients are now treated with new vasodilators, short-acting beta-blockers, and calcium channel blockers for their CAD; and new beta-blockers, ACE inhibitors, inodilators, and pacemakers/defibrillators for CHF. Finally, blood conservation in vascular surgery has incorporated many of the cardiac surgical techniques of autotransfusion and cell processing, as well as newer coagulation monitors and hemostatic agents like aprotinin.

The fields of bioethics, health policy, and health law have also become prominent in recent years and directly apply to high-risk patients undergoing extensive vascular surgical procedures. Therefore, a chapter written by an acknowledged expert, Gail A. Van Norman, MD, from the University of Washington, was added. She points out that anesthesiologists have always been prominent in dealing with issues of biomedical ethics. These contributions cover many of the most problematic ethical challenges of the 20th century, including mechanical ventilation during the polio epidemics, discontinuing life-sustaining care, abuses by medical researchers, and the development of institutional review boards to protect human subjects. Dealing with elderly, vascular surgical patients leads to ethical conflicts over autonomy and choice, competency, surrogate decision-making, limiting medical treatments (eg, DNR), allocation of scarce medical resources, end-of-life issues, and even assisted suicide. These areas all require our careful attention since they are particularly common and problematic in the care of the elderly vascular patient.

The editors gratefully acknowledge the contributions made by the authors of the individual chapters. They are the true experts who have made the field of vascular anesthesia come alive at the academic medical centers and are the teachers of our young colleagues practicing anesthesiology around the world. This book would not have been possible without their hard work and expertise.

Our sincere appreciation also goes to our administrative team of Daniel Alkofer, Connie Schenck, and Norma Kaplan, whose long hours helped make this text a reality. In addition, thanks are in order to the secretaries and assistants of the contributing authors who sent us the original manuscripts from their institutions. We would also like to thank Natasha Andjelkovic and Allan Ross of Elsevier who have made the transition from Churchill Livingstone to Elsevier so easy for all of us.

Joel A. Kaplan, MD
Carol L. Lake, MD, MBA, MPH
Michael J. Murray, MD, PhD

CONTENTS

Physiology and Pathophysiology of the Peripheral Circulation

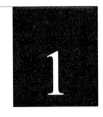

Danja Strümper, MD
Marcel E. Durieux, MD, PhD
Paul Roekaerts, MD, PhD

THIS chapter reviews the physiology of the peripheral circulation in health and in the setting of cardiovascular disease. Much of basic cardiovascular physiology has been known for many years and is well described in standard textbooks, including textbooks of anesthesia, and only a few key concepts are repeated here. Over the past 10 years, however, a wealth of new information has become available through cellular and molecular studies. Frequently, this new information has expanded the clinician's understanding; at times it has forced the reconsideration of some concepts that were accepted as dogma. Throughout this chapter, therefore, emphasis is placed on *cellular and molecular vascular physiology*, always keeping in mind in the presentation that this book is intended for the practicing clinician.

Introduction

The process of distributing oxygen and nutrients to the tissues and removing waste products from the tissues is regulated precisely. Major differences exist in the blood flow to various organs. For example, whereas inactive muscle receives 4 mL/min/100 g, the adrenal glands receive 300 mL/min/100 g. Despite these hundredfold differences in perfusion, under normal conditions supply closely matches demand; blood flow to each tissue is maintained such that tissue requirements are met, but little luxury perfusion takes place. The major exceptions to this rule are kidney and skin. The kidney receives very high blood flow (360 mL/min/100 g), much in excess of its metabolic requirements, for the specific purpose of allowing a large blood volume to be filtered each minute. Skin blood flow under cool conditions is very low (3 mL/min/100 g) but can be regulated over a wide range to allow dissipation of heat.

Redistribution of cardiac output (CO) among organs and tissues in the presence of modest changes in requirements is largely regulated at the local level. For example, blood flow to muscle may increase more than fourfold after a change from rest to exercise as a result of such local regulation. A variety of acute and long-term mechanisms are responsible for closely matching blood flow to metabolic need at organ, tissue, and cellular levels. This is observed most clearly in the brain, in which regional perfusion is tightly coupled to the rapidly changing metabolic activities in various areas. Under such conditions of relative stability, the main role of systemic regulatory

systems is restricted to maintaining constant CO and blood pressure.

In contrast, when major insults occur (hypoxia, hypovolemia) or major redistribution is necessary (as in the setting of heavy exercise), redistribution of blood flow can no longer be handled only at the local level. Major changes in CO occur, and blood flow at the organ level is profoundly redistributed, driven by central regulatory systems. Under circumstances of hypoxia or hypotension, the local responses at times may even be counterproductive and are likely to play a significant role in the pathophysiology of disease processes such as sepsis.

This chapter focuses on the interplay of various regulatory systems that together are responsible for maintenance of cellular metabolic homeostasis, both under normal conditions and in conditions of systemic insults and disease. After a brief review of vascular anatomy and physics, the mechanisms underlying short-term and longer term regulation of tissue blood flow are discussed. These largely take place at the tissue level itself. The vascular responses under two conditions of stress (hypoxia and ischemia) are then described. These two pathologic states were chosen as examples because they are common endpoints of a variety of processes, and, in addition, are of obvious clinical relevance. Finally, the functioning and malfunctioning of these systems in the setting of various cardiovascular disease states are discussed. At the end of the chapter, a brief review of the actions of anesthetics on the circulatory system is provided.

Anatomy of the Peripheral Circulation

In this section, the structure of the vascular system is briefly reviewed. The various types of vessels and the relation of their anatomic structure to their function are discussed. Specific attention is paid to the main cellular components of the vessel wall: the endothelium and the vascular smooth muscle.

Types of Vessels

The peripheral circulatory system can be anatomically divided into arteries, arterioles, capillaries, venules, veins, and lymphatics (Figure 1-1).

The *arteries* distribute the blood to the organs and function under high pressure (mean 100 mmHg). Large phasic pressure changes are created in the left ventricle. The elastic properties of the aorta and large arteries allow them to expand rapidly as the stroke volume of blood enters. This expansion permits

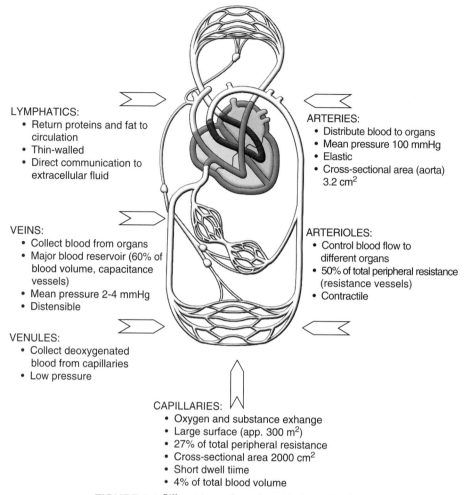

LYMPHATICS:
- Return proteins and fat to circulation
- Thin-walled
- Direct communication to extracellular fluid

ARTERIES:
- Distribute blood to organs
- Mean pressure 100 mmHg
- Elastic
- Cross-sectional area (aorta) 3.2 cm^2

VEINS:
- Collect blood from organs
- Major blood reservoir (60% of blood volume, capacitance vessels)
- Mean pressure 2-4 mmHg
- Distensible

ARTERIOLES:
- Control blood flow to different organs
- 50% of total peripheral resistance (resistance vessels)
- Contractile

VENULES:
- Collect deoxygenated blood from capillaries
- Low pressure

CAPILLARIES:
- Oxygen and substance exhange
- Large surface (app. 300 m^2)
- 27% of total peripheral resistance
- Cross-sectional area 2000 cm^2
- Short dwell tiime
- 4% of total blood volume

FIGURE 1-1 Different types of vessels and their specifications.

them to store blood transiently; the blood is then passed onward during diastole, thereby maintaining blood flow (Windkessel effect). The arteries are the vessels most susceptible to atherosclerosis.

The smallest branches of the arteries, the *arterioles*, have relatively thick muscular walls, function as the major site of resistance (*resistance vessels*), and can be considered as regulating valves that control the blood flow to different tissues. Arterioles determine up to 50% of the total peripheral resistance (TPR). In hypertension, their contractile state is increased.

The *capillaries* facilitate the oxygen and substance exchange to the tissue by diffusion and ultrafiltration through their large surface (approximately 300 m^2). Distribution within the capillary bed is regulated by precapillary sphincters, which contain some smooth muscle. Even if their diameter is much smaller than that of the arterioles (5 to 7 μm, just sufficient to accommodate red cells), they contribute less than 30% of the TPR because of their large total number, approximately 5×10^9, resulting in a cross-sectional area of 2000 cm^2 (which should be compared with the 3.2 cm^2 cross section of the aortae). Capillaries are short. As a result, even though capillary flow is sluggish (0.05 cm/s), the dwell time of red cells in a capillary

is on the order of only several seconds, and only 4% of the total blood volume is contained within this vascular bed.

Venules form the low-pressure collecting system for venous (deoxygenated) blood leaving the capillaries.

The *veins* collect blood from the organs and form the major blood reservoir (approximately 60% of blood volume). Because of their distensibility, they can accommodate large changes in blood volume with rather small changes in pressure (*capacitance vessels*). They, as well as the lung and portal circulation, belong to the low-pressure system (2 to 4 mmHg).

Finally, *lymphatics* are thin-walled channels in direct communication with extracellular fluid. They serve to return proteins and fat to the circulation but are not connected in sequence with the main blood vessels of the body.

This classic division of the various components of the vascular tree is based largely on anatomic considerations. Functionally, it has become clear that a considerable overlap exists among various segments. For example, later in this chapter, how arterioles take an active part in the diffusion of nutrients and metabolic gases to the tissues is described. Another example of overlapping function is regulation of blood supply to capillaries not only by feeding arterioles but also by precapillary sphincters.

Structure of the Vessel Wall

The walls of arteries and veins consist basically of three layers: *tunica intima*, *tunica media*, and *tunica externa* (*adventitia*) (Figure 1-2). Their structure varies throughout the vascular tree, largely determined by function and strain (caused by blood pressure). For example, two types of arteries can be histologically distinguished: those close to the heart and those located peripherally. Arteries close to the heart contain numerous elastic fibers and membranes in their wall (*elastic arteries*), whereas arteries located peripherally are enriched in smooth muscle cells (*muscular arteries*), which surround the vascular pipe in a spiral pattern.

The *intima* consists of the endothelium, a coherent single layer of flat cells (to be described in more detail later), and the subendothelial connective tissue, which contains fine collagen fibers and elastic nets. In addition, longitudinally directed smooth muscle cells occur in elastic arteries. The subendothelial connective tissue is missing at the arteriolar and capillary level. Transport vesicles, transepithelial channels, and covered and uncovered pores exist in and between the endothelial cells—which are otherwise connected closely by tight gap junctions—and facilitate transport of substances, particles, and leukocytes.

The *media* is composed of predominantly circularly arranged smooth muscle cells, collagen, and elastic fibers. The amount of each component depends on vessel function and is specific for particular vascular segments. The media absorbs the circular and longitudinal stress generated by mean blood pressure and the arterial pressure wave, and therefore facilitates regular blood flow.

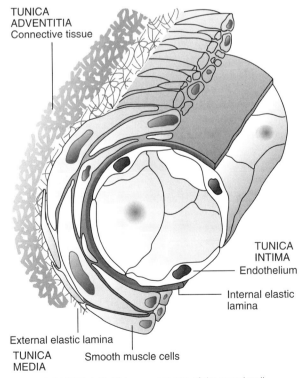

FIGURE 1-2 Major components of the vessel wall.

TUNICA ADVENTITIA Connective tissue

TUNICA INTIMA Endothelium

Internal elastic lamina

External elastic lamina

TUNICA MEDIA Smooth muscle cells

The *adventitia* is a dense network of collagen fibers with a variable content of elastic nets. It contains the vasa vasorum and nerve fibers and fixes the vessel in the surrounding tissue.

The most important cellular components of the vessel wall are the *endothelium* and the *vascular smooth muscle*.

ENDOTHELIUM. The vascular endothelium, a continuous cellular monolayer lining the blood vessels, is now known to be much more than a purely anatomic entity or a passive barrier between blood and tissue. Instead, the endothelium is an important organ with a variety of functions. It plays a range of important homeostatic roles. It participates in highly active metabolic and regulatory systems, including control of primary hemostasis, blood coagulation and fibrinolysis, platelet and leukocyte interactions with the vessel wall, lipoprotein metabolism, presentation of histocompatibility antigens, regulation of vascular tone and growth, and regulation of blood pressure. It possesses numerous receptors and releases compounds that either directly or through the release of other compounds actively participate in the regulation of vascular tone and contribute to vascular permeability.

Many crucial vasoactive endogenous compounds such as prostacyclin, thromboxane, bradykinin, nitric oxide, endothelin, angiotensin, endothelium-derived hyperpolarizing factor, and free radicals are formed in the endothelial cells to control the functions of vascular smooth muscle cells and of circulating blood cells. Gap junctions facilitate exchange of metabolites, ions, and other messenger molecules among endothelial cells and smooth muscle cells and regulate cell growth. Endothelial substances act primarily locally and exhibit relaxing, constricting, or mitogenic effects. In fact, most factors exert relaxing as well as constricting effects, depending on basal vessel tone, concentration, region within the vascular bed, distribution of receptor subtypes, and interaction with other transmitters. Interpretation of effects is even more difficult as studies examining this field use different methodologies (e.g., different preparation techniques, different vascular regions, different species, different preconstricting agents, different agonists and antibodies). All of this makes simplistic statements about the roles of various compounds in vascular regulation difficult to make and frequently untrue.

Considering the size of the vascular tree, the endothelium is a small organ. If all of the vessels were put together (arteries, arterioles, capillaries, veins, and lymphatics), they would stretch to a length of 600 miles, yet their endothelial lining would weigh only 1.5 kg. However, the endothelium has an enormous surface area; the endothelial cells lining the vascular tree would cover an area equivalent to an entire football field.

VASCULAR SMOOTH MUSCLE. The vascular smooth muscle occupies the middle portion of the blood vessel wall. Smooth muscle cells are arranged in muscle bundles, each of which forms an effector unit. *Nexus junctions* are sites for electrical coupling between cells. Other junctions serve to transmit tension information to the regulatory system.

These cells have a low resting transmembrane potential (−40 to −60 mV). Excitation occurs as a result of induced alterations in this membrane potential. Levels of intracellular calcium determine the contractile state of vascular smooth muscle. Many vasoactive substances, compounds elaborated by endothelial cells (such as endothelium-derived relaxing factor), as well as temperature, alter the force of muscular contraction by changing intracellular calcium concentrations. Norepinephrine and other vasoactive hormones may induce depolarization and increase the frequency of contraction. However, pharmacologic effects can clearly occur without changes in membrane depolarization, indicating that alterations in membrane permeability, resulting in changes in calcium levels, are important.

A variable degree of basal tone is maintained by a low rate of sympathetic nerve discharge, controlling precapillary sphincters. It should be realized that the degree of sympathetic control varies greatly among regions. This is most clearly shown by the effect of sympathectomy. Regions such as skin have powerful sympathetic control but a low resting tone and, therefore, show little effect of sympathectomy. In brain and heart, resting tone is greater but is in part regulated by metabolic autoregulation; these organs therefore still demonstrate a significant degree of intrinsic tone after sympathectomy.

Blood

Blood can be considered a "liquid tissue." It consists of plasma (intercellular fluid) and corpuscles (cells). Blood serves many functions, but its first task is substance transport. It supplies the cells of the body with nutrients and oxygen and removes metabolites and carbon dioxide. It distributes the products of endocrine glands throughout the body and coordinates—together with the nervous system—organ function. In addition, it is greatly involved in temperature regulation and host defense.

In adults, the total blood volume amounts to approximately $\frac{1}{12}$ of the body weight and consists of 45% corpuscular and 55% fluid components. The fluid part—the plasma—contains approximately 8% protein, of which about half is albumin. Albumin determines the colloid osmotic pressure and serves as a transport medium. In addition, the plasma contains fibrinogen and immunoglobulins.

The corpuscular part of the blood can be divided into erythrocytes, leukocytes, and platelets. The total blood volume of approximately 5 L contains 25 billion *erythrocytes* with a total surface area of 3000 to 4000 m^2. This considerable surface is important for their role in transporting oxygen and carbon dioxide. The iron-bound hemoglobin forms 95% of the dry weight of an erythrocyte. Its average life span is 120 days. *Leukocytes* can be divided into granulocytes (neutrophil, eosinophil, and basophil according to their staining properties), lymphocytes, and monocytes, with a relatively fixed percentage distribution. Most of the leukocytes in fact reside outside the bloodstream, where they are responsible for a major part of the host defense in different tissues and organs. They are able to perform ameboid movements, cross capillary walls, and move within tissues or back into the bloodstream. Their life span varies between days and years but is usually shorter than that of erythrocytes. *Platelets* are poorly staining and very sensitive particles with an average life span of 5 to 10 days. Endothelial lesions lead to aggregation and breakdown of platelets, thereby initiating the coagulation process (see Chapter 15).

Physics of the Peripheral Circulation

In a sense, physical laws couple the structure of the vessel wall to its functional effects. This section briefly reviews some of the major concepts in vascular physics: tension and stress in the vessel wall, filtration and diffusion, and the physical determinants of blood flow through the vascular tree.

Tension and Stress in Vascular Walls

It is important to differentiate between *stress* and *tension* within the vessel wall. Stress (σ) refers to the force *per unit wall area* in a circumferential direction and is calculated as

$$\sigma = rp/h$$

where r = internal radius, p = internal pressure, and h = wall thickness. Tension (t) refers to the force *per unit wall length* and is calculated as

$$t = \sigma h = rp$$

A vessel with a smaller radius has a mechanical advantage in terms of the tension that can be borne by the vessel wall; a capillary with its very small diameter and relatively thick wall can support greater intravascular pressures with low stress, whereas the aorta, with its large radius and relatively thin wall, is subjected to a higher tension. Even greater wall tension occurs in the setting of aortic aneurysms.

Blood vessels do not obey Hooke's law (which states that in stretched elastic material, tension is proportional to the degree of elongation). Instead, when blood vessels are stretched, they increasingly resist stretch. Thus, blood vessels develop a higher tension as they are distended (becoming stiffer or less compliant). The mechanism behind this property derives from their histologic structure. Initial stretching affects only elastic fibers (which obey Hooke's law). At a certain point, however, collagen fibers (fibrous tissue) are stretched to straight fibers, resulting in a stiffer vessel. At this point, small increases in length induce great changes in tension.

The peripheral circulation has a critical closing pressure; at low perfusion pressures flow stops completely, although arterial pressure is still higher than venous pressure (Figure 1-3).

Diffusion

Transcapillary transport takes place through diffusion, filtration, and a number of mechanisms (such as pinocytosis) designed specifically for transfer of larger molecules. The movement of fluid in and out of the capillaries is largely governed by hydrostatic pressure and colloid osmotic pressure (filtration).

The driving force for diffusional transport is a concentration gradient. Small lipid-soluble molecules (such as carbon dioxide and oxygen) move freely through endothelial cells and capillary pores. Water and water-soluble materials move through water channels in clefts (pores or slits). For small water-soluble molecules (such as sodium chloride or glucose), pore size is not important, and diffusion is flow limited. Larger molecules (such as sucrose, with a molecular mass of 358 daltons) are limited by pore size. Macromolecules (such as antibodies) are not effectively transported by diffusion.

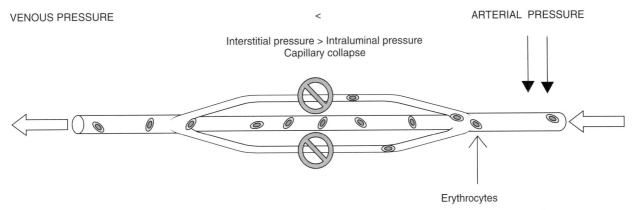

FIGURE 1-3 Critical closing pressure. If the arteriolar pressure drops below a critical value (dependent on tissue, between 10 and 30 mmHg), capillary vessels collapse (elastic tension, may be actively increased) and blood flow stops completely because interstitial pressure exceeds intraluminal pressure and the driving force to push a 7-μm erythrocyte through a 5-μm capillary is too low.

Five factors determine total diffusional flux (M): intercapillary distance, blood flow, concentration gradient for the solute, capillary permeability, and capillary surface area. The classic description of diffusion is by Fick's law:

$$M = DA/T(C_i - C_o)$$

where D = free diffusion coefficient for the substance (related to molecular weight), A = capillary surface area, T = thickness of the membrane (inversely proportional to diffusion rate), and $C_i - C_o$ = concentration difference for the substance inside to outside the vessel. Fick's law can be simplified in some settings. For example, for thin-walled vessels, it can effectively be stated as

$$M = PS(C_i - C_o)$$

where P = permeability and S = surface area of the capillary. For readily diffusible substances, for which diffusion is flow limited, it can be stated as

$$M = Q(C_a - C_v)$$

where Q is flow and $C_a - C_v$ = arteriovenous concentration difference.

Filtration

Filtration is fluid movement resulting from a hydrostatic or osmotic pressure difference across a membrane (Figure 1-4). This movement is in contrast to diffusion, which depends only on concentration gradients. Hsowever, pressure gradients can also result from concentration gradients. Plasma protein (primarily albumin and globulin) concentrations are 6 to 8 g/100 mL in blood and 0.7 to 2 g/100 mL in interstitium. These compounds are restricted in their free transport across the endothelium and therefore produce a colloid osmotic pressure, which is primarily determined by the number of molecules in solution. Seventy-five percent of the colloid osmotic pressure results from albumin (molecular weight 69,000); the remainder is due largely to globulins.

The filtration rate is determined by several factors. The *filtration coefficient* for a given capillary wall depends on the

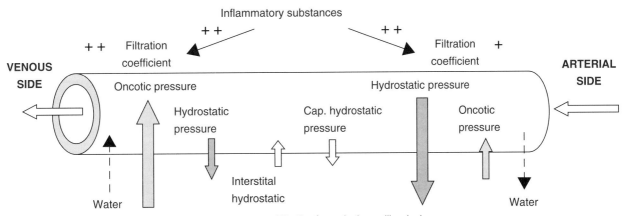

FIGURE 1-4 Filtration forces in the capillary bed.

tissue and varies under different physiologic conditions. It is usually lower on the arterial than on the venous side of the circulation because of different endothelial properties. Inflammatory substances (such as histamine) greatly enhance the filtration coefficient across the endothelium. The *capillary hydrostatic pressure* can be modified by capillary resistance vessels. The *interstitial fluid hydrostatic pressure* is usually close to zero but can be substantially positive in settings of severe edema. The final factors are *colloid osmotic pressure* in plasma and in interstitial fluid.

Starling's law describes the process of filtration:

$$FM = K(P_c + \pi_i - P_i - \pi_c)$$

where FM = fluid movement, K = filtration coefficient of capillary wall, P_c = hydrostatic pressure in the capillaries, P_i = hydrostatic pressure in interstitial fluid, π_c = oncotic pressure in the plasma, and π_i = oncotic pressure in the interstitial fluid.

Determinants of Blood Flow

This section briefly describes some of the major physical parameters determining blood flow through the vascular tree.

Blood flow can be significantly affected by *viscosity*. Plasma is a viscous solution. In addition, flow properties of blood can be affected by cellular components. Of these, erythrocytes are most important rb or rd as they form 99.9% of the circulating cell population and approximately 40% of blood volume. White blood cells may also play an important role in blood flow through the microcirculation and capillaries, especially in low-flow states (ischemia). In such a suspension, the apparent viscosity of blood changes considerably, depending upon the velocity of blood flow, the hematocrit, and the size of the blood vessel. Whereas a Newtonian fluid (such as water) shows constant viscosity at any flow velocity, blood behaves like a non-Newtonian fluid: viscosity changes with flow velocity. *Reynolds' number* (Nr) is a measure of viscous force (technically, it states the ratio of inertial over viscous forces) and varies widely through the circulation. It can be calculated as

$$Nr = VD\rho/n\varepsilon$$

where V = mean velocity, D = tube diameter, ρ = fluid density, and nε = fluid viscosity. Nr is approximately 1000 in large arteries and 10^{-3} in capillaries (where inertial forces are negligible). At low Nr, flow is essentially laminar. When Nr exceeds approximately 3000, turbulent flow occurs. In blood, because of its high viscosity, turbulence tends to be limited. However, it is responsible for such phenomena as the Korotkoff sounds and heart murmurs. Turbulent flow results in flow decreases related to viscous and kinetic losses of energy. It also increases shear stress and strain at the vascular wall and is therefore an important factor promoting atherosclerotic lesions at certain points in the arteries.

A Newtonian fluid, flowing with laminar flow through a cylinder (and neglecting inertial force and gravitational forces), exhibits a parabolic velocity profile, with greatest velocity in the center and assumed zero velocity at the boundary with the wall. As a result, in blood, the layers next to the vessel wall are relatively cell free, leading to lower hematocrits in small blood vessels (known as the Fahraeus-Lindqvist effect).

Blood flow is also influenced greatly by *vascular resistance*. Like Ohm's law for electrical currents:

$$Q = P_a - P_v/R$$

where Q = flow, P_a and P_v = arterial and venous pressures, and R = resistance. Conversely:

$$Conductance = 1/R$$

Poiseuille's law shows the influence of the combination of the various parameters discussed:

$$Q = \pi(P_1 - P_2)r^4/8nL$$

where Q = flow, π = constant, P_1 and P_2 = upstream and downstream pressures, respectively, r = vessel radius, n = viscosity, and L = vessel length. This formula shows the enormous influence of radius: a 16-fold increase in flow takes place if radius doubles. Flow is halved if viscosity or length of the tube doubles. Poiseuille's law explains why a 14-gauge intravenous catheter is so much better for volume resuscitation than an 18-gauge (and much longer) central venous catheter.

If those factors that influence resistance are considered separately, resistance in blood can be calculated from Poiseuille's law:

$$R = 8Ln/\pi r^4$$

However, as is usual in biologic systems, the situation in the vascular bed is more complicated, as the pressure-flow relationship is nonlinear. As pressure increases, the vessel dilates and, therefore, flow increases exponentially; as pressure rises, resistance falls.

Short-Term Regulation Of The Peripheral Circulation

The goal of short-term cardiovascular regulation is to provide an optimal blood supply throughout the body under resting as well as under changing environmental and stress conditions. Blood flow has to be distributed because a maximal blood supply to all organs would overtax the capacity of the heart. A minimum supply of blood to all organs has to be maintained, cardiac function and vascular tone optimized, and blood flow diverted toward active organ systems (muscles, heart, lung, brain), sometimes at the expense of other organs (gastrointestinal tract, kidneys, skin). In essence, blood supply to individual organs is mainly controlled by changes in vascular diameter at the arteriolar level. However, a vast number of mechanisms exist that act in concert (or at times against each other) to bring about the appropriate level of vasoconstriction. Because most of these pathways are regulated by receptor-activated signaling systems, the major signaling compounds and associated signaling pathways are reviewed.

Central Nervous System Regulation

Central nervous control of the circulation is mainly coordinated in the medulla oblongata, where the neuronal afferents from pressure and volume receptors (see later) enter the central nervous system (CNS). These afferents are integrated with afferents from the respiratory system and, in addition, receive input from pain and thermal receptors in the reticular formation by so-called circulation-controlling neurons. These, in turn, are connected to higher systems (such as the hypothalamus and cortex) and convert peripheral as well as central afferent input into sympathetic and parasympathetic efferent activity to the heart and vascular system. Some parts of the cerebral cortex, such as the top integration level, can regulate vegetative functions (sympathetic activity) in an anticipatory manner.

Neuronal reflex systems regulate the blood pressure for short-term stabilization and to attenuate fluctuations, for example, in response to changes in posture. In addition, these regulatory systems play critical roles in the response to systemic insults such as hypovolemia.

The central reflex system consists of pressure receptors located in the carotid sinus and aortic arch and, together with afferents from volume receptors, transmits through the glossopharyngeal and vagus nerves on the afferent side and through the sympathetic systems and vagus nerve on the efferent side. The relationship between nerve traffic and carotid sinus pressure is sigmoid in shape. The slope (gain) between impulse frequency and mean blood pressure is maximal at a normal mean arterial pressure, and this level is tightly controlled. In contrast, pressures below 50 mmHg are not sensed. These receptors are also sensitive to the rate of change of pressure.

Cardiopulmonary or volume receptors play an important role in short- and long-term volume regulation. They are located in the low-pressure system of the circulation—vena cava, both atria, and the pulmonary arteries—and can be differentiated into A-type and B-type receptors: the A-type receptors react mainly to atrial contraction and the more important B-type receptors react to passive atrial filling. Activation of these receptors induces release of natriuretic peptides—ANP, BNP, and CNP. ANP and BNP are synthesized in the atrium and CNP in endothelial cells. ANP inhibits renin and aldosterone secretion, endothelin production, proliferation of vascular smooth muscle cells, and myocardial hypertrophy; it also has sympatholytic properties.[1,2] It can be considered an endogenous antagonist of the renin-angiotensin-aldosterone system (RAAS).

Transducing the nerve impulses that form the output of the CNS regulatory system to changes in heart rate and resistance of the peripheral circulation is the task of adrenergic and cholinergic signaling systems. Norepinephrine released from sympathetic nerve endings and acetylcholine released from vagal efferents act on cognate receptor systems in the heart and vessel wall.

ADRENERGIC SYSTEMS. The vasoconstrictive adrenergic system maintains the resting tone of arterioles. It exerts strong control over capacitance vessels and thereby has the ability to alter preload. Its functional role is the short-term homeostasis of blood pressure and flow, including the reflex adjustments that arise from baroreceptor and chemoreceptor stimulation.

The division of adrenoceptors into two types—α and β—was first proposed by Ahlquist in 1948. To date, nine subtypes have been characterized using radioligand binding studies and confirmed by functional studies and molecular cloning. Adrenoceptors are present not only in pre- and postjunctional nerve endings but also in the endothelium. Cocks and Angus

showed that α_2-agonist–induced vascular relaxation was eliminated by removal of the endothelium.[3] Activation of endothelial α_2-adrenoceptors (coupled to G_i proteins) stimulates the release of nitric oxide, thereby attenuating vasoconstriction caused by activated postjunctional α_1-adrenoceptors.[4-6] $\alpha_{2A/D}$-Adrenoceptors are the primary subtype involved in mediating endothelium-dependent relaxation.[7] In contrast to pre- and postjunctional α_2-adrenoceptors, cyclic adenosine monophosphate (cAMP) is not involved in the cascade of endothelial α_2-adrenoceptor intracellular signaling.[8] Activation of endothelial β-adrenoceptors, predominantly β_2-adrenoceptors, promotes nitric oxide production (with increased cAMP and cyclic guanosine monophosphate [cGMP]) and release, leading to vasodilation (Figure 1-5).[9-11]

The distribution of the different adrenoceptors depends critically on their location within the vasculature. α-Adrenoceptors are predominant in renal and skin vessels, whereas β-adrenoceptors predominate in splanchnic and skeletal muscle vasculature. Distribution of the norepinephrine-sensitive α_2-adrenoceptors in arteries of the human limbs decreases from distal to proximal, and α_2-adrenoceptor–mediated responses are absent in larger arteries. Large coronary vessels possess both α- and β-adrenoceptors, whereas small vessels of the coronary circulation possess only β-adrenoceptors. Cerebral vessels express only a limited number of α-adrenoceptors, decreasing further with diminishing vessel diameter (human pial arteries do not respond to nerve stimulation). This difference explains, in part, why the cerebral circulation is largely exempted from vasoconstriction after sympathetic stimulation (such as in the setting of hypovolemia). Table 1-1 provides an overview of the different types of adrenoceptors and their signaling pathways (see Figure 1-5). Although much is known about distribution, regulation, and signaling pathways, the clinical implications of these findings are largely unclear.

α_1-Adrenoceptors. α_1-Adrenoceptors play a pivotal role in the regulation of vascular tone. They can be divided into three subtypes: α_{1A}, α_{1B}, and α_{1D}.[12-16] They signal mainly through $G_{q/11}$ proteins and thereby stimulate phospholipase C, thus increasing levels of inositol triphosphate (IP_3) and diacylglycerol (DAG). This increase in IP_3 and DAG results in intracellular calcium release from nonmitochondrial pools and activation of protein kinase C.[17-19] In addition, activation of other signaling pathways (calcium influx, arachidonic acid release, phospholipase D, and mitogen-activated protein kinase) has been demonstrated.[18] Regulation of the subtypes differs; prolonged exposure to the α_1-agonist phenylephrine elicited a downregulation of the α_{1A}- and α_{1B}-adrenoceptors but a time- and concentration-dependent upregulation of the α_{1D}-adrenoceptor.[20] At the moment it is not clear whether such differential sensitivity has clinical implications. Although in vitro and in vivo studies have not yielded uniform results, it has been suggested that α_{1A}- and α_{1D}-adrenoceptors predominate in regulation of vascular smooth muscle tone at the postjunctional level.[21]

α_2-Adrenoceptors. α_2-Adrenoceptors can also be divided into three subtypes: $\alpha_{2A/D}$, α_{2B}, and α_{2C}.[22] Pharmacologic studies have shown that different α_2-adrenoceptor antagonists possess different potency and/or affinity for the different α_2-adrenoceptor

- α_2- Adrenoceptor
- β_3- Adrenoceptor
- A_1- Adenosine receptor

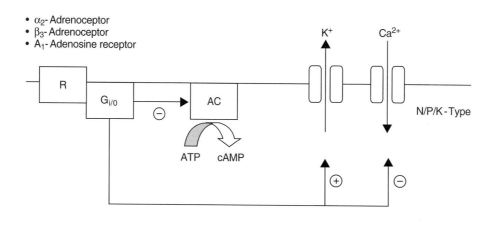

- $\beta_{1/2/3}$- Adrenoceptor
- $A_{2A/B}$- Adenosine receptor

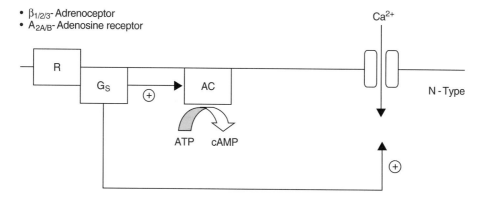

- $\alpha_{1A/1B/1D}$- Adrenoceptor
- A_3- Adenosine receptor
- M_3-Muscarinic receptor

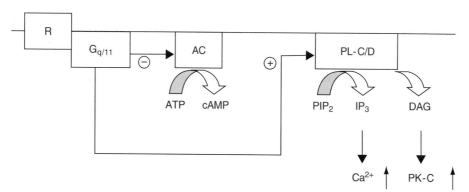

FIGURE 1-5 G protein–coupled receptor signaling pathways: R, receptor; G_i, G_S, $G_{q/11}$, coupled G protein; AC, adenylate cyclase; ATP, adenosine triphosphate; cAMP, cyclic adenosine monophosphate; PL-C/D, phospholipase-C/D; PIP_2, phosphatidylinositol bisphosphate; IP_3, inositol triphosphate; DAG, diacylglycerol; PK-C, protein kinase C; K^+ and Ca^{2+}, channels; +, stimulation; −, inhibition.

subtypes, allowing a degree of selective inhibition.[23-26] α_2-Adrenoceptors predominantly couple to G_i proteins, thus inhibiting adenylate cyclase, opening voltage-gated calcium channels,[27] and activating potassium channels.[27-29] They are also involved in sodium/hydrogen exchange and activation of phospholipases A_2, C, and D.[27] Although α_{2C}-adrenoceptors are not downregulated by exposure to agonists, $\alpha_{2A/D}$- and α_{2B}-adrenoceptors are as a result of desensitization, internalization, and sequestration.[30,31]

Although α_2-adrenoceptors (primarily $\alpha_{2A/D}$, mediating central negative feedback control of blood pressure) are found in almost all vascular tissue at the prejunctional level (although predominating in veins), they are virtually absent in arterial vessels at the postjunctional level.[32-35]

β-Adrenoceptors. β-Adrenoceptors can be divided into three subtypes: β_1, β_2, and β_3.[15] The pharmacology of β_3-adrenoceptors is distinct from that of β_1- and β_2-adrenoceptors.[36,37] All three subtypes couple to G_s proteins, thus activating adenylate

TABLE 1-1
Adrenoceptors and Their Signaling Mechanisms

Adrenoceptor	Coupled G Protein	Intracellular Transduction
α_1	Predominantly $G_{q/11}$ protein	Stimulation of phospholipase C, inositol triphosphate ⇑, diacylglycerol ⇑, intracellular Ca^{2+} release, activation of phospholipase C
α_2	G_i protein	Inhibition of adenylate cyclase, inhibition of voltage-gated Ca^{2+} channels, activation of K^+ channels
β_{1-3}	G_s protein (G_i protein)	Activation of adenylate cyclase, cAMP ⇑, protein kinase A ⇑, Ca^{2+} influx ⇑

cAMP, cyclic adenosine monophosphate.

cyclase, increasing cAMP, and facilitating calcium influx.[38-41] However, β-adrenoceptors (the β_3 subtype in particular) have been found to couple to G_i as well.[42,43] Termination of signaling involves protein binding, desensitization, and sequestration of the G protein–coupled receptor.[44,45]

In most vascular smooth muscle, postjunctional β_2-adrenoceptors predominate. Exceptions are coronary and cerebral arteries, in which β_1-adrenoceptors are the most prominent subtype.[46-48] β-Adrenoceptor–mediated relaxation markedly depends on the preexisting tone of the vessel, such as that induced by α-adrenoceptor–mediated constriction.[47,49]

CHOLINERGIC SYSTEMS. Five muscarinic receptors have been cloned (M_1 to M_5). The functional significance of the M_5 subtype is still unclear, but the other subtypes play major roles in a variety of signaling systems, ranging as widely as bronchial tone, consciousness, learning, and cardiac control. The role of muscarinic receptors in the heart is relatively straightforward; a single subtype is primarily involved, the M_2 receptor, which is located primarily on cardiac atrial tissue and to a lesser degree on ventricular tissue. It couples to a G_K protein (a G_i subtype) and induces opening of a potassium channel, thereby stabilizing the membrane potential (see Figure 1-5). This results in profound decreases in heart rate and modest decreases in inotropic state. In the peripheral vasculature M_3 is the dominant subtype; it causes nitric oxide– and endothelium-derived hyperpolarizing factor–mediated endothelium-dependent vasodilation.

Local Regulation

Local regulation of blood flow essentially serves two major purposes. In the first place, it matches the blood flow into a tissue region with the local metabolic demand (*flow-metabolism coupling*). In the second place, it adapts regional blood flow to changes in arterial pressure (*autoregulation*). In the presence of increased systemic pressure, limiting flow protects the tissue; when systemic pressure decreases, the microvasculature dilates to allow sufficient blood flow for its metabolic needs. Obviously, these two major roles are interwoven, and the same signaling systems play a role in both. Indeed, they are almost two sides of the same coin. For practical reasons, however, they are discussed separately. In addition, the primary signaling sys-

tems responding to vascular injury, which is also a local event, are discussed.

FLOW-METABOLISM COUPLING. The main role of the local regulatory mechanisms is to match regional blood flow with metabolism. A variety of compounds have been suggested to play a role in coupling metabolism with flow at the tissue level. No single factor has met all requirements for being the primary coupling agent, and it appears most likely that some combination of metabolic intermediates acts together (Table 1-2).

Adenosine. One of the best-studied candidates for a role in matching perfusion and metabolism is *adenosine*. Adenosine is a ubiquitous nucleoside that plays an important role within the cardiovascular system. It is formed intra- and extracellularly from two different substrates (adenosine monophosphate and S-adenosylhomocysteine).[50] It is an end product of adenosine triphosphate metabolism, and adenosine levels increase when the energetic state of the cell decreases. Therefore, it is released by metabolically stressed cells and acts most prominently under hypoxic conditions.[51] It acts on G protein–coupled receptors, four subtypes of which (P_1-purinoceptors) have been characterized and cloned thus far: A_1, A_{2A}, A_{2B}, and A_3, which are coupled to various G protein subtypes (see Figure 1-5).[52-56] Table 1-3 summarizes the various adenosine receptors, the coupled G proteins, and the intracellular signaling transduction pathways.

Adenosine acts in the human vasculature predominantly through endothelial A_2 receptors, inducing relaxation.[57-60] It is a potent coronary microvessel dilator[61,62] and can modulate α_1-but not α_2-adrenoceptor–mediated vasoconstriction of coronary microvessels.[63] In other regions of the vasculature, adenosine can produce dilatation or constriction, depending on vascular basal tone and region within the vasculature. Furthermore, adenosine has a concentration-dependent biphasic response—vasoconstriction at low concentrations (10^{-6} mol/L) and vasodilation at high concentrations. The constrictive effect may be indirect: stimulation and degranulation of periarteriolar mast cells by adenosine with subsequent release of histamine and thromboxane have been proposed to explain adenosine-induced vasoconstriction.[64,65]

Although research has been hampered by the fact that adenosine is metabolized rapidly and is also taken up into cells, the compound is likely to play an important role in flow-metabolism coupling in some organs. In the heart, a strong correlation has been established among myocardial oxygen

TABLE 1-2
Putative Mediators of Flow-Metabolism Coupling

Adenosine
Oxygen
pH
Carbon dioxide
Lactate
Nitric oxide
Potassium
Glucose
Fatty acids
Vitamins
Phosphate
Osmolarity
Prostaglandins

TABLE 1-3

Adenosine Receptors and Their Signaling Mechanisms

Adenosine Receptor	Coupled G Protein	Intracellular Transduction
A_1	G_i and G_o protein[217,218]	Inhibition of adenylate cyclase, activation of phospholipase C,[219,220] opening of K_{ATP}^+ channels,[221] and inhibition of N-, P-, and Q-type Ca^{2+} channels[222,223]
$A_{2A/B}$	G_S protein[224]	Stimulation of adenylate cyclase,[225,226] activation of N-type Ca^{2+} channels[227]
A_3	G_i and G_q protein[228,229]	Activation of phospholipase C/D,[220,230] inhibition of adenylate cyclase[231,232]

consumption, release of adenosine, and coronary blood flow.[66] However, antagonism of adenosine's action does not always result in significant changes in coronary perfusion. In the brain, a role for adenosine appears well established during oxygen supply-demand mismatch. In contrast, it does not appear to be of major importance in flow regulation in skeletal muscle.[67] Together, the available data suggest that adenosine is of significant importance in metabolic flow regulation, but its role may be of relevance primarily under conditions of hypoxia.

Oxygen. *Oxygen* has been suggested to be of relevance in flow-metabolism coupling and appears to be a logical candidate because lack of oxygen would indicate that an increase in blood flow would be in order. Blood vessels in various organs (brain, muscle, heart) dilate when the partial pressure of oxygen in arterial blood (PaO_2) decreases below 40 mmHg. Because the arteriolar wall is exposed to high oxygen tensions on the luminal side, it has been suggested that the oxygen gradient between the arteriolar lumen and surrounding tissue is the determining factor in inducing vasodilation. However, under conditions of normal exercise, tissue oxygen tensions do not drop to the level at which oxygen-dependent vasodilation plays a significant role. At this time, therefore, it seems likely that oxygen is not the major mediator, but it may play a role in modulating vessel responsiveness to other metabolites. The role of oxygen tension in the vascular response to systemic hypoxia is discussed subsequently.

Carbon dioxide, lactate, pH. Compounds associated with the increase in hydrogen ion concentration resulting from anaerobic metabolism (*carbon dioxide* and *lactate*), as well as *pH* itself, have been considered as putative metabolic vasodilators (Figure 1-6). The circulation of the brain is highly sensitive to changes in carbon dioxide levels, and this effect appears to be mediated by changes in cerebrospinal fluid pH. The time course of these changes, however, is too slow to explain cerebral flow-metabolism matching. Other tissues do not exhibit such sensitivity. Skeletal muscle perfusion in particular is poorly sensitive to changes in carbon dioxide level, and the change in hydrogen ion concentration during exercise is considered too small to play a significant role. Interestingly, patients with McArdle's syndrome, who are incapable of muscle glycolysis because of absence of phosphorylase, show normal vascular dilation in

response to exercise despite the absence of any changes in pH, carbon dioxide, or lactate. Thus, it appears unlikely that compounds related to anaerobic metabolism play a major role in control of local blood flow. The mechanisms underlying the effects of decreased pH on vascular tone are discussed later.

Nitric oxide. Endothelial compounds, in particular *nitric oxide*, are likely to play an important role in flow-metabolism coupling. Endothelial cells are induced to produce and release nitric oxide—the key compound in endothelium-mediated vasorelaxation (see Figure 1-6)—by a variety of neuronal (norepinephrine, acetylcholine, adenosine triphosphate, substance P), humoral (catecholamines, vasopressin, angiotensin II, insulin), and inflammation- and coagulation-related (serotonin, adenosine diphosphate, thrombin) stimuli.[5,68] In addition, increased shear on the endothelium induces nitric oxide release. These compounds activate different endothelial cell membrane receptors, which are predominantly coupled to G_i proteins. The calcium-dependent nitric oxide synthase converts L-arginine and oxygen into nitric oxide and L-citrulline, using several cofactors (e.g., reduced nicotinamide adenine dinucleotide phosphate [NADPH]).[69] Nitric oxide is released abluminally (where it relaxes adjacent vascular smooth muscle cells) and intraluminally (where it binds to proteins and blood cells and is therefore able to act at locations distant from the production site). Nitric oxide increases the activity of soluble guanylate cyclase in vascular smooth muscle, thereby increasing the amount of cGMP.[70,71] cGMP relaxes muscle by decreasing intracellular calcium concentrations by several mechanisms. It activates a calcium-dependent adenosine triphosphatase, which shifts cytoplasmic calcium back into the sarcoplasmic reticulum.[72,73] It also inhibits calcium efflux from the sarcoplasmic reticulum by phosphorylating IP_3 and opens potassium channels, inducing hyperpolarization and concomitant decreases in calcium levels.[72-76] cGMP is also capable of inhibiting G protein function[77-79] and phospholipase C activation.[80] In addition to its vasodilating properties, nitric oxide is capable of inducing apoptosis and can either increase or decrease (depending on the nitric oxide concentration) the permeability of the endothelium.[81-84]

In skeletal muscle, blocking nitric oxide release or its effects decreases functional hyperemia, and addition of the nitric oxide precursor L-arginine enhances it, suggesting that the compound is of relevance in matching metabolism and flow.[85] Potentially more important may be the role of nitric oxide in dilating the larger upstream arteries after microvascular blood flow increases. Increased downstream flow increases the shear rate in larger arteries. Increased shear stress results in increased release of nitric oxide, which then dilates the feeding artery. In this manner, nitric oxide allows flow through larger arteries to adapt to changes in microvascular resistance. Without this mechanism, any effect of metabolic mediators on microvascular flow would of necessity be limited.

Other compounds. A variety of other compounds have been suggested to be of relevance in flow-metabolism coupling. *Potassium* efflux from cells is increased during metabolic activity, and potassium could therefore be a signal that increased flow is required. This may be of greatest importance in skeletal muscle and possibly in the early response in the brain, but it seems less likely to be of importance in other organs. Lack of

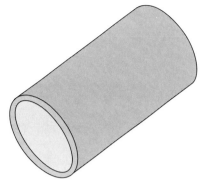

VASODILATION:
- Lack of oxygen
- Carbon dioxide, lactate, low pH
- Nitric oxide
- Prostaglandin I_1
- Lack of glucose, amino acids, fatty acids, vitamins
- Decreased vessel stretch
- Tachykinin, substance P, neurokinin A and B, calcitonin gene-related peptide

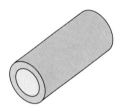

VASOCONSTRICTION:
- Angiotensin II
- Endothelin
- Superoxide
- Thromboxane

FIGURE 1-6 Effects of different compounds on vascular tone.

nutrients, such as *glucose, amino acids, fatty acids*, or even *vitamins* (such as the vitamin B deficiency in beriberi) may result in vasodilation (see Figure 1-6). Inorganic *phosphate* may play a role in regulating flow in muscle tissue. Significant roles for changes in *osmolarity* or for *prostaglandins* appear unlikely.

AUTOREGULATION. Historically, autoregulation (i.e., the local adaptation of vascular resistance to changes in systemic pressure in order to maintain constant flow) has often been considered a myogenic event; it was felt that increased vessel stretch resulting from increased systemic pressure would result in a reflex constriction of the vascular smooth muscle. The opposite would happen if decreased systemic pressure decreased vessel stretch (see Figure 1-6). Although this myogenic response may play a role, newer findings make it more likely that autoregulation is primarily mediated by a number of signaling compounds, with the balance between dilatory and constricting signaling determining the final state of the vessel. In this section, some of the compounds likely to play a role are discussed. Emphasis is on the constricting agents, as dilatory compounds have already been mentioned. Local angiotensin systems and endothelin are probably the most important.

Angiotensin II. Angiotensin was primarily considered a systemic hormone but is now known to be generated at the local level as well. Its precursor, angiotensinogen, is produced in the liver and cleaved by renin to angiotensin I (ATI).[86] Renin is an enzyme released by the kidney in response to increased sympathetic activity. The intermediate product, ATI, is converted by angiotensin-converting enzyme (ACE) to the end product angiotensin II (ATII), which was long thought to be the most potent vasoconstrictor occurring naturally in the body (see Figure 1-6). Binding of ATII to endothelial AT_1 receptors (two subtypes are known) leads to profound vasoconstriction, by several mechanisms. ATII enhances endothelin secretion, consumes NADPH (which is needed for nitric oxide synthase) to produce free radicals, and reinforces catecholamine release

from presynaptic receptors.[5,87-89] Furthermore, at the systemic level it induces thirst signaling in circulation-controlling neurons in the medulla oblongata and promotes aldosterone release from the adrenal glands to increase sodium resorption in the renal distal tubules.

Endothelin. Endothelin is a polypeptide released by vascular endothelial cells. Of the three known isoforms (ET-1, ET-2, ET-3), ET-1 is the most important and the only one that can be produced by vascular endothelial cells. It binds to G protein–coupled ET_A and ET_B receptors, causing a profound calcium-induced vasoconstriction (primarily on small vessels) (see Figure 1-6). The compound is approximately 100 times more potent than ATII. Approximately 75% of the synthesized peptide is secreted abluminally, where it binds preferentially to ET_A receptors on smooth muscle cells, inducing vasoconstriction and cell proliferation. In contrast, stimulation of endothelial ET_A receptors causes nitric oxide– and prostaglandin I2 (PGI_2)–mediated vasodilation. At low concentrations, vasoconstriction and nitric oxide– and endothelium-derived hyperpolarization factor–induced relaxation are in balance.[90] Moreover, ET-1 can increase endothelial permeability, stimulate adhesion molecule production, and exert chemotactic effects on monocytes.

Other compounds. Hyperpolarization of the vascular smooth muscle cell causes relaxation. This can be induced in different ways: by inhibition of voltage-gated calcium channels, thereby reducing the amount of free intracellular calcium, or, perhaps even more important, by activation of potassium channels facilitating potassium-calcium exchange.[91] At the microvascular level, where myoendothelial junctions are present, electrical coupling may occur.[92-94] Because some of these mechanisms are independent of nitric oxide or prostacyclins, an *endothelium-derived hyperpolarization factor* (EDHF) has been postulated. Some endothelium-derived, hyperpolarizing, short-lived metabolites of arachidonic acid, as well as other short-lived molecules such as carbon monoxide, hydroxyl radicals, and hydrogen peroxide, have been suspected, but *the* EDHF has not yet been found.[95-98]

Afferent capsaicin-sensitive motor neurons produce and release vasoactive peptides: *tachykinin, substance P, neurokinin A and B,* and *calcitonin gene–related peptide* (CGRP). In general, these cause vasodilation because of nitric oxide and EDHF release (see Figure 1-6).

INJURY RESPONSES. Vascular injury triggers a complex series of local signaling events, which have classically been divided into inflammatory and coagulatory responses. Later research, however, makes clear that major overlap exists between these two systems.[99] Complex interactions and amplification exist on both cellular and humoral levels during inflammation and coagulation (see Chapter 15). A broad spectrum of cells, mediators, pathways, and reaction cascades are inseparably interwoven. This section only suggests the complexity of interactions of blood and endothelial cells, their effects on the peripheral vasculature during inflammation, and two of the major mediators involved: thrombin and the eicosanoids.

Polymorphonuclear leukocytes play a central role in inflammation as well as in coagulation. They can initiate and amplify coagulation and modulate inflammatory cell responses. Release of superoxide influences vascular tone (primarily by inactivation of nitric oxide).[100] Furthermore, the reaction of superoxide with nitric oxide can lead to the formation of the potent free radical peroxynitrite and inhibit PGI_2 synthesis in endothelial cells, leading to vasoconstriction (see Figure 1-6).[101,102]

Endothelial cells and leukocytes interact during inflammation primarily by expression of adhesion molecules and release of cytokines. Through mechanisms mediated by the transcription factor *nuclear factor κB* (NF-κB) (see later), endothelial cells produce chemokines (interleukin-8 [IL-8] and monocyte chemoattractant protein 1 [MCP-1]) that attract leukocytes into inflammatory sites.[103-105] Initial adhesion of leukocytes to the vascular wall is mediated by different molecules of the selectin family, such as P-selectin, E-selectin, and L-selectin, whereas firm leukocyte adhesion is mediated by molecules of the immunoglobulin superfamily, such as intercellular adhesion molecule (ICAM)-1, -2, and -3 and vascular cell adhesion molecule 1 (VCAM-1).[20,106-108]

NF-κB plays a key role in these events. It is a transcription factor that remains in the cytoplasm of quiescent cells in an inactivated state. Several factors, such as cytokines (including tumor necrosis factor [TNF], IL-1, and lipopolysaccharide), viruses, hydrogen peroxide, linoleic acid, growth factors (e.g., platelet-derived growth factor [PDGF], basic fibroblast growth factor), and blood-derived factors (e.g., thrombin) can activate NF-κB, thus stimulating the inflammatory response.[109-113] NF-κB is involved in synthesis of adhesion molecules (ICAM-1, VCAM-1, E-selectin), inflammatory cytokines (IL-1, IL-6, IL-8, TNF), growth factors, and chemokines. In addition, it amplifies their signaling.[114] Its role in the response to low oxygen tensions is described later.

Thrombin. Thrombin is well known as a key intermediate in the coagulation cascade.[115] It also influences a number of other cells, including endothelial and smooth muscle cells.[116,117] Thrombin is a proteinase that binds to a G_I protein–coupled receptor, which it activates in an unusual manner: by "clipping"

off a short receptor segment (hence the receptor is named proteinase-activated receptor 1 [PAR-1]). The main intracellular signaling pathways include inhibition of cAMP, stimulation of phospholipase C, increase of IP_3 and DAG, mobilization of intracellular calcium, and activation of protein kinase C.[118,119] Other intracellular signaling pathways identified include the G protein subtypes $G_{q/11}$, G_{12}, and G_{13}; numerous mitogen-activated kinases (MAPs); and phospholipase D and A_2.[120-126]

Relative expression and function of PAR-1 on endothelial and smooth muscle cells depend on the specific vessel. Whereas removal of the endothelium leads to a strong thrombin-induced vasoconstriction in human coronary vessels because of calcium influx in the underlying smooth muscle cell, contractile responses still prevail in human umbilical and placental vessels, even with intact endothelium.[127-132] Furthermore, thrombin stimulates the expression of tissue factor and adhesion molecules (ICAM-1, VCAM-2, and E-selectin), endothelial cell contraction with increased permeability, and procollagen synthesis in smooth muscle cells and facilitates the production and release of promitogenic factors (PDGF, ET-1)—all of these steps associated with inflammation, coagulation, wound healing, and angiogenesis.[116,117,133-139] Because PAR-1–deficient mice show no differences in cardiac function and blood pressure compared with normal mice,[140] it is assumed that thrombin does not play a major role in the regulation of cardiovascular function but functions in the control of local blood flow following tissue damage.

Eicosanoids. The eicosanoids include prostaglandins (PGs), prostacyclins (PGI_2), thromboxane (TXs), leukotrienes (LTs), and hydroxyeicosatetraenoic acids (HETEs) derived from different polyunsaturated fatty acids. Derivatives of the most prominent 20-carbon fatty acid arachidonic acid are the most common and biologically important eicosanoids. Arachidonic acid is a component of the cellular membrane, is released by different phospholipases (predominantly phospholipase A_2) or lipases, and is metabolized by cyclooxygenases (COX-1, COX-2), lipoxygenases, or cytochrome P-450–dependent enzymes. Whereas COX-1 is present in the majority of tissues, COX-2 is absent under normal conditions but markedly enhanced during inflammation. The products PGI_2, PGE_2, and thromboxane have only a short half-life (seconds to minutes) and exert different actions on the vascular bed. Although PGI_2 causes vasodilation by activation of adenylate cyclase, with subsequent increases in cAMP levels, its major biologic effect is inhibition of platelet aggregation. PGI_2 analogs were shown to have cytoprotective, antiproliferative, and mitogen-suppressive properties and are able to reduce microvascular hydraulic permeability at plasma concentrations below those causing vasodilation.[141] Thromboxane is predominantly produced in platelets but also, in small amounts, in vascular endothelial cells. It counteracts the effects of PGI_2 and causes vasoconstriction and platelet aggregation (see Figure 1-6). Release of prostaglandin I_1 and nitric oxide causes substantial endothelium-dependent relaxation.[127,128]

Longer Term Regulation Of The Peripheral Circulation

The mechanisms described previously are fast feedback systems that match changes in metabolism to blood flow, protect against rapid changes in systemic pressure, or initiate responses to injury, with response times between seconds or minutes. However, in the presence of more prolonged changes in metabolic requirement, different mechanisms come into play to match flow and metabolism. The need for these other mechanisms derives from the fact that short-term metabolic control is often not able to compensate completely for changes in metabolic requirement. For example, a doubling of arterial pressure (initially inducing a massive increase in peripheral flow) results in a rapid counterregulatory response, which, within a few minutes, reduces flow back to approximately normal. However, flow does not return to exactly normal but remains elevated by a modest degree. Such remaining differences from normal can be compensated for by longer term regulatory mechanisms, playing themselves out over a time course of days to weeks. These obviously become of most relevance when metabolic demands of an organ change chronically. A typical example relevant to clinical practice is the obstruction of a coronary artery, which immediately but permanently changes oxygen supply downstream of the obstruction.

The main mechanism by which longer term regulation of flow-metabolism matching takes place is changes in tissue vascularity. Existing microvasculature may be recruited. In addition, angiogenic processes may result in development of new blood vessels.[142] It appears that a prolonged decrease in tissue oxygen tension may be the primary signal indicating the need for increased blood supply over time. The molecular mechanisms underlying this process are discussed later. Hypoxia induces changes in gene transcription and subsequent production of a variety of growth factors and other proteins, which in turn induce angiogenesis. The end result of this activity is the development of a collateral circulation supplying the area of need. A primary role has been attributed to *vascular endothelial growth factor* (VEGF). This compound, isolated from ischemic tissue, is now known to be largely responsible for the massive angiogenic activity in tumor tissue. VGEF antagonists are being studied as antitumor agents, with promising initial results. In addition to VGEF, *angiotensin II* can activate mitogenic protein kinases and induce expression of diverse growth factors (PDGF, insulin-like growth factor, basic fibroblast growth factor, and heparin-binding epidermal growth factor), leading to structural changes of the smooth muscle cells and altering vasodilator susceptibility.[143-145] *Thrombin* also, as mentioned previously, can induce signaling of mediator systems geared to longer term remodeling of the vasculature.

Important for the anesthesiologist is the realization that with increasing age or cardiovascular disease these mechanisms of longer term regulation may no longer function appropriately. Such patients may, therefore, have unnoticed but potentially detrimental gaps between tissue metabolic demand and blood supply, gaps that may become apparent only during the stresses of anesthesia and surgery.

Vascular responses to systemic insults

The previous sections have been concerned primarily with regulation in response to local events: adaptation of regional flow to metabolic requirements and to local injury. However, the vasculature also has to respond appropriately to systemic insults. These responses are of great importance for anesthesiologists as clinicians are frequently confronted with patients exhibiting systemic hypotension, hypovolemia, or hypoxia. From the following discussion, two major issues emerge. First, the microvascular response to these various insults, all of which eventually lead to decreased cellular oxygen availability, is similar irrespective of the inciting event. Second, the response of the microvasculature is frequently suboptimal. Although the existence of significant overlap will become apparent, the responses to ischemia and hypoxia are discussed separately.

Ischemia

Ischemia at the cellular level can have a variety of origins, ranging from systemic hypovolemia to localized thrombosis in the heart or brain. The role of ischemia in sepsis has been underappreciated. Significant "sludging" of blood, with resultant small vessel plugging, takes place in septic patients. Disseminated intravascular coagulation and reductions in deformability of red blood cells (in part induced by an inflammatory response) appear to play major roles.[146] Despite these various scenarios of ischemia, the response of the microvasculature to lack of perfusion is similar irrespective of the initiating mechanism. It is important to realize that, whereas control of flow-metabolism matching under nonpathologic conditions is usually accomplished at the local level, major insults such as hypovolemia require redistribution of flow among organs, which is regulated by central systems. It is not possible to differentiate completely the response to ischemia from the response to hypoxia, as one implies the other. The effects of hypoxia on the vasculature are discussed later.

SYSTEMIC RESPONSES TO CENTRAL HYPOVOLEMIA. Although the focus of this section is on the microvasculature, some current concepts about central regulation of the vasculature in the setting of systemic hypovolemia are briefly reviewed. Graded hemorrhage results in a biphasic cardiovascular response.[147] During phase I, systemic blood pressure is well maintained, a result of increases in peripheral resistance (related to increased sympathetic vasomotor activity) and heart rate (related to increased cardiac sympathetic stimulation and decreased vagal tone), mediated by arterial baroreceptors. Despite these compensatory responses, CO decreases. It remains important to realize this fact, as it is not easily established from routine monitoring modalities. The systolic variation of the arterial pressure wave observed during positive-pressure respiration may well be the most sensitive index of the CO response to hemorrhage.[148] During phase I, blood flow is selectively redistributed among the organ systems such that perfusion to heart, brain, and kidney is maintained (Figure 1-7).

When hemorrhage continues to approximately 30% of blood volume, phase II is reached. At this point the system decompensates; peripheral resistance, arterial pressure, and heart rate decrease, CO falls precipitously, and conscious subjects usually faint. At times, a brief stabilization of systemic blood pressure is observed when the pressure has decreased by approximately 50%. This is thought to result from cerebral ischemia, which induces a massive, but temporary, stimulation of the sympathetic nervous system. The mechanisms underlying failure of compensation during phase II are still being investigated. It is clear that sympathetic vasomotor drive suddenly fails and cardiac vagal stimulation increases, but the signaling pathways are not completely understood. Opiate receptor stimulation may play a major role (see Figure 1-7). The ability of naloxone to increase arterial pressure during hemorrhage in animals has been well established, and this effect is known to be mediated primarily by increased sympathetic outflow.[149] Subsequent studies have shown that naloxone can prevent the failure of sympathetic drive occurring during phase II and that this effect

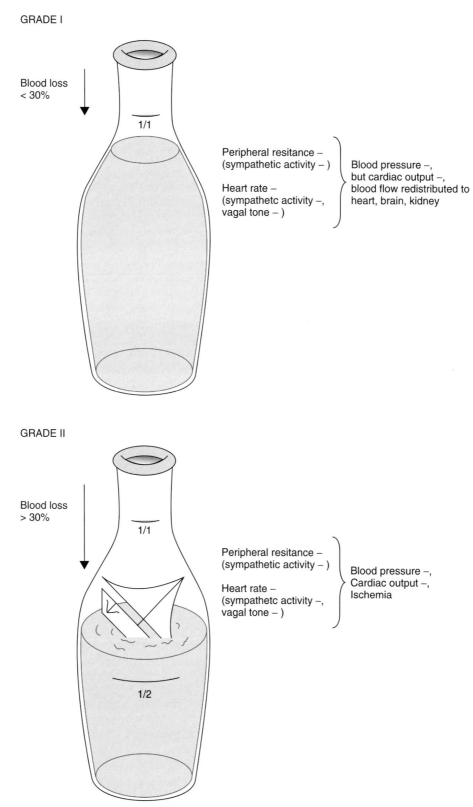

GRADE I

Blood loss
< 30%

1/1

Peripheral resitance –
(sympathetic activity –)

Heart rate –
(sympathetc activity –,
vagal tone –)

Blood pressure –,
but cardiac output –,
blood flow redistributed to
heart, brain, kidney

GRADE II

Blood loss
> 30%

1/1

1/2

Peripheral resitance –
(sympathetic activity –)

Heart rate –
(sympathetc activity –,
vagal tone –)

Blood pressure –,
Cardiac output –,
Ischemia

FIGURE 1-7 Systemic responses to central hypovolemia at different stages.

is due to blockade of δ_1 opiate receptors in the brainstem.[150] It, therefore, appears that the development of phase II is largely dependent on central opiate receptor signaling. However, as major species differences have been described in this regard, these findings should not be extrapolated to humans at this time. Central nitric oxide signaling and peripheral cannabinoid signaling may also play pathophysiologic roles. Other signaling mechanisms, although maybe not involved in the pathophysiology of phase II, may potentially be useful in treatment. CNS administration of inhibitors of 5-hydroxytryptamine 1A (5-HT$_{1A}$) serotonin receptors or α_2-adrenergic receptors can prevent development of phase II. Potentially more clinically relevant are findings that intravenous administration of adrenocorticotropic hormone fragments effectively reversed hemorrhagic hypotension in several animal species.[151]

It is of great importance to realize that the clear distribution in phases that is observed in conscious animals and humans is profoundly modified by anesthetics. Inhaled anesthetics, as well as propofol, ketamine, and dexmedetomidine, interfere with the compensatory mechanisms of phase I.[152,153] In contrast, and somewhat surprising in view of the role of opiate receptors in the development of phase II, fentanyl and alfentanil do not affect phase I.[152]

MICROVASCULAR RESPONSES TO ISCHEMIA. Because of technical issues, determining the microvascular responses to ischemia has lagged far behind the study of systemic cardiovascular effects. In order to measure microcirculatory flow, techniques such as in vivo microscopy, radiolabeled microspheres, and electromagnetic flow probes have been used. However, these techniques have significant limitations. In vivo microscopy is limited to investigation of selected tissues only (primarily skin and muscle), which are known not to be representative of other organs. Radiolabeled microspheres can provide only a snapshot of flow distribution. Flow probes can determine organ flow but not show true microvascular distribution. More recent techniques, such as optical spectroscopy, allow determination of true microcirculatory flow, oxygen tension, single-erythrocyte hemoglobin, and even the energetic state of small tissue samples.[154] Although such techniques also have limitations (the types of tissues that can be studied being a major one), they are likely to provide new, important insights into the regulatory mechanisms of the microcirculation.

Studies indicate that, at the microcirculatory level, not all vessels are created equal. When regional myocardial oxygenation is imaged using reduced nicotinamide adenine dinucleotide (NADH) videofluorimetry, uniform fluorescence is observed. During a period of ischemia, fluorescence increases (because of high NADH levels) but remains uniform. During this period, the microvasculature attempts to maximize blood flow by vasodilation. However, during reperfusion a different pattern is observed; a heterogenous, patchy fluorescence distribution develops, indicating that some microcirculatory units return to normoxia in advance of other units. The same units are also the first to become dysoxic during tachycardia and have been termed *microcirculatory weak units* (MWUs).[155] MWUs have been found to be localized close to venules, whereas the better oxygenated units are found close to arterioles. A similar pattern has been observed in other organs, including gut and kidney. In contrast, ischemia in muscle does not reveal evidence of MWUs. It appears that arteriolar-venular shunting of the limited supply of oxygenated blood during ischemic episodes may play a role in the development of MWUs. This observation is supported by findings that capillary oxygen tension is less than venular oxygen tension under ischemic conditions. For example, during hemorrhagic shock, venous oxygen tension declines to a plateau level, whereas capillary oxygen tension continues to decline.[156]

The concept of microcirculatory maldistribution based on shunting has major implications for the management of shock. Few data are available on hemorrhagic shock, but septic shock has been found to be associated with a similar pattern of MWUs, as is ischemia. Indeed, the profound microvascular shunting during septic shock probably explains why maximizing the oxygen-carrying capacity of the blood and increasing blood pressure can still be associated with cellular hypoxia. Gastric tonometry data have confirmed persistent tissue acidosis in the presence of adequate systemic oxygen-carrying capacity.[157] Use of vasopressors has historically not been successful in management of these types of shock, and this is understandable because further arteriolar constriction induced by these compounds would be likely to worsen the maldistribution already present. Thus, compounds that have microvascular dilatory capacity (pentoxifylline, dopexamine) might be more beneficial, as they might decrease the degree of shunting and make microvascular perfusion more homogenous. Alternatively, resuscitation fluids with oxygen-carrying capacity might be useful.

Hypoxia

As stated previously, tissue hypoxia is an integral part of ischemia. In addition, hypoxia can be induced by systemic events (drowning, mishaps during anesthesia), or it can occur on the tissue level (shunting in sepsis, as described previously). In either case, hypoxia results in two major effects: decreases in tissue oxygen tension and an increase in anaerobic metabolism, with subsequent decreases in pH. The cell-signaling events resulting from these two effects are discussed.

Oxygen supply at the microvascular level is more complex than previously assumed. It consists of both a convective (i.e., blood flow) component and a diffusion component. The latter takes place not only at the capillaries but also at the level of arterioles. The result of this complex system is a remarkably homogenous distribution of oxygen supply. The acute actions of hypoxia are in many ways similar to those observed after ischemia. Shunting is likely to play a major role, and hypoxia results in an inhomogenous distribution of blood supply, similar to that described previously for ischemia. Ince and Sinaasappel have suggested four potential mechanisms underlying this shunting[154]: (1) Blood might be shunted through arteriovenous anastomoses; (2) oxygen may diffuse directly from arterioles to venules in close proximity; (3) a form of microvascular steal might develop in which certain microcirculatory units selectively dilate, leaving other units underperfused; and (4) off-load time for oxygen in low-saturation states may be sufficiently prolonged that the red cell dwell time in the capillary is insufficient. Some evidence exists for each of these hypotheses, and it is likely that several of them may be responsible for the observed effects of hypoxia at the microvascular level.

The next two sections provide an overview of the current understanding of the molecular mechanisms underlying the vascular responses to decreased oxygen tension and pH.

CELLULAR SIGNALING RESPONSES TO DECREASED OXYGEN TENSION. The microvascular response to hypoxia appears to be largely mediated by signaling in endothelial cells.[158] It is important to realize that the partial pressure of oxygen (PO_2), even when above nonischemic levels, acts as a true cellular mediator. In other words, the microvascular response to hypoxia is not due to breakdown of normal signaling events in the absence of oxygen. Instead, decreased oxygen tensions induce responses through well-regulated and well-defined signaling cascades. This response is exemplified by the fact that various tissues behave differently to decreased oxygen tensions. Whereas in many tissues vasodilation is the primary response, in lung and kidney vasoconstriction takes place. In the lung, vasoconstriction leads to the well-known effect of hypoxic pulmonary vasoconstriction, which optimizes ventilation-perfusion matching.

The sensor for decreased oxygen tension has not yet been identified with certainty. On the basis of several lines of evidence, a thus far undefined heme-containing protein in the endothelium appears the most likely candidate. Carbon monoxide and nitric oxide, both of which bind with high affinity to heme, block oxygen sensitivity, as do heme biosynthesis blockers and transition metals (cobalt, nickel), which can take the place of iron in heme but lack its oxygen-binding capability. The second messenger systems are similarly not defined in detail, but protein kinases appear to play an important role as their inhibition blocks oxygen sensitivity.

As previously discussed, decreases in oxygen tension are unlikely to be the sole mechanism of immediate local control of blood flow. However, they play a major role in longer term adaptive changes of the microvasculature. These changes are induced by the expression of several growth factors and other compounds induced by decreases in oxygen tension. The genes controlled in this manner by hypoxia are regulated by a number of transcription factors, which are activated by the oxygen sensor and its downstream signaling pathways.[158] The most important of these transcription factors are the *hypoxia-inducible transcription factor 1* (HIF-1), transcription factor *AP-1*, and *NF-κB*. The latter is regulated indirectly; it is normally inactivated by a chaperone protein (IκBα). Decreased oxygen tension induces phosphorylation of IκBα, which targets it for degradation. NF-κB is then able to translocate to the nucleus and induce gene transcription.

The end result of this activity is transcription of a number of major growth factors. *Platelet-derived growth factor B* (PDGF-B) is a major mitogen and known to induce both constriction and proliferation of vascular smooth muscle. Its RNA is greatly upregulated by hypoxic conditions ($PO_2 < 40$ mmHg).[159] *Endothelin-1* (ET-1) is a major vasoconstrictor and is released at $PO_2 < 30$ mmHg in culture models.[160] Other genes expressed in response to low oxygen tensions are *insulin-like growth factor, vascular endothelial growth factor,* and *cyclooxygenase-2* (COX-2), the latter primarily regulated by NF-κB. In contrast, levels of the vasodilator nitric oxide are decreased by hypoxia; endothelial *nitric oxide synthase* levels are greatly decreased by exposure to low (but physiologic) oxygen tensions.[161] Similar findings have been observed for inducible nitric oxide syn-

thase. Nitric oxide levels exert a major influence over the response to decreased oxygen tensions. The increases in PDGF-B and ET-1 induced by hypoxia are largely depressed by the presence of nitric oxide. In contrast, in the presence of a nitric oxide synthesis inhibitor, hypoxia-induced increases in PDGF-B and ET-1 are greatly enhanced. Expression of several other antimitogenic factors is inhibited by hypoxia.

This increased expression of mitogenic compounds and inhibition of antimitogenic compounds induce major and, at times, permanent changes in the vasculature, particularly well described in the pulmonary circulation. The media and adventitia thicken, and more matrix is deposited. Smooth muscle formation is excessively stimulated, and muscle cells may peripherally extend into distal arterioles. The result is pulmonary hypertension that may be clinically significant.

CELLULAR SIGNALING RESPONSES TO DECREASED pH. Acidosis induces vasodilation. As is the case with the response to decreased oxygen tension, the underlying mechanisms have not been completely elucidated, but a significant degree of understanding has emerged.[162] Undoubtedly, the *nitric oxide* pathway plays a major role, particularly in the CNS. CO_2-dependent dilation of brain arteries is attenuated by nitric oxide synthase inhibitors, but these findings are somewhat species specific.[163] Interestingly, the source of this nitric oxide has not been convincingly demonstrated. Removal of the endothelium does not affect cerebrovascular responsiveness to CO_2. This suggests that the nitric oxide does not derive from an endothelial source. Instead, neuronal nitric oxide synthase may be more important in this regard.[164] Increased *prostanoid* production may also transduce the change in pH to vasodilation, as cyclooxygenase inhibitors abolish pH-dependent vasodilation.[165]

Although the pH sensor has not yet been identified, it appears that both intracellular pH and extracellular pH play a role. The vasodilatory response to decreased pH seems mediated by extracellular pH changes. In contrast, intracellular changes in hydrogen ion concentration appear able to blunt excessive reactions to profound extracellular acidosis.

Disease processes

The versatile and complex systems and cellular interactions described in this chapter are vulnerable to disease. Balance may be disrupted by numerous endogenous and exogenous factors. These include psychological and physical stress, pathologic states characterized by vasospasm, inflammation, leukocyte and platelet adhesion and aggregation, thrombosis, abnormal vascular proliferation, atherosclerosis, and hypertension. Endothelial cells in particular are the site of action of many drugs and exogenous substances (e.g., compounds derived from tobacco smoke, alcohol). Various assays have been used to test for endothelial dysfunction: direct measurement of nitric oxide, or of its metabolites, in plasma and urine; functional measurement of vascular nitric oxide–dependent responses; and assays of different circulating markers. In numerous pathologic conditions (e.g., atherosclerosis, hypertension, congestive heart failure, hyperhomocysteinemia, diabetes, renal failure, transplantation, cirrhosis), endothelial dysfunction has been shown to exist. Some of these issues, as well as the role of nutritional factors and drug treatment, are discussed in this section.

Aging

During aging (and in connective tissue disorders), changes in the interface among collagen fibrils, elastic fibers, and smooth muscle lead to changes in the viscoelasticity of the vessel wall. With advancing age, the accumulation of physical insults to the arterial wall (changes in pressure, flow, and diameter) may induce fragmentation of the medial elastic network, thereby leading to cardiovascular dysfunction. Physical factors have been shown to alter medial cell activity, inducing medial hypertrophy and other changes. Their potential contribution to changes in extracellular matrix proteins (perhaps mediated by integrins) has been less extensively studied. Metabolic factors may also be involved in age-related elastic fiber fragmentation. Oxidative stress in the arterial wall increases with age and leads to an increase in the production of cytokines, which stimulate the activity of elastases. Changes in elastic fiber composition may be associated with a greater propensity for calcification. Elastic fiber architecture can be modified by three reactions, namely elastolysis, elastocalcinosis, and production of new elastin fibers. These changes in the elastic network may have a number of consequences. Dilation may shift some of the strain to collagen, resulting in increases in the elastic modulus and impedance of the arterial wall. In turn, these changes may modify ventricle-artery coupling, leading to left ventricular hypertrophy (an independent risk factor for cardiovascular morbidity and mortality in elderly individuals). The increase in dilation and flow profile changes may also increase the susceptibility of the arterial wall to atheroma formation.

Despite these changes, the vasodilator response to nitrovasodilators remains intact. However, aging may be associated with loss of endothelium-dependent vasorelaxation. Several studies have now suggested that increasing age is associated with coronary endothelial dysfunction.[166,167] Brachial artery responses have been used as a predictor of coronary artery responses.[168] Using brachial artery ultrasonography, it was shown that aging was associated with progressive endothelial dysfunction.[169] These investigators found that in men, flow-mediated dilation was preserved in subjects younger than 40 years of age but declined thereafter at 0.21% of diameter dilation per year. In women, dilation was stable until the early 50s, after which it declined by 0.49% per year. The mechanisms leading to the loss of endothelium-derived relaxing factor (EDRF)–mediated vasodilation are not yet understood but may be related to age-related decreases in EDRF production or responsiveness, increased degradation of EDRF in the blood vessel wall, or increased production or responsiveness to vasoconstricting factors.

Atherosclerosis

The vascular endothelium secretes factors that not only modulate blood vessel tone but also participate in the development and progression of atherosclerosis through their effects on platelet adhesion and aggregation, thrombogenicity, and cell proliferation. Altered activities of these substances in patients with risk factors for cardiovascular disease (e.g., hypercholesterolemia, hypertension, diabetes, aging, postmenopausal status, smoking, and infections) appear to underlie the atherosclerotic process. There is increasing evidence from both preclinical studies and clinical trials that nitric oxide plays a pivotal role in the pathophysiology of arteriosclerosis.

Acetylcholine and bradykinin (both endothelium-dependent vasodilators) stimulate not only release of nitric oxide but probably release of other endothelium-derived relaxing and constricting factors as well. They may also have direct smooth muscle effects. Studies examining the effects of acetylcholine in the coronary circulation have reported depressed dilator responses in patients with hypertension, hypercholesterolemia, diabetes, and other risk factors for atherosclerosis (e.g., smoking and age > 60 years).[170-181] In these trials, the abnormality in epicardial acetylcholine response appears to correlate with the magnitude to which low-density lipoprotein (LDL) is oxidizable in the blood. This suggests that patients with greater oxidant stress in the vessel wall have greater disturbance of endothelial stimulatory function. In addition, the severity of epicardial and coronary microvascular dysfunction in response to acetylcholine correlates with the number of risk factors to which patients are exposed, with function being more depressed in those exposed to several risk factors. This implies that combined or repeated injury to the vascular endothelium is able to precipitate greater damage. The evidence suggests that the abnormal stimulatory activity of endothelium-dependent agonists is secondary to reduced nitric oxide availability. Thus, the effect of the nitric oxide synthase inhibitor N^G-monomethyl-L-arginine (L-NMMA) on coronary epicardial arteries and on the microcirculation is reduced, both at rest and after acetylcholine, in patients with risk factors for atherosclerosis or in those with established atherosclerosis. These patients have diminished resting and stimulated bioactivity of nitric oxide.

The mechanisms underlying the depression of nitric oxide activity have not been studied in detail in humans. Experimental animal models of atherosclerosis, hypercholesterolemia, hypertension, and diabetes have demonstrated that among the many biologic changes that appear in the vessel wall in these conditions, reduced bioavailability of nitric oxide in a setting of increased superoxide anion levels seems to be a uniform underlying abnormality. Increased free radicals in the vascular wall, generated from oxidized LDL, can, for example, oxidize nitric oxide to nitrite, nitrate, and peroxynitrite. The last is known to be toxic to tissues, leading to generation of more free radicals and to activation of cytokines.[182]

Several other mechanisms have been proposed for the observed abnormalities of nitric oxide in patients with risk factors for atherosclerosis. Among these are effects of these risk factors on second messenger pathways involving G proteins.[173,174] A direct effect of oxygen free radicals in downregulating endothelial nitric oxide synthase has also been demonstrated.[183] Reduction in cofactors for endothelial nitric oxide synthase, such as tetrahydrobiopterin, has been proposed as another important condition downregulating production of nitric oxide.[184,185]

A number of different strategies for improving endothelial nitric oxide availability have been explored. These include modification of risk factors such as (1) treatment of hypercholesterolemia and hypertension, (2) antioxidant therapy, (3) postmenopausal estrogen replacement, (4) L-arginine therapy, and (5) ACE inhibition. It is likely that future therapy will be targeted to improving vascular endothelial function by several of the strategies already outlined to achieve a long-term impact on atherosclerosis and its adverse manifestations.

Hypertension

EDRF plays a major role in the regulation of systemic vascular resistance. It is, therefore, conceivable that endothelial vasodilatory dysfunction could contribute to hypertension.

Indeed, endothelial dysfunction has been demonstrated in animal and human hypertension.[186-188] Depending on the experimental model, the reduction in endothelium-dependent relaxation is due to attenuation of nitric oxide activity or to the augmented elaboration of an endothelium-derived contracting factor (possibly a prostanoid). Data suggest that the endothelial dysfunction is secondary and reversible with the treatment of hypertension.[189,190] Conversely, infusions of nitric oxide synthase antagonists produced marked increases in blood pressure in experimental animals.[191] These inhibitors have been considered nonspecific, and the effect on blood pressure could conceivably be due to an effect on the neuronal nitric oxide synthase. However, more definitive data on a primary role of nitric oxide in the regulation of blood pressure were provided by the report that inactivation of the mouse endothelial nitric oxide synthase gene by homologous recombination produced mice that were significantly hypertensive.[192]

Several studies have provided evidence for endothelial vasodilatory dysfunction in hypertensive humans.[193,194] In these studies, forearm blood flow was measured by strain gauge plethysmography in response to intra-arterial infusions of endothelium-dependent and -independent vasodilators. In young patients with mild essential hypertension, endothelium-independent vasodilation was relatively undisturbed. By contrast, cholinergic vasodilation (presumably endothelium dependent) was attenuated. Whether this is a primary or secondary phenomenon is not known. Preliminary evidence suggests that this endothelial deficit may precede the appearance of essential hypertension.[195] In young normotensive individuals with hypertensive parents, cholinergic forearm vasodilation is impaired; by contrast, endothelium-independent vasodilation is normal.

Diabetes Mellitus

Attenuated endothelium-dependent relaxation upon acetylcholine administration has been reported in aortas from various diabetic animals, including rabbits with alloxan-induced diabetes and rats with genetically or streptozotocin-induced diabetes.[196-199] The exact mechanism underlying this decreased vasodilatory response of the vascular endothelium is unclear. Current hypotheses include enhanced release of constricting prostanoids, decreased bioactivity of EDRF related to free radical formation during high D-glucose metabolism, and attenuated formation of EDRF in endothelial cells from diabetic individuals.[200] On the other hand, early stages of diabetes mellitus are associated with increased blood flow and reduced peripheral resistance.[201-203] Findings suggest that hyperglycemia initially increases vascular relaxation through enhanced nitric oxide synthase related to changes in cell redox potential.[204] In agreement with this hypothesis, increased superoxide anion production has been found during hyper-

glycemia in cultured endothelial cells and vascular tissue.[205-207] Thus, diabetes-induced changes in vascular reactivity may represent a time-dependent phenomenon in which in the early stages of diabetes increased relaxation occurs, whereas in the longer term reduced vasodilatation and increased vasoconstriction take place.[208] The molecular mechanisms and mediators of this switch in vessel reactivity are still unclear.

Hyperglycemia induces increases in endothelial superoxide anion production in a concentration-dependent manner.[209] On the one hand, superoxide anions help in the adaptation of endothelial cells by elevating calcium and activating the nitric oxide synthase signaling cascade. On the other hand, superoxide anions disrupt endothelial vascular control by scavenging nitric oxide and inducing hyperactivity of smooth muscle cells. In addition, superoxide anion negatively affects endothelial prostacyclin synthesis, resulting in enhanced production of vasoconstrictory prostanoids such as prostaglandin H_2 and 15-hydroxyeicosatetraenoic acid.[210,211] Finally, superoxide anion–derived hydrogen peroxides represent potential mediators for changes in endothelial cell function during hyperglycemia.[212] These forms of reactive oxygen are produced from superoxide anions by superoxide dismutases that are, in part, upregulated during hyperglycemia.

In contrast to superoxide anions, which upregulate endothelial calcium-dependent signaling cascades, peroxides have been shown to attenuate endothelial calcium cascades and, in turn, reduce endothelial nitric oxide production.[209,213] Thus, besides the production of superoxide anions, the conversion to other reactive oxygen species through antioxidative enzymes might be crucially involved in alterations of the vascular response during hyperglycemia. Increased formation of superoxide might thus represent the key phenomenon for adaptation or dysfunction of vascular cells during hyperglycemia. Superoxide anions might mediate the early adaptation of endothelial cells to ensure vascular control by increased nitric oxide production in order to overcome the increased degradation of nitric oxide. However, in progressive stages of diabetes mellitus, superoxide anions or hydrogen peroxides might also disrupt intercellular cross talk between the endothelial cells and the smooth muscle, increase smooth muscle sensitivity, and alter prostanoid synthesis. Although the mechanisms involved in this switch of vascular responsibility are unclear, there is increasing evidence that changes in the enzymatically controlled balance of superoxide anions and hydrogen peroxides might account for alterations in vascular responsiveness during diabetes mellitus.

Effects of Anesthetics

Although the effects of anesthetics on the vascular system are well known to anesthesiologists, the mechanisms underlying these actions are not well understood.[214] In part, this results from the fact that a large number of regulatory mechanisms interact to maintain homeostasis. Within the arterial wall, vasoreactivity involves the endothelium and the vascular smooth muscle. In vivo, arterial vasoreactivity is also regulated by neuronal, hormonal, and metabolic factors. In vitro, however, the direct action of anesthetic agents on the vessel can be studied only in the absence of such factors. In the present section, the actions of inhaled, injected, and local anesthetics on the vasculature are briefly reviewed. Further studies are required to enable a better understanding of the mechanisms and the site of action of these vascular effects of anesthetics. For example, the investigation of the effects of anesthetic agents on vascular reactivity in diseases associated with endothelial dysfunction may indirectly provide insight into the role of the endothelium.

Volatile Anesthetics

In vitro studies with arterial rings have shown that inhalation anesthetics directly decrease endothelium-independent contraction induced by various pharmacologic agents. This direct effect of anesthetics results from a decrease in intracellular calcium concentration, mainly caused by an inhibition of transsarcoplasmic calcium influx. Volatile anesthetics decrease endothelium-dependent vasorelaxation at a site or sites within the nitric oxide signaling pathway, located downstream from the nitric oxide–related receptors and upstream from guanylyl cyclase. They may also decrease endothelium-independent vasorelaxation by inhibiting nitric oxide activation of guanylate cyclase.

Intravenous Anesthetics

Intravenous anesthetics, such as propofol, barbiturates, ketamine, and etomidate, also decrease vasoconstriction by various degrees. Propofol is the most potent inhibitor of vasoconstriction, thiopental the least potent. All these compounds have been shown to inhibit in some circumstances both endothelium-dependent and -independent vasorelaxation.

Local Anesthetics

Local anesthetics have biphasic effects on the circulation, both in vitro and in vivo.[215,216] In low concentrations they induce vasoconstriction, whereas in higher concentrations vasodilation occurs. The mechanisms of these effects are not known, but they appear to hold for all local anesthetics studied. The main exception is cocaine, which shows constrictive activity throughout the concentration range, probably resulting from its inhibitory effect on norepinephrine reuptake.

Conclusions

A vast amount of new information on the physiology of the vasculature has become available. However, the relevance of much of this information to clinical practice has not yet been well defined in many instances. Several issues explain this situation. First, the field is in a state of rapid expansion, and not all the relevant variables, receptor types, mediators, and signaling pathways are known yet. Second, and more important, the physiology of the vascular system is infinitely more complex than had been imagined. Not only are the variety of mediators and their signaling pathways staggering, but also it has become clear that different segments of the vascular tree may exhibit remarkably different, even opposite responses to the same mediator. This not only makes it difficult to integrate the available information into a coherent whole but also poses a major challenge to the design of therapeutics. Only highly selective drugs, targeted to very specific receptor subtypes, are likely to have easily controlled actions.

It may, therefore, take a number of years before many of the findings described in this chapter translate to therapeutic interventions in the operating room or intensive care unit. However, the availability of such a large number of potential therapeutic targets suggests that it is only a matter of time before their clinical relevance is realized.

REFERENCES

1. Burnett JC Jr, Granger JP, Opgenorth TJ: Effects of synthetic atrial natriuretic factor on renal function and renin release, *Am J Physiol* 247:F863, 1984.
2. Azevedo ER, Newton GE, Parker AB, et al: Sympathetic responses to atrial natriuretic peptide in patients with congestive heart failure, *J Cardiovasc Pharmacol* 35:129, 2000.
3. Cocks TM, Angus JA: Endothelium-dependent relaxation of coronary arteries by noradrenaline and serotonin, *Nature* 305:627, 1983.
4. Angus JA, Cocks TM, Satoh K: The alpha adrenoceptors on endothelial cells, *Fed Proc* 45:2355, 1986.
5. Vanhoutte PM, Miller VM: Alpha₂-adrenoceptors and endothelium-derived relaxing factor, *Am J Med* 87:1S, 1989.
6. Richard V, Tanner FC, Tschudi M, et al: Different activation of L-arginine pathway by bradykinin, serotonin, and clonidine in coronary arteries, *Am J Physiol* 259:H1433, 1990.
7. Bockman CS, Jeffries WB, Abel PW: Binding and functional characterization of alpha₂-adrenergic receptor subtypes on pig vascular endothelium, *J Pharmacol Exp Ther* 267:1126, 1993.
8. Bockman CS, Gonzalez-Cabrera I, Abel PW: Alpha₂-adrenoceptor subtype causing nitric oxide–mediated vascular relaxation in rats, *J Pharmacol Exp Ther* 278:1235, 1996.
9. Dawes M, Chowienczyk PJ, Ritter JM: Effects of inhibition of the L-arginine/nitric oxide pathway on vasodilation caused by beta-adrenergic agonists in human forearm, *Circulation* 95:2293, 1997.
10. Ferro A, Queen LR, Priest RM, et al: Activation of nitric oxide synthase by beta 2-adrenoceptors in human umbilical vein endothelium in vitro, *Br J Pharmacol* 126:1872, 1999.
11. Gray DW, Marshall I: Novel signal transduction pathway mediating endothelium-dependent beta-adrenoceptor vasorelaxation in rat thoracic aorta, *Br J Pharmacol* 107:684, 1992.
12. Schwinn DA, Lomasney JW, Lorenz W, et al: Molecular cloning and expression of the cDNA for a novel alpha₁-adrenergic receptor subtype, *J Biol Chem* 265:8183, 1990.
13. Cotecchia S, Schwinn DA, Randall RR, et al: Molecular cloning and expression of the cDNA for the hamster alpha₁-adrenergic receptor, *Proc Natl Acad Sci USA* 85:7159, 1988.
14. Perez DM, Piascik MT, Graham RM: Solution-phase library screening for the identification of rare clones: isolation of an alpha 1D-adrenergic receptor cDNA, *Mol Pharmacol* 40:876, 1991.
15. Bylund DB, Eikenberg DC, Hieble JP, et al: International Union of Pharmacology nomenclature of adrenoceptors, *Pharmacol Rev* 46:121, 1994.
16. Ford AP, Williams TJ, Blue DR, et al: Alpha₁-adrenoceptor classification: sharpening Occam's razor, *Trends Pharmacol Sci* 15:167, 1994.
17. Hein L, Kobilka BK: Adrenergic receptor signal transduction and regulation, *Neuropharmacology* 34:357, 1995.
18. Zhong H, Minneman KP: Alpha₁-adrenoceptor subtypes, *Eur J Pharmacol* 375:261, 1999.
19. Garcia-Sainz JA, Vazquez-Prado J, del Carmen Medina L: Alpha₁-adrenoceptors: function and phosphorylation, *Eur J Pharmacol* 389:1, 2000.
20. Yang M, Ruan J, Voller M, et al: Differential regulation of human alpha₁-adrenoceptor subtypes, *Naunyn Schmiedebergs Arch Pharmacol* 359:439, 1999.
21. Flavahan NA, Cooke JP, Shepherd JT, et al: Human postjunctional alpha₁- and alpha₂-adrenoceptors: differential distribution in arteries of the limbs, *J Pharmacol Exp Ther* 241:361, 1987.
22. Bylund DB, Blaxall HS, Iversen LJ, et al: Pharmacological characteristics of alpha₂-adrenergic receptors: comparison of pharmacologically defined subtypes with subtypes identified by molecular cloning, *Mol Pharmacol* 42:1, 1992.
23. Nahorski SR, Barnett DB, Cheung YD: Alpha-adrenoceptor-effector coupling: affinity states or heterogeneity of the alpha 2-adrenoceptor? *Clin Sci (Lond)* 68(Suppl 10):39s, 1985.

24. Bylund DB, Ray-Prenger C, Murphy TJ: Alpha$_{2A}$- and alpha$_{2B}$-adrenergic receptor subtypes: antagonist binding in tissues and cell lines containing only one subtype, *J Pharmacol Exp Ther* 245:600, 1988.

25. Starke K: Alpha-adrenoceptor subclassification, *Rev Physiol Biochem Pharmacol* 88:199, 1981.

26. Alabaster VA, Keir RF, Peters CJ: Comparison of potency of alpha$_2$-adrenoceptor antagonists in vitro: evidence for heterogeneity of alpha$_2$-adrenoceptors, *Br J Pharmacol* 88:607, 1986.

27. Cotecchia S, Kobilka BK, Daniel KW, et al: Multiple second messenger pathways of alpha-adrenergic receptor subtypes expressed in eukaryotic cells, *J Biol Chem* 265:63, 1990.

28. Wise A, Watson-Koken MA, Rees S, et al: Interactions of the alpha$_{2A}$-adrenoceptor with multiple Gi-family G-proteins: studies with pertussis toxin–resistant G-protein mutants, *Biochem J* 321(Pt 3):721, 1997.

29. Surpranant A, Horstman DA, Akbarali H, et al: A point mutation of the alpha$_2$-adrenoceptor that blocks coupling to potassium but not calcium currents, *Science* 257:977, 1992.

30. Eason MG, Liggett SB: Subtype-selective desensitization of alpha$_2$-adrenergic receptors. Different mechanisms control short and long term agonist-promoted desensitization of alpha 2C10, alpha 2C4, and alpha 2C2, *J Biol Chem* 267:25473, 1992.

31. Heck DA, Bylund DB: Differential down-regulation of alpha$_2$-adrenergic receptor subtypes, *Life Sci* 62:1467, 1998.

32. Starke K: Presynaptic alpha-autoreceptors, *Rev Physiol Biochem Pharmacol* 107:73, 1987.

33. Langer SZ: Twenty-five years since the discovery of presynaptic receptors: present knowledge and future perspectives, *Trends Pharmacol Sci* 18:95, 1997.

34. Muller-Schweinitzer E: Alpha-adrenoceptors, 5-hydroxytryptamine receptors and the action of dihydroergotamine in human venous preparations obtained during saphenectomy procedures for varicose veins, *Naunyn Schmiedebergs Arch Pharmacol* 327:299, 1984.

35. Guimaraes S, Nunes JP: The effectiveness of alpha$_2$-adrenoceptor activation increases from the distal to the proximal part of the veins of canine limbs, *Br J Pharmacol* 101:387, 1990.

36. Molenaar P, Malta E, Jones CR, et al: Autoradiographic localization and function of beta-adrenoceptors on the human internal mammary artery and saphenous vein, *Br J Pharmacol* 95:225, 1988.

37. Rohrer DK, Chruscinski A, Schauble EH, et al: Cardiovascular and metabolic alterations in mice lacking both beta$_1$- and beta$_2$-adrenergic receptors, *J Biol Chem* 274:16701, 1999.

38. Dixon RA, Kobilka BK, Strader DJ, et al: Cloning of the gene and cDNA for mammalian beta-adrenergic receptor and homology with rhodopsin, *Nature* 321:75, 1986.

39. Frielle T, Collins S, Daniel KW, et al: Cloning of the cDNA for the human beta$_1$-adrenergic receptor, *Proc Natl Acad Sci USA* 84:7920, 1987.

40. Emorine LJ, Marullo S, Briend-Sutren MM, et al: Molecular characterization of the human beta$_3$-adrenergic receptor, *Science* 245:1118, 1989.

41. Brown AM: Regulation of heartbeat by G protein–coupled ion channels, *Am J Physiol* 259:H1621, 1990.

42. Asano T, Katada T, Gilman AG, et al: Activation of the inhibitory GTP-binding protein of adenylate cyclase, Gi, by beta-adrenergic receptors in reconstituted phospholipid vesicles, *J Biol Chem* 259:9351, 1984.

43. Chaudhry A, MacKenzie RG, Georgic LM, et al: Differential interaction of beta$_1$- and beta$_3$-adrenergic receptors with Gi in rat adipocytes, *Cell Signal* 6:457, 1994.

44. Luttrell LM, Ferguson SS, Daaka Y, et al: Beta-arrestin–dependent formation of beta$_2$-adrenergic receptor–Src protein kinase complexes, *Science* 283:655, 1999.

45. Bunemann M, Lee KB, Pals-Rylaarsdam R, et al: Desensitization of G-protein–coupled receptors in the cardiovascular system, *Annu Rev Physiol* 61:169, 1999.

46. O'Donnell SR, Wanstall JC: Responses to the beta$_2$-selective agonist procaterol of vascular and atrial preparations with different functional beta-adrenoceptor populations, *Br J Pharmacol* 84:227, 1985.

47. Begonha R, Moura D, Guimaraes S: Vascular beta-adrenoceptor–mediated relaxation and the tone of the tissue in canine arteries, *J Pharm Pharmacol* 47:510, 1995.

48. Edvinsson L, Owman C: Pharmacological characterization of adrenergic alpha and beta receptors mediating the vasomotor responses of cerebral arteries in vitro, *Circ Res* 35:835, 1974.

49. Guimaraes S: Further study of the adrenoceptors of the saphenous vein of the dog: influence of factors which interfere with the concentrations of agonists at the receptor level, *Eur J Pharmacol* 34:9, 1975.

50. Sparks HV Jr, Bardenheuer H: Regulation of adenosine formation by the heart, *Circ Res* 58:193, 1986.

51. Schwartz LM, Bukowski TR, Ploger JD, et al: Endothelial adenosine transporter characterization in perfused guinea pig hearts, *Am J Physiol* 279:H1502, 2000.

52. Tucker AL, Linden J: Cloned receptors and cardiovascular responses to adenosine, *Cardiovasc Res* 27:62, 1993.

53. Linden J: Cloned adenosine A3 receptors: pharmacological properties, species differences and receptor functions, *Trends Pharmacol Sci* 15:298, 1994.

54. Fredholm BB, Abbracchio MP, Burnstock G, et al: Nomenclature and classification of purinoceptors, *Pharmacol Rev* 46:143, 1994.

55. Olah ME, Stiles GL: Adenosine receptor subtypes: characterization and therapeutic regulation, *Annu Rev Pharmacol Toxicol* 35:581, 1995.

56. Fredholm BB, Arslan G, Halldner L, et al: Structure and function of adenosine receptors and their genes, *Naunyn Schmiedebergs Arch Pharmacol* 362:364, 2000.

57. McCormack DG, Clarke B, Barnes PJ: Characterization of adenosine receptors in human pulmonary arteries, *Am J Physiol* 256:H41, 1989.

58. Reviriego J, Alonso MJ, Ibanez C, et al: Action of adenosine and characterization of adenosine receptors in human placental vasculature, *Gen Pharmacol* 21:227, 1990.

59. Sabouni MH, Hussain T, Cushing DJ, et al: G proteins subserve relaxations mediated by adenosine receptors in human coronary artery, *J Cardiovasc Pharmacol* 18:696, 1991.

60. Kemp BK, Cocks TM: Adenosine mediates relaxation of human small resistance-like coronary arteries via A2B receptors, *Br J Pharmacol* 126:1796, 1999.

61. Habazettl H, Conzen PF, Vollmar B, et al: Dilation of coronary microvessels by adenosine induced hypotension in dogs, *Int J Microcirc Clin Exp* 11:51, 1992.

62. Habazettl H, Vollmar B, Christ M, et al: Heterogeneous microvascular coronary vasodilation by adenosine and nitroglycerin in dogs, *J Appl Physiol* 76:1951, 1994.

63. DeFily DV, Patterson JL, Chilian WM: Endogenous adenosine modulates alpha$_2$-but not alpha$_1$-adrenergic constriction of coronary arterioles, *Am J Physiol* 268:H2487, 1995.

64. Doyle MP, Linden J, Duling BR: Nucleoside-induced arteriolar constriction: a mast cell–dependent response, *Am J Physiol* 266:H2042, 1994.

65. Shepherd RK, Linden J, Duling BR: Adenosine-induced vasoconstriction in vivo. Role of the mast cell and A3 adenosine receptor, *Circ Res* 78:627, 1996.

66. Berne RM, Rubio R: Coronary circulation. In Berne RM, Sperelakis N, Geiger SR (eds): *Handbook of physiology*, Bethesda, Md, 1979, American Physiological Society, 873.

67. Koch LG, Britton SL, Metting PJ: Adenosine is not essential for exercise hyperaemia in the hindlimb of conscious dogs, *J Physiol (Lond)* 429:63, 1990.

68. Bassenge E, Heusch G: Endothelial and neuro-humoral control of coronary blood flow in health and disease, *Rev Physiol Biochem Pharmacol* 116:77, 1990.

69. Michel T, Feron O: Nitric oxide synthases: which, where, how, and why? *J Clin Invest* 100:2146, 1997.

70. Rapoport RM, Murad F: Endothelium-dependent and nitrovasodilator-induced relaxation of vascular smooth muscle: role of cyclic GMP, *J Cyclic Nucleotide Protein Phosphor Res* 9:281, 1983.

71. Mayer B, Pfeiffer S, Schrammel A, et al: A new pathway of nitric oxide/cyclic GMP signaling involving *S*-nitrosoglutathione, *J Biol Chem* 273:3264, 1998.

72. Lincoln TM: Cyclic GMP and mechanisms of vasodilation, *Pharmacol Ther* 41:479, 1989.

73. Lincoln TM, Cornwell TL: Intracellular cyclic GMP receptor proteins, *FASEB J* 7:328, 1993.

74. White KA, Marletta MA: Nitric oxide synthase is a cytochrome P-450 type hemoprotein, *Biochemistry* 31:6627, 1992.

75. Forstermann U, Pollock JS, Schmidt HH, et al: Calmodulin-dependent endothelium-derived relaxing factor/nitric oxide synthase activity is present in the particulate and cytosolic fractions of bovine aortic endothelial cells, *Proc Natl Acad Sci USA* 88:1788, 1991.

76. Chen XL, Rembold CM: Cyclic nucleotide–dependent regulation of Mn^{2+} influx, (Ca^{2+})i, and arterial smooth muscle relaxation, *Am J Physiol* 263:C468, 1992.

77. Hirata M, Kohse KP, Chang CH, et al: Mechanism of cyclic GMP inhibition of inositol phosphate formation in rat aorta segments and cultured bovine aortic smooth muscle cells, *J Biol Chem* 265:1268, 1990.

78. Holzmann S: Endothelium-induced relaxation by acetylcholine associated with larger rises in cyclic GMP in coronary arterial strips, *J Cyclic Nucleotide Res* 8:409, 1982.

79. Light DB, Corbin JD, Stanton BA: Dual ion-channel regulation by cyclic GMP and cyclic GMP–dependent protein kinase, *Nature* 344:336, 1990.

80. Rapoport RM: Cyclic guanosine monophosphate inhibition of contraction may be mediated through inhibition of phosphatidylinositol hydrolysis in rat aorta, *Circ Res* 58:407, 1986.

81. Rumbaut RE, McKay MK, Huxley VH: Capillary hydraulic conductivity is decreased by nitric oxide synthase inhibition, *Am J Physiol* 268:H1856, 1995.

82. Kubes P: Nitric oxide affects microvascular permeability in the intact and inflamed vasculature, *Microcirculation* 2:235, 1995.

83. Kubes P: Nitric oxide–induced microvascular permeability alterations: a regulatory role for cGMP, *Am J Physiol* 265:H1909, 1993.

84. Arnhold S, Antoine D, Blaser H, et al: Nitric oxide decreases microvascular permeability in bradykinin stimulated and nonstimulated conditions, *J Cardiovasc Pharmacol* 33:938, 1999.

85. Sagach VF, Kindybalyuk AM, Kovalenko TN: Functional hyperemia of skeletal muscle: role of endothelium, *J Cardiovasc Pharmacol* 20:S170, 1992.

86. Johnston CI, Risvanis J: Preclinical pharmacology of angiotensin II receptor antagonists: update and outstanding issues, *Am J Hypertens* 10:306S, 1997.

87. Griendling KK, Ushio-Fukai M, Lassegue B, et al: Angiotensin II signaling in vascular smooth muscle. New concepts, *Hypertension* 29:366, 1997.

88. Harrison DG: Endothelial function and oxidant stress, *Clin Cardiol* 20 (11 Suppl 2):II-11, 1997.

89. Warnholtz A, Nickenig G, Schulz E, et al: Increased NADH-oxidase-mediated superoxide production in the early stages of atherosclerosis: evidence for involvement of the renin-angiotensin system, *Circulation* 99:2027, 1999.

90. Nakashima M, Vanhoutte PM: Age-dependent decrease in endothelium-dependent hyperpolarizations to endothelin-3 in the rat mesenteric artery, *J Cardiovasc Pharmacol* 22(Suppl 8):S352, 1993.

91. Nelson MT, Patlak JB, Worley JF, et al: Calcium channels, potassium channels, and voltage dependence of arterial smooth muscle tone, *Am J Physiol* 259:C3, 1990.

92. Beny JL, Gribi F: Dye and electrical coupling of endothelial cells in situ, *Tissue Cell* 21:797, 1989.

93. Beny JL, Pacicca C: Bidirectional electrical communication between smooth muscle and endothelial cells in the pig coronary artery, *Am J Physiol* 266:H1465, 1994.

94. Marchenko SM, Sage SO: Electrical properties of resting and acetylcholine-stimulated endothelium in intact rat aorta, *J Physiol (Lond)* 462:735, 1993.

95. Campbell WB, Harder DR: Endothelium-derived hyperpolarizing factors and vascular cytochrome P450 metabolites of arachidonic acid in the regulation of tone, *Circ Res* 84:484, 1999.

96. Randall MD, Kendall DA: Involvement of a cannabinoid in endothelium-derived hyperpolarizing factor-mediated coronary vasorelaxation, *Eur J Pharmacol* 335:205, 1997.

97. Niederhoffer N, Szabo B: Involvement of CB1 cannabinoid receptors in the EDHF-dependent vasorelaxation in rabbits, *Br J Pharmacol* 126:1383, 1999.

98. Mombouli JV, Vanhoutte PM: Endothelium-derived hyperpolarizing factor(s): updating the unknown, *Trends Pharmacol Sci* 18:252, 1997.

99. Spiess BD: *The relationship between coagulation, inflammation and endothelium—a pyramid towards outcome*, Philadelphia, 2000, Lippincott Williams & Wilkins.

100. Katusic ZS: Superoxide anion and endothelial regulation of arterial tone, *Free Radic Biol Med* 20:443, 1996.

101. Murphy MP, Packer MA, Scarlett JL, et al: Peroxynitrite: a biologically significant oxidant, *Gen Pharmacol* 31:179, 1998.

102. Palluy O, Bonne C, Modat G: Hypoxia/reoxygenation alters endothelial prostacyclin synthesis—protection by superoxide dismutase, *Free Radic Biol Med* 11:269, 1991.

103. Martin T, Cardarelli PM, Parry GC, et al: Cytokine induction of monocyte chemoattractant protein-1 gene expression in human endothelial cells depends on the cooperative action of NF-kappa B and AP-1, *Eur J Immunol* 27:1091, 1997.

104. Shono T, Ono M, Izumi H, et al: Involvement of the transcription factor NF-kappaB in tubular morphogenesis of human microvascular endothelial cells by oxidative stress, *Mol Cell Biol* 16:4231, 1996.

105. Lukacs NW, Strieter RM, Elner V, et al: Production of chemokines, interleukin-8 and monocyte chemoattractant protein-1, during monocyte: endothelial cell interactions, *Blood* 86:2767, 1995.

106. McIntyre TM, Modur V, Prescott SM, et al: Molecular mechanisms of early inflammation, *Thromb Haemost* 78:302, 1997.

107. Miyasaka M, Kawashima H, Korenaga R, et al: Involvement of selectins in atherogenesis: a primary or secondary event? *Ann NY Acad Sci* 811:25, 1997.

108. Libby P, Galis ZS: Cytokines regulate genes involved in atherogenesis, *Ann NY Acad Sci* 748:158, 1995.

109. Schreck R, Albermann K, Baeuerle PA: Nuclear factor kappa B: an oxidative stress–responsive transcription factor of eukaryotic cells (a review), *Free Radic Res Commun* 17:221, 1992.

110. Hennig B, Toborek M, Joshi-Barve S, et al: Linoleic acid activates nuclear transcription factor-kappa B (NF-kappa B) and induces NF-kappa B–dependent transcription in cultured endothelial cells, *Am J Clin Nutr* 63:322, 1996.

111. Toborek M, Barger SW, Mattson MP, et al: Linoleic acid and TNF-alpha cross-amplify oxidative injury and dysfunction of endothelial cells, *J Lipid Res* 37:123, 1996.

112. Obata H, Biro S, Arima N, et al: NF-kappa B is induced in the nuclei of cultured rat aortic smooth muscle cells by stimulation of various growth factors, *Biochem Biophys Res Commun* 224:27, 1996.

113. Anrather D, Millan MT, Palmetshofer A, et al: Thrombin activates nuclear factor-kappaB and potentiates endothelial cell activation by TNF, *J Immunol* 159:5620, 1997.

114. Siebenlist U, Franzoso G, Brown K: Structure, regulation and function of NF-kappa B, *Annu Rev Cell Biol* 10:405, 1994.

115. Davie EW, Fujikawa K, Kisiel W: The coagulation cascade: initiation, maintenance, and regulation, *Biochemistry* 30:10363, 1991.

116. Daniel TO, Gibbs VC, Milfay DF, et al: Thrombin stimulates c-*sis* gene expression in microvascular endothelial cells, *J Biol Chem* 261:9579, 1986.

117. Hattori R, Hamilton KK, Fugate RD, et al: Stimulated secretion of endothelial von Willebrand factor is accompanied by rapid redistribution to the cell surface of the intracellular granule membrane protein GMP-140, *J Biol Chem* 264:7768, 1989.

118. Babich M, King KL, Nissenson RA: Thrombin stimulates inositol phosphate production and intracellular free calcium by a pertussis toxin-insensitive mechanism in osteosarcoma cells, *Endocrinology* 126:948, 1990.

119. Hung DT, Wong YH, Vu TK, et al: The cloned platelet thrombin receptor couples to at least two distinct effectors to stimulate phosphoinositide hydrolysis and inhibit adenylyl cyclase, *J Biol Chem* 267:20831, 1992.

120. Baffy G, Yang L, Raj S, et al: G protein coupling to the thrombin receptor in Chinese hamster lung fibroblasts, *J Biol Chem* 269:8483, 1994.

121. Benka ML, Lee M, Wang GR, et al: The thrombin receptor in human platelets is coupled to a GTP binding protein of the G alpha q family, *FEBS Lett* 363:49, 1995.

122. Offermanns S, Toombs CF, Hu YH, et al: Defective platelet activation in G alpha(q)-deficient mice, *Nature* 389:183, 1997.

123. Seasholtz TM, Majumdar M, Kaplan DD, et al: Rho and Rho kinase mediate thrombin-stimulated vascular smooth muscle cell DNA synthesis and migration, *Circ Res* 84:1186, 1999.

124. Carbajal JM, Gratrix ML, Yu CH, et al: ROCK mediates thrombin's endothelial barrier dysfunction, *Am J Physiol* 279:C195, 2000.

125. McNicol A, Robson CA: Thrombin receptor–activating peptide releases arachidonic acid from human platelets: a comparison with thrombin and trypsin, *J Pharmacol Exp Ther* 281:861, 1997.

126. Cheng J, Baldassare JJ, Raben DM: Dual coupling of the alpha-thrombin receptor to signal-transduction pathways involving phosphatidylinositol and phosphatidylcholine metabolism, *Biochem J* 337:97, 1999.

127. Ku DD, Zaleski JK: Receptor mechanism of thrombin-induced endothelium-dependent and endothelium-independent coronary vascular effects in dogs, *J Cardiovasc Pharmacol* 22:609, 1993.

128. Ku DD, Dai J: Expression of thrombin receptors in human atherosclerotic coronary arteries leads to an exaggerated vasoconstrictory response in vitro, *J Cardiovasc Pharmacol* 30:649, 1997.

129. deBlois D, Drapeau G, Petitclerc E, et al: Synergism between the contractile effect of epidermal growth factor and that of des-Arg9-bradykinin or of alpha-thrombin in rabbit aortic rings, *Br J Pharmacol* 105:959, 1992.

130. Antonaccio MJ, Normandin D, Serafino R, et al: Effects of thrombin and thrombin receptor activating peptides on rat aortic vascular smooth muscle, *J Pharmacol Exp Ther* 266:125, 1993.

131. Antonaccio MJ, Normandin D: Role of Ca^{2+} in the vascular contraction caused by a thrombin receptor activating peptide, *Eur J Pharmacol* 256:37, 1994.

132. Tay-Uyboco J, Poon MC, Ahmad S, et al: Contractile actions of thrombin receptor–derived polypeptides in human umbilical and placental vasculature: evidence for distinct receptor systems, *Br J Pharmacol* 115:569, 1995.

133. Bartha K, Brisson C, Archipoff G, et al: Thrombin regulates tissue factor and thrombomodulin mRNA levels and activities in human saphenous vein endothelial cells by distinct mechanisms, *J Biol Chem* 268:421, 1993.

134. Henn V, Slupsky JR, Grafe M, et al: CD40 ligand on activated platelets triggers an inflammatory reaction of endothelial cells, *Nature* 391:591, 1998.

135. Garcia JG, Siflinger-Birnboim A, Bizios R, et al: Thrombin-induced increase in albumin permeability across the endothelium, *J Cell Physiol* 128:96,. 1986.

136. Lum H, Malik AB: Mechanisms of increased endothelial permeability, *Can J Physiol Pharmacol* 74:787, 1996.

137. Dabbagh K, Laurent GJ, McAnulty RJ, et al: Thrombin stimulates smooth muscle cell procollagen synthesis and mRNA levels via a PAR-1 mediated mechanism, *Thromb Haemost* 79:405, 1998.

138. Garcia JG, Patterson C, Bahler C, et al: Thrombin receptor activating peptides induce Ca^{2+} mobilization, barrier dysfunction, prostaglandin synthesis, and platelet-derived growth factor mRNA expression in cultured endothelium, *J Cell Physiol* 156:541, 1993.

139. Golden CL, Nick HS, Visner GA: Thrombin regulation of endothelin-1 gene in isolated human pulmonary endothelial cells, *Am J Physiol* 274:L854, 1998.

140. Darrow AL, Fung-Leung WP, Ye RD, et al: Biological consequences of thrombin receptor deficiency in mice, *Thromb Haemost* 76:860, 1996.

141. Gryglewski RJ, Chlopicki S, Swies J, et al: Prostacyclin, nitric oxide, and atherosclerosis, *Ann NY Acad Sci* 748:194; discussion 206, 1995.

142. Beck L, D'Amore PA: Vascular development: cellular and molecular regulation, *FASEB J* 11:365, 1997.

143. Seewald S, Seul C, Kettenhofen R, et al: Role of mitogen-activated protein kinase in the angiotensin II–induced DNA synthesis in vascular smooth muscle cells, *Hypertension* 31:1151, 1998.

144. Inagami T, Kambayashi Y, Ichiki T, et al: Angiotensin receptors: molecular biology and signalling, *Clin Exp Pharmacol Physiol* 26:544, 1999.

145. Gibbons GH: Cardioprotective mechanisms of ACE inhibition. The angiotensin II–nitric oxide balance, *Drugs* 54(Suppl 5):1, 1997.

146. Hinshaw LB: Sepsis/septic shock: participation of the microcirculation: an abbreviated review, *Crit Care Med* 24:1072, 1996.

147. Evans RG, Ventura S, Dampney EA, et al: Neural mechanisms in the cardiovascular responses to acute central hypovolaemia, *Clin Exp Pharmacol Physiol* 28:479, 2001.

148. Preisman S, Pfeiffer U, Lieberman N, et al: New monitors of intravascular volume: a comparison of arterial pressure waveform analysis and the intrathoracic blood volume, *Intensive Care Med* 23:651, 1997.

149. Holaday JW: Cardiovascular effects of endogenous opiate systems, *Annu Rev Pharmacol Toxicol* 23:541, 1983.

150. Ludbrook J, Ventura S: The decompensatory phase of acute hypovolaemia in rabbits involves a central d_1-opioid receptor, *Eur J Pharmacol* 252:113, 1994.

151. Bertolini A, Ferrari W, Guarini S: The adrenocorticotropic hormone (ACTH)–induced reversal of hemorrhagic shock, *Resuscitation* 18:253, 1989.

152. van Leeuwen AF, Evans RG, Ludbrook J: Effects of halothane, ketamine, propofol and alfentanil anesthesia on circulatory control in rabbits, *Clin Exp Pharmacol Physiol* 17:781, 1990.

153. Blake DW, Ludbrook J, van Leeuwen AF: Dexmedetomidine and haemodynamic responses to acute central hypovolaemia in conscious rabbits, *Clin Exp Pharmacol Physiol* 27:801, 2000.

154. Ince C, Sinaasappel M: Microcirculatory oxygenation and shunting in sepsis and shock, *Crit Care Med* 27:1369, 1999.

155. Ince C, Ashruf JF, Avontuur JA: Heterogeneity of the hypoxic state in rat heart is determined at the capillary level, *Am J Physiol* 264:H294, 1993.

156. Sinaasappel M, van Iterson M, Ince C: Microvascular oxygen pressure in the pig intestine during haemorrhagic shock and resuscitation, *J Physiol (Lond)* 514:245, 1999.

157. van der Meer TJ, Wang H, Fink MP: Endotoxemia causes ileal mucosal acidosis in the absence of mucosal hypoxia in a normodynamic porcine model of septic shock, *Crit Care Med* 23:1217, 1995.

158. Faller DV: Endothelial cell responses to hypoxic stress, *Clin Exp Pharmacol Physiol* 26:74, 1999.

159. Kourembanas S, Hannan R, Faller DV: Oxygen tension regulates the expression of platelet-derived growth factor-B chain gene in human endothelial cells, *J Clin Invest* 86:670, 1990.

160. Kourembanas S, Marsden PA, Mcquillan LP, et al: Hypoxia induces endothelin gene expression and secretion in cultured human endothelium, *J Clin Invest* 88:1054, 1991.

161. Phelan MW, Faller DV: Hypoxia decreases constitutive nitric oxide synthase transcript and protein in cultured endothelial cells, *J Cell Physiol* 167:469, 1996.

162. Aalkjaer C, Peng HL: pH and smooth muscle, *Acta Physiol Scand* 161:557, 1997.

163. Irikura K, Maynard KI, Lee WS, et al: L-NNA decreases cortical hyperemia and brain cGMP levels following CO_2 inhalation in Sprague-Dawley rats, *Am J Physiol* 267:H837, 1994.

164. Wang Q, Pelligrino DA, Baughman VL, et al: The role of neuronal nitric oxide synthase in regulation of cerebral blood flow in normocapnia and hypercapnia in rats, *J Cereb Blood Flow Metab* 15:774, 1995.

165. Wang Q, Pelligrino DA, Paulson OB, et al: Comparison of the effects of NG-nitro-L-arginine and indomethacin on the brain, *Brain Res* 641:257, 1994.

166. Egashira K, Inou T, Hirooka Y, et al: Effects of age on endothelium-dependent vasodilation of resistance coronary artery by acetylcholine in humans, *Circulation* 88:77, 1993.

167. Cohn JN, Finkelstein SM: Abnormalities of vascular compliance in hypertension, aging and heart failure, *J Hypertens Suppl* 10:S61, 1992.

168. Anderson TJ, Uehata A, Gerhard MD, et al: Close relation of endothelial function in the human coronary and peripheral circulations, *J Am Coll Cardiol* 26:1235, 1995.

169. Celermajer DS, Sorensen KE, Spiegelhalter DJ, et al: Aging is associated with endothelial dysfunction in healthy men years before the age-related decline in women, *J Am Coll Cardiol* 24:471, 1994.

170. Quyyumi AA, Mulcahy D, Andrews NP, et al: Coronary vascular nitric oxide activity in hypertension and hypercholesterolemia. Comparison of acetylcholine and substance P, *Circulation* 95:104, 1997.

171. Casino PR, Kilcoyne CM, Quyyumi AA, et al: Investigation of decreased availability of nitric oxide precursor as the mechanism responsible for impaired endothelium-dependent vasodilation in hypercholesterolemic patients, *J Am Coll Cardiol* 23:844, 1994.

172. Panza JA, Casino PR, Badar DM, et al: Effect of increased availability of endothelium-derived nitric oxide precursor on endothelium-dependent vascular relaxation in normal subjects and in patients with essential hypertension, *Circulation* 87:1475, 1993.

173. Gilligan DM, Guetta V, Panza JA, et al: Selective loss of microvascular endothelial function in human hypercholesterolemia, *Circulation* 90:35, 1994.

174. Panza JA, Garcia CE, Kilcoyne CM, et al: Impaired endothelium-dependent vasodilation in patients with essential hypertension. Evidence that nitric oxide abnormality is not localized to a single signal transduction pathway, *Circulation* 91:1732, 1995.

175. Quyyumi AA, Dakak N, Mulcahy D, et al: Nitric oxide activity in the atherosclerotic human coronary circulation, *J Am Coll Cardiol* 29:308, 1997.

176. Quyyumi AA, Dakak N, Andrews NP, et al: Nitric oxide activity in the human coronary circulation. Impact of risk factors for coronary atherosclerosis, *J Clin Invest* 95:1747, 1995.

177. Quyyumi AA, Cannon RO 3rd, Panza JA, et al: Endothelial dysfunction in patients with chest pain and normal coronary arteries, *Circulation* 86:1864, 1992.

178. Egashira K, Inou T, Hirooka Y, et al: Impaired coronary blood flow response to acetylcholine in patients with coronary risk factors and proximal atherosclerotic lesions, *J Clin Invest* 91:29, 1993.

179. Ludmer PL, Selwyn AP, Shook TL, et al: Paradoxical vasoconstriction induced by acetylcholine in atherosclerotic coronary arteries, *N Engl J Med* 315:1046, 1986.

180. Vita JA, Treasure CB, Nabel EG, et al: Coronary vasomotor response to acetylcholine relates to risk factors for coronary artery disease, *Circulation* 81:491, 1990.

181. Anderson TJ, Meredith IT, Charbonneau F, et al: Endothelium-dependent coronary vasomotion relates to the susceptibility of LDL to oxidation in humans, *Circulation* 93:1647, 1996.

182. Witztum JL: The oxidation hypothesis of atherosclerosis, *Lancet* 344:793, 1994.

183. Arnal JF, Munzel T, Venema RC, et al: Interactions between L-arginine and L-glutamine change endothelial NO production. An effect independent of NO synthase substrate availability, *J Clin Invest* 95:2565, 1995.

184. Schini Kerth VB, Vanhoutte PM: Nitric oxide synthases in vascular cells, *Exp Physiol* 80:885, 1995.

185. Harrison DG, Sayegh H, Ohara Y, et al: Regulation of expression of the endothelial cell nitric oxide synthase, *Clin Exp Pharmacol Physiol* 23:251, 1996.

186. Hirata Y, Hayakawa H, Suzuki E, et al: Direct measurements of endothelium-derived nitric oxide release by stimulation of endothelin receptors in rat kidney and its alteration in salt-induced hypertension, *Circulation* 91:1229, 1995.

187. Luscher TF, Vanhoutte PM, Raij L: Antihypertensive treatment normalizes decreased endothelium-dependent relaxations in rats with salt-induced hypertension, *Hypertension* 9:III193, 1987.

188. Lockette W, Otsuka Y, Carretero O: The loss of endothelium-dependent vascular relaxation in hypertension, *Hypertension* 8:II61, 1986.

189. Luscher TF, Raij L, Vanhoutte PM: Endothelium-dependent vascular responses in normotensive and hypertensive Dahl rats, *Hypertension* 9:157, 1987.

190. Shultz PJ, Raij L: Effects of antihypertensive agents on endothelium-dependent and endothelium-independent relaxations, *Br J Clin Pharmacol* 28(Suppl 2):151s, 1989.

191. Ribeiro MO, Antunes E, de Nucci G, et al: Chronic inhibition of nitric oxide synthesis. A new model of arterial hypertension, *Hypertension* 20:298, 1992.

192. Huang PL, Huang Z, Mashimo H, et al: Hypertension in mice lacking the gene for endothelial nitric oxide synthase, *Nature* 377:239, 1995.

193. Panza JA, Quyyumi AA, Brush JE Jr, et al: Abnormal endothelium-dependent vascular relaxation in patients with essential hypertension, *N Engl J Med* 323:22, 1990.

194. Linder L, Kiowski W, Buhler FR, et al: Indirect evidence for release of endothelium-derived relaxing factor in human forearm circulation in vivo. Blunted response in essential hypertension, *Circulation* 81:1762, 1990.

195. Taddei S, Mattei P, Virdis A, et al: Forearm vasodilation in response to acetylcholine is increased by potassium in essential hypertensive patients, *J Hypertens Suppl* 11(Suppl 5):S144, 1993.

196. Tesfamariam B, Jakubowski JA, Cohen RA: Contraction of diabetic rabbit aorta caused by endothelium-derived PGH2-TxA2, *Am J Physiol* 257:H1327, 1989.

197. Meraji S, Jayakody L, Senaratne MP, et al: Endothelium-dependent relaxation in aorta of BB rat, *Diabetes* 36:978, 1987.

198. Oyama Y, Kawasaki H, Hattori Y, et al: Attenuation of endothelium-dependent relaxation in aorta from diabetic rats, *Eur J Pharmacol* 132:75, 1986.

199. Kamata K, Miyata N, Kasuya Y: Impairment of endothelium-dependent relaxation and changes in levels of cyclic GMP in aorta from streptozotocin-induced diabetic rats, *Br J Pharmacol* 97:614, 1989.

200. Taylor AA: Pathophysiology of hypertension and endothelial dysfunction in patients with diabetes mellitus, *Endocrinol Metab Clin North Am* 30:983, 2001.

201. Mogensen CE: Glomerular filtration rate and renal plasma flow in short-term and long-term juvenile diabetes mellitus, *Scand J Clin Lab Invest* 28:91, 1971.

202. Kohner EM, Hamilton AM, Saunders SJ, et al: The retinal blood flow in diabetes, *Diabetologia* 11:27, 1975.

203. Houben AJ, Schaper NC, Slaaf DW, et al: Skin blood cell flux in insulin-dependent diabetic subjects in relation to retinopathy or incipient nephropathy, *Eur J Clin Invest* 22:67, 1992.

204. Williamson JR, Chang K, Frangos M, et al: Hyperglycemic pseudohypoxia and diabetic complications, *Diabetes* 42:801, 1993.

205. Maziere C, Auclair M, Rose Robert F, et al: Glucose-enriched medium enhances cell-mediated low density lipoprotein peroxidation, *FEBS Lett* 363:277, 1995.

206. Graier WF, Simecek S, Kukovetz WR, et al: High D-glucose–induced changes in endothelial Ca²⁺/EDRF signaling are due to generation of superoxide anions, *Diabetes* 45:1386, 1996.

207. Tesfamariam B, Cohen RA: Free radicals mediate endothelial cell dysfunction caused by elevated glucose, *Am J Physiol* 263:H321, 1992.

208. Wascher TC, Graier WF, Bahadori B, et al: Time course of endothelial dysfunction in diabetes mellitus, *Circulation* 90:1109, 1994.

209. Graier WF, Hoebel BG, Paltauf Doburzynska J, et al: Effects of superoxide anions on endothelial Ca²⁺ signaling pathways, *Arterioscler Thromb Vasc Biol* 18:1470, 1998.

210. Tesfamariam B, Brown ML, Deykin D, et al: Elevated glucose promotes generation of endothelium-derived vasoconstrictor prostanoids in rabbit aorta, *J Clin Invest* 85:929, 1990.

211. Tesfamariam B, Brown ML, Cohen RA: 15-Hydroxyeicosatetraenoic acid and diabetic endothelial dysfunction in rabbit aorta, *J Cardiovasc Pharmacol* 25:748, 1995.

212. Ceriello A, dello Russo P, Amstad P, et al: High glucose induces antioxidant enzymes in human endothelial cells in culture. Evidence linking hyperglycemia and oxidative stress, *Diabetes* 45:471, 1996.

213. Elliott SJ, Doan TN: Oxidant stress inhibits the store-dependent Ca(2+)-influx pathway of vascular endothelial cells, *Biochem J* 292:385, 1993.

214. Boillot A, Haddad E, Vallet B, et al: Effets des agents anesthésiques sur la vasomotricité artérielle, *Ann Fr Anesth Reanim* 18:415, 1999.

215. Johns RA, DiFazio CA, Longnecker DE: Lidocaine constricts or dilates rat arterioles in a dose-dependent manner, *Anesthesiology* 65:141, 1985.

216. Blair M: Cardiovascular pharmacology of local anesthetics, *Br J Anaesth* 47:247, 1975.

217. Freissmuth M, Schutz W, Linder ME: Interactions of the bovine brain A1-adenosine receptor with recombinant G protein alpha-subunits. Selectivity for rGi alpha-3, *J Biol Chem* 266:17778, 1991.

218. Munshi R, Pang IH, Sternweis PC, et al: A1 adenosine receptors of bovine brain couple to guanine nucleotide–binding proteins Gi1, Gi2, and Go, *J Biol Chem* 266:22285, 1991.

219. Abebe W, Mustafa SJ: A1 adenosine receptor–mediated Ins(1,4,5)P3 generation in allergic rabbit airway smooth muscle, *Am J Physiol* 275:L990, 1998.

220. Parsons M, Young L, Lee JE, et al: Distinct cardioprotective effects of adenosine mediated by differential coupling of receptor subtypes to phospholipases C and D, *FASEB J* 14:1423, 2000.

221. Liang BT: Direct preconditioning of cardiac ventricular myocytes via adenosine A1 receptor and KATP channel, *Am J Physiol* 271:H1769, 1996.

222. Noguchi J, Yamashita H: Adenosine inhibits voltage-dependent Ca²⁺ currents in rat dissociated supraoptic neurones via A1 receptors, *J Physiol (Lond)* 526:313, 2000.

223. Ambrosio AF, Malva JO, Carvalho AP, et al: Inhibition of N-, P/Q- and other types of Ca²⁺ channels in rat hippocampal nerve terminals by the adenosine A1 receptor, *Eur J Pharmacol* 340:301, 1997.

224. Marala RB, Mustafa SJ: Direct evidence for the coupling of A2-adenosine receptor to stimulatory guanine nucleotide–binding-protein in bovine brain striatum, *J Pharmacol Exp Ther* 266:294, 1993.

225. Stefanovic V, Vlahovic P, Savic V, et al: Adenosine stimulates 5′-nucleotidase activity in rat mesangial cells via A2 receptors, *FEBS Lett* 331:96, 1993.

226. MacEwan DJ, Kim GD, Milligan G: Agonist regulation of adenylate cyclase activity in neuroblastoma × glioma hybrid NG108-15 cells transfected to co-express adenylate cyclase type II and the beta₂-adrenoceptor. Evidence that adenylate cyclase is the limiting component for receptor-mediated stimulation of adenylate cyclase activity, *Biochem J* 318:1033, 1996.

227. Li SN, Wong PT: The adenosine receptor agonist, APNEA, increases calcium influx into rat cortical synaptosomes through N-type channels associated with A2a receptors, *Neurochem Res* 25:457, 2000.

228. Palmer TM, Gettys TW, Stiles GL: Differential interaction with and regulation of multiple G-proteins by the rat A3 adenosine receptor, *J Biol Chem* 270:16895, 1995.

229. Atkinson MR, Townsend-Nicholson A, Nicholl JK, et al: Cloning, characterisation and chromosomal assignment of the human adenosine A3 receptor (*ADORA3*) gene, *Neurosci Res* 29:73, 1997.

230. Abbracchio MP, Brambilla R, Ceruti S, et al: G protein–dependent activation of phospholipase C by adenosine A3 receptors in rat brain, *Mol Pharmacol* 48:1038, 1995.

231. Zhao Z, Francis CE, Ravid K: An A3-subtype adenosine receptor is highly expressed in rat vascular smooth muscle cells: its role in attenuating adenosine-induced increase in cAMP, *Microvasc Res* 54:243, 1997.

232. Zhao Z, Makaritsis K, Francis CE, et al: A role for the A3 adenosine receptor in determining tissue levels of cAMP and blood pressure: studies in knock-out mice, *Biochim Biophys Acta* 1500:280, 2000.

Pharmacologic Treatment of Hypertension, Heart Failure, and Ischemic Heart Disease

2

Imre Redai, MD
Riva R. Akerman, MD
Berend Mets, MB, ChB, PhD

CARDIOVASCULAR disease continues to be a leading cause of morbidity and mortality in developed countries. Maladaptive changes induced by sympathetic nervous system activation are responsible for much of the morbidity associated with hypertension, ischemic heart disease, and congestive heart failure. These disease states are characterized by widespread activation of associated neurohumoral and cytokine systems, leading to a progressive remodeling of the heart, the vascular tree, and the microcirculation. Pharmacologic therapy is, therefore, largely targeted at counteracting these maladaptive changes. This chapter gives a brief overview of the underlying pathologic processes of these diseases, followed by a discussion of current approaches to therapy. Strategies for the prevention, cessation, and reversal of the unfavorable changes in the cardiovascular system at the molecular, cellular, and organ system levels are discussed. Finally, there is a discussion of the effects of these pharmacologic agents on vascular response and vasoregulatory reflexes and mechanisms and the implications of these for anesthetic management of patients with hypertension, ischemic heart disease, and congestive heart failure.

Neurohumoral Changes in Hypertension, Ischemic Heart Disease, and Heart Failure

Essential Hypertension: The Renin-Angiotensin-Aldosterone System and Sympathetic Activation

More than 90% of all cases of hypertension are still classified as primary or essential hypertension. However, a variety of factors have been identified as possible causes of or contributors to the development of hypertension. These include renin, its product angiotensin II, angiotensin II receptors, and aldosterone. Associated ion fluxes in renal tubular and vascular smooth muscle cells have also been implicated.

Hypertensive patients are categorized into three main groups according to the defect in their renin-angiotensin-aldosterone regulation. Hypertensive patients with a low circulating renin concentration are presumed to have altered sensitivity to angiotensin II, resulting in elevated mineralocorticoid secretion and sodium retention. In about half of all hypertensive patients, renal release of renin and adrenal secretion of aldosterone are unaffected by sodium restriction, and plasma renin activity remains normal or high irrespective of salt intake. However, these patients, also known as nonmodulators, do respond to salt restriction in their diet with a decrease in blood pressure because the kidneys' ability to retain sodium is also defective. A further subset of patients present with increased renin secretion and elevated plasma renin levels secondary to chronic activation of sympathetic outflow, primarily directed toward the kidneys and the skeletal muscle vasculature. Sympathetic activation leads to renin release, which, in turn, increases vascular resistance and renal tubular sodium reabsorption.

Increased plasma norepinephrine concentrations secondary to spillover from sympathetic neuroeffector junctions and increased sympathetic nerve traffic have been shown in patients with essential hypertension.[1] The most likely mechanism relating hypertension and chronic sympathetic activation involves an angiotensin II–mediated increase in sympathetic outflow.[2] Increased angiotensin II activity may be seen in the setting of either high or low plasma renin concentration; altered angiotensin II receptor sensitivity may be a factor. The role of altered baroreflex responses in hypertension is more controversial. On the one hand, the heart rate response to baroreceptor stimulation is markedly impaired; on the other hand, baroreceptor-mediated peripheral sympathetic excitation and inhibition remain unchanged even in the setting of severe hypertension.[3] This central modulating effect of angiotensin II on the baroreflex control of heart rate in hypertension may account for the increase in blood pressure without an associated reflex bradycardia.[4]

The association between insulin resistance and hypertension has long been established. Insulin resistance and hyperinsulinemia lead to sympathetic activation and sodium retention. However, chronic sympathetic activation may precede the development of hyperinsulinemia and altered glucose metabolism by several years.[5] Continued neural vasoconstriction in skeletal muscle impairs glucose delivery and ultimately reduces glucose uptake, leading to insulin resistance.[6]

With aging, the arteries progressively stiffen, dilate, and lengthen. The decades of cyclic stress destroy the orderly structure of the elastic laminae, which are then replaced by collagen fibers, leading to thickening of the arterial wall. Loss of elastic laminae causes cystic medial degeneration and weakening of the arterial wall, which can lead to dissection or rupture. The higher peak and pulse pressures and the accelerated rate of change of pressure observed in hypertension result in earlier fracture and thinning of the elastic layers and in accelerated remodeling of the arterial wall.[7]

Endothelial dysfunction may also contribute to the altered reactivity of vascular smooth muscle. Reduced activity of nitric oxide (NO) and increased activity of endothelin-1 (an endothelium-derived vasoconstrictor) have been reported in essential hypertension.[8]

Ischemic Heart Disease and Its Effect on Cardiovascular Reflexes

Imbalance between myocardial oxygen supply and demand because of inadequate perfusion results in myocardial ischemia. Flow-limiting narrowing of the epicardial conductance arteries related to arteriosclerosis, spasm, luminal thrombi, or emboli reduces oxygen supply. Autoregulation in intramyocardial resistance arterioles may be inadequate, compromising oxygen supply. Myocardial oxygen demand may increase acutely with stress or exertion. Chronically increased workload and associated myocardial hypertrophy, as seen in hypertension or aortic stenosis, increase myocardial oxygen demand at rest. Commonly, it is the combination of increased demand and reduced supply that manifests as frank myocardial ischemia. Inadequate myocardial perfusion sufficient to cause ischemia may cause a variety of biochemical, electrochemical, and mechanical dysfunctions clinically manifested as angina, arrhythmias, and loss of pump function.

Cardiac sympathetic and parasympathetic afferents and efferents play a major role in determining the heart rate and myocardial contractility, thus affecting myocardial oxygen demand. Sympathetic afferents also carry the stimuli evoked by ischemia that are experienced as angina. Myocardial ischemia often results in activation or disruption of cardiac reflex responses. As the sympathetic and parasympathetic innervation of the ventricles is not homogenous, systemic response is determined by the location of ischemia. Ischemia of the inferoposterior wall, richly innervated by vagal afferents, often results in bradycardia and hypotension. Ischemia of the anterior wall, an area predominantly supplied by sympathetic afferents, more frequently evokes tachycardia and hypertension.[9] Local changes induced by ischemia (e.g., pH $\leq$ 6.8, tissue K^+ > 12 mM, accumulation of adenosine and other substances) may alter or disrupt conduction in epicardial or myocardial neural tissue. Cardiac reflexes are interrupted, with vagal afferents running intramyocardially more vulnerable than the epicardially distributed sympathetics. Autodenervation, the interruption of afferent sympathetic fibers by ischemia, may explain the phenomenon of painless ischemia. Efferent denervation, if complete, results in loss of sympathetic stimulation and reduced inotropy distal to the lesion; if incomplete, an imbalance of activating and inhibiting stimuli may arise, which contributes to the development of arrhythmias often seen with myocardial ischemia. Disruption of nerve supply results in denervation supersensitivity, an exaggerated response to stimulating agents such as catecholamines. The resulting autonomic and electrophysiologic changes increase the incidence of ventricular arrhythmias.[10]

Myocardial infarction has a profound effect on autonomic regulation. Baroreflex sensitivity and heart rate variability are both reduced following coronary occlusion and return to normal only about 3 months after the event. Interestingly, the period of altered autonomic regulation coincides with the period of

increased risk of sudden cardiac death following myocardial infarction. It appears that after myocardial infarction, heightened sympathetic activity favors the development of, whereas parasympathetic activity is protective against, ventricular arrhythmias.[11]

Myocardial infarction induces a sequence of reparative events. Inflammatory cells migrate to the site of the infarct, releasing cytokines and various proteases. Myofibroblasts, cells with structural characteristics of both smooth muscle cells and fibroblasts that are involved in wound healing and contraction, appear and persist for several years after the infarction. Endothelial cells may undergo apoptosis, resulting in loss of blood supply.[12] Thus, proliferative and degenerative processes act in conjunction to produce remodeling of the injured myocardium. Furthermore, myofibroblasts synthesize and secrete angiotensin II, which, together with the altered forces affecting the myocardium, contributes to the global remodeling of the postinfarction heart.[13]

Heart Failure, Neuroendocrine Activation, and Myocardial Remodeling

Any progressive structural or functional disorder that impairs the ability of the ventricle to fill with or eject blood limits the ability of the heart to generate flow adequate for the metabolic requirements of the body and ultimately results in heart failure.[14]

Systolic dysfunction, primarily an impairment of myocardial contractility, constitutes 60% to 80% of all cases of heart failure. In approximately two thirds of these patients, the instigating cause is ischemic heart disease. Unfortunately, these patients have the worst prognosis: about one third are not expected to survive beyond 3 months, and mortality among the remainder is about 10% annually.[15] Although hypertension, valvular disease, myocarditis, and various toxins have been identified as possible causes of systolic dysfunction, for the majority of patients with nonischemic systolic dysfunction, the precipitating cause remains unclear.

Diastolic dysfunction affects the remaining 20% to 40% of patients. In these patients the systolic ejection function of the ventricle is preserved. However, the diastolic relaxation of the myocardium is restricted, which results in impaired diastolic filling. Although the majority of patients with diastolic dysfunction present without a well-defined myocardial abnormality, structural changes related to aging (such as aortic stiffening), hypertension, restrictive and hypertrophic cardiomyopathies, and infiltrative myocardial processes might be involved. It is not uncommon for elements of systolic and diastolic dysfunction to be present in the same patient.[14]

The elevated end-diastolic volume associated with systolic dysfunction or increased end-diastolic pressure seen in diastolic dysfunction tends to increase ventricular wall stress. Remodeling of the heart results in hypertrophy of the left ventricle, which normalizes wall stress according to Laplace's law. However, these changes are achieved at a cost. The number of capillaries does not increase in parallel with the developing myocyte hypertrophy, and microvascular abnormalities and elevated wall tension further limit blood flow. This condition leads to a state of energy starvation, and the myocardial fibers contract more slowly on an altered, flattened force-velocity curve. Although initially this change allows the cardiac fibers to contract at a lower energy cost, it ultimately leads to a reduced cardiac output followed by pump failure.[16] Furthermore, expression of messenger RNA (mRNA) of the slow-contracting β-myosin heavy chain is increased from 77% to 93% in patients with dilated cardiomyopathy.[17]

Collagenase activation results in the disruption of the collagenous network of the heart. New collagen is synthesized and the rearrangement of collagen support allows myocardial fiber elongation, slippage, and, ultimately, ventricular dilatation. This continued remodeling results in an enlarged, hypertrophied ventricle with worsened performance, increased oxygen consumption, and impaired subendocardial blood flow that is at increased risk for ventricular arrhythmias.[18] It is generally accepted that the progressive remodeling of the myocardium after the initial myocardial insult plays no compensatory role and that the process of hypertrophy and dilatation is maladaptive and harmful.[19] Experimental data support this notion. Two animal models, one consisting of transgenic mice overexpressing the $G\alpha_q$ inhibitor peptide, the other involving knockout mice lacking endogenous epinephrine and norepinephrine production, were designed. Both animals lack the ability to respond with left ventricular hypertrophy to chronic pressure overload. However, despite the lack of ability to compensate for increased wall stress, there was less deterioration in heart function over time than in control animals.[20]

Neuroendocrine activation ensues at the earliest stages of heart failure. Elevated levels of circulating norepinephrine, atrial natriuretic peptide, endothelin-1, and arginine vasopressin, as well as increased local production of angiotensin II, induce myocyte hypertrophy and proliferation. Both norepinephrine and angiotensin II were shown to have trophic effects and, together with mechanical stretch, play an important role in early remodeling of the ventricle.[21] The increased plasma norepinephrine level correlates with the development of heart failure, ischemic events, and cardiovascular mortality.[22]

Various changes in myocardial and vascular gene expression are associated with the development of heart failure.[23] Loss of the potassium channel responsible for the early, transient current (I_{to}) results in prolonged repolarization. When this defect was corrected, using an adenoviral shuttle vector containing a potassium channel genetic construct, both the repolarization time and the contraction velocity returned to control values.[24] Expression and function of sarcoplasmic reticulum Ca^{2+} adenosine triphosphatase (ATPase) are also reduced by the sustained elevation of plasma norepinephrine levels seen in patients with heart failure. A vicious circle ensues in which the diminished intracellular calcium handling leads to worsening heart function, which in turn causes a further elevation of plasma norepinephrine and, thus, a further reduction in sarcoplasmic reticulum Ca^{2+}-ATPase activity.[16] A parallel downregulation has been reported for phospholamban and calsequestrin, two proteins with a key role in intracellular Ca^{2+} handling and regulation of myofiber contraction and relaxation. Thus, it appears that proteins responsible for calcium handling and movement in the sarcoplasmic reticulum are sensitive to the elevated circulating catecholamine levels observed in heart failure.[23]

Expression and function of cardiac receptors in human heart failure have been extensively studied. Although chronic α_{1C}-adrenergic receptor stimulation has a direct hypertrophic effect on myocardial cells, the α_1-receptor concentration remains unchanged. The elevated catecholamine levels characteristic of human heart failure induce the downregulation of β_1-receptors but do not affect the number of β_2-receptors. Furthermore, there is an associated increase in $G\alpha_i$ subunit levels, resulting in further inhibition of adenylyl cyclase activity.[25] The number of angiotensin II receptors also increases from the early stages of cardiac remodeling and remains increased throughout the development of end-stage heart failure.[26]

Tumor necrosis factor-α (TNF-α) is a proinflammatory cytokine with cytolytic and negative inotropic effects. The nonfailing myocardium does not express TNF-α, whereas the failing human myocardium produces significant quantities.[27] Plasma levels of TNF-α and interleukin-6 are also increased. A correlation has been found between TNF-α levels, neurohumoral activation, and progression or stage of heart failure.[27] Multicenter studies (Randomized Enbrel North American Strategy to Study Antagonism of Cytokines [RENAISSANCE]) are under way to examine the link between cytokine expression in the failing human heart and myocardial remodeling. Early reports from patients with severe heart failure treated with the soluble TNF-α receptor blocker etanercept show not only a reduction in circulating TNF-α levels but also a significant improvement in functional status.[28] By contrast, inotropic agents such as milrinone and dobutamine have no effect upon, or actually increase, circulating TNF-α levels; despite the short-term clinical improvement seen with these agents, this deleterious effect on TNF-α levels may ultimately cause worsening heart failure.[29]

Progressive cell loss in the heart occurs not only as part of natural aging but also in all forms of cardiomyopathy, in ischemic heart disease, and in hypertensive myocardial hypertrophy. Myocyte death occurs through apoptosis or cell necrosis, and the combination of the two could markedly decrease the number of functioning cells in the heart.[12] Necrotic cell death and resultant scarring account for the loss of nearly 10% of functional myocardium in patients with end-stage heart failure. In the same patients, about 0.25% of all myocytes show histologic signs of ongoing apoptosis; this is a more than 200-fold increase compared with healthy control subjects.[30] The process of programmed cell death is completed in 20 minutes to 24 hours; thus, loss of heart tissue over time through apoptosis is considerable even when apoptotic cell numbers at any given time are small.

Mechanical and neurohumoral factors present in heart failure may induce apoptosis.[31] Isometric stretch of papillary muscle or pressure overload of the left ventricle by aortic banding was shown to initiate apoptosis. Exposing isolated adult cardiomyocytes in culture to angiotensin II or atrial natriuretic peptide results in a fourfold increase in the percentage of apoptotic cells. Furthermore, chronic ischemia and repeated reperfusion injury are associated with multiple alterations of the intra- and extracellular milieu that may initiate programmed cell death.

The long-held view that cardiac myocytes are terminally differentiated cells incapable of division has been questioned. Mitotic myocytes have been found even in normal human hearts and the rate of mitosis increases nearly 10-fold in heart failure. Thus, loss and gain of myocardial cells happen simultaneously in myocardial remodeling.[32]

Continued sympathetic stimulation and the associated neuro-humoral changes induce unfavorable changes in the peripheral vascular tone. There is a significant attenuation of endothelial NO production, which correlates with the severity of heart failure. Endothelial dysfunction is further reflected in reduced response to vasodilatory substances such as atrial natriuretic peptide and adrenomedullin. Apoptotic changes of the vascular endothelium and the subintimal region may predispose to atheromatous degeneration and contribute to worsening function. Thus, in addition to myocardial remodeling, continuous vascular remodeling is taking place in heart failure.[33]

The Role of β-Adrenergic Receptor Blockade in the Treatment of Hypertension, Ischemic Heart Disease, and Heart Failure

The first synthetic β-adrenergic receptor–blocking compounds appeared in the late 1950s.[34] They were synthesized shortly after Ahlquist presented his theory on sympathetic receptors. These drugs were specifically designed to interfere with pathologic changes in sympathetic regulation in hypertension and heart disease.

β-Adrenergic Receptors and Associated Signaling Pathways

Adrenergic receptors belong to the family of G protein–coupled receptors[20] (Figure 2-1). Adrenergic receptors have been divided into two main groups: α- and β-receptors. Three subtypes of β-adrenergic receptors have been cloned. The β_1-receptor, which constitutes 75% to 80% of all adrenergic receptors in the heart, is predominantly found on the postsynaptic folds of cardiac sympathoeffector junctions. This distribution suggests that the primary physiologic role of the β_1-receptor is in the sympathetic adrenergic neural regulation of cardiac rate and contractility. The β_2-receptor is more widespread. In the heart, where it is mainly extrajunctional, it constitutes about 10% of all adrenergic receptors. β_2-Receptors are also found in peripheral blood vessels, bronchi, kidneys, and myometrium. The β_2-receptor appears to be responsible for the systemic response to circulating catecholamines. Norepinephrine and epinephrine are the two main intrinsic agonists of the β-adrenergic receptor. Although their agonist potency is equal on the β_1-receptor, norepinephrine has little, if any, effect on β_2-receptors.

G proteins are guanine nucleotide–binding regulatory proteins. They are heterotrimers composed of three subunits: α, β, and γ. Several subtypes of stimulatory and inhibitory G proteins have been described and cloned. In the resting state, the heterotrimers are associated with the G protein binding site, which is located on the intracellular domain of the transmembrane receptor. The conformational change following receptor activation induces splitting of the G protein complex into Gα and Gβγ subunits. These subunits dissociate from the receptor to interact with adenylyl cyclases, protein kinases, phospholipases, and ion channels. Second messengers or ion fluxes generated by

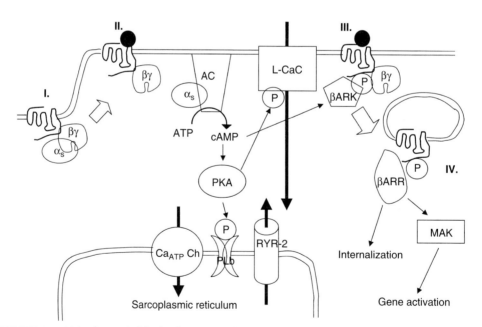

FIGURE 2-1 Molecular events following β-receptor activation in the heart. **I**, The resting β-receptor is coupled to the heterotrimeric G_s protein. **II**, Following ligand (●) binding, the Gαs subunit dissociates from the receptor–G protein complex and activates adenylyl cyclase (AC). AC catalyzes conversion of ATP to cAMP. cAMP in turn activates protein kinase A (PKA) and β-adrenoceptor kinase 1 (βARK). Activated PKA phosphorylates (P) L-type calcium channels (L-CaC) and phospholamban (PLb). Conductivity of L-type calcium channels increases (*thick black arrows* represent calcium fluxes), enhancing ryanodine-2 receptor (RYR-2) opening and efflux of calcium from the sarcoplasmic reticulum. Phosphorylated PLb disengages from the sarcoplasmic reticulum calcium ATPase pump (Ca_{ATP} Ch), which in turn enhances sarcoplasmic calcium uptake. **III**, Activation of βARK leads to the phosphorylation of the G protein binding site on the β-receptor. **IV**, Binding of β-arrestin (βARR) to the phosphorylated receptor initiates receptor internalization and activation of mitogen-activated kinases (MAK).

these targets of G proteins cause activation or inhibition of intracellular signaling pathways, thereby determining the response of the individual cell. The primary effector G protein associated with β-receptors is $G\alpha_s$. When released following activation of the β-receptor, $G\alpha_s$ stimulates adenylyl cyclase, resulting in an increase in intracellular cyclic adenosine monophosphate (cAMP) levels.

Continued stimulation of β-receptors results in a reduced response of the target cell. This adaptive mechanism is known as desensitization (see Figure 2-1). Two main mechanisms of receptor desensitization have been outlined. Receptor down-regulation involves a net loss of receptors secondary to reduced synthesis and increased degradation of receptor mRNA and protein. Phosphorylation of the intracellular G protein binding site of the receptor results in the inability to form new complexes with G protein heterotrimers. This uncoupling of the receptor from G proteins may result from phosphorylation by protein kinase A, a cAMP-dependent enzyme, or by β-adrenergic receptor kinase 1 (βARK1), which is activated by the $\beta\gamma$ subunits of the G protein complex. Phosphorylation of agonist-occupied β-receptors enhances affinity of the receptors for cytosolic β-arrestins, proteins responsible for uncoupling and internalization of a number of G protein–linked receptors. The binding of β-arrestin to the receptor then either induces receptor internalization or stimulates mitogen-activated protein kinases responsible for inducing cell hypertrophy, proliferation, or apoptosis.

Chronic sympathetic stimulation and elevated catecholamine levels in heart failure lead to desensitization of both β_1- and β_2-receptors. β_1- receptors appear to be downregulated and internalized selectively, presumably because of their postjunctional location, and the ratio of β_2- to β_1- receptors in the heart increases. However, elevated βARK1 levels lead to increased phosphorylation and uncoupling from G proteins of both receptors. This not only results in attenuation of cAMP-dependent signaling through both receptors but also may enhance coupling to β-arrestin–dependent pathways of cell hypertrophy, apoptosis, and myocardial remodeling.[20]

General Characteristics of β-Receptor Antagonists

β-Receptor antagonists show striking similarities to the parent catecholamine compounds. However, in β-receptor antagonists, the original two-carbon distance between the amino terminal and the aryl group of catecholamines is extended to a three- or four-atom length. This change abolishes sympathomimetic activity while still allowing docking of the molecule to the β-receptor.

β-Receptor antagonists with equal affinity to both β_1- and β_2-receptors are classified as nonselective; typical examples are propranolol, nadolol, carvedilol, timolol, and labetalol. When the need for β_1-selective antagonists was recognized, drugs such as metoprolol, atenolol, acebutolol, and esmolol were developed. These drugs have a higher affinity for the β_1-receptor, but in the individual patient their effect on β_2-receptors may be significant. Several β-receptor antagonists are actually weak partial agonists with a high affinity for the β-receptor. They stimulate the β-receptor in the absence of a potent agonist such as epinephrine or isoproterenol but antagonize the effect of the agonist

when it is present. This feature is also known as intrinsic sympathomimetic activity; pindolol and acebutolol are typical examples. Celiprolol is a β_1-selective antagonist with β_2-agonist properties. Some drugs, such as labetalol and carvedilol, were found to have antagonist effects on both β- and α-receptors. Sotalol has unique antiarrhythmic properties not related to its β-receptor antagonist activity.

The majority of β-receptor antagonists are highly lipophilic and well absorbed from the gut. They undergo significant first-pass metabolism in the liver and their bioavailability is 25% to 40%. This high, but variable, first-pass metabolism results in significant variability in drug plasma and tissue levels in individual patients. However, because clinical endpoints such as reduction of heart rate and blood pressure are easily determined, establishing the appropriate therapeutic drug dose is seldom a problem. Reducing hepatic blood flow (because of inhaled anesthetics or surgical stress) increases the bioavailability and plasma concentration of lipophilic β-blockers. Smoking increases hepatic biotransformation of propranolol.

Absorption of hydrophilic β-receptor antagonists such as nadolol and atenolol is only about 30% to 50%. The absorbed drug passes through the portohepatic circulation unaltered, and elimination is predominantly renal; caution is advised when these drugs are administered to patients with poor or worsening renal function. Esmolol is an intravenously administered ultra-short-acting β-receptor antagonist. It contains an ester link that is hydrolyzed by red blood cell esterases. Esmolol has distribution and elimination half-lives of 1.3 and 8 to 10 minutes, respectively, and its volume of distribution is 2 L/kg; these parameters are unaffected by general anesthesia or use of chronic β-blocker therapy.[35] Esmolol has an active metabolite, which is 500 times less potent than the parent compound. It is excreted by the kidney, and clinically significant accumulation of this metabolite has not been reported. The pharmacologic characteristics of β-receptor antagonists are summarized in Table 2-1.

Cardiovascular Effects of β-Receptor Antagonists

HEALTHY SUBJECTS. β-Receptor antagonists slow the heart rate and reduce myocardial contractility. As parasympathetic innervation determines the tone of the normal resting adult heart, the changes of basal heart rate and stroke volume in a healthy person are unremarkable. However, β-receptor antagonists attenuate stress- or exercise-induced increases in heart rate and cardiac output.

β-Receptor antagonists reduce the rate of sinus node depolarization and slow conduction in atrial and atrioventricular (AV) nodal tissue. They prolong the functional refractory period of the AV node and suppress the rate of depolarization of ectopic pacemakers. These effects are more pronounced in states of sympathetic activation.[36]

Blood pressure is not altered significantly by β-receptor antagonists in healthy individuals. Peripheral blockade of β_2-receptors by nonselective β-receptor antagonists results in vasoconstriction. The concomitant reduction in cardiac output results in a compensatory increase of sympathetic activity, resulting in peripheral α_1-receptor activation. However, this increase in peripheral vascular resistance is short lived, and vascular resistance soon returns to or below normal levels.[37]

TABLE 2-1

The Pharmacokinetic Characteristics, Recommended Daily Oral Doses, and Intravenous Doses of β-Receptor Antagonist Drugs

Drug	Selectivity	Features	Absorption (%)	First-Pass Metabolism (%)	Protein Bound (%)	Elimination	Half-Life (hours)	Oral Dose (mg daily)	IV Dose (mg) Repeat Interval
Acebutolol	Yes	ISA	~100	60	26	Liver	3-4	200-800	NA
Atenolol	Yes	None	50	10	3	Kidney	5-8	50-100	2.5 mg/5 min (max 10 mg)
Carvedilol	No	α_1 block, memb	~100	60-75	98	Liver	6-10	12.5-50	NA
Celiprolol	Yes	ISA	30-70	Minimal	30	Renal	4-6	200-600	NA
Esmolol	Yes	None	NA	NA	50	Erythrocyte esterase	8 min	NA	50-100 mg/0.05-0.3 mg/kg/min infusion
Labetalol	No	α_1 block	~100	70	50	Liver	6-8	400-1200	5-20 mg/5-10 min
Metoprolol	Yes	None	~100	60	5-10	Liver	3-4	100-400	5 mg/2 min (max 15 mg)
Nadolol	No	None	37	Minimal	30	Kidney	20-24	80-320	NA
Oxprenolol	No	ISA	70-90	20-65	80-90	Liver	1.5-4	120-480	1-2 mg (max 5 mg)
Pindolol	No	ISA	~100	10-15	40	Liver/kidney	3-4	15-45	0.1-0.4 mg
Propranolol	No	memb	~100	~75	90	Liver	3-5	40-320	0.5-1 mg (max 3 mg)
Sotalol	No	Class III	~100	10	Minimal	Kidney	7-15	160-320	0.2-0.5 mg/kg/hr
Timolol	No	None	~100	50	80	Liver	3-5	15-60	NA

α_1 block, α_1-adrenergic receptor antagonist activity; Class III, class III antiarrhythmic action; ISA, intrinsic sympathomimetic activity; memb, membrane-stabilizing activity, NA, not applicable.

HYPERTENSIVE PATIENTS. β-Receptor antagonists are effective in reducing blood pressure in hypertensive patients.[38] Although the therapeutic use of β-blockers in hypertension is well established, the mechanism is still poorly understood. It appears that different mechanisms may be responsible for similar reductions in blood pressure achieved by different β-receptor antagonists. β-Receptor antagonists suppress plasma renin activity, but no correlation was found between the reduction in blood pressure and the drop in renin activity. When compared with each other, different β-receptor antagonists appear to have different effects on cardiac output, renal blood flow, and peripheral β_2-receptor downregulation. Changes in cardiac output, circulating blood volume, or angiotensin-mediated vasoconstriction do not fully explain the antihypertensive effect of β-receptor antagonists. Interference with vasoconstrictor nerve activity through blockade of either central or peripheral prejunctional β-adrenergic receptors is believed to be the most likely explanation for the blood pressure–lowering effect of these drugs.[39]

Reduction of peripheral vascular resistance by α_1-receptor antagonism (labetalol, carvedilol) or partial β_2-agonist activity (celiprolol) may contribute to the antihypertensive effect of selected β-blockers. These added features may improve peripheral tissue perfusion, but there is no difference between these drugs and the rest of the β-receptor antagonists in overall efficiency of maintaining blood pressure reduction in hypertensive patients.

PATIENTS WITH ISCHEMIC HEART DISEASE. β-Receptor antagonists reduce the frequency and the severity of attacks in patients suffering from exertional angina. They reduce the risk of progression to myocardial infarction and improve long-term survival following acute myocardial infarction.[40]

Exercise and stress lead to sympathetic activation, manifested by tachycardia and increased contractility. By reducing tachycardia and depressing contractility, β-receptor antagonists are effective in preventing the associated increase in myocardial oxygen demand. The reduction in heart rate also increases diastolic perfusion time and enhances subendocardial capillary blood flow. Thus, β-blockers maintain the balance between myocardial oxygen supply and demand. All β-blockers appear to be equally effective in the treatment of exertional angina. However, their use is contraindicated in patients with Prinzmetal's (vasospastic) angina, as β-blocker therapy may lead to unopposed α-receptor activity and worsening of the symptoms.

β-Blockers are also useful in blunting reflex tachycardias associated with vasodilator drug therapy and are often combined with nitrates or dihydropyridine calcium channel blockers for this reason. Furthermore, the reduction in heart rate induced by β-blocker therapy may increase left ventricular end-diastolic wall tension, which may increase myocardial oxygen demand and compromise subendocardial blood flow. Combination therapy with nitrates reduces preload and prevents the deleterious effects of β-blocker–induced bradycardia.

PATIENTS WITH CONGESTIVE HEART FAILURE. It was known since the 1970s that chronic β-receptor antagonist therapy improves functional status and exercise tolerance of patients with dilated cardiomyopathy.[41] In light of the more recent appreciation of the deleterious effects of chronic sympathetic stimulation on myocardial remodeling, attention has been directed toward the use of β-receptor antagonists in congestive heart failure.[14]

When β-receptor antagonist therapy is initiated in patients with congestive heart failure, there is an initial reduction in contractility resulting in a decrease of the ejection fraction.

Patients with borderline cardiac function may poorly tolerate even small reductions in cardiac performance, and advancement of β-receptor antagonist therapy in these patients should be attempted gradually and with caution. However, when therapy is established and maximized, cardiac performance and the patient's well-being improve, and overall mortality is reduced by 30% to 60%.[42,43] β-Receptor antagonist therapy is now recommended for all patients with symptomatic heart failure who are in stable condition.[14]

Functional improvement related to treatment with β-receptor antagonists in patients with dilated cardiomyopathy is associated with changes in myocardial gene expression. In a heart failure model, selective reductions of myocardial TNF-α and interleukin-1β expression also accompanied the functional improvement achieved with β-receptor antagonist treatment.[44] Patients with dilated cardiomyopathy who were treated with metoprolol or carvedilol and had an improvement in left ventricular ejection fraction also had increases in sarcoplasmic reticulum Ca^{2+}-ATPase mRNA and α-myosin heavy-chain mRNA and a decrease in β-myosin heavy-chain mRNA.[17] This association of clinical improvement with suppression of markers of myocardial remodeling offers biochemical evidence for beneficial changes induced on the cellular level by long-term β-blocker therapy in patients with heart failure.

It is still unclear how β-receptor blockade improves myocardial function. As described earlier, β-receptor stimulation and activation of βARK1 lead to phosphorylation and desensitization of the β-receptor. Blocking β-receptors may lead to a normalization of βARK1 levels and an increase in the number of functional β-receptors. Furthermore, phosphorylated β-receptors activate pathways involved in cell hypertrophy, proliferation, and apoptosis. Interruption of these pathways is crucial for arresting and reversing myocardial remodeling.[20] Inhibition of βARK1 using genetic manipulation results in prevention or reversal of cardiac failure in numerous animal models. This suggests that the uncoupling of cardiac β-receptors from G proteins and adenylyl cyclase by continued sympathetic stimulation in heart failure is not beneficial but rather harmful.[45]

Side Effects Associated with β-Receptor Antagonists

Life-threatening bradycardia with β-receptor antagonists is rare. However, β-receptor antagonists should be used with extreme caution in patients with impaired AV conduction (partial or complete AV block). Combining β-blockers with drugs that slow AV conduction (such as verapamil) is not recommended. Significant bradycardia associated with β-blockers is usually treated with atropine.

Fatigue and inability to perform exercise are common side effects of β-blocker therapy. During exercise, the maximum achievable work is reduced by approximately 10% to 15%.[46] Patients with limited myocardial reserve are the most vulnerable. As discussed previously, β-receptor antagonists may exacerbate heart failure in the setting of cardiomyopathy or myocardial infarction. Clinically significant acute heart failure induced by β-blockers is usually treated with β-agonists. Glucagon has non-β-receptor-mediated positive inotropic and chronotropic effects and has been used successfully in β-blocker-induced heart failure.

Prolonged use of β-blockers results in increases in the numbers and sensitivity of β-receptors. This leads to a rebound effect: abrupt discontinuation of β-blockers has been associated with an increased risk of sudden death resulting from arrhythmias and exacerbation of ischemic symptoms. If the drug has to be stopped, it should be stopped gradually. When perioperative oral intake is restricted, patients should be switched to an intravenous β-receptor antagonist.[47]

Currently used selective β-receptor antagonists still retain a significant effect on $β_2$-receptors. This may induce bronchospasm in patients with reactive airways disease, and β-blockers are usually avoided in asthmatics. However, the benefits of β-receptor antagonism use outweight the risks following myocardial infarction in patients with chronic obstructive airway disease.[48] Celiprolol, which has intrinsic $β_2$-stimulating activity, has been promoted for use in patients with reactive airways disease. However, the advantages of its use over selective $β_1$-antagonists without intrinsic sympathomimetic activity are yet to be proved.[49]

Long-term β-blocker therapy reduces mortality following myocardial infarction in patients with insulin-dependent diabetes.[48] However, recognition of hypoglycemia may become difficult in the presence of β-receptor antagonists by the masking of tachycardia commonly associated with low blood glucose levels. Recovery from hypoglycemia is also slower in the presence of β-blockade. Thus, although clearly beneficial, β-blockers should be used with appropriate caution in patients with insulin-dependent diabetes.

β-Blockers adversely affect the lipid profile. High-density lipoprotein (HDL) cholesterol is reduced and serum triglyceride levels increase. In hypercholesterolemic patients, $β_1$-selective drugs are likely to affect plasma lipids adversely to a lesser extent than nonselective ones. Furthermore, celiprolol, secondary to its partial $β_2$-agonist properties, has been shown to improve the lipid pattern.[50]

Insomnia, nightmares, and worsening of depression were associated with β-adrenoceptor antagonist therapy. Male impotence and erectile dysfunction may adversely affect quality of life.

Perioperative Use of β-Receptor Antagonists

High-cardiac-risk surgery such as major vascular surgery results in activation of the sympathetic nervous system and increased plasma catecholamine levels. The associated increases in heart rate, contractility, and peripheral vascular resistance increase myocardial oxygen demand. Should oxygen supply be jeopardized because of coronary artery disease, blood loss, impaired pulmonary oxygen uptake, perioperative metabolic derangement, or a combination of these, the resulting myocardial supply-demand imbalance leads to myocardial ischemia. Furthermore, hyperdynamic circulation increases the shear stress over atheromatous plaques in coronary arteries. This condition may result in plaque rupture and acute thrombotic occlusion of the artery.[51]

Sympatholytic effects of β-blockade should counteract these unwanted effects and may prevent the development of perioperative myocardial ischemia. It is well established that chronic β-blocker therapy should be continued perioperatively.[52] A single oral dose of a β-receptor antagonist reduces myocardial ischemic events associated with laryngoscopy, endotracheal intubation, and emergence from anesthesia.[53] Studies have presented evidence for the beneficial effects of perioperative β-receptor blockade in selected populations of patients undergoing major noncardiac surgery. Atenolol, when administered to patients with a history of coronary artery disease undergoing major noncardiac surgery prior to induction of anesthesia and continued until 7 days postoperatively, reduced the incidence of ischemic events in the first 48 hours by 50%.[54] A large multicenter trial in patients undergoing major vascular surgery who were found to have significant wall motion abnormalities on preoperative dobutamine stress echocardiography showed that bisoprolol, when started at least 1 week preoperatively and continued for 30 days postoperatively, reduced the combined incidence of cardiac death and nonfatal myocardial infarction by a factor of 10.[55] Although these studies certainly support the use of β-receptor antagonists in high-risk patients, the benefits of routine use of these drugs in intermediate-risk patients remain to be established.[56]

Perioperative β-blockade may not be suitable for all patients. Those with limited left ventricular reserve may experience clinical heart failure following even low doses of β-blockers. In patients with asthma or chronic obstructive airway disease, the risks of inducing exacerbation of the airway reactivity should be weighed against the benefits of myocardial protection. Patients with significant sinus node dysfunction or conduction abnormalities should also be treated with caution.

The Role of Nitrovasodilators in the Treatment of Ischemic Heart Disease and Heart Failure

Nitrate-containing compounds have been used for medicinal purposes for more than 150 years, although their mechanism of action has been elucidated relatively recently. Nitroglycerin (NTG) was discovered in 1847 by Ascanio Sobrero, who observed a severe headache produced by small amounts of the substance on the tongue. In 1867, T. Lauder Brunton first administered amyl nitrite to relieve angina, and in 1879, William Murrell first described the use of sublingual NTG in the relief and prophylaxis of anginal pain.[57] Murad discovered the release of NO from NTG in 1977, and in 1980, Furchgott et al noted the importance of endothelium in the vasodilation caused by acetylcholine (ACh) and described an unstable relaxing substance, which they called endothelium-derived relaxing factor (EDRF). In 1987, Ignarro et al proposed that NO and EDRF were identical. The importance of NO as a cardiovascular signaling molecule is evidenced by the awarding of the Nobel Prize in Medicine or Physiology to Murad, Furchgott, and Ignarro in 1998.[58]

An Overview of Nitric Oxide and Nitric Oxide Synthase

NO is a small, reactive molecule.[59] Endogenous NO is produced in a two-step sequential oxidation of L-arginine to L-citrulline by nitric oxide synthase (NOS). NOS is a heme-containing metalloenzyme containing two functional parts: the reductase domain, involved in the reduction of reduced nicotinamide adenine dinucleotide phosphate (NADPH) and transfer of electrons, and the oxygenase domain, where the reactive center of the enzyme is located. The dimeric arrangement of NOS allows electron transfer to take place between the reductase and oxygenase domains of the two subunits. Tetrahydrobiopterin (THB)

bound to the oxygenase domain stabilizes the dimeric structure of the enzyme, supports the binding of L-arginine, affects the conformation of the heme iron, and participates in the redox function of the domain.[60] In the absence of THB, NOS catalyzes formation of superoxide anion (O_2^-) and may be a source of peroxynitrile synthesis.

Three isoforms of NOS have been isolated and characterized. Neuronal NOS (nNOS or NOS I) and endothelial NOS (eNOS or NOS III) are both constitutive enzymes, expressed in cells and tissues at all times. Inducible NOS (iNOS or NOS II) is expressed only in selected tissues (e.g., lung epithelial cells) and is typically synthesized in response to inflammatory mediators.[61] Hypoxia and laminar shear stress upregulate eNOS mRNA production and eNOS synthesis, which leads to increased NO production and release.

NO is an important endogenous messenger for a variety of physiologic functions, including cardiovascular regulation, immune function, penile erection, and long-term memory.[62] In the myocardium, NO has a direct chronotropic effect mediated by activation of the inward pacemaker current I_f.[63] NO appears to advance parasympathetic and inhibit sympathetic activation both in healthy subjects and in patients with chronic heart failure.[64] NO-induced increases in myocardial cyclic guanosine monophosphate (cGMP) concentration result in antagonism of β-receptor stimulation, reduced calcium influx, decreased contractility, reduced myocardial oxygen consumption, and opening of ATP-dependent potassium channels (K_{ATP}).[65] Endothelial dysfunction associated with reduced synthesis and enhanced elimination of NO has been observed in heart failure as well as in atherosclerotic and hypertensive vascular remodeling. Peripheral endothelial basal NO release is preserved or enhanced in patients with chronic heart failure; however, ACh-induced vasodilation is markedly impaired in the same patients. Elevated circulating TNF and cytokine levels frequently observed in patients with heart failure impair eNOS function and reduce NO release.

NO diffuses into vascular smooth muscle cells and binds to the ferroheme prosthetic group of soluble guanylate cyclase (sGC), inducing a conformational change and enhancing conversion of GTP to cGMP; activated cGMP causes vascular smooth muscle relaxation and inhibition of platelet aggregation[66] (Figure 2-2). NO in nanomolar concentrations accelerates cGMP formation by several hundredfold.[62] cGMP activates a cGMP-dependent protein kinase, which mediates vasodilation through reduced intracellular calcium levels and dephosphorylation of myosin light chain. The cGMP-independent effects of NO involve S-nitrosylation of cysteine residues in proteins and formation of dinitrosyl-iron complexes. Whereas heme binding of NO is rapidly reversible, nitrosylation reactions result in long-lasting effects.

NO plays an important cardioprotective role associated with late-phase ischemic preconditioning. Ischemic preconditioning, whereby brief ischemic insults render the heart resistant to subsequent ischemic damage, is a biphasic phenomenon. The late phase develops after 12 hours and lasts for 3 to 4 days and confers protection against both myocardial stunning and infarction. NO is one of the trigger molecules initiating late-phase preconditioning. Rapid calcium influx associated with reperfusion activates iNOS and increases NO production. The

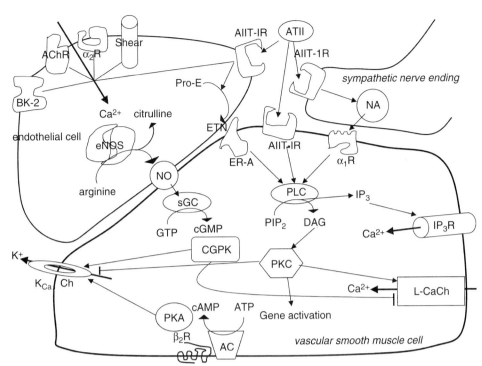

FIGURE 2-2 Mechanisms regulating the tone of vascular smooth muscle. *Vasodilatory mechanisms* are represented on the left side of the figure. Bradykinin (BK-2), acetylcholine (AchR), α_2-adrenergic receptors (α_2R), angiotensin II type 1 (AIIT-1) receptor stimulation and shear stress increase calcium influx to the endothelial cell. Calcium-dependent endothelial nitric oxide synthase (eNOS) is activated and NO synthesis from arginine is increased. NO diffuses into the smooth muscle cell and activates soluble guanylyl cyclase (sGC), which converts GTP to cGMP. cGMP activates cGMP-dependent protein kinase (CGPK). Phosphorylation by CGPK inactivates L-type calcium channels (L-CaCh) and activates calcium-dependent potassium channels (K_{ca}Ch). This leads to decreased calcium availability in the cell and to hyperpolarization of the sarcolemma. Calcium-dependent potassium channels also are activated by protein kinase A (PKA). *Vasoconstrictive mechanisms* are illustrated on the right side of the figure. Angiotensin II type 1 receptor activation augments endothelin (ETN) production from preproendothelin (Pro-E) in the endothelial cell and noradrenaline release from the sympathetic nerve terminal. Stimulation of endothelin receptors (ER-A), angiotensin II type 1 receptors, and α_1-adrenergic receptors (α_1R) on vascular smooth muscle cells activates phospholipase C (PLC). PLC cleaves phosphoinositol diphosphate (PIP$_2$) into inositol triphosphate (IP$_3$) and diacylglycerol phosphate (DAG). IP$_3$ activates IP$_3$-dependent calcium channels (IP$_3$R), increasing calcium influx. DAG activates protein kinase C (PKC). PKC activates L-type calcium channels and inhibits calcium-dependent potassium channels. PKC activation is also involved in expression of genes associated with proliferation and hypertrophy.

NO produced reacts with O_2^- to form peroxynitrile anion, which initiates the protein kinase and gene expression cascade characteristic of ischemic preconditioning. Ischemia induces iNOS expression, and iNOS-generated NO appears to be a major cardioprotective contributor in the effector phase of late ischemic preconditioning.[67] There has been much interest in the therapeutic use of exogenous NO donors such as NTG to mimic these late-phase preconditioning effects. In survivors of acute myocardial infarction, intermittent therapy with transdermal NTG patches initiated 1 week after the ischemic event was found to improve left ventricular function and prevent remodeling.[68] These effects were noted predominantly in patients with depressed left ventricular function. Interestingly, increasing the dose of NTG led to a less pronounced effect on left ventricular remodeling, possibly because of an increase in nitrate tolerance at higher doses. In a study in conscious rabbits, pretreatment with intravenous NTG in the absence of ischemia protected against myocardial stunning 24 hours later through a protein kinase C (PKC)-dependent mechanism.[69] This effect of

NTG took place in the absence of significant hemodynamic changes, and the degree of protection conferred by NTG was equivalent to that seen in the late phase of ischemic preconditioning. In another study, patients given intravenous NTG 24 hours before undergoing coronary angioplasty were found to have significant attenuation of myocardial ischemia compared with control subjects as assessed by regional left ventricular wall motion, ST-segment changes, and chest pain.[78] This finding has important implications, as the prophylactic administration of nitrates may be part of a future therapeutic approach to ischemic cardioprotection.

General Characteristics of the Nitrovasodilators

Organic nitrates such as glyceryl trinitrate or NTG are esters of nitric acid, and organic nitrates such as sodium nitroprusside (SNP) are esters of nitrous acid. Organic nitrates with low molecular mass are somewhat volatile, and NTG in its pure form is explosive.[71]

Although the nitrovasodilator drugs in clinical use differ in their individual pharmacologic profiles, they share a common molecular mechanism of therapeutic action: the release of NO from the nitrate molecule. The various compounds release NO in different ways, depending on chemical structure. Compounds with lower oxidation states of nitrogen such as SNP, nitrosamines, and nitrosothiols release NO nonenzymatically by one-electron reduction, whereas organic nitrates such as NTG require a complex enzymatic reduction necessitating free sulfhydryl groups to release NO.[72,73] Evidence for the involvement of an enzymatic process in the biotransformation of nitrates to NO comes from the observation that when vascular smooth muscle and endothelial cells are denatured, conversion of NTG to NO is reduced up to 90%.[72] Reduction of SNP leads to release of NO and cyanide (CN^-); however, the NO released from SNP is such a potent vasodilator that clinically effective doses of SNP usually do not produce toxic amounts of CN^-.[73] CN^- is metabolized to thiocyanate in the liver, and thiocyanate is eliminated by the kidneys.

Orally administered nitrates attain varied peak plasma levels despite achieving comparable degrees of vasodilation. Therefore, nitrates are dosed according to their clinical and hemodynamic effects rather than plasma concentration.[74] Most organic nitrates are substantially metabolized by hepatic enzymes. Isosorbide-5-mononitrate is an exception, exhibiting a longer half-life and better bioavailability than its parent compound, isosorbide dinitrate. Transdermal NTG avoids first-pass inactivation by the liver and has superior absorption and more reliable plasma concentrations compared with NTG ointment.[75] Sublingual NTG (SL NTG) has a half-life of 1 to 3 minutes, achieving peak plasma concentrations within 4 minutes of administration. SNP must be administered as an intravenous infusion, with an onset of action within 30 seconds and peak effect within 2 minutes of initiation of the infusion; the hypotensive effect is abolished within 3 minutes of discontinuing the infusion. Both SNP and NTG are among the first-line parenteral drugs used to treat hypertensive emergencies.[38]

Nitrates appear to exert a greater vasodilatory effect upon vessels characterized by abnormal endothelial function.[74] This effect contrasts with that of endogenous compounds such as acetylcholine, histamine, bradykinin, ATP, and thrombin, which require an intact endothelium in order to dilate blood vessels; in the presence of damaged endothelium, some of these endogenous vasodilators actually become vasoconstrictors.[76]

Organic nitrates such as NTG are predominantly venodilators, preferentially reducing preload with little or no effect on afterload, especially at low concentrations. The mechanism of this "venoselectivity" is unknown; it may be explained by enrichment of the NO-producing enzyme in venous smooth muscle cells.[77] At higher concentrations, the nitrovasodilators exert an anti-ischemic effect by simultaneously decreasing myocardial oxygen demand and increasing myocardial oxygen supply. NTG decreases myocardial oxygen demand by increasing venous capacitance and, thus, decreasing venous return to the heart (i.e., preload). This reduction in cardiac preload leads to reduced left and right ventricular diastolic pressure and cavity size, which in turn results in reductions in diastolic wall stress and myocardial oxygen consumption. NTG dilates arteriolar resistance vessels, resulting in decreased systemic blood pressure and systolic wall tension (i.e., afterload), with an increase in aortic compliance and minimal effect on heart rate. Pulmonary vascular resistance and cardiac output are usually slightly decreased. The reduction of ventricular diastolic pressure improves the transmural distribution of myocardial perfusion by decreasing extrinsic diastolic compression of subendocardial vessels.[78] Although total myocardial blood flow remains unaffected, an NTG-mediated decrease in preload has been found to maintain normal transmural distribution favoring the endocardium in the setting of infrarenal aortic occlusion.[79]

NTG significantly increases blood flow to diseased regions of the myocardium, although total myocardial blood flow may not change.[80] The coronary dilation produced by nitrovasodilators is seen mainly in larger epicardial coronary arteries more than 200 µm in diameter, with minimal effect on coronary resistance vessels less than 100 µm in diameter; this selective vasodilation of large coronary arteries without impairment of autoregulation in the coronary microcirculation prevents the coronary steal phenomenon that occurs with other, nonselective vasodilators such as dipyridamole.

In a study comparing the effects of intravenous NTG, amlodipine, and atenolol on platelet function in vivo using whole-blood flow cytometry, an antiplatelet effect was seen only with NTG. The increase in intracellular cGMP caused by NO liberated from NTG was found to inhibit and reverse platelet aggregation by inhibition of fibrinogen binding and prevention of the oxidation of arachidonic acid and its conversion to proaggregatory compounds. Nitrates also inhibited platelet degranulation as measured by decreased expression of P-selectin on the platelet surface both at rest and in response to stimulation by agonists such as adenosine diphosphate (ADP) and thrombin. However, platelet responsiveness to nitrates may be altered in patients with coronary artery disease because of the functionally abnormal endothelium often seen in these patients. Moreover, the antiplatelet effect of nitrates may be attenuated by the increased catecholamine levels seen in the setting of acute myocardial infarction or nitrate-induced hypotension. This study did not evaluate the efficacy of oral nitrates or the long-term effects of nitrate tolerance on platelet function.[81] Reduced platelet responsiveness to the antiplatelet effects of nitrovasodilators in patients with symptomatic ischemic heart disease compared with nonischemic patients has been demonstrated. This finding might result from the activation of systemic inflammation seen in ischemic heart disease, resulting in inactivation of platelet cGMP and increased superoxide production.[82]

Nitrovasodilators in the Treatment of Ischemic Heart Disease

The use of nitrates in the early phase of anterior myocardial infarction may significantly reduce infarct size through improved myocardial blood flow to infarct and noninfarct border zones, sustained integrity of the myocardial collagen matrix, and decreased preload and afterload.[83] The preload reduction induced by nitrovasodilators causes a central-to-peripheral redistribution of blood volume and resultant decrease in left ventricular filling pressures. However, nitrates in high doses may reduce diastolic arterial pressure below a critical level necessary for coronary perfusion and actually increase mortality.

Myocardial ischemia maximally dilates coronary arterioles, and NTG has no further dilating effect on these vessels. This effect is demonstrated in the finding that intracoronary injection of NTG was ineffective in relieving anginal pain despite significant increases in coronary sinus blood flow, suggesting that blood flow increased only in arterioles not already maximally dilated by ischemia. On the other hand, intravenous injection of NTG rapidly relieved anginal pain in the same patients in association with decreases in arterial blood pressure and coronary sinus blood flow, probably reflecting a decrease in myocardial oxygen consumption. Thus, NTG-induced coronary vasodilation does not significantly contribute to the antianginal effect of NTG.[84] However, whereas in pharmacologic concentrations NTG dilates large coronary arteries without affecting the microvascular bed, the suprapharmacologic dose of intracoronary NTG (a bolus of 75 μg) may induce a concomitant dilation of the coronary arteriolar resistance bed.[78] In fact, Brown et al noted a reduction in estimated stenosis flow resistance of 38% in severely diseased segments of coronary arteries.[78] SL NTG, unlike intracoronary NTG, has been shown to increase coronary artery diameter only minimally; isosorbide dinitrate (ISDN) spray, however, resulted in increases in coronary artery diameter comparable to those with intracoronary NTG and thus may be the drug of choice for routine administration in coronary angiographic procedures.[85]

The role of intravenous NTG in the prophylaxis of perioperative myocardial ischemia remains controversial. In patients with stable angina undergoing noncardiac surgery, prophylactic infusion of NTG at a dose of 1 μg/kg/min significantly reduced the incidence of intraoperative myocardial ischemia as evidenced by ischemic ST-segment changes on Holter monitoring compared with an intravenous NTG dose of 0.5 μg/kg/min.[86] However, no difference was found between an intravenous NTG infusion at 0.5 μg/kg/min and placebo in prevention of ischemic electrocardiographic (ECG) changes in patients undergoing coronary artery bypass grafting (CABG).[87] A later study also observed no reduction in the incidence of perioperative myocardial ischemia in coronary patients undergoing noncardiac surgery who received a prophylactic NTG infusion at 1 μg/kg/min compared with control subjects.[88] The disparity between the studies may be due to the presence of more severe coronary artery disease and probably worse left ventricular function in patients in the first study, and the hemodynamic benefit of NTG may correlate with the degree of left ventricular function at baseline. Patients with left ventricular failure exhibit more uniform improvement in degree of myocardial ischemia and fewer deleterious hemodynamic responses with NTG than those without left ventricular failure; this has also been demonstrated in the setting of acute myocardial infarction.[89] Furthermore, onset of perioperative ischemic ECG changes in patients receiving NTG took place at higher heart rates than in the control group; this may indicate a therapeutic effect of NTG in increasing the heart rate threshold at which myocardial ischemia is manifest.[88]

Intravenous NTG frequently has been used intraoperatively to treat hypertension that may result in myocardial ischemia in patients with coronary artery disease. During anesthesia for CABG, intravenous NTG, infused at 1 μg/kg/min, has been shown to reduce significantly arterial and central venous pressures as well as systemic vascular resistance and stroke work index without a concomitant change in cardiac index or heart rate.[90] A study comparing the effects of intravenous NTG in patients before and during CABG showed some hemodynamic differences in awake and anesthetized patients. In awake patients, stroke volume, cardiac index, and pulmonary capillary wedge pressure decreased; arterial blood pressure decreased only slightly secondary to compensatory increases in heart rate and systemic vascular resistance, and no change in myocardial oxygen consumption was observed. In anesthetized patients, arterial blood pressure and systemic vascular resistance decreased without a change in heart rate or cardiac index, and calculated myocardial oxygen consumption decreased in conjunction with an increase in coronary sinus oxygen content.[91] Relief of myocardial ischemia with NTG has been demonstrated by a reversal of coronary lactate production to extraction; however, excessive hypotension can occur with NTG infusion, leading to reductions in coronary perfusion pressure, blood flow, and lactate extraction.[92]

A widely cited but flawed meta-analysis had shown a reduction in mortality with nitrates in the setting of acute myocardial infarction, but this notion has been challenged.[93] Two large randomized clinical trials were performed to determine the effect of nitrates on morbidity and mortality in patients with known or suspected acute myocardial infarction.[94,95] The Gruppo Italiano per lo Studio della Sopravvivenza nell' Infarto Miocardico (GISSI-3) trial showed no benefit of transdermal NTG even with early drug administration and continued therapy for 6 weeks, whereas angiotensin-converting enzyme (ACE) inhibitors decreased both mortality and severe left ventricular dysfunction up to 6 months after randomization. However, the combination of nitrates plus ACE inhibitors was found to be safe and effective, with an even greater effect in elderly and female patients.[94,95] The Fourth International Study of Infarct Survival (ISIS-4) showed that, unlike oral captopril, oral mononitrate failed to cause a significant reduction in 5-week mortality or confer any later survival advantage, although fewer deaths were seen on days 0 to 1 after acute myocardial infarction with nitrate therapy.[96] In fact, there is some evidence indicating that long-term nitrate therapy may *increase* the number of adverse cardiac events in patients with myocardial infarction, possibly secondary to reflex neurohumoral activation in response to nitrates (see Rebound Ischemia later).[97] It should be borne in mind that many patients in the placebo arm of both GISSI-3 and ISIS-4 received open-label nitrates at the discretion of the physician in charge, potentially obscuring a beneficial nitrate effect.

Few clinical studies have been performed comparing long-acting nitrates with β-blockers or calcium channel blockers in the treatment of stable angina. A meta-analysis showed no significant difference between these drug classes as measured by number of angina episodes, exercise tolerance, and adverse events; there were not enough studies to assess differences in long-term survival.[98] The use of a long-acting nitrate is a class I recommendation in the management of chronic stable angina, either in conjunction with a β-blocker if initial treatment with β-blockade has not been successful or as initial therapy for patients in whom β-blockers are contraindicated.[40] SL NTG or NTG spray is also a class I recommendation for immediate relief of anginal pain. These formulations can also be used prophylactically before exercising. When the effects of 50- and 100-mg doses of sustained-release isosorbide mononitrate (SR ISMN) were compared in patients with stable angina, the higher nitrate dose was associated with greater improvement in quality of life and New York Heart Association (NYHA) angina classification without significantly more side effects.[99] Compounds with pharmacologic properties similar to those of organic nitrates such as molsidomine (a sydnonimine) and nicorandil (a potassium channel activator) may prove to be beneficial in the management of chronic stable angina.

The role of nitrovasodilators in the treatment of unstable angina remains controversial. Although there is insufficient evidence to demonstrate whether the nitrovasodilators decrease mortality and incidence of acute myocardial infarction when used in the therapy of unstable angina, nitrates play a critical role in the symptomatic relief of chest pain in these patients. Intravenous NTG can effectively relieve symptoms of angina even in patients refractory to other agents, including oral or topical nitrates. In addition to their favorable effect on myocardial oxygen supply and demand, nitrates may exert an antianginal effect by prevention of platelet aggregation at the site of endothelial injury; this antiplatelet effect, mediated by the NO pathway, may provide added benefit to patients receiving aspirin therapy, in whom the antiplatelet effect is mediated by the cyclooxygenase pathway. However, studies in patients with unstable angina showed that nitrate therapy in the absence of concurrent aspirin or heparin therapy did not lead to a decreased incidence of revascularization. Because concurrent use of intravenous NTG and heparin may cause heparin resistance, the partial thromboplastin time must be watched closely in this setting.[100] During the acute phase of unstable angina, intravenous NTG is the nitrate formulation of choice because of ease of both upward titration and rapid discontinuation. Intravenous NTG is generally used continuously for the first 24 to 72 hours in patients with acute unstable angina, with gradual tapering and institution of long-acting intermittent nitrate therapy. Although nitrate tolerance develops, it can be overcome with escalating doses of intravenous NTG in the short term; there is no role for intermittent nitrate therapy in the treatment of acute unstable angina (see Tolerance and Rebound Ischemia later).

In patients with atypical vasospastic angina, the vasodilatory effect of NTG on atherosclerotic or nonatherosclerotic large epicardial coronary arteries may be especially helpful in relieving coronary vasospasm; however, calcium channel blockers such as nifedipine remain the treatment of choice for variant angina.

Unlike the organic nitrates, nitrites such as isoamyl nitrite (ISAN) do not seem to manifest tolerance to the beneficial hemodynamic effects, even after prolonged infusion. One possible explanation may be that different enzymatic regulation exists for the nitrates and nitrites. Alternatively, the more pronounced afterload reduction seen with nitrites (without significant tachycardia) may lead to sustained reduction of left ventricular end-diastolic pressure.[101] ISAN is approved in the United States for treatment of angina, although it is rarely used. The beneficial effects of ISAN on left ventricular end-diastolic pressure and afterload, combined with the lack of observed tolerance, make ISAN a potentially attractive agent for treatment of congestive heart failure. ISAN must be administered by inhalation because of its volatility, and it has a fast onset and short duration of action.

Nitrovasodilators in the Treatment of Heart Failure

Although they are commonly used in the treatment of chronic congestive heart failure (CHF), organic nitrates are not approved by the Food and Drug Administration for this purpose, and nitrates are not recommended for routine use in the American College of Cardiology–American Heart Association guidelines for the management of chronic adult heart failure.[14] The combination of a nitrate plus hydralazine is recommended only for patients who cannot tolerate ACE inhibitors and who remain symptomatic after being treated with digitalis, a β-blocker, and diuretics.[14] This recommendation stems from the Veterans Administration Heart Failure Trials (V-HeFT), in which ACE inhibitors clearly conferred a survival advantage over direct vasodilators in patients with chronic heart failure, while a nitrate-hydralazine combination conferred a survival advantage only over placebo.[102] Nonetheless, the favorable hemodynamic profile of NTG makes it an ideal drug for treatment of CHF. Acutely, the reduction in preload and afterload without significant associated tachycardia is clearly beneficial. The decrease in left ventricular preload leads to a decrease in secondary pulmonary hypertension and, thus, decreased shortness of breath. Moreover, NTG-induced venodilation and subsequent reduction in left ventricular volume have been reported to decrease the severity of mitral regurgitation (MR), an important fact given the large number of CHF patients with coexisting MR. The V-HeFT studies demonstrated improvement in both maximum oxygen consumption and left ventricular ejection fraction in response to therapy with ISDN plus hydralazine; these effects were both superior to the effect of an ACE inhibitor.[102] High-dose NTG has also significantly improved maximal treadmill exercise time.[103] There is evidence to suggest that even small nonvasodilating doses of NTG may actually enhance endogenous, endothelium-dependent vasodilation.[103] Therefore, there is substantial evidence indicating significant symptomatic improvement from the addition of nitrovasodilators to standard CHF therapy; more studies are needed to evaluate the impact of the addition of nitrovasodilators to standard CHF therapy on mortality.

Patients with chronic CHF frequently have decreased vascular responsiveness to nitrates. One possible theory to explain this apparent nitrate resistance in CHF is that capacitance vessels may already be maximally stretched and, thus, unable to dilate further in response to nitrates; this is supported by the increased right atrial pressure seen in nonresponders. Alternatively, increased amounts of sodium and water within the vascular wall may impair the vascular response to nitrates. Whatever the reason, CHF patients generally require higher doses of nitrovasodilators than patients with ischemic heart disease to achieve the same hemodynamic effect. The small transdermal patch sizes available limit the effectiveness of this type of nitrate regimen. Oral isosorbide mononitrate may be more suitable in the treatment of chronic CHF, as it does not undergo first-pass hepatic metabolism, is available in once-daily and high-dose controlled-release preparations, and yields more persistent hemodynamic effects.[103]

Atrial natriuretic peptide (ANP) is under investigation as an alternative vasodilator for use in decompensated CHF. ANP is produced by the myocardium in response to increased wall stress, hypertrophy, and volume overload. ANP also induces vascular relaxation by increasing cGMP levels, but by activation of particulate, rather than soluble, guanylate cyclase; thus, tissues tolerant to nitrate-induced vasodilation may still respond to ANP.[76] Like NTG, ANP reduces both preload and afterload without causing significant tachycardia, thus increasing cardiac output and improving symptoms of CHF. The Vasodilation in the Management of Acute CHF (VMAC) study showed a greater reduction in pulmonary capillary wedge pressure with nesiritide (Natrecor), a recombinant human brain natriuretic peptide (BNP), than with standard therapy plus NTG or placebo. Both BNP and NTG caused comparable symptomatic improvement of dyspnea over placebo. Side effect profiles of the two drugs were similar, although headache and abdominal pain were seen more frequently with NTG.[104]

Side Effects Associated with Nitrovasodilator Therapy

The organic nitrates are generally well tolerated; the side effects that occur are mainly due to drug actions on the cardiovascular system. Headache and flushing are common because of arteriolar dilation, and in fact this side effect was first recognized in the 1800s in explosives workers. NTG-induced headaches generally respond to acetaminophen. The decrease in afterload may cause orthostatic hypotension with dizziness, weakness, and, possibly, syncope. Hypotension may be especially severe in patients with autonomic dysfunction, even at low nitrate doses. SL NTG may rarely cause bradycardia and hypotension, probably secondary to activation of the Bezold-Jarisch reflex.

Nitrates are contraindicated in patients taking sildenafil (Viagra). Sildenafil inhibits cGMP-specific phosphodiesterase 5 (PDE5), causing an increase in cGMP; in combination with the increase in cGMP caused by organic nitrates, profound hypotension can result. Nitrates in any form should not be given within 24 hours of the last dose of sildenafil.

Nitrates are also contraindicated in idiopathic hypertrophic subaortic stenosis (IHSS) because of the potential to increase left ventricular outflow tract obstruction and precipitate syncope. Nitrates can also precipitate syncope in patients with severe aortic stenosis and should be used with caution in these patients.

NTG causes a transient increase in intracranial pressure with intravenous bolus injection in both awake and anesthetized patients. Prior administration of barbiturates does not appear to attenuate this phenomenon.[105] Therefore, NTG should be administered cautiously to patients with decreased intracranial compliance.

Rarely, SNP administration can cause severe acidosis because of toxic accumulations of CN^-, usually with infusions greater than 5 µg/kg/min. Accumulation of CN^- can be prevented by administration of thiosulfate, which is the limiting factor in CN^- metabolism. ISAN can be used to treat cyanide toxicity associated with SNP. Infusion of SNP longer than 24 to 48 hours is associated with an increased risk of thiocyanate tox-

icity, heralded by nausea, anorexia, fatigue, disorientation, and psychosis. High levels of thiocyanate may uncommonly cause hypothyroidism secondary to inhibition of iodine uptake by the thyroid gland.

The nitrovasodilators cause a decrease in arterial partial pressure of oxygen (Po_2) without significant changes in arterial Pco_2, pH, mixed venous Po_2, or base excess.[106] This reduction in Pao_2 is probably caused by an increase in ventilation-perfusion mismatch related to pharmacologic pulmonary vasodilation of poorly ventilated lung units. SNP has been shown to inhibit hypoxic pulmonary vasoconstriction (HPV) more than NTG because of its more intense vasodilator effect.[107] Because there is evidence of an increased incidence of hypoxemia as well as patchy airway obstruction in the setting of acute myocardial infarction, the existence of a greater number of lung units with ventilation-perfusion inequality may make these patients particularly susceptible to nitrate-induced hypoxemia.[108] However, in patients undergoing CABG, NTG-induced hypoxemia did not cause myocardial ischemia, as evidenced by a simultaneous decrease in coronary sinus lactate concentration.[109] Fortunately, patients with advanced lung disease are unlikely to be affected by the pulmonary vasodilator effects of the nitrovasodilators as they tend to have pulmonary vessels that are already maximally distended and poorly responsive to alveolar hypoxia.[110]

There are conflicting reports about the effect of SNP administration on renal blood flow. In postoperative CABG patients, SNP was found to decrease renal vascular resistance in proportion to an increase in cardiac output, in parallel with decreases in pulmonary and systemic vascular resistance. Decreases in renal blood flow shown in some studies may be explained by failure to maintain left atrial pressure, causing a decrease in blood pressure below the renal range of autoregulation.[111]

UNIQUE SIDE EFFECTS OF NITRATE DRUGS: THE PHENOMENA OF TOLERANCE AND REBOUND ISCHEMIA

Tolerance. The development of tolerance, in which there is a blunted response to the hemodynamic effects of nitrates, occurs shortly after the onset of therapy with nitrates and is often the limiting factor in their therapeutic usefulness. Tolerance occurs with all forms of nitrate administration. There is also concern about cross-tolerance to other endothelium-dependent and -independent vasodilators. The mechanism behind the phenomenon of nitrate tolerance is the subject of intense research.

"True" tolerance is thought to arise from an inability of vascular smooth muscle to convert NTG to NO and usually occurs after 3 days of treatment. The four mechanisms commonly cited to account for true vascular tolerance are desensitization of guanylyl cyclase, increased phosphodiesterase activity causing increased cGMP breakdown, depletion of intracellular sulfhydryl groups, and impaired NTG biotransformation.[112] The concept of intracellular sulfhydryl group depletion causing nitrate tolerance has gone out of favor, as administration of thiols increases nitrate responsiveness in both tolerant and nontolerant states.

Proposed mechanisms for tolerance extraneous to the vessel wall, known as pseudotolerance, include intravascular volume expansion and neurohumoral activation. Nitrate-induced changes in Starling forces across capillary beds cause an increase in plasma volume, which may counteract the nitrate-induced reduction in preload; however, administration of diuretics has not been shown to eliminate tolerance.[113] In addition, most of the intravascular fluid shift takes place within an hour of initiating therapy with NTG, with preservation of NTG-induced reduction of pulmonary capillary wedge pressure; after infusion of NTG for 24 to 48 hours, pulmonary capillary wedge pressure rises to pretreatment value without additional increases in intravascular volume, suggesting involvement of other mechanisms. Nitrate therapy is associated with increases in plasma renin activity, aldosterone, and vasopressin in the first 24 to 48 hours after starting NTG, during which time epicardial coronary arteries continue to respond to NTG. However, after return of neurohumoral parameters to normal, epicardial coronary vasodilation is absent, suggesting a mechanism of nitrate tolerance intrinsic to the tolerant vasculature.[112]

There is growing evidence for increased levels of O_2^- anions in tolerant tissue causing chemical inactivation of NO released from NTG before it is able to activate sGC in vascular smooth muscle. O_2^- rapidly binds to NO to form peroxynitrite ($ONOO^-$), which has a less pronounced effect on sGC. Additional support for this hypothesis lies in the virtual elimination of tolerance in in vitro animal models by preincubation of tolerant vessels with superoxide dismutase.[112] Antihypertensive agents with antioxidant properties such as hydralazine and carvedilol have been shown to prevent nitrate tolerance induced by oxygen free radicals; there may also potentially be a role for vitamins C and E. The primary source of O_2^- appears to be a membrane-bound reduced nicotinamide adenine dinucleotide (NADH) oxidase, which is modulated by angiotensin II. In fact, both ACE inhibitors and AT_1 receptor antagonists decrease O_2^- production and prevent nitrate tolerance in vivo.[114]

Another theory of nitrate tolerance holds that locally produced endothelin-1 (ET-1) enhances sensitivity to a number of vasocontrictive substances such as angiotensin II, serotonin, phenylephrine, and KCl by a PKC-mediated mechanism. PKC inhibitors abolish this hypersensitivity to vasoconstrictors.[112] In addition, the ET-1 receptor antagonist bosentan in high doses partly decreases O_2^- production and improves response to NTG; however, treatment with bosentan is not as effective as treatment with AT_1 receptor antagonists.[114]

Rebound ischemia. In order to prevent the onset of tolerance, long-acting nitrates are generally prescribed in an intermittent dosing regimen, with a daily drug-free interval of 8 to 12 hours. Although this dosing regimen is effective in preventing nitrate tolerance, studies have shown a decrease in anginal threshold and increases in rebound ischemia, myocardial infarction, and sudden death during the nitrate-free period. Many workers in the explosives industry who were chronically exposed to high nitrate levels at work experienced the "Sunday heart attack" upon "withdrawal" over the weekend.[58] Twelve hours after removal of a transdermal NTG or placebo patch, patients in the placebo group exhibited better exercise tolerance than patients receiving active nitrate therapy; this is known as the zero hour effect.[115] Withdrawal of transdermal NTG has been associated with worsening endothelial dysfunction, as evidenced by an increase in vasoconstriction more than five times greater than

in a control group.[116] The reason for this worsening in the setting of NTG withdrawal may be an NTG-induced hypersensitivity to vasoconstrictors (see Tolerance) unopposed by the vasodilatory actions of NTG itself. Removal of NTG patches has also been associated with significant constriction of large coronary arteries in response to ACh. ACh can induce vasodilation by stimulating endothelial NO release, but ACh also causes vasoconstriction by its actions at muscarinic M_3 receptors on vascular smooth muscle cells. It is unknown whether this ACh-mediated vasoconstriction is indicative of endothelial dysfunction or smooth muscle cell hypersensitivity to vasoconstrictors.[117] Given the increased ischemic risk during the nitrate-free period, it may be advisable to use a β-blocker or calcium channel blocker in conjunction with intermittent nitrate therapy in order to provide 24-hour prophylaxis against ischemic cardiac events.[100]

Perioperative Uses of the Nitrovasodilators

SNP is frequently used to induce controlled hypotension to reduce bleeding during surgery. SNP in conscious dogs without depressed cardiac function has been shown to decrease stroke volume markedly while having little effect on myocardial contractility. SNP significantly decreased blood flow to all areas of the myocardium as well as to liver, spleen, and intestine without affecting their vascular resistances; by contrast, SNP significantly decreased vascular resistances of cerebral and renal tissues without affecting their blood flow. The reflex adaptations and autoregulation of the various vascular beds may account for the lack of toxicity seen with SNP-induced controlled hypotension.[118]

NTG bolus injection has been described as a safer and less invasive alternative to adenosine-induced temporary asystole or electrically induced ventricular fibrillation to control blood pressure during endovascular stenting of thoracic aortic aneurysms.[119] SNP can be used to decrease blood pressure in acute aortic dissection, but it should be administered in conjunction with a ß-blocker in order to prevent an increased rate of rise in aortic pressure. As mentioned earlier, both intravenous NTG and SNP are first-line agents in the therapy of hypertensive emergencies.

Although the evidence remains unclear, NTG continues to be widely used in the perioperative management of patients with coronary artery disease. Nitrates are certainly useful in the symptomatic relief of postoperative chest pain. Future studies should better elucidate the role of the nitrovasodilators in the prevention and management of perioperative ischemia.

Inhibitors of the Renin-Angiotensin System in the Treatment of Hypertension, Ischemic Heart Disease, and Heart Failure

Inhibition of ACE in a normotensive experimental animal has little effect on the blood pressure of the animal. It was the realization of the beneficial effect of ACE inhibition in human hypertension that led to a breakthrough in the development and clinical introduction of ACE inhibitors. The importance of these drugs in the management of CHF was discovered much later.

An Overview of the Renin-Angiotensin System and Its Role in Hypertension and Cardiac Remodeling

Renin is a protease enzyme that is synthesized, stored, and released in the circulation by the juxtaglomerular cells of renal afferent arterioles (Figure 2-3). Renin release is determined by the state of arterial fullness, which is a function of cardiac output and peripheral vascular resistance.[120] Changes in arterial filling are reflected in increases and decreases of the pressure in the afferent renal arterioles, which in turn inhibit or stimulate renin release. This prostaglandin-dependent mechanism is known as the intrarenal baroreceptor pathway.[121] Arterial filling also determines baroreflex and renal sympathetic efferent activities. Increased renal sympathetic activity increases norepinephrine release, which stimulates β_1 receptors on the juxtaglomerular cells, resulting in renin release. Renin release is also regulated by the chloride flux across the macula densa. The macula densa is a group of specialized epithelial cells in the distal portion of the thick ascending limb of Henle that is interposed between the afferent and efferent arterioles. An increase in chloride flux across the macula densa induces release of

adenosine, which, by activating adenosine A_1 receptors on juxtaglomerular cells, inhibits renin release. A decrease in chloride flux induces release of prostaglandin from the macula densa, which stimulates renin secretion from juxtaglomerular cells. This chloride ion–dependent regulation of renin secretion is known as the macula densa pathway.[121]

Renin release is regulated by two major feedback mechanisms: (1) local increase of angiotensin II concentration following renin release stimulates angiotensin AT_1 receptors on juxtaglomerular cells, which directly inhibits further renin release, and (2) the activation of the renin-angiotensin system elicits physiologic responses resulting in increased blood pressure and reduced urine output. When blood pressure increases and arterial fullness normalizes, glomerular filtration rate also increases, reducing proximal tubular NaCl reabsorption. Afferent arteriolar pressure increases, while renal nerve sympathetic activity decreases, and chloride flux across the macula densa increases. These changes, in turn, restore renin release to baseline levels (see Figure 2-3).

Renin has a plasma half-life of 15 minutes. Angiotensinogen, its primary substrate, is an α_2-globulin synthesized

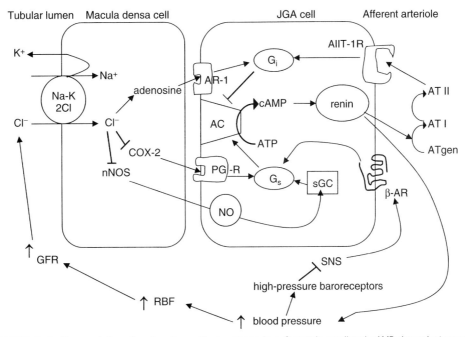

FIGURE 2-3 The regulation of renin release. Renin release is a G protein–mediated cAMP-dependent process. Macula densa cells are sensitive to changes in chloride flux in the distal tubule. Increasing chloride influx through the sodium-potassium-chloride symporter (Na-K-2Cl) leads to the augmentation of adenosine release and the inhibition of COX-2–dependent prostaglandin and nNOS-dependent NO synthesis. Reduced chloride flux results in the opposite effect. Renin is synthesized and stored in the juxtaglomerular (JGA) cells of the afferent arteriole. Prostaglandin receptor (PG-R) and β-adrenergic receptor (β-AR) activation and NO binding to soluble guanylyl cyclase (sGC) activate the stimulatory G_s protein, and adenosine-1 receptor (AR-1) and angiotensin II type 1 receptor (AIIT-1R) activate the inhibitory G_i protein. G proteins in turn activate or inhibit adenylyl cyclase (AC), which determines cellular cAMP levels. The renin released into the circulation converts angiotensinogen (ATgen) to angiotensin I (AT I), which is then further converted into angiotensin II (AT II). Locally produced AT II inhibits further renin release. This is known as the short-loop feedback regulation of renin release. Circulating renin increases systemic blood pressure, which activates high-pressure baroreceptors and decreases renal sympathetic activity (SNS) reducing juxtaglomerular β-receptor activity. Renal blood flow (RBF) and glomerular filtration rate (GFR) increase, resulting in increased distal tubular delivery of chloride ions and shifting macula densa output toward the adenosine pathway. This is known as the long-loop feedback regulation of renin release.

in the liver. Renin cleaves a 10-amino-acid peptide known as angiotensin I from angiotensinogen. This decapeptide has minimal physiologic activity and rapidly undergoes further enzymatic modification by ACE, which removes a dipeptide from the carboxyl terminal. The resulting product, angiotensin II, is responsible for the majority of the physiologic effects. Angiotensin II itself is then further cleaved by either aminopeptidase, resulting in angiotensin III, or carboxypeptidase, resulting in angiotensin (1-7) (1-7 stands for amino acids 1 to 7 of the original angiotensinogen peptide). Further degradation of angiotensin peptides by nonspecific peptidases results in the hexapeptide angiotensin IV.

ACE is a zinc-containing carboxypeptidase. It is a nonspecific peptidyldipeptide hydrolase, cleaving not only angiotensin I but also a number of circulating vasoactive peptides such as bradykinin. The majority of ACE exists in membrane-bound form on the luminal surface of the vascular endothelium. ACE is continuously removed from the endothelial surface. Circulating ACE represents this shed fraction of the enzyme pool. However, it is the endothelial uptake of circulating renin and endothelium-bound ACE that is mainly responsible for conversion of angiotensinogen to angiotensin I and angiotensin II.[122]

Angiotensin II binds to specific, G protein–coupled cell surface receptors. Angiotensin II type 1 (AT_1) receptors predominate in the adult and are responsible for the physiologic effects of angiotensin II. Stimulation of AT_1 activates phospholipases A_2 and C, resulting in inhibition of adenylyl cyclase, opening of calcium channels, and activation of tyrosine kinases. Angiotensin II type 2 (AT_2) receptor is most abundant in fetal life, and its expression is limited in adult tissues. However, AT_2 receptor protein is present in the heart and its expression is equal to that of the AT_1 receptor in the adult ventricle. Upregulation of AT_2 has been observed following myocardial infarction. The physiologic effects of AT_2 stimulation are characteristically opposite to those of AT_1 stimulation and involve activation of tyrosine phosphatase, opening of potassium and inactivation of calcium channels, stimulation of NO production, and induction of apoptotic pathways. Angiotensin III binds to AT_1 and AT_2. Specific AT_4 receptors for angiotensin (1-7) and angiotensin IV have also been identified.[123] These receptors are believed to utilize NO-dependent pathways to oppose vascular and renal effects of AT_1 stimulation.[124]

The binding of angiotensin II to AT_1 receptors on vascular smooth muscle cells induces vasoconstriction and an acute increase in blood pressure (see Figure 2-2). Angiotensin II augments peripheral norepinephrine release and inhibits norepinephrine uptake by stimulation of presynaptic AT_1 receptors on sympathetic nerve terminals. In addition, angiotensin II increases central sympathetic outflow, attenuates baroreceptor reflex, and enhances release of vasopressin from the neurohypophysis and of catecholamines from the adrenal medulla.

Angiotensin II is linked to the production of endothelin, a potent endothelium-derived vasoconstrictor. There is a dose-dependent increase in endothelin formation with increasing doses of angiotensin II, and vasoconstriction can be prevented with either an endothelin receptor antagonist or an AT_1 receptor antagonist.[125] Angiotensin II acutely stimulates NO release from vascular endothelial cells, and prolonged exposure inhibits inducible NOS and either stimulates or has no effect on endothelial NOS expression in vascular cells. On the other hand, NO downregulates AT_1 receptors by a cGMP-dependent mechanism.

The delicate balance between the vasoconstrictive angiotensin-endothelin and vasodilatory NO systems is expressed not only in immediate receptor-mediated events but also in enzyme and receptor expression and regulation and may have an important role in vascular and cardiac remodeling as well.[126] There is evidence that angiotensin II increases vascular oxidative stress by accelerated production of reactive oxygen species through the activation of membrane-bound NADH and NADPH oxidases. These oxygen radicals increase inactivation and degradation of NO, causing impairment of endothelium-dependent vasodilatation. Peroxynitrile, a product of reaction between oxygen radicals and NO, further contributes to vasoconstriction and vascular injury.[127]

Chronic stimulation of AT_1 results in activation of multiple intracellular cascades involved in gene expression, leading to cellular hypertrophy and growth. Cardiac and vascular smooth muscle cells express increased levels of platelet-derived growth factor and transforming growth factor β, which are potent inducers of RNA and protein synthesis. Extracellular matrix proteins such as collagens and fibronectin accumulate in cardiac and vascular interstitium. This leads to cardiac hypertrophy, remodeling, vascular thickening, atherosclerosis, and glomerulosclerosis.[128] Increased renin and angiotensin II activity was also detected in the vicinity of inflammatory cells in atherosclerotic lesions, and angiotensin II was shown to increase plasminogen activator inhibitor levels in vascular tissue. These inflammatory and prothrombotic features of angiotensin II further damage vascular wall integrity and may lead to circulatory compromise of parenchymal organs.[129]

Angiotensin II utilizes a number of mechanisms to reduce the urinary excretion of sodium and water while increasing the excretion of potassium. It has a variable effect on glomerular filtration rate (GFR). Whereas low concentrations of angiotensin II preferentially constrict renal efferent arterioles and increase GFR, high concentrations and increased renal sympathetic activity result in afferent arteriolar and glomerular mesangial cell constriction leading to a reduction in GFR. Angiotensin II directly augments proximal tubular sodium resorption by enhancing Na^+-H^+ exchange. It redirects blood flow from the vasa recta, reducing renal medullary blood flow and limiting medullary sodium elimination. Stimulation of AT_1 receptors on adrenal zona glomerulosa cells results in aldosterone release, which increases sodium reabsorption and potassium excretion in the distal tubules.[130]

Angiotensin II is a powerful dipsogen. The circumventricular organs and the lamina terminalis of the anteroventral third ventricle of the brain have abundant angiotensinergic innervation and are rich in AT_1 receptors. Connections to the brainstem, hypothalamus, and limbic system ensure interactions with baroreceptor, neurohumoral, and behavioral mechanisms responsible for regulation of volume status and thirst. It appears that activation of angiotensinergic nerve fiber systems in the vicinity of the anteroventral third ventricle is responsible for immediate and brief dipsogenic responses and that elevated circulating angiotensin II levels elicit a slower but more prolonged thirst. Angiotensin II also causes an increase in sodium appetite and intake.[131] Although these mechanisms are extremely useful in restoring adequate circulating blood volume in acute hypovolemic states such as hemorrhage, prolonged elevated angiotensin II levels, characteristic in pathologic conditions such as heart failure, can lead to continued thirst, increased sodium intake, and unwanted fluid accumulation.

Angiotensin-Converting Enzyme Inhibitors

GENERAL CHARACTERISTICS OF ACE INHIBITORS. The first orally effective and clinically useful ACE inhibitor, captopril, was synthesized in 1975.[132] It was designed to mimic the binding characteristics of a naturally occurring nonapeptide ACE inhibitor, which was originally purified from a Brazilian viper venom.

The active site of ACE has three main binding sites: a positively charged pocket to bind the terminal carboxyl group of angiotensin I, an intermediate pocket forming hydrogen bonds with the carboxyl terminal amide bond, and a zinc-containing pocket responsible for the enzymatic activity. The zinc ion embedded in this pocket is suitably located to polarize the penultimate carbamino group, making it susceptible to hydrolytic cleavage.[133] Succinyl-L-proline was the original prototype molecule. Subsequent modifications led to the development of the three major chemical groups of ACE inhibitors currently in clinical use. First, the carboxyl terminal was changed to a mercapto group. This alteration increased the binding to zinc (and thus the inhibitory potency) without loss of specificity or an increase in toxicity. The resulting drug is captopril. Substituting glutaryl for succinyl led to the development of the first tripeptide analogs, enalapril and lisinopril, in the 1980s. Finally, hydroxyphosphinyl substitution of the second

carboxyl in the tripeptide analogs yielded fosinopril in the late 1980s.[132] Ester linkage of ACE inhibitors results in prodrugs with favorable oral absorption and bioavailability. However, these prodrugs are often two to three magnitudes less potent than the active metabolites and have to undergo enzymatic transformation in the liver to be converted into the active form.

All currently marketed ACE inhibitors are equally effective in blocking the enzyme and have similar therapeutic and adverse effects. Potency, bioavailability, elimination, and tissue distribution vary among the drugs and are the main basis for differences in prescription preference. The pharmacokinetic characteristics of the 10 oral ACE inhibitors currently marketed in the United States are summarized in Table 2-2. The hydrolyzed form of enalapril, enalaprilat, is available for intravenous administration. Its usual dose is 0.625 to 5 mg over 5 minutes repeated every 6 hours if needed. Time to onset is 15 to 30 minutes, and a precipitous decrease in blood pressure may occur in high-renin states. Intravenous enalaprilat should be used with caution in acute myocardial infarction.[38]

PHARMACOLOGIC EFFECTS OF ACE INHIBITORS

Effects on normotensive subjects. ACE inhibitors are highly selective for ACE. They suppress the formation of angiotensin II from angiotensin I and inhibit the enzymatic breakdown of bradykinin. Inhibition of angiotensin II formation interferes with renin regulation, and plasma renin levels rise. Furthermore, alternative pathways of angiotensin I metabolism result in increased levels of angiotensin (1-7). However, in a normotensive, sodium-repleted subject, ACE inhibitors have little effect on blood pressure; in a normotensive subject, ACE inhibitor administration results in a significant drop in blood pressure only in the setting of sodium depletion.[134] Bronchial reactivity to

---

TABLE 2-2

Names, Pharmacokinetic Characteristics and Recommended Daily Doses of Angiotensin-Converting Enzyme Inhibitors

Name	Trade Name	Chemical Structure	Prodrug	Bioavailability (%)	Time to Peak Plasma Concentration (hours)*	Half-Life (hours)	Elimination	Usual Daily Dose in Hypertension (mg)†‡	Starting Dose in Heart Failure (mg)
Benazepril	Lotensin	Dicarboxyl	Yes	37	1-2 (1/2)	11	Renal	5 to 40 (1-2)	
Captopril	Capoten	Sulfhydryl	No	75 (50)§	1	2	Renal	25 to 150 (2-3)	6.25
Enalapril	Vasotec	Dicarboxyl	Yes	60	3-4 (1)	11 (1.3)‖	Renal	5 to 40 (1-2)	2.5
Fosinopril	Monopril	Phosphinyl	Yes	36	3	11.5	Renal and hepatic	10 to 40 (1-2)	5
Lisinopril	Prinivil, Zestril	Dicarboxyl	No	30	7	12	Renal	5 to 40 (1)	2.5 to 5
Moexipril	Univasc	Dicarboxyl	Yes	13 (?)	1.5	2 to 12	Renal	7.5 to 15 (2)	
Perindopril	Aceon	Dicarboxyl	Yes	75 (50)§	3-7	3 to 10¶	Renal	2 to 16 (1-2)	
Quinalapril	Accupril	Dicarboxyl	Yes	60	2 (1)	2¶	Renal and feces (2:1)	5 to 80 (1-2)	
Ramipril	Altace	Dicarboxyl	Yes	55	3 (1)	9 to 18	Renal	1.25 to 20 (1-2)	
Trandolapril	Mavik	Dicarboxyl	Yes	10-70	4-10	10	Renal and feces (1:2)	1 to 4 (1)	0.5

*Of active metabolite and (prodrug).
†(Daily frequency of administration).
‡From reference 38.
§(Bioavailability when drug is taken with meal).
‖Half-life of active metabolite and (prodrug).
¶Terminal half-lives of over 24 hours related to tissue argiotensin-converting enzyme binding have been reported.

histamine and kinins remains unchanged in asthmatics and in patients with chronic obstructive pulmonary disease. ACE inhibitors have no effect on glucose or lipid metabolism.

Effects on hypertensive subjects. With the exception of primary hyperaldosteronism, ACE inhibitors are effective in lowering the blood pressure in hypertension. Although only patients with high pretreatment plasma renin activity and elevated angiotensin II levels respond to ACE inhibitor therapy rapidly (and initial doses of ACE inhibitors should be reduced in these patients), after several weeks of treatment a reduction in blood pressure is also observed in hypertensive patients with normal or low initial plasma renin activity. Several possible mechanisms have been implicated in the blood pressure reduction seen in these patients: increased natriuresis, an increase in the compliance of large arteries, and inhibition of tissue angiotensin II production with consequent reduction of peripheral vascular resistance. Renal blood flow increases, but as both the afferent and efferent arterioles dilate, GFR and filtration fraction decrease. Resting heart rate, baroreflex function, and cardiovascular responses to change in posture and exercise are minimally affected. Aldosterone secretion is only mildly reduced, and potassium retention is seldom a problem.[121]

Although current guidelines do not consider ACE inhibitors as initial drug choices for the treatment of hypertension, they may have additional benefits for patients in the setting of diabetic nephropathy, heart failure, and following myocardial infarction.[38] Regression of hypertensive myocardial hypertrophy, small artery remodeling, and diabetic nephropathy have all been shown in clinical trials.[135–137]

Effects in patients with ischemic heart disease. ACE inhibitors reduce overall mortality after myocardial infarction when treatment is started early following the ischemic event.[138] Treatment with an ACE inhibitor has been shown to improve baroreflex control and to reduce sympathetic activity after uncomplicated myocardial infarction. The inhibition of sympathetic nerve activity may contribute to the beneficial effect of ACE inhibitor drugs in myocardial infarction.[139] This effect is particularly pronounced in patients with diabetes and hypertensive patients. ACE inhibitors should be started in the acute phase of myocardial infarction, and therapy should be continued for the long term in patients with persistent systolic ventricular dysfunction.

Patients at high risk of cardiovascular events also benefit from treatment with ACE inhibitors.[140] ACE inhibitor therapy over 5 years significantly reduced the risks of death, myocardial infarction, and stroke in patients with vascular disease or diabetes who had one additional cardiovascular risk factor even in the absence of systolic left ventricular dysfunction. An improvement in endothelial NO-endothelin balance, a reduction in oxygen radical production, and ACE inhibitor–induced reduction of plasminogen activator inhibitor activity may play a role in the improved survival of these patients.[141] Direct evidence for the beneficial effect of ACE inhibitor therapy on endothelial function is the observation that ACh-induced vasoconstriction of diseased coronary arteries was markedly attenuated in patients following 6 months of quinapril therapy.[142]

Effect in patients with congestive heart failure. ACE inhibition is indicated for all patients with symptomatic left ventricular dysfunction.[14] Randomized clinical trials involving patients with asymptomatic, moderate, and severe left ventricular dysfunction have shown beneficial effects of ACE inhibitors both in reduction of mortality and in improvement in cardiac function.[143-145] Left ventricular dilation and remodeling following myocardial infarction are also limited by ACE inhibitors.[146]

The deleterious consequences of the increased accumulation and expression of renin, ACE, and angiotensin II in the failing ventricle have already been discussed in detail. ACE inhibitor therapy is effective in interrupting and reversing the hypertrophic and apoptotic processes of myocardial remodeling.[147]

ACE inhibitors exert beneficial effects in heart failure both locally in the myocardium and through their systemic effects. ACE inhibitors reduce peripheral vascular resistance and increase venous capacitance. The initial drop in blood pressure soon returns toward pretreatment levels unless the patient is hypertensive at the start of ACE inhibitor therapy. Heart rate is unchanged or decreased. Decreased renovascular resistance leads to increased renal blood flow and natriuresis. Pulmonary artery pressure and pulmonary capillary wedge pressure are decreased, significantly reducing subjective discomfort related to pulmonary congestion and increasing exercise tolerance.[148]

Chronic ACE inhibitor therapy in patients with CHF leads to reduced plasma norepinephrine levels, attenuated central sympathetic outflow, and increased vagal tone.[149,150] These favorable changes in autonomic regulation may contribute to the reduction in sudden cardiac death attributed to ACE inhibitor therapy in this population of patients.

SIDE EFFECTS OF ACE INHIBITOR THERAPY. ACE inhibitors are well tolerated, and serious side effects are rare.[151] Side effects include hypotension, renal failure, electrolyte disturbances, cough, and angioneurotic edema.

Patients with high plasma renin activity may respond with a sudden drop in blood pressure and orthostatic changes after the first dose of an ACE inhibitor. Diuretics may result in salt depletion, and this may also result in an exaggerated response to ACE inhibitors. Patients taking diuretics or multiple antihypertensive medications and patients with heart failure should receive a smaller than usual initial dose of an ACE inhibitor.

ACE inhibition may lead to acute renal failure in patients with bilateral renal artery stenosis or stenosis of the artery to a single kidney and, therefore, is contraindicated in these patients. Serum potassium levels should be carefully monitored in patients with chronic renal failure or when ACE inhibitors are combined with potassium-sparing diuretics or potassium replacement therapy.

ACE inhibition results in a dry, irritating cough in up to 20% of patients. The incidence is similar regardless of which drug is used, and it occurs more often in women. It appears most commonly within the first 6 months after starting ACE inhibitors and occasionally leads to discontinuation of the drug. Pulmonary accumulation of bradykinin is believed to be responsible for this adverse effect. Some patients may experience a maculopapular rash, which usually responds to a brief course of antihistamines.

Angioneurotic edema is a potentially life-threatening side effect of ACE inhibitor therapy. The incidence is about 0.1% to 0.5%, and it is more common in African-Americans. The median time to occurrence is within the first 6 months of starting ACE inhibitor therapy. However, it may develop within hours after the first dose of the drug and is characterized by swelling of the lips, nasal and oral mucosa, tongue, and in more severe cases the hypopharynx and the larynx. Less than 20% of patients with ACE-induced angioneurotic edema develop airway obstruction leading to respiratory distress. Among those who develop acute airway obstruction, mortality is estimated to range from 5% to 20%. The most common causes are inhibition of complement 1-esterase and bradykinin accumulation; less frequently, tissue-specific antibodies have been implicated.[152]

Administration of ACE inhibitors during the second and third trimesters of pregnancy results in growth retardation, oligohydramnios, fetal pulmonary hypoplasia, and fetal and neonatal death. When pregnancy is diagnosed, ACE inhibitors should be discontinued and replaced by an alternative antihypertensive drug.

Rare but serious side effects of ACE inhibitor therapy are neutropenia and liver damage. Loss of taste is most common with captopril and is usually reversible by switching to another ACE inhibitor.[121]

Angiotensin II-Receptor Antagonists

GENERAL CHARACTERISTICS. Angiotensin II-receptor antagonists were developed from N-benzylimidazole-5-acetic acid derivatives.[153] The drugs in clinical use closely resemble the active core of angiotensin II, are highly selective for the AT_1 receptor, and are devoid of agonist activity. Because of their slow dissociation, they demonstrate sustained inhibition of the receptor even in the presence of high angiotensin II concentrations.

Angiotensin II-receptor antagonists inhibit the biologic effects attributed to AT_1-receptor stimulation. Angiotensin II–induced rapid and slow pressor responses and vascular smooth muscle contraction are inhibited, as well as aldosterone, adrenal medullary catecholamine, and vasopressin release. Angiotensin II-receptor antagonists also inhibit sympathetic adrenergic transmission and myocardial and vascular smooth muscle hypertrophy and hyperplasia.

Although angiotensin II-receptor blockade and ACE inhibition both lead to a physiologic reduction in the effects of angiotensin II, they differ in several key aspects. Angiotensin II-receptor blockers directly and effectively inhibit activation of AT_1 receptors; ACE inhibitors prevent angiotensin II formation by ACE, whereas angiotensin II that is produced in small but significant amounts by chymase (an enzyme that is present in the left ventricle of human hearts) remains pharmacologically active. Although both drugs stimulate renin release, circulating angiotensin II levels are low with ACE inhibition and are high with angiotensin II-receptor inhibitors. In the former case, angiotensin (1-7) may play a role in the pharmacologic effect; in the latter, activation of AT_2 and AT_4 receptors by increased angiotensin II and angiotensin II breakdown products may contribute with antiproliferative and vasodilatory actions. Increased bradykinin levels and associated activation of NO pathways may have a beneficial effect on endothelial function with ACE inhibition; angiotensin II-receptor blockers lack this effect.[154]

The pharmacologic and pharmacokinetic characteristics of angiotensin II-receptor inhibitors currently available in the United States are summarized in Table 2-3.

PHARMACOLOGIC EFFECTS OF ANGIOTENSIN II-RECEPTOR INHIBITORS. Angiotensin II-receptor antagonists have little if any effect on blood pressure in normotensive subjects. In hypertensive patients, the blood pressure–reducing efficiency of angiotensin II-receptor antagonists is similar to that of ACE inhibitors. Different angiotensin II-receptor antagonists produce comparable blood pressure reductions with similar response rates in patients (45% to 55%) when used at their recommended doses. The combination of hydrochlorothiazide and angiotensin II antagonists significantly improves the antihypertensive effect and response rate (55% to 70%).[155]

As physiologically active plasma levels of angiotensin II persist in patients with heart failure despite long-term ACE inhibitor therapy,[156] there is ongoing interest in angiotensin II-inhibitor therapy in the treatment of CHF. Initial studies comparing an angiotensin II-receptor antagonist (losartan) with an ACE inhibitor (captopril) showed no significant difference in overall mortality or sudden death. Furthermore, fewer patients discontinued angiotensin II-antagonist therapy because of an adverse effect of the drug as compared with ACE inhibitors.[157] Addition of valsartan to the treatment regimen of patients in heart failure has reduced the incidence of hospitalization for heart failure with no change in overall mortality. It also resulted

---

TABLE 2-3

Names, Pharmacokinetic Characteristics, and Recommended Daily Doses of Angiotensin II AT$_1$-Receptor Inhibitors

Name	Trade Name	Prodrug	Bioavailability	Time to Peak Plasma Concentration (hours)	Half-Life	Elimination	Usual Daily Dose in Hypertension* (mg)
Candesartan	Atacand	Yes	Less than 50%	3 to 4	9 hours	Renal and biliary (1:2)	4 to 32 (1-2)
Eprosartan	Teveten	No	Less than 50%	1 to 2	5-9 hours	Renal and biliary	400 to 800 (1-2)
Irbesartan	Avapro	No	70%	2	11-15 hours	Renal and biliary (1:4)	150 to 300 (1)
Losartan	Cozaar	No†	Less than 50%	1‡	2.5 hours§	Renal and biliary	25 to 100 (1-2)
Telmisartan	Micardis	No	Less than 50%	1/2 to 1	1 day	Biliary	40 to 80 (1)
Valsartan	Diovan	No	Less than 50%	2 to 4	9 hours	Mainly biliary	80 to 320 (1)

*(Daily frequency of administration).
†Losartan has an active metabolite (EXP 3174), which is more potent than the parent drug.
‡3 hours for EXP 3174.
§6-9 hours for EXP 3174.

in significant improvements in signs and symptoms of heart failure and quality of life. However, a subgroup of patients receiving a combination of valsartan, an ACE inhibitor, and a β-blocker showed increases in mortality and morbidity. This combination is not recommended until further studies elucidate this issue.[158]

A differential effect of ACE inhibitors and angiotensin II-receptor inhibitors on coronary circulation in dilated cardiomyopathy has been demonstrated in a study in which enalaprilat, but not losartan, improved transmural myocardial perfusion at rest and during induced tachycardia. This difference on coronary circulation is believed to be secondary to the effect of enalaprilat on bradykinin metabolism.[159]

SIDE EFFECTS OF ANGIOTENSIN II-RECEPTOR ANTAGONISTS. Adverse effects of these drugs are similar to those discussed in the ACE inhibitor section. The drugs should be administered with caution to patients with high plasma renin activity or chronic renal failure and to those taking potassium-sparing diuretics. Angiotensin II-receptor antagonists should be avoided in patients with renovascular disease and in pregnant women. However, cough is absent and angioneurotic edema is less frequent than with ACE inhibitors.[121]

Vasopeptidase Inhibitors

Vasopeptidase inhibitors exert their pharmacologic effect by inhibiting several enzymes involved in vasoactive peptide metabolism.[160] Target enzymes identified for inhibition include neutral endopeptidase (NEP), the enzyme responsible for cleavage and inactivation of natriuretic peptides, endothelin-converting enzyme, and TNF-α–converting enzyme.

Omapatrilat, a drug with dual ACE-NEP inhibitor activity, has been shown to be more effective than ACE inhibitors alone in controlling hypertension in volume overload. Inhibition of NEP increases natriuretic peptide levels, which results in natriuresis and reduction of fluid overload and its associated subjective symptoms. Omapatrilat was comparable to lisinopril in the treatment of CHF and improved the NYHA functional status of patients with advanced heart failure more effectively than lisinopril.[161]

Omapatrilat has a side effect profile similar to that of ACE inhibitors. An increase in serum creatinine levels was three times less frequent than with lisinopril, but dizziness and gastrointestinal side effects (vomiting, diarrhea) were more common. Of note, the incidence of angioneurotic edema with omapatrilat is currently estimated as 0.7%, which is significantly higher than that observed with ACE inhibitor therapy.[162]

Perioperative Use of Drugs Affecting the Renin-Angiotensin System

Patients treated with ACE inhibitors or angiotensin-receptor antagonists may respond with more profound hypotension to induction of general anesthesia than patients receiving other forms of antihypertensive therapy.[163,164] Intraoperative hypotension refractory to treatment with ephedrine and/or phenylephrine was reported with both drug groups. ACE inhibitors appear to decrease the vasoconstrictive response to α-adrenergic agents in some patients even when baroreflex sensitivity is preserved.[165] Administration of a vasopressin agonist drug was

suggested to treat acute hypotension in patients receiving angiotensin II-antagonist or ACE inhibitor therapy.[164,166] The incidence of anesthesia induction–related hypotension can be significantly reduced by discontinuing ACE inhibitors the evening before surgery.[167]

Preoperative oral enalapril or sublingual captopril has been reported to blunt the hypertensive response to laryngoscopy and intubation.[168,169] However, this effect is unpredictable, and hypotension may remain sustained after induction of anesthesia. Furthermore, the heart rate response to airway instrumentation is not obtunded by ACE inhibitors, which makes these drugs less favorable than β-blockers. Chronic ACE inhibitor therapy has no added benefits for obtunding pressor or heart rate response to laryngoscopy compared with other antihypertensive modalities.[170]

Enalaprilat has been used to control intraoperative hypertension. It is most useful when a slow and gradual onset of effect and a sustained reduction of blood pressure are desired.[171] Pretreatment of patients undergoing abdominal aortic cross-clamping with oral captopril resulted in an increased incidence of intraoperative hypotension and did not prevent postoperative hypertension and tachycardia. However, captopril-treated patients had a significantly increased intraoperative urine output.[172] The combination of captopril with SNP does not confer any significant advantage in patients undergoing spine fusion with deliberate hypotension when compared with SNP alone.[173]

Familiarity with side effects of ACE inhibitor therapy is important. Cough in these patients may be a frequent finding during preoperative assessment. Anesthesiologists are also involved in emergency airway management of patients with angioneurotic edema.

Digitalis Glycosides and Their Use in the Treatment of Heart Failure

The use of digitalis glycosides in the treatment of heart failure was first reported in the late 18th century.[174] Digitalis glycosides are alkaloids found in the leaves of some plants, such as the garden plant foxglove (*Digitalis purpurea*). Digoxin and digitoxin are the two cardiac glycosides currently in clinical use in the United States. Although initially believed to exert their beneficial effects by control of heart rate in atrial fibrillation and by positive inotropic action, later developments have pointed toward a more subtle mechanism: modulation of sympathetic and parasympathetic autonomic nervous system activity.[175]

Mechanism of Action and Pharmacology of Digitalis Glycosides

Digitalis glycosides are potent inhibitors of sodium-potassium-ATPase (Na-K-ATPase), the pump responsible for maintaining membrane potential and intracellular ion homeostasis by exchanging intracellular sodium for extracellular potassium. Digitalis glycosides bind to a specific binding site on the extracellular portion of the α subunit of the ion pump. Binding of the glycoside stabilizes the ion channel in its phosphorylated form, inhibiting the dephosphorylation and conformational change necessary for expulsion of sodium ions. This leads to accumulation of intracellular sodium.[176]

Intracellular calcium concentration is a function of the cytoplasmic sodium concentration. Inhibition of the Na-K-ATPase and accumulation of sodium in cardiac myocytes reduce the electrochemical potential driving the sodium-calcium exchanger, resulting in increased intracellular calcium levels. The surplus calcium exerts a prolonged effect on troponin, enhancing contraction. Elevated intracellular calcium levels also enhance diastolic relaxation. Increased cytosolic calcium activates calcium-dependent kinases responsible for the phosphorylation of phospholamban. Phospholamban is a key regulator of sarcoplasmic reticular calcium uptake; it inhibits calcium-dependent ATPase activity and calcium uptake into the sarcoplasmic reticulum. Phosphorylation of phospholamban releases this inhibition, allowing rapid uptake of calcium from the sarcoplasm to the sarcoplasmic reticulum. Rapid removal of calcium is important for diastolic relaxation. Furthermore, more calcium is pumped into the sarcoplasmic reticulum, where it becomes available for release with subsequent contractions. Increased intracellular calcium concentrations increase the rate of spontaneous diastolic depolarization and augment delayed afterdepolarization, which may result in increased automaticity in ventricular muscle fibers.

Digitalis glycosides inhibit renal proximal tubular Na-K-ATPase, which increases sodium and chloride delivery to the distal portions of the nephron, reducing renin release and increasing urine output.[177]

Inhibition of Na-K-ATPase of autonomic nervous system cells by digitalis glycosides may result in sympathomimetic or sympatholytic effects. When administered to healthy subjects, digitalis glycosides produce mild sympathetic activation by sensitizing carotid sinus nerves. This augmentation of cardiopulmonary baroreflex control is unique to digitalis glycosides, as neither β-receptor agonists nor phosphodiesterase inhibitors have been found to have any effect on baroreflex activity.[178] Healthy subjects respond to digitalis glycosides with increases in systolic, diastolic, and mean arterial blood pressure and decreases in heart rate and right atrial pressure. However, forearm vascular resistance and muscle sympathetic nerve activity remain unchanged.[179] Digitalis glycosides increase ventilatory responses to hypoxia by 50% but do not affect the response to hypercapnia.[180]

When administered to patients with chronic heart failure, digitalis glycosides produce significant sympathoinhibition in addition to their direct positive inotropic effects on the myocardium. Systolic and pulse pressures increase, and mean arterial pressure remains unchanged. The heart rate decreases, right atrial and pulmonary artery diastolic pressures decrease, and the cardiac index increases. There is a decrease in forearm vascular resistance and a profound and sustained decrease in muscle sympathetic nerve activity.[179] This sympathoinhibition following digitalis administration in patients with heart failure precedes any observed hemodynamic action of the drug. Furthermore, acute digitalization of such patients rapidly normalizes impaired baroreflex-mediated mechanisms.[175] Chronic digitalis administration to patients with heart failure restores the ability of these patients to increase ejection fraction with exercise.[181]

Digitalis glycosides also increase vagal tone. Combined with sympathetic inhibition, this results in prolongation of the effective refractory period and a decrease in conduction velocity of atrioventricular nodal tissue. With higher concentrations of digitalis, the combination of direct tissue effects of the drug plus indirect vagal stimulation may result in bradycardia and heart block.

Administration of digitalis to patients with heart failure significantly reduces serum renin activity as well as norepinephrine and aldosterone levels.[182]

Digoxin

Intravenous digoxin produces pharmacologic effects in 5 to 30 minutes. When it is taken orally, the onset of effect occurs in about 1 hour, with maximum effect 2 to 6 hours later. Oral bioavailability is 60% to 75%, and absorption is delayed when the drug is taken with food. Intramuscular injection of digoxin is not recommended as absorption is erratic and muscle necrosis may ensue. The usual oral dose is 0.125 to 0.25 mg. In the past, an intravenous loading dose of 0.5 to 1.0 mg was given in three divided doses (half of the loading dose initially, followed by a quarter of the loading dose at 4- to 8-hour intervals). The use of newer, more effective intravenous inotropic agents and antiarrhythmic medications has largely replaced the need for rapid intravenous loading with digoxin in clinical practice.

Digoxin is approximately 25% protein bound in the plasma but is bound extensively in parenchymal organs and to a lesser extent in the skeletal muscle. Accumulation of digoxin in fat is minimal, and dosing is based on the lean body mass. Volume of distribution is 5 to 7 L/kg, and the terminal elimination half-life is 30 to 40 hours; the elimination half-life may extend beyond 100 hours in anuric patients, as 60% to 75% of digoxin is normally excreted unchanged by the kidney. Dialysis is ineffective in removing digoxin; only about 3% is removed during 5 hours of hemodialysis. When converting oral to intravenous dosing, a 33% decrease from the oral dose is recommended.

Amiodarone, verapamil, captopril, diltiazem, nifedipine, quinidine, and cyclosporine may all increase blood levels of digoxin, whereas thyroxine reduces blood levels.

Digitoxin

Digitoxin is less hydrophilic than digoxin. It is available only in the tablet form in the United States. Its absorption, although almost complete, is slower than that of digoxin. When it is taken orally, the onset of effect occurs in about 2 hours and the maximum effect is reached in 8 to 12 hours. The usual dose is 0.05 to 0.2 mg daily.

Digitoxin is 90% protein bound. It is metabolized in the liver with an elimination half-life of 5 to 7 days. Its metabolites are inactive; they are excreted by the kidney.

Diltiazem, verapamil, and quinidine may increase serum levels of digitoxin, whereas barbiturates and phenytoin increase its metabolism in the liver and reduce serum levels.

The Use of Digitalis Glycosides in Heart Failure

The use of digitalis glycosides in heart failure, although a common practice, remains somewhat controversial. When atrial fibrillation is present, the reduction in heart rate seen with digitalis use is clearly beneficial. However, the use of digitalis in patients with chronic heart failure and sinus rhythm remains under scrutiny.

Digoxin, in a large, prospective, randomized trial, did not reduce mortality when added to preexisting treatment in patents with heart failure. However, it reduced the rate of hospitalization for worsening heart failure. Although there was a trend toward a reduction of death rate related to worsening heart failure, this was counterbalanced by an increased incidence of death from other cardiac causes, presumably arrhythmias.[183]

Digoxin is unique among drugs used in the treatment of heart failure, having both positive inotropic and sympatholytic effects. The positive inotropic effects are well recognized as deleterious when it is used for long-term therapy, but the sympatholytic effects have been proved to be exceptionally beneficial in these patients.[184] It is also recognized that the positive inotropic and arrhythmogenic effects of digoxin become manifest at higher serum concentrations (>1.2 ng/mL), whereas autonomic nervous system effects can be detected at much lower serum levels (>0.5 ng/mL). Indeed, no correlation between improvement in the treadmill exercise capacity of patients with heart failure and serum digoxin levels has been found, although patients taking placebo performed significantly worse.[185] Thus, it appears that inhibition of sympathetic outflow and renin activity, rather than a positive inotropic effect, is the reason for the beneficial effect of digoxin in heart failure. Controversy surrounds the use of digoxin following acute myocardial infarction. Available studies suggest increased mortality in this population of patients.[186,187] However, because of the lack of adequate prospective, randomized trials, the risks and benefits of digoxin use following myocardial infarction still remain unknown.

Adverse Effects of Digitalis Glycosides

Digitalis glycosides may cause various arrhythmias and conduction disturbances. Prolongation of the PR interval and ST-segment depression are common with digitalis glycosides, and digitalis use should be considered when interpreting routine ECG studies. Sinus bradycardia, AV conduction delays of any degree, atrial tachycardias (often associated with slow pulse rate related to coexisting AV block), accelerated junctional rhythm, and ventricular premature contractions (initially often in the form of bigeminy and deteriorating to ventricular tachycardia and fibrillation) have all been described. Hypoxia, hypokalemia, hypomagnesemia, and hypercalcemia sensitize the myocardium to the arrhythmogenic effects of digitalis glycosides. Potassium administration in the absence of a high-degree AV block may be beneficial even when serum potassium concentrations are in the normal range, as binding of digoxin to the Na-K-ATPase is antagonized by a high potassium concentration. Ventricular arrhythmias are treated with lidocaine or phenytoin, drugs with minimal effect on AV conduction. Cardioversion in the presence of digitalis often results in provoking arrhythmias, and the drug should be withheld for 24 hours prior to planned cardioversion. Should cardioversion be necessary, the lowest effective energy should be used. Cardioversion is not recommended in the treatment of digitalis-induced arrhythmias.

Gastrointestinal side effects include anorexia, nausea, vomiting, and diarrhea. Nausea, although often present, is an unreliable sign of excessive digitalis dosage. Central nervous system effects of digitalis include apathy, fatigue, malaise, visual disturbance (changes in color vision), and, less frequently, depression or psychosis. Rarely, skin rashes associated with eosinophilia, thrombocytopenia, and intestinal ischemia may be associated with digitalis use.

Future Perspectives

Following many years of investigation, circulating endogenous glycosides of hypothalamic and adrenal origin have been identified: ouabain, marinobufagenin, and cardenolide.[188] These steroid-based substances are presumed to play a role in sodium and volume regulation. The serum concentration of ouabain is elevated with increased sodium intake, hypoxia, and physical exercise and is chronically elevated in some patients with hypertension associated with low serum renin levels. Marinobufagenin is a specific antagonist of α_1-type Na-K-ATPase, found in renal tubular cells. Interestingly, serum levels of marinobufagenin increase acutely after myocardial infarction. Although endogenous glycosides increase renal sodium excretion, prolonged administration in experimental animals results in the development of hypertension. Agonist and antagonist substances have been synthesized, and novel approaches in the treatment of hypertension and heart failure may become available utilizing the endogenous glycoside system.

The Pharmacology of Diuretics and Their Role in the Treatment of Hypertension and Congestive Heart Failure

Diuretics have been used as the first-line treatment of both hypertension and CHF. An increase in urine flow and elimination of excess solute were thought to be beneficial. However, in light of the newer concepts of cardiac and vascular remodeling, the role of diuretics in the treatment of these conditions may undergo reevaluation.

Mechanism of Action and Pharmacologic Effects of Diuretics

Diuretics are traditionally classified according to their site of action. Loop diuretics inhibit the Na^+-K^+-$2Cl^-$ symporter in the thick ascending loop of Henle. Thiazide diuretics inhibit the Na^+-Cl^- symporter, predominantly in the distal convoluted tubules. Both symporters belong to the same 12-transmembrane-domain, electroneutral, cation-coupled-chloride cotransporter family of membrane proteins. Potassium-sparing diuretics either inhibit renal epithelial sodium channels (e.g., amiloride) or antagonize the action of aldosterone (e.g., spironolactone).[121] Osmotic diuretics and carbonic anhydrase inhibitors are not used in the treatment of hypertension and chronic heart failure and are not discussed in this chapter.

Loop Diuretics

The Na^+-K^+-$2Cl^-$ symporter in the thick ascending loop of Henle is the last resorptive mechanism available to the kidney for sodium conservation. Sodium escaping resorption in the proximal tubules is easily reabsorbed here. However, tubules distal to the thick ascending limb have a limited resorptive capacity for sodium. Thus, blockade of the Na^+-K^+-$2Cl^-$ symporter by loop diuretics is highly effective in increasing sodium and water elimination.

The $Na^+-K^+-2Cl^-$ symporter exploits the electrochemical gradient for sodium ion generated by the Na-K-ATPase located on the basolateral surface of the tubule cells. The sodium and chloride entering the tubule cell exit through the basolateral surface; the former is expelled by the Na-K-ATPase, and the latter leaves through a chloride channel. Potassium ions return to the tubule lumen through an apical potassium channel. The apical surface is impermeable to chloride ions. This difference in chloride conductance between the apical and basolateral cell membranes produces a potential difference between the tubule lumen and the peritubular interstitium, enhancing the resorption of cations such as calcium and magnesium.

Inhibition of the $Na^+-K^+-2Cl^-$ symporter increases not only sodium and chloride elimination but also the excretion of calcium and magnesium, as inhibiting the symporter abolishes the potential difference between the lumen and the peritubular interstitium. Increased delivery of sodium ions to the distal tubules enhances potassium and hydrogen ion exchange and results in hypokalemia and alkalosis. Furthermore, as sodium resorption in the medullary part of the thick ascending loop is primarily responsible for the establishment of the hypertonic gradient in the renal medulla, interference with sodium resorption ultimately results in loss of the ability to concentrate (or to dilute) urine, and urine osmolality becomes identical to plasma osmolality.[189]

Inhibition of chloride uptake in macula densa cells by loop diuretics causes activation of cyclooxygenase-2 (COX-2) and a prostaglandin-mediated increase in renin release.[190] Both nonsteroidal anti-inflammatory drugs and selective COX-2 inhibitors attenuate loop diuretic–induced diuresis, saluresis, and renin release.[191] Initial rises in serum catecholamine levels and plasma renin activity are common following the introduction of loop diuretics.[192] This is most commonly due to hypovolemia-induced baroreflex activation, although in patients with severe heart failure there actually are reductions in catecholamine levels and plasma renin activity when hemodynamic conditions have improved.[193,194] Administration of loop diuretics often results in an immediate increase in venous capacitance, reduction of ventricular filling volume, and relief of congestive symptoms. These effects precede the diuretic effect of these drugs and are due to COX-2–mediated prostaglandin release.[195] Loop diuretics have no direct venodilatory effect.[196]

The pharmacologic characteristics of loop diuretics are summarized in Table 2-4. It is of interest that in spite of the low bioavailability of furosemide, the oral and intravenous bolus doses are equal in efficacy. Gradual absorption from the gut probably results in a better time course of delivery to the renal tubules. Similarly, continuous infusion of furosemide results in a better diuretic response than administration of the same dose of the drug as a bolus injection.[193]

In severe heart failure, oral absorption of loop diuretics is limited by edema of the gut wall and reduced splanchnic blood flow. Efficacy of the drug is limited by reduced renal blood flow, resulting in reduced glomerular filtration and tubular secretion of these drugs.

Thiazide Diuretics

The class of diuretics commonly known as thiazides inhibits the Na^+-Cl^- symporter on the apical surface of distal convoluted tubule cells. This symporter is responsible for resorption of 5% to 10% of filtered sodium; therefore, the expected diuretic effect, even with full inhibition of the symporter, is moderate. It is of note that although the original drugs inhibiting the Na^+-Cl^- symporter were all benzothiadiazide derivatives, some newer members of the group are in fact not thiazides in chemical structure.

The Na^+-Cl^- symporter, similar to the $Na^+-K^+-2Cl^-$ symporter, utilizes the electrochemical gradient of the sodium ion to facilitate sodium and chloride resorption. The resorbed sodium is then actively expelled from tubule cells by Na^+-K^+-ATPase on the basolateral surface while chloride exits through chloride channels. The binding site for thiazide diuretics on the symporter is poorly characterized at present, but it is likely to involve both the sodium and the chloride binding sites.[197]

Inhibition of sodium resorption in the distal convoluted tubules increases Na^+-K^+ and Na^+-H^+ exchange, resulting in hypokalemia and alkalosis. The Na^+-Cl^- symporter does not alter the potential between the lumen and the interstitium, and there is no facilitation of calcium or magnesium resorption. Calcium excretion actually decreases with chronic administration of thiazide diuretics; however, hypercalcemia is not a significant problem with thiazide diuretics. On the other hand, thiazide diuretics produce a significant loss of magnesium and magnesium replacement may facilitate calcium excretion in hypertensive patients.[198]

Thiazide diuretics have no direct effect on renal renin release as their site of action is distal to the macula densa. However, systemic hypovolemia may still result in sympathetic activation and increased renin and aldosterone levels.[199]

The pharmacologic characteristics of thiazide diuretics are summarized in Table 2-5.

TABLE 2-4

The Pharmacologic Characteristics of Loop Diuretics Currently Available for Clinical Use in the United States

Generic Name	Trade Name	Chemical Structure	Bioavailability (%)	Onset Time of Oral Dose (hours)	Half-Life (hours)	Duration of Action (hours)	Usual Daily Dose (mg)*
Bumetanide	Bumex	Sulfonamide	80	0.5-1	1-1.5	4-6	0.5-2 (10)
Ethacrynic acid	Edecrin	Phenoxyacetate	100	0.5	1	6-8	50-100 (400)
Furosemide	Lasix	Sulfonamide	60-70	1-2	1.5	6-8	20-80 (400)
Torsemide	Demadex	Sulfonylurea	80	1	3.5	6-8	10-20 (200)

*Maximum recommended daily dose in patients with adequate renal function in parentheses.

TABLE 2-5

The Pharmacologic Characteristics of the Thiazide Diuretics Currently Available for Clinical Use in the United States

Generic Name	Bioavailability (%)	Onset Time of Oral Dose (hours)	Half-Life (hours)	Duration of Action (hours)	Elimination	Usual Daily Dose
Bendroflumethiazide	100	2	3-4	18	30% renal	2.5-10 mg
Chlorthalidone	60	2.6	40-60	48-72	Renal	25-100 mg
Chlorothiazide	Variable*	2	0.75-2	6-12	Renal	0.5-2 g
Hydrochlorothiazide	70	2	6-15	6-12	Renal	25-100 mg
Hydroflumethiazide	50	2	2; 17†	6-12	65% renal	25-200 mg
Indapamide	90	2	14	24	70% renal	1.25-5 mg
Methyclothiazide		2		24	Renal	2.5-10 mg
Metolazone (Zaroxolyn)‡	65	4	70	Long	80% renal	2.5-20 mg
Metolazone (Mykrox)‡	90	2	14	Long	80% renal	0.5-1 mg
Polythiazide	100	2	24	Long	25% renal	1-4 mg
Trichlormethiazide			2-7	6-12	Renal	1-4 mg

*The bioavailability of chlorothiazide is dose dependent but poor in general.
†Biphasic half-life: α half-life, 2 hours; β half-life, 17 hours.
‡The two formulations of metolazone are not interchangable. Mykrox has more rapid absorption and onset of action and shorter duration.

Potassium-Sparing Diuretics

Inhibition of the Na^+-K^+ exchange in the late distal tubules and the proximal collecting ducts prevents the unwanted urinary loss of potassium that occurs with the use of thiazides or loop diuretics. This pharmacologic effect may be achieved either through inhibition of renal epithelial sodium channels or by antagonism of the cytosolic aldosterone receptor.

INHIBITORS OF RENAL EPITHELIAL SODIUM CHANNELS. Apical membrane epithelial sodium channels of cells in the late distal tubules and proximal collecting ducts allow sodium ion influx from the tubular lumen into the cytoplasm. This influx of positive ions creates a lumen-negative potential and reverses the local electrochemical gradient for potassium ions. The apical membrane of the epithelial cells is permeable to potassium ions, which leads to potassium loss from the cells. As the basolateral membrane Na^+-K^+-ATPase continuously extrudes sodium from the cell, a counterflux of sodium and potassium ions occurs between the apical and basolateral surfaces. This mechanism results in net sodium gain and potassium loss in the distal part of the tubule system. Under normal circumstances, this sodium gain and potassium loss are minimal. When a thiazide or loop diuretic is administered, the increased distal sodium flux markedly augments potassium excretion.

Amiloride and triamterene, two organic bases, exert their effect by binding to the luminal aspect of epithelial sodium channels (ENaCs). This occupancy of the sodium binding site is competitive, and the effects of amiloride and triamterene can be reversed by a high-salt diet. The blockade of sodium transport hyperpolarizes the tubule cell and decreases the apical excretion not only of potassium but of calcium, magnesium, and hydrogen ions as well.[121]

Amiloride is poorly absorbed, with an oral bioavailability of only 20%. Peak serum concentrations are achieved 3 to 4 hours after administration. Serum half-life is 6 hours, whereas the biologic half-life is about 20 hours. Amiloride is eliminated unchanged by the kidney. The usual dose of amiloride is 5 mg once daily.

Triamterene is better absorbed from the gut than amiloride. Its oral bioavailability is 30% to 70% and peak plasma concentration is reached in 2 to 4 hours. The half-life of triamterene is 4 hours. Triamterene is extensively metabolized. Its metabolite, 4-OH-triamterene sulfate, is equipotent with the parent drug and is eliminated through the kidney. The usual dose is 100 mg twice daily, and the total daily dose should not exceed 300 mg.

ALDOSTERONE RECEPTOR ANTAGONISTS. Aldosterone is the main mineralocorticoid hormone. When aldosterone enters the cell, it binds to a cytosolic mineralocorticoid receptor protein. The aldosterone-receptor complex then translocates to the nucleus and initiates transcription of mRNA encoding aldosterone-induced peptides, among them the serum and glucocorticoid-inducible kinase, a protein kinase involved in phosphorylation of a number of ion channels. This leads to activation of channels involved in sodium resorption, most notably ENaC, basolateral Na^+-K^+-ATPase, apical potassium channels, and the Na^+-Cl^- symporter. Nontranscriptional effects of aldosterone also play a role, as reflected in the biphasic nature of the epithelial sodium resorptive response to aldosterone. The early response takes place in the first ½ to 3 hours and is characterized by a two- to threefold increase in sodium resorption. This initial response is followed by the late phase, which lasts about 24 hours and leads to a 20-fold increase in sodium resorption. Although there is no transcriptional activity during the early phase, even in the late phase, redistribution and activation of preexisting channels are more likely to be responsible for the increase in resorptive capacity than synthesis of new ion channels.[200]

Spironolactone (Aldactone) competitively inhibits binding of aldosterone to its receptor. It is most effective when serum or local aldosterone levels are high. Chronically elevated aldosterone levels result in hypertension. Initially, aldosterone induces water and sodium retention, increasing intravascular volume and cardiac output. Tissue autoregulation subsequently responds to perfusion in excess of local metabolic needs with vasoconstriction. This process redirects the excess volume to the central circulation, thereby increasing renal perfusion. This leads to increases in renal sodium and water excretion and restoration of intravascular volume and cardiac output toward normal. However, higher peripheral resistance persists, and hypertension develops.[201] Antagonizing the effects of aldosterone can break this vicious circle.

Spironolactone is rapidly absorbed, with a bioavailability of more than 90%. It undergoes significant first-pass metabolism. About a third of the oral dose is converted to canrenone, which has approximately one third of the activity of the parent compound. Spironolactone achieves its peak plasma levels in about 1 to 1.5 hours and has a plasma half-life of 1 hour. Canrenone attains its peak serum concentration in 2 to 4 hours and has a half-life between 13 and 24 hours. Elimination of spironolactone and canrenone is by the kidneys. The usual daily dose of spironolactone is 25 to 200 mg, which can be divided or administered as a single dose.

Diuretics in the Treatment of Hypertension

Thiazide diuretics have been used for the treatment of elevated blood pressure since the mid-1950s, and they have remained first-line drugs in the treatment of hypertension ever since.[38,202] In equipotent doses, thiazide diuretics are considered to be equally effective in the treatment of hypertension. When used in low or high doses, hydrochlorothiazide was associated with reduced incidences of stroke, total cardiovascular events, and mortality compared with placebo or no treatment; however, only low-dose thiazide regimens reduce the rate of myocardial ischemic events.[203] Furthermore, low-dose thiazide therapy appears to be as effective as high-dose thiazide therapy in reducing arterial blood pressure. When thiazides were compared with β-receptor antagonists or calcium channel blockers, no significant differences in mortality and cardiovascular morbidity were demonstrated, and the magnitude of blood pressure reduction was also similar.[204] Regression of left ventricular hypertrophy associated with hypertension secondary to thiazide treatment was comparable to that with ACE inhibitor, calcium channel blocker, or β-receptor antagonist therapy.[205] Thiazide diuretics are well tolerated, and withdrawal of patients because of adverse effects from treatment is less frequent than with other antihypertensive drugs.[203] Thiazide diuretics remain the standard against which newer agents are tested.[206]

Because of their short half-life, loop diuretics are used less frequently in the treatment of uncomplicated hypertension. However, they are as effective as thiazide diuretics in reducing blood pressure in hypertension, and their use in elderly patients with heart failure, coronary artery disease, and elevated creatinine levels is on the rise.[207,208]

Chronic antihypertensive therapy with even small doses of thiazides or loop diuretics may lead to excessive loss of potassium. However, hypokalemia is easily detectable and usually easy to manage by adding a potassium-sparing diuretic. The use of potassium-sparing diuretics rather than potassium supplementation not only is more cost effective but also counteracts the effects of elevated aldosterone levels often associated with thiazide-induced hypokalemia.[199]

Diuretics in the Treatment of Congestive Heart Failure

Diuretics are essential in the symptomatic management of patients with congestive heart failure. When fluid retention is resolved, treatment with diuretics is continued to prevent recurrence of fluid retention. Diuretics are seldom used as monotherapy in CHF, and are usually combined with an ACE inhibitor or a β-receptor antagonist.[184] Compared with placebo, loop diuretics alone or in combination with a thiazide reduce mortality and relapse rate and improve exercise capacity in patients with CHF.[209] There are no data available on the long-term effect of loop diuretics on the natural course of heart failure. However, in the majority of patients, discontinuation of diuretic treatment results in worsening heart failure, necessitating restarting the drug.[210]

Patients with heart failure may become resistant to the effect of loop diuretics. The importance of this phenomenon is that high diuretic requirements are independently associated with mortality, sudden death, and pump failure.[211] Development of resistance may be due to reduced bioavailability. Orally administered furosemide is notoriously unreliably absorbed in worsening heart failure, and switching the patient to a better absorbed drug such as torsemide may result in improved diuresis.[212] However, in the majority of patients, loop diuretic resistance is the result of an aldosterone-induced increase in the amount and activity of the Na^+-Cl^- symporter in the distal convoluted tubules, resulting in increased sodium and water resorption.[213] Addition of a thiazide diuretic such as metolazone or an aldosterone antagonist such as spironolactone restores natriuresis and diuresis in these patients.[214,215]

Aldosterone has emerged as a key mediator in the pathogenesis of heart failure. In addition to the traditional and well-known role of aldosterone in promoting sodium retention, aldosterone and aldosterone-induced proteins are expressed by the failing myocardium and may play a role in maladaptive myocardial remodeling and cardiac fibrosis. Although spironolactone is effective in abolishing aldosterone-induced myocardial changes in laboratory animals, unlike ACE inhibitors and angiotensin II–receptor antagonists.[216] In addition, spironolactone attenuates superoxide anion formation by endothelial cells, which results in improvement in NO-mediated vasodilation.[217]

In the Randomized Aldactone Evaluation Study (RALES), addition of spironolactone to preexisting therapy (ACE inhibitor, loop diuretic, and, in most cases, digoxin) reduced mortality by 30% over a period of 24 months. The incidence of worsening heart failure was also reduced by more than a third in the study group, and a significantly larger number of patients experienced symptomatic improvement. Serum potassium levels were mildly elevated in the treatment group (by an average of 0.3 mmol/L), and the incidence of serious hyperkalemia was 2%.[218] This study not only established spironolactone as a drug for treatment of heart failure but also galvanized research efforts for elucidating the aldosterone-related pathomechanism in heart failure.

Adverse Effects of Diuretics

Loop diuretics can cause hypokalemia and alkalosis. Hypokalemia may lead to arrhythmias, particularly when associated with hypomagnesemia or digitalis use. However, chronic hypokalemia per se is not associated with an increased incidence of intraoperative arrhythmias.[219] Minimizing the dose of the drug and adding a potassium-sparing diuretic are usually sufficient for correction of hypokalemia.

Overzealous treatment with loop diuretics may result in intravascular volume depletion, dizziness, reduced GFR, and even circulatory collapse. Hyponatremia is usually the result of repletion of lost solute with liberal amounts of water. Hyperglycemia, hyperuricemia, and unfavorable changes in lipid profile are unwanted metabolic effects of loop diuretics. Loop diuretics are ototoxic, and this effect is synergistic with the ototoxic effect of aminoglycoside antibiotics.

Thiazides can similarly cause hypokalemic alkalosis with hypomagnesemia. Excessive use of diuretics may result in severe hyponatremia. However, calcium elimination is not increased, and hydrochlorothiazide has been shown to slow cortical bone loss in postmenopausal women.[220]

Although thiazide diuretics impair glucose tolerance, long-term treatment of hypertensive patients with thiazide diuretics has not been shown to promote the development of diabetes in these patients.[221]

Erectile dysfunction is a frequent reason for discontinuing the drug. Skin rashes and photosensitivity, gastrointestinal symptoms (cramping, nausea, constipation), and headaches may occur.

Potassium-sparing diuretics may cause hyperkalemia. Concurrent use of ACE inhibitors or nonsteroidal anti-inflammatory drugs increases the risk. Amiloride and triamterene may cause headaches, nausea, and vomiting. Triamterene causes photosensitization and reduces glucose tolerance. A common side effect of spironolactone in men is gynecomastia; in women, deepening of the voice, hirsutism, and menstrual irregularities may occur. Triamterence can reduce sexual libido in both genders. Exacerbation of peptic ulcer disease has been described, and spironolactone should be avoided in such patients. Headaches, drowsiness, and diarrhea are minor side effects. Rarely, skin rashes and blood dyscrasias may occur.

Calcium Channel Blocking Drugs for the Treatment of Hyertension and Ischemic Heart Disease

Calcium channel blocking drugs were introduced to clinical practice in the 1960s.[222] Calcium channel antagonists are among the most commonly prescribed drugs for the treatment of hypertension, ischemic heart disease, and cardiac arrhythmias. Although they are effective in reducing blood pressure and alleviating symptoms of myocardial ischemia, their long-term use may not result in the benefits seen with β-receptor antagonists or ACE inhibitors in the same populations of patients.[223]

Calcium Channels in the Cardiovascular System

The cytosolic calcium concentration at rest is about five magnitudes lower than the extracellular calcium concentration. This concentration gradient, combined with the negative charge of the cell compared with the extracellular space, provides a powerful electrochemical force that drives calcium ions into the cells through selective or nonselective ion channels.[224] A number of voltage-gated, calcium-selective ion channels

were described and characterized. All calcium channels consist of a pore-forming α_1 subunit, which is characterized by a primary structure of four repetitive domains (also called motifs), each consisting of six putative transmembrane segments. The fourth transmembrane segment serves as the voltage sensor of the calcium channel, and the fifth and sixth segments form the ion channel pore, the sixth segment being responsible for the voltage-dependent inactivation.[225] Cardiac and smooth muscle L-type calcium channels all contain the α_{1C} subunit type. Although the basic functional and pharmacologic characteristics of calcium ion transport are determined by the α_1 subunit, three other modulatory subunits complete the ion channel: the intracellular β subunit and the disulfide-linked $\alpha_2\delta$ subunits.[226] Phosphorylation of various subunits increases calcium current. Amino acid residues for phosphorylation are present on all four subunits. Subunits α_1 and β were identified as substrates of the cAMP-dependent protein kinase A, and subunits α_1 and $\alpha_2\delta$ are targets for the diacylglycerol-dependent PKC[227] (Figure 2-2).

Two types of voltage-gated calcium channels have been found in the plasma membrane of myocardial and vascular smooth muscle cells: the L-type (long-lasting) and the T-type (transient). L-type channels open at a membrane potential of −40 to −30 mV, with a maximum calcium flux at membrane potentials of 0 to +10 mV, and their opening is sustained.[228] L-type calcium channels are predominant in adult cells. They contribute to the plateau phase of the action potential and are responsible for initiation of excitation-contraction coupling in atrial and ventricular myocytes. This is due to their arrangement in the transverse tubular system in close proximity to the calcium-sensitive ryanodine-2 receptors, which are responsible for release of calcium from the sarcoplasmic reticulum (see later). Calcium entry through L-type channels contributes to sinus nodal pacemaker activity and is essential for conduction in the AV nodal tissue.[224] Calcium entry through L-type calcium channels is responsible for at least 50% of the vascular smooth muscle tone. Furthermore, L-type calcium channels associated with ryanodine receptors and calcium-activated potassium channels may play a significant role in vasodilatory regulation of vascular tone.[229] In brief, localized calcium influx in this arrangement results in release of calcium from the smooth muscle sarcoplasmic reticulum, activation of potassium channels, and hyperpolarization. This membrane hyperpolarization results in smooth muscle relaxation and vasodilation. Association with NO-mediated cGMP release and protein kinase G, and with β-receptor–mediated increase in cAMP with subsequent activation of protein kinase A, increases L-type calcium influx and activation of calcium-sensitive potassium channels. On the other hand, PKC, the phosphorylase associated with α-adrenergic, endothelin, and angiotensin II receptors, inhibits calcium-sensitive potassium channels. Thus, the physiologic effect of calcium influx in smooth muscle cells is determined not only by the quantity of calcium ions but also by their exact location in the cell.[229]

T-type calcium channels open at a membrane potential of −70 to −60 mV, which is lower than that of L-type channels.[228] T-type channel opening is transient, and these channels become refractory soon after the initial membrane depolarization. T-type channels are predominant in the developing (fetal) heart and are believed to have a role in cell growth and differentiation.[224]

T-type channels, which open at a lower membrane potential, have an important role in initiating sinus nodal pacemaker activity. However, T-type channels constitute less than 10% of all calcium channels in the adult heart and are not found in the transverse tubule system; thus, their contribution to excitation-contraction coupling is probably negligible. T-type calcium channels are found in increased amounts on ventricular myocardial cells in dilated cardiomyopathy, and this reexpression of fetal calcium channels may be a factor in myocardial remodeling.[230]

Although extracellular calcium is abundant, the majority of calcium participating in excitation-contraction coupling originates from well-organized subcellular sources. Cardiac muscle cells store calcium ions for rapid release in the sarcoplasmic reticulum, and vascular muscle cells have calcium available in their endoplasmic reticulum. Release of calcium from these intracellular stores is coupled to ryanodine-2 receptors or to inositol triphosphate (IP_3) receptors. Ryanodine-2 receptors respond to the sudden, localized increase of intracellular calcium concentration secondary to L-type calcium channel opening and calcium influx (calcium sparks), and IP_3 receptors mediate calcium release in response to phospholipase C activation by α-adrenergic or angiotensin II receptors.[231] IP_3-dependent calcium release and influx are responsible for the other 50% of vascular smooth muscle tone. Calcium released from the sarcoplasmic or endoplasmic reticulum is available for rapid but limited increase of intracellular calcium concentration in well-defined areas of the cell, and highly effective ATP-driven calcium pumps are in place to return the calcium ions rapidly to their storage compartments. Influx of extracellular calcium is relegated to initiation of excitation-contraction coupling in cardiac myocytes but remains an important contributor in determining resting tone of vascular smooth muscle cells.[231]

Mechanism of Action and Pharmacology of Calcium Channel Antagonist Drugs

The currently available calcium channel antagonist drugs are all inhibitors of the L-type calcium channel. The basic chemical structure of the calcium channel antagonists determines their binding site on the calcium channel. The phenylalkylamines, a prototype of which is verapamil, preferentially bind to a pair of glutamate residues on segment 6 of domains III and IV of the α_{1C} subunit on the intracellular side of the cell membrane. Rapid depolarization causes an increased rate of binding of the drug to both open and inactivated channels and increased decay of the calcium current during depolarization because of progressive block of open channels and slow recovery of inactivated channels. This binding results in a frequency-dependent enhancement of calcium channel blockade by phenylalkylamine drugs and is the basis of the antiarrhythmic action of verapamil. Benzothiazepines, of which the only agent in clinical use is diltiazem, binds to the extracellular side of transmembrane segment 6 of domains III and IV of the calcium ion pore α_{1C} subunit. Diltiazem produces more tonic block than verapamil but less than the dihydropyridine drugs. On the other hand, the frequency dependence of the block is seven times more than that of the dihydropyridines but only a quarter of that of verapamil.[226] Dihydropyridines, a typical example being nifedipine, have the highest affinity for the inactivated state of the calcium channel of the three groups, resulting in a steeply voltage-dependent block with little frequency dependence. Their binding site is on the extracellular surface of the α_{1C} subunit, but in a deeper, more hydrophobic location than the benzothiazepine binding site, and is located on transmembrane segments 5 and 6 of domains III and IV. It has been suggested that binding of a dihydropyridine-type antagonist results in stabilizing the ion channel with a single calcium ion bound in a blocking position in the pore.[226]

The phenylalkylamine, benzothiazepine, and dihydropyridine binding sites are allosterically linked and binding of one type of drug inhibits subsequent binding of either of the other two types to the receptor.[232]

The pharmacokinetic properties of calcium channel blockers used in the treatment of ischemic heart disease and hypertension are summarized in Table 2-6.

Clinical Effects of Calcium Channel Blockers
L-TYPE CALCIUM CHANNEL ANTAGONISTS
Normal subjects. Calcium channel blockers are peripheral vasodilators. The most potent vasodilators are the dihydropyridines; the least effective are bepridil and diltiazem. Verapamil is intermediate in vasodilating potency. All calcium channel blockers preferentially dilate arteries and precapillary arterioles. However, nicardipine augments transcapillary leak,

---

TABLE 2-6

The Pharmacokinetic Characteristics and Recommended Daily Doses of Calcium Channel Antagonist Drugs

Drug	Bioavailability (%)	Protein Binding (%)	Metabolism	Excretion	Half-Life (hours)	Daily Dose (mg)
Verapamil	20-35	95	95%; liver	Renal	3-7	120-480
Diltiazem	40	70-80	Liver	Renal	3-4.5	120-480
Bepridil	60	99	~100%; liver	Renal	26-64	200-400
Amlodipine	52-88	97.5	90%; liver	Renal	35-60	2.5-10
Felodipine	15	99	99.5%; liver	Renal	11-16	2.5-10
Isradipine	16-18	95	100%; liver	Renal; GI	8-12	5-20
Nicardipine	35	>95%	99%; liver	Renal	8	60-120
Nifedipine	45-56	95	~100%; liver	Renal; GI	2	30-120
Nisoldipine	4-8	99	~100%; liver	Renal; GI	7-12	20-40

GI, gastrointestinal.

and nifedipine increases the permeability of postcapillary venules, both effects resulting in peripheral edema.[233]

Hypertensive patients. When administered acutely to hypertensive subjects, short-acting calcium antagonists of both the dihydropyridine and nondihydropyridine class increase heart rate to the same extent for comparable reductions in mean arterial pressure. However, the increase in serum norepinephrine levels is more pronounced with dihydropyridine drugs. The increase in serum norepinephrine levels is in direct correlation with the increase in heart rate and in inverse correlation with the change in mean arterial pressure. This suggests a nonspecific effect of vasodilation on baroreflex activity.[234]

When short-acting calcium antagonists are used for an extended period of time, the heart rate increase is markedly attenuated with dihydropyridine-type drugs and there is an actual decrease in resting heart rate with nondihydropyridine drugs. However, there is no difference in the increase of plasma norepinephrine between the two drug groups. Furthermore, the correlation between norepinephrine levels, heart rate, and blood pressure changes, as seen when the drugs are administered acutely, is not present with chronic administration of the drugs, suggesting some readjustment in baroreflex activity with long-term use of calcium antagonists.[234]

When long-acting calcium antagonists are used for long-term treatment, heart rate remains unchanged compared with the pretreatment value with dihydropyridine drugs, but it is significantly decreased with nondihydropyridine drugs. Plasma norepinephrine levels are increased in patients using dihydropyridine drugs and are decreased in patients using nondihydropyridine drugs. Thus, use of short-acting calcium antagonists, regardless of their chemical structure, results in chronically elevated norepinephrine levels; only the long-acting formulations of nondihydropyridine drugs appear to have the beneficial effect of reducing serum norepinephrine levels as well as blood pressure.[234] Peripheral sympathetic nerve activity at rest or with activity is unchanged by chronic treatment with a short-acting dihydropyridine, nondihydropyridine, or a long-acting dihydropyridine drug.[235]

An overview of controlled trials of dihydropyridine calcium antagonists showed a 39% decrease in the incidence of stroke and a 28% decrease in the occurrence of major cardiovascular events compared with the effect of placebo. When calcium channel blocker–based therapy (dihydropyridine and nondihydropyridine) was compared with β-blocker– or diuretic-based therapy for hypertension, patients receiving calcium channel blockers showed a reduced overall incidence of stroke but an increased incidence of events related to coronary heart disease. No difference was noted between the treatment groups regarding the incidence of heart failure and overall death rates from cardiovascular or noncardiovascular causes.[236] Adverse cardiovascular events appear to be associated with the use of a short- rather than long-acting calcium channel antagonist.[237] Coronary heart disease risk may be reduced in patients receiving ACE inhibitor–based antihypertensive therapy compared with patients receiving dihydropyridine calcium channel blockers, but the risks of stroke and overall and cardiovascular death appear to be similar between the two treatment modalities.[236] Furthermore, reduction of hypertension-associated left ventricular hypertrophy and improvement in diastolic filling were

identical in hypertensive patients who were treated for 12 months with either enalapril or a slow-release nifedipine preparation.[238] In view of the equivocal results of large clinical trials and published meta-analyses, cost and quality-of-life issues may be the decisive factors in choosing between calcium channel blockers and other equally effective antihypertensive medications.[239]

Patients with ischemic heart disease. Calcium antagonists are effective in the treatment of both classic angina pectoris and vasospastic (Prinzmetal's) angina. Calcium antagonists prolong angina-free exercise time, decrease the frequency of anginal episodes, and decrease the need for supplementary NTG in patients with stable angina pectoris.[223] Monotherapy with a calcium channel blocker appears to be as effective as monotherapy with a β-receptor antagonist and even as the combination of the two drugs.[240] However, it has been recognized since the late 1980s that administration of short-acting formulations of calcium antagonists may be deleterious following acute coronary syndromes.[241] Studies since the initial observations have concluded that administration of calcium channel blockers of any class worsens outcome in patients with prior myocardial infarction complicated by CHF. However, when diltiazem or verapamil was administered to patients recovering from myocardial infarction without pulmonary congestion, both mortality and reinfarction rates were significantly reduced.[242] No similar evidence is available for dihydropyridine-type calcium antagonists in patients after myocardial infarction.

Today, the administration of a β-receptor antagonist remains the treatment of choice in unstable angina. However, careful addition of a calcium channel antagonist may be beneficial should the patient remain unstable in spite of adequate β-blockade.[243] There is no role for short-acting calcium channel blockers in the treatment of acute myocardial infarction.[244] Proposed mechanisms for the possible adverse effects of calcium antagonists in acute myocardial infarction include sympathetic activation with secondary tachycardia, proischemia, and negative inotropy. It has been shown that administration of nicardipine resulted in significantly increased coronary artery wall stress compared with esmolol in patients with coronary artery disease. This difference may result in an increased risk of plaque rupture and coronary artery occlusion in the setting of acute myocardial infarction.[245]

Progressive atherosclerosis is a characteristic feature of coronary artery disease. Dihydropyridines were long believed to have beneficial effects on the progress of atherosclerotic lesions. Amlodipine was shown in laboratory experiments to reduce smooth muscle proliferation and to have antioxidant activity. Clinical studies with amlodipine have shown reduction in progression of arterial medial wall thickening, and the need for angioplasty or surgical revascularization was also reduced.[246] Furthermore, amlodipine reduces exercise-induced platelet activation in patients with chronic stable angina.[247] It may also be of clinical importance that amlodipine-treated patients have experienced a significantly reduced incidence and extent of postischemic dysfunction compared with patients treated with isosorbide mononitrate. This difference was attributed to reduced postischemic myocardial calcium influx, which prevents reperfusion injury and stunning.[248] However, this effect of amlodipine was not reproducible in an animal model of myocardial ischemia-reperfusion.[249]

Patients with congestive heart failure. As discussed previously, calcium channel blockers worsen clinical outcome when administered to patients with CHF following myocardial infarction. However, patients with nonischemic heart failure may actually benefit from a calcium channel blocker as amlodipine has reduced both sudden cardiac death and mortality resulting from pump failure in these patients.[250] L-type calcium channel numbers and calcium currents have been shown to be reduced in myocytes obtained from failing hypertrophied hearts.[227] Whether calcium channel blockade has a beneficial effect on calcium channel downregulation similar to the effect of β-receptor antagonism on β-receptor downregulation in heart failure is yet to be established.

T-TYPE CALCIUM CHANNEL ANTAGONISTS. Mibefradil, a mixed T- and L-type calcium channel antagonist with 10 to 20 times higher selectivity for the T-type channel, was briefly marketed in the 1990s. It was an effective vasodilator and has been used in the treatment of hypertension and ischemic heart disease. Mibefradil reduced heart rate, but in contrast to verapamil and diltiazem, it had no negative inotropic effects and actually improved cardiac function.[251] Addition of mibefradil to preexisting β-blocker therapy in patients with ischemic heart disease has improved exercise tolerance and decreased the number of weekly anginal attacks.[252] Mibefradil has been found to be more effective in improving exercise tolerance than diltiazem.[253] Mibefradil may be beneficial in patients experiencing acute myocardial infarction, as it reduces reperfusion injury and the extent of myocardial damage associated with acute coronary occlusion. These beneficial effects may be attributed to a mechanism resulting in activation of K_{ATP} channels, the final common mediator of ischemic preconditioning-related cardioprotection.[249] Mibefradil is a potent inhibitor of cytochrome P-450 CYP3A4 and interferes with the metabolism of at least 26 other drugs. Concurrent use of mibefradil with β-blockers, digoxin, verapamil, diltiazem, and dihydropyridine calcium channel blockers may result in severe bradycardia, myocardial depression, and hypotension.[254] These unwanted side effects resulted in the withdrawal of mibefradil from the U.S. market in January 1998. However, the beneficial effect of T-type calcium channel blockers is well recognized, and drugs with fewer side effects may find a role in the future in the treatment of hypertension and ischemic heart disease.[253]

Side Effects of Calcium Channel Blockers

CARDIOVASCULAR SIDE EFFECTS. The use of calcium channel blockers may result in excessive vasodilatation leading to flushing, headache, dizziness, hypotension, and nausea. Peripheral edema is most characteristic for dihydropyridine drugs and is secondary to increased microvascular permeability.[233]

Inhibition of AV conduction by verapamil may result in bradycardia and asystole in susceptible patients. It is more common after intravenous administration of the drug. It may also exacerbate conduction disturbances associated with digitalis toxicity and its use is contraindicated when digitalis toxicity is suspected.[255] Diltiazem may have similar effects on AV conduction. Combination of verapamil or diltiazem with amiodarone or a β-blocker may result in profound inhibition of sinus node function or AV conduction in susceptible individuals. Bepridil prolongs the QT_C interval and may induce torsades de pointes in the setting of hypokalemia. Because of this side effect, bepridil is indicated for use only in patients with angina refractory to medical and surgical management.[256]

Concerns about increased morbidity and mortality with the use of calcium channel blockers in patients with ischemic heart disease were discussed in detail previously. All calcium channel blockers are negative inotropes, but clinically significant worsening of myocardial failure is observed only with acute administration of verapamil or diltiazem.

OTHER SIDE EFFECTS. Constipation observed with calcium channel blockers is secondary to gastrointestinal smooth muscle relaxation and reduced motility. Calcium channel blocker use may be associated with an increased incidence of gastrointestinal bleeding necessitating hospital admission in elderly hypertensive patients.[257] Earlier concerns about the association of calcium channel blocker use and increased incidence of cancer have not been substantiated by large surveys.[258] Verapamil and diltiazem inhibit cytochrome P-450 CYP3A, causing interference with the metabolism of several drugs including midazolam, carbamazepine, and cyclosporine. Verapamil decreases the clearance and the volume of distribution of digoxin, resulting in increased serum levels.

Miscellaneous Drugs Used in the Treatment of Hypertension

A variety of drugs are used in the treatment of hypertension, exploiting mechanisms ranging from blockade of central or ganglionic sympathetic outflow to inhibition of peripheral α-adrenergic receptors and direct relaxation of vascular smooth muscle. The pharmacology of these drugs is briefly reviewed in this section.

Clonidine

Clonidine, originally developed as an imidazoline-based topical vasoconstrictor, was later found to have not only α_1-but also α_2-adrenergic agonist activity. Clonidine has central and peripheral stimulatory effects on α_1-and α_2-receptors and is 200 times more potent on α_2-than α_1-receptors.

Clonidine stimulates postsynaptic α_2-receptors in the medulla and hypothalamus, leading to decreased sympathetic and increased parasympathetic outflow, which results in bradycardia and a reduction in blood pressure.[259] However, when the drug is first administered to a patient, vasoconstriction and hypertension related to peripheral α_1-receptor stimulation may precede the hypotensive effect. This phenomenon is more pronounced with intravenous administration of clonidine. Peripheral presynaptic α_2-receptor stimulation decreases norepinephrine release and contributes to the hypotensive effect.[260] Clonidine administration reduces plasma norepinephrine, renin, and aldosterone levels.[261-263] Baroreflex sensitivity is unaltered and orthostatic hypotension is unlikely after clonidine administration.[264]

Clonidine reduces blood pressure, heart rate, and stroke volume within 30 to 60 minutes after oral administration. Systemic venodilation coupled with blockade of central sympathetic outflow results in orthostatic effects.[265] Although the peripheral vascular resistance continues to decrease, cardiac output usually returns to baseline over 4 to 6 weeks with continued administration of clonidine. There is no evidence of decreased myocardial contractility or increased pulmonary vascular resistance following oral administration of clonidine.[266] In patients with CHF, clonidine has been found to reduce heart rate, systemic vascular resistance, and pulmonary arterial wedge pressure with only a small decrease in cardiac index.[267] Clonidine does not interfere with exercise-induced increases in cardiac output and oxygen consumption.[268] α_2-Receptor stimulation suppresses insulin secretion, and clonidine may suppress hypoglycemia-induced signs of adrenergic response.[269] However, it does not appreciably interfere with diabetic control and is considered to be safe for diabetic patients.[270]

The pharmacokinetic characteristics of clonidine are summarized in Table 2-7. Common side effects of clonidine are drowsiness and xerostomia. Marked bradycardia and sexual dysfunction have been reported. Withdrawal reactions (headache, anxiety, sweating, tremor, tachycardia and abdominal cramps) and rebound hypertension following abrupt discontinuation of clonidine are common.[271]

Clonidine is used to provide sedation and to control cardiovascular responses during withdrawal in alcoholics and heroin addicts.[272,273] It has a beneficial effect on chronic diarrhea accompanying diabetic autonomic dysfunction.[274] The peripheral stimulatory effects of clonidine are used to control severe idiopathic orthostatic hypotension. In patients with this problem, the central sympathetic regulatory mechanisms are absent and the only observable effect of clonidine is peripheral vasoconstriction.[275]

Central and spinal α_2-adrenergic stimulation has sedative, anxiolytic, and analgesic effects, and these characteristics of clonidine are utilized in anesthetic practice. Hemodynamic stability improved and circulating catecholamine levels were reduced when clonidine was administered to patients undergoing coronary artery bypass surgery.[276] It reduces the minimal alveolar concentration of volatile anesthetics, and is a useful adjuvant in neuraxial anesthesia.[277-279] Clonidine in doses of 1 to 2 μg/kg is effective in preventing postoperative shivering.[280, 281]

Transdermal administration of clonidine reduces the incidence and severity of unwanted side effects and withdrawal reactions.[282] Two to three days are needed to achieve a steady state after the patch is applied. Removal of the patch results in a gradual decrease of serum concentration over approximately 1 week.[283]

Guanidine Derivatives

Guanfacine and guanabenz are guanidine derivative antihypertensive drugs with structural and functional similarity to clonidine. Guanabenz is extensively metabolized and may be safer in patients with renal failure but it is more problematic in cirrhotic individuals.[284] Side effects of the guanidine derivatives are similar to those of clonidine but milder, and withdrawal symptoms occur less frequently.[285] The pharmacokinetic characteristics and recommended dosing of the guanidine derivatives are presented in Table 2-7.

α-Methyldopa

α-Methyldopa has little effect on the blood pressure in normotensive subjects but was found to be very effective in lowering blood pressure in hypertensive subjects.[286] It is converted to α-methylnorepinephrine, which inhibits dopa decarboxylase and replaces norepinephrine in presynaptic norepinephrine stores. However, central α_2-receptor stimulation by the metabolite is principally responsible for the hypotensive effect of α-methyldopa.[287] The L isomer is solely responsible for the pharmacologic effect.

α-Methyldopa is well tolerated by patients. The changes in cardiac output and heart rate are minimal. Should any orthostatic hypotension develop, it is mainly due to a reduction in preload secondary to venodilation. Although treatment with α-methyldopa reverses left ventricular hypertrophy associated with hypertension, this effect does not correlate with the extent of blood pressure reduction.[288] Rebound hypertension is unusual after the discontinuation of the drug, and α-methyldopa has minimal effects on baroreflex regulation in the awake or anesthetized patient.[289]

In addition to the side effects associated with other centrally acting α_2-agonists, acquired hemolytic anemia and liver dysfunction may occur in patients taking α-methyldopa and the drug is contraindicated in patients with cirrhosis or active liver disease. A positive direct Coombs test was noted

---

TABLE 2-7

The Pharmacokinetic Characteristics and Recommended Daily Doses of Some Drugs Used for the Treatment of Hypertension

Drug	Bioavailability (%)	Protein Binding (%)	Metabolism (%)	Excretion	Half-Life (hours)	Daily Dose
Clonidine	~100	30-40	40-60, liver	Renal	10-20	0.15-0.45 mg
Guanfacine	~80	70	55, liver	Renal	14	1-2 mg
Guanabenz	20-30	10	~100, liver	GI, renal	3-4	8-32 mg
α-Methyldopa	8-62	83	Liver	Renal	1.5-2	1-2 g; max 4 g
Prazosin	~100	97	>90, liver	Renal	2-4	6-15 mg
Terazosin	~100	>95	~90, liver	GI, renal	12	1-10 mg
Doxazosin	~100	98	~95, liver	GI, renal	22	1-16 mg
Alfuzosin	~100	90	~95, liver	GI	9	5-10 mg
Tamsulosin	~100	99	~89, liver	Renal	12	0.4 mg
Indoramin	~100	92	~95	GI, renal	4	50-200 mg
Urapidil	~100	80	85-90	GI, renal	4.7	60-120 mg
Hydralazine	26-55	90	100; liver	Renal	1	25-200 mg

GI, gastrointestinal.

in 10% to 20% of patients receiving α-methyldopa therapy. This effect may delay or interfere with crossmatching blood for transfusion, and the blood bank should be notified about this possibility as soon as possible. Patients with carotid sinus hypersensitivity or sinus node dysfunction may experience severe bradycardia and sinus arrest. Hyperprolactinemia with gynecomastia and galactorrhea has been reported with α-methyldopa use. The pharmacokinetic characteristics and recommended dosing of α-methyldopa are presented in Table 2-7.

Reserpine

Reserpine is an alkaloid of the shrub *Rauwolfia serpentina*. It binds irreversibly to synaptic storage vesicles in adrenergic and serotoninergic nerve terminals, inhibiting both vesicular uptake and release of neurotransmitters. The dysfunctional nerve terminals are unable to release any neurotransmitter at all, and only synthesis of new storage vesicles following discontinuation of reserpine restores function to baseline.[290]

Reserpine reduces both cardiac output and peripheral vascular resistance. Orthostatic hypotension may occur but is usually mild and transient. With chronic use of the drug salt and water retention occurs, which blunts the antihypertensive effect of the drug. This is also known as "pseudotolerance." Addition of a small dose of a thiazide diuretic is effective in overcoming pseudotolerance. Reserpine interferes minimally with baroreceptor function under general anesthesia.[289]

The most common side effect of reserpine is drowsiness. Depression, which is rare but may develop into a suicidal reaction, may start insidiously and reserpine should be discontinued immediately should signs of depression occur.[291]

α$_1$-Adrenoceptor Antagonists Used in Chronic Hypertension

The piperazinyl quinazoles are a family of drugs developed for their selective antagonism of the α$_1$-receptor. Prazosin was the first of a series of piperazinyl quinazoles with various pharmacokinetic but similar pharmacodynamic properties. Originally developed as a phosphodiesterase inhibitor, prazosin was found to be a 1000 times more potent inhibitor of the α$_1$-receptor than of the α$_2$-receptor.[292]

The cardiovascular effects of these drugs are a combination of arteriolar dilatation and an increase of capillary and venous capacitance resulting in a reduction of venous return. Depression of baroreceptor function results in significant blunting of reflex tachycardia.[293] Caution is necessary when the patient takes the first dose of an α$_1$-antagonist as significant postural hypotension, even syncope, may occur. This event is usually prevented by taking the first dose at bedtime and by slowly increasing the dosage. The favorable hemodynamic effects made piperazinyl quinazoles a popular choice in the treatment of hypertension in the 1980s. However, hypertensive patients receiving α$_1$-antagonist therapy demonstrated increased cardiovascular mortality, especially the development of CHF, compared with other treatment modalities, and piperazinyl quinazoles are no longer recommended as first-line treatment for hypertension.[38,294,295]

Piperazinyl quinazoles inhibit α$_1$-receptors in the smooth muscle of the bladder neck and prostatic urethra and improve urinary flow in patients with benign prostatic hyperplasia.[296] These drugs continue to be prescribed for hypertensive males with prostatism.[297]

The most significant side effects of α$_1$-antagonists are related to postural hypotension: dizziness, headache, drowsiness, and nausea. The pharmacokinetic characteristics and recommended daily doses of some piperazinyl quinazoles are summarized in Table 2-7.

Indoramin and urapidil are two selective α$_1$-receptor inhibitors developed for the treatment of hypertension. A urapidil-induced drop in blood pressure may result in baroreflex-mediated increases in heart rate and cardiac output.[298]

Hydralazine

Hydralazine is a direct-acting arteriolar vasodilator. Its mechanism of action is unknown. It has little, if any, effect on large-capacitance arteries or veins.

Vasodilation and hypotension induced by hydralazine result in baroreflex activation and compensatory release of catecholamines and renin. Heart rate and contractility increase with increased metabolic demand on the myocardium. As coronary perfusion is not augmented by hydralazine, patients with significant coronary artery stenosis may develop myocardial ischemia following administration of hydralazine. Furthermore, hydralazine may induce myocardial ischemia in the absence of significant hypotension or tachycardia, presumably by coronary arteriolar dilation and steal.[299]

Hydralazine, when taken orally, is extensively metabolized by the liver, by acetylation in the bowel wall, and by conjugation in the plasma with circulating ketoacids. Systemic bioavailability is a function of bowel wall acetylation of the drug; it is approximately 35% in slow acetylators and about half of that in fast acetylators. Dosing, thus, is adjusted to pharmacologic effect. The pharmacokinetics of hydralazine is unaltered in patients with CHF.[300] The pharmacokinetic characteristics and recommended dosing of hydralazine are presented in Table 2-7.

The use of hydralazine in the treatment of hypertension has decreased over the past decades. It is no longer recommended as first-line treatment in patients with heart failure, and up to half of the patients failed to tolerate the drug because of its unwanted side effects.[14,15] However, combining hydralazine with nitrates in these patients is beneficial; it prevents the development of tolerance to nitrates, which may contribute to the reduced mortality in patients with CHF when the drugs are used in combination.[301]

Headache, nausea, flushing, palpitation, and dizziness are common with hydralazine and are due to peripheral vasodilation. Myocardial ischemia may develop in susceptible patients (see earlier) and the drug should be used with caution in patients at risk for coronary artery disease. Tachyphylaxis often develops, necessitating escalating dosing or addition of another drug such as a diuretic or a β-receptor antagonist. Hydralazine inhibits DNA methylation and can cause drug-induced lupus syndrome in a dose-related fashion.[302] Lupus syndrome secondary to hydralazine use is more common in females and slow acetylators.[303] Hydralazine is also associated with a polyneuropathy, which is dose dependent and related to depletion of pyridoxine stores.[304]

Summary

Although most of the drugs in clinical use for the treatment of hypertension, ischemic heart disease, and CHF have been around for a long time, their mechanism of action is only beginning to be truly understood. The combination of evidence based medicine and a greater understanding of the pathophysiology of these diseases continues to result in broader applications for these agents. As research continues to evolve in the area of cardiac physiology and pharmacology, these drugs are finding more and more novel therapeutic uses, both perioperatively and in long-term management.

REFERENCES

1. Mancia G, Grassi G, Giannattasio C, et al: Sympathetic activation in the pathogenesis of hypertension and progression of organ damage, *Hypertension* 34:724, 1999.
2. DiBona G: Nervous kidney: interaction between renal sympathetic nerves and the renin-angiotensin system in the control of renal function, *Hypertension* 36:1083, 2000.
3. Grassi G, Cattaneo BM, Seravalle G, et al: Baroreflex control of sympathetic nerve activity in essential and secondary hypertension, *Hypertension* 31:68, 1998.
4. Reid IA: Interactions between ANG II, sympathetic nervous system, and baroreceptor reflexes in regulation of blood pressure, *Am J Physiol* 262:E763, 1992.
5. Masuo K, Mikami H, Ogihara T, et al: Sympathetic nerve hyperactivity precedes hyperinsulinemia and blood pressure elevation in young, nonobese Japanese population, *Am J Hypertens* 10:77, 1997.
6. Julius S, Gundrandsson T, Jamerson K, et al: The interconnection between sympathetics, microcirculation and insulin resistance in hypertension, *Blood Press* 1:9, 1992.
7. O'Rourke M: Arterial stiffness, systolic blood pressure, and the logical treatment of arterial hypertension, *Hypertension* 15:339, 1990.
8. Panza JA: High-normal blood pressure—more "high" than "normal," *N Engl J Med* 345:1337, 2001.
9. Robertson D, Hollister AS, Forman MB, et al: Reflexes unique to myocardial ischemia, *J Am Coll Cardiol* 5:99B, 1985.
10. Zipes DP: Influence of myocardial ischemia and infarction on autonomic innervation of the heart, *Circulation* 82:1095, 1990.
11. Barron HV, Lesh MD: Autonomic nervous system and sudden cardiac death, *J Am Coll Cardiol* 27:1053, 1996.
12. Anversa P, Kajstura J: Myocyte cell death in the diseased heart, *Circ Res* 82:1231, 1998.
13. Katwa LC, Campbell SE, Tyagi SC, et al: Cultured myofibroblasts generate angiotensin peptides de novo, *J Mol Cell Cardiol* 29:1375, 1997.
14. Hunt SA, Baker DW, Chin MH, et al: ACC/AHA guidelines for the evaluation and management of chronic heart failure in the adult: executive summary, *Circulation* 104:2996, 2001.
15. Cleland JGF, John J, Dhawan J, et al: What is the optimal medical management of ischaemic heart failure? *Br Med Bull* 59:135, 2001.
16. Alpert NR, Leavitt BJ, Ittleman FP, et al: A mechanical analysis of the force-frequency relation in non-failing and progressively failing human myocardium, *Basic Res Cardiol* 93(Suppl 1):23, 1998.
17. Lowes BD, Gilbert EM, Abraham WT, et al: Myocardial gene expression in dilated cardiomyopathy treated with beta-blocking agents, *N Engl J Med* 346:1357, 2002.
18. Cohn JN: Structural basis for heart failure: ventricular remodeling and its pharmacological inhibition, *Circulation* 91:2504, 1995.
19. Francis GS: Pathophysiology of chronic heart failure, *Am J Med* 110:37S, 2001.
20. Rockman HA, Koch WJ, Lefkowitz RJ: Seven-transmembrane-spanning receptors and heart function, *Nature* 415:206, 2002.
21. Francis GS, McDonald KM, Cohn JN: Neurohumoral activation in preclinical heart failure: remodeling and the potential for intervention, *Circulation* 87(Suppl IV):90, 1993.
22. Benedict CR, Shelton B, Johnstone DE, et al: Prognostic significance of plasma norepinephrine in patients with asymptomatic left ventricular dysfunction, *Circulation* 94:690, 1996.
23. Swynghedauw B: Molecular mechanisms of myocardial remodeling, *Physiol Rev* 79:215, 1999.
24. Nuss HB, Johns DC, Kääb S, et al: Reversal of potassium channel deficiency in cells from failing hearts by adenoviral gene transfer: a prototype for gene therapy for disorders of cardiac excitability and contractility, *Gene Ther* 3:900, 1996.
25. Brodde O-E: β_1- and β_2-adenoceptors in human heart: properties, function and alterations in chronic heart failure, *Pharmacol Rev* 43:203, 1991.
26. Regitz-Zagrosek V, Friedel N, Heymann A, et al: Regulation, chamber localization and subtype distribution of angiotensin II receptors in human hearts, *Circulation* 91:1461, 1995.
27. Torre-Amione G, Kapadia S, Benedict C, et al: Proinflammatory cytokine levels in patients with depressed left ventricular ejection fraction: a report from the Studies of Left Ventricular Dysfunction (SOLVD), *J Am Coll Cardiol* 27:1201, 1996.
28. Feldman AM, Combes A, Wagner D, et al: The role of tumor necrosis factor in the pathophysiology of heart failure, *J Am Coll Cardiol* 35:537, 2000.
29. Milani RV, Mehra MR, Endres S, et al: The clinical relevance of circulating tumor necrosis factor–α in acute decompensated chronic heart failure without cachexia, *Chest* 110:992, 1996.
30. Olivetti G, Abbi R, Quaini F, et al: Apoptosis in the failing human heart, *N Engl J Med* 336:1131, 1997.
31. Haunstetter A, Izumo S: Apoptosis: basic mechanisms and implications for cardiovascular disease, *Circ Res* 82:1111, 1998.
32. Kajstura J, Leri A, Finato N, et al: Myocyte proliferation in end-stage cardiac failure in humans, *Proc Natl Acad Sci USA* 95:8801, 1998.
33. Nakamura M: Peripheral vascular remodeling in chronic heart failure: clinical relevance and new conceptualization of its mechanisms, *J Card Fail* 5:127, 1999.
34. Stapleton MP: Sir James Black and propranolol. The role of the basic sciences in the history of cardiovascular pharmacology, *Tex Heart Inst J* 24:336, 1997.
35. de Bruijn NP, Reves JG, Croughwell N, et al: Pharmacokinetics of esmolol in anesthetized patients receiving chronic β-blocker therapy, *Anesthesiology* 66:323, 1987.
36. Hoffman BB: Catecholamines, sympathomimetic drugs, and adrenergic receptor antagonists. In Hardman JG, Limbird LE (eds): *Goodman and Gilman's the pharmacological basis of therapeutics*, ed 10, New York, 2001, McGraw-Hill, 215.
37. Man in't Veld AJ, Van den Meiracker AH, Schalekamp MA: Do betablockers really increase peripheral vascular resistance? Review of the literature and new observations under basal conditions, *Am J Hypertens* 1:91, 1988.
38. Sheps SG, Black HR, Cohen JD, et al: The sixth report of the Joint National Committee on prevention, detection, evaluation, and treatment of high blood pressure, *Arch Intern Med* 157:2413, 1997.
39. van den Meiracker AH, Man in't Veld AJ, Boomsma F, et al: Hemodynamic and beta-adrenergic receptor adaptations during long-term beta-adrenoceptor blockade. Studies with acebutolol, atenolol, pindolol, and propranolol in hypertensive patients, *Circulation* 80:903, 1989.
40. Gibbons RJ, Chatterjee K, Daley J, et al: ACC/AHA/ACP-ASIM guidelines for the management of patients with chronic stable angina, *J Am Coll Cardiol* 33:2097, 1999.
41. Waagstein F, Hjalmarson Å, Varnauskas E, et al: Effect of chronic betaadrenergic receptor blockade in congestive cardiomyopathy, *Br Heart J* 37:1022, 1975.
42. Bristow MR, Gilbert EM, Abraham WT et al: Carvedilol produces doserelated improvements in left ventricular function and survival in subjects with chronic heart failure, *Circulation* 94:2807, 1996.
43. Hjalmarson Å, Goldstein S, and the MERIT-HF Study Group: Effect of metoprolol CR/XL in chronic heart failure: Metoprolol CR/XL Randomised Intervention Trial in Congestive Heart Failure (MERIT-HF), *Lancet* 353:2001, 1999.
44. Prabhu SD, Chandrasekar B, Murray DR, et al: β-Adrenergic blockade in developing heart failure: effects on myocardial inflammatory cytokines, nitric oxide, and remodeling, *Circulation* 101:2103, 2000.
45. Lefkowitz RJ, Rockman HA, Koch WJ: Catecholamines, cardiac β-adrenergic receptors, and heart failure, *Circulation* 101:1634, 2000.
46. Gullestad L, Hallen J, Medbo JI, et al: The effect of acute vs chronic treatment with beta-adrenoceptor blockade on exercise performance, haemodynamic and metabolic parameters in healthy men and women, *Br J Clin Pharmacol* 41:57, 1996.

47. Frishman WH: β-Adrenergic blocker withdrawal, *Am J Cardiol* 59:26F, 1987.
48. Gottlieb SS, McCarter RJ, Vogel RA, et al: Effect of beta-blockade on mortality among high-risk and low-risk patients after myocardial infarction, *N Engl J Med* 339:489, 1998.
49. Salpeter S, Ormiston T, Salpeter E: Cardioselective beta-blockers for reversible airway disease, *Cochrane Database Syst Rev* (1):CD002992, 2002.
50. Fogari R, Zoppi A, Corradi L, et al: Beta-blocker effects on plasma lipids during prolonged treatment of hypertensive patients with hypercholesterolemia, *J Cardiovasc Pharmacol* 33:534, 1999.
51. Dawood MM, Gutpa DK, Southern J, et al: Pathology of fatal perioperative myocardial infarction: implications regarding pathophysiology and prevention, *Int J Cardiol* 57:37, 1996.
52. Ponten J, Biber B, Bjuro T, et al: β-Receptor blocker withdrawal. A preoperative problem in general surgery? *Acta Anaesthesiol Scand Suppl* 76:32, 1982.
53. Stone JG, Foëx P, Sear JW, et al: Myocardial ischemia in untreated hypertensive patients: effect of a single small oral dose of a beta-adrenergic blocking agent, *Anesthesiology* 68:495, 1988.
54. Wallace A, Leyug B, Tateo I, et al: Prophylactic atenolol reduces postoperative myocardial ischemia, *Anesthesiology* 88:7, 1998.
55. Poldermans D, Boersma E, Bax JJ, et al: The effect of bisoprolol on perioperative mortality and myocardial infarction in high-risk patients undergoing vascular surgery, *N Engl J Med* 341:1789, 1999.
56. Howel SJ, Sear JW, Foëx P: Perioperative β-blockade: a useful treatment that should be greeted with cautious enthusiasm, *Br J Anaesth* 86:161, 2001.
57. Murrell W: Nitro-glycerine as a remedy for angina pectoris, *Lancet* 1:80, 1879.
58. Marsh N, Marsh A: A short history of nitroglycerin and nitric oxide in pharmacology and physiology, *Clin Exp Pharmacol Physiol* 27:313, 2000.
59. Stamler JS, Singel DJ, Loscalzo J: Biochemistry of nitric oxide and its redox-activated forms, *Science* 258:1898, 1992.
60. Grover JT, Wang CCY: Nitric oxide synthase: models and mechanisms, *Curr Opin Chem Biol* 4:687, 2000.
61. Stuehr DL: Mammalian nitric oxide synthases, *Biochim Biophys Acta* 1411:217, 1999.
62. Mayer B, Hemmens B: Biosynthesis and action of nitric oxide in mammalian cells, *Trends Biochem Sci* 22:477, 1997.
63. Musialek P, Lei M, Brown HF, et al: Nitric oxide can increase heart rate by stimulating the hyperpolarization-activated inward current, I(f), *Circ Res* 81:60, 1997.
64. Chowdhary S, Ng GA, Nuttal SL, et al: Nitric oxide and cardiac parasympathetic control in human heart failure, *Clin Sci* 102:397, 2002.
65. Kelly RA, Balligand JL, Smith TW: Nitric oxide and cardiac function, *Circ Res* 79:363, 1996.
66. O'Byrne S, Shirodaria C, Millar T, et al: Inhibition of platelet aggregation with glyceryl trinitrate and xanthine oxidoreductase, *J Pharmacol Exp Ther* 292:326, 2000.
67. Dawn B, Bolli R: Role of nitric oxide in myocardial preconditioning, *Ann NY Acad Sci* 962:18, 2002.
68. Mahmarian JJ, Moyé LA, Chinoy DA, et al: Transdermal nitroglycerin patch therapy improves left ventricular function and prevents remodeling after acute myocardial infarction, *Circulation* 97:2017, 1998.
69. Banerjee S, Tang XL, Qui Y, et al: Nitroglycerin induces late preconditioning against myocardial stunning via a PKC-dependent pathway, *Am J Physiol* 277:H2488, 1999.
70. Leesar MA, Stoddard MF, Dawn B, et al: Delayed-preconditioning mimetic action of nitroglycerin in patients undergoing coronary angioplasty, *Circulation* 103:2935, 2001.
71. Kerins DM, Robertson RM, Robertson D: Drugs used in the treatment of myocardial ischemia. In Hardman JG, Limbird LE (eds): *Goodman and Gilman's the pharmacological basis of therapeutics*, ed 10, New York, 2001, McGraw-Hill, 843.
72. Feelisch M, Kelm M: Biotransformation of organic nitrates to nitric oxide by vascular smooth muscle and endothelial cells, *Biochem Biophys Res Commun* 180:286, 1991.
73. Harrison DG, Bates JN: The nitrovasodilators. New ideas about old drugs, *Circulation* 8:1461, 1993.
74. Darius H: Role of nitrates for the therapy of coronary artery disease patients in the years beyond 2000, *J Cardiovasc Pharmacol* 34(Suppl 2):S15, 1999.
75. Hashimoto S, Yamauchi E, Kobayashi A, et al: The pharmacokinetics of trinitroglycerin and its metabolites in patients with chronic stable angina, *Br J Clin Pharmacol* 50:373, 2000.
76. Waldman SA, Murad F: Cyclic GMP synthesis and function, *Pharmacol Rev* 39:163, 1987.
77. Bauer JA, Fung HL: Arterial versus venous metabolism of nitroglycerin to nitric oxide: a possible explanation of organic nitrate venoselectivity, *J Cardiovasc Pharmacol* 28:371, 1996.
78. Brown BG, Bolson E, Petersen RB, et al: The mechanism of nitroglycerin action: stenosis vasodilation as a major component of the drug response, *Circulation* 64:1089, 1981.
79. Hummel BW, Raess DH, Gewertz BL, et al: Effect of nitroglycerin and aortic occlusion on myocardial blood flow, *Surgery* 92:159, 1982.
80. Horwitz LD, Gorlin R, Taylor WJ, et al: Effects of nitroglycerin on regional myocardial blood flow in coronary artery disease, *J Clin Invest* 50:1578, 1971.
81. Knight CJ, Panesar M, Wilson DJ, et al: Different effects of calcium antagonists, nitrates, and β-blockers on platelet function. Possible importance for the treatment of unstable angina, *Circulation* 95:125, 1997.
82. Chirkov YY, Holmes AS, Willoughby SR, et al: Stable angina and acute coronary syndromes are associated with nitric oxide resistance in platelets, *J Am Coll Cardiol* 37:1851, 2001.
83. Jugdutt BI, Khan MI, Jugdutt SJ, et al: Impact of left ventricular unloading after late reperfusion of canine anterior myocardial infarction on remodeling and function using isosorbide-5-mononitrate, *Circulation* 92:926, 1995.
84. Ganz W, Marcus HS: Failure of intracoronary nitroglycerin to alleviate pacing-induced angina, *Circulation* 46:880, 1972.
85. Pfister M, Seiler C, Fleisch M, et al: Nitrate-induced coronary vasodilatation: differential effects of sublingul application by capsule or spray, *Heart* 80:365, 1998.
86. Coriat P, Daloz M, Bousseau D, et al: Prevention of intraoperative myocardial ischemia during noncardiac surgery with intravenous nitroglycerin, *Anesthesiology* 61:193, 1984.
87. Thompson IR, Mutch WAC, Culligan JD: Failure of intravenous nitroglycerin to prevent intraoperative myocardial ischemia during fentanyl-pancuronium anesthesia, *Anesthesiology* 61:385, 1984.
88. Dodds TM, Stone GJ, Coromilas J, et al: Prophylactic nitroglycerin infusion during noncardiac surgery does not reduce perioperative ischemia, *Anesth Analg* 76:705, 1993.
89. Bussmann WD, Schofer H, Kurita A, et al: Nitroglycerin in acute myocardial infarction. X. Effect of small and large doses of nitroglycerin on sigma ST segment deviation—experimental and clinical results, *Clin Cardiol* 2:106, 1979.
90. Kaplan JA, Dunbar RW, Jones EL: Nitroglycerin infusion during coronary artery surgery, *Anesthesiology* 45:14, 1976.
91. Moffitt EA, Sethna DH, Gray RJ, et al: Myocardial and systemic effects of nitroglycerin, given awake and during anesthesia in coronary patients, *Can Anaesth Soc J* 30:352, 1983.
92. Sethna DH, Moffitt EA, Bussell JA, et al: Intravenous nitroglycerin and myocardial metabolism during anesthesia in patients undergoing myocardial revascularization, *Anesth Analg* 61:828, 1982.
93. Yusuf S, Collins R, MacMahon S, et al: Effect of intravenous nitrates on mortality in acute myocardil infarction: an overview of randomized trials, *Lancet* 1:1088, 1988.
94. GISSI-3 Investigators: GISSI-3: effects of lisinopril and transdermal glyceryl trinitrate singly and together on 6-week mortality and ventricular function after acute myocardial infarction, *Lancet* 1:1115, 1994.
95. GISSI-3 Invastigators: Six-month effects of early treatment with lisinopril and transdermal glyceryl trinitrate singly and together withdrawn six weeks after acute myocardial infarction: the GISSI-3 trial, *J Am Coll Cardiol* 27:337, 1996.
96. ISIS-4 Collaborators: ISIS-4: A randomised factorial trial assessing early oral captopril, oral mononitrate, and intravenous magnesium sulphate in 58, 050 patients with suspected acute myocardial infarction, *Lancet* 1:669, 1995.
97. Kanamasa K, Hayashi T, Takenada T, et al: Chronic use of continuous dosing of long-term nitrates does not prevent cardiac events in patients with severe acute myocardial infarction, *Cardiology* 94:139, 2000.
98. Heidenreich PA, McDonald KM, Hastic T, et al: Meta-analysis of trials comparing β-blockers, calcium antagonists, and nitrates for stable angina, *JAMA* 281:1927, 1999.
99. Zwinderman AH, Cleophas TJ, van der Sluijs H, et al: Comparison of 50-mg and 100-mg sustained-release isosorbide mononitrate in the treatment of stable angina pectoris: effects on quality-of-life indices, *Angiology* 50:963, 1999.
100. Thadani U, Opie LH: Nitrates for unstable angina, *Cardiovasc Drug Ther* 8:719, 1994.

101. Bauer JA, Nolan T, Fung H-L: Vascular and hemodynamic differences between organic nitrates and nitrites, *J Pharmacol Exp Ther* 280:326, 1997.

102. Cohn JN, Archibald DG, Ziesche S, et al: Effect of vasodilator therapy on mortality in chronic congestive heart failure: results of a Veterans Administration cooperative study, *N Engl J Med* 314:1542, 1986.

103. Elkayam U, Karaalp IS, Wani OR, et al: The role of organic nitrates in the treatment of heart failure, *Prog Cardiovasc Dis* 41:255, 1999.

104. Publication Committee for the VMAC Investigators: Intravenous nesiritide vs nitroglycerin for the treatment of decompensated congestive heart failure. A randomized controlled trial, *JAMA* 287:1531, 2002.

105. Dohi S, Matsumoto M, Takahashi T: The effects of nitroglycerin on cerebrospinal fluid pressure in awake and anesthetized humans, *Anesthesiology* 54:511, 1981.

106. Mookherjee S, Fuleihan D, Warner RA, et al: Effects of sublingual nitroglycerin on resting pulmonary gas exchange and hemodynamics in man, *Circulation* 57:106, 1978.

107. Casthely PA, Lear S, Cottrell JE, et al: Intrapulmonary shunting during induced hypotension, *Anesth Analg* 61:231, 1982.

108. Kochukoshy KN, Chick TW, Jenne JW: The effect of nitroglycerin in gas exchange on chronic obstructive pulmonary disease, *Am Rev Respir Dis* 111:177, 1975.

109. Toraman F, Kopman EA, Çalişirişçi Ü, et al: Nitroglycerin-induced hypoxemia does not produce myocardial ischemia, *J Cardiothorac Vasc Anesth* 11:861, 1997.

110. Hales CA, Westphal D: Hypoxemia following the administration of sublingual nitroglycerin, *Am J Med* 65:911, 1978.

111. Maseda J, Hilberman M, Derby GC, et al: The renal effects of sodium nitroprusside in postoperative cardiac surgical patients, *Anesthesiology* 54:284, 1981.

112. Münzel T, Kurz S, Heitzer T, et al: New insights into mechanisms underlying nitrate tolerance, *Am J Cardiol* 77(Suppl C):24C, 1996.

113. Kelly RA, Smith TW: Nitric oxide and nitrovasodilators: similarities, differences, and interactions, *Am J Cardiol* 77(Suppl C):2C, 1996.

114. Kurz S, Hink U, Nickenig G, et al: Evidence for causal role of the renin-angiotensin system in nitrate tolerance, *Circulation* 99:3181, 1999.

115. DeMots H, Glasser SP: Intermittent transdermal nitroglycerin therapy in the treatment of chronic stable angina, *J Am Coll Cardiol* 13:786, 1989.

116. Azevedo ER, Schofield AM, Kelly S, et al: Nitroglycerin withdrawal increases endothelium-dependent vasomotor response to acetylcholine, *J Am Coll Cardiol* 37:505, 2001.

117. Caramori PR, Adelman AG, Azevedo ER, et al: Therapy with nitroglycerin increases coronary vasoconstriction in response to acetylcholine, *J Am Coll Cardiol* 32:1969, 1998.

118. Dumont L, Lamoureux C, Lelorier J, et al: Intravenous infusion of nitroprusside: effects upon cardiovascular dynamics and regional blood flow distribution in conscious dogs, *Arch Int Pharmacodyn* 261:109, 1983.

119. Bernard EO, Schmid ER, Lachat ML, et al: Nitroglycerin to control blood pressure during endovascular stent-grafting of descending thoracic aortic aneurysms, *J Vasc Surg* 31:790, 2000.

120. Schrier RW, Abraham WT: Hormones and hemodynamics in heart failure, *N Engl J Med* 341:577, 1999.

121. Jackson EK: Renin and angiotensin. In Hardman JG, Limbird LE (eds): *Goodman and Gilman's the pharmacological basis of therapeutics*, ed 10, New York, 2001, McGraw-Hill, 809.

122. Hilgers KF, Veelken R, Muller DN, et al: Renin uptake by the endothelium mediates vascular angiotensin formation, *Hypertension* 38:243, 2001.

123. Swanson G, Hanesworth JM, Sardinia M, et al: Discovery of a distinct binding site for angiotensin II (3-8), a putative angiotensin IV receptor, *Regul Pept* 40:409, 1992.

124. Ardaillou R: Angiotensin II receptors, *J Am Soc Nephrol* 10(Suppl 11):S30, 1999.

125. Lüscher TF: Endothelial dysfunction: the role and impact of the renin-angiotensin system, *Heart* 84(Suppl I):i20, 2000.

126. Millatt LJ, Abdel-Rahman EM, Siragy HM: Angiotensin II and nitric oxide: a question of balance, *Regul Pept* 81:1, 1999.

127. Sowers JR: Hypertension, angiotensin II and oxidative stress, *N Engl J Med* 346:1999, 2002.

128. Kim S, Iwao H: Molecular and cellular mechanisms of angiotensin II–mediated cardiovascular and renal diseases, *Pharmacol Rev* 52:11, 2001.

129. Rosendorff C: The renin-angiotensin system and vascular hypertrophy, *J Am Coll Cardiol* 28:803, 1996.

130. Timmermans PB, Wong PC, Chiu A, et al: Angiotensin II receptors and angiotensin II-receptor antagonists, *Pharmacol Rev* 45:205, 1993.

131. Fitzsimmons JT: Angiotensin, thirst, and sodium appetite, *Physiol Rev* 78:583, 1998.

132. Cushman DW, Ondetti MA: History of the design of captopril and related inhibitors of angiotensin-converting enzyme, *Hypertension* 17:589, 1991.

133. Ondetti MA, Rubin B, Cushman DW: Design of specific inhibitors of angiotensin-converting enzyme: new class of orally active antihypertensive agents, *Science* 196:441, 1977.

134. Brunner HR, Nussberger J, Waeber B: Effects of angiotensin-converting enzyme inhibition: a clinical point of view, *J Cardiovasc Pharmacol* 7(Suppl 4):S73, 1985.

135. Dahlof B, Pennert K, Hansson L: Reversal of left ventricular hypertrophy in hypertensive patients: a metaanalysis of 109 treatment studies, *Am J Hypertens* 5:95, 1992.

136. Sihm I, Schroeder AP, Aalkjaer C, et al: Regression of media-to-lumen ratio in human subcutaneous arteries and left ventricular hypertrophy during treatment with an angiotensin-converting enzyme inhibitor–based regimen in hypertensive patients, *Am J Cardiol* 76:38E, 1995.

137. Lewis EJ, Hunsicker LG, Bain RP, et al: The effect of angiotensin-converting-enzyme inhibition on diabetic nephropathy, *N Engl J Med* 329:1456, 1993.

138. ACE Inhibitor Myocardial Infarction Collaborative Group: Indications for ACE inhibitors in the early treatment of acute myocardial infarction. Systematic overview of individual data from 100,000 patients in randomized trials, *Circulation* 97:2202, 1998.

139. Hirosaka M, Yuasa F, Yuyama R, et al: Effect of angiotensin-converting enzyme inhibitor on cardiopulmonary baroreflex sensitivity in patients with acute myocardial infarction, *Am J Cardiol* 86:1241, 2000.

140. Yusuf S, Sleight P, Pogue J, et al: Effects of an angiotensin-converting enzyme inhibitor ramipril, on cardiovascular events in high-risk patients. The Heart Outcomes Prevention Evaluation Study Investigators, *N Engl J Med* 342:145, 478 (erratum), 2000.

141. Mancini GBJ: Role of angiotensin-converting enzyme inhibition in the reversal of endothelial dysfunction in coronary artery disease, *Am J Med* 105:40S, 1998.

142. Mancini GBJ, Henry GC, Macaya C, et al: Angiotensin-converting enzyme inhibition with quinapril improves endothelial vasomotor dysfunction in patients with coronary artery disease: the TREND (Trial on Reversing Endothelial Dysfunction) study, *Circulation* 94:258, 1996.

143. SOLVD Investigators: Effect of enalapril on mortality and the development of heart failure in asymptomatic patients with reduced left ventricular ejection fractions, *N Engl J Med* 327:685, 1768 (erratum), 1992.

144. Cohn JN, Johnson G, Ziesche S, et al: A comparison of enalapril with hydralazine–isosorbide dinitrate in the treatment of congestive heart failure, *N Engl J Med* 325:303, 1991.

145. CONSENSUS Trial Study Group: Effects of enalapril on mortality in severe congestive heart failure: results of the Cooperative North Scandinavian Enalapril Survival Study (CONSENSUS), *N Engl J Med* 316:1429, 1987.

146. Pfeffer MA, Braunwald E, Moyé LA, et al: Effect of captopril on mortality and morbidity in patients with left ventricular dysfunction after myocardial infarction: results of the Survival and Ventricular Enlargement Trial, *N Engl J Med* 327:669, 1992.

147. Greenberg B, Quinones MA, Koilpillai C, et al: Effects of long-term enalapril therapy on cardiac structure and function in patients with left ventricular dysfunction. Results of the SOLVD echocardiographic substudy, *Circulation* 91:2573, 1995.

148. The Captopril-Digoxin Multicenter Research Group: Comparative effects of therapy with captopril and digoxin in patients with mild-to-moderate heart failure, *JAMA* 259:539, 1988.

149. Grassi G, Cattaneo BM, Seravalle G, et al: Effects of chronic ACE inhibition on sympathetic nerve traffic and baroreflex control of circulation in heart failure, *Circulation* 96:1173, 1997.

150. Osterziel KJ, Dietz R: Improvement of vagal tone by ACE inhibition: a mechanism of cardioprotection in patients with mild-to-moderate heart failure, *J Cardiovasc Pharmacol* 27(Suppl 2):S25, 1996.

151. Kostis JB, Shelton B, Gosselin G, et al: Adverse effects of enalapril in the Studies of Left Ventricular Dysfunction (SOLVD), *Am Heart J* 131:350, 1996.

152. Agostoni A, Cicardi M, Cugno M et al: Angioedema due to angiotensin-converting enzyme inhibitors, *Immunopharmacology* 44:21, 1999.

153. Siegl PK: Discovery of losartan, the first specific non-peptide angiotensin II-receptor antagonist, *J Hypertens* 11(3 Suppl):S19, 1993.

154. Siragy H: Angiotensin II-receptor blockers: review of the binding characteristics, *Am J Cardiol* 84:3S, 1999.

155. Conlin PR, Spence JD, Williams B, et al: Angiotensin II antagonists for hypertension: are there differences in efficacy? *Am J Hypertens* 13:418, 2000.

156. Jorde UP, Ennezat PV, Lisker J, et al: Maximally recommended daily doses of angiotensin-converting enzyme (ACE) inhibitors do not completely prevent ACE-mediated formation of angiotensin II in chronic heart failure, *Circulation* 101:844, 2000.

157. Pitt B, Poole-Wilson PA, Segal R, et al: Effect of losartan compared with captopril on mortality in patients with symptomatic heart failure: randomised trial—the Losartan Heart Failure Survival Study ELITE II, *Lancet* 355:1582, 2000.

158. Cohn JN, Tognioni G: A randomized trial of the angiotensin-receptor blocker valsartan in chronic heart failure, *N Engl J Med* 345:1667, 2001.

159. Nikolaidis LA, Dovespike A, Huerbin R, et al: Angiotensin-converting enzyme inhibitors improve coronary flow reserve in dilated cardiomyopathy by a bradykinin-mediated, nitric oxide–dependent mechanism, *Circulation* 105:2785, 2002.

160. Burnett JC: Vasopeptidase inhibition: a new concept in blood pressure management, *J Hypertens* 17(1 Suppl):S37, 1999.

161. Rouleau JL, Pfeffer MA, Stewart DJ, et al: Comparison of vasopeptidase inhibitor omapatrilat, and lisinopril on exercise tolerance and morbidity in patients with heart failure: IMPRESS randomised trial, *Lancet* 356:615, 2000.

162. Messerli FH, Nussberger J: Vasopeptidase inhibition and angio-edema, *Lancet* 356:608, 2000.

163. Colson P, Saussine M, Seguin JR, et al: Hemodynamic effects of anesthesia in patients chronically treated with angiotensin-converting enzyme inhibitors, *Anesth Analg* 74:805, 1992.

164. Brabant SM, Bertrand M, Eyraud D, et al: The hemodynamic effects of anesthetic induction in vascular surgical patients chronically treated with angiotensin II-receptor antagonist, *Anesth Analg* 89:1388, 1999.

165. Licker M, Schweizer A, Hohn L: Cardiovascular responses to anesthetic induction in patients chronically treated with angiotensin-converting enzyme inhibitors, *Can J Anaesth* 47:433, 2000.

166. Meersschaert K, Brun L, Gourdin M, et al: Terlipressin-ephedrine versus ephedrine to treat hypotension at the induction of anesthesia in patients chronically treated with angiotensin-converting enzyme inhibitors: a prospective, randomized, double-blinded, crossover study, *Anesth Analg* 94:835, 2002.

167. Coriat P, Richter C, Douraki T, et al: Influence of chronic angiotensin-converting enzyme inhibition on anesthetic induction, *Anesthesiology* 81:299, 1994.

168. Yates AP, Hunter DN: Anaesthesia and angiotensin-converting enzyme inhibitors. The effect of enalapril on perioperative cardiovascular stability, *Anaesthesia* 43:935, 1988.

169. McCarthy GJ, Hainsworth M, Lindsay K, et al: Pressor responses to tracheal intubation after sublingual captopril. A pilot study, *Anaesthesia* 45:243, 1990.

170. Sear JW, Jewkes C, Tellez JC, et al: Does the choice of antihypertensive therapy influence haemodynamic responses to induction, laryngoscopy and intubation? *Br J Anaesth* 73:303, 1994.

171. Mets B, Miller ED: Renin-angiotensin-aldosterone system: ACE inhibitors. In Prys-Roberts C, Brown BR (eds): *International practice of anaesthesia: successor to general anaesthesia*, ed 6, London, 1997, Butterworth-Heinemann Medical, 1.

172. Kataja JH, Kaukinen S, Viinamaki OV, et al: Hemodynamic and hormonal changes in patients pretreated with captopril for surgery of the abdominal aorta, *J Cardiothorac Anesth* 3:425, 1989.

173. Porter SS, Asher M, Fox DK: Comparison of intravenous nitroprusside, nitroprusside-captopril, and nitroglycerin for deliberate hypotension during posterior spine fusion in adults, *J Clin Anesth* 1:87, 1988.

174. Withering W: *An account of the foxglove, and some of its medical uses: with practical remarks on dropsy, and other diseases*, Birmingham, England. 1785, M Swinney,

175. Ferguson DW: Digitalis and neurohormonal abnormalities in heart failure and implications for therapy, *Am J Cardiol* 69:24G, 1992.

176. Joubert PH, Grossmann M: Local and systemic effects of Na$^+$/K$^+$ ATPase inhibition, *Eur J Clin Invest* 31(Suppl 2):1, 2001.

177. Nelson JA, Nechay BR: Effects of cardiac glycosides on renal adenosine triphosphatase activity and Na$^+$ reabsorption in dogs, *J Pharmacol Exp Ther* 175:727, 1970.

178. Schobel HP, Oren RM, Roach PJ, et al: Contrasting effects of digitalis and dobutamine on baroreflex sympathetic control in normal humans, *Circulation* 84:1118, 1991.

179. Ferguson DW, Berg WJ, Sanders JS, et al: Sympathoinhibitory responses to digitalis glycosides in heart failure patients. Direct evidence from sympathetic neural recordings, *Circulation* 80:65, 1989.

180. Schobel HP, Ferguson DW, Clary MP, et al: Differential effects of digitalis on chemoreflex responses in humans, *Hypertension* 23:302, 1994.

181. Morisco C, Cuocolo A, Romano M, et al: Influence of digitalis on left ventricular functional response to exercise in congestive heart failure, *Am J Cardiol* 77:480, 1996.

182. Khoury AM, Davila DF, Bellabarba G, et al: Acute effects of digitalis and enalapril on the neurohormonal profile of patients with severe congestive heart failure, *Int J Cardiol* 57:21, 1996.

183. Garg R, Gorlin R, Smith T et al, For the Digitalis Investigation Group: The effect of digoxin on mortality and morbidity in patients with heart failure, *N Engl J Med* 336:525, 1997.

184. Lonn E, McKelvie R: Drug treatment in heart failure, *Br J Med* 320:1188, 2000.

185. Adams KF Jr, Gheorghiade M, Uretsky BF: Clinical benefits of low serum digoxin concentrations in heart failure, *J Am Coll Cardiol* 39:946, 2002.

186. Bigger JT, Fleiss JL, Rolniczky LM, et al: Effect of digitalis treatment on survival after acute myocardial infarction, *Am J Cardiol* 55:623, 1985.

187. Reicher-Reiss H, Jonas M, Boyko V, et al: Are coronary patients at higher risk with digoxin therapy? An ongoing controversy, *Int J Cardiol* 68:137, 1999.

188. Schöner W: Endogenous cardiac glycosides, a new class of steroid hormones, *Eur J Biochem* 269:2440, 2002.

189. Russell JM: Sodium-potassium-chloride cotransport, *Physiol Rev* 80:211, 2000.

190. Stichtenoth DO, Wagner B, Frölich JC: Effect of selective inhibition of the inducible cyclooxygenase on renin release in healthy volunteers, *J Invest Med* 94:290, 1998.

191. Kammerl MC, Nüsing RM, Richthammer W, et al: Inhibition of COX-2 counteracts the effect of diuretics in rats, *Kidney Int* 60:1684, 2001.

192. Francis GS, Bendict C, Johnstone DE, et al: Comparison of neuroendocrine activation in patients with left ventricular dysfunction with and without congestive heart failure. A substudy of the Studies of Left Ventricular Dysfunction (SOLVD), *Circulation* 82:1724, 1990.

193. Dormans TPJ, van Meyel JJM, Gerlag PGG, et al: Diuretic efficacy of high-dose furosemide in severe heart failure: bolus injection versus continuous infusion, *J Am Coll Cardiol* 28:376, 1996.

194. Johnson W, Omland T, Hall C, et al: Neurohormonal activation rapidly decreases after intravenous therapy with diuretics and vasodilators for class IV heart failure, *J Am Coll Cardiol* 39:1623, 2002.

195. Gerber JG: Role of prostaglandins in the hemodynamic and tubular effects of furosemide, *Fed Proc* 42:1707, 1983.

196. Harada K, Ohmori M, Fujimura A, et al: No evidence of a direct venodilatory effect of furosemide in healthy human subjects, *J Clin Pharmacol* 36:271, 1996.

197. Monroy A, Plata C, Hebert SC, et al: Characterization of the thiazide-sensitive Na$^+$-Cl$^-$ cotransporter: a new model for ions and diuretics interaction, *Am J Physiol* 279:F161, 2000.

198. Sullivan JM, Dluhy RG, Wacker WE, et al: Interrelationship among thiazide diuretics and calcium, magnesium, sodium, and potassium balance in normal and hypertensive man, *J Clin Pharmacol* 18:530, 1978.

199. Weber MA, Drayer JIM, Rev A, et al: Disparate patterns of aldosterone response during diuretic treatment of hypertension, *Ann Intern Med* 87:558, 1977.

200. Stockand JD: New ideas about aldosterone signaling in epithelia, *Am J Physiol* 282:F559, 2002.

201. Lifton RP, Gharavi AG, Geller DS: Molecular mechanisms of human hypertension, *Cell* 104:545, 2001.

202. Freis ED: Studies in hemodynamics and hypertension, *Hypertension* 38:1, 2001.

203. Wright JM: Choosing a first-line drug in the management of elevated blood pressure: What is the evidence? 1: Thiazide diuretics, *CMAJ* 163:57, 2000.

204. Wright JM, Lee CH, Chambers GK: Systematic review of antihypertensive therapies: does the evidence assist in choosing a first-line drug? *CMAJ* 161:25, 1999.

205. Schmieder RE, Martus P, Klingbeil A: Reversal of left ventricular hypertrophy in essential hypertension. A meta-analysis of randomized double-blind studies, *JAMA* 275:1507, 1997.

206. McInnes GT: Debate: Does it matter how you lower blood pressure? *Curr Control Trials Cardiovasc Med* 2:63, 2001.

207. van der Heijden M, Donders SH, Cleophas TJ, et al: A randomized, placebo-controlled study of loop diuretics in patients with essential hypertension: the bumetanide and furosemide on lipid profile (BUFUL) clinical study report, *J Clin Pharmacol* 38:630, 1998.

208. Onder G, Gambassi G, Landi F, et al: Trends in antihypertensive drugs in the elderly: the decline of thiazides, *J Hum Hypertens* 15:291, 2001.

209. Faris R, Flather M, purcell H, et al: Current evidence supporting the role of diuretics in heart failure: a meta analysis of randomised controlled trials, *Int J Cardiol* 82:149, 2002.

210. Grinstead WC, Francis MJ, Marks GF, et al: Discontinuation of diuretic therapy in stable congestive heart failure secondary to coronary artery disease or idiopathic dilated cardiomyopathy, *Am J Cardiol* 73:881, 1994.

211. Neuberg GW, Miller AB, O'Connor CM, et al: Diuretic resistance predicts mortality in patients with advanced heart failure, *Am Heart J* 144:31, 2002.

212. Murray MD, Deer MM, Fergusson JA, et al: Open-labeled randomized trial of torsemide compared to furosemide therapy for patients with heart failure, *Am J Med* 111:513, 2001.

213. Abdallah JG, Schrier RW, Edelstein C, et al: Loop diuretic infusion increases thiazide-sensitive Na$^+$/Cl$^-$cotransporter abundance: role of aldosterone, *J Am Soc Nephrol* 12:1335, 2001.

214. Marone C, Muggli F, Lahn W, et al: Pharmacokinetic and pharmacodynamic interaction between furosemide and metolazone in man, *Eur J Clin Invest* 15:253, 1985.

215. Laragh JH, Sealey JE: K$^+$ depletion and the progression of hypertensive disease or heart failure. The pathogenic role of diuretic-induced aldosterone secretion, *Hypertension* 37:806, 2001.

216. Funder J: Mineralocorticoids and cardiac fibrosis: the decade in review, *Clin Exp Pharmacol Physiol* 28:1002, 2001.

217. Bauersachs J, Heck M, Fraccarollo D, et al: Addition of spironolactone to angiotensin-converting enzyme inhibition in heart failure improves endothelial vasomotor function. Role of vascular superoxide anion formation and endothelial nitric oxide synthase expression, *J Am Coll Cardiol* 39:351, 2002.

218. Pitt B, Zannad F, Remme WJ, et al: The effect of spironolactone on morbidity and mortality in patients with severe heart failure, *N Engl J Med* 341:709, 1999.

219. Vitez TS, Soper LE, Wong KC: Chronic hypokalemia and intraoperative dysrhythmias, *Anesthesiology* 63:130, 1985.

220. Reid IR, Ames RW, Orr-Walker BJ, et al: Hydrochlorothiazide reduces loss of cortical bone in normal postmenopausal women, *Am J Med* 109:362, 2000.

221. Gress TW, Nieto FJ, Shahar E, et al: Hypertension and antihypertensive therapy as risk factors for type 2 diabetes mellitus. Atherosclerosis Risk in Communities Study, *N Engl J Med* 342:905, 2000.

222. Fleckenstein A: History of calcium antagonists, *Circ Res* 52(Suppl I):3, 1983.

223. Abernethy DR, Schwartz JB: Calcium-antagonist drugs, *N Engl J Med* 341:1447, 1999.

224. Katz AM: Calcium channel diversity in the cardiovascular system, *J Am Coll Cardiol* 28:522, 1996.

225. Hering S, Berjukow S, Aczél S, et al: Ca^{2+} channel block and inactivation: common molecular determinants, *Trends Pharmacol Sci* 19:439, 1998.

226. Hockerman GH, Peterson BZ, Johnson BD, et al: Molecular determinants of drug binding and action on L-type calcium channels, *Annu Rev Pharmacol Toxicol* 37:361, 1997.

227. Mukherjee R, Spinale FG: L-type calcium channel abundance and function with cardiac hypertrophy and failure: a review, *J Mol Cell Cardiol* 30:1899, 1998.

228. Bean BP: Two kinds of calcium channels in canine atrial cells, *J Gen Physiol* 86:1, 1985.

229. Jaggar JH, Wellman GC, Heppner TJ, et al: Ca^{2+} channels, ryanodine receptors and Ca^{2+}-activated K$^+$ channels: a functional unit for regulating arterial tone, *Acta Physiol Scand* 164:577, 1998.

230. Sen L, Smith TW: T-type Ca$^+$ channels are abnormal in genetically determined cardiomyopathic hamster hearts, *Circ Res* 75:149, 1994.

231. Niggli E: Localized intracellular calcium signaling in muscle: calcium sparks and calcium quarks, *Annu Rev Physiol* 61:311, 1999.

232. Striessnig J, Grabner M, Mitterdorfer J, et al: Structural basis of binding to L Ca$^+$ channels, *Trends Pharmacol Sci* 19:108, 1998.

233. Taherzedeh M, Das AK, Warren JB: Nifedipine increases microvascular permeability via direct local effect on postcapillary venules, *Am J Physiol* 275:H1388, 1998.

234. Grossman E, Messerli FH: Effect of calcium antagonists on plasma norepinephrine levels, heart rate and blood pressure, *Am J Cardiol* 80:1453, 1997.

235. Binggeli C, Corti R, Sudano I, et al: Effects of chronic calcium channel blockade on sympathetic nerve activity in hypertension, *Hypertension* 39:892, 2002.

236. Neal B and the Blood Pressure Lowering Treatment Trials Collaboration: Effects of ACE inhibitors, calcium antagonists, and other blood-pressure-lowering drugs: results of prospectively designed overviews of randomized trials, *Lancet* 359:1955, 2000.

237. Alderman MH, Cohen H, Roqué R, et al: Effect of long-acting and short-acting calcium antagonists on cardiovascular outcomes in hypertensive patients, *Lancet* 349:594, 1997.

238. Devereux RB, Palmieri V, Sharpe N, et al: Effects of once-daily angiotensin-converting enzyme inhibition and calcium channel blockade–based antihypertensive treatment regimens on left ventricular hypertrophy and diastolic filling in hypertension, *Circulation* 104:1248, 2001.

239. Opie LH: Calcium channel blockers in hypertension: reappraisal after new trials and major meta-analyses, *Am J Hypertens* 14:1074, 2001.

240. Pehrsson SK, Ringqvist I, Ekdahl S, et al: Monotherapy with amlodipine or atenolol versus their combination in stable angina pectoris, *Clin Cardiol* 23:763, 2000.

241. Gibson RS: Current status of calcium channel blocking drugs after Q-wave and non–Q-wave myocardial infarction, *Circulation* 80(Suppl IV):IV107, 1989.

242. Gibson RS, Hansen JF, Messerli F, et al: Long-term effects of diltiazem and verapamil on mortality and cardiovascualr events in non–Q-wave acute myocardial infarction without pulmonary congestion: post hoc subset analysis of Multicenter Diltiazem Trial and the Second Danish Verapamil Infarction Trial studies, *Am J Cardiol* 86:275, 2000.

243. Lubsen J: Medical management of unstable angina. What have we learned from the randomized trials? *Circulation* 82(3 Suppl):II182, 1990.

244. Opie LH: Calcium channel antagonists should be among the first-line drugs in the management of cardiovascular disease, *Cardiovasc Drugs Ther* 10:455, 1996.

245. Williams MJA, Low CJS, Wilkins GT, et al: Randomised comparison of the effects of nicardipine and esmolol on coronary artery wall stress: implications for the risk of plaque rupture, *Heart* 84:377, 2000.

246. Miller AB: Effect of lipid-lowering agents, angiotensin-converting enzyme inhibitors, and calcium antagonists on coronary disease risk, *Am J Cardiol* 88(Suppl M):21, 2001.

247. Sanguini V, Gallu M, Sciarra L, et al: Effect of amlodipine on exercise-induced platelet activation in patients affected by chronic stable angina, *Clin Cardiol* 22:575, 1999.

248. Rinaldi CA, Linka AZ, Masani ND, et al: Randomized, double-blind crossover study to investigate the effects of amlodipine and isosorbide mononitrate on the time course and severity of exercise-induced myocardial stunning, *Circulation* 98:746, 1998.

249. Schulz R, Post H, Jalowy A, et al: Unique cardioprotective action of the new calcium antagonist mibefradil, *Circulation* 99:305, 1999.

250. O'Connor CM, Carson PE, Miller AB, et al: Effect of amlodipine on mode of death among patients with advanced heart failure in the PRAISE trial, *Am J Cardiol* 82:881, 1998.

251. Bernink PJLM, Prager G, Schelling A, et al: Antihypertensive properties of the novel calcium antagonist mibefradil (Ro 40-5967), *Hypertension* 27:426, 1996.

252. Alpert JS, Korbin I, DeQuattro V, et al: Additional antianginal and anti-ischemic efficacy of mibefradil in patients pretreated with a beta-blocker for chronic stable angina pectoris, *Am J Cardiol* 79:1025, 1997.

253. Lee DS, Goodman S, Dean DM, et al: Randomized comparison of T-type versus L-type calcium channel blockade on exercise duration in stable angina: results of the Posicor Reduction of Ischemia During Exercise (PRIDE) trial, *Am Heart J* 144:60, 2002.

254. Mullins ME, Horowith Z, Linden DHJ, et al: Life-threatening interactions of mibefradil and β-blockers with dihydropyridine calcium channel blockers, *JAMA* 280:157, 1998.

255. Brogden RN, Benfield P: Verapamil: a review of its pharmacological properties and therapeutic use in coronary artery disease, *Drugs* 51:792, 1996.

256. Hollingshead LM, Faulds D, Fitton A: Bepridil. A review of its pharmacological properties and therapeutic use in stable angina pectoris, *Drugs* 44:835, 1992.

257. Kaplan RC, Heckbert SR, Koepsell TD, et al: Use of calcium channel blockers and risk on hospitalized patients with gastrointestinal tract bleeding, *Arch Intern Med* 160:1849, 2000.

258. Stahl M, Bulpitt CJ, Palmer AJ, et al: Calcium channel blockers, ACE inhibitors, and the risk of cancer in hypertensive patients: a report from the Department of Health Hypertension Care Computing Project (DHCCP), *J Hum Hypertens* 14:299, 2000.

259. Kobinger W, Walland A: Blood circulation studies with 2-(2, 6-dichlorophenylamino)-2-imidazoline hydrochloride, *Arzneimittelforschung* 17:292, 1967.

260. Langer SZ: Presynaptic regulation of the release of catecholamines, *Pharmacol Rev* 32:337, 1980.

261. Mitchell HC, Pettinger WA: Dose-response of clonidine on plasma catecholamines in the hypernoradrenergic state associated with vasodilator β-blocker therapy, *J Cardiovasc Pharmacol* 3:647, 1981.

262. Wing LMH, Reid JL, Davies DS, et al: Pharmacokinetic and concentration effect relationship of clonidine in essential hypertension, *Eur J Clin Pharmacol* 12:463, 1977.

263. Niarchos AP, Baer L, Radichevich I: Role of renin and aldosterone suppression in the antihypertensive mechanism of clonidine, *Am J Med* 65:614, 1978.

264. Muzi M, Goff D, Kampine J, et al: Clonidine reduces sympathetic activity but maintains baroreflex responses in normotensive humans, *Anesthesiology* 77:864, 1992.

265. Brest AN: Hemodynamic and cardiac effects of clonidine, *J Cardiovasc Pharmacol* 2:S39, 1980.

266. Pettinger WA: Pharmacology of clonidine, *J Cardiovasc Pharmacol*, 2:S21, 1980.

267. Magorien RD, Hermiller JB, Unverferth DV, et al: Regional hemodynamic effects of clonidine in congestive heart failure, *J Cardiovasc Pharmacol* 7:91, 1985.

268. Muir AL, Burton JL, Lawrie DM: Circulatory effects at rest and exercise of clonidine, an imidazoline derivative with hypotensive properties, *Lancet* 2:181, 1969.

269. Langer J, Panten U, Zielmann S: Effects of α-adrenoceptor antagonists on clonidine-induced inhibition of insulin secretion by isolated pancreatic islets, *Br J Pharmacol* 79:415, 1983.

270. Guthrie GP, Miller RE, Kotchen TA: Clonidine in patients with diabetes and mild hypertension, *Clin Pharmacol Ther* 34:713, 1983.

271. Houston MC: Abrupt cessation of treatment in hypertension: consideration of clinical features, mechanisms, prevention and management of the discontinuation syndrome, *Am Heart J* 102:415, 1981.

272. Bond WS: Psychiatric indications for clonidine: the neuropharmacologic and clinical basis, *J Clin Psychopharmacol* 6:81, 1986.

273. Gold MS, Redmond DE, Kleber HD: Clonidine blocks acute opiate withdrawal symptoms, *Lancet* 2:599, 1978.

274. Fedorak RN, Field M, Chang EB: Treatment of diabetic diarrhea with clonidine, *Ann Intern Med* 102:197, 1985.

275. Robertson D, Goldberg MR, Hollister AS, et al: Clonidine raises blood pressure in severe idiopathic orthostatic hypotension, *Am J Med* 74:193, 1983.

276. Flacke JW, Bloor BC, Flacke WE, et al: Reduced narcotic requirements by clonidine with improved hemodynamic and adrenergic stability in patients undergoing coronary bypass surgery, *Anesthesiology* 67:11, 1987.

277. Bloor BC, Flacke WE: Reduction in halothane anesthetic requirements by clonidine, an α₂ adrenergic agonist, *Anesth Analg* 61:741, 1982.

278. El-Kerdawy HM, Zalingen EE, Bovill JG: The influence of the α₂-adrenoceptor agonist, clonidine, on the EEG and on the MAC of isoflurane, *Eur J Anaesthesiol* 17:105, 2000.

279. Klimscha W, Chiari A, Krafft P, et al: Hemodynamic and analgesic effects of clonidine added repetitively to continuous epidural and spinal blocks, *Anesth Analg* 80:322, 1995.

280. Vanderstappen I, Vandermeersch E, Vanacker B, et al: The effect of prophylactic clonidine on postoperative shivering. A large prospective double-blind study, *Anaesthesia* 51:351, 1996.

281. Sia S: I.V. clonidine prevents post-extradural shivering, *Br J Anaesth* 81:145, 1998.

282. Lowenthal DT, Matzek KM, MacGregor TR: Clinical pharmacokinetics of clonidine, *Clin Pharmacokinet* 14:287, 1988.

283. Langley MS, Heel RC: Transdermal clonidine: a preliminary review of its pharmacodynamic properties and therapeutic efficacy, *Drugs* 35:123, 1988.

284. Lasseter KC, Shapse D, Pascucci VL, et al: Pharmacokinetics of guanabenz in patients with impaired liver function, *J Cardiovasc Pharmacol* 6:S766, 1984.

285. Sorkin EM, Heel RC: Guanfacine. A review of its pharmacodynamic and pharmacokinetic properties and therapeutic efficacy in the treatment of hypertension, *Drugs* 31:301, 1986.

286. Sjoerdsma A: Methyldopa, *Br J Clin Pharmacol* 13:45, 1982.

287. Van Zwieten PA, Thoolen MJ, Timmermans PB: The hypotensive activity and the side effects of methyldopa, clonidine and guanfacine, *Hypertension* 6(SII):28, 1984.

288. Fouad FM, Nakashima Y, Tarazi RC, et al: Reversal of left ventricular hypertrophy in hypertensive patients treated with methyldopa. Lack of association with blood pressure control, *Am J Cardiol* 49:795, 1982.

289. Ryhanen P, Hanhela R, Jouppila R, et al: Circulatory changes during and after surgical anesthesia in hypertensive patients treated with clonidine, methyldopa and reserpine, *Int Surg* 69:29, 1984.

290. Giachetti A, Hollenbeck RA, Shore PA: Localization and binding of reserpine in the membrane of adrenomedullary amine storage granules, *Naunyn Schmiedebergs Arch Pharmacol* 283:263, 1974.

291. Ambrosino SV: Depressive reactions associated with reserpine, *NY State J Med* 74:860, 1974.

292. Hess HJ: Prazosin: Biochemistry and structure-activity studies, *Postgrad Med* 5:S9, 1975.

293. Sasso EH, O'Connor DT: Prazosin depression of baroreceptor function in hypertensive man, *Eur J Clin Pharmacol* 22:7, 1982.

294. Cohn JN, Archibald DG, Ziesche S, et al: The effect of vasodilator therapy on mortality in chronic congestive heart failure: results of a Veterans Administration cooperative study, *N Engl J Med* 314:1547, 1986.

295. ALLHAT: Hypertension and α-adrenergic blockers: preliminary ALLHAT results, *CMAJ* 163:437, 2000.

296. Kirby RS, Coppinger SW, Corcoran MO, et al: Prazosin in the treatment of prostatic obstruction. A placebo-controlled study, *Br J Urol* 60:136, 1987.

297. Mehta SS, Wilcox CS, Schulman KS: Treatment of hypertension in patients with comorbidities: results from the study of hypertensive prescribing practices (SHyPP), *Am J Hypertens* 12:333, 1999.

298. Kobrin I, Ventura HO, Messerli FH, et al: Immediate hemodynamic effects of urapidil in patients with essential hypertension, *Am J Cardiol* 55:722, 1985.

299. Packer M, Meller J, Medina N, et al: Provocation of myocardial ischemic events during initiation of vasodilator therapy for severe chronic heart failure. Clinical and hemodynamic evaluation of 52 consecutive patients with ischemic cardiomyopathy, *Am J Cardiol* 48:939, 1981.

300. Mulrow JP, Crawford MH: Clinical pharmacokinetics and therapeutic use of hydralazine in congestive heart failure, *Clin Pharmacokinet* 16:86, 1989.

301. Bauer JA, Fung HL: Concurrent hydralazine administration prevents nitroglycerin induced hemodynamic tolerance in experimental heart failure, *Circulation* 84:35, 1991.

302. Yung RL, Richardson BC: Role of T-cell DNA methylation in lupus syndromes, *Lupus* 3:487, 1994.

303. Cush JJ, Goldings EA: Drug-induced lupus: clinical spectrum and pathogenesis, *Am J Med Sci* 290:36, 1985.

304. Raskin NH, Fishman RA: Pyridoxine-deficiency neuropathy due to hydralazine, *N Engl J Med* 273:1182, 1965.

Imaging of the Vasculature

3

Brian A. Aronson, MD

VASCULAR IMAGING can be divided into two categories; physiologic and anatomic. Physiologic imaging measures the biologic significance of vascular flow to specific body regions. Techniques include: sphygmomanometry, plethysmography, pulse volume recordings, Doppler, and ultrasonography. Invasive physiologic imaging can be performed using direct pressure measurements across vascular segments. Anatomic imaging focuses on demonstrating the anatomic characteristics of blood vessels using contrast angiography. More recently, ultrasonography, magnetic resonance (MR) angiography, and computed tomography (CT) angiography represent noninvasive approaches to anatomic vascular imaging.

Physiologic noninvasive studies are usually performed as screening tests to evaluate vascular disease. When these physiologic noninvasive tests suggest significant vascular disease, confirmation with anatomic tests is indicated. Contrast angiography is the anatomic study of choice, although duplex ultrasonography, MR angiography (MRA), and CT angiography (CTA) are widely accepted for presurgical evaluation.

Physiologic Noninvasive Testing

Sphygmomanometry

Cuff blood pressure measurement is the simplest way to evaluate the physiologic significance of peripheral vascular disease. A simple bedside evaluation comparing the blood pressure in the arms and the legs, known as the ankle brachial index, is very sensitive for detecting peripheral vascular disease. An ankle brachial index less than 0.9 indicates the presence of disease[1] (Figure 3-1).

A variation on sphygmomanometry is the segmental limb pressure examination. Blood pressure cuffs are placed on the arms and on the legs above the knee, below the knee, and at the ankle. Pressure drops across these segments are a helpful indicator of the location of significant peripheral vascular disease. In general, a drop of 20 mmHg across a specific segment is an indicator of significant disease that would then warrant anatomic imaging.[2]

Arterial Doppler

When an ultrasound beam is focused on the red cells in flowing blood, the frequency of the reflected echoes varies with the velocity and direction of blood flow. Doppler ultrasonography uses this principle to detect flowing blood, to measure and dis-

play various velocity characteristics, and to estimate blood flow. Advanced duplex Doppler imaging combines real-time imaging with Doppler ultrasound. A particular vessel can be imaged and a point in that vessel selected for Doppler measurement of flow velocity and associated characteristics. Important clinical examples are carotid artery evaluation and determination of the patency of arterial supply to a transplanted organ. Color-flow Doppler imaging is another advance combining anatomic display and velocity data in an easily comprehended form. Color is used to represent flow wherever it occurs in the displayed ultrasound image. Varying intensities of red or blue echoes represent magnitude and direction of velocities of flow to or from the transducer.

Doppler waveform analysis is based on the knowledge of the appropriate waveform given the site interrogated. In general, visceral arterial blood supply gives a low-resistance waveform and muscular body parts demonstrate a high-resistance waveform.

The typical low-resistance waveform pattern is a short time to peak velocity during systole followed by a high level of diastolic flow. A high-resistance pattern is a short time to peak velocity followed by a rapid decrease to baseline and reversal of flow in diastole. The high-resistance bed with stenosis initially shows loss of the reversal of flow in diastole, which progressively worsens to delayed time to peak with increased velocities at the stenosis and increased diastolic flow and then, ultimately, to a rounded low-velocity waveform as occlusion occurs. The best way to understand this is from the physical diagnosis term "pulsus parvus et tardus" (small and late).

The low-resistance bed with stenosis initially shows a less crisp waveform known as spectral broadening. This pattern is caused by turbulent flow manifesting as multiple flow velocities. As stenosis worsens, velocity increases and diastolic flow decreases. Ultrasound evaluation has application in the evaluation of the carotid arteries, renal arteries, mesenteric arteries, and the aorta. Identifying these structures with ultrasound and then subjecting them to Doppler interrogation allows accurate identification of lesions.

Changes in the Doppler waveform indicate significant disease. An increase in velocity also indicates the level of stenosis. Specific velocity criteria can be applied to correlate with ratios of anatomic stenosis.[3]

Initially, Doppler evaluation was done alone; however, now it is done in concert with gray scale and color-flow ultrasound imaging or duplex ultrasonography. The techniques also improve the ability of Doppler to detect significant disease. The anatomic imaging provided by the duplex ultrasound allows

Acknowledgment: Contributions made by Peter Hentzen, MD and Albert Seow, MD.

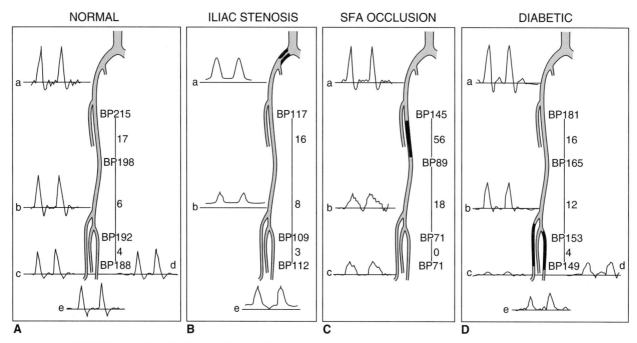

FIGURE 3-1 Example of noninvasive blood flow study of the lower extremity. **A,** Normal blood flow examination with triphasic waveforms. The high thigh blood pressure is normally greater than the other pressures because of the relative smaller size of the blood pressure cuff compared with the diameter of the upper thigh. **B,** An aortoiliac stenosis causes loss of reverse flow in early diastole on the waveform and a gradient between the brachial artery and high thigh pressure cuff. **C,** A femoral popliteal occlusion causes a gradient between the high thigh and above-knee cuff of more than 30 mmHg. The waveform below the occlusion has loss of reverse flow in diastole and blunting of the systolic peak. **D,** Infrapopliteal occlusive disease is inferred by a combination of abnormal waveforms on the tibial arteries and a pressure gradient. The presence of diabetic-related vascular calcifications can cause a false-negative test result. a, femoral; b, popliteal; c, anterior tibialis; d, posterior tibialis; e, dorsalis pedis; SFA, superficial femoral artery. (Modified from Gerlock AJ, Giyanani VL, Krebs C: *Applications of Noninvasive Vascular Techniques,* Philadelphia, 1988, WB Saunders.)

accurate placement of the Doppler gate to evaluate the waveform and velocity accurately. In addition, direct correlations between diameter of the vessel wall and region of stenosis to velocities can be made at the time of screening (Figure 3-2).

Ultrasound

Clinical ultrasound imaging begins with pulses of sound energy created when a crystal in the transducer is pulsed electrically. As the wave of sound energy passes through the patient, a small percentage is reflected at various interfaces between and within the body tissues. After transmitting the pulse, the transducer also receives the reflected sound energy and uses these echoes to form a display. In the commonly used B-mode imaging, echoes of various magnitudes are received from various positions in the patient as the transducer scans a two-dimensional (2D) slice of the patient. The magnitudes are assigned shades of gray, and a computer displays each point in the appropriate spatial orientation, generating the ultrasound image. This image is, therefore, an anatomic representation based on the reaction of sound energy to the various tissues in the body and to interfaces between the tissues. Blood and other body fluids appear echoless or black because fluid does not reflect sound waves and returns no echo. Thus, ultrasound is an excellent modality for vascular imaging. Ultrasound imaging can demonstrate size and course of major blood vessels, demonstrate presence of calcium (by its total absorption of sound waves), differentiate

blood in a vessel or aneurysm from thrombus (by its solid appearance), and visualize and characterize soft tissue masses associated with or adjacent to blood vessels.

Because of the short time it takes to send out a pulse of sound energy and receive the echo, real-time imaging, within certain mechanical and electronic constraints, is possible. A real-time image is a motion picture of rapidly acquired sequenced images from specially designed transducers that allow moving parts to be more easily studied and facilitate acquisition of diagnostic static images.

Computed Tomography

Several advances in CTA have occurred since its inception in 1992. The most notable was the advent of the multislice acquisition technique, which drove the technology to a point at which resolution could be achieved at or near that of conventional angiography for several applications. In addition, larger sections of the body can be imaged more rapidly than with helical single-slice CT scanners. CT allows images to be obtained without the invasive arterial catheterization used in conventional angiography (Figure 3-3). This eliminates the risk of hemorrhage from arterial puncture and allows those with a coagulopathy or receiving anticoagulation therapy to be studied without reservation or delay.

Multislice CT gives greater longitudinal resolution than single-slice CT and allows postprocessing of images so that

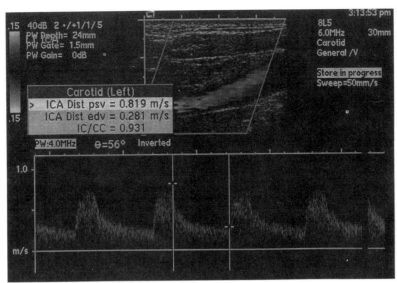

FIGURE 3-2 Carotid duplex ultrasonography.

quality 2D and 3D images can be created from the axial data and unwanted background information may be deleted.[4] Scans are obtained rapidly because several overlapping axial images are obtained at once so that the patient's motion and respiratory motion effects on the images are substantially decreased. Also, a greater amount of the body can be imaged during a single injection of contrast material.

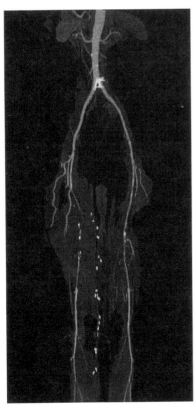

FIGURE 3-3 Computed tomography angiogram of abdominal aorta and bilateral lower extremities. Note the right superficial femoral occlusion.

Images are obtained after bolus injection of contrast material into a peripheral vein, and scanning is initiated when the arterial system of interest is optimally opacified.

CTA is now an important method to evaluate the abdominal aorta for an aneurysm or a dissection to expedite emergency surgical planning. The pulmonary arteries are commonly studied to look for possible emboli. Renal arteries and mesenteric arteries can be evaluated for stenosis or vasculitis. Other applications commonly used include the aortic arch for traumatic abnormalities as well as the circle of Willis in the brain for areas of stenosis or aneurysm. Carotid arteries and peripheral vessels are also studied for atherosclerotic plaque causing areas of stenosis.

In the evaluation of traumatic thoracic aortic injury, CTA is an invaluable asset. Not only is it accurate in depicting the anatomic boundary of a dissection, but also other associated injuries can be diagnosed such as rib or sternal fractures and lung abnormalities (pneumothorax, hemothorax, or contusion).[5] The study can be completed and interpreted in a matter of minutes, which is crucial in the event of thoracic aortic injury as mortality substantially increases with each minute between injury and surgical repair. Typically, a specialized team (physician, nurse, and specially trained technologist) is needed to perform conventional angiography. There is also a substantial risk of extending the aortic dissection or transection during conventional angiography with wires or catheters directly inserted into an injured major vessel, which is not a complication shared by CTA.

CTA has also become important in the urgent diagnosis of pulmonary embolus.[6] The examination is low risk, rapid, and, with the improved technology and resolution afforded by multislice acquisition, very sensitive and specific for central pulmonary artery occlusions. However, there is still a role for conventional angiography for treatment purposes and evaluation of the small distal branches that are not well demonstrated on CTA.

Abdominal aortic aneurysms can be initially evaluated or serially studied by CTA. This gives an accurate depiction not only of the size of the aortic lumen but also of the outer diameter of the aorta and the degree of mural thrombus, which cannot be seen by conventional angiography.

Renal vessels can be evaluated for stenosis with CTA and 3D images can be created, which eliminates problems with overlapping vessels that may be encountered with the 2D images of conventional angiography. CT can also evaluate renal parenchyma and perfusion.

CTA can be used to diagnose emergently cerebral aneurysms associated with subarachnoid hemorrhage for rapid operative planning. Other vascular malformations such as arteriovenous malformations, venous and cavernous malformations, and capillary telangiectasias can be evaluated but are probably better characterized by conventional angiography or MRA.

Magnetic Resonance Angiography

Magnetic resonance imaging (MRI) and MRA have revolutionized the noninvasive diagnosis of vascular pathology from the circle of Willis to runoffs of the lower extremities. Using MRA and the advances in CT technology with the advent of multidetector CTs producing CT angiograms, it is now possible to perform high-quality diagnostic vascular imaging in less than a minute of actual scan time, obviating the need for the invasive procedure of catheter angiography. These new noninvasive techniques are faster, able to be rendered into 3D formats, are of equivalent diagnostic accuracy, and are done without the morbidity and mortality associated with conventional catheter angiography. These new imaging techniques are replacing catheter angiography as screening methods, which can more safely characterize vascular pathology in large populations, thereby allowing the identification of pathologic vascular lesions in a larger population of patients.

The ultimate appearance of the MRA depends upon the particular imaging technique used; blood within vessels may appear bright or dark. On non–flow-sensitive spin-echo images, blood vessels are normally dark. Spin-echo pulse sequences utilize a pair (90° and 180°) of section-selective radiofrequency (RF) pulses to create an MR signal. Blood flowing out of the plane of the section during the time interval between successive RF pulses results in an absence of signal, which is called a flow void. In a fast spin-echo sequence, a long train of echoes is acquired using a series of 180° RF pulses resulting in even more pronounced washout effects than with conventional spin-echo imaging. This technique is employed in order to produce a dark-blood MRA, using the minimum intensity pixel projection computer algorithm.[7]

Gradient-echo pulse sequences are used to produce bright-blood MRAs. Utilizing this technique, only a single RF pulse is applied during each sequence repetition, resulting in no signal loss related to washout effects. Data for images on which blood is bright can be acquired as a series of overlapping thin sections (sequential 2D) or as one or more thick (3D) volumes. The basic bright-blood technique is called time of flight (TOF). This method relies on blood flowing into the volume of interest producing positive flow contrast, while the background tissues are saturated continuously by the repeated application of RF pulses, causing them to remain dark compared with the bright inflowing blood. Saturation pulses can be applied in variable thickness slabs in any plane in order to eliminate the signal

selectively from unwanted vessels. In this way, arterial inflow can be saturated in the pelvis with a superior saturation slab, yielding a venogram of the pelvic veins. Postprocessing of the 2D or 3D gradient-echo sequence source images produces the 3D depiction of the vessels of interest. Using bright-blood MR techniques, the images are processed with an algorithm that produces a maximum intensity pixel projection. This 3D projection can then be manipulated and viewed from any perspective on a workstation, with the further capability of being able to perform reformatted images in any plane desirable in order to evaluate further vascular lesions or vessel origins.[8]

With advances in gradient technology, an increasingly preferred method for MRA of the body is the combination of breath-hold 3D gradient-echo sequences with short repetition time (TR) and short echo time (TE) during the intravenous administration of gadolinium chelate.[9] The gadolinium shortens the T1 of the blood from 1200 down to 50 msec, causing the blood to appear very bright irrespective of flow direction or flow velocity. The timing of the contrast injection must be correct in order to ensure synchronization between the transit of the intravascular gadolinium through the volume of interest and MR scanning. Many techniques have been used in order to accomplish correct timing, including empirical estimation of transit time, administering a small test bolus of contrast agent to determine the time delay between injection and arrival of the contrast agent bolus in the target vessel, automated detection of contrast bolus passage, and MR fluoroscopy to observe contrast passage directly.[10]

The carotid bifurcation can be evaluated using several different MR techniques, including 2D TOF, 3D TOF, and contrast-enhanced MRA. The aorta is best imaged by contrast-enhanced MRA (Figure 3-4). The main renal arteries are well imaged using MRA. Peripheral angiography can now be performed using contrast-enhanced MRA and stepping-table techniques, which rival conventional angiography in accuracy.[11] Whole-body 3D MRA has been performed from the carotid bifurcation to the ankle in 72 seconds with the aid of intravenous gadolinium and utilizing the stepping-table platform.[12] Conventional pulmonary angiography has largely been replaced by multidetector CTA, with pulmonary MRA still an area of active work. The role of coronary MRA is still investigational at this time, with the roles of coronary artery screening and CTA yet to be defined, leaving conventional coronary angiography as the "gold standard" for some years to come.

Nuclear Medicine

Imaging of the vasculature by injection of radionuclides has some current utility in clinical practice, and future developments promise even greater applications. Radionuclides are usually injected in small amounts into a peripheral arm vein, making the scanning ideal for outpatients. The small injection volume and low levels of radiation are much more physiologic than the large amounts of contrast material required by conventional contrast studies. The most commonly used agents are technetium pertechnetate ($^{99m}TcO_4$), ^{99m}Tc-labeled human serum albumin (^{99m}Tc-HSA), and ^{99m}Tc-labeled red blood cells (^{99m}Tc-RBC). The imaging device is a sophisticated gamma camera in which an array of photomultiplier tubes detects gamma emissions from the radionuclide, pinpoints their loca-

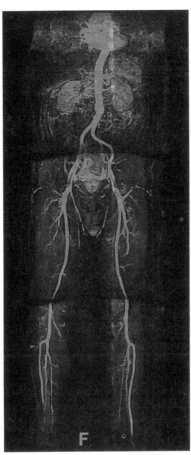

FIGURE 3-4 Magnetic resonance angiogram of whole aorta and lower extremities.

tion, and forms an image of the vessels or organs of interest based on the quantity of radiation received from each point of the image. A computer system attached to the gamma camera allows further processing over time and can measure perfusion, blood flow, and transit time.[13]

For angiography, a bolus injection into an arm vein can be followed by first-pass imaging as the radionuclide passes from the veins through the heart and lungs to the vessels of interest. Blood pool imaging 10 to 15 minutes later is based on an equilibrium of the radionuclide spread through the vascular system. Radionuclide angiography can demonstrate patency and blood flow but has low resolution, approximately 4 mm, and can give little anatomic detail. For this reason it has little role in planning vascular surgery. Specialized applications, such as arterial injection with 22-gauge needles and radionuclide angiography following conventional angiography, are not yet widely employed.

Radionuclide venography is performed with injection of ^{99m}Tc-labeled macroaggregated albumin (^{99m}Tc-MAA), ^{99m}Tc-labeled microspheres, or ^{99m}Tc-RBC into a dorsal foot vein. Tourniquets around the ankle force the agent into the deep venous system. Imaging over the legs can demonstrate obstruction and collateral flow but no filling defects. It is not adequate for venous morphology, and acute obstruction is difficult to differentiate from chronic. This study, therefore, has not displaced the venous duplex ultrasound or venogram in the diagnosis of

deep vein thrombosis. However, newer agents specific for acute thrombus have some clinical utility but have remained less utilized in the acute setting. The main emerging role of radionuclide imaging is evaluation of the end organ. Cardiac and brain scintigraphy and positron emission tomography are examples. Renal scintigraphy manipulated by drugs also has marked utility in evaluating the significance of vascular lesions.

Radiologic Anatomy and Pathology

Arteriosclerosis is the generic inclusive term that describes thickening and hardening of the arterial wall. The pathologic forms that are responsible for radiologic and clinical changes include the following: (1) hyaline and proliferative arteriosclerosis that results in diffuse arteriolar narrowing, (2) hypertensive arteriosclerosis that results in luminal dilation and tortuosity related to loss of resilience of arterial walls, and (3) atherosclerosis. Atherosclerosis is the most common pathologic process involving most arteries. In this disease, discrete localized raised plaques (atheromas) involve the intima of large and medium-sized arteries. Although involvement can be localized clinically and even radiologically to a single site, more often it is diffuse, with different manifestations at different sites. These lesions can be present along one wall of a vessel or can become circumferential. They may undergo a variety of degenerative changes, such as calcification. Hemorrhage occurring into a plaque may result in further luminal compromise or vascular occlusion. Ulceration of the plaque can initiate thrombosis and distal embolization.

The atherosclerotic process can also cause degeneration of elastic elements in the media, resulting in arterial dilation and aneurysm formation. Most common in the aorta, this dilation may be fusiform or saccular and can range from strictly focal to a remarkably diffuse dilation. Diffuse dilation without focal aneurysm formation is termed *arteria magna.*

The effects of atherosclerosis on arteries result in a variety of appearances. Plain film findings include calcification as well as certain contour abnormalities. Changes in aortic contour may be seen as the aorta is outlined by air in the lungs. When calcification occurs in a plaque, it delineates the location of the intima. Therefore, the distance from the calcification to the outer margin of the vessel measures the thickness of the intima, media, and adventitia. This may be helpful in the plain film diagnosis of thoracic aortic dissection. In the abdomen and extremities, where the outer walls of blood vessels blend with the surrounding soft tissue, contours can be appreciated only by inference; for example, lateral displacement of the proximal left ureter can result from a large abdominal aortic aneurysm.

Angiographic findings of atherosclerosis vary from smooth diffuse narrowing to grossly irregular vessels to marked dilation. Vessels can be occluded or may contain short or long areas of stenosis. Localized aneurysmal dilation can be fusiform (concentrically dilated) or saccular (protruding from one wall). Finally, as contrast material defines only the actual patent lumen, aneurysms that are lined with clot may simulate a relatively normal aortic lumen. Ultrasound, CT, or MRI can usually detect an aneurysm with thrombus surrounding the patent lumen.

Great Vessel Pathology

CONGENITAL VARIATIONS. Anomalies of the great vessels frequently occur.[14] Variations can result in vessels with common origins, ranging from one origin for all four vessels to separate origins for each one. Ectopic origins occur as well. The most common is an ectopic right subclavian artery, with this vessel arising distal to the left subclavian artery and passing to the right behind the esophagus, creating an extrinsic defect on its posterior wall as seen during upper gastrointestinal examination. The anomaly is asymptomatic but can cause a radiographic appearance that may be confusing unless the presence of the anomaly is appreciated.

Coarctation of the aorta occurs in the descending aorta and results in several classic radiographic findings. These include rib notching, left ventricular hypertrophy, and poststenotic dilation. Rib notching results from erosions of the undersurface of the posterior ribs produced by enlarged and tortuous intercostal vessels that serve as collateral circulation from the aortic branches proximal to the coarctation to those that are distal (Figure 3-5).

Other anomalies include a right-sided aortic arch and a double aortic arch or aortic ring. The former indents the esophagus and trachea on the right, and the latter results in anterior tracheal and posterior esophageal indentation.

A double arch may cause dysphagia. Another common aortic anomaly is a patent ductus arteriosus that results in flow from the aorta through the ductus to the left pulmonary artery, a left-to-right shunt.

ATHEROSCLEROTIC AORTIC ANEURYSM. Atherosclerotic aneurysms are the most common pathology in the thoracic aorta. Most occur in men in the sixth to seventh decades, and there is a high incidence of associated cardiovascular disease.[15,16] The most common cause of death related to atherosclerotic aneurysm is rupture. Most commonly, aneurysms involve the distal aortic

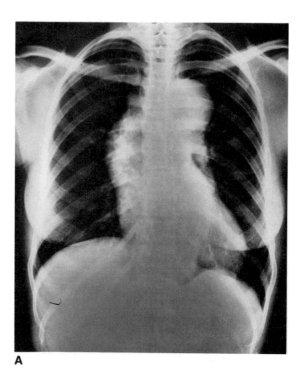

A

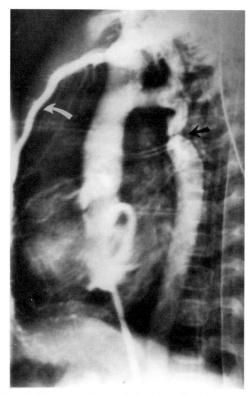

FIGURE 3-5 Thoracic angiogram, lateral view, showing coarctation of the aorta distal to the left subclavian artery (*black arrow*). Note the hypertrophied internal mammary artery providing collateral flow (*white arrow*).

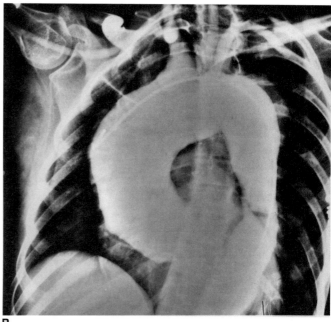

B

FIGURE 3-6 A, Radiographic view of frontal chest showing marked ectasia of the thoracic aorta. It is important not to confuse this appearance with a discrete aneurysm or mediastinal mass. **B,** Angiogram of the same patient. There is diffuse ectasia of the thoracic aorta, explaining the fullness on the chest film. Uncoiling of the descending aorta is present as well. This contributes to the bulge behind the heart on the left. Uncoiling is a common finding in older patients.

arch and descending aorta; they rarely occur in the ascending aorta.[17] They may be saccular, fusiform, or diffusely ectatic, and there may be associated calcification (Figure 3-6). Plain films outline one wall of the aneurysm against the air-filled lung. Air prevents the use of transthoracic ultrasound in evaluating thoracic aneurysms because air attenuates the sound waves. Contrast-enhanced CT accurately demonstrates the aneurysm and its lumen. MRI can also demonstrate the aneurysm, however, without the need for contrast material.

AORTIC TRANSECTION. Aortic transections are almost all due to blunt, nonpenetrating trauma. The likely etiology is that shearing forces at areas of fixation of the aorta occur because of blunt direct trauma or rapid deceleration as occurs in motor vehicle accidents. The intima tears, and a false aneurysm results, causing the media and adventitia to bulge. Complete tears through the aortic wall also occur, usually resulting in massive mediastinal hemorrhage and often death. The most common site is the aortic isthmus at the attachment of the ligamentum arteriosum, the remains of the ductus arteriosus. Here the aorta is fixed to the pulmonary artery. The next most common site is the ascending aorta, followed by the distal descending aorta.[18]

Radiographic plain film findings include widening of the mediastinum related to mediastinal hemorrhage. Other findings related to mediastinal hemorrhage include loss of sharpness or obliteration of the aortic knob and the "apical cap" sign. This is produced by mediastinal blood dissecting over the apex of the left lung between the chest wall and the parietal pleura, producing a dense "cap" over that lung.[19,20] These findings occur with venous hemorrhage as well and, therefore, are not diagnostic only of arterial bleeding. When a pseudoaneurysm occurs, it simulates a left-sided mediastinal mass, displacing the trachea to the right. If a nasogastric tube is present in the esophagus, it too is displaced to the right.[20]

Angiographic findings include irregularity of the aortic wall in the area of intimal injury. Occasionally, an intimal flap is seen. If the pseudoaneurysm is patent, its lumen is demonstrated as well (Figure 3-7). Finally, when small pseudoaneurysms occur and are smooth in contour, differentiation from a ductus diverticulum can occasionally be a problem.

CT findings include direct and indirect signs. Direct signs are aortic contour irregularity, intraluminal filling defect, pseudoaneurysm, and contrast extravasation. Indirect signs include mediastinal hematoma, rib fractures, pleural effusion, and lung contusion (Figure 3-8).

MISCELLANEOUS ANEURYSMS. Mycotic aneurysm is an aneurysm that forms secondary to infection. The normal arterial intima is resistant to infection, and it is generally felt that prior arterial damage must be present for a mycotic aneurysm to occur. The most frequent source of damage is atherosclerosis.[21] Mycotic aneurysms are almost always saccular but are indistinguishable from other saccular aneurysms. They rarely calcify. Luetic aneurysm, now a rarity, was once among the most common causes of aneurysms of the ascending aorta, with curvilinear calcification as a distinguishing feature. Since the advent of antibiotics, the incidence of all mycotic aneurysms has markedly decreased. Sinus of Valsalva aneurysm is a rare congenital condition usually involving the right aortic sinus. Acquired aneurysms of the aortic sinuses can occur as well.

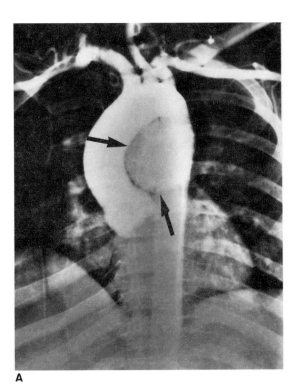

A

B

FIGURE 3-7 A, Thoracic aortogram, frontal projection, showing post-traumatic saccular aneurysm (*arrows*). **B,** Thoracic aortogram, lateral view.

AORTIC DISSECTION. Aortic dissection is a widening of the aorta resulting from pathology of the media. Dissection may result from Marfan's syndrome, in which the mesodermal components of the media are easily disrupted, or from a combination of hypertension and the normal degenerative changes in the aortic wall that occur with aging.

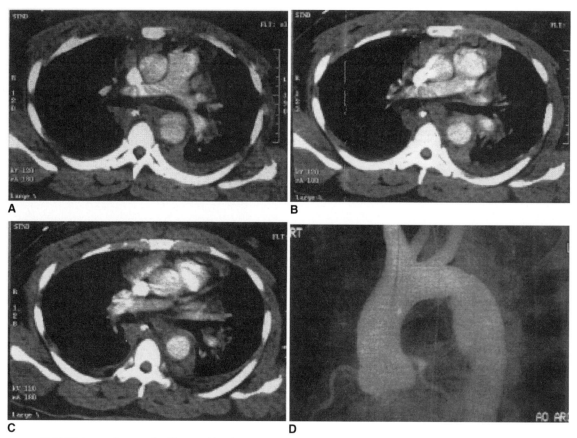

FIGURE 3-8 Images of a 33-year-old male unrestrained driver involved in a motor vehicle accident. **A** to **C,** Three consecutive images from a contrast-enhanced computed tomographic scan through the distal aortic arch demonstrate dilated aorta and an intimal flap with abrupt decrease in aortic caliber distally (i.e., pseudoaneurysm). **D,** Aortogram confirms the pseudoaneurysm with intimal flap. (Courtesy of Dr. Albert Seow.)

Because of medial degeneration, blood entering a defect in the intima separates the intima from the media or splits the damaged media itself. This false channel, or dissection, can extend down the aorta, sometimes occluding branches as it advances. Sometimes the intima tears again at a more distal point and blood from the false lumen reenters the true lumen.

Plain film findings of aortic dissection are only suggestive and include increased space between intimal calcification, if present, and the outer margin of the aorta related to hemorrhage in the media. This is also appreciated on CT scans. CT and MRI are quite helpful in demonstrating the true and false lumen. As a consequence, many centers feel that good-quality imaging may provide enough information for the surgeon to operate without angiography and its added risks of catheter trauma and additional contrast load (Figure 3-9).

The angiographic findings depend on whether or not the false lumen is patent. If it is, contrast in both lumina is separated by the intima, which appears as a black line when seen tangentially. When the false lumen is thrombosed, only the true lumen is opacified. In these cases, differentiation from an atherosclerotic aneurysm with thrombus is difficult.

The true lumen may be markedly narrowed and distorted by the false lumen. Dissections can even extend into branches of

the aorta, sometimes occluding them. Dissection involving the root of the aorta can result in aortic insufficiency by disrupting the aortic valve annulus. Finally, the dissection may extend into the pericardium, in which case pericardial fluid is present. A plain film shows an enlarged cardiac shadow; ultrasound, CT, or MRI shows the fluid collection itself.

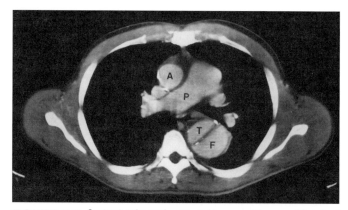

FIGURE 3-9 Contrast-enhanced computed tomographic scan of the chest demonstrates type B dissection. An intimal flap can be seen separating the true lumen (T) from the false lumen (F). A, ascending aorta; P, main pulmonary artery.

THORACIC OUTLET SYNDROME. The paths taken by both sub-clavian arteries and veins make them susceptible to compression from adjacent structures, including cervical ribs, the first rib, the clavicle, and the scalene muscles, causing pain, swelling, paresthesia, and weakness. Laterally, the axillary artery can be compressed between the head of the humerus and the pectoralis minor muscle. Neoplasm arising in the axilla or the apex of the lung, fibrosis from previous radiation therapy, previous lung trauma, and primary vascular diseases such as Takayasu's arteritis may compromise the thoracic outlet as well.

Arterial compressions are best demonstrated by placing the patient in the position that produces symptoms and obliterates the pulse. This is usually hyperabduction. Occasionally, long-standing compression results in aneurysm formation. Thrombus formation within these aneurysms can result in embolization to the fingers (Figure 3-10).

GREAT VESSEL ATHEROSCLEROSIS. The most common disease affecting the great vessels is atherosclerosis. The earliest report linking stroke with extracranial atherosclerosis is credited to Gowers, who, in 1875, described a patient with right hemiplegia and blindness in the left eye. He attributed this syndrome to occlusion of the left carotid artery in the neck.[22]

Because the carotid bifurcations lie just under the skin, they are easily imaged in great detail by modern ultrasound equipment, allowing excellent morphologic definition of lesions (Figure 3-11). Angiography also provides excellent images of the carotid bifurcations as well as the origins of the great vessels. With increasing frequency these images are being obtained with digital subtraction. The images that are produced intra-arterially are superior to those from intravenous injections, but they require that a catheter be placed in the aortic arch or, on occasion, in the vessel in question. The hemodynamic effects of vessel narrowing can also be evaluated by a variety of noninvasive tests. These include evaluation of ophthalmic artery pressure, which decreases with a significant decrease in blood flow, evaluation of flow across the lesion by duplex Doppler examination, and color-flow Doppler testing. MRA of the intra- and extracranial vasculature combined with hemodynamic information now enables clinicians to obtain enough information noninvasively to make clinical decisions.

Pathologically, lesions of the extracranial vessels can be divided into stenosis leading to occlusion and discrete plaque, both ulcerative and nonulcerative. There is an extensive body of literature that tries to answer the question of the significance of a specific lesion. As 30% to 50% of patients develop strokes with no history of previous transient ischemic attacks or any other warning signal, it is important to identify the patients with lesions that predispose to stroke.[23] Asymptomatic carotid stenosis was the original lesion associated with stroke.

SUBCLAVIAN STEAL. A specific syndrome, subclavian steal, occurs when there is stenosis or occlusion of the left subclavian artery proximal to the left vertebral artery. In these patients, the demand for blood flow to the left upper extremity during exercise or strenuous work exceeds the supply from the narrowed subclavian artery. Excess demand results in the sumping or "stealing" of blood from the vertebral artery to compensate for the poor flow from the subclavian artery. This causes

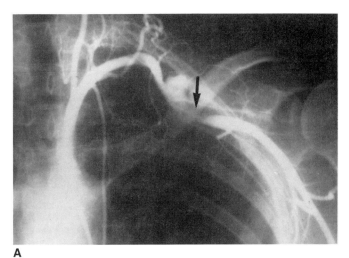

A

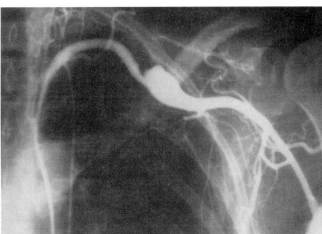

B

FIGURE 3-10 A, Left subclavian arteriogram. There is narrowing of the artery where it traverses the scalene triangle (*arrow*). The arm is hyperabducted and elevated. This was also the position of symptoms. An aneurysm is noted proximal to the stenosis, which can be a source for distal emboli. These aneurysms result from repeated trauma from adjacent structures. **B,** Same patient, neutral position. The narrowing is no longer present.

reversal of blood flow down the vertebral artery and out the distal subclavian artery, diverting blood from the brain. As a result, these patients suffer from dizziness and syncope (Figure 3-12). Angioplasty of an appropriate lesion, or an extra-anatomic vascular graft, reverses the situation and alleviates the symptoms.

Abdominal Aortic Pathology

Atherosclerosis is the most common pathologic process involving the aorta and most other arteries. The most common site of involvement is the distal aorta, below the renal arteries. Radiologically, the pathology ranges from aneurysm formation to occlusion.

ANEURYSM. Abdominal aortic aneurysms can be fusiform or saccular and can range from strictly focal to diffuse dilation, almost always involving only the infrarenal aorta (Figure 3-13). The intima of the aneurysm may be completely or incompletely

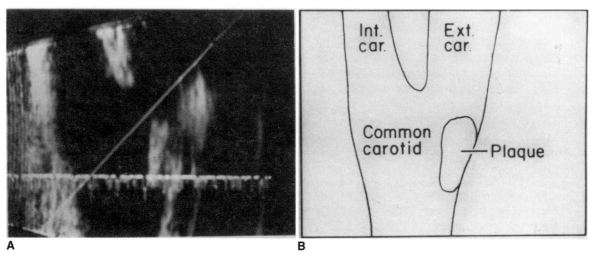

FIGURE 3-11 A and **B,** Duplex Doppler ultrasound examination demonstrates a plaque on the wall of the common carotid artery.

calcified. Plain radiographs show this calcification, if present, but cannot differentiate a patent lumen from intraluminal thrombus. The primary diagnostic modality for imaging an abdominal aortic aneurysm is ultrasonography, which is a noninvasive technique that reliably images an aneurysm in all its dimensions and easily differentiates blood from intraluminal clot (Figure 3-14). Follow-up ultrasonography is reliable for detecting interval enlargement. The generally accepted surgical wisdom is that the typical aneurysm expands at a rate of 0.4 to 0.5 cm per year and that rupture occurs at a substantial rate between 4 and 5 cm (23.4% in one study) and even below 4 cm (9.5% in the same study).[24] A population-based study challenged

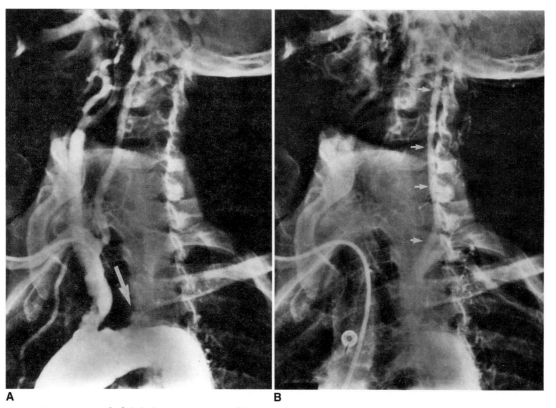

FIGURE 3-12 A, Subclavian steal syndrome. Eighty-year-old woman with recurrent dizziness. Thoracic aortogram performed through the right axillary artery demonstrates complete occlusion of the left subclavian artery just distal to its origin (*arrow*). **B,** Later film from the same study demonstrates delayed filling of the left subclavian and axillary arteries. These vessels fill by "stealing" blood from the vertebral artery (*arrows*), which in turn has filled from the cerebral circulation.

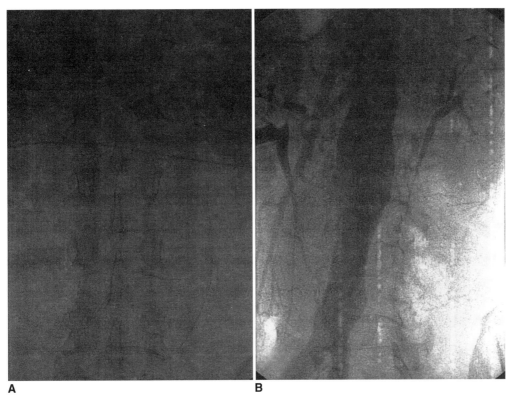

FIGURE 3-13 Abdominal aortic aneurysm. **A,** Plain film. **B,** Digital subtraction angiography.

these data with a mean expansion rate of only 0.2 cm per year and only 24% expanding at 0.4 cm or more per year. Risk of rupture was also less, with a 0% 5-year risk for aneurysms less than 5 cm and 25% for those greater than 5 cm. All aneurysms were at least 5 cm at the time of rupture.[25]

CT can give an accurate image of an aortic aneurysm with serial cross-sectional images. Intravenous contrast injection allows accurate demonstration of the lumen and differentiation from thrombus (Figure 3-15). Calcification in the wall of the aneurysm is easily seen, as is periaortic inflammatory reaction or fibrosis, which can complicate surgical resection. CT can usually determine the relationship of the neck of the aneurysm to the renal arteries, which is an important surgical landmark (Figure 3-16). Extreme aortic tortuosity, however, can result in

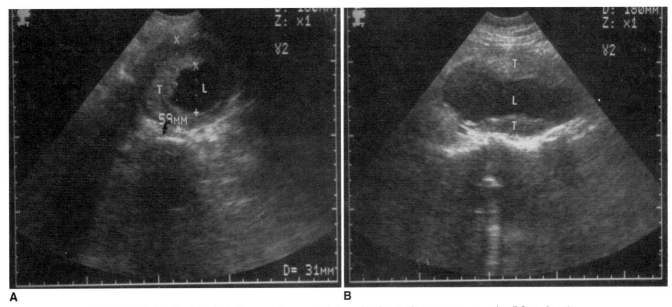

FIGURE 3-14 A, Abdominal ultrasound image, axial view, showing aortic aneurysm measuring 5.9 cm in antero-posterior diameter. Ultrasonography readily differentiates the lumen (L) from thrombus (T). **B,** Longitudinal view demonstrates the length of the aneurysm and again demonstrates patent lumen (L) surrounded by thrombus (T).

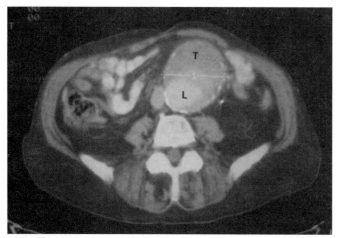

FIGURE 3-15 Abdominal computed tomographic scan. The axial image was made through an aortic aneurysm measuring 7.63 cm in diameter. Note intimal calcifications in the wall of the aneurysm. L, contrast density in patent lumen; T, unopacified thrombus within the aneurysm.

misleading information. Ultrasound may have the same limitation, and this is often a reason for resorting to angiography.

In most instances, MRI can differentiate flowing blood from thrombus in an aneurysm and gives an accurate picture of the aneurysm. Sometimes turbulent flow can simulate thrombus, but changing parameters of the scan can help differentiate between them, all this without contrast injection or ionizing radiation.[26]

Aortography may be required if other, less invasive studies have not demonstrated the neck of the aneurysm or are necessary for surgical planning. Aortography opacifies the lumen of the aorta, and unless there is calcification in the aortic wall, comparison with ultrasound is necessary to determine the presence of luminal thrombus and the true size of the aneurysm. Most abdominal aortic aneurysms are fusiform, with a concentrically dilated lumen. A saccular aneurysm, a localized outpouching of one wall of the aorta, is uncommon. Kinking at the neck of the aneurysm, a common finding, may make determination of renal artery involvement difficult and require oblique or lateral filming.

STENOSIS AND OCCLUSION. Atherosclerosis commonly results in compromise of the vascular lumen. Although occasionally such narrowing of the aorta may be so diffuse and smooth as to simulate other less common pathologies such as arteritis or fibrosis, atherosclerotic narrowing is usually irregular, with mural filling defects and plaque formation. Such plaques are often eccentric and may be present on only one wall, more often the posterior wall. When viewed en face, posterior plaques may not narrow the luminal diameter but only result in variations in density of the contrast material. Oblique or lateral views of the aortogram can assess the significance of the contrast density variations. Atherosclerosis of the abdominal aorta can progress to complete occlusion, but this often has some component of thrombosis as well, perhaps initiated by lesions in the iliac arteries. Originally described by Leriche, abdominal aortic occlusion almost universally spares the renal arteries, although the interior mesenteric artery is frequently involved.[27]

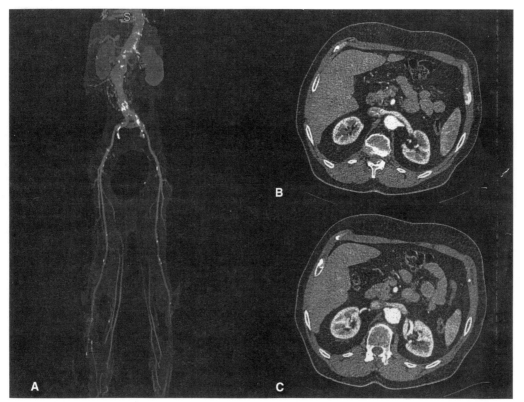

FIGURE 3-16 Computed tomographic angiogram of same patient as in Figure 3-13. **A,** Multi-image reformat. **B,** Axial section showing left renal artery. **C,** Axial section showing right renal artery.

Although most often related to atherosclerosis, compromise of the aortic lumen may be due to other entities. The false lumen of a dissection, almost always originating in the thoracic aorta, can cause smooth narrowing of the abdominal aorta and may extend into the iliac or renal arteries, narrowing or occluding them (Figure 3-17). Takayasu's disease and other forms of arteritis can involve the aorta as well, often combining areas of stenosis with aneurysms. Perivascular fibrosis can have several different causes, such as radiotherapy or idiopathic retroperitoneal fibrosis, and can cause narrowing of the abdominal aorta.

Renal Artery Pathology

Atherosclerosis is the most common lesion compromising the renal artery. It often occurs at the orifice and is almost always in the proximal portion of the artery. Usually localized, lesions may be multiple or bilateral and range from plaques to stenosis to complete occlusion. Usually associated with aortic disease, plaques may extend from the aorta into the renal artery. MRA, CTA, ultrasonography, and renal scintigraphy can evaluate flow in renal arteries. Angiography remains the gold standard to evaluate lesions identified on screening examinations.

Renal artery stenosis and occlusion may cause hypertension through the renin-angiotensin system, and bilateral renal artery stenosis may manifest as renal failure. Fibromuscular dysplasia involving the renal arteries is seen most often in females, usually in a younger age group than atherosclerosis. There are multiple pathologic types with various angiographic patterns, some of which give localized areas of stenosis.[28] The most common type, however, medial fibroplasia with aneurysm, is characterized by multiple areas of stenosis alternating with aneurysmal dilation, the "string of beads" appearance (Figure 3-18). The lesions usually occur in the distal two thirds of the artery and may be bilateral.

Penetrating or blunt trauma to the kidneys may be minor with preserved renal function and require no therapy or may be major with extravasation of blood and urine and can be associated with shock. Intravenous pyelography and CT evaluate renal function, hemorrhage, and additional organ involvement. Major injuries can then be evaluated by renal arteriography to determine the extent of the renal trauma, to look for multiple renal arteries, and to evaluate the other kidney. After evaluating the location, nature, and severity of injury, appropriate therapy can be chosen. Accurate diagnosis is required to eliminate unnecessary surgical exploration that may result in nephrectomy.

Emboli to the renal artery can cause occlusion of the main renal artery or branches. They typically produce a concave filling defect on angiography and are easy to miss clinically because the remaining kidney easily compensates for any loss in renal function. After renal transplantation, nuclear renal scan and Doppler ultrasound are used to evaluate flow in the transplanted artery. Before renal artery surgical or intra-arterial therapy, arteriography is usually performed. Arteriovenous malformation, most often after biopsy or post-traumatic, can be diagnosed or suggested by ultrasonography if it is large enough.

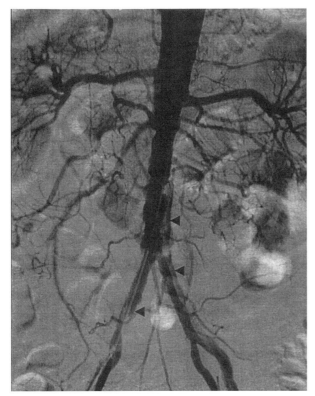

FIGURE 3-17 Aortic dissection extending into both common iliac arteries (*arrowheads*).

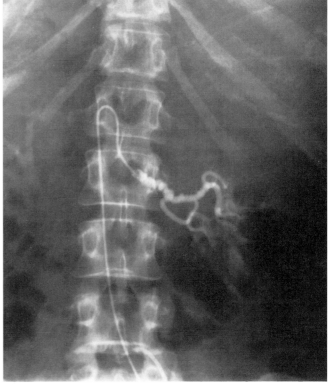

FIGURE 3-18 Left renal arteriogram. Alternating stenoses and aneurysms give classic "string of beads" appearance of fibromuscular hyperplasia.

At angiography, the direct communication between the artery and vein is demonstrated, and embolization can be definitive therapy.

Celiac and Mesenteric Pathology

ANOMALIES. Anomalies of the celiac and mesenteric systems are frequent. The left gastric artery commonly gives off the arterial supply to the left lobe of the liver, and the right hepatic artery originates as a major branch of the proximal superior mesenteric artery (SMA) in 20% of patients.

ATHEROSCLEROSIS. As in other vascular systems, the most common lesion involving the celiac and mesenteric circulation is atherosclerosis. Stenosis or occlusion usually involves the origin of the vessels and is most common in the inferior mesenteric artery, followed by superior mesenteric and then celiac arteries (Figure 3-19). These three arteries are connected by such efficient collateral pathways that symptomatic chronic mesenteric insufficiency is said to require compromise of two of the three vessels. An aortogram in the lateral projection demonstrates the origin of the celiac and mesenteric arteries to best advantage. The frontal projection demonstrates the course of these arteries, the major collateral pathways, and the origin and course of the inferior mesenteric artery. The presence of major mesenteric collaterals is itself suggestive of significant disease at the origins of the vessels. Stenosis at the superior surface of the proximal celiac artery, in younger patients without other signs of atherosclerosis, is thought to be due to pressure from the crura of the diaphragm and/or the celiac ganglion. This has been called the *celiac compression syndrome.*[29] If no other cause for the symptoms is found, surgical correction may be helpful.

MESENTERIC ISCHEMIA. Acute mesenteric occlusion by thrombosis or embolus is clinically an event with nonspecific symptoms, including pain, bowel ileus, and blood in the stool. Plain films of the abdomen may show an ileus pattern with diffusely dilated, air-filled loops of bowel. SMA occlusion typically results in dilation of the small intestine and right colon, whereas inferior mesenteric occlusion results in left colon ileus. If the vascular compromise has progressed to bowel infarction, there may be a thickening of the bowel wall, with hemorrhage and edema thickening the valvulae conniventes. It is important to appreciate, however, that patients with extensive ischemia and even infarction may have normal plain films. At angiography, the occlusion is usually in the proximal portion of the SMA. Thrombosis is usually associated with aortic atherosclerosis and occurs near the origin. Emboli often originate from the heart, for example, in patients with atrial fibrillation, postmyocardial infarction, or valve replacements, and may be multiple. They usually lodge proximally but may be present in branches as well (Figure 3-20). In addition to confirming the diagnosis, angiography guides the surgeon to possible therapy.

Nonocclusive mesenteric ischemia is an entity in which low flow in the mesenteric circulation causes ischemic changes in the bowel. The clinical setting is usually in patients with hypotensive episodes or in postmyocardial infarction patients with low cardiac output. In these situations, the mesenteric blood flow is "sacrificed" in favor of cardiac and cerebral flow, and bowel ischemia and even necrosis may result. Angiography confirms the absence of anatomic obstruction and may show diffuse narrowing of the SMA and branches (Figure 3-21). Areas of vascular spasm may be present and may give a beaded appearance to smaller branches.[30]

Angiographic therapy may be employed after the diagnosis is made.[31] Vasodilating drugs infused into the SMA may relieve the ischemia and prevent necrosis. Papaverine is infused at 30 to 40 mg/hr followed by repeated angiography at 12 to 24 hours and clinical reevaluation. Papaverine should be used carefully in patients with coronary artery disease.

Pelvic Pathology

Although nuclear medicine scans, ultrasonography, Doppler, CT, and MRI can evaluate arterial flow, angiography of pelvic and lower extremity atherosclerosis remains the gold standard from which to select therapy. Angiographic findings fall into the typical patterns. Focal aneurysmal dilatation of iliac arteries occurs—unilaterally, more often bilaterally, and often in conjunction with aortic aneurysm. Plaques involving any of the pelvic vessels can cause irregularity, focal or diffuse areas of stenosis, or obstruction. Calcification commonly occurs, and the abundance of collateral circulation allows many of these lesions to remain asymptomatic. Emboli from the heart or from aortic lesions, when large enough, lodge in iliac vessels, the filling defect creating a concave border to the contrast material in the vessel. Emboli frequently lodge at bifurcations such as the common iliac and the common femoral arteries.

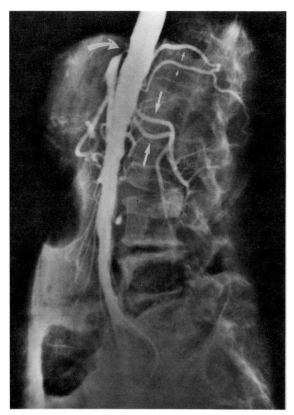

FIGURE 3-19 Lateral abdominal aortogram for bowel ischemia shows marked stenosis (*curved arrow*) at the origin of the celiac artery with poststenotic dilation. The origin of the superior mesenteric artery is not well seen. Lumbar (*small arrows*) and renal (*larger arrows*) arteries are shown.

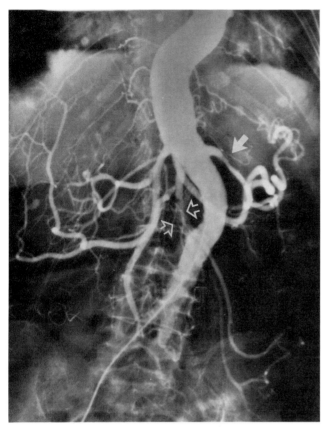

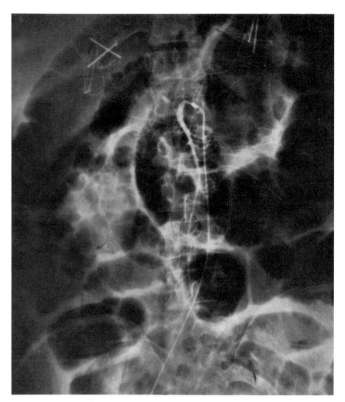

FIGURE 3-20 Abdominal aortogram demonstrates a tortuous aorta obscuring the origins of the major branches. Oblong filling defect (*open arrows*) in the proximal superior mesenteric artery represents an embolus in this patient with symptoms of intestinal ischemia and a cardiac source for emboli. Superior mesenteric artery branches fill slowly past the embolus. Note moderate stenosis in the proximal left renal artery (*solid arrow*).

FIGURE 3-21 Superior mesenteric arteriogram demonstrates diffusely narrowed superior mesenteric artery including all its branches. Flow is very slow. Diffusely dilated, air-filled large and small bowel indicate ileus, helping to confirm the diagnosis of bowel ischemia. Similar arteriographic findings may be seen in shock or following vasopressin infusion for gastrointestinal bleeding.

The possibility of microsurgical techniques to improve pudendal blood supply in patients with impotence has contributed to the importance of diagnostic angiography in the pelvis. Atherosclerosis affects the major pelvic vessels and can lead to stenosis and obstruction of minor but essential vessels supplying the corpora cavernosa. Lesions of the aorta, common iliac, and hypogastric arteries should be addressed by interventional radiologic or surgical techniques prior to attempting therapy of the distal vessels. Selective arteriography of the internal pudendal artery, when properly performed, can assess the adequacy of the pudendal blood supply and determine appropriate therapy.

Upper Extremity

Upper extremity vascular disease is infrequent compared with that in the lower extremities. Atherosclerosis itself affects the upper extremities much less frequently than the lower and, when it does occur, is often asymptomatic because of the good collateral circulation in the upper limbs.

Angiographic findings of atherosclerosis are the same as those in the rest of the body, that is, irregular arterial walls, stenosis, occlusion, and aneurysm. Emboli can affect the upper extremities as well as the lower, again the main source being the heart. Thrombus in an aneurysm of the subclavian artery can be

another source for upper extremity emboli. Larger emboli usually obstruct the brachial artery at its bifurcation, whereas smaller emboli often involve the digital arteries. The angiographic manifestations of vascular trauma to the upper extremities are similar to those of the lower extremities.

Lower Extremity

ATHEROSCLEROSIS. Again, atherosclerosis is the most common lesion affecting the lower extremities. The spectrum of pathologic and radiologic changes is similar to that in other parts of the body—localized plaques, irregular vessel walls, and progression from eccentric or concentric stenosis to occlusion, short or long (Figure 3-22). Aneurysm in the lower extremities is unusual except for popliteal artery aneurysm. This is a focal aneurysm in the popliteal fossa that is often bilateral and becomes symptomatic owing to occlusion or production of distal emboli. Although atherosclerotic lesions are often focal in nature, they are usually multifocal, with involvement at several levels from the aorta distally. Diffuse involvement, however, is not unusual. One of the most common sites of obstruction is in the distal superficial femoral artery where it enters the adductor canal. Mechanical trauma to the vessel may be the predisposing factor at this site. The distal runoff vessels and the popliteal artery are other common areas of obstruction, but almost every site can be involved. Of note is the often remarkably symmetrical nature of the atherosclerotic

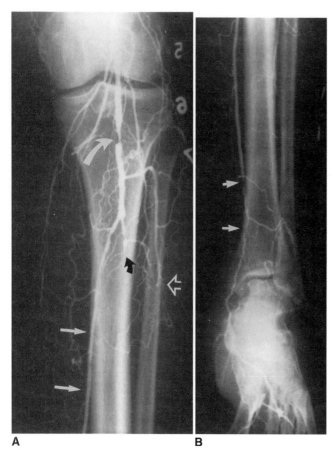

A **B**

FIGURE 3-22 A, Peripheral arteriogram demonstrates marked stenosis of the distal popliteal artery (*white curved arrow*), occlusion of the anterior tibial (*open arrow*) and peroneal (*black arrow*) arteries, and patency of the posterior tibial artery (*straight arrows*). **B,** Continuation of posterior tibial artery, which gives major blood supply to the foot. Some areas of stenosis (*arrows*) are seen. Collaterals attempt to supply the dorsal surface of the foot.

involvement, for example, bilateral occlusions at the same sites and similar patterns of distal runoff. Diabetes is generally a major predisposing factor to the development of atherosclerosis and particularly to disease in small peripheral vessels not amenable to surgical therapy.

Lower extremity arteriography is used for planning therapy in symptomatic atherosclerotic disease. The location and extent of focal lesions and their number and distribution, the nature of the arterial inflow vessels, and the quality of the distal runoff all affect therapy. With clinical and arteriographic information a decision can be made concerning the appropriate therapy—transluminal angioplasty, surgery, or both.

EMBOLIZATION. Embolization commonly affects the lower extremities, sudden onset of symptoms being the key to clinical suspicion. Thrombotic occlusion of a previously stenotic lesion may also give symptoms of sudden onset. Arteriography is often important in differentiation. An embolus classically causes obstruction with a concave edge to the column of contrast material, and there are few collateral vessels. Acute thrombosis occurs at a preexisting atherosclerotic lesion, usually a stenosis, which has resulted in previous significant col-

lateral vascular supply. Stenosis can be a differentiating point, but an embolus can also lodge in a preexisting stenosis, and accurate differentiation is not always possible. The source for emboli is usually the heart, but aortic aneurysms with intraluminal clot and ulcerated atheromatous plaques can also cause embolization.

Trauma

Necessity for evaluation of the vasculature after trauma is dependent on the proximity of the trauma to the vessels and the clinical examination. Vascular surgeons vary in their criteria for requesting arteriography. Findings on the arteriogram include spasm, vessel wall irregularity, obstruction, and laceration or transection with hematoma or pseudoaneurysm. Post-traumatic arterial spasm may give a severe arterial injury the appearance of a minor abnormality as extravasation may not be appreciated, or convert transection, with potentially significant hemorrhage, into the appearance of arterial occlusion. Therefore, some sources suggest that any of the subtle arteriographic signs of arterial injury need to be evaluated by surgical exploration. Others advocate careful clinical and radiologic follow-up in certain cases.[32]

Pseudoaneurysm results from an area of chronic hemorrhage that has developed an organized, fibrotic wall. A pseudoaneurysm communicates with the vascular lumen but is not surrounded by any vessel layers. It usually occurs at anastomoses and may result from infection, technical problems, or breakdown of graft materials. Infection of a pseudoaneurysm may also occur after its formation. It is easily suspected clinically, and arteriographic confirmation and evaluation of distal vasculature may be helpful before therapy.

Venous Pathology

VENOUS THROMBOSIS—ACUTE AND CHRONIC. The diagnosis of acute venous thrombosis has been simplified with advances in ultrasound image quality. The common femoral, proximal superficial femoral, and popliteal veins are easily seen and examined for acute thrombosis. The normal vein is easily compressed by the examining transducer, and changes in diameter with respiration can easily be appreciated. The acutely thrombosed vein is not compressible, nor does the diameter change with respiration.

When ultrasound results are equivocal or when the femoral and popliteal veins are normal by ultrasound, and the calf, thigh, or pelvic veins need to be evaluated, or when the distinction between acute and chronic thrombosis must be made, venography is performed.

Acute clot is seen as an intraluminal filling defect (Figure 3-23). When extensive thrombosis exists, associated edema of the soft tissue of the calf compresses the deep veins so that all blood flow is through the superficial veins. In these cases, differentiation between compression of the deep system by the surrounding edema and complete thrombosis cannot be made. Finally, ascending venography does not visualize the deep pelvic veins that are often a silent source of thrombi causing pulmonary emboli.

When thrombosis persists, veins either become obliterated and thus do not fill or recanalize over time to varying degrees. Veins that completely recanalize may look normal. Partial

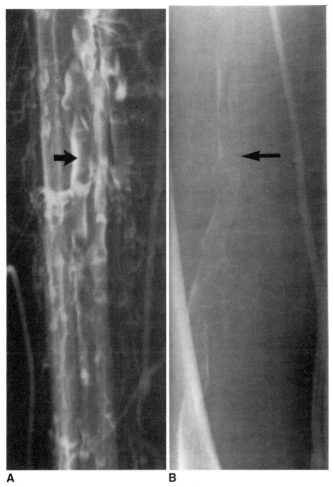

A   **B**

FIGURE 3-23 A, Ascending venogram. Clot outlined by contrast material fills the deep veins of the calf (*arrow*). **B,** Ascending venogram. Clot fills the superficial femoral vein. Contrast material can be seen between the clot and vessel wall (*arrow*).

prudent to perform them for patients in this group. Patients in the intermediate group may require a pulmonary angiogram to exclude or support the diagnosis of pulmonary embolus when the clinical findings are confusing or if the patient cannot tolerate anticoagulation and vena cava filter placement is being considered. Finally, pulmonary angiography may be performed to define the full extent and location of clot when patients with worsening clinical findings are being considered for embolectomy.

The angiographic diagnosis of pulmonary embolus requires that the clot be visualized, as complete occlusion of vessels can occur from a variety of causes (Figure 3-24). These include scarring from previous infection as well as neoplasm. To make the diagnosis of intravascular clot, an intraluminal filling defect with contrast outlining the clot within the vessel must be seen.

PULMONARY ARTERIOVENOUS FISTULA. These lesions are congenital. They are direct communications between pulmonary arteries and veins with dilation of the affected vessels. They are often multiple and associated with skin and mucous membrane telangiectasia as components of Osler-Weber-Rendu disease. The complications of pulmonary arteriovenous fistulas include hemoptysis, brain abscess, cyanosis, and polycythemia.[34] Plain film findings include a "mass" with large vessels leading to it. The diagnosis is obvious at angiography, and the current therapy is percutaneous embolization.[35]

CONGENITAL VARIATIONS. The most common anomaly is a persistent left superior vena cava (SVC) (Figure 3-25). This entity usually occurs in the presence of a normal SVC but may exist alone or together with other cardiac anomalies.[36]

On plain films, the left SVC may appear as a bulge below the aortic arch or as a left paramediastinal density. The diagnosis is easily achieved by venous angiography or noninvasively by MRI. It is important to appreciate the presence of this

recanalization results in the thread and string sign. The walls of these veins are also irregular. Multiple channels may be seen, and collateral circulation may be visualized when partial occlusion is present.

PULMONARY EMBOLUS. With the advent of improved CT technology CTA has nearly replaced diagnostic pulmonary angiography. Limitations of CTA technique, however, restrict the imaging of small vessel involvement and angiography remains the gold standard. Noninvasive testing often confuses the clinical picture, and the lack of true specificity in many instances makes the angiogram the definitive test. Plain film findings are often nonspecific, including pleural effusions, scattered infiltrates, and atelectasis. Some patients with pulmonary emboli have a normal chest radiograph.

Patients are divided into four groups on the basis of radionuclide lung scans and chest films—normal, low probability, intermediate, and high probability.[33] It is generally accepted that normal scans exclude emboli. It has been shown that a low-probability scan in the presence of strong clinical findings of embolization should be questioned. Because pulmonary angiograms are highly accurate and relatively safe, it is usually

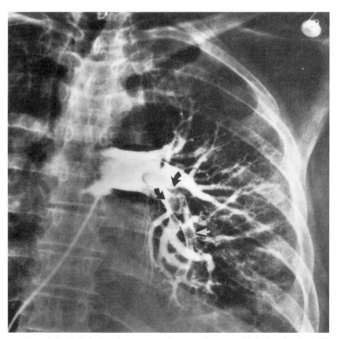

FIGURE 3-24 Left pulmonary angiogram shows multiple intraluminal filling defects diagnostic of pulmonary emboli (*arrows*).

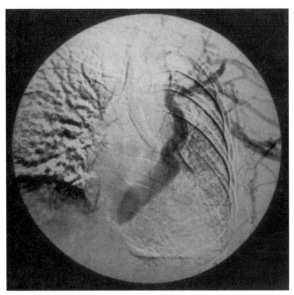

FIGURE 3-25 Digital subtraction venogram of the left upper extremity. Left-sided vena cava is demonstrated.

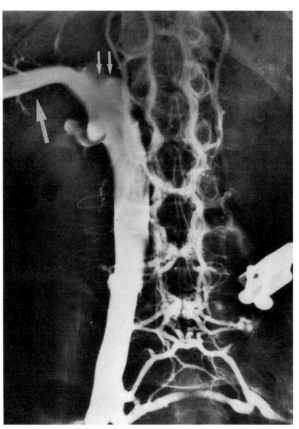

FIGURE 3-26 Obstruction of inferior vena cava (*small arrows*) within the liver. Venous flow from the abdomen and lower extremities enters a lower hepatic vein (*large arrow*) and the vertebral venous plexus. Blood in these collaterals makes its way to the superior vena cava and to the heart.

anomaly, as central catheters placed in the left subclavian vein or left internal jugular vein may descend in the mediastinum to the left to enter the heart rather than on the right side if they enter a left-sided vena cava.

SUPERIOR VENA CAVA SYNDROME. Obstruction of the SVC produces a classic syndrome. It consists of swelling of the face and neck, distention of neck veins, headache, and cyanosis. Most cases result from neoplasm, but large aortic aneurysms and mediastinal fibrosis can cause obstruction as well. Finally, infected and/or clotted central venous catheters can lead to SVC obstruction. The collateral route for blood flow from an obstructed SVC is through the azygous system.

INFERIOR VENA CAVA PATHOLOGY. The inferior vena cava (IVC) can be effectively studied by ultrasonography, CT, and MRI, demonstrating occlusion or thrombosis and any adjacent masses. Cavography is necessary when findings are equivocal or more details about the obstructing lesion or the collateral circulation are needed. Cavography is often performed before pulmonary angiography to exclude thrombus in the IVC. Angiographic changes in the IVC include localized displacement, narrowing intrinsic or extrinsic defects, occlusion, and thrombosis. Diffuse narrowing may also be seen. Obstruction of the IVC is most often in its lower portion, resulting from extension of thrombus into the IVC from extrinsic or intrinsic pelvic masses or fibrosis surrounding the IVC. Collateral routes are many and varied, including ascending lumbar, vertebral, azygous, gonadal, renal, abdominal wall, hemorrhoidal, and portal veins (Figure 3-26).

Following placement of IVC filters for prevention of pulmonary emboli, plain radiographs can demonstrate filter position and exclude migration or tilting. Ultrasonography and CT can detect patency of the IVC . Cavography may be necessary to confirm or exclude thrombus on the superior edge of the filter, requiring placement of another filter.

CHRONIC VENOUS STASIS. Valvular insufficiency of the lower extremity is a common health problem.[37] Competent valves allow efficient function of the pumping effect of the calf muscles; that is, contraction results only in cephalic flow. When valves are incompetent, blood flows both up and down as the muscle pump contracts and relaxes. When only the superficial vein valves are involved, the result of insufficiency is superficial varicosities (varicose veins). When the valves of the deep system are incompetent, resulting reflux produces a chain of events leading to chronic venous stasis.

Incompetence of valves can occur as a result of a primary valve defect, possibly congenital, or can result when recurrent thrombophlebitis destroys the valves. In these patients, obliteration of the vein lumen can also occur, resulting in obstruction. Increased pressure, from either valve incompetence or obstruction of the lumen, is directed at the perforating vein valves, which also become incompetent. Elevated pressure is then transmitted to the capillary bed and superficial veins, resulting in extravasation of fluid and red cells into the subcutaneous tissue and causing induration, swelling, discoloration, and edema. The degree of obstruction can be appreciated by ascending venography, and the degree of reflux can be appreciated by descending venography (Figure 3-27).

Venous occlusion of an upper extremity is usually asymptomatic because of excellent collateral pathways. Symptomatic axillary vein occlusion is often associated with thrombosis brought on by vigorous upper body exercise such as weight lifting and

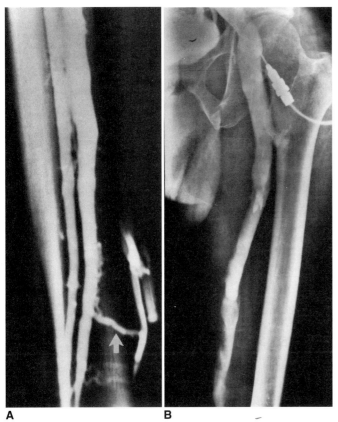

A   **B**

FIGURE 3-27 A, Ascending venogram. The deep system fills as a tourniquet prevents antegrade filling of superficial veins. There is retrograde flow into a superficial vein through an incompetent perforator (*arrow*). **B,** Descending venogram. A 5F catheter has been placed into the common femoral vein. The patient is semierect. Contrast material is injected as the patient performs the Valsalva maneuver. Contrast material refluxes freely down the superficial femoral vein in a patient with chronic venous stasis, indicating incompetence of the superficial femoral vein valves.

swimming—the effort thrombosis syndrome. This entity is usually seen in patients with hypertrophied thoracic and upper extremity musculature as a result of strenuous work or exercise. Some have advocated the use of lytic therapy in this entity, as these patients usually have some persisting disability if the vein does not recanalize.

PORTAL HYPERTENSION. Portal venous hypertension is usually secondary to chronic progressive liver disease and has multiple manifestations, some of which require vascular evaluation. When resistance to blood flow through the liver reaches a certain point, portal-systemic collaterals open, diverting the portal blood to the systemic circulation and decompressing the portal system. Major collateral pathways exist in several different areas. Left gastric and short gastric veins can drain through esophageal veins to the azygous system, resulting in esophageal and/or gastric varices. The inferior mesenteric vein can drain through the hemorrhoidal veins to the iliac veins. Veins from the spleen can drain into retroperitoneal and renal veins. The umbilical vein from the left portal vein may recanalize and dilate, producing the "caput medusa" sign, described as a clinical finding in cirrhosis.

Imaging studies (ultrasonography, CT, MRI) can easily detect these enlarged veins and collaterals. Duplex Doppler is able to evaluate the direction of flow in large veins. Angiography, however, is usually performed prior to creation of a portal-systemic shunt or when failure of such a shunt is suggested.

When a large volume of contrast material is injected into the celiac or splenic artery of a normal patient, the spleen is perfused, and there is opacification of the splenic vein, the portal vein, and its branches. Injection into the SMA, sometimes after injection of vasodilating drugs, results in mesenteric venous filling and opacification of the superior mesenteric vein, the portal vein, and branches. In a patient with suspected portal hypertension prior to creating a shunt, angiography confirms portal hypertension and patency of the major veins. There may be poor portal vein opacification because of increased resistance in the liver. There may be reversal of flow in the splenic vein or the superior or inferior mesenteric veins. Any or all of the portal-systemic collaterals mentioned previously may be demonstrated.

Transjugular portography can be used to evaluate portal hypertension by hepatic pressure evaluations and wedged hepatic contrast (CO_2 is best) injection to fill portal veins in a retrograde fashion. Direct visualization of the portal system by splenoportography (injection of contrast material directly into the spleen) is no longer used. Transhepatic portography is not commonly used for routine diagnosis in portal hypertension (Figure 3-28).

Evaluation of patients after portocaval, mesocaval, or splenorenal shunts when failure is suspected is most commonly performed arterially. A patent shunt opacifies the IVC. When the shunt fails, recurrent portal-systemic collaterals are demonstrated. Alternatively, through femoral veins and IVC, the shunt itself may be catheterized. Patency or a partially compromised

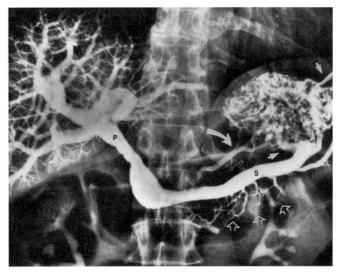

FIGURE 3-28 Transhepatic splenic and portal venogram. Catheter is placed through the liver, into a portal vein branch, and out into the splenic vein. Splenic vein (S), portal vein (P), and all intrahepatic portal branches are patent. Pancreatic branches (*open arrows*) and short gastric branches to the fundus of the stomach (*solid arrows*) are well demonstrated. Contrast material is seen in the coronary or left gastric vein from the stomach as well (*curved arrow*).

shunt can be demonstrated. If the shunt is narrowed, angioplasty may be attempted to reestablish flow.

REFERENCES

1. Braun MA, Nemcek AA Jr, Vogelzang RL: *Interventional radiology procedure manual*, sec 1, chap 1, New York, 1997, Churchill Livingstone, 3.
2. Strandness DE Jr, Van Breda A: *Vascular diseases: surgical and interventional therapy*, vol I, sec IV, 11, New York, 1994, Churchill Livingstone, 145.
3. Kaufman JA, Hartnell GG, Trerotola SO (eds): *Noninvasive vascular imaging: with ultrasound, computed tomography, and magnetic resonance; part 1, tutorial*, 7, Fairfax, VA, 1997, Society of Cardiovascular & Interventional Radiology, 97.
4. Hu H, He HD, Foley WD, Fox SH: Four multidetector-row helical CT: image quality and volume coverage speed, *Radiology* 215:55, 2000.
5. Kuhlman JE, Pozniak MA, Collins J, Knisely BL: Radiographic and CT findings of blunt chest trauma: aortic injuries and looking beyond them, *Radiographics* 18:1085, 1998.
6. Vassilios R, Bersille PM: Multidetector row spiral CT pulmonary angiography: comparison with single detector row spiral CT, *Radiology* 221:606, 2001.
7. Edelman RR, Chien D, Kim D: Fast selective black blood MR imaging, *Radiology* 181:655, 1991.
8. Saloner D: MRA: principles and display. In Higgins CB, Hricak H, Helms CA (eds): *Magnetic resonance imaging of the body*, ed 3, Philadelphia, 1997, Lippincott-Raven, 1345.
9. Prince MR: Body MR angiography with gadolinium contrast agents, *Magn Reson Imaging Clin North Am* 14:11, 1996.
10. Prince MR: Contrast-enhanced MR angiography: theory and optimization, *Magn Reson Imaging Clin North Am* 6:257, 1998.
11. Meaney JF, Ridgway JP, Chakraverty S, et al: Stepping-table gadolinium-enhanced digital subtraction MR angiography of the aorta and lower extremity arteries: preliminary experience, *Radiology* 211:59, 1999.
12. Goyen M, Quick HH, Debatin JF, et al: Whole-body three-dimensional MR angiography with a rolling table platform: initial clinical experience, *Radiology* 224:270, 2002.
13. Ennis JT, Dowsett DJ: *Vascular radionuclide imaging. a clinical atlas*, Chichester, UK, 1983, John Wiley & Sons.
14. Neuhaser EBD: The roentgen diagnosis of double aortic arch and other anomalies of the great vessels, *Am J Roentgenol* 56:1, 1946.
15. Joyce JW, Farbairn JF II, Kinhcaid OW, Juergens JL: Aneurysms of the thoracic aorta: a clinical study with special reference to diagnosis, *Circulation* 29:176, 1964.
16. McNamara JJ, Pressler VN: Natural history of arteriosclerotic thoracic aortic aneurysms, *Ann Thorac Surg* 26:468, 1978.
17. Steinberg I: The arteriosclerotic thoracic aorta: clinical and roentgen observations, *Angiology* 7:405, 1956.
18. Sevitt S: The mechanisms of traumatic rupture of the thoracic aorta, *Br J Surg* 64:166, 1977.
19. Sanborn JC, Heitzman CR, Markarian B: Traumatic rupture of the thoracic aorta: roentgen pathologic correlations, *Radiology* 95:293, 1970.
20. Tisnado J, Fong YT, Als A, Roach JF: A new radiographic sign of acute traumatic rupture of the thoracic aorta: displacement of the nasogastric tube to the right, *Radiology* 125:603, 1977.
21. Singh H, Parkhurst GF: Bacterial aortitis, *NY State J Med* 72:2779, 1972.
22. Gowers WR: On a case of simultaneous embolism of central retinal and middle cerebral arteries, *Lancet* 2:794, 1875.
23. Moore W: Fundamental considerations in cerebral vascular disease. In Rutherford RD (ed): *Vascular surgery*, ed 3, Philadelphia, 2000, WB Saunders, 1294
24. Darling RC, Messina CR, Brewster DC, Ottinger LW: Autopsy study of unoperated abdominal aortic aneurysms: the case for early resection, *Circulation* 56(Suppl 2):161, 1977.
25. Nevitt MP, Ballard DJ, Hallet JW Jr: Prognosis of abdominal aortic aneurysms. A population-based study, *N Engl J Med* 321:1009, 1989.
26. Dumoulin CL, Hart HR: Magnetic resonance angiography, *Radiology* 161:717, 1986.
27. Beckwith R, Huffman ER, Eiseman B, Blount SG Jr: Chronic aortoiliac thrombosis: a review of 65 cases, *N Engl J Med* 258:721, 1958.
28. Ekelund L, Gerlock J, Molin J, Smith C: Roentgenologic appearance of fibromuscular dysplasia, *Acta Radiol Diagn* 19:433, 1978.
29. Rob C: Surgical diseases of the celiac and mesenteric arteries, *Arch Surg* 93:21, 1966.
30. Siegelman SS, Sprayregen S, Boley SJ: Angiographic diagnosis of mesenteric arterial vasoconstriction, *Radiology* 112:533, 1974.
31. Boley SJ, Sprayregen S, Veith FJ, et al: An aggressive roentgenologic and surgical approach to acute mesenteric ischemia. In Nyhus LM (ed): *Surgery annual*, vol 5, New York, 1973, Appleton-Century-Crofts, 335
32. Sclafani SJ, Cooper R, Shaftan GW, et al: Arterial trauma: diagnostic and therapeutic angiography, *Radiology* 161:165, 1986.
33. Pope CF, Sostman HD: Venous thrombosis and pulmonary embolus. In Putnam CE, Ravin CE (eds): *Textbook of diagnostic imaging*, Philadelphia, 1988, WB Saunders, 592
34. Higgins CB, Wexler L: Clinical and angiographic features of pulmonary arteriovenous fistulas in children, *Radiology* 119:171, 1976.
35. Terry PB, Barth KH, Kaufman SL, White RI: Balloon embolization for treatment of pulmonary artery fistulas, *Med Intell* 302:1189, 1980.
36. Campbell M, Deuchar DC: Left-sided superior vena cava, *Br Heart J* 16:423, 1954.
37. Train JS, Schanzer H, Pierce EC II, et al: Radiological evaluation of the chronic venous stasis syndrome, *JAMA* 258:941, 1987.

Endovascular Procedures

Brian A. Aronson, MD

A S endovascular techniques have become more accepted, there has been a rapid increase in the number of fluoroscopically guided endovascular procedures. Interventional radiologists, vascular surgeons, and interventional cardiologists all perform procedures in this manner. The success of these procedures has increased, and the techniques are becoming more widely utilized.

These procedures are performed mainly in three locations: the interventional radiology suite, the cardiac catheterization laboratory, and the operating room. It is essential that all personnel staffing rooms where these procedures are performed have a basic understanding of radiation safety to protect themselves and others.

It is beyond the scope of this chapter to explain the physics behind radiation safety, but a brief discussion of protection of personnel in a radiology suite is in order.

Radiation Safety

An important concern for those working around fluoroscopy is radiation safety. No one federal department governs the medical use of x-rays. Instead, multiple public and private organizations have created standards for the use of x-ray equipment.[1] The Center for Devices and Radiological Health within the Food and Drug Administration regulates equipment design. The Occupational Safety and Health Administration places limits on radiation doses for employees in the workplace, and each state department of health and human services places additional regulations. Although this diversity of responsibility for x-ray regulation seems dispersed, it is actually quite uniform because of the recommendations of the National Council on Radiation Protection and Measurements.

Other organizations also publish recommendations. Specifically, the International Commission on Radiation Protection and the International Council on Radiation Protection and Units are two well-known organizations. It is beyond the scope of this chapter to review these limitations specifically; suffice it to say here that doses should always be kept as low as reasonably achievable, which is a basic principle of radiation use. The monitoring of radiation dose to workers is the specific responsibility of the radiation safety officer at each institution.

Basically, an x-ray beam diverges from its source as it passes through space, and this reduces the intensity (Figure 4-1). Therefore, the first measure of protection from radiation is distance. As the distance from a radiation source is doubled, the radiation decreases to one fourth.[2] Although this relationship strictly holds for a point source of radiation, it is also applicable as a means of protection from radiation exposure during endovascular procedures. This is known as the inverse square law. The farther away from the source of the radiation, the lower the dose delivered.

Another way to limit radiation exposure of personnel is to limit the time of fluoroscopy and diagnostic number of angiography runs. This is related to the needs of the operator; however, some basic observations can be made. For example, pulsed fluoroscopy rather than continuous fluoroscopy can reduce the amount of time of x-ray exposure.[3] It is important to note, however, that as endovascular procedures become more sophisticated, larger doses of radiation are necessary.

Probably the most important principle of radiation safety is shielding. Shielding occurs at the source of the radiation as well as from lead shielding worn by people within the fluoroscopy room. A 0.5-mm lead equivalent can reduce the intensity of the radiation beam by approximately 90%.[4] With distance away from the patient and appropriate shielding, the fluoroscopy dose to health professionals can be limited.

Finally, it is essential that all professionals who routinely expose themselves to radiation wear monitors. It is important that radiation dose over time be known to everyone who works within the radiation field. Dose must be monitored at all sites where people work and the accumulated dose monitored over time.

Endovascular Technique

All endovascular techniques can be thought of as entailing five generic elements. First, access to the vascular system must be achieved. Frequently, multiple access sites are necessary for complex endovascular procedures. Second, diagnostic angiography must be performed to reconfirm the site of the endovascular pathology. Third, guide wire and catheter position across the pathologic segment to be treated must be ascertained. Fourth, the therapeutic intervention is carried out. And fifth, access site management is performed. Although most endovascular procedures are straightforward, marked difficulty can be encountered in any one of these procedural segments. When difficulty is encountered, procedure times are prolonged.

Anesthesia Requirements for Endovascular Procedures

Most endovascular techniques, especially those in the angiography suite or the cardiac catheterization laboratory, usually

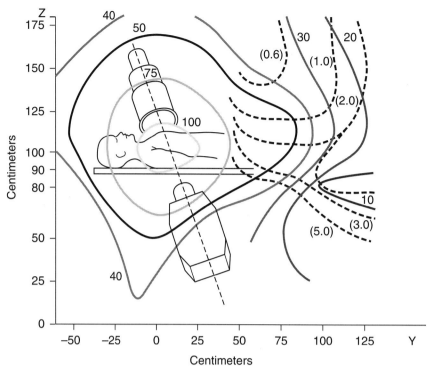

FIGURE 4-1 Isoexposure curves with a rotating C-arm system. (From Tilkian AG, Daily EK: *Cardiovascular procedures, diagnostic techniques and therapeutic procedures*, St. Louis, 1986, Mosby, 456.)

require conscious sedation only. Most endovascular procedures such as iliac artery stent or balloon angioplasty require only a short time to complete. On occasion, however, endovascular procedures can become complex and require quite long procedure times. At this point, the anesthesiologist becomes a critical part of the team in order to maintain the patient safely in an appropriate position for the procedure.

Only a few endovascular procedures require prolonged immobilization. Transjugular intrahepatic portal systemic shunt (TIPS) procedures require at least 90 minutes and frequently 3 to 4 hours to complete. Traditionally, these have been performed under general anesthesia. Neuroendovascular interventional procedures such as endovascular aneurysm coiling and arterial venous malformation therapy frequently require prolonged immobilization and deep anesthesia.

Endovascular Procedures in the Interventional Radiology Suite

Endovascular procedures encompass both arterial and venous revascularizations. Arterial revascularizations tend to focus on crossing occlusive or highly stenotic lesions with guide wire and catheter techniques and then angioplasty using balloon dilatation or assisted angioplasty using metal stents.

Among the most common endovascular procedures are those related to dialysis access. These procedures include percutaneous dialysis graft thrombectomy and thrombolysis as well as venous angioplasty and stenting. Most procedures last approximately 1 hour and can be performed under local anesthesia alone; however, occasional complex procedures requiring recanalization and central vein reconstruction can require several hours. The patient's tolerance for the endovascular pro-

cedure wanes significantly as procedure times increase. The need for deeper conscious sedation or support from the appropriate level of anesthesia personnel is a growing concern in the interventional radiology community.

Most interventional radiology suites are inadequately equipped for the administration of anesthesia. This can make appropriate anesthesia difficult. Space becomes a major issue with poor accessibility to the patient because of heavy ceiling- or floor-mounted equipment and possibly reduced staffing with a limited number of nurses and technologists.

Endovascular Procedures in the Operating Room

The operating room is particularly favorable for anesthesia; however, it is much less favorable for the interventional radiologist. Although general anesthesia and deep conscious sedation can easily be performed safely in the operating room setting, the use of portable fluoroscopy equipment markedly increases the scatter radiation and hence the radiation dose to the health professionals. Radiation dose is of particular concern because the patient having an endovascular procedure in the operating room most likely has a complex procedure and hence is likely to require a large radiation exposure to complete the procedure.

Very complex endovascular procedures can, on occasion, require conversion to an open procedure. Emergency conversion of an endovascular procedure frequently represents a catastrophic event requiring aggressive critical care support as well as anesthesia. The anesthesiologist should always be aware that endovascular catastrophe and emergency conversion to an open operation are possibilities.

Percutaneous Transluminal Angioplasty

Percutaneous transluminal angioplasty is the mainstay of endovascular techniques. It can be applied to a variety of anatomic vascular beds as well as a variety of clinical conditions. As technology has improved, supplementation of balloon dilatation with endovascular stents, mechanical atherectomy, and pharmacologic manipulation has improved technical success.[5] (Figure 4-2).

Positioning for angioplasty is related to the site of access. Most access for central and peripheral vascular interventions is through the common femoral artery at the groin, requiring supine positioning. On occasion, alternative access sites are required because of specific issues related to the patient. Standard alternative access sites are the axillary, brachial, and popliteal arteries. Positioning requirements change for each of these access sites. The axillary artery requires the supine position with the arm above the head. Brachial artery access requires supine positioning with the arm directly extended. Popliteal artery access requires prone positioning. Different positions affect the placement of anesthetic equipment.

The time required to perform an angioplasty procedure varies. As alluded to earlier, difficulty in any of the five steps throughout the procedure can add significant time to the procedure itself. In general, however, aortoiliac angioplasty is usually achieved successfully in 1 to 2 hours. Lower extremity angioplasty frequently requires somewhat more time, but 2 to 3 hours is a reasonable expectation. Subclavian artery and carotid artery interventions can be performed relatively quickly in the 1- to 2-hour range; however, the potential for a neurologic complication may markedly increase the length of the procedure.[6]

Complications of Angioplasty

The most common complication of angioplasty involves the access site.[7] Hematoma at the access site can be small and limited to the surrounding area or extend along body planes. Especially at the usual common femoral artery access site, large hematomas can occur and extend into the retroperitoneum with significant blood loss.

A worsening scenario similar to hematoma is the pseudoaneurysm with persistent flow through the access artery into the hematoma. The pseudoaneurysm represents a more difficult clinical challenge often requiring a second procedure for correction.

Postaccess arterial venous fistula is also a well-known complication. It is thought that this results from a through-and-through

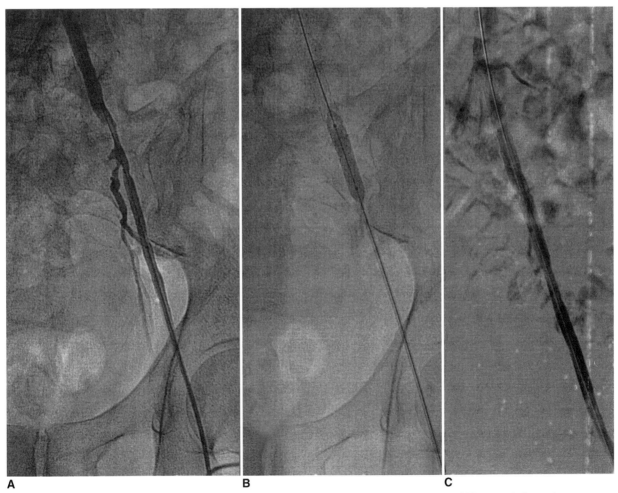

A   **B**   **C**

FIGURE 4-2 Iliac artery primary stent angiography: **A,** Preprocedure. **B,** Balloon expandable stent deployment. **C,** Postprocedure.

puncture of the artery that also enters the vein, thereby causing a variation on the post-traumatic arterial venous fistula. Occasionally, this fistula can lead to high-output cardiac failure (Figure 4-3).

Complications at the site of intervention or secondary to guide wire and catheter techniques also occur. Specifically, endovascular dissection, spasm, acute thrombosis, and arterial rupture have been well described (Figure 4-4A and B).[7] Although these are rare, when they do occur complex interventions are frequently required with a marked prolongation of the procedure. In addition, if the endovascular technique is unable to reverse these complications, conversion to an open procedure may be necessary. The anesthesiologist must always be aware that conversion to an open procedure is a possibility.

Complications distal to the intervention site, secondary to distal embolization of bits of fractured plaque or thrombus, also occur. Again, addressing these complications can be time consuming and ultimately require conversion to an open procedure.

Cholesterol embolism is a devastating complication related to cholesterol crystals beneath the atherosclerotic plaque.[5] Little can be done to address this issue. It is evident by classical findings on the trunk and lower extremities. The classical finding is livedo reticularis, painful small cyanotic patches on the skin.

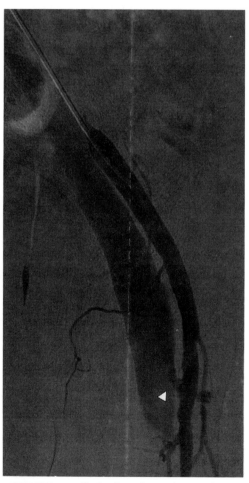

FIGURE 4-3 Postangiography arteriovenous fistula.

Renal failure is always a concern after iodine contrast agent administration. Angiographic control for endovascular interventions is a particular risk because of the extensive imaging requirements. Support for contrast-induced nephropathy is not an uncommon clinical need.

Endovascular Stent Graft

Advances in stent technology have allowed the development of stent grafts. This technique uses a premanufactured covered stent to exclude aneurysms and traumatically injured segments of vessel (Figure 4-5).

Because the device is an endovascular graft rolled on a self-expanding stent, it requires large access sites. The aortic device can require access sites of 22F or larger, limiting access to the common femoral approach. In addition, it requires open visualization at the arterial access site. The cutdown procedure at the common femoral artery adds complexity to the access portion of the procedure and adds time to the total procedure length.

The procedure itself should be well planned after extensive diagnostic evaluation before the patient is brought to the operating room. Contrast injection remains necessary to control deployment of the device.

Currently approved aortic devices are bifurcated and deploy from the aorta into both common iliac arteries, which requires secondary access at the contralateral common femoral artery to deploy the contralateral limb of the graft. This access site is smaller than the primary access site and frequently can be managed in a percutaneous fashion. Some operators prefer a third access site from the left upper extremity for contrast injection during deployment of the device.

After the aortic and ipsilateral limbs are deployed, it is necessary to steer a guide wire through the contralateral limb acceptance site into the aortic graft. Although there is some learning curve in this technique, it is usually not difficult. Once the second guide wire is in position, the contralateral limb can be safely deployed.

Some difficulties can be encountered in deploying the aortic device with poor expansions of the stent or failure to release from the delivery system. These issues have improved as technology improves but still remain a concern. These factors may add additional time to the procedure and ultimately require conversion to an open procedure.

As technology improves, the delivery systems are less cumbersome and require less time to deploy. At this time the procedure requires 2 to 4 hours. Because of the potential for emergency open conversion, nearly all patients undergo this procedure under general anesthesia in a room in which aortofemoral or aortoiliac bypass grafting can be performed.

Potential complications from these procedures are acute occlusion of the aorta, aortoiliac injury and laceration, failure of deployment of the device, maldeployment of the device, and access site complications.[8]

Complications related to deployment of the device are failure of the device to deploy, which may be addressed from an endovascular approach but more than likely requires conversion to an open procedure, and misplacement of the device, which occludes a visceral artery such as a renal artery. Arterial occlusion may also be dealt with through an endovascular

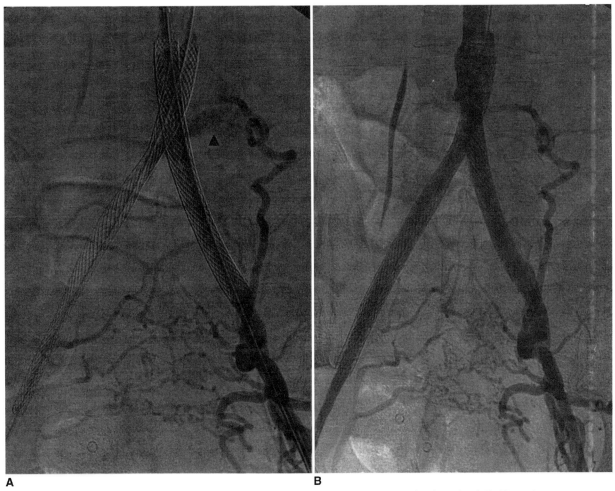

A   **B**

FIGURE 4-4 Iliac artery rupture during balloon angioplasty. **A,** Contrast extravasation (*arrowhead*). **B,** After endovascular repair with a stent graft.

approach but is more likely to require conversion to an open procedure.[8]

Other complications include endoleaks, which more accurately reflect failure of the device and are identified in a delayed fashion. In addition, groin complications similar to those with angioplasty can be encountered. Acute aneurysm rupture is also a feared complication, which requires conversion to an open procedure.

Thrombolytic Therapy

Acute thrombotic or embolic occlusions of the arterial tree can be managed effectively with a variety of thrombolytic medications delivered into the clot through an infusion catheter. The technique centers on a diagnostic angiogram, which confirms the location of the acute thrombus. Using a guide wire and catheter technique, the infusion catheter is embedded within the thrombus and direct infusion of thrombolytic drugs carried out. Although two methods are described, the pulse spray technique and the drip-infusion technique, most centers utilize the drip-infusion technique.

Pulse spray of acute thrombus is performed with the operator pulsing small amounts of thrombolytic medication into the clot over 20-minute intervals with frequent contrast injection to evaluate progress. This technique is tedious for operators and personnel and may require 1 to 2 hours and yield mixed results.

The drip-infusion technique is somewhat more favorable for the operator and personnel; however, it takes quite a bit more time. The time within the procedure room is usually limited to the diagnostic angiography plus an additional placement of the infusion catheter. Drip infusion, over 7 to 24 or more hours, is then completed in the intensive care unit. The patient usually returns to the angiography suite for interval evaluation at approximately 8-hour intervals. After completion of thrombolytic therapy, a focal lesion may be identified that can then be treated with endovascular angioplasty.

Complications of thrombolytic therapy are related to the coagulopathy that is induced. Access site hematoma, extending into the retroperitoneal space, and bleeding at other sites, including intracranial hemorrhage and gastrointestinal hemorrhage, can be life threatening.[9]

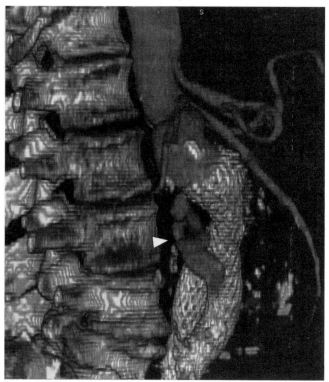

FIGURE 4-5 Computed tomographic angiogram showing bifurcated aortic endograft with posterior endoleak (*arrowhead*).

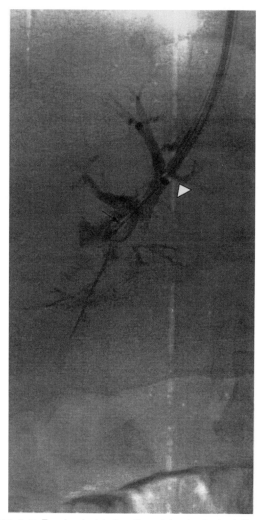

FIGURE 4-6 Transjugular intrahepatic portal systemic shunt. Needle tip in portal vein (*arrow*). Steel directioning canula in hepatic vein (*arrowhead*).

Transjugular Intrahepatic Portal Systemic Shunt

The TIPS procedure is utilized in the setting of portal hypertension. Patients who do not respond to medical management to control variceal bleeding or recurrent ascites qualify for this procedure. This procedure does, however, place additional load on the heart by increasing venous return. Therefore, patients with preprocedure heart failure are not candidates for this procedure. On occasion, patients are brought to the angiography area for an emergency TIPS because of failure of endoscopic techniques for gastrointestinal hemorrhage.

The procedure is performed through the right internal jugular vein. The first step in the procedure is to measure right atrial pressure. If right atrial pressure is too high (higher than portal pressure), no TIPS can be created. This does not mean that the procedure is terminated; rather, the portosystemic shunt is not created. Access via the liver through the portal vein is still obtained and an attempt is made at coil embolization of the bleeding varices.

After standard hepatic venography and pressure evaluation, a large steel directioning canula is inserted into the right hepatic vein. The steel canula is then directed anteriorly and a thin-walled long needle advanced through the canula through the substance of the liver into the portal vein (Figure 4-6). This is then confirmed to be in an appropriate position by contrast injection and, using a guide wire catheter exchange technique, a catheter is advanced into the portal vein. Portal vein imaging is then performed.

If the patient is a favorable candidate, the TIPS is then created with a balloon catheter followed by transhepatic stent deployment (Figure 4-7). Usually the pressure in the portal system is reduced and the portal systemic pressure gradient is reduced to less than 5 mmHg. This effectively treats the varices by removing their pressure heads. Very large varices can be additionally controlled with the coil embolization technique. The coil embolization technique alone can be carried out in a setting in which the patient is not a candidate for the TIPS shunt.

Potential complications of this procedure are perforation of the liver with intra-abdominal bleeding, injury to the portal vein, liver laceration, acute congestive heart failure, failure of the procedure with uncontrollable variceal bleeding, and death.[10]

The puncture from the hepatic vein to the portal vein requires control of the patient's respiration to stabilize the liver. For this reason, most TIPS procedures are performed under general anesthesia.[11] The procedure takes from 2 to 4 hours to complete. In patients with marked ascites or unusual liver anatomy, it may take even longer. In addition, coil embolization

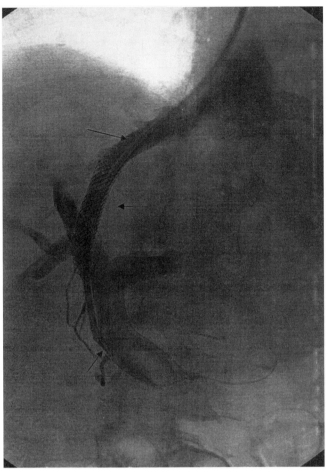

FIGURE 4-7 Transjugular intrahepatic portal systemic shunt. Hepatic vein (*top arrow*), TIPS stent (*middle arrow*), portal vein (*bottom arrow*).

of varices can be technically difficult, adding several hours to the procedure.

Inferior Vena Cava Filter Placement

Inferior vena cava filter placement is performed in the setting of deep vein thrombosis of the lower extremities of a patient who has not responded to anticoagulation therapy, or in whom anticoagulation therapy is contraindicated, to prevent pulmonary embolism.

Access is achieved through the right internal jugular vein, the right common femoral vein, or alternative sites—in specific circumstances, either the antecubital vein or other locations. These alternative sites require careful selection of a device.

The procedure consists of obtaining access and then performing an inferior venacavogram. The cavogram assesses intracaval clot, location of the renal veins, and anatomic variation such as duplicated inferior vena cava. In the setting of the duplicated inferior vena cava, two inferior vena cava filters are required. In the setting of intracaval thrombus, if it extends to the level of the renal veins, suprarenal placement of the filter has to be performed. In addition, if the patient's inferior vena cava is quite large (>28 mm), careful choice of the filter device is necessary (Figure 4-8). After the inferior venacavogram is performed, the inferior vena cava filter is deployed below the

level of the renal veins except in specific clinical situations. The procedure usually takes 30 to 60 minutes.

Acute complications of inferior vena cava filter placement are unusual. However, acute caval thrombosis is a consideration. In addition, embolization of the deep vein thrombosis with acute pulmonary embolism can still occur in this setting. If there is large clot burden in the femoral and iliac veins, manipulation can cause acute embolism.[12] Most complications, however, are delayed and related to caval thrombosis or failure of the inferior vena cava filter.

Dialysis Access Management

Maintaining dialysis access is the mainstay of modern interventional radiology practice. Treatment of thrombus or malfunctioning dialysis shunts encompasses a broad range of endovascular skill.

The clotted shunt is a particular problem. Current techniques to restore flow include three main approaches: (1) thrombolytic therapy, (2) thrombectomy, and (3) combination of 1 and 2. Thrombolytic therapy involves thrombolytic medications that dissolve the clot within the graft. Mechanical thrombectomy macerates the clot, allowing it to flow safely back into the venous system, and open thrombectomy removes clot from the graft. The endovascular techniques focus on mechanical thrombectomy and thrombolytic therapy.

Thrombolytic therapy is quite successful and safe. Procedure time is approximately 1 hour to achieve restoration of flow. A post-thrombolysis shuntogram is performed to evaluate the arterial and venous anastomoses as well as the outflow veins. Depending on these findings, additional interventions may take up to an additional 2 hours to effect balloon dilatation and possibly stent placement (Figure 4-9).

Mechanical thrombectomy is similar to thrombolytic therapy. Mechanical thrombectomy takes approximately the same amount of time as thrombolytic therapy. A post-thrombectomy shuntogram is performed to evaluate the causative issues.

Potential complications of graft management include embolization of clot material with pulmonary embolism; embolization of clot into the arterial inflow site with distal arterial embolization; and complications of the thrombolytic therapy itself. Delayed manifestation of an infected graft is also a concern.[13]

Complications of a balloon angioplasty within the graft are acute graft rupture or thrombosis, which may require aggressive management but can usually be controlled from an endovascular approach (Figure 4-10).

Peripheral and Central Venous Interventions

Deep vein thrombosis in the lower extremities, while posing significant risk of pulmonary embolism, also manifests as a specific clinical entity. The postphlebitic syndrome with venous stasis and swollen legs is of particular concern. In an attempt to improve the postphlebitic syndrome, thrombolytic therapy for deep vein thrombosis has been applied. Thrombolytic therapy is likely to be effective only in the first 2 to 3 weeks after clot formation. After this time, valvular

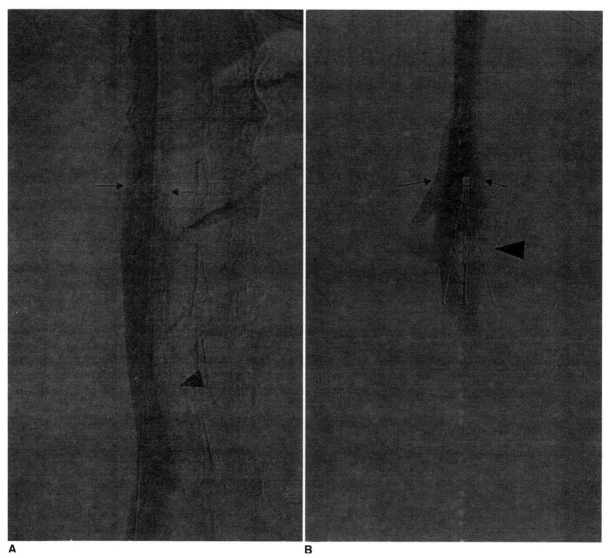

A   B

FIGURE 4-8 Inferior vena cava (IVC) filter placement. **A,** Thrombus in left common iliac vein and lower IVC (*arrow-head*). Inflow defect at renal veins (*arrows*). **B,** IVC filter (*arrowhead*) with proximal tip at renal vein inflow (*arrows*).

damage and organization of the clot make the technique less successful.

In this procedure, the thrombosed segment of vein is reached in a retrograde fashion usually from a popliteal venous approach. Drip-infusion technique is then utilized. Infusions for up to 1 week are required to clear the venous clot. The potential complications of the technique are dislodgment of the clot with pulmonary embolism and potential death and complications of thrombolytic therapy with hemorrhage in various parts of the body.[14]

Venous reconstruction can also be performed. Central vein stenosis in the upper and lower extremities can easily be identified during venography. Using angioplasty and stenting technique, restoration of flow through the central veins can be achieved. Difficulties can be encountered when recanalizing the central veins and procedures may be prolonged, requir-ing several hours to complete. Potential complications of central vein reconstruction are low but include central vein laceration and thrombus embolization with pulmonary embolism.[15,16]

Miscellaneous Endovascular Procedures
Acute Hemorrhage Embolization

In the acutely traumatized or symptomatic patient with acute bleeding, the injured vessel can frequently be identified and occluded using coil or particulate embolization techniques. These patients are usually unstable at presentation, requiring aggressive resuscitation and medical support during the per-formance of the procedure. On occasion, these procedures can be prolonged because of the requirement for subselective catheterization.

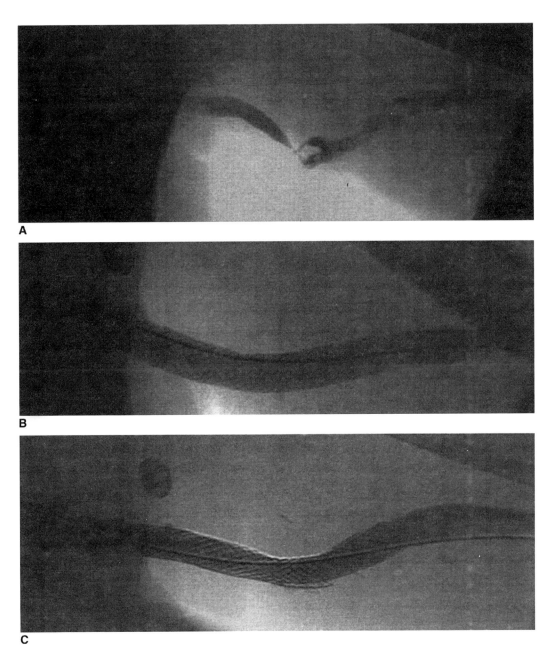

FIGURE 4-9 Upper arm dialysis graft with venous anastomosis stenosis. **A,** Stenosis. **B,** Angioplasty with stent deployment. **C,** Restored patency.

Gastrointestinal Procedures

Mesenteric ischemia without signs of peritonitis may be treated with vasodilator therapy. This approach is particularly useful in the setting of nonocclusive mesenteric ischemia. Gastrointestinal hemorrhage can be addressed using the transcatheter embolization technique. Procedures can be prolonged because of the requirement for subselective catheterization.

Neurointerventional Therapy

Endovascular techniques for the treatment of carotid artery disease, intracranial aneurysms, and arterial venous malformations, and transcatheter techniques for other intracranial

pathology such as tumors have improved over the past 10 to 15 years. These procedures require high-grade biplane angiography equipment and can be performed only in selected centers. There is an absolute requirement for stillness of the patient for many of these procedures because of the delicate nature of the technique. General anesthesia with neuromuscular blockade and controlled ventilation is essential for the success of many of these techniques. Neurointerventional endovascular procedures are never quick. Procedure times from 2 to 12 hours may be required.

Complications include acute subarachnoid hemorrhage and acute vessel thrombosis, both of which can result in stroke and

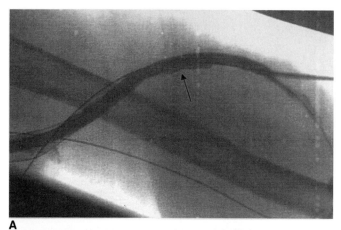

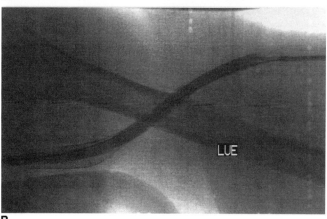

FIGURE 4-10 Dialysis graft rupture after angioplasty. **A,** Perigraft contrast indicates graft rupture (*arrow*). **B,** Repair with endovascular stent graft.

sudden death. In addition, prolonged radiation exposure can result in superficial burns.

Although endovascular techniques appear minimally invasive, complications can be severe, requiring prolonged endovascular procedures or conversion to open technique in an urgent way.

REFERENCES

1. Conover MB: Radiation hazards. In Tilkian AG, Daily EK: *Cardiovascular procedures; diagnostic techniques and therapeutic procedures,* St. Louis, 1986, Mosby, 451.
2. Marx MV: Radiation exposure in interventional radiology. In Ansell G, Bettmann MA, Kaufman JA, Wilkins RA (eds): *Complications in diagnostic imaging and interventional radiology,* ed 3, part 2, Cambridge, MA, 1996, Blackwell Science, 133.
3. FDA Public Health Advisory: Avoidance of serious x-ray induced skin injuries to patients during fluoroscopically guided procedures. U.S. Food and Drug Administration: *Medical bulletin,* USFDA, September 30, 1994.
4. Geise RA, Morain RL: Radiation management in interventional radiology. In Wilfrido R. Castaneda-Zuniga: *Interventional radiology,* ed 3, vol 1, Baltimore 1997, Lippincott, Williams & Wilkins, 1.
5. LaBerge JM, Darcy MD (eds): *Peripheral vascular interventions,* Fairfax, VA, 1994, Society of Cardiovascular & Interventional Radiology.
6. Kachel R: Current status and future possibilities of balloon angioplasty in the carotid artery. In Connors JJ III, Wojak JC (eds): *Interventional neuroradiology: strategies and practical techniques,* Philadelphia, 1999, WB Saunders, 473.
7. Wilkinson LS, Wilkins RA: Complications of percutaneous angioplasty. In Ansell G, Bettmann MA, Kaufman JA, Wilkins RA (eds): *Complications in diagnostic imaging and interventional radiology,* ed 3, part 4, Cambridge, MA, 1996, Blackwell Science, 346.
8. Fox LA, Powell A: Troubleshooting techniques for abdominal aortic aneurysm endograft placement: when things go wrong, *Tech Vasc Interv Radiol* 4:213, 2001.
9. McNamara TO, Dong P, Chen J, et al: Bleeding complications associated with the use of rt-PA versus r-PA for peripheral arterial and venous thromboembolic occlusions, *Tech Vasc Interv Radiol* 4:92, 2001.
10. Sawhney R, Wall SD: TIPS complications, *Tech Vasc Interv Radiol* 1:80, 1998.
11. Tongprasert S, Torralba SM: Anesthesia for interventional radiology, *Adv Anesth* 19:127, 2001.
12. Nicholson AA: Inferior vena cava filters. In Dyet JF, Nicholson AA, Ettles DF, Wilson SE: *Textbook of endovascular procedures,* New York, 2000, Churchill Livingstone, 234.
13. Aruny JE: Maintaining native arteriovenous fistulas for dialysis access, *Tech Vasc Interv Radiol* 2:199, 1999.
14. Semba CP, Galloway I, Earnshaw JJ: Lower limb venous interventions. In Dyet JF, Nicholson AA, Ettles DF, Wilson SE: *Textbook of endovascular procedures,* New York, 2000, Churchill Livingstone, 209.
15. Gray RJ: Angioplasty and stents for peripheral and central venous lesions, *Tech Vasc Interv Radiol* 2:189, 1999.
16. Gaines P, Kafie FE, Wilson SE: Upper limb venous and superior vena cava intervention. In Dyet JF, Nicholson AA, Ettles DF, Wilson SE: *Textbook of endovascular procedures,* New York, 2000, Churchill Livingstone, 222.

Preoperative Cardiac Evaluation before Major Vascular Surgery

5

Lee A. Fleisher, MD

THE patient presenting for major vascular surgery continues to represent a diagnostic dilemma with respect to the appropriate degree of preoperative evaluation. It is now well established that such patients have a high degree of significant coronary artery disease, the majority of which is silent in nature.[1] For these patients, cardiac complications represent the greatest source of both perioperative and long-term morbidity and mortality.[2,3]

On the basis of these facts, numerous investigators have advocated the use of preoperative evaluation and perioperative cardiac interventions as a means of reducing perioperative risk.[4-6] Despite initial enthusiasm and evidence to support such an approval, there are two forces opposing the use of extensive testing. Several authors have questioned the need for extensive diagnostic testing because of a decrease in the incidence of perioperative fatal and nonfatal myocardial infarction (MI).[7-9] In particular, perioperative β-blocker therapy was shown to reduce cardiac morbidity and mortality significantly in two randomized clinical trials.[10,11] The question remains whether this decrease in complication rate is a function of improved preoperative evaluation or perioperative management and whether simply providing routine β-blocker therapy to all patients would be sufficient to prevent major morbidity and mortality. Compounding this clinical controversy are issues related to medical economics. There is increasing emphasis on reducing perioperative cost by reducing preoperative testing. Yet, cardiologists frequently view the preoperative evaluation as a period in which they can identify additional patients with both symptomatic and asymptomatic disease in whom life-prolonging diagnostic evaluations and interventions can be performed. Therefore, there are competing economic incentives surrounding the preoperative evaluation.

This review focuses on the value of preoperative testing as a means of effecting perioperative and long-term interventions that improve patients' health. Both short-term (perioperative) and long-term perspectives are taken in the discussion because the answer may change depending on the perspective used; that is, preoperative cardiac testing and interventions may demonstrate a benefit only if a long-term perspective is taken. Each specific operation is discussed, and the overall strategies advocated in the American Heart Association/American College of Cardiology and American College of Physician Guidelines are reviewed.[12-14]

Carotid Endarterectomy

The extent of preoperative evaluation for a patient undergoing carotid endarterectomy (CEA) has changed dramatically over the years. The major complication following CEA has traditionally been cardiovascular in nature, primarily MI.[15,16] The other primary issue in such patients is related to the nature of the surgery itself, that is, the risk of stroke. In determining the indication for CEA, the clinician must balance the risks of perioperative death and cardiovascular complications against the potential benefit of reducing the risk of sustaining a future stroke. Large-scale studies demonstrating superiority of surgical therapy depended on the institutional perioperative cardiac complication rate. With advances in perioperative care, the literature would suggest that the perioperative cardiac risk has dramatically decreased.[17]

The question remains whether there is a subset of patients in whom an extensive preoperative evaluation is warranted. As already described, the key question is, what potential perioperative interventions would be contemplated in the patient with carotid disease? If extensive coronary artery disease is detected, coronary revascularization might be considered. From a patient's perspective, a stroke is associated with a much worse quality of life than a perioperative MI. For other types of major vascular surgery, coronary revascularization would be considered before the noncardiac surgery. In the case of CEA, the risk of stroke during cardiopulmonary bypass is sufficiently high that CEA is performed before coronary artery bypass grafting (CABG) surgery in many patients.[18-21] The question remains whether selected patients are candidates for a combined procedure.

When combined coronary revascularization and CEA surgery was initially evaluated, perioperative morbidity and mortality were extremely high, limiting the usefulness of such an approach.[18] In fact, a meta-analysis published in 1999 suggested that staged procedures are associated with lower risk than combined procedures.[21] More recent studies have indicated that a combined procedure can be performed safely in selected high-risk patients.[19,22-28] Current clinical judgment suggests that the indications for a combined procedure are unstable or highly symptomatic coronary artery disease and carotid disease.[22] Yet, the utilization of off-pump coronary artery bypass may change the decision if it is truly associated with lower neurologic risk.[29,30]

On the basis of the available evidence, the initial evaluation of the patient for CEA should include a determination of whether highly symptomatic coronary artery disease is present. Specifically, symptoms consistent with unstable angina or angina with minimal exercise and signs of left ventricular dysfunction denote such a population. For those patients, further cardiovascular testing and potentially a combined carotid-cardiac operation should be considered. For patients who have an excellent exercise tolerance, even in the presence of chronic stable angina, further diagnostic evaluation is not required before carotid surgery because coronary revascularization would not be required preoperatively. Patients with carotid disease should be considered at high risk, and long-term evaluation and management of atherosclerotic disease should be considered.

Aortic Surgery

The patient undergoing aortic surgery is the best studied and defined with regard to the value of preoperative cardiovascular evaluation and testing. Aortic surgery is usually either elective or emergent (e.g., a ruptured aneurysm). For emergent procedures, no preoperative evaluation is possible except for an abbreviated history. For elective procedures, perioperative morbidity and mortality have traditionally been considered high and interventions are frequently contemplated. In fact, three decision algorithms have been published evaluating the value of diagnostic testing and coronary revascularization before abdominal aortic surgery.[31-33]

In addition to considering coronary revascularization, changes in monitoring may be contemplated on the basis of the probability and extent of coronary artery disease. Several randomized trials attempted to address issues of outcome in vascular surgery patients with respect to the use of a pulmonary artery (PA) catheter. For patients undergoing aortic surgery, a PA catheter was not associated with improved outcomes compared with those of patients who had a central venous pressure catheter if the ejection fraction was greater than 50% in one small study or if the patient had a negative cardiovascular workup or prior coronary intervention in a second study.[34,35] Polanczyk and colleagues performed a variation on a case-control study (using a propensity index) to determine whether the use of a PA catheter was associated with worse outcomes for noncardiac surgery.[36] No difference in cardiac events was noted, but an increased incidence of congestive heart failure was detected in the PA catheter group. Aortic surgery was excluded from this study, making it difficult to generalize to these patients. However, many clinicians believe that a PA catheter does have added benefit if extensive coronary artery disease is present. Therefore a negative work-up may have value and be cost-effective in identifying low-risk patients in whom pulmonary catheter monitoring may be of no or minimal benefit.

In determining the need for cardiac evaluation in aortic surgery, there may be differences between aneurysmal and occlusive disease. Patients with occlusive disease clearly have extensive atherosclerosis, but the intraoperative course may be better tolerated because the cross-clamp is rarely placed above the renal arteries and many patients may have extensive collateral vessels. Aneurysmal disease is commonly related to atherosclerosis but may also be due to nonatherosclerotic processes. Therefore, atherosclerosis may be minimal in some patients, but the intraoperative course may be more "stressful" because of the absence of collaterals and the potential for a suprarenal or supraceliac cross-clamp. All of these factors must be incorporated into the decision to undertake further evaluation.

Infrainguinal Bypass Surgery

The patient undergoing infrainguinal revascularization represents a unique diagnostic dilemma. Diffuse atherosclerotic disease is a hallmark of such patients.[1] However, many clinicians view infrainguinal surgery as less risky than aortic surgery. The absence of a cross-clamp on the aorta and a nonintraabdominal procedure led some to classify this procedure as lower risk than aortic surgery. Counterbalancing the less invasive nature of the surgery is the high probability of diffuse atherosclerotic disease. In several comparative studies of infrainguinal versus aortic surgery, the rates of cardiac morbidity and mortality were similar in the two groups.[3,37,38] Patients undergoing aortic surgery have more intraoperative myocardial ischemia, whereas patients undergoing infrainguinal surgery have more risk factors, such as congestive heart failure. The patients also have a high incidence of long-term cardiac morbidity and mortality after discharge home.[39] Therefore, it may be prudent to continue performing preoperative cardiac testing in patients undergoing infrainguinal surgery because of their overall high perioperative and long-term cardiovascular risk.

Unlike aortic and carotid surgery, infrainguinal surgery is frequently performed on an urgent basis. Although many patients undergo revascularization for claudication pain, a substantial number of individuals have surgery for nonhealing ulcers or pain at rest. The potential changes in perioperative management are less well defined for the patient requiring infrainguinal bypass surgery. One alternative operation is undergoing amputation as an initial procedure. However, amputation is associated with the highest perioperative and long-term risk because of the inability to rehabilitate and the sedentary lifestyle.[40] Many clinicians, therefore, believe that revascularization is a more prudent option in most patients.

The decision to perform coronary revascularization prior to infrainguinal surgery is in part dependent on the urgency of the surgery. As previously noted, most of the surgeries are of an urgent nature and therefore coronary bypass grafting is not a viable option. As discussed later in the chapter, percutaneous transluminal coronary angioplasty (PTCA) performed immediately prior to noncardiac surgery may not confer major beneficial effects. Yet, in a highly symptomatic patient with signs of left ventricular dysfunction, the use of PTCA may be beneficial. However, evidence suggests that the use of a coronary stent within 30 days of noncardiac surgery is associated with high rates of complications, including death.[41] PTCA may allow easier management during the perioperative period, but there is no evidence to suggest that such an approach reduces cardiac complications. Use of more invasive monitoring in high-risk patients has also been considered. In two randomized trials to address this issue in infrainguinal surgery, there was no difference in the rate of cardiac complications in those who routinely had PA catheters inserted compared with those who had them placed only if indications existed.[42,43] In one study, there was a lower rate of graft thrombosis in the patients without a PA catheter, but other maneuvers such as the use of regional anesthesia may obviate this effect.[42]

Therefore, the decision to perform diagnostic testing in the patient undergoing infrainguinal revascularization surgery depends upon the potential benefit of further defining coronary artery disease. In patients with unstable angina or angina at minimal exercise, further testing might identify patients with high-risk anatomy in whom coronary revascularization would be appropriate. This evaluation may occur preoperatively in patients undergoing elective procedures or postoperatively in urgent cases.

Clinical Risk

In 1977, Goldman and colleagues published their landmark article studying 1001 patients undergoing noncardiac surgical procedures, excluding transurethral resection of the prostate (TURP).[44] The authors excluded this surgery because of their impression of a low morbidity rate when performed under spinal anesthesia. They identified nine risk factors and gave each factor a certain number of points (Goldman Cardiac Risk Index or CRI). An MI and S_3 gallop were identified as the most significant risk factors. By adding up the total number of points, patients were placed in one of four classes. The patient's class could then be compared with the rates of morbidity and mortality from the original cohort.

The CRI was subsequently validated in another cohort of patients; however, it has not been found to be predictive in patients undergoing major vascular surgery.[45,46] Multiple studies have demonstrated that major vascular surgery is associated with a higher rate of morbidity and mortality than nonvascular surgery.[44,47-49] In order to rectify this problem, Detsky and colleagues proposed a modification of the CRI for vascular patients.[50]

Although both of these indices were extremely useful when initially proposed, perioperative care has changed significantly in the intervening years. Goldman classes III and IV continue to represent a high-risk cohort; however, mortality has been lower than originally reported.[51] In addition, many vascular surgery patients would be classified as low risk but would benefit from further risk stratification.[46] Significant changes in the medical care of the patient with coronary artery disease have had profound impact on the perioperative period.

In an attempt to update the original index, Goldman and colleagues at Brigham and Women's Hospital studied 4315 patients older than 50 years undergoing elective major noncardiac procedures in a tertiary-care teaching hospital.[52] Six independent predictors of complications were identified and included in a Revised Cardiac Risk Index: high-risk type of surgery, history of ischemic heart disease, history of congestive heart failure, history of cerebrovascular disease, preoperative treatment with insulin, and preoperative serum creatinine greater than 2.0 mg/dL. Rates of major cardiac complication with 0, 1, 2, or 3 of these factors were 0.5%, 1.3%, 4%, and 9%, respectively, in the derivation cohort and 0.4%, 0.9%, 7%, and 11%, respectively, among 1422 patients in the validation cohort.

A primary issue with all of these indices from the anesthesiologist's perspective is that a simple estimate of risk does not help in refining perioperative management but may provide information to assess the probability of risk. In contrast, the anesthesiologist is most concerned with defining the cardiovascular risk factors and symptoms or signs of unstable cardiac disease states such as myocardial ischemia, congestive heart failure, valvular heart disease, and significant cardiac arrhyth-

mias. Guidelines on Perioperative Cardiovascular Evaluation for Noncardiac Surgery from the American Heart Association/American College of Cardiology acknowledge the contribution of the numerous risk indices related to preoperative cardiac evaluation; however, they primarily approached the question of clinical risk on the basis of three distinct categories: major, intermediate, and minor.[14]

Clinical Evaluation of the Patient

The clinical evaluation of the patient must begin by identification of major clinical risk factors (Table 5-1). The *major clinical predictors* of increased perioperative cardiovascular risk are unstable coronary syndromes such as recent MI with evidence of important ischemic risk and unstable or severe angina; decompensated congestive heart failure, significant arrhythmias (high-grade atrioventricular block, symptomatic arrhythmias in the presence of underlying heart disease, supraventricular arrhythmias with uncontrolled ventricular rate), and severe valvular disease.

Patients with acute coronary syndromes, such as unstable angina or decompensated congestive heart failure of ischemic origin, are at high risk of developing further decompensation, myocardial necrosis, and death during the perioperative

---

TABLE 5-1

Clinical Predictors of Increased Perioperative Cardiovascular Risk (Myocardial Infarction, Congestive Heart Failure, Death)

Major

Unstable coronary syndromes
Recent myocardial infarction* with evidence of important ischemic risk with clinical symptoms or noninvasive study
Unstable or severe angina (Canadian class III or IV)†
Decompensated congestive heart failure
Significant arrhythmias
High-grade atrioventricular block
Symptomatic ventricular arrhythmias in the presence of underlying heart disease
Supraventricular arrhythmias with uncontrolled ventricular rate
Severe valvular disease

Intermediate

Mild angina pectoris (Canadian class I or II)
Prior myocardial infarction by history or pathologic Q waves
Compensated or prior congestive heart failure
Diabetes mellitus
Chronic renal insufficiency

Minor

Advanced age
Abnormal ECG (left ventricular hypertrophy, left bundle branch block, ST-T abnormalities)
Rhythm other than sinus (e.g., atrial fibrillation)
Low functional capacity (e.g., inability to climb one flight of stairs with a bag of groceries)
History of stroke
Uncontrolled systemic hypertension

*The American College of Cardiology National Database Library defines recent MI as greater than 7 days but less than or equal to 1 month (30 days).
†Campeau L: Grading of angina pectoris, *Circulation* 54:522, 1976.
ECG, electrocardiogram.
From Eagle KA, Berger PB, Calkins H, et al: *J Am Coll Cardiol* 39:542, 2002.

period.[53] Such patients should not undergo noncardiac surgery except in the most emergent of circumstances. If this surgery is truly emergent, stabilization by pharmacologic and mechanical interventions such as intra-aortic balloon pump counterpulsation is warranted.

Patients with a prior MI have coronary artery disease, although a small group of patients may sustain an MI from a nonatherosclerotic mechanism. Traditionally, risk assessment for noncardiac surgery was based upon the time interval between the MI and surgery. Multiple studies have demonstrated an increased incidence of reinfarction if the MI was within 6 months of surgery.[54-56] With improvements in perioperative care, this difference has decreased.[57]

However, the importance of the intervening time interval may no longer be valid in the current era of thrombolytics, angioplasty, and risk stratification after an acute MI. Although many patients with an MI may continue to have myocardium at risk for subsequent ischemia and infarction, other patients may have their critical coronary stenosis either totally occluded or widely patent. The American Heart Association/American College of Cardiology Task Force on Perioperative Evaluation of the Cardiac Patient Undergoing Noncardiac Surgery has advocated that patients with an MI less than 6 weeks old as the group at highest risk; after that period, risk stratification is based upon the presentation of disease (i.e., those with active ischemia being at highest risk).[14]

Intermediate predictors of increased risk are the factors that have been associated with higher perioperative risk in multiple studies. The guidelines currently consider mild angina pectoris, prior MI, compensated or prior congestive heart failure, chronic renal insufficiency, and diabetes mellitus as intermediate risk factors.

Minor predictors of risk are those associated with coronary artery disease, but their relationship with perioperative cardiac complications is not well established. These include advanced age, abnormal electrocardiogram, rhythm other than sinus, low functional capacity, history of stroke, and uncontrolled systemic hypertension.

Guidelines for Preoperative Testing for Coronary Artery Disease

Multiple algorithms have been published regarding the use of preoperative cardiovascular testing prior to vascular surgery; however, there have been no studies to evaluate their validity.[12-14,58,59] The American College of Cardiology and American Heart Association have updated their Guidelines on Perioperative Cardiovascular Evaluation for Noncardiac Surgery and have reaffirmed their original algorithm on the basis of expert opinion and the accumulating evidence.[12,14] The approach that the guideline takes is the integration of clinical risk factors, exercise capacity, and the surgical procedure into the decision process.

Nine basic steps are advocated (Figure 5-1). First, the clinician must evaluate the urgency of the surgery and the appropriateness of a formal preoperative assessment. Next, the clinician determines whether the patient has undergone a previous revascularization procedure or coronary evaluation. If the evaluation was negative, the patient should proceed to surgery. The patients with unstable coronary syndromes should be identified

and appropriate treatment instituted. Finally, the decision to undergo further testing depends upon the interaction of the clinical risk factors (see Table 5-1), surgery-specific risk (Table 5-2), and functional capacity (Table 5-3). The authors of the guideline suggest that all patients undergoing aortic or infrainguinal bypass surgery should be considered at high surgical risk, and, therefore, further evaluation should be considered. Patients undergoing carotid surgery should be considered at moderate risk.

The American College of Physicians guideline attempts to apply the evidence-based approach.[13] The initial decision point is the assessment of risk using the Detsky modification of the CRI. If patients are in class II or III, they are considered at high risk. If they are in class I, the presence of other clinical factors according to work by Eagle and colleagues or Vanzetto and colleagues is used for further stratification of risk.[60,61] Those with multiple markers for cardiovascular disease according to these risk indices and those undergoing major vascular surgery are considered appropriate for further diagnostic testing by either dipyridamole imaging or dobutamine stress echocardiography.

There has been a great deal of nonrandomized evidence to support a Bayesian approach to testing. The algorithm proposed in the American Heart Association/American College of Cardiology guidelines has been prospectively tested. Bartels and colleagues employed an algorithm similar to the guidelines in which testing was reserved for selected patients and reported low rates of morbidity and mortality.[62] Despite the guidelines' suggestion that all patients undergoing high-risk vascular surgery require testing, most investigators have shown that testing is indicated only in selected patients. Eagle and colleagues evaluated the implications of the prior probability of disease based upon clinical criteria in determining the predictive value of preoperative testing.[60] Patients without clinical risk factors (angina, Q waves, ventricular ectopic activity being treated, diabetes, age older than 70 years) had only a 3% incidence of perioperative morbidity, and noninvasive testing could not further stratify risk. Similarly, patients with three or more clinical risk factors had 50% morbidity and noninvasive testing did not further discriminate risk. Preoperative dipyridamole thallium imaging was, however, useful in the group at moderate risk (one or two risk factors). This concept, whereby the probability of a disease outcome after testing is a function of the probability of disease before testing and the sensitivity and specificity of the test, is an application of Bayes' theorem. It helps explain differences in predictive values reported between consecutive and selective series of patients.

Paul and colleagues evaluated the ability of these clinical risk factors to predict angiographic severity of coronary artery disease in patients undergoing vascular surgery.[63] Using the cohort of patients at the Cleveland Clinic who underwent angiography, they demonstrated that critical three-vessel and/or left main disease was present in only 5% of low-risk patients (no risk factors) and 43% of high-risk patients (more than two risk factors). The authors developed a clinical predictive rule whereby the absence of angina, prior MI, or history of congestive heart failure is associated with a 94% predictive value for being free of critical coronary disease.

Two studies illustrate the reduced value of noninvasive testing when consecutive surgical patients (i.e., nonselected) are

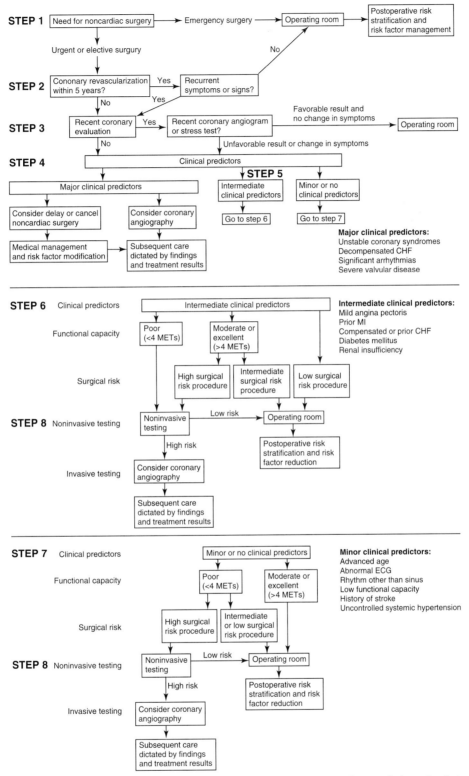

FIGURE 5-1 The American Heart Association/American College of Cardiology Task Force on Perioperative Evaluation of Cardiac Patients Undergoing Noncardiac Surgery has proposed an algorithm for decisions regarding the need for further evaluation. It is one of multiple algorithms proposed in the literature. It is based upon expert opinion and incorporates eight steps. First, the clinician must evaluate the urgency of the surgery and the appropriateness of a formal preoperative assessment. Next, he or she must determine whether the patient has had a previous revascularization procedure or coronary evaluation. The patients with unstable coronary syndromes should be identified, and appropriate treatment should be instituted. The decision to have further testing depends on the interaction of the clinical risk factors, surgery-specific risk, and functional capacity. CHF, congestive heart failure; ECG, electrocardiogram; MET, metabolic equivalent; MI, myocardial infarction. (Adapted from Eagle KA, Berger PB, Calkins H, et al: *J Am Coll Cardiol* 39:542, 2002.)

TABLE 5-2

Cardiac Risk* Stratification for Noncardiac Surgical Procedures

High	(Reported cardiac risk often >5%)
	Emergent major operations, particularly in the elderly
	Aortic and other major vascular
	Peripheral vascular
	Anticipated prolonged surgical procedures associated with large fluid shifts and/or blood loss
Intermediate	(Reported cardiac risk generally <5%)
	Carotid endarterectomy
	Head and neck
	Intraperitoneal and intrathoracic
	Orthopedic
	Prostate
Low[†]	(Reported cardiac risk generally <1%)
	Endoscopic procedure
	Superficial procedure
	Cataract
	Breast

*Combined incidence of cardiac death and nonfatal myocardial infarction.
[†]Do not generally require further preoperative cardiac testing.
From Eagle KA, Berger PB, Calkins H, et al: *J Am Coll Cardiol* 39:542, 2002.

studied. Mangano and colleagues studied 60 consecutive patients undergoing vascular surgery and reported a positive predictive value of 27% for adverse cardiac events, a negative predictive value of 82%, and no net discriminative ability of the test.[64] Baron and colleagues studied the largest (457) consecutive population of patients undergoing abdominal aortic surgery and were also unable to demonstrate an association between thallium redistribution and perioperative cardiac morbidity.[65] Both studies illustrate the low positive predictive value and significant incidence of morbidity in patients with negative test results if consecutive patients are studied.

The additive value of diagnostic testing is best illustrated by Vanzetto and colleagues.[61] They observed a cohort of consecutive abdominal aortic surgery patients and performed dipyridamole thallium imaging in patients with more than two clinical or electrocardiographic cardiac risk variables. The results of the test were not made available to the clinicians. Major cardiac events occurred in 23% of patients with a reversible thallium defect and 1% of patients without a reversible thallium defect in clinically high-cardiac-risk patients. In addition,

the greater the number of clinical risk factors, the higher the incidence of cardiac events in the patients with a reversible defect.

L'Italien et al constructed a Bayesian model using clinical risk factors and the results of dipyridamole thallium imaging (Figure 5-2).[66] The pretest (baseline) probability of an event can be calculated in a manner similar to cardiac risk indices, in which clinical risk factors are each associated with a certain numerical weight that can be added to determine overall risk. The results of dipyridamole thallium imaging can then be used to modify the risk and determine the post-test probability of an event. In this manner, clinical risk factors can be used to determine whether the test will raise the probability of morbidity above some threshold for action.

Noninvasive Cardiovascular Stress Testing

Multiple noninvasive diagnostic tests have been proposed to evaluate the extent of coronary artery disease before noncardiac surgery. The exercise electrocardiogram (ECG) has been the traditional method of evaluating individuals for the presence of coronary artery disease. It represents the least invasive and most cost-effective method of detecting ischemia, with reasonable sensitivity (68% to 81%) and specificity (66% to 77%) for identifying coronary artery disease. The goal of the test is to provoke ischemia through exercise by causing an increase in myocardial oxygen demand relative to myocardial oxygen supply. Electrocardiographic signs of myocardial ischemia and clinical signs of left ventricular dysfunction are considered positive. However, as outlined previously, patients with good exercise tolerance rarely benefit from further testing. Therefore, information regarding maximal heart rate (HR), exercise level, and blood pressure during the test must be provided.

A significant number of high-risk patients either are unable to exercise or have contraindications to exercise. In surgical patients, this phenomenon is most evident in patients with claudication or an abdominal aortic aneurysm undergoing vascular surgery, both of which are associated with a high rate of perioperative cardiac morbidity. Therefore, pharmacologic stress testing has become popular, particularly as a preoperative test in vascular surgery patients.

Pharmacologic stress for the detection of coronary artery disease can be divided into two categories: (1) those that result in coronary artery vasodilatation and (2) those that increase myocardial oxygen demand. Examples of coronary vasodila-

TABLE 5-3

Estimated Energy Requirement for Various Activities*

1 MET	Can you take care of yourself?	4 METs	Climb a flight of stairs or walk up a hill?
	Eat, dress, or use the toilet?		Walk on level ground at 4 mph or 6.4 km/hr?
	Walk indoors around the house?		Run a short distance?
	Walk a block or two on level ground at 2-3 mph or 3.2-4.8 km/hr?		Do heavy work around the house like scrubbing floors or lifting or moving heavy furniture?
	Do light work around the house like dusting or washing dishes?		Participate in moderate recreational activities like golf, bowling, dancing, doubles tennis, or throwing a baseball or football?
		>10 METs	Participate in strenuous sports like swimming, singles tennis, football, basketball, or skiing?

*Adapted from the Duke Activity Status Index and American Heart Association Exercise Standards.
MET, metabolic equivalent.
From Eagle KA, Berger PB, Calkins H, et al: *J Am Coll Cardiol* 39:542, 2002.

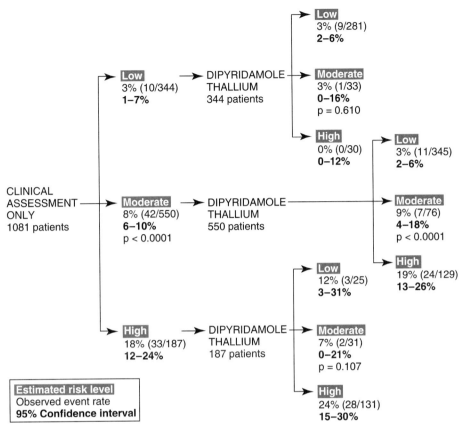

FIGURE 5-2 Suggested algorithm and results for using clinical variables and dipyridamole thallium results sequentially to stratify risk in 1081 patients. Values shown are the event rates (nonfatal myocardial infarction or cardiac death) and associated 95% confidence intervals. Clinical variables include advanced age (>70 years), history of angina, history of myocardial infarction, history of diabetes, history of congestive heart failure, and prior coronary bypass grafting. Dipyridamole thallium variables were ischemic electrocardiographic changes, fixed defects, and reversible defects. Cut points defining low, moderate, and high risk correspond to post-test probabilities of 0% to 5%, 5% to 15%, and greater than 15%, respectively, for both models. See text for detailed discussion of algorithm. (From L'Italien GJ, Paul SD, Hendel RC, et al: *J Am Coll Cardiol* 27:779, 1996.)

tors are dipyridamole and adenosine. Dipyridamole works by blocking adenosine reuptake and increasing adenosine concentration in the coronary vessels. Adenosine is a direct coronary vasodilator. After infusion of the vasodilator, flow is preferentially distributed to areas distal to normal coronary arteries, with minimal flow to areas distal to a coronary stenosis. A radioisotope, such as thallium or technetium 99m sestamibi, is then injected. Normal myocardium shows up on initial imaging, whereas areas of myocardial necrosis or areas distal to a significant coronary stenosis demonstrate a defect. After a delay of several hours, or after infusion of a second dose of technetium 99m sestamibi, the myocardium is again imaged. The initial defects that remain as defects are consistent with old scar, and the defects that demonstrate normal activity on subsequent imaging are consistent with areas at risk for myocardial ischemia. Several authors have shown that the presence of a redistribution defect on dipyridamole thallium or technetium imaging in patients undergoing peripheral vascular surgery is predictive of postoperative cardiac events.[4,5,67-69]

In order to increase the predictive value of the test, several strategies have been suggested. The redistribution defect can be quantitated, with larger areas of defect being associated with increased risk. In addition, both increased lung uptake and left ventricular cavity dilation have been shown to be markers of ventricular dysfunction with ischemia. Fleisher and colleagues demonstrated that the delineation of "low-" and "high-" risk thallium scans (larger area of defect, increased lung uptake, and left ventricular cavity dilation) markedly improved the test's predictive value.[70] They demonstrated that only patients with high-risk thallium scans were at increased risk for perioperative morbidity and long-term mortality. Therefore, the consultant must provide greater detail regarding the test result than simply a "yes-no" answer.

The ambulatory ECG (AECG or Holter) provides a means of continuously monitoring the ECG for significant ST-segment changes during the preoperative period. A positive test is the presence of significant ST-segment depression or elevation of at least 1-minute duration. Raby and colleagues demonstrated that the presence of silent ischemia was a strong predictor of outcome, whereas its absence was associated with a good outcome in 99% of patients.[71] Other investigators have demonstrated the value of silent AECG monitoring, although the negative predictive values have not been as high as originally reported. Fleisher and colleagues demonstrated a similar predictive value of dipyridamole thallium imaging and AECG monitoring; however, the quantity of silent ischemia could not be used to identify the patients at greatest risk who might benefit from further testing and coronary revascularization.[70] Preoperative AECG monitoring is rarely used for screening at present.

Stress echocardiography has received attention as a preoperative test.[72-76] Patients are given an infusion of dobutamine to increase both HR and inotropy. If HR cannot be raised to greater than 85% of the age-predicted maximum, atropine is given. The ECG is monitored continuously for ST-segment changes. The ECG is also monitored at discrete time points for the appearance of new or worsened regional wall motion abnormalities (RWMAs), which is considered a positive test. These RWMAs represent areas at risk for myocardial ischemia. The advantage of this test is that it is a dynamic assessment of the ability to provoke myocardial ischemia in response to increased HR, similar to what might be observed in the perioperative period. Similarly to the work with dipyridamole thallium imaging, dobutamine stress echocardiography can be further quantified. The presence of wall motion abnormalities at low HR is the best predictor of increased

perioperative risk, with large areas of defect being of secondary importance.[76]

Boersma and colleagues evaluated the utility of dobutamine stress echocardiography with respect to the extent of wall motion abnormalities and use of β-blockers during surgery.[77] They assigned one point for each of the following characteristics: age older than 70 years, current angina, MI, congestive heart failure, prior cerebrovascular event, diabetes mellitus, and renal failure. As the total of number of clinical risk factors increases, perioperative cardiac event rates also increase. Dobutamine stress echocardiography was performed only in patients with a significant number of risk factors, and the patients who demonstrated new wall motion abnormalities had higher event rates than those without new wall motion abnormalities for the same clinical risk score. When the risk of death from MI was stratified by perioperative β-blocker usage, there was no significant improvement in those without any of the prior risk factors (Figure 5-3). In those with a risk factor score between 0 and 3, which represented more than half of all patients, the rate of cardiac events was reduced from 3% to 0.9% by β-blockers. Most important, in those without at least three risk factors, constituting 17% of the population, β-blocker

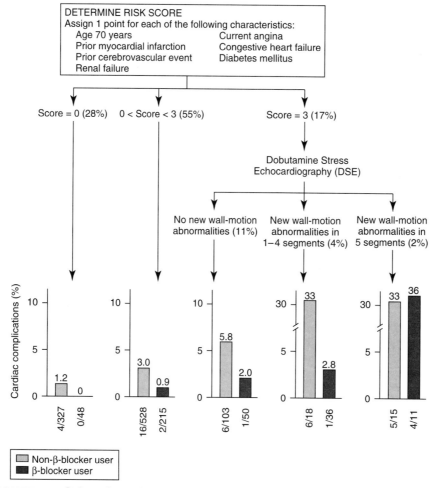

FIGURE 5-3 Perioperative cardiac risk and death in different populations of patients enrolled in a randomized controlled trial of β-blockers. Risk is defined according to clinical risk and use of β-blockers both as part of the randomized and nonrandomized cohort of individuals. (From Boersma E, Poldermans D, Bax JJ, et. al: Predictors of cardiac events after major vascular surgery: Role of clinical characteristics, dobutamine echocardiography, and beta-blocker therapy, *JAMA* 285(14):1865, 2001.)

therapy was effective in reducing cardiac events in those with new wall motion abnormalities in one to four segments (33% vs. 2.8%), having a smaller effect in those without new wall motion abnormalities (5.8% vs. 2%), but had no effect in the patients with new wall motion abnormalities in more than five segments. The group with extensive wall motion abnormalities may be the group to consider for coronary revascularization.

The question remains regarding the choice of diagnostic tests for a given patient. Several groups have published meta-analyses of preoperative diagnostic tests. Mantha et al demonstrated good predictive values of AECG monitoring, radionuclide angiography, dipyridamole thallium imaging, and dobutamine stress echocardiography.[78] Shaw et al also demonstrated good predictive values of dipyridamole thallium imaging and dobutamine stress echocardiography.[79] Both studies demonstrated the superior predictive value of dobutamine stress echocardiography; however, there was significant overlap of the confidence intervals with other tests. However, the most important determinant with respect to the choice of preoperative testing is the expertise at the local institution.

VALUE OF PREOPERATIVE STATIC VENTRICULAR FUNCTION TESTS. Baseline left ventricular systolic function can be assessed using echocardiography, radionuclide angiography, and/or contrast ventriculography. Many elderly patients complain of dyspnea. If the etiology is clearly defined (e.g., documented congestive heart failure), further testing is not warranted. In contrast, dyspnea of unknown etiology warrants a careful preoperative assessment. Left ventricular ejection fraction (LVEF) has been correlated with short- and long-term prognosis in multiple studies in patients undergoing noncardiac surgery.[46,78] The greatest risk of perioperative ischemic events is believed to be in patients with a resting LVEF less than 35%, but this has not been a consistent predictor and some studies have found that left ventricular systolic dysfunction does not predict cardiac complications after vascular surgery. Most important, a study of a large number of patients undergoing noncardiac surgery was unable to demonstrate additive value of a preoperative echocardiogram over information based upon clinical history.[80]

In addition to an assessment of ventricular function, echocardiography can provide important information regarding valvular function. Because each of the valvular lesions has different pathophysiologic implications for perioperative management and the risk of surgery in a patient with aortic stenosis is extremely high, further defining the extent of valvular insufficiency, stenotic area, and/or flow gradient is important.

Ventricular function can also be assessed using radionuclide angiography. In addition to assessment of LVEF, regional wall motion abnormalities can be discerned. During coronary angiography, contrast ventriculography can be performed. Frequently, a qualitative, rather than quantitative, assessment of LVEF is performed on the ventriculogram.

Coronary Angiography

Unlike the tests described previously, coronary angiography provides the clinician with anatomic and not functional information as well as a static ejection fraction. Although a critical stenosis delineates an area at risk for developing myocardial ischemia, the functional response to that ischemia cannot be determined. Although coronary artery disease is the substrate for a perioperative MI, the critical stenosis may not be the underlying pathophysiology. In the ambulatory population, many infarctions are the result of acute thrombosis of a noncritical stenosis. Therefore, the value of routine angiography prior to noncardiac surgery depends upon the ability to correct the lesions that cause morbidity. Eagle et al have suggested that coronary angiography be considered as the primary testing modality in the subset of patients who have multiple risk factors.[60]

Coronary Revascularization

As already described, coronary revascularization before noncardiac surgery has been proposed as a means of reducing perioperative risk. There are no randomized trials to address this issue, and such a trial would require a very large sample size and have multiple confounding issues. However, there are several large cohort studies which suggest that in patients who survive CABG, the risk of subsequent noncardiac surgery is low.[81,82] Eagle and colleagues reported a long-term analysis of patients entered into the Coronary Artery Surgery Study (CASS).[82] They observed patients randomly assigned to medical or surgical therapy for coronary artery disease for more than 10 years who subsequently underwent 3066 noncardiac operations. The rate of perioperative MI and death was reported stratified by type of surgical procedure. Intermediate-risk surgery such as CEA was associated with a combined morbidity and mortality of 1% to 5% with a small but significant improvement in outcome in patients who underwent prior revascularization. The most significant reduction was in patients undergoing major vascular surgery such as abdominal or lower extremity revascularization. In these patients, prior coronary revascularization was associated with fewer postoperative deaths (1.7% versus 3.3%, $P = 0.03$) and MIs (0.8% versus 2.7%, $P = 0.002$) compared with medically managed coronary disease. Therefore, CABG was beneficial in selected populations based upon a nonrandomized design if they had survived the initial coronary operation. Rihal et al utilized the same CASS database and found that CABG significantly improved survival in the patients with both peripheral vascular disease and triple-vessel coronary disease, especially the group with depressed ventricular function.[83]

Several small case series have demonstrated that morbidity and mortality were low after noncardiac surgery in patients who had a PTCA at some point before noncardiac surgery.[84-86] Posner and colleagues utilized an administrative data set of patients who underwent PTCA and noncardiac surgery in Washington State.[87] They matched patients with coronary disease undergoing noncardiac surgery with and without prior PTCA and looked at cardiac complications. In this nonrandomized design, they noted a significantly lower rate of 30-day cardiac complications in patients who underwent PTCA at least 90 days before the noncardiac surgery. Notably, PTCA within 90 days of noncardiac surgery was not associated with improvement in outcome. Although the explanation for these results is unknown, it can be speculated that they support the idea that PTCA performed "to get the patient through surgery" may not improve perioperative outcome because cardiac complications may not occur as a function of asymptomatic stenoses. Hassan and colleagues evaluated the value of multivessel angioplasty for subsequent noncardiac surgery in the Bypass Angioplasty Revascularization Investigation

(BARI).[88] A total of 501 patients had noncardiac surgery a median of 29 months after the most recent revascularization procedure. Mortality and nonfatal MI occurred in 4 of the 250 CABG surgery-assigned patients and 4 of the 251 angioplasty-assigned patients. Therefore, there does not appear to be an optimal choice of revascularization procedure for multivessel disease, although a larger scale study is necessary to confirm these findings.

Evidence regarding the value of coronary stent placement is currently lacking. Of importance, the outcome in 40 patients who underwent coronary stent placement less than 6 weeks before noncardiac surgery requiring general anesthesia has been reported.[41] There were 7 MIs, 11 major bleeding episodes, and 8 deaths. All deaths and MIs, as well as 8 of 11 bleeding episodes, occurred in patients subjected to surgery fewer than 14 days from stenting. Four patients died after undergoing surgery 1 day after stenting. The time between stenting and surgery appeared to be the main determinant of outcome, and the authors recommend that a minimum of 2 weeks, and preferably 4 weeks, elapse before elective surgery.

Risks versus Benefits of Coronary Revascularization

An alternative approach to determining the optimal strategy for medical care in the absence of clinical trials is construction of a decision analysis. Three decision analyses have been published on the issue of cardiovascular testing before major vascular surgery (Figure 5-4).[31-33] Two of the strategies evaluated

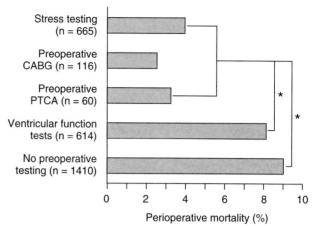

FIGURE 5-5 Perioperative mortality for patients undergoing aortic surgery according to the extent of preoperative testing and interventions within 6 months of surgery. Stress testing with or without coronary revascularization was associated with significantly less perioperative mortality than no preoperative testing, which was associated with the highest rate of perioperative mortality. *$P < 0.05$ compared with the no-testing strategy. CABG, coronary artery bypass grafting; PTCA, percutaneous transluminal angioplasty. (From Fleisher LA, Eagle KA, Shaffer T, et al: *Anesth Analg* 89:849, 1999.)

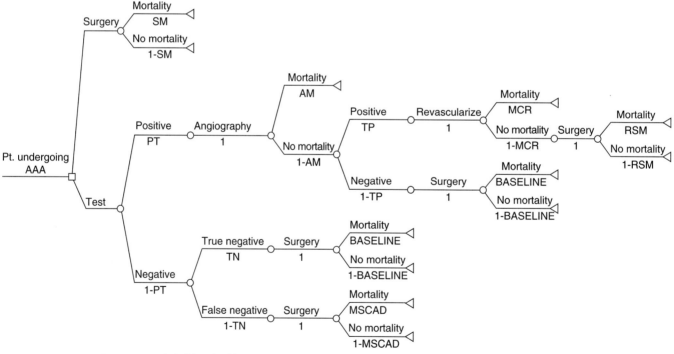

FIGURE 5-4 A decision algorithm evaluating the decision between vascular surgery alone or coronary artery revascularization before vascular surgery. There are currently no randomized trials to address the optimal strategy. By outlining the multiple decision points at which a patient can sustain mortality by choosing to undergo coronary revascularization first, the optimal strategy for preoperative evaluation can be demonstrated. Specifically, variation in mortalities at each decision point can change the optimal strategy. AAA, abdominal aortic aneurysm; AM, angiography mortality; MCR, mortality from coronary revascularization; SM, vascular surgery mortality; PT, positive test probability; TP, probability of true positive test; MSCAD, vascular surgery mortality in patients with coronary revascularization. (From Fleisher LA, Skolnick ED, Holroyd KJ, et al: *Anesth Analg* 79:661, 1994.)

short-term outcome and assumed that patients with significant coronary artery disease would undergo CABG prior to noncardiac surgery.[31,32] Both models found that the optimal decisions, sensitive to local morbidity and mortality rates, were within the clinically observed range. These models suggest that preoperative testing for the purpose of coronary revascularization is not the optimal strategy if local perioperative morbidity and mortality are low for vascular surgery. Glance included 5-year outcome and demonstrated that selective screening before vascular surgery may improve 5-year survival and be cost-effective.[33]

Administrative databases can also be utilized to evaluate the impact of preoperative testing and interventions. Fleisher and colleagues utilized the Medicare claims data to determine the relationship between preoperative testing and interventions and 1-year outcome.[39] Stress testing, with or without coronary revascularization, was associated with improved short- and long-term survival in aortic surgery (Figure 5-5). The use of stress testing with coronary revascularization was not associ-

ated with reduced perioperative mortality after infrainguinal surgery. Stress testing alone was associated with reduced long-term mortality in patients undergoing infrainguinal revascularization. Although this represents selected data from insurance claims, it does suggest that there is long-term benefit from testing, particularly in aortic surgery.

A major factor that affects the potential long-term cost-effectiveness is the patient's age. For example, an 80-year-old diabetic patient with significant comorbid diseases may gain few additional life years and may actually have a decrease in the quality of the final years on undergoing coronary revascularization. In contrast, a 55-year-old man with an abdominal aortic aneurysm who is found to have occult left main disease would have a substantial increase in both the length and quality of his life as a result of preoperative cardiovascular testing and coronary revascularization. Appropriate patients with diffuse disease or a significant left main stenosis amenable to surgery with an acceptable risk should undergo CABG before

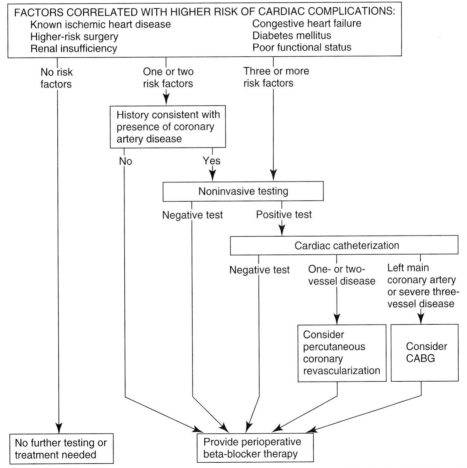

FIGURE 5-6 Strategy for assessing the risk of perioperative coronary complications in patients scheduled to undergo noncardiac surgery. The decision whether to perform noninvasive testing is based on the presence of clinical risk factors, the patient's functional status, and the type of surgery scheduled. If the result of a noninvasive test is abnormal, the decision whether to perform cardiac catheterization is based on several features. The likelihood of left main coronary artery disease or severe three-vessel disease is much higher and cardiac catheterization should be considered more strongly if ischemia is provoked at a low level of stress or persists during stress testing, if there is severe ST segment depression, if large areas of the myocardium appear to be at risk, or if ischemia is demonstrated in a patient known to have left ventricular dysfunction at rest. Coronary artery bypass grafting (CABG) and percutaneous coronary revascularization should be performed only if justified independently of the need for noncardiac surgery. (From Fleisher LA, Eagle KA: *N Engl J Med* 345:1677, 2001.)

noncardiac surgery. In this instance, the procedure is justified on the basis of long-term benefit, and performing it before major vascular surgery reduces the risk of a fatal or nonfatal perioperative MI.

Summary

The preoperative evaluation of the patient undergoing major vascular surgery should focus on identification of those with unstable symptoms and those who might benefit from further perioperative interventions. Diagnostic testing is of value in patients at moderate-to-high risk, but the specific choice of test depends on institutional factors, particularly in the current era with changes based upon the evidence regarding perioperative β-blocker therapy. The decision to undergo coronary revascularization is based upon perioperative morbidity and mortality rates for each procedure and potential long-term benefits, although the risks and benefits of different therapies are perhaps changing. One potential algorithm incorporating these changes in perioperative management into the preoperative evaluation paradigm is shown in Figure 5-6.[89]

REFERENCES

1. Hertzer NR, Bevan EG, Young JR, et al: Coronary artery disease in peripheral vascular patients: a classification of 1000 coronary angiograms and results of surgical management, *Ann Surg* 199:223, 1984.
2. Mangano DT: Perioperative cardiac morbidity, *Anesthesiology* 72:153, 1990.
3. L'Italien GL, Cambria RP, Cutler BS, et al: Comparative early and late cardiac morbidity among patients requiring different vascular surgery procedures, *J Vasc Surg* 21:935, 1995.
4. Boucher CA, Brewster DC, Darling RC, et al: Determination of cardiac risk by dipyridamole-thallium imaging before peripheral vascular surgery, *N Engl J Med* 312:389, 1985.
5. Cutler BS, Leppo JA: Dipyridamole thallium 201 scintigraphy to detect coronary artery disease before abdominal aortic surgery, *J Vasc Surg* 5:91, 1985.
6. Fleisher LA, Barash PG: Preoperative cardiac evaluation for noncardiac surgery: a functional approach, *Anesth Analg* 74:586, 1992.
7. D'Angelo AJ, Puppala D, Farber A, et al: Is preoperative cardiac evaluation for abdominal aortic aneurysm repair necessary? *J Vasc Surg* 25:152, 1997.
8. de Virgilio C, Pak S, Arnell T, et al: Cardiac assessment prior to vascular surgery: is dipyridamole-sestamibi necessary? *Ann Vasc Surg* 10:325, 1996.
9. Rosenfeld BA, Breslow MJ, Dorman T: Postoperative management strategies may obviate the need for most preoperative cardiac testing, *Anesthesiology* 84:1266, 1996 (letter).
10. Mangano DT, Layug EL, Wallace A, et al: Effect of atenolol on mortality and cardiovascular morbidity after noncardiac surgery. Multicenter Study of Perioperative Ischemia Research Group, *N Engl J Med* 335:1713, 1996.
11. Poldermans D, Boersma E, Bax JJ, et al: The effect of bisoprolol on perioperative mortality and myocardial infarction in high-risk patients undergoing vascular surgery. Dutch Echocardiographic Cardiac Risk Evaluation Applying Stress Echocardiography Study Group, *N Engl J Med* 341:1789, 1999.
12. Eagle K, Brundage B, Chaitman B, et al: Guidelines for perioperative cardiovascular evaluation of the noncardiac surgery patient. A report of the American Heart Association/American College of Cardiology Task Force on Assessment of Diagnostic and Therapeutic Cardiovascular Procedures, *Circulation* 93:1278, 1996.
13. Palda VA, Detsky AS: Perioperative assessment and management of risk from coronary artery disease, *Ann Intern Med* 127:313, 1997.
14. Eagle KA, Berger PB, Calkins H, et al: ACC/AHA guideline update for perioperative cardiovascular evaluation for noncardiac surgery—executive summary: a report of the American College of Cardiology/American Heart Association Task Force on Practice Guidelines (Committee to Update the 1996 Guidelines on Perioperative Cardiovascular Evaluation for Noncardiac Surgery), *J Am Coll Cardiol* 39:542, 2002.

15. O'Donnell TF Jr, Callow AD, Willet C, et al: The impact of coronary artery disease on carotid endarterectomy, *Ann Surg* 198:705, 1983.
16. Rihal C, Gersh B, Whisnant J, et al: Influence of coronary heart disease on morbidity and mortality after carotid endarterectomy: a population-based study in Olmsted County, Minnesota (1970-1988), *J Am Coll Cardiol* 19:1254, 1992.
17. Estes JM, Guadagnoli E, Wolf R, et al: The impact of cardiac comorbidity after carotid endarterectomy, *J Vasc Surg* 28:577, 1998.
18. Hertzer NR, Loop FD, Taylor PC, et al: Staged and combined surgical approach to simultaneous carotid and coronary vascular disease, *Surgery* 84:803, 1978.
19. Chang BB, Darling RC 3rd, Shah DM, et al: Carotid endarterectomy can be safely performed with acceptable mortality and morbidity in patients requiring coronary artery bypass grafts, *Am J Surg* 168:94, 1994.
20. Giangola G, Migaly J, Riles TS, et al: Perioperative morbidity and mortality in combined vs. staged approaches to carotid and coronary revascularization, *Ann Vasc Surg* 10:138, 1996.
21. Borger MA, Fremes SE, Weisel RD, et al: Coronary bypass and carotid endarterectomy: does a combined approach increase risk? A metaanalysis, *Ann Thorac Surg* 68:14, 1999.
22. Perler BA, Burdick JF, Williams GM: The safety of carotid endarterectomy at the time of coronary artery bypass surgery: analysis of results in a high-risk patient population, *J Vasc Surg* 2:558, 1985.
23. Mackey WC, Khabbaz K, Bojar R, et al: Simultaneous carotid endarterectomy and coronary bypass: perioperative risk and long-term survival, *J Vasc Surg* 24:58, 1996.
24. Vicaretti M, Fletcher JP, Klineberg P, et al: Combined coronary artery bypass grafting and carotid endarterectomy, *Cardiovasc Surg* 5:266, 1997.
25. Donatelli F, Pelenghi S, Pocar M, et al: Combined carotid and cardiac procedures: improved results and surgical approach, *Cardiovasc Surg* 6:506, 1998.
26. Darling RC 3rd, Dylewski M, Chang BB, et al: Combined carotid endarterectomy and coronary artery bypass grafting does not increase the risk of perioperative stroke, *Cardiovasc Surg* 6:448, 1998.
27. Char D, Cuadra S, Ricotta J, et al: Combined coronary artery bypass and carotid endarterectomy: long-term results, *Cardiovasc Surg* 10:111, 2002.
28. Bonardelli S, Portolani N, Tiberio GA, et al: Combined surgical approach for carotid and coronary stenosis. Sixty-four patients and review of literature, *J Cardiovasc Surg (Torino)* 43:385, 2002.
29. Youssuf AM, Karanam R, Prendergast T, et al: Combined off-pump myocardial revascularization and carotid endarterectomy: early experience, *Ann Thorac Surg* 72:1542, 2001.
30. Van Dijk D, Jansen EW, Hijman R, et al: Cognitive outcome after off-pump and on-pump coronary artery bypass graft surgery: a randomized trial, *JAMA* 287:1405, 2002.
31. Fleisher LA, Skolnick ED, Holroyd KJ, et al: Coronary artery revascularization before abdominal aortic aneurysm surgery: a decision analytic approach, *Anesth Analg* 79:661, 1994.
32. Mason JJ, Owens DK, Harris RA, et al: The role of coronary angiography and coronary revascularization before noncardiac surgery, *JAMA* 273:1919, 1995.
33. Glance LG: Selective preoperative cardiac screening improves five-year survival in patients undergoing major vascular surgery: a cost-effectiveness analysis, *J Cardiothorac Vasc Anesth* 13:265, 1999.
34. Isaacson IJ, Lowdon JD, Berry AJ, et al: The value of pulmonary artery and central venous monitoring in patients undergoing abdominal aortic reconstructive surgery: a comparative study of two selected, randomized groups, *J Vasc Surg* 12:754, 1990.
35. Joyce WP, Provan JL, Ameli FM, et al: The role of central haemodynamic monitoring in abdominal aortic surgery: a prospective randomized study, *Eur J Vasc Surg* 4:633, 1990.
36. Polanczyk CA, Rohde LE, Goldman L, et al: Right heart catheterization and cardiac complications in patients undergoing noncardiac surgery: an observational study, *JAMA* 286:309, 2001.
37. Krupski WC, Layug EL, Reilly LM, et al: Comparison of cardiac morbidity between aortic and infrainguinal operations. Study of Perioperative Ischemia (SPI) Research Group, *J Vasc Surg* 15:354, 1992.
38. Krupski WC, Layug EL, Reilly LM, et al: Comparison of cardiac morbidity rates between aortic and infrainguinal operations: two-year follow-up. Study of Perioperative Ischemia Research Group, *J Vasc Surg* 18:609, 1993.
39. Fleisher LA, Eagle KA, Shaffer T, et al: Perioperative and long-term mortality rates after major vascular surgery: the relationship to preoperative testing in the Medicare population, *Anesth Analg* 89:849, 1999.
40. Ashton CM, Petersen NJ, Wray NP, et al: The incidence of perioperative myocardial infarction in men undergoing noncardiac surgery, *Ann Intern Med* 118:504, 1993.

41. Kaluza GL, Joseph J, Lee JR, et al: Catastrophic outcomes of noncardiac surgery soon after coronary stenting, *J Am Coll Cardiol* 35:1288, 2000.
42. Berlauk JF, Abrams JH, Gilmour IJ, et al: Preoperative optimization of cardiovascular hemodynamics improves outcome in peripheral vascular surgery: a prospective, randomized clinical trial, *Ann Surg* 214:289, 1991.
43. Bender JS, Smith-Meek MA, Jones CE: Routine pulmonary artery catheterization does not reduce morbidity and mortality of elective vascular surgery: results of a prospective, randomized trial, *Ann Surg* 226:229, 1997.
44. Goldman L, Caldera DL, Nussbaum SR, et al: Multifactorial index of cardiac risk in noncardiac surgical procedures, *N Engl J Med* 297:845, 1977.
45. Zeldin RA: Assessing cardiac risk in patients who undergo noncardiac surgical procedures, *Can J Surg* 27:402, 1984.
46. McEnroe CS, O'Donnell TF, Yeager A, et al: Comparison of ejection fraction and Goldman risk factor analysis to dipyridamole–thallium 201 studies in the evaluation of cardiac morbidity after aortic aneurysm surgery, *J Vasc Surg* 11:497, 1990.
47. Fleisher L, Rosenbaum S, Nelson A, et al: The predictive value of preoperative silent ischemia for postoperative ischemic cardiac events in vascular and nonvascular surgical patients, *Am Heart J* 122:980, 1991.
48. Calvin JE, Kieser TM, Walley VM, et al: Cardiac mortality and morbidity after vascular surgery, *Can J Surg* 29:93, 1986.
49. Mangano DT, Browner WS, Hollenberg M, et al: Association of perioperative myocardial ischemia with cardiac morbidity and mortality in men undergoing noncardiac surgery, *N Engl J Med* 323:1781, 1990.
50. Detsky A, Abrams H, McLaughlin J, et al: Predicting cardiac complications in patients undergoing non-cardiac surgery, *J Gen Intern Med* 1:211, 1986.
51. Shah K, Kleinman B, Rao T, et al: Reduction in mortality from cardiac causes in Goldman class IV patients, *J Cardiothorac Anesth* 2:789, 1988.
52. Lee TH, Marcantonio ER, Mangione CM, et al: Derivation and prospective validation of a simple index for prediction of cardiac risk of major noncardiac surgery, *Circulation* 100:1043, 1999.
53. Shah KB, Kleinman BS, Rao T, et al: Angina and other risk factors in patients with cardiac diseases undergoing noncardiac operations, *Anesth Analg* 70:240, 1990.
54. Tarhan S, Moffitt EA, Taylor WF, et al: Myocardial infarction after general anesthesia, *JAMA* 220:1451, 1972.
55. Rao TLK, Jacobs KH, El-Etr AA: Reinfarction following anesthesia in patients with myocardial infarction, *Anesthesiology* 59:499, 1983.
56. Shah KB, Kleinman BS, Sami H, et al: Reevaluation of perioperative myocardial infarction in patients with prior myocardial infarction undergoing noncardiac operations, *Anesth Analg* 71:231, 1990.
57. Rivers SP, Scher LA, Gupta SK, et al: Safety of peripheral vascular surgery after recent acute myocardial infarction, *J Vasc Surg* 11:70, 1990.
58. Mangano DT, Goldman L: Preoperative assessment of patients with known or suspected coronary disease, *N Engl J Med* 333:1750, 1995.
59. Mangano DT: Assessment of the patient with cardiac disease: an anesthesiologist's paradigm, *Anesthesiology* 91:1521, 1999.
60. Eagle KA, Coley CM, Newell JB, et al: Combining clinical and thallium data optimizes preoperative assessment of cardiac risk before major vascular surgery, *Ann Intern Med* 110:859, 1989.
61. Vanzetto G, Machecourt J, Blendea D, et al: Additive value of thallium single-photon emission computed tomography myocardial imaging for prediction of perioperative events in clinically selected high cardiac risk patients having abdominal aortic surgery, *Am J Cardiol* 77:143, 1996.
62. Bartels C, Bechtel J, Hossmann V, et al: Cardiac risk stratification for high-risk vascular surgery, *Circulation* 95:2473, 1997.
63. Paul SD, Eagle KA, Kuntz KM, et al: Concordance of preoperative clinical risk with angiographic severity of coronary artery disease in patients undergoing vascular surgery, *Circulation* 94:1561, 1996.
64. Mangano DT, London MJ, Tubau JF, et al: Dipyridamole thallium-201 scintigraphy as a preoperative screening test. A reexamination of its predictive potential. Study of Perioperative Ischemia Research Group, *Circulation* 84:493, 1991.
65. Baron JF, Mundler O, Bertrand M, et al: Dipyridamole-thallium scintigraphy and gated radionuclide angiography to assess cardiac risk before abdominal aortic surgery, *N Engl J Med* 330:663, 1994.
66. L'Italien GJ, Paul SD, Hendel RC, et al: Development and validation of a Bayesian model for perioperative cardiac risk assessment in a cohort of 1,081 vascular surgical candidates, *J Am Coll Cardiol* 27:779, 1996.
67. Lette J, Waters D, Lapointe J, et al: Usefulness of the severity and extent of reversible perfusion defects during thallium-dipyridamole imaging for

cardiac risk assessment before noncardiac surgery, *Am J Cardiol* 64:276, 1989.
68. McPhail NV, Ruddy TD, Barber GG, et al: Cardiac risk stratification using dipyridamole myocardial perfusion imaging and ambulatory ECG monitoring prior to vascular surgery, *Eur J Vasc Surg* 7:151, 1993.
69. Tischler MD, Lee TH, Hirsch AT, et al: Prediction of major cardiac events after peripheral vascular surgery using dipyridamole echocardiography, *Am J Cardiol* 68:593, 1991.
70. Fleisher LA, Rosenbaum SH, Nelson AH, et al: Preoperative dipyridamole thallium imaging and Holter monitoring as a predictor of perioperative cardiac events and long term outcome, *Anesthesiology* 83:906, 1995.
71. Raby KE, Goldman L, Creager MA, et al: Correlation between perioperative ischemia and major cardiac events after peripheral vascular surgery, *N Engl J Med* 321:1296, 1989.
72. Davila-Roman V, Waggoner A, Sicard G, et al: Dobutamine stress echocardiography predicts surgical outcome in patients with an aortic aneurysm and peripheral vascular disease, *J Am Coll Cardiol* 21:957, 1993.
73. Lane RT, Sawada SG, Segar DS, et al: Dobutamine stress echocardiography for assessment of cardiac risk before noncardiac surgery, *Am J Cardiol* 68:976, 1991.
74. Langan ER, Youkey JR, Franklin DP, et al: Dobutamine stress echocardiography for cardiac risk assessment before aortic surgery, *J Vasc Surg* 18:905, 1993.
75. Poldermans D, Fioretti PM, Forster T, et al: Dobutamine-atropine stress echocardiography for assessment of perioperative and late cardiac risk in patients undergoing major vascular surgery, *Eur J Vasc Surg* 8:286, 1994.
76. Poldermans D, Arnese M, Fioretti PM, et al: Improved cardiac risk stratification in major vascular surgery with dobutamine-atropine stress echocardiography, *J Am Coll Cardiol* 26:648, 1995.
77. Boersma E, Poldermans D, Bax JJ, et al: Predictors of cardiac events after major vascular surgery: role of clinical characteristics, dobutamine echocardiography, and beta-blocker therapy, *JAMA* 285:1865, 2001.
78. Mantha S, Roizen MF, Barnard J, et al: Relative effectiveness of four preoperative tests for predicting adverse cardiac outcomes after vascular surgery: a meta-analysis, *Anesth Analg* 79:422, 1994.
79. Shaw LJ, Eagle KA, Gersh BJ, et al: Meta-analysis of intravenous dipyridamole-thallium-201 imaging (1985 to 1994) and dobutamine echocardiography (1991 to 1994) for risk stratification before vascular surgery, *J Am Coll Cardiol* 27:787, 1996.
80. Halm EA, Browner WS, Tubau JF, et al: Echocardiography for assessing cardiac risk in patients having noncardiac surgery. Study of Perioperative Ischemia Research Group, *Ann Intern Med* 125:433, 1996.
81. Elmore J, Hallett J, Gibbons R, et al: Myocardial revascularization before abdominal aortic aneurysmorrhaphy: effect of coronary angioplasty, *Mayo Clin Proc* 68:637, 1993.
82. Eagle KA, Rihal CS, Mickel MC, et al: Cardiac risk of noncardiac surgery: influence of coronary disease and type of surgery in 3368 operations. CASS Investigators and University of Michigan Heart Care Program. Coronary Artery Surgery Study, *Circulation* 96:1882, 1997.
83. Rihal CS, Eagle KA, Mickel MC, et al: Surgical therapy for coronary artery disease among patients with combined coronary artery and peripheral vascular disease, *Circulation* 91:46, 1995.
84. Allen J, Helling T, Hartzler G: Operative procedures not involving the heart after percutaneous transluminal coronary angioplasty, *Surg Gynecol Obstet* 173:285, 1991.
85. Gottlieb A, Banoub M, Sprung J, et al: Perioperative cardiovascular morbidity in patients with coronary artery disease undergoing vascular surgery after percutaneous transluminal coronary angioplasty, *J Cardiothorac Vasc Anesth* 12:501, 1998.
86. Huber KC, Evans MA, Bresnahan JF, et al: Outcome of noncardiac operations in patients with severe coronary artery disease successfully treated preoperatively with coronary angioplasty, *Mayo Clin Proc* 67:15, 1992.
87. Posner KL, Van Norman GA, Chan V: Adverse cardiac outcomes after noncardiac surgery in patients with prior percutaneous transluminal coronary angioplasty, *Anesth Analg* 89:553, 1999.
88. Hassan SA, Hlatky MA, Boothroyd DB, et al: Outcomes of noncardiac surgery after coronary bypass surgery or coronary angioplasty in the Bypass Angioplasty Revascularization Investigation (BARI), *Am J Med* 110:260, 2001.
89. Fleisher LA, Eagle KA: Clinical practice. Lowering cardiac risk in noncardiac surgery, *N Engl J Med* 345:1677, 2001.

Optimizing the Patient for Vascular Surgery

6

Catherine K. Lineberger, MD

IN the more than a decade since the publication of the first edition of this book, the perioperative management of all surgical patients has undergone a paradigm shift. The days when patients were admitted to the hospital for preoperative evaluation and medical preparation are over. Increasingly, even the sickest patients undergoing the most stressful surgeries are admitted only on the day of surgery. The reasons for this change have been multifactorial, but it is largely due to the influence of third-party payers' desire to minimize costs. The impact of this change remains unclear with regard to patients' outcomes and satisfaction. The new order presents challenges and opportunities to anesthesiologists and surgeons who care for these patients.

One of these challenges is minimal opportunity for the intended anesthesiologist to interact with and educate his or her patients. The bulk of preoperative evaluation and management occurs in preoperative screening clinics and is often conducted by personnel different from the intended anesthesiology team. A well-organized system can allow early evaluation of the patient and an opportunity to work up and intervene if important clinical problems are discovered, often without last-minute impact on the operating schedule. However, it deprives the patient and anesthesiologist of the opportunity to meet each other. Often a critically ill patient meets his or her anesthesiologist minutes to hours before surgery, and, depending on the setting, the anesthesiologist may not have any opportunity to meet the patient's important family members. Vascular anesthesiologists must add superb empathy and instantaneous confidence building to their lists of skills and talents in order to develop trust in the patient-anesthesiologist relationship. The value of the preoperative visit has been demonstrated in the past.[1,2] Interestingly, the authors of the first reference, written in an era of more extended preoperative hospitalization, stated that "little time is available for anesthetists to establish rapport with their patients." There is a certain irony to these words when the era in which they were written is compared with the situation today.

In keeping with the new paradigm of surgery in the 21st century, this chapter addresses the common medical problems in patients with vascular disease and emphasizes the appropriate perioperative management of these disorders.

Management of Medical Problems Commonly seen in Vascular Surgery Patients

Hypertension

Hypertension is defined as persistent elevation of the blood pressure. Normal limits for blood pressure have evolved over time. Optimal blood pressure is defined as a systolic blood pressure less than 120 mmHg and diastolic blood pressure less than 80 mmHg. Hypertension is characterized by stages, with the earliest stage of hypertension defined as systolic pressure between 140 and 159 mmHg and diastolic blood pressure between 90 and 99 mmHg.[3]

PRIMARY OR ESSENTIAL HYPERTENSION. Most patients with hypertension present with no obvious etiology for the blood pressure derangement. Approximately 95% of patients with newly diagnosed hypertension fall into this category. The specific etiology of essential hypertension is unknown but clearly involves a number of physiologic abnormalities, including the renin-angiotensin system, sympathetic nervous system, neuroendocrine system, atrial natriuretic hormones, and baroreceptor system.[4]

SECONDARY HYPERTENSION. Secondary hypertension refers to elevations in blood pressure that are attributable to specific underlying conditions. Only about 5% of patients who present with hypertension are found to have secondary hypertension, but appropriate history and examinations indicate the patients who are deserving of work-up to rule out causes of secondary hypertension. Causes of secondary hypertension include neuroendocrine tumors such as pheochromocytoma, hyperthyroidism, Cushing's syndrome, primary aldosteronism, renal artery stenosis, and intrinsic renal parenchymal disease. In the population of vascular surgery patients, renal artery stenosis and renal impairment, with activation of the renin-angiotensin system, are the more likely causes of secondary hypertension. Patients receiving multiple antihypertensive agents, whose blood pressure remains elevated, should be evaluated for the presence of renal artery stenosis, which can be treated percutaneously with stents or in some cases with renal artery revascularization.

ISOLATED SYSTOLIC HYPERTENSION AND WHITE COAT HYPERTENSION. Isolated systolic hypertension is defined by its name, that is, elevated systolic blood pressure without concomitant diastolic blood pressure elevation. Isolated systolic hypertension was once thought to be an inconsequential result of the aging of the vascular system ("benign essential hypertension") and is often undertreated. Newer evidence suggests that isolated systolic hypertension is actually a significant predictor of cardiovascular disease, cardiovascular event risk, and stroke. Many prospective trials suggest that systolic hypertension is as important as if not more important than diastolic hypertension in predicting the likelihood of cardiovascular problems.[5-8] It has been suggested that physicians need more education about this issue and that patients with isolated systolic hypertension should be treated more aggressively.[9-12]

Similarly, white coat hypertension is a frequently encountered problem, both in outpatient clinics and in the preoperative holding area. This term refers to patients whose blood pressure is elevated in the clinical setting but who record normal blood pressures in their homes or in more relaxed settings. Although patients with white coat hypertension are not at increased risk for cardiac morbidity, the presence of this phenomenon seems to be a predictor for the subsequent development of essential hypertension and left ventricular hypertrophy.[13,14]

PATHOPHYSIOLOGY. Untreated hypertension results in a number of cardiovascular findings, including concentric left ventricular hypertrophy, thickening and stiffening of arterial walls, increased systemic vascular resistance, and, initially, preserved cardiac output. Patients with long-standing untreated hypertension are at increased risk of overt or silent myocardial ischemia, congestive heart failure (CHF), and decreased left ventricular compliance. Patients with significant left ventricular hypertrophy can develop myocardial ischemia in the absence of stenotic coronary artery lesions owing to inadequate perfusion of the endocardium by perforating coronary arterioles.

Patients with untreated hypertension are at risk for developing diastolic heart failure or diastolic dysfunction. This consists of impaired ventricular relaxation, with preservation of ventricular contractility, and is often associated with left ventricular hypertrophy. Patients can present with dyspnea and other signs of CHF despite the preservation of systolic function. This phenomenon is common in elderly persons, particularly in women.[15-17]

Other implications of hypertension include a rightward shift of the cerebral autoregulatory curve causing cerebral ischemia to occur at higher blood pressures than in normal patients. Hypertensive patients are more likely to develop atherosclerotic disease of the extracranial and intracranial blood vessels and are predisposed to both hemorrhagic and embolic strokes. Continued exposure of the renal vasculature to high blood pressure induces glomerular sclerosis in the kidney, decreasing the capacity of the kidney for glomerular filtration and ultimately decreasing creatinine clearance. Autoregulation of the kidney is impaired in a manner similar to that described for the cerebral circulation.

INTRAOPERATIVE COURSE OF HYPERTENSIVE PATIENTS. Hypertensive patients, particularly those with poorly controlled hypertension, manifest blood pressure lability under the effects of anesthesia. They are more susceptible to intraoperative hypotension and often require the use of vasopressors to allow administration of amnestic doses of anesthetic. Hypertensive patients have exaggerated hemodynamic responses to painful stimuli such as airway manipulation and incision and during emergence from anesthesia. Induction of general or regional anesthesia may unmask chronic intravascular volume depletion. This hypotension may be attenuated by appropriate, judicious administration of intravenous fluid prior to induction of anesthesia and careful selection and titration of anesthetic drugs and techniques. Patients whose blood pressure is controlled and who are treated preoperatively with antihypertensive agents have a less labile intraoperative course.[4,18] Preoperative anxiety and stress may exacerbate hypertension and can be ameliorated by appropriate utilization of sedative premedicants or anxiolytics, which are described later in this chapter.

POSTOPERATIVE COURSE OF HYPERTENSIVE PATIENTS. Hypertensive patients are at increased risk of perioperative complications including pulmonary edema, myocardial ischemia, arrhythmias, hypertension, neurologic events, and renal insufficiency. The risk of these complications is increased in proportion to the degree of preoperative hypertension.[19] Goldman and Caldera pointed out that patients with inadequately controlled preoperative hypertension were no more likely to have cardiac complications but that uncontrolled blood pressure preoperatively was a marker for postoperative hypertension.[20] The significance of postoperative hypertension should not be minimized, however. Rose and colleagues found that patients who experienced postoperative hypertension and tachycardia in the postanesthesia care unit had higher rates of unplanned admission to critical care units and higher mortality than patients without these findings.[21] Their study population was largely well, consisting primarily of patients with American Society of Anesthesiologists physical status I and II. It is reasonable to infer that these risks could be higher for the typical vascular surgery patient with multiple medical problems. Given the ease of instituting and continuing β-blockade in the perioperative period, it seems prudent to treat preoperative and postoperative hypertension aggressively.

RECOMMENDATIONS FOR PREOPERATIVE MANAGEMENT OF HYPERTENSION. As already mentioned, chronic hypertension changes cerebral autoregulation, shifting the autoregulatory curve to the right. Significant decreases in cerebral blood flow can occur with higher blood pressures than in normotensive patients. Appropriate chronic antihypertensive therapy results in a leftward shift of the cerebral autoregulatory curve but generally does not restore the curve to normal.[22,23] This situation persists even after months of antihypertensive therapy, and most elective vascular surgical procedures are not amenable to months of delay for optimization of blood pressure. Given this situation, acute treatment of blood pressure for a few days prior to surgery does not restore a normal cerebral autoregulatory curve, and therefore careful management of blood pressure under anesthesia is critical to avoid ischemia of vulnerable vascular beds, such as the brain and the kidney. Caution should be taken to avoid overaggressive reduction of blood pressure to levels below the autoregulatory curves for the brain and kidneys. Many anesthesiologists follow a rule that a 25% decrease in mean arterial pressure from baseline approaches the lower limit of autoregulation and use these parameters for perioperative blood pressure control.[4]

MANAGEMENT OF ANTIHYPERTENSIVE THERAPY IN THE PREOPERATIVE PERIOD. In the early era of the development of antihypertensive agents, much concern focused on the potential disastrous consequences of severe hypotension and bradycardia in patients whose antihypertensive agents were continued until the time of surgery.[24-26] Review of these studies reveals that the anesthesia was often conducted with fixed doses of drugs and that titration of drugs was not practiced. With better understanding of the interactions between antihypertensives and anesthetics, intraoperative hypotension has become less of a problem.[27,28] Currently, fear of the consequences of abrupt withdrawal of antihypertensives, including β-receptor blockers and central α-adrenergic agonists (severe rebound hypertension, tachycardia, myocardial ischemia), has led to the recommendation that most antihypertensive medications be continued up to the time of surgery.[18,29,30]

A possible exception to this rule is for angiotensin-converting enzyme inhibitors (ACEIs) and angiotensin receptor antagonists (ARAs). Some authors have reported severe hypotension occurring under anesthesia when these drugs are given on the day of surgery and recommend withholding ACEI and ARA drugs on the day of surgery.[31,32] However, this practice has been questioned by others.[33] ACEIs have been promoted as reducing the hemodynamic stressors of laryngoscopy, intubation, and surgery, and there are reports of significant hypertension in the postoperative period in patients whose ACEI agents were withheld on the day of surgery.[31] Review of the issue shows that although continuation of ACEIs and ARAs on the day of surgery may result in more hypotension with induction of anesthesia, the hypotension can easily be treated with modest doses of pressors. Even in the studies that expressed concern about the interaction of ACEIs and anesthesia, the average dose of pressor required was small and the hypotension episodes were transient.[34] Several other studies have indicated successful treatment of ACEI- or ARA-induced hypotension with the use of vasopressin or its analogs.[35-37] Perhaps the best strategy is to appreciate the interaction of antihypertensive agents with anesthetic drugs and appropriately adapt the anesthetic strategy (monitoring and choice of drugs). In summary, most antihypertensives, including the normal morning doses, should be continued up until the time of surgery. Table 6-1 summarizes many of the commonly used antihypertensive drugs, their interactions with anesthetics, and recommendations for perioperative management of the drugs (see Chapter 2).

Coronary Artery Disease

Coronary artery disease is widely prevalent in patients presenting for vascular surgery. The associated risk factors for coronary artery disease are the same as those for peripheral vascular disease. Perioperative cardiac morbidity is the greatest cause of complications after vascular surgery.[38] Nearly 20 years ago, a series of 1000 patients scheduled for elective vascular surgery underwent coronary angiography in a study designed to decrease perioperative cardiac morbidity. Only 8% of the patients in this series had normal coronary arteries, and approximately 55% of the patients' coronary anatomy was classified as advanced or severe.[39] In the United States alone, approximately 50,000 perioperative myocardial infarctions occur each year.[40] Clearly, the vascular surgery patient comes to the operation with a high risk of having coronary artery disease. It is also clear that an episode of ischemia in the perioperative period is a strong prognostic factor for morbidity and mortality.[41-43] Therefore, a large component of optimization of the patient for vascular surgery involves risk stratification and measures to reduce the negative impact of coronary artery disease. The appropriate cardiac risk assessment for vascular surgery is described more fully in Chapter 5 and has been the subject of much discussion.[44] This chapter's focus is limited to the preparation of the patient with known coronary artery disease who is presenting for vascular surgery.

CLINICAL PRESENTATION OF CORONARY ARTERY DISEASE. The key element in optimizing patients with coronary artery disease for surgery is a carefully targeted history and physical examination with specific attention to the cardiac, vascular, and pulmonary systems. Key features of the history should include previous cardiac problems, such as hypertension, angina or myocardial infarction, heart failure, and arrhythmias. The presence or absence of modifiable risk factors for coronary artery disease and current medications should be noted. Emphasis should be placed on the functional status of the patient. The physical examination should focus on the cardiorespiratory and vascular systems and should include measurement of blood

TABLE 6-1

Therapeutics Used for Hypertension and Perioperative Management

Drug Class	Examples	Side Effects	Anesthetic Interactions	Perioperative Strategy
Diuretics				
Thiazide	Hydrochlorothiazide	Hyperuricemia Hypokalemia Hypomagnesemia Hyponatremia Hyperglycemia Hyperlipidemia	Hypokalemia-related arrhythmias Potentiation of neuromuscular blockade	Consider holding unless patient has congestive heart failure (CHF)
Loop-type	Furosemide Ethacrynic acid	Hypovolemia Same as thiazides	Same as thiazides	Same as thiazides
Potassium-sparing	Spironolactone	Hyperkalemia Hyponatremia	Same as thiazides	Same as thiazides
Adrenergic Inhibitors				
β-Receptor antagonists	Propranolol Atenolol* Metoprolol* Esmolol*	Bradycardia CHF Fatigue Bronchospasm Mask symptoms of hypoglycemia Impotence Lipid changes	↑Myocardial depressant effects of anesthetics and CEI ↓Hepatic clearance of drugs ↑Serum K⁺ after succinylcholine	Continue up to and through perioperative period

Continued

TABLE 6-1

Therapeutics Used for Hypertension and Perioperative Management—cont'd

Drug Class	Examples	Side Effects	Anesthetic Interactions	Perioperative Strategy
Adrenergic Inhibitors—cont'd				
Sympathomimetic β-receptor antagonists	Pindolol	Similar to above except less resting bradycardia and lipid changes	Similar to β-receptor antagonists	Continue up to and through perioperative period
α-Receptor antagonists	Prazosin Terazosin	Orthostatic hypotension	↓Ability to vasoconstrict in response to hypovolemia	Continue up to and through perioperative period
α-β Receptor antagonists	Labetalol	Similar to β-receptor antagonists Labetalol has intrinsic sympathomimetic activity	Similar to β-receptor antagonists	Continue up to and through perioperative period
Central α-adrenergic agonists	Clonidine Guanabenz	Sedation Bradycardia Orthostatic hypotension Rebound hypertension	Decreased minimum alveolar concentration (MAC)	Continue up to and through perioperative period
Peripheral adrenergic antagonists	Reserpine	Rarely used Orthostatic hypotension Bradycardia Depression	Decreased MAC	Continue
Angiotensin Antagonists				
Angiotensin-converting enzyme inhibitors (ACEIs)	Enalapril Captopril Lisinopril Ramipril Benazepril	Cough Hypotension Acute renal failure[†] Angioedema Hyperkalemia	↑Hyperkalemia with succinylcholine ↑Need for vasopressors on induction and after cardiopulmonary bypass	Consider holding on day of surgery unless patient has CHF
Angiotensin receptor antagonists (ARAs)	Losartan Irbesartan Valsartan	Same as ACEI, lower incidence of bradykinin-related side effects such as cough	Same as ACEI	Consider holding on day of surgery unless patient has CHF
Calcium Entry Inhibitors				
Calcium channel blockers	Diltiazem Verapamil	Bradycardia Atrioventricular block Heart failure	↑Myocardial depressant effects of anesthetics and β-receptor antagonists	Continue up to and through perioperative period
Dihydropyridines	Nifedipine Nicardipine Nimodipine	Tachycardia Dizziness ↑Myocardial ischemia	↑Myocardial depressant effects of anesthetic and β-receptor antagonists ↑Prolongation of atrioventricular conduction with β-receptor antagonists ↑Cerebral blood flow ↓MAC	Continue up to and through perioperative period
Direct Vasodilators				
	Hydralazine Minoxidil Nitroprusside	Tachycardia ↑Myocardial ischemia Lupus-like syndrome Fluid retention (hydralazine)	Potentiate anesthetic-induced hypotension	Continue up to and through perioperative period

*Cardioselective β-receptor antagonists.
[†]In the presence of renal artery stenosis.
Adapted from Domino KB: *Am J Anesth* 26:259, 1999.

pressure in both extremities, heart rate, examination of the neck for jugular venous pressure contours and carotid bruits, careful precordial and chest examination, abdominal palpation for evidence of hepatomegaly or a pulsatile abdominal mass, and examination of the extremities for the pulse examination and to rule out peripheral edema.[44]

Angina and unstable angina. Patients with coronary artery disease manifest symptoms when myocardial oxygen supply is inadequate to meet demand. Myocardial ischemia can result from severe critical stenosis of a coronary artery, thrombosis or plaque rupture, or increased myocardial oxygen demand such as with exercise. Patients with stable angina should be assessed for the degree of heart rate control, adequacy of blood pressure control, and status of other comorbid conditions such as diabetes and lung disease.

Unstable angina is defined as the new onset of severe angina that occurs frequently (≥ 3 episodes per day), accelerating angina (i.e., an increasing pattern of angina in a patient with previously stable angina), or angina that occurs at rest. Patients with unstable angina are at high risk for a myocardial infarction and in general should not undergo noncardiac or vascular surgery except in extreme situations in which the surgical condition is an immediate threat to life.

Myocardial infarction. Patients who have suffered myocardial infarctions have demonstrated the presence of coronary artery disease. Historically, these patients were thought to be at extreme risk of reinfarction and death if subjected to surgery within 3 to 6 months of the infarction.[45-47] Subsequent studies demonstrated lower risk, attributable to better perioperative monitoring and hemodynamic management.[48,49] An even more recent philosophy is that the risk of reinfarction is related to the amount of myocardium at risk for ischemia following myocardial infarction. Potentially ischemic myocardium can be quantified with functional cardiac testing such as dobutamine stress echocardiography or myocardial perfusion imaging. The results of such testing may determine that a patient has little myocardial tissue at risk following a completed infarction, which may place the patient at low risk for perioperative reinfarction despite a recent myocardial infarction.

The implications of percutaneous coronary intervention and stenting. The appropriate timing of noncardiac surgery after percutaneous transluminal coronary angioplasty (PTCA) and stenting is controversial. The superiority of coronary stenting over angioplasty alone has been demonstrated for durable patency. However, the risk of stent thrombosis in the initial poststent interval is high, and there are reports of catastrophic cardiac events occurring in patients who have undergone coronary artery stenting in preparation for noncardiac surgery, particularly within 2 weeks of stenting.[50,51] The presumed mechanism for this is partly the hypercoagulable state induced with surgery and the stress response. Recommendations are that patients who undergo coronary stenting should receive a full course of antiplatelet therapy following the stent procedure, ideally for 4 weeks.[44] The current standard of care is to use the newer antiplatelet agents such as clopidogrel for this therapy. The safety of regional anesthesia in the setting of these drugs is unclear, and the latest American Society of Regional Anesthesia and Pain Medicine consensus guidelines suggest a conservative approach.[52] This therapy has potential

implications for the ability to utilize central neuraxial anesthesia or analgesia for both aortic and peripheral vascular reconstruction.

THE PERIOPERATIVE STRESS RESPONSE AND RISK OF MYOCARDIAL ISCHEMIA. The induction of anesthesia and the trauma of surgical procedures invoke a potent stress response in the patient. Presumably, the stress response is a vestige of the "fight or flight" response to threats. However, in the patient with coronary artery disease, this response can be maladaptive and, if left unmodulated, can result in myocardial ischemia from a variety of mechanisms. Myocardial ischemia can result from imbalance in myocardial oxygen supply and demand, altered myocardial energy utilization, instability of coronary plaques, or promotion of a hypercoagulable state.[53-55] Although the neuroendocrine response to stress commences intraoperatively, the postoperative period is the time when patients are at maximal risk for deleterious effects of the stress response (Figure 6-1).

PERIOPERATIVE MEDICAL MANAGEMENT OF CORONARY ARTERY DISEASE. As indicated previously, perioperative management of the vascular surgery patient includes ensuring compliance and optimization of blood pressure and heart rate control as well as planning for anesthetic and analgesic regimens that effectively moderate the surgical stress response and provide optimal analgesia for the patient.

Nitrates. The class of drugs with the longest history in the treatment of coronary artery disease is the nitrates. They can be administered sublingually, orally, topically, or intravenously. Systemic nitrates cause systemic venodilation, decreasing preload and ventricular fiber length. They also cause coronary artery vasodilation. One of the problems with the use of nitrates is the development of tolerance, and for this reason many patients receive nitrates during the daytime only, with an abstinent period at night. Patients who are receiving chronic nitrate therapy should continue the drug until the time of surgery. The efficacy of intraoperative nitroglycerin is unclear. Several studies evaluating the efficacy of prophylactic nitroglycerin failed to demonstrate any decrease in the incidence of myocardial ischemia or death.[56-59] However, patients who have been nitrate responsive and who manifest intraoperative ischemia should receive intravenous nitroglycerin unless they are hypotensive (see Chapter 2).[44]

β-Adrenergic blockade. It is reasonable to believe that administering agents to block the specific agents of the surgical stress response might be helpful in preventing perioperative myocardial ischemia. A number of studies have been conducted to assess the efficacy of such a strategy. The cornerstone of medical management of coronary artery disease is β-receptor blockade. Several studies have assessed the efficacy of β-receptor antagonists. Many of these studies have demonstrated benefit in reducing perioperative ischemic cardiac events.[60-66] Another study found beneficial hemodynamic results from the use of perioperative β-blockade but did not find a decrease in markers of the perioperative stress response in a group of elderly orthopedic patients.[67]

The applicability of these studies to large groups of patients at risk has been difficult because of criticisms of study design and the particular features of the study populations, which are often small.[68-72] However, the demonstration of benefit in the

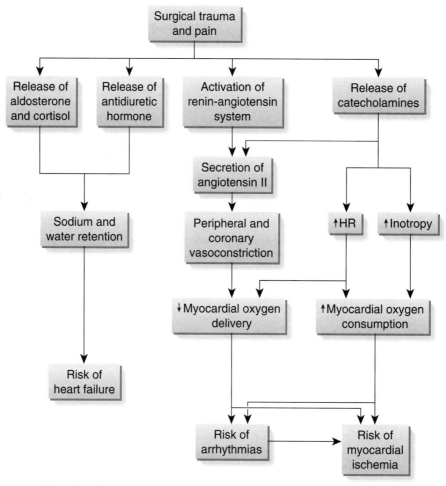

FIGURE 6-1 Hemodynamic consequences of the surgical stress response. In patients with coronary artery disease or left ventricular dysfunction, this response can be detrimental. HR, heart rate.

study by Poldermans et al and general lack of significant side effects of the cardioselective β-blockers have led to broad recommendations for their use in most of the typical patients undergoing vascular surgery.[63] In the most recent American College of Cardiology/American Heart Association (ACC/AHA) Practice Guidelines for Perioperative Cardiovascular Evaluation for Noncardiac Surgery, the use of perioperative β-blockers is a class I recommendation in patients who have symptomatic angina, hypertension, or arrhythmias that respond to β-blockers and in patients who have been demonstrated to be at high cardiac risk by preoperative evaluation who are undergoing vascular surgery.[44] The use of β-blockade is a class IIa recommendation for patients with untreated hypertension, known coronary artery disease, or major risk factors for coronary artery disease. Class I recommendations are conditions for which there is evidence and/or general agreement that the treatment is useful and effective. Class II recommendations are conditions for which there is conflicting evidence and/or a divergence of opinion about the usefulness or efficacy of a treatment. Within class II recommendations, class IIa recommendations imply that the weight of the evidence is in favor of the treatment, and in class IIb the weight of the evidence does not support the treatment.

α-Adrenergic blockade. The use of α-adrenergic agonists for perioperative cardiac protection has been studied. Although the specific results of these studies have varied regarding which aspect of cardiac outcome was positively affected, all of these studies have demonstrated some beneficial effect of α-receptor agonism. One large study of mivazerol infusion used intraoperatively and postoperatively found no decrease in the incidence of myocardial infarction but did find a reduced cardiac death rate.[73] Another smaller trial comparing two mivazerol doses with placebo found no difference in perioperative death or myocardial infarction between groups but found less ischemia in the high-risk group.[74] Two other studies that evaluated clonidine found a decrease in the incidence of perioperative myocardial ischemia.[75,76] The relative lack of data regarding α-adrenergic agonists in this setting has resulted in a class IIb recommendation for α_2-agonists.[44]

Heart Failure

CHF is an important public health problem. It affects more than 3 million patients in the United States with an annual incidence of 400,000 new cases and twice as many annual hospitalizations.[16] Unlike that of coronary heart disease and other forms of cardiovascular disease, its incidence is increasing. This increase is a consequence of the improved survival of patients experiencing myocardial infarction and the improved treatment of hypertension and other risk factors for CHF. The morbidity and mortality associated with CHF are considerable. Mortality rates within 1 year of initial hospitalization for CHF in a variety of studies in elderly persons are approximately 25%.[16] Mortality rates in younger patients range from 8% to 19%.[77-79] The survival rate in patients with CHF is inversely proportional to left ventricular function.[80]

The broadest view of the pathophysiology of heart failure is impaired ability of stroke volume to meet the needs of the peripheral circulation. When this occurs acutely, many compensatory changes occur, including tachycardia and vasoconstriction mediated by catecholamines, which produce increased ventricular filling through the Frank-Starling mechanism. Reduced renal perfusion and sympathetic activation cause the release of renin from the kidney, with activation of the renin-angiotensin system. Angiotensin II secretion results in continued vasoconstriction as well as sodium and intravascular volume retention through aldosterone stimulation. Eventually, in chronic CHF, no further improvements in contractility can occur because the ventricle is functioning on the flat portion of the Frank-Starling curve. The initial compensatory changes become detrimental.[81] Eventually, the myocardium experiences decreased β-receptor responsiveness, with less response to catecholamines, and less β_2-receptor–mediated vasodilation.[82] Clinical signs include the presence of an S_3 heart sound, jugular venous distention, peripheral edema, and pulmonary rales. Symptoms include decreased exercise tolerance, dyspnea, orthopnea, and cough. Transthoracic echocardiography is a useful diagnostic modality to assess left ventricular function and ejection fraction as well as to rule out any other cardiac pathology that may exacerbate the problem.

Heart failure can arise because of problems with systolic or diastolic function. Classic descriptions of heart failure centered predominantly on systolic dysfunction or CHF. More recently, problems with diastolic function have been described and suggest a different pathophysiologic process from "pump failure." Understanding this difference is important as the presentation, prognosis, and treatment of systolic heart failure are different from those for diastolic heart failure.[80,83] High-output failure is uncommon but should be suspected in appropriate clinical scenarios such as chronic anemia and hyperthyroidism. Vascular surgery patients may have specific reasons for high-output failure such as shunting through hemodialysis fistulas and, rarely, from large arteriovenous fistulas (e.g., aortocaval, femoral arteriovenous).

Systolic dysfunction in the vascular surgery population is usually attributable to the consequences of myocardial ischemia and infarction, although other forms of heart failure can also be a problem in this population of patients.[80] Chronic hypertension, frequently associated with left ventricular hypertrophy, can cause the diastolic heart failure variant, which is found more often in women (Figure 6-2).[84] A study of the Framingham Heart Study population found that over the past 50 years, the incidence of heart failure has declined in women but not in men.[85] Survival after the onset of heart failure has improved in both sexes over the same time interval. The gender difference in this study is believed to be related to the differ-

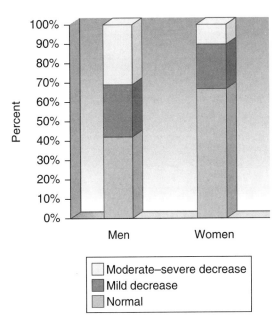

LV SYSTOLIC FUNCTION BY GENDER

FIGURE 6-2 Data demonstrating better preservation of left ventricular (LV) systolic function in women. This may account for the higher incidence of diastolic heart failure in this group. (Modified from Kitzman DW, Gardin JM, Gottdiener JA, et al: *Am J Cardiol* 87:413, 2001.)

ence in etiology of heart failure in men and women. Men typically experience heart failure after repeated episodes of myocardial ischemia or infarction (systolic heart failure), whereas in women, heart failure is more often attributed to undertreated hypertension and left ventricular hypertrophy (diastolic heart failure). The decreased incidence of heart failure in women may be accounted for by the improvements in treatment of hypertension. Overall survival has probably improved because of advances in the medical therapy of heart failure, including ACEIs and β-receptor blockade, which are the standard of care.[86-88] Table 6-2 outlines the recommended medical therapies for heart failure. The suggested use of digitalis in CHF is limited to patients with symptomatic left ventricular dysfunction or asymptomatic patients with atrial fibrillation.[89] The treatment of diastolic dysfunction is more controversial but generally includes aggressive treatment of hypertension.[90]

RATIONALE FOR USE OF ACE-I AND β-RECEPTOR ANTAGONISTS. Therapy for heart failure is intended to reduce the risk of additional ischemic injury to the failing heart, reduce the process of myocardial remodeling that occurs in response to increased afterload, and promote optimization of cardiac output by decreasing left ventricular afterload. ACEIs have widespread effects at multiple levels of the renin-angiotensin system. They inhibit the secretion of angiotensin II, promoting vasodilation and afterload reduction, which allows improvement in stroke volume and cardiac output. Angiotensin II–mediated sympathetic nervous system activation is also prevented.[81] ACEIs have been shown to prevent further deterioration in left ventricular function, which may be the mechanism

TABLE 6-2

Therapy for Heart Failure

Category of Patient	Therapy	Recommendation Class*	Level of Evidence†
At high risk for CHF	Blood pressure control	I	A
With history of vascular disease, diabetes, hypertension	ACEI	I	B
With supraventricular tachyarrhythmia	Ventricular rate control	I	B
LV dysfunction but asymptomatic	ACEI	I	A
With history of MI	ACEI	I	A
With reduced EF	ACEI	I	B
With recent MI	β-Blocker	I	A
With reduced EF	β-Blocker	I	B
LV dysfunction with current or prior symptoms	Sodium restriction	I	A
With evidence of fluid retention	Diuretic	I	A
	ACEI	I	A
	β-Blocker	I	A
	Digitalis	I	A
Patients who cannot tolerate ACEI	ARA	IIa	A
Diastolic dysfunction	Blood pressure control	I	A

Definition of recommendation class: I, conditions for which there is evidence for and/or general agreement that the treatment is useful and effective; II, conditions for which there is conflicting evidence and/or a divergence of opinion about the usefulness or efficacy of a treatment; IIa, the weight of the evidence or opinion is in favor of the treatment.

†*Levels of evidence*: A, data derived from multiple randomized clinical trials; B, data derived from single randomized trial or nonrandomized studies; C, primary source of recommendation is consensus of experts.

ACEI, angiotensin-converting enzyme inhibitor; ARA, angiotensin receptor antagonist; CHF, congestive heart failure; EF, ejection fraction; LV, left ventricular; MI, myocardial infarction.

Adapted from Hunt HA, Baker DW, Chin MH, et al: *Circulation* 104:2996, 2001.

responsible for the improvement in survival in heart failure (see Chapter 2).[91]

β-receptor blockade was initially thought to be harmful to patients with heart failure, but a series of studies has demonstrated improved morbidity and mortality in patients receiving β-receptor antagonists. The beneficial effects of β-receptor antagonists include decreasing resting heart rate, controlling arrhythmias, and countering the maladaptive effects of increased adrenergic drive found in chronic heart failure.[92] These maladaptive effects include an increase in myocardial oxygen demand, downregulation of β_1-receptors, and uncoupling of β_2-receptors, which eventually render the myocyte less responsive to catecholamines. β-Blockade reduces this response and allows better myocardial oxygen balance, resulting in improved left ventricular function and exercise tolerance (see Chapter 2).[93]

PERIOPERATIVE MANAGEMENT. Historically, the presence of heart failure was the most significant predictor of adverse cardiac events in the perioperative period.[94,95] The revision of the

ACC/AHA recommendations for perioperative management of the patient with cardiac disease undergoing noncardiac surgery classifies acute CHF as a major predictor of adverse cardiac events.[44] A past history of CHF is considered a moderate risk factor. Patients with a history of CHF should undergo careful physical examination and history to elicit their cardiac status. Elective surgery should be postponed in patients who manifest new decompensation or symptoms. ACEIs and β-blockers are the mainstay of medical therapy for CHF and should be continued up to and including the day of surgery. The concern over the use of ACEIs in the perioperative period, with severe hypotension occurring with induction of anesthesia, has not been demonstrated in one study of patients taking ACEIs for heart failure.[96] In general, the peripheral vasodilation associated with most anesthetic techniques is well tolerated by patients with impaired left ventricular function as long as perfusion pressures are reasonable. The patient should continue any medications prescribed for heart failure until the time of surgery, and provision should be made to continue these drugs postoperatively. Selection of invasive monitoring techniques should be based on the patient's condition as well as the expected surgical procedure. Careful fluid management may dictate increased levels of invasive monitoring, particularly in patients with impaired renal function and CHF. In addition, attention to providing excellent postoperative analgesia and continuing cardiac medications postoperatively can work to prevent increases in systemic vascular resistance that might be poorly tolerated or precipitate acute pulmonary congestion.

Cardiac Valvular Disease

Cardiac valvular disease is a common problem in elderly people. Rheumatic heart disease, which formerly accounted for a large amount of valve pathology, is much less of an issue in the current era.

AORTIC STENOSIS. Valvular aortic stenosis can be a result of degenerative changes in a congenitally bicuspid aortic valve (1% to 2% of the population), rheumatic heart disease, or more commonly degenerative changes in a structurally normal aortic valve.[97] Obstruction to left ventricular outflow can occur at the valvular, subvalvular, or supravalvular level, but the valvular type is the most common. Elderly patients develop stiffening, fibrosis, and calcification of the aortic valve, and the prevalence of aortic stenosis increases with age. In an observational study of patients in a long-term healthcare facility, Aronow found valvular aortic stenosis in approximately 14% of elderly men.[98] Another study found that approximately 3% of persons older than 75 years had critical aortic stenosis, defined as a valve area less than 1 cm² (normal 2.5 to 3.5 cm²).[99]

When a pressure gradient across the aortic valve exists, left ventricular pressures must increase in order to compensate and allow normal cardiac output. As a result of this obstruction, left ventricular mass increases, resulting in left ventricular hypertrophy and, eventually, decreased compliance of the left ventricle. Slow heart rates allow more complete emptying of the ventricle, and tachycardia is poorly tolerated with significant aortic stenosis because of the combination of decreased ventricular ejection time and decreased diastolic time, resulting in decreased perfusion of the thickened myocardium via epicardial arteries. In addition, left ventricular preload becomes more dependent on the atrial contraction component, so rhythms other than sinus rhythm are poorly tolerated when aortic stenosis becomes severe.

The classic symptoms of aortic stenosis are angina, CHF, and syncope. The likelihood of these symptoms increased with the severity of valve stenosis in a study by Aronow and colleagues.[100] Symptom onset is usually gradual and progressive, and the prognosis for untreated aortic stenosis when CHF develops is poor.[101,102] The intensity of the aortic murmur and other related physical examination findings, such as the presence of an aortic ejection click, are not reliable predictors of the severity of valvular aortic stenosis.[98] Careful physical examination is important to determine the presence of systolic ejection murmurs, but echocardiography is the preferred modality for the diagnosis and severity determination of aortic stenosis as well as other cardiac valvular pathology.

There is general agreement that aortic valve replacement should be considered for symptomatic severe aortic stenosis and for asymptomatic severe stenosis with evidence of left ventricular dysfunction, even in octogenarians.[97,102,103] For patients undergoing vascular surgical procedures who present with evidence of aortic stenosis, a decision about the timing of valve replacement relative to elective vascular surgery must consider the degree of urgency of the vascular procedure as well as the degree and symptoms of aortic stenosis. Surgical decisions should also consider that survival after the onset of symptoms is poor. Patients survive an average of 3 years after the onset of angina, 2 years after dyspnea occurs, and 1.5 to 2 years after CHF ensues.[104] Unfortunately, less invasive approaches to aortic stenosis such as balloon valvuloplasty have not been proved effective.[102]

One small study of approximately 50 patients with uncorrected severe aortic stenosis undergoing noncardiac surgery found only one complication in the group.[105] Although this is only one study and generalization is limited, it is possible that patients with severe aortic stenosis, particularly if asymptomatic, can undergo noncardiac surgery without prior aortic valve replacement. In rare circumstances, patients with severe symptomatic aortic stenosis who require noncardiac surgery might be candidates for aortic balloon valvuloplasty.[106] Obviously, close hemodynamic monitoring and consideration of the pathophysiology of the disease should be incorporated into the anesthetic plan for any patient with severe aortic stenosis presenting for vascular surgery.

Regarding specific measures in the perioperative period, patients with aortic stenosis should receive subacute bacterial endocarditis prophylaxis for indicated procedures.[107] Anesthetic planning should include a low threshold for invasive arterial pressure monitoring in order to ensure optimization of diastolic coronary perfusion pressure and preservation of systemic vascular resistance. Sinus rhythm should be maintained, and slow heart rates will be better tolerated as this will allow longer diastolic times, with more time for endocardial perfusion. A variety of anesthetic techniques can be used safely, although central neuraxial blocks, particularly single dose, should be used only with extreme caution in patients with severe aortic stenosis.

AORTIC REGURGITATION. As with aortic stenosis, the prevalence of aortic regurgitation increases with age. Significant aortic regurgitation was found in about a third of men older than 80 in one study.[98] Aortic regurgitation can develop as a result of degeneration of the valve leaflets, often seen with congenital bicuspid aortic valves, or as a result of pathology of the aortic root, which widens the aortic valve aperture.[102] The progression of chronic aortic regurgitation may be insidious and asymptomatic for many years. When symptoms start to develop, they usually consist of dyspnea on exertion or decreased exercise tolerance.[102]

Aortic regurgitation adds regurgitant blood to normal left ventricular volume, causing a volume overload condition. The ventricle adapts to this with dilation and eccentric hypertrophy. Initially, compliance increases so that filling pressures remain normal. Eventually, as the regurgitant volume increases, stroke volume increases to maintain forward cardiac output. After a time, ventricular wall tension increases to a point at which compliance is reduced. At this point, cardiac output decreases as the stroke volume can no longer increase. If the patient has a competent mitral valve, the pulmonary circulation is protected from the increased left ventricular pressures, but when the valve fails, pulmonary artery pressures increase. From this description, it is clear that a cornerstone of medical therapy for aortic regurgitation is afterload reduction, often accomplished with ACEIs. ACEIs can slow the rate of left ventricular dilation.[102]

Transthoracic echocardiography is a useful diagnostic and prognostic tool for patients with aortic regurgitation. The degree of ventricular dilation can be assessed, and echocardiography can assist with planning the timing of valve replacement. There is widespread agreement that valve replacement is indicated for symptomatic aortic regurgitation, regardless of end-systolic left ventricular systolic size. For the asymptomatic patient, it is felt that the onset of excessive ventricular dilation is a marker for incipient left ventricular systolic dysfunction. The dilation can be assessed with serial echocardiograms, and valve replacement surgery is indicated when ventricular end-systolic dimension exceeds 55 mm.[102] Surgery performed before the onset of irreversible left ventricular dysfunction is associated with good survival and improvement in symptoms.[108]

Patients with aortic regurgitation who are presenting for noncardiac surgery should receive appropriate antibiotic prophylaxis for endocarditis.[107] Hemodynamic monitoring should be planned with consideration of the pathophysiology of aortic regurgitation and the degree of cardiac compensation. Evidence of heart failure symptoms should prompt attention to the patient's cardiac status and delay of vascular surgery unless the surgical procedure is urgent. Most anesthetic agents have vasodilatory effects, reduce afterload, and are well tolerated. Significant bradycardia should be avoided as it can result in severe left ventricular dilation. Regional anesthesia, including central neuraxial conduction blocks, can be well tolerated in this group.

MITRAL STENOSIS. Mitral valve stenosis can arise from rheumatic heart disease or from mitral annular calcium deposition. In the United States, mitral annular calcium is a much more common etiology of mitral stenosis. Mitral annular calcium was found on echocardiography in approximately a third of elderly men in one prospective study, and mitral stenosis was found to exist in approximately 6% of these men.[98] In the same series, rheumatic mitral stenosis was found in less than 1% of the study population. Patients with mitral annular calcification with or without mitral valve stenosis have a higher incidence of atrial fibrillation, coronary disease, CHF, stroke, and transient ischemic attack than patients without mitral annular calcification.

The onset of hemodynamically significant mitral valve stenosis is progressive over many years. The predominant physiologic feature is obstruction to left ventricular filling and a pressure gradient between the left atrium and ventricle. Eventually, left atrial pressure rises to compensate for the gradient and to maintain ventricular filling. This compensatory mechanism maintains cardiac output until the mitral valve area is reduced to approximately 1.5 cm.^{2} Chronically increased left atrial pressure is transmitted to the pulmonary venous system and eventually to the pulmonary arterial circulation, resulting in pulmonary hypertension and, ultimately, right ventricular failure. Left ventricular function is usually preserved unless the patient has coexisting coronary artery disease or has dysfunction as a result of rheumatic myocarditis.[106]

Enlargement of the left atrium predisposes the patient to the development of atrial fibrillation. The loss of coordinated atrial contraction decreases ventricular filling, particularly through a stenotic mitral valve, and generally causes a decrease in cardiac output. Hemodynamic goals in caring for patients with mitral stenosis are summarized in Table 6-3, but maintenance of a slow heart rate is essential for allowing optimal time for left ventricular filling. Attempts at chemical or electrical cardioversion of patients with long-standing chronic atrial fibrillation are rarely successful, but emergent cardioversion of patients with mitral stenosis who develop acute atrial fibrillation is important to preserve cardiac output.

A cornerstone of therapy for patients with chronic atrial fibrillation is antithrombotic therapy. This has been demonstrated to decrease the risk of stroke and cerebral events.[109] Atrial fibrillation is the most common cardiac arrhythmia, and its incidence is estimated as approximately 6% of people older than 65 and 10% of patients older than 80, with or without the presence of mitral stenosis.[110] Patients undergoing major surgery who receive warfarin therapy should discontinue its use prior to surgery, with enough time for normalization of coagulation status, and patients deemed at high risk for a cerebral event should be converted to shorter acting heparin therapy in the perioperative period. The coagulation status of the patient can have impact on the choice of anesthetics, particularly regional anesthesia.

MITRAL REGURGITATION. Mitral valve regurgitation in the typical elderly vascular patient occurs as a result of ischemia with ensuing papillary muscle dysfunction or degenerative changes in the mitral valve apparatus.[111] Much as with mitral valvular stenosis, the most common cause of chronic mitral regurgitation is mitral annular calcium. A prospective study revealed echocardiographic evidence of at least mild mitral regurgitation in approximately a third of elderly patients, with greater degrees of insufficiency in patients with mitral annular calcification.[98]

Chronic mitral regurgitation is usually well tolerated as the left ventricle accommodates to volume overload more readily than to pressure overload. The regurgitant mitral valve allows a pressure pop-off to the left atrium, which dilates and increases in compliance. Ventricular function remains normal unless there is concomitant ischemic disease or cardiomyopathy. Pulmonary hypertension can occur because of prolonged increases in left atrial volume and pressure.

Patients undergoing vascular surgery who have mitral regurgitation should be carefully evaluated for the cause of the valvular dysfunction (e.g., rheumatic disease, ischemia). In the absence of evidence of CHF or pulmonary edema, surgery can proceed with planning for and understanding of the underlying hemodynamic principles. Pretreatment with the appropriate antibiotics for endocarditis prophylaxis should be undertaken.[107] Many anesthetic techniques are suitable for patients with mitral regurgitation, and as long as preload is maintained at a reasonable level, regional anesthesia, including central neuraxial blockade, is well tolerated for appropriate cases. The systemic vasodilation caused by most general anesthetic agents, as well as central neuraxial blockade, is usually well tolerated by this group of patients. Significant increases in afterload, such as cross-clamping of the aorta, increase the regurgitant fraction of the left ventricle and can be offset by appropriate use of vasodilators. Table 6-3 outlines the hemodynamic principles for the classic valve lesions.

Diabetes Mellitus

Diabetes mellitus is a chronic, multisystem disease that arises from a relative or absolute lack of insulin. The two types of diabetes, juvenile-onset or type 1 and non–insulin-dependent or type 2, have distinct differences. Patients with type 1 diabetes have suffered destruction of the islet cells in the pancreas and have an absolute deficiency of insulin. They are susceptible to the development of ketoacidosis and require exogenous insulin. Those with type 2 diabetes have insulin resistance or a relative deficiency of insulin. Obesity is commonly associated with type 2 diabetes mellitus.

Accelerated atherosclerosis is common in diabetes and accounts for the high incidence of both vascular disease and coronary artery disease in diabetics. The reason for such a high association is not entirely clear, but it is thought to be related to glycosylation of various lipoproteins that are important in

---

TABLE 6-3

Cardiac Valvular Disease and Hemodynamic Goals

Valve Lesion	Heart Rate	Preload	Afterload	Contractility
Aortic stenosis	Slow, maintain sinus rhythm	Full	High	Normal
Aortic insufficiency	Normal to increased	Normal to full	Low	Normal
Mitral stenosis	Slow, sinus rhythm optimal	Full	Normal	Normal
Mitral regurgitation	Normal to increased	Full	Low	Normal

the genesis of atherosclerosis. Other potential factors include decreased synthesis of vasodilating prostacyclins and increased platelet adhesiveness in diabetics. In addition, diabetics have a high incidence of coronary artery disease and, with the development of autonomic neuropathy, are at high risk for silent ischemia. One older study found a high incidence (7%) of postoperative death in patients with diabetes-induced autonomic dysfunction.[112] A more recent study agreed that diabetics have autonomic dysfunction but did not find an altered hemodynamic response to induction of anesthesia in these patients.[113] Diabetics have a higher risk of mortality from coronary artery disease even compared with nondiabetics who have suffered a previous myocardial infarction.[114] Diabetics also have increased morbidity and mortality compared with nondiabetics undergoing vascular surgery.[115]

Autonomic neuropathy is also associated with the development of delayed gastric emptying or gastroparesis.[116] A careful history can elicit symptoms of gastroparesis, but as a general rule, patients with other end-organ manifestations of diabetes are likely to have delayed gastric emptying. Premedication with a prokinetic drug such as metoclopramide may promote gastric emptying, but steps to avoid pulmonary aspiration of gastric contents should be included in the anesthetic plan.

Diabetes causes diffuse microangiopathy in all vascular beds. This process accounts for diabetic retinopathy and nephropathy. The basement membrane in the glomerulus becomes thickened, with the development of proteinuria. Renal failure is a devastating consequence of diabetes. Several studies have demonstrated a renoprotective effect with ACEIs and ARAs. Early institution of treatment with an ACEI or ARA is now a standard of care in diabetics to decrease the likelihood of renal failure, with or without hypertension.[117,118]

Preoperative evaluation of diabetic patients should focus on assessing the presence and severity of end-organ complications and understanding the hypoglycemic regimen prescribed for the patient. Table 6-4 describes the available oral hypoglycemic agents and their perioperative considerations. Monitoring and anesthetic choices should be predicated upon the severity of the comorbid diseases. Patients with ketoacidosis or hyperosmolar coma should not undergo surgical procedures unless they are

emergency procedures.[119] In general, given the consequences of undetected hypoglycemia in anesthetized patients, most clinicians favor tolerance of mild hyperglycemia in diabetic patients undergoing surgery. However, hyperglycemia is detrimental when patients experience neurologic injury, so tighter glycemic control may be desirable in vascular surgery patients undergoing cerebral revascularization or aortic surgery.[120,121]

Perioperative glucose management can be handled in a variety of ways. Diabetic patients, particularly those with type 1 diabetes, are best handled as first cases so that blood sugar management can be closely supervised in the operating room. In general, the neuroendocrine stress response is greater with more invasive surgery, increasing the likelihood of perioperative hyperglycemia. Those with type 2 diabetes undergoing minor outpatient procedures can usually be managed by withholding oral hypoglycemics on the day of surgery, checking a preoperative blood sugar, and administering insulin if needed. Type 1 diabetics require insulin despite their nil per os status but are also at risk of hypoglycemia without an exogenous source of carbohydrate. For minor-to-moderate surgery, normoglycemia can be accomplished by administering a portion of the normal dose of long-acting insulin subcutaneously upon arrival in the preoperative area. Table 6-5 describes the pharmacokinetics of the commonly used insulins. An intravenous infusion of 5% dextrose is started at the same time to minimize the risk of hypoglycemia. Frequent blood sugar measurements are made, and additional insulin is given as necessary. Patients under anesthesia should receive insulin intravenously, as skin blood flow and insulin absorption can vary tremendously during surgery. Patients with brittle diabetes, or who are undergoing extensive surgery, can often be managed more easily with a continuous infusion of insulin, titrated to blood glucose, which is monitored hourly.[122]

Obstructive Lung Disease and Tobacco Abuse

Tobacco use is a known risk factor for the development of coronary artery disease, peripheral vascular disease, and cerebrovascular disease. It is also closely associated with the development of chronic obstructive pulmonary disease

---

TABLE 6-4

Common Oral Hypoglycemic Agents*

Category	Examples	Method of Action	Cautions
Sulfonylureas	Glyburide Glipizide Glimepiride	Stimulate insulin release from pancreatic islet beta cells	Hyperglycemia, aplastic anemia, agranulocytosis
Biguanides	Metformin	Decrease hepatic glucose production and intestinal glucose absorption, increase insulin sensitivity	Lactic acidosis Avoid iodinated contrast material Discontinue 48 hours preoperatively
Glucosidase inhibitors	Acarbose Miglitol	Decrease intestinal absorption of glucose, inhibit pancreatic α-amylase and intestinal α-glucoside hydrolase	Modest hypoglycemic effect
Thiazolidinediones	Rosiglitazone Pioglitazone	Increase insulin sensitivity	Gastrointestinal side effects Low risk of hypoglycemia. Risk of hepatic toxicity, anemia

*All of these medications have interactions with common antihypertensive medications such as β-blockers and angiotensin-converting enzyme inhibitors, which can decrease the hypoglycemic effects of these drugs.

TABLE 6-5

Pharmacokinetics of Commonly Used Insulin Preparations

Type	Examples	Route of Administration	Onset (min)	Peak Effect (min)	Duration (hr)
Insulin lispro	Lispro	SC	<30	30–90	<6
Insulin lente	Humulin L	SC	60–180	480–720	18–24
Insulin regular	Humulin R	SC, IV	30	120–240	6–8
Insulin ultralente	Humulin U	SC	240–480	960–1080	>36
Insulin aspart	NovoLog	SC	<30	60–180	3–5
Insulin glargine	Lantus	SC	60	Unknown	24

IV, intravenous; SC, subcutaneous.

(COPD). It is not surprising that a large number of patients presenting for vascular surgery have COPD and/or a history of tobacco abuse. Patients with chronic lung disease and smokers are at increased risk for the development of postoperative pulmonary complications (PPCs). Complications include bronchospasm, diaphragmatic dysfunction, hypoxemia, atelectasis, pneumonia, and the need for postoperative ventilation. Smokers have an increased volume of tracheobronchial secretions and decreased mucociliary clearance of secretions.[123]

The pulmonary effects of general anesthesia include a decrease in closing capacity, decreased functional residual capacity, ventilation-perfusion mismatch, and impaired mucociliary clearance. The impact of the site of surgery is also important, as upper abdominal surgery, such as open abdominal aortic surgery, has the greatest negative impact on pulmonary function postoperatively through its effect on the muscles of respiration.[124] In addition, exposure to tobacco smoke causes impairment of the tracheobronchial mucociliary elevator and impairment of the antibacterial and inflammatory function of alveolar macrophages, leading to increased risk of pulmonary infection.[125,126] Tobacco smoke increases the amount of carboxyhemoglobin in the blood, which limits cellular oxygen transport. Nicotine promotes vasoconstriction and may predispose to myocardial ischemia and exacerbate hypertension.[127,128] Given the high prevalence of coronary artery disease in vascular patients, this finding is significant. Another study has found increased likelihood of wound infection and impaired wound healing and flap function in smokers.[129]

On the basis of these detrimental factors, some authors suggest cessation of smoking 6 months prior to surgery.[130] Two studies of PPCs in cardiac surgery found an increased risk of PPCs if smoking is ceased within 8 weeks of surgery.[131,132] The 8-week abstinence recommendation is supported by the facts that sputum production does not decrease until 7 to 14 days of abstinence from tobacco, and pulmonary function tests and patients' symptoms typically require 4 to 6 weeks of abstinence for improvement.

From a practical perspective, most smokers, particularly if anxious, find it very difficult to quit smoking prior to surgery, and not many vascular operations are so elective as to allow a 6-month-long abstinence period. More practical recommendations for the management of COPD and cigarette smoking would be to encourage smoking cessation if this can be achieved within the 8-week interval shown to decrease the likelihood of PPC prior to surgery.[133] If this is not possible, patients should be encouraged to abstain from nicotine beginning 24 to 48 hours before surgery in order to decrease circulating levels of carboxyhemoglobin.[130]

Patients with COPD should be assessed for the presence of superimposed infection and, if it is present, should receive antibiotics for an appropriate time interval prior to surgery. Any inhaled bronchodilators prescribed for the patient should be continued through the time of surgery. Patients who take inhaled or systemic steroids should have these drugs continued through the time of surgery. With the advent of modern bronchodilators, methylxanthines are used much less frequently, but patients who are maintained on theophylline should continue this medication through surgery. Anesthesiologists should be alert to the propensity for tachyarrhythmias with this drug as well as its interactions with other drugs and their clearance and metabolism. Patients with severe obstructive disease should be evaluated for nutritional and electrolyte disturbances, and any abnormalities should be corrected depending upon the urgency of the surgical procedure. Also, COPD patients and patients with asthma can benefit from administration of steroid therapy prior to surgery. Steroid therapy has been shown to decrease the likelihood of bronchospasm in the perioperative period and has not been demonstrated to affect the postoperative course adversely.[134] Other risk reduction strategies in the perioperative period include lung expansion maneuvers and provision of appropriate postoperative pain control.[135]

Premedication of the Vascular Surgery Patient

The setting for perioperative medical practice in the early 21st century is quite different from that in the past. However, the goals of premedication for vascular surgery have not changed. The challenge is accomplishing these goals in what is increasingly an outpatient situation.

Table 6-6 outlines the goals of premedication for the vascular surgery patient.[136] The focus on outpatient preoperative management can allow a more optimal time frame to accomplish the goal of stabilizing comorbid medical conditions. Many patients present for vascular surgery in centers far removed from their homes; but whenever possible, it is advantageous for the anesthesiologist to see the patient in the preoperative clinic as much as 2 to 4 weeks ahead of the planned surgical date. This allows adequate time for institution of therapy for comorbid conditions or for specialized medical consultation should it be required. Certain goals of premedication are unique to the vascular surgery patient.

TABLE 6-6

TABLE 6-6

Goals of Premedication in the Vascular Surgery Patient

Continue therapy of chronic medical conditions
Provide anxiolysis
Facilitate preinduction invasive procedures
Optimize cardiovascular stability
Prevent cardiorespiratory depression
In selected cases, premedication can provide the following:
Protection for patients at risk for pulmonary aspiration
Pain control for limb ischemia
Amnesia
Antisialagogue effect
Antiemetic effect
Prophylaxis against allergic reactions
Prevention of bacterial endocarditis

Modified from Clark SK, Rung GW, Hensley FA Jr: Premedication for the vascular surgery patient. In Kaplan JA (ed): *Vascular anesthesia*, New York, 1991, Churchill Livingstone, p188.

Sedative-Hypnotics

It is now unusual for patients presenting for vascular surgery to have met their anesthesiologist prior to the day of surgery. This situation can lead to a great amount of anxiety for the patient and family, who are understandably already anxious about the planned surgical procedure. Anesthesiologists have little time to establish a comfortable rapport and sense of trust, yet this is important for these patients, who are often at high risk.

A decision about whether to prescribe an oral anxiolytic that the patient can take prior to arriving at the hospital must be individualized to the needs of the patient, the surgical procedure, and the anesthesia team that is to care for the patient on the day of surgery. Many anesthesiologists enjoy having the opportunity to interact with their patients and would prefer to be able to meet the patient without the clouding effects of sedatives. Also, it is optimal if the patient can accurately answer questions about any interval changes in his or her condition, particularly if there has been a long time interval between the preoperative visit and the day of surgery. Many vascular surgery patients are elderly with associated comorbid conditions, and the effects of aging on the metabolism and elimination of sedatives should be considered.[111] The philosophy of premedication for the increasingly rare inpatient presenting for vascular surgery has also evolved over the last decade. Often, the safest way to premedicate these patients, who are usually quite ill, is to withhold sedating premedicants until the patient has arrived in the preoperative area, at which point the patient can receive medication under the direct supervision of the anesthesiologist, with appropriate monitoring and concomitant oxygen administration. One new challenge is the development of endovascular techniques for aortic reconstruction. When regional anesthesia is used, precise titration of sedation is necessary to maintain the patient in a calm but cooperative state so that she or he can cooperate with breath holding during angiography and graft deployment. Care must be taken to avoid oversedating these patients while establishing invasive monitoring and regional anesthesia.

Benzodiazepines are the most widely used form of anxiolytic. They have replaced barbiturates as the most popular form of sedative premedicant because of their greater predictability of effect and lack of antianalgesic effect. They can be administered by a variety of routes and produce sedation and amnesia in addition to anxiolysis. Toxicity of the benzodiazepines, particularly when administered without other sedatives or central nervous system depressants, is low. The various drugs in this class vary in their pharmacokinetics, and this should be considered when selecting premedication drugs. For example, the long elimination half-lives of diazepam or lorazepam may make these drugs less desirable in elderly patients or in patients presenting for carotid endarterectomy, in whom prompt and accurate postoperative neurologic assessment is important.[111]

Midazolam is the most widely used sedative preoperative medication. It offers advantages over the classic benzodiazepine diazepam in that it has a more rapid onset and shorter duration. Its solubility in water avoids the phlebitis and painful injection that were associated with diazepam and its propylene glycol solvent.[137] Its rapid onset after intravenous dosing (1 to 2 minutes) makes it an attractive choice for use in the setting of same-day admission for surgery and simplifies dose titration.

Lorazepam is another benzodiazepine with utility in vascular surgery. It is about twice as potent as midazolam and can be administered orally or parenterally. Its maximum effect is slower than that of midazolam, approximately 30 minutes after intravenous injection and about 30 to 60 minutes after oral administration.[138] It has a more extended duration than that of midazolam, which makes it an attractive choice for patients undergoing longer procedures, such as aortic aneurysm repair.

Although diazepam has a long record of use and safety as a premedicant, it has been supplanted by lorazepam and midazolam because of some of its side effects. Diazepam is solubilized in propylene glycol and causes pain on intravenous injection as well as intramuscular injection. Its onset is slow, and it has the longest elimination half-life of the benzodiazepines. Unlike those of lorazepam, its metabolites are active, and this can create prolonged sedative effects that may be undesirable in elderly patients or in situations in which early mobilization of the patient is preferred.

α_2-Adrenergic Agonists

α_2-Adrenergic agonists have been used as premedicants to promote both anxiolysis and cardiovascular stability.[139] The largest experience is with clonidine, which can be administered orally in doses of about 2 to 5 µg/kg. The effects of clonidine include sedation, dry mouth, bradycardia, and hypotension. It has been used to promote hemodynamic stability during periods of stress such as laryngoscopy and surgical stimulation. Dexmedetomidine has similar effects, but its utility as a premedicant is limited by the need for intravenous infusion.

Opioids

Approximately 15 years ago it was common for inpatients presenting for vascular surgical procedures to receive intramuscular opioids in conjunction with a sedative hypnotic as a premedication. They were then transported to the operating room without a nurse or physician and often without supplemental oxygen. The response to such premedication was variable, and many patients arrived in the operating room in an overse-dated state.

This state of affairs is no surprise if the side effects of opi-oids are considered. Opioids in usual doses are not myocardial depressants but depress respiration in a dose-responsive fash-ion. They decrease ventilatory response to hypercarbia and the carotid body response to hypoxia.[140] In addition, patients who have had bilateral carotid endarterectomy or sequential endarterectomy have a long-lasting decreased carotid chemore-ceptor response to hypoxia, which should be considered when such a patient presents for additional vascular surgery.[141]

Opioids are desirable premedicants when the patient is expe-riencing pain before the operation, such as a patient awaiting lower extremity revascularization who has rest or ischemic pain. They are also useful to reduce the pain associated with invasive monitoring procedures or placement of epidural catheters. However, unsupervised administration of opioids to patients who do not have pain, particularly the opioid naive, can be hazardous. Opioids also have other undesirable side effects, including pruritus that is mediated by histamine release and provocation of nausea by stimulation of the chemoreceptor trig-ger zone in the medulla. It should also be remembered that opi-oids and benzodiazepines are synergistic and potentiate each other's effects when given in combination.

If an opioid premedication is desired, the use of fentanyl, a synthetic opioid agonist, as a premedicant is attractive because of its rapid onset (6 to 7 minutes after intravenous dosing), which facilitates gradual dose titration. This feature, along with sparing of cardiac depressant effects, makes it useful for the outpatient presenting for vascular surgery. Fentanyl is redistrib-uted rapidly to the lungs, fat, and muscle, which accounts for its short duration. Clearance rates may be decreased in elderly patients, which can prolong the elimination and effect of fentanyl.[142]

Aspiration Prophylaxis

Vascular surgery patients are not unique in their potential risk for pulmonary aspiration of gastric contents. However, some groups of vascular surgical patients are at high risk of aspira-tion, either because of long-standing diabetes or because of cer-tain surgical conditions. Conditions such as large abdominal aortic aneurysms exert an intra-abdominal mass effect, and emergent operations for conditions such as ruptured abdominal aortic aneurysm or mesenteric ischemia affect gastrointestinal motility.

The goal in premedication for aspiration prophylaxis is to minimize the volume and increase the pH of gastric contents. This goal can be partially achieved by administration of H_2-receptor antagonists, which increase gastric pH but have no effect on gastric volume. Cimetidine, ranitidine, famotidine, and nizatidine have all been shown to increase gastric pH.[143,144] These drugs have few side effects, but some practitioners favor using drugs other than cimetidine because of its inhibition of the hepatic mixed-function oxidase system. Theoretically, this inhibition can prolong the half-life of other drugs. In addition, cimetidine is the shortest acting of the agents and requires more frequent dosing. For these reasons, ranitidine and famotidine have become more widely used for aspiration prophylaxis. They can be administered by mouth or intravenously. The

newer class of proton pump inhibitors, such as omeprazole and pantoprazole, have also been used to increase gastric pH and, like the H_2-receptor antagonists, have not been shown to decrease gastric volume reliably.[145]

Administration of clear nonparticulate antacid (sodium cit-rate, 30 mL) reliably raises the pH of gastric contents. The use of particulate antacids is not advisable because of the risk of pulmonary toxicity should they be aspirated. Nonparticulate antacids are useful to raise the pH of gastric contents acutely but have limited duration of effect, usually less than 30 min-utes. For this reason, they are most effective when used in emergency situations when doses of H_2-receptor antagonists have not had adequate time for full effect.

As mentioned earlier, diabetic patients with gastroparesis are at high risk of passive reflux and aspiration of gastric contents. The addition of a gastrokinetic agent such as meto-clopramide can promote gastric emptying. Metoclopramide is a dopamine antagonist that produces upper gastrointesti-nal motility and increases lower esophageal sphincter tone. It may be most effective when combined with H_2-receptor antagonists.[146]

Conclusion

Vascular anesthesiologists face increasing challenges as older and sicker patients present for repair of vascular surgical prob-lems. The drive toward less invasive surgical procedures means that these technologies will be offered to groups of patients who are unfit for conventional repair. Preoperative optimiza-tion of the multiple comorbid medical conditions associated with vascular disease helps to provide the best possible out-come in the postoperative period. The increasing number of patients presenting on the day of surgery can provide an enhanced opportunity to address these preoperative concerns; at the same time, it provides the anesthesiologist and the patient with the challenge of establishing a meaningful rapport in the stressful environment of the preoperative holding area.

REFERENCES

1. Egbert LD, Battit GE, Turndorf H, et al: The value of the preoperative visit by an anesthetist, *JAMA* 185:553, 1963.
2. Leigh JM, Walker J, Janaganathan P: Effect of preoperative anaesthetic visit on anxiety, *Br Med J* 2:987, 1977.
3. Sixth report of the Joint National Committee on Prevention, Detection, Evaluation and Treatment of High Blood Pressure, *Arch Intern Med* 157:2413, 1997.
4. Domino KB: Perioperative hypertension, *Am J Anesth* 26:259, 1999.
5. The Management Committee of the Australian National Blood Pressure Study: Prognostic factors in the treatment of mild hypertension, *Circulation* 69:668, 1984.
6. Hypertension Detection, and Follow-up Program Cooperative Group: Five-year findings of the Hypertension Detection and Follow-Up Program I. Reduction in mortality of persons with high blood pressure, including mild hypertension, *JAMA* 242:2562, 1979.
7. Amery A, Brixko R, Clement D, et al: Efficacy of antihypertensive drug treatment according to age, sex, blood pressure and previous cardiovascular disease in patients over the age of 60, *Lancet* 339:589, 1986.
8. Medical Research Council Working Party: MRC trial of treatment of mild hypertension: principal results, *Br Med J* 291:97, 1985.
9. Kannell WB: Elevated systolic blood pressure as a cardiovascular risk factor, *Am J Cardiol* 85:251, 2000.

10. Staessen JA, Fagard R, Lutgarde T, et al: Randomised double-blind comparison of placebo and active treatment for older patients with isolated systolic hypertension, *Lancet* 350:757, 1997.

11. Black HR: Isolated systolic hypertension in the elderly: lessons from clinical trials and future directions, *J Hypertens* 17(Suppl 5):S49, 1999.

12. Amery A, Brixko F, Clement D, et al: Mortality and morbidity results from the European Working Party on High Blood Pressure in the Elderly Trial, *Lancet* 338:1349, 1985.

13. Verdecchia P: White coat hypertension in adults and children, *Blood Press Monit* 4:175, 1999.

14. Verdecchia P, Palatini P, Schillaci G, et al: Independent predictors of isolated clinical ("white coat") hypertension, *J Hypertens* 6:1015, 2001.

15. Richardson LG, Rocks M: Women and heart failure, *Heart Lung* 30:87, 2001.

16. Kitzman DW: Diastolic heart failure in the elderly, *Heart Fail Rev* 7:17, 2002.

17. Senni M, Redfield MM: Heart failure with preserved systolic function: a different natural history? *J Am Coll Cardiol* 38:1277, 2001.

18. Prys-Roberts C, Meloche R, Foex P: Studies of anaesthesia in relation to hypertension I. Cardiovascular responses of treated and untreated patients, *Br J Anaesth* 43:122, 1971.

19. Assidao CB, Donegan JH, Whitesell RC, et al: Factors associated with perioperative complications during carotid endarterectomy, *Anesth Analg* 61:631, 1982.

20. Goldman L, Caldera DL: Risks of general anesthesia and elective operation in the hypertensive patient, *Anesthesiology* 50:285, 1979.

21. Rose DK, Cohen MM, DeBoer DM: Cardiovascular events in the postanesthesia care unit: contribution of risk factors, *Anesthesiology* 84:772, 1996.

22. Strandgaard S: Autoregulation of cerebral blood flow in hypertensive patients. The modifying influence of prolonged antihypertensive treatment on the tolerance to acute, drug-induced hypotension, *Circulation* 53:720, 1976.

23. Hoffmann WE, Miletich DJ, Albrecht RF: Cerebrovascular response to hypotension in hypertensive rats: effect of antihypertensive therapy, *Anesthesiology* 58:326, 1983.

24. Chelly JE, Rogers K, Hysing ES, et al: Cardiovascular effects of and interaction between calcium blocking drugs and anesthetic in chronically instrumented dogs I, *Anesthesiology* 64:560, 1986.

25. Hantler CB, Wilston N , Learned DM, et al: Impaired myocardial conduction in patients receiving diltiazem therapy during enflurane anesthesia, *Anesthesiology* 67:94, 1987.

26. Rogers K, Hysing ES, Merin RG, et al: Cardiovascular effects of and interaction between calcium blocking drugs and anesthetics in chronically instrumented dogs II. Verapamil, enflurane, and isoflurane, *Anesthesiology* 64:568, 1986.

27. Woodside J, Garner L, Bedford RP: Captopril reduces the dose requirement for sodium nitroprusside-induced hypotension, *Anesthesiology* 60:413, 1984.

28. Flecke JW: Alpha$_2$-adrenergic agonists in cardiovascular anesthesia, *J Cardiothorac Vasc Anesth* 5:344, 1992.

29. O'Connor DE: Accelerated acute clonidine withdrawal syndrome during coronary artery bypass surgery, *Br J Anaesth* 53:431, 1981.

30. Subramanian VB, Bowles MJ, Khurmi NS, et al: Calcium antagonist withdrawal syndrome: objective demonstration with frequency-modulated ambulatory ST-segment monitoring, *Br Med J* 286:520, 1983.

31. Coriat P, Richer C, Douraki T, et al: Influence of chronic angiotensin-converting enzyme inhibition on anesthetic induction, *Anesthesiology* 81:299, 1994.

32. Colson P, Saussine M, Seguin JR: Hemodynamic effects of anesthesia in patients chronically treated with angiotensin-converting enzyme inhibitors, *Anesth Analg* 74:805, 1992.

33. Yates AP, Hunter DN: Anaesthesia and angiotensin-converting enzyme inhibitors, *Anaesthesia* 43:935, 1988.

34. Bertrand M, Godet G, Meersschaert K, et al: Should the angiotensin II antagonists be discontinued before surgery? *Anesth Analg* 92:26, 2001.

35. Eyraud D, Mouren S, Teugels K, et al: Treating anesthesia-induced hypotension by angiotensin II in patients chronically treated with angiotensin-converting enzyme inhibitors, *Anesth Analg* 86:259, 1998.

36. Brabant SM, Bertrand M, Eyraud D, et al: The hemodynamic effects of anesthetic induction in vascular surgical patients chronically treated with angiotensin II receptor antagonists, *Anesth Analg* 88:1388, 1999.

37. Eyraud D, Brabant S, Nathalie D, et al: Treatment of intraoperative refractory hypotension with terlipressin in patients chronically treated with an antagonist of the renin-angiotensin system, *Anesth Analg* 88:980, 1999.

38. Criqui MH, Langer RD, Fronek A, et al: Mortality over a period of 10 years in patients with peripheral arterial disease, *N Engl J Med* 326:381, 1992.

39. Hertzer NR, Beven EG, Young JR, et al: Coronary artery disease in peripheral vascular patients. A classification of 1000 coronary angiograms and results of surgical management, *Ann Surg* 199:223, 1984.

40. Fleisher LA, Eagle KA: Clinical practice: lowering cardiac risk in noncardiac surgery, *N Engl J Med* 23:1677, 2001.

41. Mangano DT, Browner WS, Hollenberg M, et al: Association of perioperative myocardial ischemia with cardiac morbidity and mortality in men undergoing noncardiac surgery, *N Engl J Med* 323:1781, 1990.

42. Mangano DT, Browner WS, Hollenberg M, et al: Long-term cardiac prognosis following noncardiac surgery, *JAMA* 268:233, 1992.

43. Fleisher LA, Nelson AH, Rosenbaum SH: Postoperative myocardial ischemia: etiology of cardiac morbidity or manifestation of underlying disease? *J Clin Anesth* 7:97, 1995.

44. Eagle KA, Berger PB, Calkins H: ACC/AHA guideline update on perioperative cardiovascular evaluation for noncardiac surgery. Executive summary: report of the American College of Cardiology/American Heart Association Task Force on Practice Guidelines (Committee to Update the 1996 Guidelines on Perioperative Cardiovascular Evaluation for Noncardiac Surgery), *Circulation* 105:1257, 2002.

45. Tarhan S, Moffitt EA, Taylor WF, et al: Myocardial infarction after general anesthesia, *JAMA* 220:1451, 1972.

46. Steen PA, Tinker JH, Tarhan S: Myocardial reinfarction after anesthesia and surgery, *JAMA* 239: 2566, 1978.

47. Goldman L: Cardiac risks and complications of noncardiac surgery, *Ann Intern Med* 98:504, 1983.

48. Rao TLK, Jacobs KH, El-Etr AA: Reinfarction following anesthesia in patients with myocardial infarction, *Anesthesiology* 59:499, 1983.

49. Shah KB, Kleinman BS, Sami H, et al: Reevaluation of perioperative myocardial infarction in patients with prior myocardial infarction undergoing noncardiac operations, *Anesth Analg* 71:231, 1990.

50. Vicenzi MN, Ribitsch D, Luha O, et al: Coronary artery stenting before noncardiac surgery: more threat than safety? *Anesthesiology* 94:367, 2001.

51. Kaluza GL, Joseph J, Lee JR, et al: Catastrophic outcomes of noncardiac surgery soon after coronary stenting, *J Am Coll Cardiol* 35:1288, 2000.

52. American Society of Regional Anesthesia and Pain Medicine Consensus Statement: Regional anesthesia in the anticoagulated patient—defining the risks, *http://www.asra.com*, 2002.

53. Rosenfeld BA, Faraday N, Campbell D, et al: Hemostatic effects of stress hormone infusion, *Anesthesiology* 81:1116, 1994.

54. Rosenfeld BA, Beattie C, Christopherson R, et al: The effects of different anesthetic regimens on fibrinolysis and the development of postoperative arterial thrombosis, *Anesthesiology* 79:435, 1993.

55. Lubarsky DA, Fisher SD, Slaughter TF, et al: Myocardial ischemia correlates with reduced fibrinolytic activity following peripheral vascular surgery, *J Clin Anesth* 12:136, 2000.

56. Coriat P, Daloz M, Bousseau D, et al: Prevention of intraoperative myocardial ischemia during noncardiac surgery with nitroglycerin, *Anesthesiology* 61:193, 1984.

57. Thompson IR, Mutch WA, Culligan JD: Failure of intravenous nitroglycerin to prevent intraoperative myocardial ischemia during fentanyl-pancuronium anesthesia, *Anesthesiology* 61:385, 1984.

58. Gallagher JD, Moore RA, Jose AB, et al: Prophylactic nitroglycerin infusions during coronary artery bypass surgery, *Anesthesiology* 64:785, 1986.

59. Dodds TM, Stone JG, Coromilas J, et al: Prophylactic nitroglycerin infusion during noncardiac surgery does not reduce perioperative ischemia, *Anesth Analg* 76:705, 1993.

60. Pasternack PF, Grossi EA, Baumann FG, et al: Beta-blockade to decrease silent myocardial ischemia during peripheral vascular surgery, *Am J Surg* 158:113, 1989.

61. Mangano DT, Layug EL, Wallace A, et al: Effect of atenolol on mortality and cardiovascular morbidity after noncardiac surgery, *N Engl J Med* 335:1713, 1996.

62. Wallace A, Layug B, Tateo I, et al: Prophylactic atenolol reduces postoperative myocardial ischemia, *Anesthesiology* 88:7, 1998.

63. Poldermans D, Boersma E, Bax JJ: The effect of bisoprolol on perioperative mortality and myocardial infarction in high-risk patients undergoing vascular surgery, *N Engl J Med* 341:1789, 1999.

64. Raby KE, Brull SJ, Timimi F, et al: The effect of heart rate control on myocardial ischemia among high-risk patients after vascular surgery, *Anesth Analg* 88:477, 1999.

65. Urban MK, Markowitz SM, Gordon MA, et al: Postoperative prophylactic administration of beta-adrenergic blockers in patients at risk for myocardial ischemia, *Anesth Analg* 90:1257, 2000.

66. Boersma E, Poldermans D, Bax JJ, et al: Predictors of cardiac events after major vascular surgery. Role of clinical characteristics, dobutamine echocardiography, and beta-blocker therapy, *JAMA* 285:1865, 2001.

67. Zaugg M, Tagliente T, Lucchinetti E, et al: Beneficial effects from beta-adrenergic blockade in elderly patients undergoing noncardiac surgery, *Anesthesiology* 91:1674, 1999.

68. Howell SJ, Sear JW, Foex P: Perioperative beta-blockade: a useful treatment that should be greeted with cautious enthusiasm, *Br J Anaesth* 86:161, 2001.

69. Cruickshank JM: Beta-blockers continue to surprise us, *Eur Heart J* 21:354, 2000.

70. Auerbach AD, Goldman L: Beta-blockers and reduction of cardiac events in noncardiac surgery-clinical applications, *JAMA* 287:1445, 2002.

71. Warltier DC: Beta-adrenergic-blocking drugs: incredibly useful, incredibly underutilized, *Anesthesiology* 88:2, 1998.

72. Lee TH: Reducing cardiac risk in noncardiac surgery, *N Engl J Med* 341:1838, 1999.

73. Oliver MF, Goldman L, Julian DG, et al: Effect of mivazerol on perioperative cardiac complications during noncardiac surgery in patients with coronary heart disease: The European Mivazerol Trial (EMIT), *Anesthesiology* 91:951, 1999.

74. Mangano DT, Martin E, Motsch J, et al: Perioperative sympatholysis: beneficial effects of the alpha$_2$-adrenoreceptor agonist mivazerol on hemodynamic stability and myocardial ischemia, *Anesthesiology* 86:346, 1997.

75. Schumeier KD, Mainzer B, Cierpka J, et al: Small, oral dose of clonidine reduces the incidence of intraoperative myocardial ischemia in patients having vascular surgery, *Anesthesiology* 85:706, 1996.

76. Ellis JE, Drijvers G, Pedlow S, et al: Premedication with oral and transdermal clonidine provides safe and efficacious postoperative sympatholysis, *Anesth Analg* 79:1133, 1994.

77. Graves EJ: National hospital discharge survey: annual summary, 1993, *Vital Health Stat* 13:1, 1995.

78. Cohn JN, Johnson G: Heart failure with normal ejection fraction. The V-HeFT Study. Veterans Administration Cooperative Study Group, *Circulation* 81:III48, 1990.

79. Ramachandran S, Vasan RS, Larson MG, et al: Congestive heart failure in subjects with normal versus reduced left ventricular ejection fraction, *J Am Coll Cardiol* 33:1948, 1999.

80. Rich MW: Epidemiology, pathophysiology, and etiology of congestive heart failure in older adults, *J Am Geriatr Soc* 45:968, 1997.

81. Mirenda JV, Grissom TE: Anesthetic implications of the renin-angiotensin system and angiotensin-converting enzyme inhibitors, *Anesth Analg* 72:667, 1991.

82. Colucci WS, Ribeiro JP Rocco MB, et al: Impaired chronotropic response to exercise in patients with congestive heart failure, *Circulation* 80:314, 1989.

83. Iriarte M, Murga N, Sagastagoitia D, et al: Congestive heart failure from left ventricular diastolic dysfunction in systemic hypertension, *Am J Cardiol* 71:308, 1993.

84. Kitzman DW, Gardin JM, Gottdiener JS, et al: Importance of heart failure with preserved systolic function in patients ≥65 years of age, *Am J Cardiol* 87:413, 2001.

85. Levy D Kenchaiah S, Larson MG, et al: Long-term trends in the incidence of and survival with heart failure, *N Engl J Med* 347:1397, 2002.

86. The CONSENSUS Trial Study Group: Effects of enalapril on mortality in severe congestive heart failure: results of the Cooperative North Scandinavian Enalapril Survival Study (CONSENSUS), *N Engl J Med* 316:1429, 1987.

87. Packer M, Coats AJ, Fowler MB, et al: Effect of carvedilol on survival in severe chronic heart failure, *N Engl J Med* 344:1651, 2001.

88. Hunt HA, Baker DW, Chin MH, et al: ACC/AHA Guidelines for the Evaluation and Management of Chronic Heart Failure: executive summary: a report of the American College of Cardiology/American Heart Association Task Force on Practice Guidelines, *Circulation* 104:2996, 2001.

89. The Digitalis Investigation Group: The effect of digoxin on mortality and morbidity in patients with heart failure, *N Engl J Med* 336:525, 1997.

90. Warner JG, Metzger DC, Kitzman DW, et al: Losartan improves exercise tolerance in patients with diastolic dysfunction and a hypertensive response to exercise, *J Am Coll Cardiol* 33:1567, 1999.

91. Sear JW, Higham H: Issues in the perioperative management of the elderly patient with cardiovascular disease, *Drugs Aging* 19:429, 2002.

92. Foody JM, Farrell MH, Krumholz HM: Beta-blocker therapy in heart failure: scientific review, *JAMA* 287:883, 2002.

93. Hjalmarson A, Goldstein S, Fagerberg B, et al: Effect of controlled-release metoprolol on total mortality, hospitalizations, and well-being in patients with heart failure: the Metoprolol CR/XL Randomized Intervention Trial in Congestive Heart Failure (MERIT-HF), *JAMA* 283:1295, 2000.

94. Goldman L, Caldera DL, Nussbaum SR, et al: Multifactorial index of cardiac risk in noncardiac surgical procedures, *N Engl J Med* 297:845, 1977.

95. Detsky AS, Abrams HB, McLaughlin JR, et al: Predicting cardiac complications in patients undergoing noncardiac surgery, *J Gen Intern Med* 1:211, 1986.

96. Rycjwaert F, Colson P: Hemodynamic effects of anesthesia in patients with ischemic heart failure chronically treated with angiotensin-converting enzymes, *Anesth Analg* 84:945, 1997.

97. Carabello BA: Aortic stenosis, *N Engl J Med* 346:677, 2002.

98. Aronow WS: The older man's heart and heart disease, *Med Clin North Am* 5:1291, 1999.

99. Lindroos M, Kupari M, Heikkila J: Prevalence of aortic valve abnormalities in the elderly: an echocardiographic study of a random population sample, *J Am Coll Cardiol* 21:1220, 1993.

100. Aronow WS, Ahn C, Shirani J, et al: Comparison of the frequency of new coronary events in older persons with mild, moderate and severe valvular aortic stenosis with those without aortic stenosis, *Am J Cardiol* 81:647, 1998.

101. Aronow WS, Ahn C, Kronzon I, et al: Prognosis of congestive heart failure in patients aged ≥ 62 years with unoperated severe valvular aortic stenosis, *Am J Cardiol* 72:846, 1993.

102. Otto CM: Timing of aortic valve surgery, *Heart* 84:211, 2000.

103. Aikawa K, Otto CM: Timing of surgery in aortic stenosis, *Prog Cardiovasc Dis* 43:477, 2001.

104. Faggiano P, Aurigemma GP, Rusconi C, et al: Progression of valvular aortic stenosis in adults: literature review and clinical implications, *Am Heart J* 132:408, 1996.

105. O'Keefe JH Jr, Shub C, Rettke SR: Risk of noncardiac surgical procedures in patients with aortic stenosis, *Mayo Clin Proc* 64:400, 1989.

106. Bonow RO, Carabello B, deLeon AC Jr, et al: ACC/AHA practice guidelines: guidelines for the management of patients with valvular heart disease: Executive summary. A report of the American College of Cardiology/American Heart Association Task Force on Practice Guidelines, *Circulation* 98:1949, 1998.

107. Dajani AS, Taubert KA, Wilson W, et al: Prevention of bacterial endocarditis. Recommendations by the American Heart Association, *JAMA* 277:1794, 1997.

108. Klodas E, Enriquez Sarano M, Tajik AJ, et al: Aortic regurgitation complicated by extreme left ventricular dilation: long-term outcome after surgical correction, *J Am Coll Cardiol* 27:670, 1996.

109. Singer DE, Go AS: Antithrombotic therapy in atrial fibrillation, *Clin Geriatr Med* 17:131, 2001.

110. Feinberg WM, Blackshear JL, Laupacis A, et al: Prevalence, age distribution, and gender of patients with atrial fibrillation. Analysis and implications, *Arch Intern Med* 155:469, 1995.

111. Sear JW, Higham H: Issues in the perioperative management of the elderly patient with cardiovascular disease, *Drugs Aging* 19:429, 2002.

112. Charlson ME, MacKenzie CR, Gold JP: Preoperative autonomic function abnormalities in patients with diabetes mellitus and patients with hypertension, *J Am Coll Surg* 179:1, 1994.

113. Keyl C, Lemberger P, Palitzsch KD, et al: Cardiovascular autonomic dysfunction and hemodynamic response to anesthetic induction in patients with coronary artery disease and diabetes mellitus, *Anesth Analg* 88:985, 1999.

114. Haffner SM, Lehto S, Ronnemaa T, et al: Mortality from coronary heart disease in subjects with type 2 diabetes and in nondiabetic subjects with and without prior myocardial infarction, *N Engl J Med* 339:229, 1998.

115. Treiman GS, Treiman RL, Foran RF, et al: The influence of diabetes mellitus on the risk of abdominal aortic surgery, *Am Surg* 60:436, 1994.

116. Ishihara H, Singh H, Giesecke AH: Relationship between diabetic autonomic neuropathy and gastric contents, *Anesth Analg* 78:943, 1994.

117. Poulsen PL, Ebbehoj E, Nosadini R, et al: Early ACE-I intervention in microalbuminuric patients with type I diabetes: effects on albumin excretion, 24 hour ambulatory blood pressure, and renal function, *Diabetes Metab* 27:123, 2001.

118. Lewis EJ, Hunsicker LG, Clarke WR, et al: Renoprotective effect of the angiotensin-receptor antagonist irbesartan in patients with nephropathy due to type 2 diabetes, *N Engl J Med* 345:851, 2001.

119. Schwartz JJ, Rosenbaum SH, Graf GJ: Anesthesia and the endocrine system. In Barash PG, Cullen BF, Stoelting RK (eds): *Clinical anesthesia*, ed 4, Philadelphia, 2001, Lippincott Williams & Wilkins, p 1134.

120. Lanier WL: Glucose management during cardiopulmonary bypass: cardiovascular and neurologic implications, *Anesth Analg* 72:423, 1991.

121. Sieber FE: The neurologic implications of diabetic hyperglycemia during surgical procedures at increased risk for brain ischemia, *J Clin Anesth* 9:334, 1997.

122. Hirsch IB, McGill JB, Cryer PE, et al: Perioperative management of surgical patients with diabetes mellitus, *Anesthesiology* 74:346, 1991.

123. Bluman LG, Mosca L, Newman N, et al: Preoperative smoking habits and postoperative pulmonary complications, *Chest* 113:883, 1998.

124. Warner DO: Preventing postoperative pulmonary complications, *Anesthesiology* 92:1467, 2000.

125. Kotani N, Hashimoto H, Sessler DI, et al: Smoking decreases alveolar macrophage function during anesthesia and surgery, *Anesthesiology* 92:1268, 2000.

126. Kotani N, Kushikata R, Hashimoto H, et al: Recovery of intraoperative microbicidal and inflammatory functions of alveolar immune cells after a tobacco smoke–free period, *Anesthesiology* 94:999, 2001.

127. Woehlck HJ, Connolly LA, Cinquegrani MP, et al: Acute smoking increases ST depression in humans during general anesthesia, *Anesth Analg* 89:856, 1999.

128. Adams KF, Koch G, Chatterjee B, et al: Acute elevation of blood carboxyhemoglobin to 6% impairs exercise performance and aggravates symptoms in patients with ischemic heart disease, *J Am Coll Cardiol* 12:900, 1988.

129. Myles PS, Iacono GA, Hunt JO, et al: Risk of respiratory complications and wound infection in patients undergoing ambulatory surgery: smokers versus nonsmokers, *Anesthesiology* 97:842, 2002.

130. Swissler B: Should smokers stop smoking preoperatively—and if so, when? *Curr Opin Anesthesiol* 15:53, 2002.

131. Warner MA, Divertie MB, Tinker JH: Preoperative cessation of smoking and pulmonary complications in coronary artery bypass patients, *Anesthesiology* 60:380, 1984.

132. Warner MA, Offord KP, Warner ME, et al: Role of preoperative cessation of smoking and other factors in postoperative pulmonary complications: a blinded prospective study of coronary artery bypass patients, *Mayo Clin Proc* 64:609, 1989.

133. Schwilk B, Bothner U, Schraag S, et al: Perioperative respiratory events in smokers and nonsmokers undergoing general anaesthesia, *Acta Anesthesiol Scand* 41:348, 1997.

134. Kabalin CS, Yarnold PR, Grammer LC: Low complication rate of corticosteroid-treated asthmatics undergoing surgical procedures, *Arch Intern Med* 155:1379, 1995.

135. Smetana GW: Preoperative pulmonary evaluation, *N Engl J Med* 340:937, 1999.

136. Clark SK, Rung GW, Hensley FA Jr: Premedication for the vascular surgery patient. In Kaplan JA (ed): *Vascular anesthesia*, New York, 1991, Churchill Livingstone.

137. Reves JG, Fragen RJ, Vinik HR, et al: Midazolam: pharmacology and uses, *Anesthesiology* 62:310, 1985.

138. Bradshaw EG, Ali AA, Mulley BA, et al: Plasma concentrations and clinical effects of lorazepam after oral administration, *Br J Anaesth* 53:517, 1981.

139. Bernard JM, Bourreli B, Hommeril JL, et al: Effects of oral clonidine premedication and postoperative IV infusion on haemodynamic and adrenergic responses during recovery from anesthesia, *Acta Anaesthesiol Scand* 35:54, 1991.

140. Weil JV, McCullough RE, Kline JS: Diminished ventilatory response to hypoxia and hypercapnia after morphine in man, *N Engl J Med* 292:1103, 1975.

141. Wade J, Larson CP, Hickey RF, et al: Effect of carotid endarterectomy on carotid chemoreceptor and baroreceptor function in man, *N Engl J Med* 282:823, 1970.

142. Moyers JR, Vincent CM: Preoperative medication. In Barash PG, Cullen BF, Stoelting RK (eds): *Clinical anesthesia*, ed 4, Philadelphia, 2001, Lippincott Williams & Wilkins.

143. Stoelting RK: Gastric fluid pH in patients receiving cimetidine, *Anesth Analg* 57:675, 1978.

144. Escolano F, Castano J, Lopez R, et al: Effects of omeprazole, ranitidine, famotidine and placebo on gastric secretion in patients undergoing elective surgery, *Br J Anaesth* 69:404, 1992.

145. Rocke DA, Rout CC, Gouws E: Intravenous administration of the proton pump inhibitor omeprazole reduces the risk of acid aspiration at emergency cesarean section, *Anesth Analg* 78:1093, 1994.

146. O'Sullivan G, Sear JW, Bullingham RES, et al: The effect of magnesium trisilicate, metoclopramide and ranitidine on gastric pH, volume and serum gastrin, *Anaesthesia* 40:246, 1985.

Choice of Invasive Versus Noninvasive Surgery

Monica Myers Mordecai, MD

OVER the last two decades, the introduction of minimally invasive treatment options for a variety of vascular disease processes has made a dramatic contribution to the change in practice for vascular surgery. The ability to approach pathology from both intraluminal and extraluminal means has allowed vascular surgeons unique treatment options that were not available less than a decade ago. Intraluminal techniques, including balloon angioplasty, stenting, atherectomy, thrombectomy, and thrombolysis, have been used by interventional radiologists, cardiologists, and vascular surgeons for the diagnostic and therapeutic management of a variety of vascular disorders. Endovascular treatment now extends to aneurysmal disease states of the aorta. Parodi and colleagues first described abdominal aortic aneurysms (AAAs) treated by endovascular placement of a stented prosthetic graft.[1]

Treatment Alternatives

Conventional Surgical Repair

With the high risk of aneurysm rupture, the current standard of treatment of an AAA is open surgical repair. The natural history of an aortic aneurysm is characterized by continued expansion and rupture of the aneurysm. When considering rupture before and during hospitalization, the mortality rate for ruptured aneurysms may exceed 90%.[2] Standard surgical repair involves a major abdominal incision, exposure of the aorta, cross-clamping of the aorta, removal of the aneurysmal aorta, and replacement with a prosthetic graft. Considerable hemodynamic and metabolic stresses are associated with surgical trauma, aortic cross-clamping, large fluid shifts from blood loss, and third-space losses or shifts. Open surgical repair is curative as the aneurysm is removed and the treatment requires minimal follow-up, low risk of aortic rupture, and a proven long-term success rate. Any treatment for an aortic aneurysm must obviously involve a lower mortality rate than the risk of aneurysm rupture (see Chapter 11).

Initially, the mortality rate for elective surgical repair of nonruptured AAAs was approximately 20%, but mortality now averages 2% in single-center, 4% in multicenter, and 7% in population-based studies.[3-5] The decrease in mortality is due partly to improved surgical techniques and material, increased surgical experience, and improvements in anesthetic management, monitoring, and postoperative care. Although mortality has decreased, aortic surgery is still associated with significant morbidity and the potential for a long convalescence. Morbidity from open surgical repair may be due to myocardial infarction, renal failure, pulmonary dysfunction, hepatic failure, ischemic bowel, or stroke. Furthermore, some patients may not be eligible for the operation because the risks are considered too high. These factors have led to the investigation of alternative methods for the management of AAAs.

Endovascular Techniques

Endovascular repair of major aortic aneurysm disease is less invasive than open surgical repair and is used to treat various aortic diseases, most commonly infrarenal AAAs. The first endovascular grafts were handmade, individualized graft systems tailored by the surgeons. The procedure is usually performed in an operating room with interventional capabilities. The patient is prepared and draped for a standard surgical repair in the event that conversion to an open surgical procedure is necessary. Access is typically infrainguinal through bilateral femoral or iliac artery cutdown. Large-diameter introducer systems are placed by arteriotomy. Intravenous contrast dye and fluoroscopy are used intermittently during the procedure to define arterial structures and to confirm proper placement and function of the graft and its components. Proximal and distal grafts are anchored to the walls of the aorta and its branch vessels. The goal of treatment is to provide a new conduit of blood flow through the endoluminal graft without removing the aneurysm, effectively isolating the aneurysm from the circulation and preventing rupture.

Endovascular Devices

This area of medicine has been driven by the rapid advancement of graft system technology. The basic components of each device include a delivery system, mobile and fixed components of the prosthetic graft, and anchoring or fixation devices. Endovascular graft technology is a rapidly evolving field with a number of commercially available advanced systems used worldwide. Graft systems include AnueRx, EVT/Ancure, Excluder, Stentor, Talent, Vanguard, and Zenith, among others. Some systems have already come off the market because of failure of certain components. In the United States, the Food and Drug Administration (FDA) had strict inclusion and exclusion criteria for the systems used in the first clinical trials. Today the FDA has approved two devices for commercial use—the Ancure tube and the bifurcated endovascular grafting system by Guidant Endovascular Technologies, Inc. (Indianapolis, IN) and the

AneuRx (bifurcated) Stent Graft system by Medtronic (Minneapolis, MN).[6,7] The three main types of prosthetic stent grafts available today are the aorto-aortic tube graft, bifurcated aorto-bi-iliac graft, and aorto-uni-iliac graft. It is important to have an understanding of the devices and steps of this technically demanding procedure.

Intraoperative device-related complications are common and may affect anesthetic management. As technology improves, device-related complications are decreasing, which may be due to improvements of the devices, delivery systems, and operator use. Risk factors for device-related complications are known. Device complications are dangerous, as they may lead to conversion to an open procedure, which is associated with increased operative mortality.[8]

Advantages of Endovascular Repair of Abdominal Aortic Aneurysms

Initial studies have found that when compared with conventional, open surgical repair, endovascular stent grafting (EVSGR) has considerable advantages regarding, for example, amount of blood loss, use of an intensive care unit (ICU), length of hospitalization, and speed of recovery.[9,10] The most significant of these is the recovery, as patients with an uncomplicated hospital course return to their normal state of health and activity within days of the surgery. An endovascular approach avoids a major abdominal incision, dissection of the aorta, and aortic cross-clamping (see Chapter 11).

During conventional surgical repair, the placement of an aortic cross-clamp immediately increases afterload and systemic vascular resistance, and the heart compensates for the increased myocardial oxygen demand with an increase in coronary blood flow. Patients with limited cardiac reserve, therefore, may not tolerate the hemodynamic consequences of aortic cross-clamping. Cardiovascular complications observed in patients undergoing elective AAA repair almost always occurred at the time of infrarenal aortic cross-clamping.[11] Metabolic disturbances related to aortic cross-clamping include metabolic acidosis and release of multiple mediators associated with the stress response.[12]

Less hemodynamic and metabolic stress is found with endovascular repair than with open surgical repair.[13] Plasma catecholamine concentrations, changes in cardiovascular variables, and acid-base imbalance were all greater with open surgical repair.[14] The decreased stress response may also be due to reduced bowel ischemia, endotoxemia, and cytokine generation.[15] Each technique produced a different biologic response—endovascular repair induced an inflammatory response, whereas conventional open repair induced responses associated with extensive surgical trauma and reperfusion injury.[16]

Other advantages of endovascular repair include postoperatively improved respiratory function and analgesia control.[17] Because of the localized nature of the procedure, endovascular repair allows the possibility of regional and intravenous anesthetic alternatives to general anesthesia (Table 7-1).

TABLE 7-1

Comparisons of Conventional Open Surgical Repair and Endovascular Repair of Infrarenal Abdominal Aortic Aneurysms

Property	General Anesthesia	Regional or Local Anesthesia
Need for anatomic criteria	No	Yes
Incision	Abdominal	Inguinal
Use of intensive care unit	Yes	No
Postoperative analgesics	Significant	Minimal
Advanced to a normal diet	Days	<24 hours
Long-term success	Proven	Questionable

Selection of Patients

Anatomic Considerations for Endovascular Repair

The choice of treatment by standard surgical repair or a minimally invasive endovascular approach is currently limited by institutional practices, availability, and patient-related considerations. In large centers experienced with both techniques, the choice can be based on the anatomic features of the aneurysm and the patient's comorbid conditions. With the endovascular approach, unlike open surgical repair, the first decision in selection of patients for treatment is based on strict anatomic criteria. With the first generation of endografts, only a small percentage of patients had aneurysm anatomy that was suitable for endovascular repair. Since the introduction of the bifurcated system, approximately half of patients with infrarenal AAAs are candidates on the basis of anatomic criteria.[18,19] Criteria are specific to each system used and may change as the systems continue to evolve. The guidelines are designed to improve patients' outcomes. The breaching of anatomic criteria has led to a significant increase in the complication rate for endovascular repair.[20,21]

Preoperative evaluation must first define the anatomy of the abdominal aorta and branch vessels. The infrarenal aortic neck anatomy is crucial as this is the location for the proximal attachment site of the graft. The length is important in order to have the greatest area of graft in contact with normal aorta for attachment and seal. Aortic curvature in this area presents both immediate and late concerns. Angulation makes placement more difficult and also increases force on the prosthetic graft, increasing the potential for distal migration of the graft. The presence of an aortic branch vessel may allow continued flow into the aneurysm sac. The iliac artery anatomy in regard to tortuosity, aneurysm formation, and diameter is also critical as these vessels hold the larger diameter delivery systems (Table 7-2).

When the determination is made that the aneurysm is amenable to treatment by less invasive options, selection of patients is determined, weighing risks and benefits of nontreatment versus treatment with invasive or noninvasive repair based on patients' comorbidities. The preoperative evaluation for each treatment option is essentially identical. Preoperative evaluation to determine and quantify cardiac,

TABLE 7-2

Anatomic Consideration for Endovascular Repair of Infrarenal Aortic Aneurysms

Infrarenal aorta
　Aortic neck diameter
　Aortic neck length
　Aortic intraluminal disease at attachment sites
　Aortic neck angulation
Common iliac arteries
　Stenosis
　Aneurysm
　Tortuosity

---

pulmonary, and renal function; to allow optimization of medical therapies; and to assess risk factors known to increase perioperative morbidity and mortality is essential (see Chapters 5 and 6). A small percentage of patients have prohibitive risk for open surgical repair. The designation of "unfit" for open surgical repair and "unfit" for anesthesia is often not well defined. The American Society of Anesthesiologists (ASA) classification is a generalization of overall medical status and was never intended as a measure of perioperative risk stratification. The Society of Vascular Surgery/International Society of Cardiothoracic Surgery-North American chapter has defined age, cardiac function, pulmonary function, and renal function as the predictors of medical risk for elective aneurysm repair.[22]

Intraoperative Management

Because of the technical aspects of the endovascular graft systems and the procedure, endovascular repair of an aortic aneurysm presents unique challenges to intraoperative management and development of a safe anesthetic plan. The procedure is less invasive than open surgical repair and less likely to induce hemodynamic stress, yet it may still be associated with many of the same risks and complications as aortic surgery, such as massive sudden blood loss because of aortic rupture.

The goals of intraoperative management should be to provide hemodynamic stability while preserving cardiac and renal blood flow and the maintenance of intravascular volume, adequate oxygenation, and body temperature.

In addition to the patient's history and physical examination, preoperative measures include premedication and explanation of intraoperative events to reduce the patient's anxiety. After the patient is brought to the operating room, appropriate catheters for hemodynamic monitoring should be placed, in addition to large-bore intravenous access. An arterial catheter is required for continuous blood pressure monitoring and can also be used to collect samples for arterial blood gases, hematocrit, and activated coagulation times as needed. Because of the systemic nature of atherosclerosis, before placement of a radial arterial catheter, blood pressure should be checked in both arms to detect any differences. Central venous access should be considered to provide central delivery of vasopressors and to determine and maintain intravascular volume. When local anesthesia is used, a central venous catheter may not be necessary. In

patients with poor left ventricular function or renal failure, a pulmonary artery catheter or transesophageal echocardiography can provide a more accurate assessment of intravascular volume and cardiac function. A Foley catheter is required as an additional measure of volume status and function. Temperature should also be closely followed and maintained as patients are prepared for a full open procedure, which leaves a large surface area exposed.

The operation requires close intraoperative fluid management with early replacement of preoperative deficits and maintenance of intravascular volume. An initial dose of heparin, 5000 units, is administered intravenously before the arterial incision. With the first generation of endovascular delivery systems, significant blood loss could occur during placement and manipulation of the systems. Advances have improved the hemostatic valves and other components, which have decreased blood loss during the procedure.

Postoperative Care

Postoperative recovery after endovascular surgery usually does not require the use of an ICU. The patients are typically advanced to a regular diet and are ambulatory on the first postoperative day. Analgesic requirements are minimal and can be managed with nonsteroidal anti-inflammatory medications or small boluses of narcotic. Postimplantation syndrome related to a systemic inflammatory response to the graft material may occur postoperatively, manifesting with fever, leukocytosis, and increased C-reactive protein concentrations.[23,24] Hyperpyrexia can be associated with tachycardia, which warrants continued monitoring of hemodynamic variables in patients with cardiac disease. With an uncomplicated perioperative course, the average length of hospital stay is less than 5 days.

Anesthetic Techniques

As reported in 1991 by Parodi et al, the first intraluminal grafts were performed under local or limited epidural anesthesia.[1] For the experimental procedure, these investigators selected five high-risk patients with serious comorbidity, such as severe chronic obstructive pulmonary disease, acute stroke, severe asthma, or an ejection fraction less than 20%. Parodi et al suggested that the transfemoral approach allowed the procedure to be performed under local or limited epidural anesthesia without the morbidity of a high regional block or general inhalation anesthetic. Various anesthetic techniques for the management of endovascular surgery have since been reported, including general, combined general and regional, epidural, combined spinal-epidural anesthesia, bilateral paravertebral blocks, and local anesthesia with sedation (see Chapters 9 and 11).

Most institutions initially performed endovascular surgery under general anesthesia. For both surgeons and anesthesiologists, this choice was probably related to the uncertainties inherent in performing a new surgical technique. For example, according to a report of clinical experience at one institution, EVSGR procedures were performed under general anesthesia until acceptable operating room times and a low risk of surgical complications could be determined; after the first seven operations, most were done under local anesthesia.[25]

A safe anesthetic can be administered by a vigilant and capable anesthesiologist using any of the techniques mentioned previously. The question is whether any particular anesthetic technique is superior in achieving the goals of anesthetic management; that is, providing hemodynamic stability with minimal use of inotropic agents, maintaining intravascular volume without excessive volume administration, and preserving cardiac, pulmonary, renal, and cerebral blood function.

General Anesthesia

For the induction and maintenance of general anesthesia, the choice of medications and means of hemodynamic monitoring are based on the patient's cardiac function (see Chapter 9). Patients with preserved left ventricular function generally tolerate the depressant effects of intravenous and inhaled anesthetic agents with appropriate compensatory mechanisms. General anesthesia typically consists of a balanced technique with a low-dose inhalation agent and narcotics. Muscle relaxants are typically not necessary. For patients with compromised left ventricular function, a narcotic-based technique provides greater hemodynamic stability. General anesthesia provides airway control throughout the procedure, allows stable hemodynamic management, can accommodate for variations in duration of the operation, eliminates the possibility of movement of the patient, and allows control of respiratory movement during fluoroscopy. Furthermore, the patient would be anesthetized for placement of additional intravascular catheters, and any issues of the patient's toleration of supine positioning on the operating table during long operations would be avoided. In the limited nonrandomized, retrospective studies of anesthetic technique, general anesthesia was associated with more hypotensive episodes, increased fluid requirements, and increased use of inotropic support compared with regional or local anesthesia.[25-27]

Regional Anesthesia

Spinal, epidural, and combined spinal-epidural techniques have been used for endovascular surgery. The sensory level of anesthetic blockade needed is below the T10 dermatome and provides anesthesia for the infrainguinal surgical field and for peritoneal retraction, if needed, for iliac artery exposure. The block can be performed in the low lumbar region. The level of sensory anesthesia required for endovascular surgery has fewer hemodynamic side effects than the high thoracic level needed for open surgical repair.

The advantages of epidural anesthesia over other regional techniques include the ability to titrate the local anesthetic slowly to achieve the appropriate sensory level and accommodate variations in duration of the procedure. Also, slow titration of an epidural anesthetic allows compensatory mechanisms to minimize hemodynamic changes. Spinal anesthesia is more difficult to titrate slowly to a specific level and would be inadequate if the operation were unexpectedly prolonged.

Advantages of Regional Anesthesia

Some institutions base the choice of anesthetic on the surgical approach, with regional anesthesia used for the iliac approach and local anesthesia for the femoral approach[25] (see Chapter 9). Regional anesthesia has a proven advantage over general anesthesia in regard to postoperative pulmonary function. General anesthesia with mechanical ventilation can cause decreased lung volume, ventilation-perfusion mismatch, decreased functional residual capacity, atelectasis, impaired ciliary function with thickened secretions predisposing to postoperative pulmonary dysfunction, and infections.[28] The benefits of regional anesthesia for patients with compromised myocardial function remain controversial because of difficulty in demonstrating differences in morbidity and mortality.

In attempting to identify differences in outcome, many studies have compared general anesthesia with combined general-epidural anesthesia for surgical procedures associated with significantly more surgical trauma or that require a higher thoracic level of anesthesia than would be required for endovascular surgery. Hemodynamic effects related to increased venous capacitance and decreased preload of a low lumbar epidural titrated slowly are minimal. If blood pressure is maintained, myocardial function should not be significantly affected. Regional anesthesia has been reported in a series of 21 patients with no periods of clinically significant hypotension during the procedure.[29] The use of vasopressors and median fluid balance was lower with the use of regional versus general anesthesia for endovascular repair of aortic aneurysms.[25]

Other benefits of regional over general anesthesia include a shorter hospital stay after the operation.[30] Intraoperative blood loss has been reported to be lower in patients undergoing regional versus general anesthesia. For endovascular repair, the intraoperative blood loss appears to be unchanged with regional anesthesia.[24,25,30] Because of the low level of anesthesia required for this procedure, the theoretical disadvantages of regional anesthesia, such as difficulty of control of hemodynamics in a bleeding patient with a high sympathectomy or postoperative fluid overload when the block recedes, are not present. The incidence of thrombotic events in peripheral grafts, coronary arteries, and lower extremity veins is lower with regional than with general anesthesia. This finding probably results from the attenuation of the hypercoagulable state in patients undergoing peripheral vascular procedures.

Potential disadvantages with regional anesthesia include difficulties in keeping the patient comfortable while intravascular catheters are being placed and in having the patient tolerate supine positioning on the operating table during long operations.

Risk of Epidural Hematoma

In patients undergoing peripheral vascular surgery while receiving intraoperative heparin, regional anesthesia can be safely performed, with a low risk of spinal or epidural hematoma.[31] Theoretical concerns about placement of a catheter in a patient who will be intraoperatively anticoagulated should not restrict the use of regional anesthesia if results of coagulation tests performed at the time of placement of the block or epidural catheter and before removal of the catheter are normal. Neurologic function should be monitored postoperatively.

Local Anesthesia

For the transfemoral approach, local anesthesia is well tolerated and provides greater hemodynamic stability than other anesthetic techniques, as demonstrated by decreased use of inotropic agents. Intravenous sedation regimens include titration of benzodiazepines with or without continuous infusions of propofol or narcotics. Modifications in surgical technique and catheter technology have simplified parts of the procedure, for example, by decreasing clamping time, leg ischemia, and pain for patients. Henretta et al first demonstrated the feasibility of local anesthesia with intravenous sedation as a safe alternative in a clinical series of 47 patients.[32] Their series had 48 consecutive patients. Only one patient was excluded because of severe esophageal stricture. In one patient, the anesthesia technique had to be converted to a general anesthetic because of the need for a retroperitoneal approach for iliac artery repair. Only one patient was admitted to the ICU. A retrospective nonrandomized analysis of 91 patients found local anesthesia superior to both general and epidural anesthesia, with evaluation based on decreased fluid requirements, decreased operating time, decreased use of inotropic agents, and decreased hospital stay.[25]

As with any surgical procedure with local or regional anesthesia, preparations must be made for switching to a general anesthesia in the event of conversion to open surgical techniques or if further access to the iliac arteries is needed (Table 7-3).

Should Endovascular Surgery Lower the Threshold for Elective Aneurysm Repair?

With a less invasive treatment option, the question could be considered if there is any benefit of endovascular repair of smaller aneurysms. Using mathematical models to assess long-term benefits of treatment and nontreatment, indications for aneurysm repair have not changed since the introduction of this technique.[33] The delay of treatment of smaller aneurysms does not change the characteristics of the aneurysm or make the patient unsuitable for endovascular repair. In aneurysms smaller than 7 cm, there is no correlation between aneurysm size and suitability for endovascular repair.[34]

Complications of Endovascular Aortic Surgery

The development of endoluminal therapies has introduced new treatment options but has also created complex issues regarding patients' care. There are many ethical, scientific, and practice issues that must be considered with the introduction of a new surgical procedure. The new treatment should have morbidity and mortality rates equal to or lower than those of current therapies. With small clinical studies having wide variation in outcome parameters, larger prospective studies are needed. EUROSTAR (EUROpean collaborators on Stent-graft Techniques for abdominal aortic Aneurysm Repair), established in 1996 as a voluntary registry of more than 90 centers for the purpose of combining and studying a large database on outcome, now contains information on more than 3000 patients. There are also three prospective European trials currently under way, attempting to evaluate selection of patients and treatment alternatives: the UK EVAR (endovascular aneurysm repair), the Dutch DREAM trial (Dutch Randomized Endovascular Aneurysm Management), and the French ACE project (Aneurysme Chirurgie de l'aorte contre Endoprothèse).

Major perioperative complications have been reported with EVSGR placement including aneurysm rupture, myocardial infarction, cardiac arrhythmia, pneumonia, respiratory failure, renal failure related to dye load or acute occlusion, and peripheral embolization including a fatal cerebral embolization. These complications with endovascular repair are infrequent. Device-related complications include arterial injury during placement of the introducer systems, inability to advance the delivery sheath, inability to deploy the device, device occlusion or stenosis, migration, and endoleak formation. Device-related complications may lead to conversion to an open procedure, which is associated with increased operative mortality.[35-37]

Systemic and Device-Related Complications

When compared with open surgical repair, endovascular repair has the immediate advantages of decreased morbidity and mortality; the major disadvantage of endovascular repair is the inability to ensure long-term success of the grafts. The durability of the graft material has been investigated. In an analysis of explanted devices from the EUROSTAR registry, the woven polyester sleeves had evidence of yarn shifting, distortion, damage, and filament breakage leading to the formation of holes in the fabric and structural failure of the metallic frame. The conclusion is that the biomaterials within the devices studied require further improvement.[38]

TABLE 7-3

Comparison of General, Epidural, and Local Anesthesia for Endovascular Aneurysm Repair

Anesthetic Technique	n	Fluid Administration (mL)	Vasopressor Use (%)	Operating Time (min)
Local anesthesia	63	100 ± 147	8	100
Epidural infusion	8	1460 ± 446	25	125
General anesthesia	19	1950 ± 590	50	172

From Bettex DA, Lachat M, Pfammatter T: *Eur J Vasc Endovasc Surg* 21:179, 2001.

Endovascular repair of AAAs requires continued close surveillance because of the frequent need for secondary interventions. The risk of late failure is 3% per year, and the continued presence of the risk of aneurysm rupture is 1% per year.[39] With this treatment, the aneurysm is isolated from the normal circulation. *Endoleak* is a term used to describe persistent communication between normal circulation and the aneurysm sac after placement of the graft. Endoleaks are classified by the site of flow into the aneurysm sac. The types of endoleaks include type I, caused by an inadequate seal at the proximal or distal segments of the endoprosthesis; type II, from branch flow through patent accessory renal, inferior mesenteric, hypogastric, lumbar, or sacral arteries; and type III, a midgraft leak through a fabric hole or from an inadequate seal between graft components. The potential to increase aneurysm size or increase intraluminal pressure could lead to aneurysm rupture. The natural history and management are somewhat controversial. Type I and III endoleaks are usually considered major complications, representing failure of treatment correlating with a higher risk of aneurysmal rupture and conversion to open surgical repair. The significance of type II endoleaks is still under investigation, and they may require intervention only if there is an increase in aneurysm size.[40,41] In a study population of 1023 patients, secondary interventions were performed in 18% of patients with a mean period of 21 months after initial graft placement.[42]

What is the Role of Endovascular Repair in Patients Considered Unfit for Conventional Open Repair?

The limited life span of this group of patients makes it difficult to assess long-term outcomes of this procedure. The life expectancy of any patient with significant comorbidity should be greater than 1 year to realize any benefit from the procedure. In a study of 381 patients considered unfit for open repair or anesthesia, patients with significant comorbidity had higher mortality rates from non–aneurysm-related complications, with cardiac events the most significant. Whether mortality is due to an effect of treatment or a natural progression of the patient's disease is not known; however, the mortality rate was greater than the mortality rate associated with the natural history of AAAs greater than 5 cm. The presence of symptoms and anatomic ease of endovascular treatment are additional considerations in this population. With both early and late mortality increased in high-risk patients, patients with significant comorbidity may benefit from endovascular repair only if the aneurysm size is greater than 6 cm (Figure 7-1).[43-45]

Summary

Anesthetic management for major vascular surgery is one of the most complex areas of practice in anesthesiology. Repair of aortic aneurysms involves significant hemodynamic and

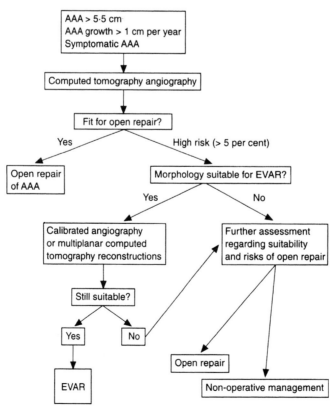

FIGURE 7-1 Protocol for assessment of abdominal aortic aneurysms (AAAs) being considered for surgical repair. EVAR, endovascular repair. (From Woodburn KR, Chant H, Davies JN, et al: *Br J Surg* 88:77, 2001.)

metabolic stresses, particularly in a population of patients that is usually elderly and has multiple comorbid conditions such as ischemic heart disease, hypertension, chronic pulmonary disease, diabetes mellitus, and renal dysfunction. The introduction of endovascular repair of AAAs has presented a unique treatment option to approximately half of patients presenting for aneurysm repair. The immediate benefits of reducing early morbidity, blood loss, length of stay, and recovery have been proved. The long-term success of the endovascular prosthetic grafts is concerning because of the need for lifelong surveillance, secondary interventions, and continued risk of aneurysm rupture.

As the technology of this rapidly evolving surgery continues to develop, materials and structural designs are hoped to resolve these issues. Indications for EVSGR placement now extend well beyond elective AAA repair to include repair of ruptured abdominal aneurysms in patients with contained bleeding, thoracoabdominal aneurysms, and aortic injuries caused by blunt trauma.[46-48] Many of these operations are performed under local anesthesia. Even when surgical and anesthetic techniques are less invasive, patients have a high incidence of severe coexisting diseases and continue to require complex management throughout the perioperative period.

REFERENCES

1. Parodi JC, Palmaz JC, Barone HD: Transfemoral intraluminal graft implantation for abdominal aortic aneurysms, *Ann Vasc Surg* 5:491, 1991.
2. Ernst CB: Abdominal aortic aneurysm, *N Engl J Med* 328:1167, 1993.
3. Crawford ES, Saleh SA, Babb JW III, et al: Infrarenal abdominal aortic aneurysm. Factors influencing survival after operation performed over a 25-year period, *Ann Surg* 193:699, 1993.
4. Katz DJ, Stanley JC, Zelenock GB: Operative mortality rates for intact and ruptured abdominal aortic aneurysms in Michigan: an eleven-year statewide experience, *J Vasc Surg* 19:804, 1994.
5. Zarins CK, White RA, Schwarten D, et al: AneuRx stent graft versus open surgical repair of abdominal aortic aneurysms: multicenter prospective clinical trial, *J Vasc Surg* 29:292, 1999.
6. Abel D, Shulman M: The FDA and regulatory issues in graft development, *Semin Vasc Surg* 12:74, 1999.
7. Lipsitz EC, Ohki T, Veith FJ: Overview of techniques and devices for endovascular abdominal aortic aneurysm repair, *Semin Intervent Cardiol* 5:21, 2000.
8. Laheij RJF, van Marrecwijk CJ: The evolving technique of endovascular tenting of abdominal aortic aneurysm: time for reappraisal, *Eur J Vasc Endovasc Surg* 22:436, 2001.
9. May J, White GH, Yu W, et al: Results of endoluminal grafting of abdominal aneurysms are dependent on aneurysm morphology, *Ann Vasc Surg* 10:254, 1996.
10. Brewster DC, Geller SC, Kaufman JA, et al: Initial experience with endovascular aneurysm repair: comparison of early results with outcome of conventional open repair, *J Vasc Surg* 27:992, 1998.
11. Dunn E, Prager RL, Fry W, Kirsh MM: The effect of abdominal aortic cross-clamping on myocardial function, *J Surg Res* 22:463, 1997.
12. Gelman S: The pathophysiology of aortic cross-clamping and unclamping, *Anesthesiology* 82:1026, 1995.
13. Baxendale BR, Baker DM, Hutchison A, et al: Haemodynamic and metabolic response to endovascular repair of infrarenal aortic aneurysm, *Br J Anaesth* 77:581, 1996.
14. Thompson JP, Boyle JR, Thompson MM, et al: Cardiovascular and catecholamine responses during endovascular and conventional abdominal aortic aneurysm repair, *Eur J Vasc Endovasc Surg* 17:326, 1999.
15. Elmarasy NM, Soong CV, Walker SR, et al: Sigmoid ischemia and the inflammatory response following endovascular abdominal aortic aneurysm repair, *J Endovasc Ther* 7:21, 2000.
16. Swartbol P, Norgren L, Albrechtsson U, et al: Biological responses differ considerably between endovascular and conventional abdominal aortic aneurysm repair, *Eur J Vasc Endovasc Surg* 12:18, 1996.
17. Boyle JR, Thompson JP, Thompson MM, et al: Improved respiratory function and analgesia control after endovascular repair, *J Endovasc Surg* 4:62, 1997.
18. Schumacher H, Eckstein HH, Kallinowski F, Allenberg JR: Morphometry and classification of abdominal aortic aneurysm: patient selection for endovascular and open surgery, *J Endovasc Surg* 4:39, 1997.
19. Woodburn KR, Chant H, Davies JN, et al: Suitability for endovascular aneurysm repair in an unselected population, *Br J Surg* 88:77, 2001.
20. Adelman MA, Rockman CB, Lamparello PJ, et al: Endovascular abdominal aortic aneurysm (AAA) repair since the FDA approval. Are we going too far? *J Cardiovasc Surg* 43:359, 2002.
21. Stanley BM, Semmens JB, Mai Q, et al: Evaluation of patient selection guidelines for endoluminal AAA repair with the Zenith Stent-Graft: the Australian experience, *J Endovasc Ther* 8:457, 2001.
22. Hollier LH, Taylor LM, Oschner J: Recommended indications for operative treatment of abdominal aortic aneurysms. Report of a subcommittee of the Joint Council of the Society for Vascular Surgery and the North American Chapter of the International Society for Cardiovascular Surgery, *J Vasc Surg* 15:1046, 1992.
23. Blum U, Voshage G, Lammer J, et al: Endoluminal stent-grafts for infrarenal abdominal aortic aneurysms, *N Engl J Med* 336:13, 1997.
24. Eberle B, Weiler N, Duber C, et al: Anesthesia in endovascular treatment of aortic aneurysm. Results and perioperative risks, *Anaesthesist* 45:931, 1996.
25. Bettex DA, Lachat M, Pfammatter T, et al: To compare general, epidural and local anaesthesia for endovascular aneurysm repair (EVAR), *Eur J Vasc Endovasc Surg* 21:179, 2001.
26. Greiff JM, Thompson MM, Langham BT: Anaesthetic implications of aortic stent surgery, *Br J Anaesth* 75:779, 1995.
27. Baker AB, Lloyd G, Fraser TA, et al: Retrospective review of 100 cases of endoluminal aortic stent-graft surgery from an anaesthetic perspective, *Anaesth Intensive Care* 25:378, 1997.
28. Tisi GM: Preoperative identification and evaluation of the patient with lung disease, *Med Clin North Am* 71:399, 1987.
29. Aadahl P, Lundbom J, Hatlinghus S, Myhre HO: Regional anesthesia for endovascular treatment of abdominal aortic aneurysms, *J Endovasc Surg* 4:56, 1997.
30. Cao P, Giordano G, De Rango P, et al: Epidural anesthesia reduces length of hospitalization after endoluminal abdominal aortic aneurysm repair, *J Vasc Surg* 30:651, 1999.
31. Yeager MP, Fillinger MP, Lundberg J: Cardiothoracic and vascular surgery. In Brown DL (ed): *Regional anesthesia and analgesia*. Philadelphia, 1996, WB Saunders, 512.
32. Henretta JP, Hodgson KJ, Mattos MA, et al: Feasibility of endovascular repair of abdominal aortic aneurysms with local anesthesia with intravenous sedation, *J Vasc Surg* 29:793, 1999.
33. Finlayson SRG, Birkmeyer JD, Fillinger MF, Cronenwett JL: Should endovascular surgery lower the threshold for repair of abdominal aortic aneurysms? *J Vasc Surg* 29:973, 1999.
34. Armon MP, Yusef SW, Latief K, et al: Anatomical suitability of abdominal aortic aneurysms for endovascular repair, *Br J Surg* 84:178, 1997.
35. Moskowitz DM, Kahn RA, Marin ML, Hollier LH: Intraoperative rupture of an abdominal aortic aneurysm during a endovascular stent-graft procedure, *Can J Anaesth* 46:887, 1999.
36. May J, White GH, Waugh R, et al: Adverse events after endoluminal repair of abdominal aortic aneurysms: a comparison during two successive periods of time, *J Vasc Surg* 29:32, 1999.
37. May J, White GH, Yu W, et al: Conversion from endoluminal to open repair of abdominal aortic aneurysms: a hazardous procedure, *Eur J Vasc Endovasc Surg* 14:4, 1997.
38. Guidoin R, Marois Y, Douville Y, et al: First-generation aortic endografts: analysis of explanted Stentor devices from the EUROSTAR Registry, *J Endovasc Ther* 7:105, 2000.
39. Harris PL, Vallabhaneni SR: Incidence and risk factors of late rupture, conversion, and death after endovascular repair of infrarenal aortic aneurysms: the EUROSTAR experience, *J Vasc Surg* 32:739, 2000.
40. van Marrewijk C, Buth J, Harris PL, et al: Significance of endoleaks after endovascular repair of abdominal aortic aneurysms: the EUROSTAR experience, *J Vasc Surg* 35:461, 2002.
41. Veith FJ, Baum RA, Ohki T, et al: Nature and significance of endoleaks and endotension: summary of opinions expressed at an international conference, *J Vasc Surg* 35:1029, 2002.
42. Ahn SS, Ro KM: The EUROSTAR series: the need for secondary interventions. In Branchereau A, Jacobs M (eds) *Surgical and endovascular treatment of aortic aneurysms*. Armonk, NY, 2000, Futura, 163.

43. Riambau V, Leheij RJ, Garcia-Madrid C, et al: The association between co-morbidity and mortality after abdominal aortic aneurysm endografting in patients ineligible for elective open surgery, *Eur J Vasc Endovasc Surg* 22:265, 2001.

44. Buth J, van Marrewijk CJ, Harris PL, et al: Outcome of endovascular abdominal aortic aneurysm repair in patients with conditions considered unfit for an open procedure: a report on the EUROSTAR experience, *J Vasc Surg* 35:211, 2002.

45. Scott RA, Ashton HA, Lamparelli MJ, et al: A 14-year experience with 6 cm as a criterion for surgical treatment of abdominal aortic aneurysm, *Br J Surg* 86:1317, 1999.

46. Lachat M, Pfammatter T, Turina M: Transfemoral endografting of thoracic aortic aneurysm under local anesthesia: a simple, safe, and fast track procedure, *Vasa* 28:204, 1999.

47. Lachat M, Pfammatter T, Bernard E, et al: Successful endovascular repair of a leaking abdominal aortic aneurysm under local anesthesia, *Swiss Surg* 7:86, 2001.

48. Ruchat P, Capasso P, Chollet-Rivier M, et al: Endovascular treatment of aortic rupture by blunt chest trauma, *J Cardiovasc Surg* 42:77, 2001.

Cardiovascular Monitoring

David L. Reich, MD
Alexander Mittnacht, MD

PATIENTS undergoing anesthesia and surgery fall into various risk categories that depend upon underlying medical conditions and the physiologic trespass inherent in the surgical procedure. Patients undergoing vascular surgery constitute a challenging subset. Patients often present with significant comorbid conditions, and cardiovascular function is often compromised. Anesthetic management must, therefore, be tailored to provide state-of-the-art perioperative care in order to reduce complications. If surgery is of an urgent or emergency nature, it may not be possible preoperatively to optimize the medical condition. Even when medical management is superb, these high-risk patients are more likely to have hemodynamic instability in the perioperative period.[1] It is, therefore, crucial to measure physiologic parameters in order to maintain stable hemodynamic conditions. Devices range from those that are completely noninvasive, such as electrocardiography (ECG), pulse oximetry, or the blood pressure cuff, to those that are quite invasive, such as the pulmonary artery catheter (PAC). Less invasive technologies, such as transesophageal echocardiography (TEE) and noninvasive cardiac output monitors, continue to find an increasing role in the perioperative monitoring of patients with vascular disease. The ultimate goal of hemodynamic monitoring is to improve patients' outcomes with minimal risk. Generally, this means use of the least invasive forms of monitoring that are consistent with safe anesthetic care. Minimal monitoring standards have been established by the American Society of Anesthesiologists and should be employed in all vascular patients.[2] The purpose of this chapter is to illustrate a means of determining the appropriate level of monitoring for the patient with vascular disease.

Electrocardiography

ECG is one of the standard clinical modalities used to monitor patients in the perioperative setting. Current technology allows much more sophisticated data processing, and modern ECG devices have little resemblance to those used a few decades ago. During vascular surgery, the continuous online monitoring of a five-lead ECG has been a standard for years. Beyond its usefulness for the intraoperative recognition of arrhythmias, one of the major indications is for the intraoperative diagnosis of myocardial ischemia.

Etiology of Arrhythmias

Arrhythmias are common during vascular surgery, and their causes are numerous.[3] They are most common during endotracheal intubation or extubation and occur more frequently in patients with preexisting cardiac disease. The major factors contributing to the development of perioperative arrhythmias are as follows:

1. Anesthetic agents. Halogenated hydrocarbons, such as halothane and enflurane, are known to produce arrhythmias, probably by a reentrant mechanism.[4] The effect of volatile anesthetics on the QT interval has been shown in numerous studies, and associated changes in the QT interval can be the cause of potentially hazardous arrhythmias.[5-7] Halothane has also been shown to sensitize the myocardium to endogenous and exogenous catecholamines. Drugs that block the reuptake of norepinephrine, such as cocaine and ketamine, can facilitate the development of epinephrine-induced arrhythmias. The Food and Drug Administration has issued a "black box" warning regarding the use of droperidol because of its potentially proarrhythmic effect related to QT prolongation.

2. Abnormal arterial blood gases or electrolytes. Hyperventilation is known to reduce serum potassium. If the preoperative potassium is low, it is possible to reduce serum potassium into the 2 mEq/L range and perhaps precipitate severe cardiac arrhythmias.

3. Endotracheal intubation. This may be the most common cause of arrhythmias during surgery and is often associated with hemodynamic alterations.

4. Reflexes. Vagal stimulation may produce sinus bradycardia and allow ventricular escape mechanisms to occur. In vascular surgery, these reflexes may be related to traction on the peritoneum or direct pressure on the vagus nerve during carotid surgery. Stimulation of the carotid sinus can also lead to arrhythmias.

5. Central nervous system stimulation and dysfunction of the autonomic nervous system.

6. Preexisting cardiac disease. Patients with known cardiac disease have a much higher incidence of arrhythmias during anesthesia than patients without known disease.

7. Central venous cannulation. The insertion of catheters or wires into the central circulation often leads to arrhythmias, especially when the endocardium of the right ventricle is stimulated.

Etiology of Conduction Defects

Conduction defects occasionally occur during vascular surgery. They can result from the passage of a PAC through the right ventricle or can be a manifestation of myocardial ischemia.

133

Because high-grade conduction defects (second- and third-degree atrioventricular [AV] block) often have deleterious effects on hemodynamic performance, their intraoperative recognition is important.

Etiology of Myocardial Ischemia

Factors that predispose to the development of perioperative myocardial ischemia include the presence of preexisting coronary artery disease, and perioperative events that affect the myocardial oxygen supply-demand balance. Because coronary artery disease is often present in vascular surgical patients, perioperative monitoring for ischemia is essential. Modern ECG devices allow online continuous ST trend analysis, and crucial events can be automatically recorded. In the vascular surgery setting, the five-electrode system has become the standard for perioperative ischemia monitoring. The use of five electrodes allows the recording of the six standard bipolar limb leads as well as one precordial unipolar lead, which in general is placed in the V_5 position. Usually, leads II and V_5 are monitored continuously and the combined sensitivity to detect ischemia is about 80%. Anterolateral leads, such as V_5, are more sensitive to ischemia of the left anterior descending coronary artery (LAD) distribution, and right ventricular ischemia is more likely to be manifest in lead II. Using a 12-lead tracing, the combination of V_4 and V_5 increased sensitivity to about 90%, but lead II is considered to be superior for the detection of atrial arrhythmias.[8]

In a recent study by Landsberg et al, using a 12-lead ECG to detect perioperative myocardial ischemia, V_3 was most sensitive to ischemia (86.8%), followed by V_4 (78.9%) and V_5 (65.8%).[9] However, because V_4 was closest to the isoelectric baseline, it was considered the most suitable for ischemia monitoring in the perioperative setting.

The importance of monitoring patients for ischemic events postoperatively was shown by Mangano et al.[10] This study of the perioperative period found that postoperative ischemic episodes were the most severe, longer in duration, and without clinical symptoms in the majority of cases. Patients followed up for ischemia as long as 1 week postoperatively showed a maximum number of recorded ischemic events on postoperative day 3.[11]

Diagnostic Techniques

STANDARD AND PRECORDIAL LEAD SYSTEMS. The small electric currents produced by the electrical activity of the heart spread throughout the body, which behaves as a conductor. This electrical activity enables the surface ECG to be recorded at many sites. The standard leads are bipolar leads because they measure differences in potential between pairs of electrodes. The leads are placed on the extremities, and the polarities correspond to the conventions of Einthoven's triangle (Figure 8-1). Additional information regarding the heart's electrical activity is obtained by placing electrodes closer to the heart in the region of the thorax. If the three standard leads are connected through resistances of 5000 ohms each, a common central terminal with zero potential is obtained. When this common electrode is used with another active electrode, the potential difference between them represents the actual potential. In the unipolar lead system, the standard leads form the

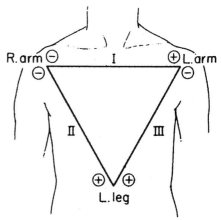

FIGURE 8-1 Einthoven's triangle indicating the polarities of the bipolar limb leads. (From Griffin RM, Kaplan JA: ECG lead systems. In Thys DM and Kaplan JA [ed]: *The ECG in anesthesia and critical care*, ed 1, New York, 1987, Churchill Livingstone, 18.)

neutral electrode and an exploring electrode is placed on the chest wall.

THE THREE-ELECTRODE SYSTEM. As the name implies, this system utilizes only three electrodes to record the ECG. In such a system, the ECG is observed along one bipolar lead between two of the electrodes, while the third electrode serves as a ground. A selector switch allows sequential monitoring of the electrodes without changing their location. The main advantage of the three-electrode system is its simplicity, but it provides a less complete reflection of myocardial electrical activity.

THE MODIFIED THREE-ELECTRODE SYSTEM. Numerous modifications of the standard bipolar limb lead system have been developed. Some of these are displayed in Figure 8-2. They are used in an attempt to maximize P-wave height for the diagnosis of atrial arrhythmias or to increase the sensitivity of the ECG for the detection of anterior myocardial ischemia. In clinical studies, these modified three-electrode systems have been shown to be as sensitive as or more sensitive than the standard V_5 lead system for the intraoperative diagnosis of ischemia.

THE FIVE-ELECTRODE SYSTEM. The use of five electrodes allows the recording of the six standard bipolar limb leads as well as one precordial unipolar lead. Generally, the unipolar lead is placed in the V_5 position, along the anterior axillary line in the fifth intercostal space (Figure 8-3). Thus, by adding only two electrodes to the ECG system, up to seven different leads can be simultaneously monitored. This allows clinicians to monitor several areas of the myocardium for ischemia or to diagnose atrial and ventricular arrhythmias more easily.

INVASIVE ECG. The electrical potentials of the heart can also be measured from body cavities adjacent to the heart (the esophagus or trachea) or from within the heart itself.

ESOPHAGEAL ECG. The concept of esophageal ECG is not new, and numerous studies have demonstrated the usefulness of this approach in the diagnosis of complicated arrhythmias. A prominent P wave is usually displayed in the presence of atrial depolarization and its relationship to the ventricular electrical activity can be examined. The esophageal electrode is incorporated into an esophageal stethoscope and connected to conventional ECG wires. To observe a bipolar esophageal ECG, the electrodes are connected to the right and left arm terminals

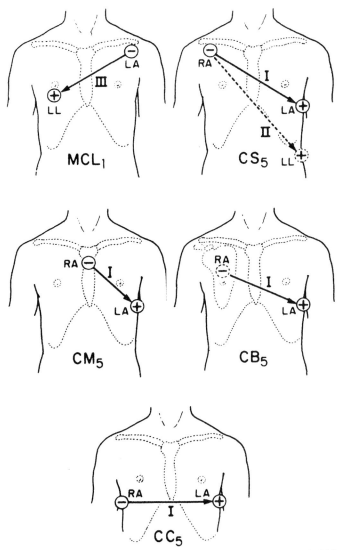

FIGURE 8-2 Modified bipolar limb leads. (From Griffin RM, Kaplan JA: ECG lead systems. In Thys DM and Kaplan JA [ed]: *The ECG in anesthesia and critical care*, ed 1, New York, 1987, Churchill Livingstone, 19.)

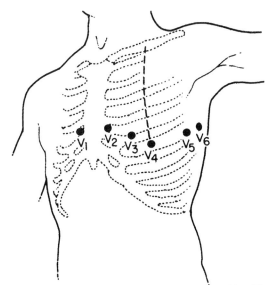

FIGURE 8-3 Standard precordial unipolar lead positions. (From Thys DM: The normal ECG. In Thys DM and Kaplan JA [ed]: *The ECG in anesthesia and critical care*, ed 1, New York, 1987, Churchill Livingstone, 6.)

and lead I is selected on the monitor. In 20 cardiac patients, Kates et al observed that 100% of atrial arrhythmias were correctly diagnosed with the esophageal lead (using intracavitary ECG as the standard), and lead II led to a correct diagnosis in 54% of the cases and V_5 in 42% of the cases.[12]

ENDOTRACHEAL ECG. The endotracheal ECG allows monitoring of the ECG when it is impractical or impossible to monitor the surface ECG. The endotracheal ECG consists of a standard endotracheal tube in which two electrodes have been embedded. This device may be most useful in pediatric patients for the diagnosis of atrial arrhythmias.[13]

MULTIPURPOSE PULMONARY ARTERY CATHETER. Chatterjee et al first described the use of a modified balloon-tipped flotation catheter for recording intracavitary electrograms.[14] The multipurpose PAC that is presently available has all of the features of a standard PAC. In addition, three atrial and two ventricular electrodes have been incorporated into the catheter. These electrodes allow the recording of intracavitary ECG and the estab-

lishment of atrial or AV pacing (although rates of capture are higher with endocardial pacing wires). The diagnostic capabilities with this catheter are varied (see later) because atrial, ventricular, or AV nodal arrhythmias and conduction blocks can be demonstrated.

Recording and Interpretation

BASIC REQUIREMENTS. The function of the ECG is to detect, amplify, display, and record the ECG signal. The ECG is usually displayed on an oscilloscope, and most monitors offer nonfade storage oscilloscopes to facilitate wave recognition. These offer no advantages over the use of direct-writing recorders that enable accurate interpretation of difficult ECGs and provide a written record for the patient's chart. All ECG monitors for use in patients with cardiac disease should, thus, also have paper or electronic recording capabilities. The recorder is needed to make accurate diagnoses of complex arrhythmias as well as to allow careful analysis of all the ECG waveforms. In addition, the recorder allows differentiation of real ECG changes from oscilloscope artifacts.

ARTIFACTS

Patient. The electrical signal that is generated by the heart and is monitored by the ECG is a very weak signal amounting to only 0.5 to 2 millivolts at the skin surface. It is, therefore, imperative that the skin be prepared optimally to avoid signal loss at the skin-electrode interface. The skin should be clean, and it is best to abrade the skin lightly to remove part of the stratum corneum, which can be a source of high resistance to the measured voltages. To avoid the problem of muscle artifact, electrodes should be placed over bony prominences whenever possible. Muscle movement, especially in the form of shivering, can produce significant ECG artifact.

Electrodes and leads. Loose electrodes and broken leads may produce a variety of artifacts that may simulate arrhythmias, Q waves, or inverted T waves.[15] Pregelled, disposable electrodes are usually used in the operating room. It is important that all the electrodes be moist, uniform, and not past the expiration date. To ensure good contact between the electrode and the skin, the electrical resistance of the skin should be minimized (i.e., the skin rubbed with alcohol) and excess body hair removed. Some ECG monitors have built-in cable testers that enable a lead to be tested by connecting the cable's distal end into the monitor. A high resistance causes a large voltage drop indicating that the lead is faulty. The main source of artifact from ECG leads is loss of the integrity of the lead insulation. A lack of insulation enhances interference by other electrical fields in the operating room, such as 60-Hz alternating current and electrocautery. Any damaged ECG lead should be discarded for this reason. Lead movement can also lead to artifact.

Electrocautery remains the most important source of ECG interference in the operating room, and it usually completely obliterates the ECG tracing. Electrocautery has three component frequencies.[16] The radiofrequency between 800 and 2000 kHz causes most of the interference, coupled with 60-Hz alternating-current frequency and 0.1- to 10-Hz low-frequency noise from intermittent contact of the electrosurgical unit with the patient's tissues. Preamplifiers may be modified to suppress radiofrequency interference.

Monitoring system. Most ECG monitors have filters to decrease environmental artifacts. They can usually operate in two modes. The first is the monitoring mode, which operates in the frequency response range of 0.5 to 50 Hz. The monitoring mode eliminates artifacts such as wandering baseline, but no clinical judgment can be made about the height of QRS or degree of ST-segment depression or elevation when the device is in this mode. Monitors may also operate in a diagnostic mode that has a greater frequency response of 0.05 to 100 Hz. In the patient with vascular disease, this mode should be utilized whenever possible because it allows the diagnosis of myocardial ischemia.

Automatic Recording

Holter monitoring has been utilized by a number of investigators to document the perioperative incidence of arrhythmias and myocardial ischemia. In Holter monitoring, ECG information from one or two bipolar leads is recorded by a small device. Up to 48 hours of ECG signals can be collected. Subsequently, the recording is processed by a playback system and the ECG signals are analyzed. On most modern systems, the playback unit includes a dedicated computer for rapid analysis of the data and automatic recognition of arrhythmias. Holter monitoring has been used to study the perioperative incidence of arrhythmias in cardiac and vascular surgical patients.[17-20]

Computer-Assisted Electrocardiogram Interpretation

During prolonged visual observation of the ECG on the oscilloscope, certain arrhythmias go undetected. This was clearly demonstrated by Romhilt et al, who showed that coronary care unit nurses failed to detect serious ventricular arrhythmias in 84% of their patients.[21] In a similar study, Holmberg et al found that, in their coronary care unit, the detection rate for ventricular tachycardia was as low as 42%.[22] Modern ECG monitoring devices have built-in computer processing devices that allow computer-assisted detection, interpretation, and storage of arrhythmias or ischemic events.[23] The accuracy of computer-assisted interpretation has been shown to vary among manufacturers; however, some programs have shown highly accurate results when compared with the interpretation by experienced cardiologists.[24,25] Online display of numerical values of ST-segment analysis facilitates easy detection of ischemic events and trends that can be recorded. Generally, the position of the ST segment is measured 60 to 80 msec following the J point, although some ECG devices allow individual adjustment by the clinician. This automated recording of arrhythmias or ischemic events also aids in the post hoc analysis of major perioperative events (e.g., when a patient's unstable condition requires the physician's complete attention).

Pulse Oximetry

Pulse oximetry has been criticized for being widely accepted without demonstration of its efficacy in improving outcomes.[26] Outcome studies of pulse oximetry are inconsistent, and the numbers of patients that must be studied are prohibitively large.[27-29] The vast majority of clinicians have nevertheless accepted pulse oximetry as an intraoperative monitoring standard, and this is reflected in current practice parameters.

The absorbance spectra of oxyhemoglobin and reduced hemoglobin significantly differ. Oxyhemoglobin absorbs most infrared light (940 nm) and transmits most red light (660 nm). Reduced hemoglobin absorbs more red light and transmits infrared light. Tissue and blood vessels also absorb red and infrared light, however, at a constant rate. It is the pulsatile component of the light absorbance that the pulse oximeter uses to calculate the arterial oxygen concentration. There are multiple sources of artifact and interference with pulse oximetry signal acquisition. These include diminished tissue perfusion (limb ischemia, hypothermia, vasoconstricting drugs), ambient light, intravenous dyes, carboxyhemoglobin, and methemoglobin.[30] Reich et al showed that there is a high incidence of pulse oximetry failure in the vascular surgery setting.[31] Another disadvantage of pulse oximetry is that the partial pressure of oxygen in arterial blood (Pao_2) must fall below 100 mmHg before the device begins to detect any change and below 60 mmHg before rapid changes occur. Thus, the device is not sensitive to changes in Pao_2 over wide ranges with clinical relevance.

Blood Pressure

Blood pressure (BP) is the most commonly used method of assessing the cardiovascular system. The magnitude of the BP is directly related to the cardiac output (CO) and the systemic vascular resistance (SVR). This is roughly analogous to Ohm's law of electricity (voltage = current × resistance), where BP is analogous to voltage, CO to flow, and SVR to resistance. Thus, an increase in the BP may reflect an increase in CO, SVR, or both. Although the BP is one of the easiest cardiovascular variables to measure, it gives only indirect information about the patient's cardiovascular status. Mean arterial pressure (MAP) is probably the most useful parameter to measure in assessing organ perfusion, except for the heart, where diastolic blood pressure (DBP) is most important. MAP is measured directly by integrating the arterial waveform tracing over time or using the formula: MAP = (SBP + [2 × DBP]) ÷ 3, where SBP is systolic blood pressure. The pulse pressure is the difference between SBP and DBP. Anesthesia for vascular surgery is frequently complicated by lability of BP related to several factors, including the nature of vascular surgery itself. Sudden losses of significant blood volumes may occur at almost any time. The vascular surgical population also includes many patients with labile hypertension and atherosclerotic heart disease. Thus, a safe and reliable method is required for the accurate measurement of BP during vascular surgery.

Noninvasive Blood Pressure

The Riva-Rocci occlusive cuff for the sphygmomanometric measurement of BP was described in 1896, and Harvey Cushing promoted the measurement of BP during anesthesia for neurosurgical procedures in 1903. A sphygmomanometer consists of an elastic bladder surrounded by an unyielding cuff that evenly distributes the pressure in the bladder to the encircled extremity. The elastic bladder is filled with air until a suprasystolic pressure is applied to the extremity, and then the air is slowly released. For accurate BP measurement, two conditions must be met: (1) the cuff must be 20% wider than the diameter of the extremity; and (2) the bladder must be attached to a calibrated aneroid or mercury manometer. If the cuff is applied too loosely or tightly, this also results in inaccuracy.[32,33]

METHODS OF SPHYGMOMANOMETRY

Palpatory technique. One of the easiest methods of obtaining the SBP is to locate a pulse, inflate a proximal cuff until the pulse is absent, and then slowly deflate the cuff until the first pulse is palpated. Variations on this technique include using a Doppler probe or a pulse oximeter to indicate when the first pulse is present. In children younger than 1 year, the limb can be observed for flushing that occurs when the cuff pressure is less than SBP.[34] Unfortunately, only the SBP is accurately measured by this method.

Korotkoff sounds. Korotkoff sound auscultation is the most traditional and widespread method of BP determination outside the operating room for vascular patients. As the cuff is deflated from a suprasystolic pressure, a stethoscope is placed over a distal artery. The sound of blood rushing into the empty arterial tree creates Korotkoff sounds when the cuff pressure is less than systolic pressure.[35] The sounds disappear when the cuff pressure is less than the diastolic pressure.

An accurate determination of BP by this method requires that the cuff be deflated slowly. Otherwise, the systolic pressure is underestimated and the diastolic pressure is either overestimated or underestimated. However, there are other potential sources of inaccuracy with this technique. Atherosclerosis may result in stiffening of the artery that prevents the cuff from completely occluding the artery, even at suprasystolic pressures ("lead pipe syndrome"), causing overestimation of the SBP. Hypotensive states, such as hypovolemic shock, and vasopressor infusions may result in hypoperfusion of the extremity with underestimation of the BP.[36]

OSCILLOMETRY. Von Recklinghausen introduced the oscillotonometer in 1931. The device consists of a double-cuff system with a proximal cuff for occlusion of arterial inflow and a distal cuff to measure arterial pulsations. The distal cuff begins

to pulsate when the proximal cuff deflates below systolic pressure, and maximal oscillations occur when the proximal cuff is at MAP. The diastolic pressure is, however, not easily determined by this method.[37]

Automated oscillometric BP devices are available from numerous manufacturers. These devices differ from oscillotonometers in that there is only one cuff. A solenoid valve controls the deflation of the cuff, holding the cuff volume momentarily constant, so that the amplitude of the oscillation may be recorded. As the cuff deflates from a suprasystolic pressure, the oscillations are measured for at least two cardiac cycles at multiple cuff pressures. A computer then analyzes the pattern of oscillations at different cuff pressures. Systolic pressure is defined at the point of rapidly increasing oscillation, and diastolic pressure is defined at rapidly decreasing oscillation. MAP is the cuff pressure associated with maximal oscillation.[38]

Automated oscillometric BP determination has been favorably compared with invasively determined BP in both adults and neonates.[39,40] However, the cycle times are prolonged when the oscillations are irregular (as in atrial fibrillation or with movement of the patient) or slow (sinus bradycardia). These devices usually remain accurate during hypotension but may fail when there is severe hypovolemia or vasoconstriction.

PHOTOPLETHYSMOGRAPHY. The Peñaz principle involves the measurement of an arterial pressure waveform by unloading the arterial wall of the finger.[41] Although not currently available, a functional product (the Finapres) consisted of a finger pressure cuff and an infrared photoplethysmograph. A servo control mechanism varied the pressure in the finger cuff to maintain constant infrared absorbance distal to the cuff. The pressure waveform generated in the finger cuff correlated with the arterial pressure waveform. The Finapres device correlated with arterial pressure measured by the auscultatory method and direct intra-arterial measurement.[42-45]

There remain concerns that this device may result in digital nerve injury or ischemic injury. However, the device has been used for prolonged periods without adverse sequelae.[46] Moderate degrees of peripheral vasoconstriction are associated with some inaccuracy, but severe vasoconstriction (as with high vasopressor doses) and severe peripheral vascular disease hinder the use of this technique (Figure 8-4).[47,48]

DOPPLER METHOD. The Doppler effect is the change in frequency of a waveform that is reflected from a moving surface. This principle can be applied to detect the motion of an arterial wall distal to an inflated cuff. Doppler measurement of SBP closely correlated with, but slightly underestimated, intra-arterial measurement in one pediatric study.[49] The advantages of this technique are that it is useful in pediatrics and in adults with low-flow states and that the technique may be automated. The disadvantage is that MAP and DBP are not easily obtained and that motion, electrocautery, and Doppler probe dislocation interfere with accurate measurements.[50]

ADVANTAGES AND DISADVANTAGES OF NONINVASIVE PRESSURE

MONITORING. Noninvasive BP measurement techniques are advantageous in that they are technically easy to perform, easily automated, generally accurate, and carry a negligible infectious risk. However, several risks still remain. There is the potential for electrical macroshock with electrical devices. Prolonged or too frequent cuff inflation may result in tissue

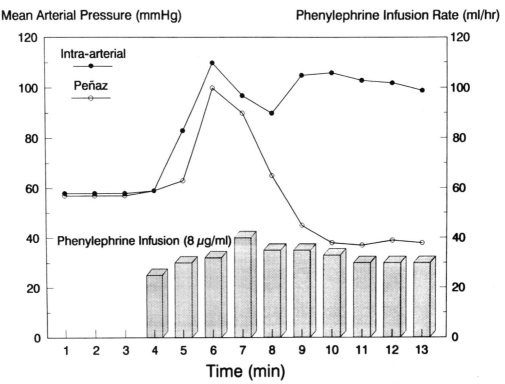

Mean Arterial Pressure (mmHg)

Phenylephrine Infusion Rate (ml/hr)

Time (min)

FIGURE 8-4 Mean arterial pressures derived from a radial arterial cannula and a Peñaz finger photoplethysmography device before and during a phenylephrine infusion in a single patient. The curves demonstrate the inaccuracy of the Peñaz device during periods of vasoconstriction. (Modified from Kurki T, Smith NT, Head N: *J Clin Monit* 3:6, 1987.)

ischemia or nerve damage. Ulnar nerve palsy has been reported with an automated device that compressed the nerve against the ulnar groove.[51]

There is also the potential for inaccurate or delayed BP readings for the reasons mentioned before.[52] Vascular surgical patients may be especially susceptible to these errors because of slower or irregular heart rates (from associated cardiovascular disease) and rigid peripheral arteries (from atherosclerosis). Thus, there remains that risk that the patient may be inappropriately managed because of erroneous or delayed information.

Invasive Pressure Monitoring

GENERAL. In vascular anesthesia, pressures inside the blood vessels or cardiac chambers are commonly measured. Arterial pressure is gauged by placing a catheter into a peripheral artery while other catheters, placed in the central circulation, measure central venous or intracardiac pressures. Pressure waves in the arterial and venous tree represent the transmission of forces generated in the cardiac chambers. Measurement of these forces requires the conversion of mechanical energy into electronic signals. Electromechanical transducers accomplish this function. Other components of a system for intravascular pressure measurement include the intravascular catheter, fluid-filled tubing and connections, an electronic analyzer, and a display system. The accurate reproduction of intravascular pressures is determined by the dynamic response (or frequency response) of the transducer-tubing assembly and the frequency content of the pressure waveform. The following paragraphs briefly describe these concepts and review the various factors that influence them.

FREQUENCY CONTENT. Pressure waves generated in the heart are complex rather than simple sine waves. These complex waves can be described mathematically as a summation of a series of simple sine waves of differing amplitude and frequency. The process used to extract sine waves from complex waves is called Fourier analysis (Figure 8-5). The fundamental frequency, or first harmonic, describes the number of times that the pressure fluctuation occurs per second and is a measure of the heart rate. At a heart rate of 120 bpm, the fundamental frequency is 2 Hz, and at a heart rate of 60 bpm it is 1 Hz. It has been shown that the essential information of an arterial waveform is contained within the first 10 harmonics of the wave (10×1 Hz = 10 Hz for a heart rate of 60 bpm and 10×2 Hz = 20 Hz for a heart rate of 120 bpm). A general principle of intravascular pressure measuring systems states that accurate reproduction of a complex waveform requires that the frequency response remain constant throughout the range of frequencies found in the measured wave.

DYNAMIC RESPONSE. The dynamic response depends on the natural frequency and damping coefficient of the pressure transmission system (catheter, tubing, stopcocks, transducer assembly); the dynamic response of a pressure measurement system is thus evaluated by measuring these two characteristics. Systems with less-than-optimal natural frequency or damping produce erroneous pressure recordings. This situation is usually manifested by overestimation of systolic pressures in the systemic arterial tree and amplification of artifacts, such as catheter whip, a pressure swing produced by the motion of the catheter tip.

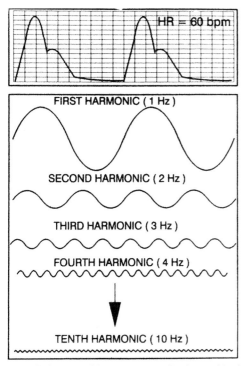

FIGURE 8-5 An intra-arterial pressure recording is noted in the graph at the top. Below, the arterial waveform is broken down into sine waves of increasing frequency. The arterial waveform can be accurately reconstructed from sine waves with frequencies from the first to the tenth harmonics.

were artifactually increased. Large air bubbles interfere with the transmission of the pressure wave and primarily increase damping.

DAMPING COEFFICIENT. In most systems, oscillations decay over time because of frictional losses or damping. In pressure measurement systems, the role of damping is to ensure that, as the input frequency increases, the frequency response remains constant while the system's natural frequency is approached. Damping is often expressed as a damping coefficient. A damping coefficient of zero indicates that no damping is achieved, and a coefficient of one signifies that a system is critically damped. As the damping coefficient increases, the frequency response at the natural frequency decreases and the response time is increased. The ideal damping coefficient is in part determined by the system's natural frequency.

Most pressure measuring systems used in anesthesia today are underdamped with coefficients in the range 0.1 to 0.2. With the addition of energy to the system, the response time is rapid but some overshoot occurs. The damping of a pressure measuring system can be gauged by observing the response to a rapid flush of the system, known as the fast flush test (Figure 8-6). In a system with a low damping coefficient, the fast flush test results in several oscillations above and below the true pressure before the pressure waveform stabilizes. In an adequately damped system, the baseline is reached after one oscillation, whereas in an overdamped system, the baseline is reached after a delay and without oscillations.

NATURAL FREQUENCY. The frequency at which the ratio of output amplitude (signal plus distortion) over input amplitude (pure signal) is largest is called the natural frequency. Ideally, the natural frequency of a system should be as high as possible. Usually, a system's frequency response remains constant at lower frequencies but then gradually increases with increasing input frequency until the maximal frequency response is reached at the natural frequency of the system. The optimal natural frequency is, in part, determined by the heart rate. If a patient's heart rate is 120 bpm, the fundamental frequency of the arterial waveform is 2 Hz. Accurate pressure measurements, at this heart rate, require a constant frequency response up to at least 20 Hz (10th harmonic). Therefore, the natural frequency of the measuring system should preferably exceed 20 Hz if an artifact-free waveform is to be obtained.

In clinical practice, the natural frequency of bare transducers is normally in the range 100 to 500 Hz, but that of the catheter-tubing assembly can be considerably lower. It decreases significantly with increasing length of tubing and in the presence of small air bubbles. Boutros and Albert demonstrated that with a change in the length of low-compliance tubing from 6 inches to 5 feet, the natural frequency decreased from 34 to 7 Hz.[53] As a result of the reduced natural frequency, the systolic pressures measured with the longer tubing exceeded reference pressures by 17.3%. The effects of small air bubbles on the dynamic response of pressure measurement systems were studied by Shinozaki et al.[54] They noted that with the inclusion of small air bubbles (0.05 to 0.25 mL) in the pressure tubing, the natural frequency decreased and the measured SBPs

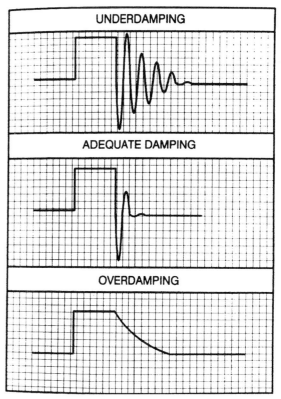

FIGURE 8-6 The fast flush test is demonstrated in three different systems. The middle graph represents the optimal damping for accurate pressure measurement.

Hunziker studied the damping coefficients and natural frequencies of seven commercially available disposable transducers.[55] Each transducer was investigated with long tubing (60-inch pole mount) or short tubing (12-inch patient mount) before and after insertion of a small air bubble (0.03 mL) into the tubing. Lengthening of the tubing and inclusion of the air bubble resulted in marked decreases in natural frequency and increases in damping coefficient. Only one of the transducers had adequate dynamic response and accuracy in both the pole-mounted and patient-mounted version. All systems were severely underdamped, and most led to systematic overestimation of the systolic arterial pressure. Several devices that can be included in a pressure monitoring system to adjust the damping coefficient have been described.[56,57] They are not commonly used, however.

Many of the problems described could be avoided by the use of catheters with pressure-sensing transducers at their tip. Although these catheters eliminate the problems associated with fluid-filled tubing, they cannot be rezeroed once inserted and they are expensive and fragile.

Arterial Pressure Monitoring

Although numerous methods of noninvasive BP measurement are clinically available, all of these require the detection of flow past an occlusive cuff. These noninvasive methods tend to underestimate SBP and overestimate DBP regardless of the technique. In addition, none, except the Peñaz technique, generates an arterial waveform. Direct intra-arterial monitoring remains the "gold standard" against which all noninvasive techniques are compared.[58]

ADVANTAGES. Vascular surgery is frequently complicated by wide swings in BP related to shifts in intravascular volume and superimposed cardiovascular disease. Intra-arterial monitoring provides a beat-to-beat indication of arterial pressure and waveform. Multiple arterial blood gases may also be obtained. Intra-arterial monitoring is indicated in all patients undergoing major vascular surgery. It is also indicated in those undergoing minor vascular surgery if significant cardiopulmonary or metabolic diseases coexist. The arterial waveform tracing provides much more information than timely BP measurements. The slope of the upstroke correlates with dP/dT, which gives a rough indication of myocardial contractility. An increase in SVR results in both an increase in the slope of the upstroke and a decrease in the slope of the downstroke. The acute changes that occur in the tracing with arrhythmias give a visual estimate of the hemodynamic consequences of events such as the loss of atrial systole. In addition, hypovolemia is suggested when a large respiratory variation and a narrowed pulse pressure are observed on the arterial pressure tracing.[59-61]

SITES

Radial and ulnar arteries. During vascular surgery, the radial artery is the one most commonly selected because of its superficial location, easy accessibility, and the presence of collateral circulation. Prior to cannulating the radial artery for monitoring purposes, it is, however, necessary to ascertain the adequacy of the collateral circulation and the absence of proximal obstructions. The ulnar artery provides the majority of blood flow to the hand in about 90% of humans.[62] The radial and ulnar arteries are connected by a palmar arch that provides collateral flow

to the hand in the event of radial artery occlusion. The palmar circulation is routinely checked using an Allen test prior to radial arterial cannulation. The Allen test is performed by occluding both radial and ulnar arteries by compression and exercising the hand until it is pale. The ulnar artery is then released (with the hand open loosely), and the time until the hand regains its normal color is noted.[63] With a normal collateral circulation, the color returns to the hand in about 5 seconds. If, however, the hand takes longer than 15 seconds to return to its normal color, cannulation of the radial artery is relatively contraindicated.[64] The hand may remain pale if the fingers are hyperextended or widely spread apart even in the presence of a normal collateral circulation.[65] Variations on the Allen test include using a Doppler probe or pulse oximeter to document collateral flow.[66-68] If the Allen test demonstrates that the hand is dependent on the radial artery for adequate filling and other cannulation sites are not available, the ulnar artery may be selected.

The predictive value of the Allen test has been challenged. In a large series of children in whom radial arterial catheterization was performed without a preliminary Allen test, there was an absence of complications.[69] Slogoff et al cannulated the radial artery in 16 patients with poor ulnar collateral circulation (assessed using the Allen test) with no complications.[70] In contrast, Mangano and Hickey reported a case of hand ischemia requiring amputation in a patient with a normal preoperative Allen test.[71] Thus, the predictive value of the Allen test is questionable.[72]

Another factor that may influence the choice of which extremity to use for intra-arterial monitoring is the presence of a proximal arterial cutdown site. Monitoring of the radial artery distal to a brachial arterial cutdown site may result in damped waveforms or vascular thrombosis and, thus, is not recommended.[73] Other factors that influence the site of cannulation in vascular surgery include the site of surgery, the vessels that will require clamping to obtain vascular control, any history of ischemia or prior surgery of the limb, and the presence of arteriovenous hemodialysis shunts, if any.

Brachial or axillary arteries. The brachial artery lies medial to the bicipital tendon in the antecubital fossa in close proximity to the median nerve. The complications from brachial artery monitoring are lower than those following brachial artery cutdown for cardiac catheterization.[74] Still, there is little, if any, collateral flow to the hand should brachial artery occlusion occur. Therefore, other sites should be chosen, if possible. Brachial artery pressure tracings resemble those in the femoral artery, with less systolic augmentation than radial artery tracings.[75]

The axillary artery may be cannulated by the Seldinger technique near the junction of the deltoid and pectoral muscles. This site has been recommended for long-term catheterization in the intensive care unit and in patients with peripheral vascular disease.[76,77] Because the tip of the 15- to 20-cm catheter may lie in the aortic arch, the use of the left axillary artery is recommended to minimize the chance of cerebral embolization during flushing.

Femoral and dorsalis pedis arteries. The femoral artery is a less attractive choice for arterial monitoring in patients with vascular disease than in the cardiac surgical population. Aortic inflow obstruction may decrease the arterial pressure in the femoral artery, or the femoral artery may be the site of the surgery itself. The use of this site remains controversial because of the high rate of ischemic complications and pseudoaneurysm formation following diagnostic angiographic and cardiac catheterization procedures as well as data indicating a higher risk of catheter-associated infection compared with the use of other cannulation sites.[78]

Dorsalis pedis arterial monitoring is contraindicated in surgery for lower extremity revascularization. However, in vascular surgery performed elsewhere, dorsalis pedis or posterior tibial artery cannulation can be a reasonable alternative to radial arterial catheterization. The systolic pressure is usually 10 to 20 mmHg higher in the dorsalis pedis artery than in the radial or brachial arteries, wherein the diastolic pressure is 15 to 20 mmHg lower.[79]

In patients undergoing thoracoabdominal aortic reconstruction, femoral arterial monitoring may be required in addition to monitoring arterial pressure in one of the upper extremities. In these operations, one of the femoral arteries may be perfused using partial left or right heart bypass in order to preserve spinal cord and visceral organ blood flow. It is important to measure the distal aortic pressure by monitoring the femoral (or dorsalis pedis) artery in the other leg in order to optimize the distal perfusion pressure. Unfortunately, it is still not clear whether the incidence of paraplegia, hepatic dysfunction, or renal failure is less with distal perfusion and what the optimal pressure for distal perfusion should be (See Chapter 11).[80-82]

Superficial temporal artery. The superficial temporal artery is a branch of the external carotid artery that passes anterior to the ear. It has a variable course that may be determined with a Doppler probe.[83] The artery may be quite tortuous and difficult to cannulate. The tip of the catheter must be positioned carefully so that embolization through the internal carotid to the cerebral circulation does not occur. This approach is not recommended in the vascular patient with carotid occlusive or cerebrovascular disease. Superficial temporal artery catheterization is rarely performed.

COMPLICATIONS

Hemorrhage. Any arterial monitoring catheter carries the potential risk of death from exsanguination if the catheter becomes disconnected. The use of Luer-Lok (instead of tapered) connections and monitors with low-pressure alarms should decrease the risk of this complication.[84] Stopcocks are an additional source of occult hemorrhage because of the potential for loose connections or inadvertent changes in the position of the control lever that would open the system to the atmosphere.

Thrombosis and distal ischemia. Thrombosis of the radial artery following cannulation has been extensively studied. Factors that correlate with an increased incidence of thrombosis include prolonged duration of cannulation, larger catheters, and smaller radial artery size (i.e., a greater proportion of the artery is occupied by the catheter).[85-87] The incidence of thrombosis is not affected by the technique of cannulation but is lowered with aspirin pretreatment.[88,89] Bedford recommended removing arterial catheters with continuous aspiration of the catheter by syringe, during proximal and distal occlusion of the vessel, in order to remove accumulated thrombus.[90] The association

between radial artery thrombosis and ischemia of the hand, however, is less certain. As noted previously, an abnormal Allen test was not associated with hand complications following radial artery cannulation, and, despite the frequent use of radial artery cannulation, hand complications are rarely reported.[70,91] The incidence of distal ischemia would be expected to be higher in vascular patients with generalized atherosclerosis. The hand should be closely examined at regular intervals in patients with axillary, brachial, radial, or ulnar arterial catheters. Because thrombosis may appear several days after the catheter has been removed, the examinations should be continued through the postoperative period.[92] Although recanalization of the thrombosed artery can be expected in an average of 13 days, the collateral blood flow may be inadequate during this period.[93] Any evidence of hand ischemia should be aggressively investigated and promptly treated in order to prevent morbidity.[94] The treatment plan should involve consultation with a vascular, hand, or plastic surgeon. Treatment has traditionally been conservative. However, fibrinolytic agents such as streptokinase, heparin, antiplatelet agents, stellate ganglion blockade, and surgical intervention are modalities that should be considered.

Embolization. Particulate matter or air that is forcefully flushed into an arterial catheter can move proximally as well as distally within the artery. Cerebral embolization is most likely from axillary or temporal sites but is also possible with brachial and radial catheters.[95] Emboli from the right arm are more likely to reach the cerebral circulation than those from the left arm because of anatomy and direction of blood flow in the aortic arch. Other factors that influence the likelihood of cerebral embolization include the volume of flush solution and the rapidity of injection.[96]

Hematoma and neurologic injury. Hematoma formation may occur at any arterial puncture or cannulation site and is particularly common with coagulopathy. If a large hematoma develops, the resultant pressure may result in compression of the artery and distal ischemia or compression of an adjacent nerve, resulting in a neuropathy. Nerve damage is especially likely if the nerve and artery lie in a fibrous sheath (such as the brachial plexus) or a limited tissue compartment such as the forearm. Hematoma formation should be prevented by the application of direct pressure following arterial punctures and the correction of any underlying coagulopathy.

Vascular surgical patients often require anticoagulation in the perioperative period. Surgical consultation should be obtained if massive hematoma formation or neurologic dysfunction develops. Surgical exploration may be necessary if conservative measures are ineffective.

Direct nerve injuries may also result from needle trauma during attempts at arterial cannulation. The median nerve is in close proximity to the brachial artery, and the axillary artery lies within the brachial plexus sheath.

Late vascular complications. Incomplete disruption of the wall of an artery may eventually result in pseudoaneurysm formation. The wall of the pseudoaneurysm is composed of fibrous tissue that continues to expand. If the pseudoaneurysm ruptures into a vein or if both a vein and artery are injured simultaneously, an arteriovenous fistula results. The treatment for these lesions is surgical repair or percutaneous stent implantation.[97-99]

Inaccurate pressure readings. Despite the great advantages of intra-arterial monitoring, it does not always give accurate pressure readings. The monitoring system may be incorrectly zeroed and calibrated, or the transducers may not be level with the patient. The waveform is dampened if the catheter is kinked or partially thrombosed. In vasoconstricted patients or those in hypovolemic shock, the brachial and radial artery pressures may not reflect the true central aortic pressure. Another possible etiology for inaccurate readings is unsuspected arterial stenosis proximal to the monitored artery, as occurs with thoracic outlet syndrome and subclavian stenosis. Unsuspected Raynaud syndrome also yields unreliable pressure readings from peripheral arteries. Concomitant use of a noninvasive BP measurement system aids in recognizing instances in which the invasive measurement is incorrect. A cuff placed on the same arm as a brachial or radial artery catheter can be slowly deflated until the first systole is detected on the arterial waveform tracing. This procedure gives a good indication of the systolic pressure and is a useful method for checking the accuracy of invasive BP measurement.

Infection risk. One complication that is common to all forms of invasive monitoring is the risk of infection. The infectious organism may contaminate the catheter prior to insertion (poor manufacturing standards), during insertion (poor aseptic technique), or after final placement (bacteremia, poor aseptic technique, or infection at the insertion site). As one example of poor aseptic technique, contaminated blood gas syringes have been linked with arterial catheter infections.[100] Other factors that are associated with catheter infection include nondisposable transducer domes, dextrose flush solution, and duration of insertion.[101-103]

Vascular surgical patients frequently undergo implantation of prosthetic graft materials for revascularization. Any infection of these foreign bodies necessitates removal of the graft. Thus, it is essential that strict aseptic technique be used during placement of any monitoring catheter in order to prevent catheter-related sepsis. Whenever infection at the cannulation site is identified, the catheter must be removed. The catheter is a foreign body, which is not sterilized with antibiotic therapy.

Central Venous Pressure Monitoring

Advantages

Central venous pressure (CVP) catheters are used to measure the filling pressure of the right ventricle, give an assessment of the intravascular volume status, and assess right ventricular function. The distal end of the catheter must lie within one of the large intrathoracic veins or the right atrium. Although water manometers have been used in the past, in modern practice, the electronic system is preferred because it allows observation of the right atrial waveform, providing additional information. In any pressure monitoring system, it is necessary to have a reproducible landmark (such as the midaxillary line) as a zero reference. This reference is especially important in monitoring venous pressures because small changes in transducer height produce proportionately larger errors compared with arterial pressure monitoring.

The right atrial waveform has three upward deflections (a, c, and v waves) and two downward deflections (x and y descents) (Figure 8-7). The a wave is produced by atrial systole, occur-

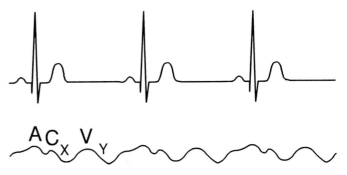

FIGURE 8-7 The atrial waveform concomitant with the ECG.

ring after the P wave on the ECG but before the first heart sound. This is followed shortly by the c wave, which occurs as the tricuspid valve closes and bulges upward into the right atrium. As ventricular systole continues, the tricuspid valve is pulled away from the right atrium by the contracting ventricle. This causes the x descent. The v wave is a complex phenomenon that occurs as blood fills the atrium prior to the opening of the tricuspid valve at the end of systole. The y descent occurs as the tricuspid valve opens, the myocardium relaxes, and blood begins to fill the right ventricle during early diastole.[104] The right atrium waveform may be useful in the diagnosis of pathologic cardiac conditions that are not uncommon in the vascular surgical patient. The onset of an irregular rhythm and the loss of the a wave suggest atrial flutter or fibrillation. Junctional (nodal) rhythm results in "cannon a waves" as the atrium contracts against a closed tricuspid valve (Figure 8-8). These waves may also be present in complete heart block and ventricular arrhythmias. Cannon v waves occur if there is a significant degree of tricuspid regurgitation. Large v waves may also appear on the right atrial waveform if the ventricle becomes noncompliant because of ischemia or right ventricular failure.[105]

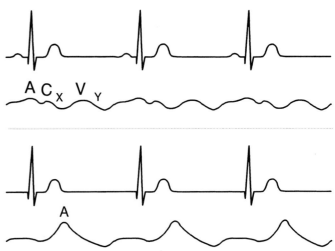

FIGURE 8-8 The normal ECG and atrial waveform are demonstrated above. The ECG below has no P waves and the atrial waveform has cannon A waves.

Indications

CVP monitoring in the vascular surgical patient is mainly performed as an indicator of intravascular volume. The accuracy and reliablility of CVP monitoring depend on many factors, including the functional status of the right and left ventricles, the presence of pulmonary disease, and ventilatory factors such as positive end-expiratory pressure (PEEP). The CVP correlates with left heart filling pressures only in patients with good left ventricular and pulmonary function.[106]

Sites

The technique for percutaneous central venous cannulation has been well described elsewhere.[107] Briefly, the cannulation may be accomplished by catheter-through-the-needle, catheter-over-the-needle, or catheter-over-a-wire (Seldinger) techniques. A modification of the Seldinger technique is preferred when the vein is cannulated by a small (18 or 20 gauge) catheter over the needle. The small catheter is then connected to a transducer or a manometer to confirm that a venous waveform is present. The small catheter is then exchanged over a wire for a larger central venous monitoring catheter. Alternatively, blood may be aspirated from the small catheter and visually compared with an arterial blood sample to confirm venous placement of the small catheter.[108] The use of ultrasound-guided central venous cannulation has been shown to increase the success rate and decrease the rate of complications.[109-114]

INTERNAL JUGULAR VEIN. Anesthesiologists often prefer the internal jugular vein to other approaches. It is a clean area that is easily accessible during most vascular procedures. The incidence of successfully reaching the superior vena cava is high with right internal jugular cannulation because of the straight path followed by the catheter.[115] The technique is relatively contraindicated in patients with previous neck surgery and absolutely contraindicated with local infection or superior vena caval obstruction. The risk of hematoma formation is increased with anticoagulation. If severe carotid occlusive disease is present, caution must be exercised in palpating for landmarks so as not to dislodge a plaque and cause a stroke.

EXTERNAL JUGULAR VEIN. The external jugular vein is another means of reaching the central circulation. However, the success rate is lower because of the tortuous path that the vein follows to the intrathoracic veins. In addition, a valve is usually present at the point where the external jugular perforates the fascia to empty into the subclavian vein. However, a success rate as high as 90% was reported using a J-wire to slide past obstructions to the central circulation.[116] The main advantage of this technique is that there is no need to advance a needle into the deeper structures of the neck.

SUBCLAVIAN VEIN. The subclavian vein is readily accessible from supraclavicular or infraclavicular approaches and has been used for decades for central venous access.[117] The success rate is higher than with the external jugular approach but lower than with the right internal jugular approach.[118] The subclavian vein is less frequently cannulated by anesthesiologists because of the higher incidence of complications (see later). However, this may be the cannulation sight of choice in carotid artery surgery, when CVP monitoring is indicated.

ANTECUBITAL VEINS. Another route for central venous monitoring is through the basilic or cephalic veins. The advantages of this approach are the low likelihood of complications and ease of access intraoperatively if the arm is exposed. The major disadvantage is that it is difficult to ensure placement of the catheter into a central vein. Studies have indicated that blind advancement results in central venous cannulation in 59% to 75% of attempts.[119,120] Unsuccessful attempts are most frequently due to failure to advance the catheter past the shoulder or cannulation of the ipsilateral internal jugular vein. Turning the head to the ipsilateral side may help to prevent internal jugular placement of the catheter.[121]

FEMORAL VEIN. The femoral vein is rarely cannulated in the adult patient for monitoring in the perioperative period but is not uncommonly used for vascular access for rapid volume infusion. However, the cannulation is technically simple and the success rate is high. Overall, the literature reports a higher rate of catheter sepsis and thrombophlebitis with this approach; yet, in subgroups of patients, this might be the only available venous access and some studies indicate a comparable rate of infectious risk in these patients.[122-124] Patients with the superior vena caval syndrome who require central venous monitoring require the femoral approach in order to obtain true central pressures. A long catheter is required in order to reach the mediastinal portion of the inferior vena cava in the adult patient.

Complications

ARTERIAL PUNCTURE. Inadvertent arterial puncture during central venous cannulation is not uncommon. The two reasons why this occurs are (1) that all of the veins commonly used for cannulation lie in close proximity to arteries (except the external jugular and cephalic) and (2) that the venous anatomy is quite variable. Localized hematoma formation is the usual consequence. Hematoma formation may be minimized if a small-gauge needle (e.g., 22 gauge) is used initially to localize the vein. If a large-bore catheter is to be inserted ($\geq$4F), the vein is first cannulated with an 18- or 20-gauge catheter. Venous placement is confirmed by comparison with an arterial sample or by transducing the waveform, and then the small catheter is exchanged over a wire for the larger catheter using the Seldinger technique.[125]

A massive hematoma may form if the arterial puncture is large, direct pressure is not applied, or the patient is receiving anticoagulants or has a coagulopathy. In the neck, a hematoma may lead to tracheal obstruction requiring intubation. In the arm or leg, venous obstruction may occur. Arteriovenous fistula is also a reported complication of central venous cannulation.[126,127] Hemothorax is a potential complication if the subclavian artery is lacerated during cannulation. Symptoms of hypovolemia predominate because of the large volume necessary to fill the hemithorax. Hemothorax may also occur if an indwelling catheter erodes through a venous structure into the pleural cavity.

PNEUMOTHORAX OR HYDROTHORAX. If the pleural cavity is entered and lung tissue is punctured during a cannulation attempt, a pneumothorax may result. Tension pneumothorax is possible if air continues to accumulate because of a "ball-valve" effect. Pneumothorax is most common with subclavian punctures and occurs only rarely with internal jugular cannulation.[128] If the catheter tip is placed extravascularly in the pleural cavity or erodes into this position, the fluid that is infused into the catheter accumulates in the pleural cavity.[129] Auscultation, percussion, and radiography of the chest are used to make the diagnosis.

CHYLOTHORAX. Injury to the thoracic duct resulting in chylothorax has been reported following left internal jugular cannulation.[130,131] The anatomic relationships of the thoracic duct make chylothorax a potential complication of left subclavian catheterization as well (Figure 8-9).[132] This is a serious complication that may require surgical treatment or the application of PEEP.[133,134] Chylothorax is one of the reasons why right internal cannulation is preferred over left.[135]

PERICARDIAL EFFUSION OR TAMPONADE. If the right atrium or ventricle is perforated during central venous cannulation, pericardial effusion or tamponade may result.[136] The likelihood of this complication is increased when inflexible guide wires or catheters are used. Pericardial tamponade is a rare, but potentially fatal, complication of central venous catheterization.[137,138]

EMBOLISM. Air embolism is a potentially fatal complication that is possible whenever there is negative pressure in a portion of the venous system that is open to the atmosphere.[139-141] Embolization is likely when patients are in the semiupright or sitting position or if there is a strong inspiratory effort. Thus, air embolism may be prevented by using positional maneuvers, such as the Trendelenburg position, to ensure positive venous pressure in the vessel to be cannulated. When the central venous catheter is placed, it is important to ensure that the catheter is firmly attached to its connecting tubing. The com-

plication may even occur after the catheter has been removed but the subcutaneous tract has failed to close.[142]

Catheter fragments may be sheared off by the inserting needle and embolize to the right side of the heart and pulmonary circulation. This complication is especially likely when catheter-through-the-needle cannulation kits are used. This problem can be avoided by not withdrawing the catheter through the needle. During unsuccessful catheterization, the needle and catheter must be simultaneously withdrawn. The catheter fragment position within the right-sided circulation determines whether surgery or percutaneous transvenous techniques are necessary for its removal.[143]

NERVE INJURY. The brachial plexus, stellate ganglion, and phrenic nerve all lie in close proximity to the internal jugular vein. A needle may injure the nerves during cannulation attempts.[144-146] Horner's syndrome has been reported following internal jugular cannulation.[147]

Pulmonary Artery Catheterization
Advantages

Perioperative monitoring with the flow-directed PAC has been a major advance in the care of the vascular surgical patient. Since it was introduced in the 1970s, PAC use has increased the amount of diagnostic information that can be obtained at the bedside in the critically ill patient.[148] Specific information that is available with the PAC includes pulmonary artery systolic pressure, pulmonary artery diastolic (PAD) pressure, mean pulmonary arterial pressure (MPAP), pulmonary capillary wedge pressure (PCWP), mixed venous oxygen sampling, and intermittent thermodilution CO determinations. Specialized catheters are also available that measure right ventricular ejection fraction, continuous mixed venous oxygen saturation, and continuous thermodilution CO.

The reason for measuring PCWP and PAD pressure is that they are estimates of left atrial pressure (LAP), which, in turn, is an estimate of left ventricular end-diastolic pressure (LVEDP). LVEDP is an index of left ventricular end-diastolic volume (LVEDV), which truly reflects left ventricular preload.[149] The relationship between LVEDP and LVEDV is described by the left ventricular compliance curve. This curve is nonlinear and is affected by many factors, such as ventricular hypertrophy and myocardial ischemia.[150,151] The CVP indicates right-sided filling pressures, which are indirect (and often inaccurate) estimates of left heart filling pressures (Figure 8-10). Vascular surgical patients have a high incidence of coronary artery and pulmonary disease, and CVP is even less likely to accurately reflect left-sided filling pressures in this population.[152] However, even the PCWP and PAD pressures do not accurately measure the LVEDP in the presence of pulmonary vascular disease, PEEP, or mitral valvular disease.[153-155]

The PCWP waveform is analogous to the right atrial (CVP) waveform described earlier. The a, c, and v waves are similarly timed to the cardiac cycle. Cannon a waves occur during nodal rhythm and complete heart block. Large v waves have been described during mitral regurgitation and during episodes of myocardial ischemia.[156] The etiology of large v waves during myocardial ischemia is probably a decrease in diastolic ventricular compliance. However, large v waves did not correlate with

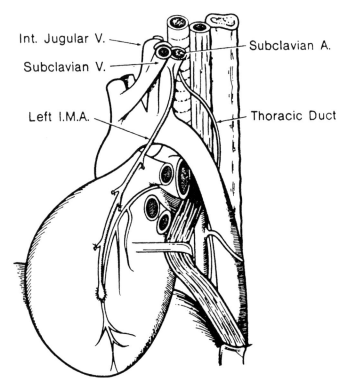

Int. Jugular V.
Subclavian V.
Left I.M.A.
Subclavian A.
Thoracic Duct

FIGURE 8-9 The complex anatomic relationship among the internal jugular vein, subclavian vein, left internal mammary artery (IMA), and the thoracic duct is diagrammed. (From DiLello F, Werner P, Kleinman E, et al: *Ann Thorac Surg* 44:660, 1987.)

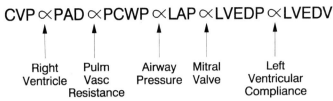

$$CVP \propto PAD \propto PCWP \propto LAP \propto LVEDP \propto LVEDV$$

| Right Ventricle | Pulm Vasc Resistance | Airway Pressure | Mitral Valve | Left Ventricular Compliance |

FIGURE 8-10 The relationships among central venous pressure (CVP), pulmonary artery diastolic pressure (PAD), pulmonary capillary wedge pressure (PCWP), left atrial pressure (LAP), left ventricular end-diastolic pressure (LVEDP), and left ventricular end-diastolic volume (LVEDV) are shown. The arrows indicate factors that adversely affect the reflection of left ventricular preload in the parameters noted to the left of the figure.

other determinants of ischemia in a study of vascular surgical patients with coronary artery disease (Figure 8-11).[157]

Indications and Contraindications

INDICATIONS. There has been an ongoing debate about whether PAC monitoring improves outcome in critically ill patients. The data gathered by Connors et al, in a large series of intensive care unit patients, demonstrated a higher mortality with PAC monitoring.[158,159] Randomized trials involving patients with myocardial infarction seemed to confirm these data, whereas earlier prospective studies of surgical patients showed improved outcome.[160-163] A meta-analysis by Barone et al found only four adequately randomized prospective studies, and the use of the PAC did not improve outcome in vascular surgery patients.[164]

A number of studies looked at how the catheter was used and how the data were interpreted. The results showed inadequate training and misinterpretation of PAC-acquired data even by senior physicians.[165,166] In general, the data indicate that probably not all critically ill patients benefit from PA catheterization. During this era of increased cost awareness, the role of

the PAC and the selection of surgical patients for whom PAC placement is beneficial may have to be reevaluated.[167,168]

The indications for PAC monitoring, therefore, tend to vary widely among institutions and among different intensive care and operating room settings within institutions. National organizations, such as the American Society of Anesthesiologists, have published practice parameters to guide practitioners in the appropriate use of this technology. (http://www.asahq.org/practice/pulm/pulm_artery.html) Using an evidence-based medicine approach, it is certainly not established whether PAC monitoring, or any less invasive form of CO monitoring, reduces morbidity or mortality.

A generally accepted list of indications for the PAC in the vascular surgical population is shown in Table 8-1.

CONTRAINDICATIONS

Absolute

1. Severe tricuspid or pulmonic valvular stenosis
2. Right atrial or right ventricular masses (tumor, clot)
3. Tetralogy of Fallot

Relative

1. Severe arrhythmias
2. Coagulopathy
3. Newly inserted pacemaker wires

Sites

The considerations regarding the insertion site for PAC are the same as for CVP catheters (see earlier). The right internal jugular approach remains the most convenient because of the direct path between this vessel and the right atrium. The PAC is inserted with pressure monitoring of the distal lumen to guide its placement. Figure 8-12 indicates the waveforms encountered during flotation of the catheter from the right atrium into the pulmonary artery.

Complications

The complications associated with PAC placement include almost all of those detailed in the section on CVP placement (see earlier). However, neither atrial nor ventricular perforation has been reported with balloon-tipped catheters. Additional complications that are unique to the PAC are detailed here.

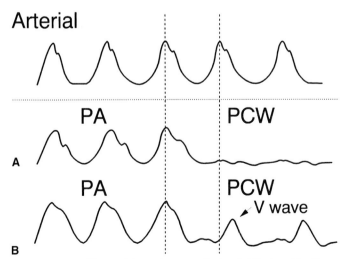

Arterial

FIGURE 8-11 The arterial waveforms are displayed at the top of the figure. In **A,** a normal pulmonary arterial and pulmonary capillary wedge tracing are diagrammed. In **B,** the widened pulmonary arterial waveform and corresponding pulmonary capillary wedge tracing are shown in a patient with large V waves.

TABLE 8-1

Indications for the Pulmonary Artery Catheter in the Vascular Surgical Population

1. Major vascular procedures involving large fluid shifts and/or blood loss in patients with ventricular dysfunction or valvular heart disease.
2. Patients with recent myocardial infarctions or unstable angina.
3. Patients in hypovolemic, cardiogenic, or septic shock, or with multiple organ failure.
4. Massive trauma cases.
5. Patients with right heart failure, COPD, pulmonary hypertension, or pulmonary embolism.
6. Patients requiring inotropes or intra-aortic balloon counterpulsation.
7. Patients undergoing surgery of the aorta requiring cross-clamping.
8. Patients undergoing hepatic transplantation.
9. Patients with massive ascites.
10. Planned endovascular repairs of the aorta with a high risk of conversion to an open repair.

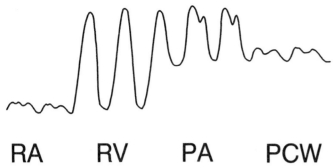

RA RV PA PCW

FIGURE 8-12 The waveforms encountered during flotation of a pulmonary artery catheter from the right atrium, through the right ventricle and the pulmonary artery to the pulmonary capillary wedge position.

ARRHYTHMIAS. The most common complication associated with PAC insertion is transient arrhythmias, especially premature ventricular contractions.[169,170] However, fatal arrhythmias have also been rarely reported.[171] Intravenous lidocaine has been used in attempts to suppress these arrhythmias with mixed results.[172,173] A positional maneuver entailing 5° head-up and right lateral tilt was associated with a definite decrease in malignant arrhythmias (compared with the Trendelenburg position) during PAC insertion.[174]

CONDUCTION DEFECTS. Complete heart block may develop during pulmonary artery catheterization in patients with existing left bundle-branch block.[175-177] This potentially fatal complication is most likely due to pressure from the catheter tip on the ventricular septum, causing transient right bundle-branch block. The incidence of right bundle-branch block was 3% in a prospective series of patients undergoing PAC.[178] However, none of the patients with existing left bundle-branch block developed complete heart block in that series. In another study of 47 patients with a left bundle-branch block, there were 2 cases of complete heart block, but only in patients with recent onset of left bundle-branch block.[179] Pacemaker capabilities (external pacemaker or pacing PAC) should be immediately available when catheterizing patients with a left bundle-branch block.

ENDOBRONCHIAL HEMORRHAGE. Iatrogenic rupture of the PA has become more common since the advent of PAC monitoring in the intensive care unit and the operating room.[180-183] The incidence of PA-induced endobronchial hemorrhage is 0.064% to 0.20%.[184,185] Hannan et al reported a 46% mortality rate in a review of 28 cases of PA-induced endobronchial hemorrhage, but the mortality was 75% in the anticoagulated patients.[186] From these reports, several risk factors have emerged: advanced age, pulmonary hypertension, mitral stenosis, coagulopathy, distal placement of the catheter, and balloon hyperinflation. In the majority of cases, the right pulmonary artery is affected.[187]

It is important to consider the etiology of the hemorrhage when forming a therapeutic plan. If the hemorrhage is minimal and a coagulopathy coexists, correction of the coagulopathy may be the only necessary therapy. Protection of the uninvolved lung is of prime importance. Tilting the patient toward the affected side and performing an endobronchial intubation are maneuvers that are useful to protect the contralateral lung.[188] Strategies proposed to stop the hemorrhage include the application of PEEP, placement of bronchial blockers, rigid or flexible bronchoscopy, injection of clotted blood through the PAC, hyperinflation of the PAC balloon, and pulmonary resection.[189,190]

The clinician is obviously at a disadvantage unless the site of hemorrhage is known. A chest radiograph usually indicates the general location of the lesion. A small amount of radiographic contrast dye may help to pinpoint the lesion if active hemorrhage is present. Although the etiology of endobronchial hemorrhage may be unclear, the bleeding site must be unequivocally located before surgical treatment is attempted.

PULMONARY INFARCTION. An early report suggested that there was a 7.2% incidence of pulmonary infarction with PAC use.[191] However, continuously monitoring the PA waveform and keeping the balloon deflated when not determining the PCWP (to prevent inadvertent wedging of the catheter) were not standard practice at that time. Distal migration of PACs may also occur intraoperatively because of changes in the heart's size, softening of the catheter, uncoiling of the catheter, and changes in the patient's position.

CATHETER KNOTTING. Knotting of a PAC usually occurs as a result of coiling of the catheter within the right ventricle.[192,193] Insertion of an appropriately sized guide wire under fluoroscopic guidance may aid in unknotting the catheter.[194-196] Alternatively, the knot may be tightened and withdrawn percutaneously along with the introducer if no intracardiac structures are entangled.[197]

VALVULAR DAMAGE. Withdrawal of the catheter with the balloon inflated may result in injury to the tricuspid or pulmonic valves.[198-200] Septic endocarditis has also resulted from an indwelling PAC.[201]

THROMBOCYTOPENIA. Mild thrombocytopenia has been reported in dogs and humans with indwelling PACs.[202] This probably results from increased platelet consumption. Heparin-coated PACs might trigger heparin-induced thrombocytopenia.[203,204] This disease is associated with high morbidity and mortality and is due to an immune reponse to heparin that results in thrombotic events and a consumption thrombocytopenia.[205,206]

Special Pulmonary Artery Catheters

CONTINUOUS MIXED VENOUS OXYHEMOGLOBIN SATURATION MONITORING. Modifications of the PAC have made it possible to continuously measure mixed venous oxyhemoglobin saturation (Svo_2). A fiberoptic light source at the tip of the PAC uses reflectance spectrophotometry to measure Svo_2. It has been shown that Svo_2 can be useful as a surrogate of CO when hemoglobin concentration and oxygen consumption are stable.[207]

Theory. The Fick equation states that oxygen consumption equals the CO multiplied by the difference between the arterial and mixed venous oxygen contents:

$$Q = Vo_2/(Cao_2 - Cvo_2) \times 10$$

where Q is CO in L/min, Vo_2 is oxygen consumption in mL O_2/min, Cao_2 is arterial oxygen content in mL O_2/100 mL blood, Cvo_2 is mixed venous oxygen content in mL O_2/100 mL blood, and 10 is a factor to convert units to L/min. This equation is used again later in the calculation of CO using the direct Fick method.

The effect of dissolved oxygen is negligible in the mixed venous blood. Thus, mixed venous oxygen saturation closely correlates with mixed venous oxygen content. A decrease in mixed venous oxygen saturation indicates one of the following:

1. Decreased cardiac output
2. Decreased arterial oxygen content
3. Increased oxygen consumption
4. Decrease in oxygen-carrying capacity (as occurs with decreased hemoglobin)

Clinical applications. This form of monitoring has never become standard in the perioperative and critical care settings despite many years of clinical use. The most important reasons why the use of continuous Svo_2 monitoring has not been more prevalent in the operating room include (1) a poor correlation between CO and Svo_2, (2) an ongoing debate about the benefit of the routine use of a PAC in cardiac surgery patients, and (3) the higher costs of these PACs.[208-212] There remain many physicians who believe that continuous mixed venous oxygen saturation monitoring provides an effective early warning sign of impending hemodynamic compromise.

PACING CATHETERS

Electrode catheters. The multipurpose PAC (originally produced by Baxter Edwards, Santa Ana, CA) contains five electrodes for bipolar atrial, ventricular, or AV sequential pacing. With appropriate filtering, the catheter may also be used for recording intracardiac ECG. The intraoperative success rates for atrial, ventricular, and AV sequential capture have been reported as 80%, 93%, and 73%, respectively.[213]

Pacing wire catheters. The Paceport and A-V Paceport catheters (Edwards Lifesciences Corporation, Irvine, CA) have lumina for the introduction of a ventricular wire (Paceport) or both atrial and ventricular wires (A-V Paceport) for temporary transvenous pacing. The success rate for ventricular pacing capture was 96% for the Paceport.[214] The success rates for atrial and ventricular pacing capture prior to cardiopulmonary bypass were 98% and 100%, respectively, in a study of the A-V Paceport.[215] The additional risk of atrial or ventricular perforation is present with thin pacing wires but has not yet been reported in the literature.

Cardiac Output

The measurement of CO is an essential component of the hemodynamic monitoring of the vascular patient. The original devices that measured CO required highly invasive techniques, and pulmonary artery catheterization has remained one of the most common methods used. Among all the specific information that can be gathered with the PAC, CO is an essential parameter for calculating the bulk of the derived hemodynamic indices. In addition to providing information that has implications for the management of preload, afterload, heart rate, and contractility, CO reflects the status of the entire circulatory system. Using the PAC, multiple CO values can be obtained at frequent intervals using an inert indicator and without blood withdrawal.

There is a clear preference and trend toward less invasive procedures, and CO monitoring is no exception. Technologies such as TEE have gained widespread acceptance in cardiac and high-risk noncardiac procedures. In the following review, only methods that are currently applicable in the operating room or are under investigation for such application are described.

Thermodilution

PRINCIPLES OF THE MEASUREMENT. CO measurement using the cold injectate thermodilution method has been the gold standard in the clinical setting for the last three decades. The thermodilution method, like all other indicator dilution techniques, is based on the observation that, for a known amount of indicator introduced at one point in the circulation, the same amount of indicator should be detectable at a downstream point. Stewart and Hamilton established that the amount of indicator detected at the downstream point was equal to the product of CO and the change in indicator concentration over time.[216] CO is, therefore, calculated using the following equation:

$$CO = I \times 60 / \int C \, dt$$

where CO is cardiac output, I is amount of indicator injected, $\int C \, dt$ is the integral of indicator concentration over time, and 60 converts seconds to minutes.

If the indicator is injected as a bolus, a recording of the indicator concentration over time produces a curve with a rapid upslope and a more gradual exponential decline. The area under the curve represents the denominator in the Stewart-Hamilton equation, and CO is equal to the amount of injected indicator divided by the area under the curve.

The concept of a thermal indicator was introduced by Fegler in 1954 and was first applied in humans by Branthwaite and Bradley in 1968.[217,218] Early efforts with this technique were hampered by the need to place a thermistor in the pulmonary artery. With the subsequent development of the balloon-tipped flow-directed PAC, placement of the catheter in the pulmonary artery became simple. Today, thermodilution is the most commonly applied CO measurement technique.[219,220] For the measurement of CO by thermodilution, the Stewart-Hamilton equation needs to be modified to take the particular characteristics of the thermal indicator into account. It becomes:

$$CO = [V(Tb - Ti) \times K1 \times K2] \times 60 / \int_0^\infty \Delta TB(t) \, dt$$

where CO is cardiac output (L/min), V is volume of injectate (mL), Tb is initial blood temperature (°C), Ti is initial injectate temperature (°C), K1 is density factor and K2 is a computation constant (that takes catheter deadspace, heat change in transit, injection rate, and units into account), and $\int_0^\infty \Delta TB(t) \, dt$ represents the integral of blood temperature change over time.

ACCURACY AND PRECISION

Accuracy. The accuracy of the thermodilution technique has been evaluated by comparing its results with those obtained by other methods of CO determination, either in vitro or in vivo. In vitro, a variety of mechanical models have been used to produce precisely controlled blood flows.[221,222] Under those strictly controlled conditions, the accuracy of the thermodilution CO measurements has varied from ±7% to ±13%. In vivo, the accuracy of the thermodilution technique has been tested in comparisons with the direct Fick method, electromagnetic flow measurements, and the indocyanine green method in numerous experiments.[223] In comparisons with the direct Fick method, correlation coefficients of 0.96 were obtained in two studies, but thermodilution has been found to overestimate total aortic electromagnetic flow, including coronary flow, by 3% when either iced or room-temperature injectate was used.[224-226]

In comparisons between thermodilution and indocyanine green, some authors have found excellent correlations over a wide range of outputs, whereas others have observed that thermodilution systematically overestimates dye dilution–determined CO.[227-229] Both of these techniques, however, are based on the same principle, and the accuracy of both is contingent upon a large number of conditions being met. In general, it is accepted that, under optimal circumstances, the error in accuracy of the thermodilution CO technique is ±10%.

Factors that influence accuracy. Deviation from optimal measurement technique markedly influences accuracy. If the delivered amount of indicator is smaller than the volume for which the cardiac computer has been programmed, the CO value is erroneously elevated. Similar errors occur when the volume of the indicator does not correspond to the volume indicated by the computation constant. Loss of volume occurs when the syringes are incompletely filled or when the proximal injection port of the PAC is located within the introducer sheath. Injection in this location results in loss of indicator to the side arm of the introducer and falsely elevated CO values.

When more indicator is delivered than the computer was programmed for, the opposite is observed. Wetzel and Latson observed variations of up to 80% in measured CO when the rate of administration of room-temperature peripheral crystalloid infusions was intermittently and rapidly altered.[230] Under those circumstances, the errors were due to fluctuations in baseline blood temperature.

Other errors are occasionally observed in the presence of unusual conditions within the circulation. For instance, in patients with intracardiac shunts, the CO cannot be measured by the thermodilution technique. Loss of indicator or rapid recirculation results in erroneously elevated values.[231]

PRECISION. The reproducibility of the thermodilution method has also been tested in vivo and in vitro. In vitro, Mackenzie et al have compared thermodilution CO measurements with absolute flows measured in an artificial circulation.[232] They concluded that the reproducibility of the results was poor and that the ability to detect changes in flow rates was limited. In vivo, reproducibility can be assessed by obtaining a large number of thermodilution CO values and calculating their standard deviation. Hoel established that to reach 95% probability of being within 5% of the true CO requires seven injections.[233] With three injections there was an 89% probability of being within 10% of the true CO.

The reproducibility of the technique was also examined by Stetz et al, who reviewed 14 publications on the use of thermodilution in clinical practice.[234] They concluded that with the use of commercial thermodilution devices, a minimal difference of 12% to 15% (average 13%) between determinations was required to be statistically significant, provided that each determination was obtained by averaging three measurements. If each determination was the result of only a single measurement, a minimal difference of 20% to 26% (average 22%) was required for statistical significance. They also noted that thermodilution, direct Fick, and indocyanine green were equally accurate and that the accuracy was not influenced by the use of iced versus room-temperature indicator.

Stevens et al have studied the effects of the respiratory cycle on thermodilution CO in critically ill patients.[235] They prospectively studied 32 patients in a randomized scheme comparing three thermodilution CO measurements at peak inspiration, at end-exhalation, or randomly in spontaneously breathing and mechanically ventilated patients. These investigators confirmed that injections at specific times in the respiratory cycle resulted in less variability but possibly decreased accuracy. They nevertheless concluded that, in clinical practice, the improvement in reproducibility was more important than the decrease in accuracy. The effects of injectate volume and temperature on the variability of thermodilution CO have also been studied in critically ill patients.[236] Six combinations of injectate volume (3, 5, and 10 mL) and temperature (0°C and room temperature) were studied in 18 adult, intubated patients. The best reproducibility was obtained with the 10-mL injections at 0°C or room temperature. In summary, the precision of the thermodilution CO technique is not very good, and every attempt should be made to keep the rate and duration of the indicator injection as constant as possible.

LIMITATIONS. The tail end of the temperature curve can be influenced by spontaneous temperature variations in the PA. Extrapolation of that portion of the curve is, therefore, essential. Various manufacturers have handled this problem differently, and inconsistent results can sometimes be observed when switching from one CO computer to another.[237]

The PAC is not without problems, and the list of reported complications is long (see earlier). In addition, the determination of CO remains intermittent, and frequent measurements can lead to fluid overload. Complications have also been attributed to the rapid injection of cold indicator into the right atrium. Slowing of the heart rate was described by Nishikawa and Dohi.[238] In a prospective study, Harris et al observed that, with the use of iced injectate, a decrease in heart rate of more than 10% occurred in 22% of the determinations.[239]

CONTINUOUS THERMODILUTION CARDIAC OUTPUT. Pulmonary arterial catheters with the ability to measure CO continuously were introduced into clinical practice in the 1990s. The method that has gained the most clinical use functions by mildly heating the blood in a pseudorandom stochastic fashion. In vitro as well as in vivo studies have shown that a good correlation exists between this method and other measures of CO.[240-245] Bolus thermodilution CO still holds its place as the gold standard of CO measurements in the clinical setting, but its accuracy is adversely affected by imprecise technique, it introduces extra intravenous volume, and the measurements are labor intensive. Continuous CO (CCO) catheters should alleviate these problems and provide a continuous CO trend.[246] Despite this, their routine use in cardiac surgery patients has not been shown to improve outcome, and they are more expensive than standard PACs.

Other Techniques for Measuring Cardiac Output

THE DIRECT FICK METHOD. In the direct Fick method, CO is determined from the oxygen consumption and the difference between the arterial and mixed venous oxygen content (see earlier). Although the direct Fick method is often mentioned as a gold standard for the measurement of CO, it is not widely used in clinical practice because of inherent difficulties related to the measurement of oxygen consumption.

The measurement and its validation. Oxygen consumption is equal to the product of the expired air volume and the difference between the oxygen content in the inspired and expired gas. The expired air volume can be measured by a variety of means, and the difference between the inspired and expired oxygen concentration is determined by gas analysis. For the calculation of the arteriovenous oxygen content difference, arterial and mixed venous blood samples are obtained. The oxygen consumption and arteriovenous oxygen content difference must be measured at steady state because the Fick principle is valid only when tissue oxygen uptake is equal to lung oxygen uptake.[247] The accuracy and reproducibility of the direct Fick CO technique have been determined in a variety of animal and human experiments. They have usually been found to be high.[248-260]

Limitations. The major limitations of the direct Fick technique are related to errors in sampling and analysis or to inability to maintain steady-state hemodynamic and respiratory conditions.[261,262] To minimize errors in sampling, it must be certain that the venous blood is truly mixed venous blood and that the blood samples represent average, rather than instantaneous, samples.

The most serious errors in the measurement of CO by the direct Fick technique result from changes in pulmonary volumes. Indeed, the methods used to measure oxygen consumption determine the uptake of oxygen by the lungs rather than by the blood. Because lung volumes can change, the oxygen consumption by the tissues is not necessarily being measured.

INDICATOR DILUTION. Indicator dilution technique for the measurement of CO, originally performed using indocyanine (green) dye, has seen a renaissance with the introduction of lithium chloride as the indicator.[263] Currently, a lithium chloride solution is injected through a central venous catheter and a lithium-selective electrode that is connected to a standard intra-arterial cannula measures plasma concentrations. With this method, unlike thermodilution measurements of CO, no PAC needs to be inserted. Only intra-arterial and central venous catheters are required. Comparisons with standard techniques have been promising.[264,265]

One of the problems in using indicator dilution techniques is that recirculation of the marker occurs before the first-pass curve is completed (Figure 8-13).[266] The overlapping of several curves interferes with the exact integration of the area under the dye concentration versus time curve, which is needed for the exact calculation of CO.

PULSE CONTOUR. Another method of CO measurement is arterial pulse contour analysis. Arterial pulse waveforms are analyzed and allow the calculation of CO. Pulse waveforms are derived from invasive arterial catheters. The notion that stroke volume (SV) can be quantified from the pulse pressure dates back to observations by Erlanger and Hooker in 1904 and assumes that the rate of blood flow from the arterial to the venous system is proportional to the rate of arterial pressure decline.[267]

Validation studies have shown varying results when compared with acknowledged techniques.[268-270] New methods of

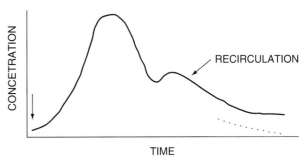

FIGURE 8-13 *An indicator thermodilution curve with the recirculation peak noted. The dotted line indicates the extrapolation necessary for accurate cardiac output determination.*

signal processing have been introduced with the goal of achieving better correlation with accepted methods of CO measurements.[271-274] Drawbacks of this technique include the need to calibrate the system against a standard technique, such as transpulmonary bolus thermodilution, its invasive nature, and nonlinearity related to changing compliance of the arterial system. Damped arterial waveforms and arrhythmias may lead to false results, and aortic pathology and body position must be considered when calculating CO with this technique.[275] One group attempted to measure pulse contour CO noninvasively using pulse wave tracings from digital plethysmography.[276]

THORACIC BIOIMPEDANCE. Thoracic impedance devices provide continuous noninvasive estimates of CO. The first attempts at measuring CO by thoracic electrical impedance date back to 1966, when Kubicek et al presented an empirical equation for the calculation of left ventricular SV.[277] To measure thoracic electrical impedance, an alternating current of low amplitude and high frequency is introduced and simultaneously sensed by two sets of electrodes placed around the neck and xyphoid process. Changes in thoracic impedance are induced by ventilation and pulsatile blood flow. For the measurement of SV, only the cardiac-induced pulsatile component is analyzed (dZ/dt). Commercial systems have been introduced with improved software for advanced signal processing, but validation studies show highly inconsistent results. Although some studies trying to validate bioimpedance CO measurements found good agreement between thermodilution and bioimpedance CO, this is not the conclusion of all investigators.[278-289]

In a prospective study, Shoemaker et al compared the bioimpedance technique with standard thermodilution CO in emergency patients.[290] The correlation was promising ($r = 0.85$) but the accuracy was not, suggesting that the bioimpedance technique may be useful for trend analysis rather than absolute values.[291] More promising data, such as those from a study by Sageman et al on aortocoronary bypass patients, suggest that bioimpedance can be a valid equivalent to thermodilution measurements of CO in this group of patients.[292]

Factors that may interfere include pulmonary edema, large pleural effusions, and intracardiac shunts. Intraoperatively, lead placement may infringe on the surgical field. There may also be significant variability between different thoracic electrical impedance devices.[293] The advantage of the bioimpedance technique is the continuous online display of noninvasive data that may lead to prompt recognition of hemodynamic changes in patients.

GAS TECHNOLOGY. Noninvasive monitoring of CO using the carbon dioxide rebreathing method is based upon the Fick principle (see earlier). Substituting CO_2 production for oxygen consumption, capnographic measurement of CO_2 concentrations may be used to provide a noninvasive Fick estimate of CO. The rebreathing technique is used to estimate mixed venous partial pressure of carbon dioxide (pCO_2). In the clinical setting, patients are sedated and mechanically ventilated, and capnometry equipment is attached to a processor that calculates CO.[294]

Studies comparing the CO_2 rebreathing method with standard measures of CO have yielded conflicting results.[295-298] A study by Binder and Parkin in postoperative cardiac surgical patients compared the CO_2 method with the thermodilution method and showed a good correlation.[299] In contrast, van Heerden et al, using a different device, found that CO measurements in cardiac surgery patients were overestimated using the CO_2 rebreathing technique.[300]

CARDIAC OUTPUT MEASUREMENTS USING ULTRASOUND TECHNOLOGY. SV and CO measurements can be accomplished using different echocardiographic techniques. Early attempts were made using M-mode echocardiographic dimensions and results were promising.[301,302] Two-dimensional (2D) echocardiography measurements depend on adequate imaging and calculate volume dimensions from 2D data using a geometric assumption of chamber size and shape. With the introduction of three-dimensional (3D) echocardiography, it should be possible to overcome some of the problems encountered with this mathematical approach and to determine and visualize true chamber size.[303] A different technique uses Doppler echocardiography to determine CO. Unlike CO measurements derived from 2D echocardiography, those obtained with Doppler echocardiography are less dependent on geometric assumptions.

Doppler ultrasound. Ultrasound can be used for the measurement of CO based on the Doppler principle. Information on blood flow is obtained by applying Doppler frequency shift analysis to echoes reflected by the moving red blood cells. Blood flow velocity, direction, and acceleration can be instantaneously determined. From this information, SV and CO are calculated using the following formula:

$$SV = VTI \times CSA$$

where VTI is the Doppler velocity-time integral (i.e., the area under the Doppler spectral display curve) and CSA is the cross-sectional area at the site of flow measurement. SV is then multiplied by heart rate to calculate the CO. Blood flow in the human heart can be described by the continuity equation, which states that the flow measured at one cross-sectional area of the heart is equal to the flow measured at another cross section (as long as there is no intracardiac shunting). Theoretically, CO may be measured at all anatomic sites in which a cross-sectional area is determined and a Doppler beam positioned. Depending on the velocity being measured, pulsed-wave Doppler or continuous-wave Doppler technology is applied. The ultrasound signals can be transmitted and detected using transthoracic, transesophageal, suprasternal, or transtracheal

transducers. In clinical practice, CO measurements can be made at the aortic, pulmonary artery, or mitral valve positions.[304-308]

The degree of accuracy in comparative studies has been promising.[309-318] Technical limitations include the quality of the imaging, the accuracy of the valve or outflow tract area calculations, and the degree of alignment between the ultrasound beam and the direction of blood flow. Because the cross-sectional area is determined from 2D images, converting measurements of the radius to calculate area leads to exponential increases in any errors. Calculation of the cross-sectional area at the mitral valve site gives varying results because the orifice is not constant throughout the cardiac cycle.[319] In addition, the Doppler beam must be as parallel to the blood flow as possible. Angles greater than 30° between the ultrasound beam and the direction of blood flow lead to increased error despite angle correction algorithms.

Two-dimensional volume determination. 2D echocardiography allows the calculation of CO using the following formula:

$$CO = (EDV - ESV) \times HR$$

where CO is cardiac output, EDV is end-diastolic volume, ESV is end-systolic volume, and HR is heart rate. SV is calculated from 2D short-axis views using echocardiography. Reliable estimation of CO depends on adequate imaging that allows exact tracing of the endocardial border. Echo-derived cardiac index (CI) showed a good correlation with simultaneously measured CI using the standard thermodilution method.[320-322]

Automated border detection. Automated border detection (ABD) is an endocardial tracking algorithm superimposed on B-mode (2D) images. ABD is commercially available on some modern TEE machines and allows semiautomated measurement of left ventricular areas. The blood-endocardial interface is detected and continuously displayed (Figure 8-14). End-diastolic area, end-systolic area, and fractional area of contraction are also displayed. Computer processing of the 2D data (using a single-plane modification of Simpson's rule) allows an estimation of left ventricular volumes and ejection fraction.[323,324] Validation studies comparing ABD with conductance catheter volume measurement or thermodilution showed promising results.[325-329] Absolute measurements of left ventricular dimensions tend to be systematically underestimated by ABD techniques; however, ABD might still be useful for detecting CO trends rather than absolute values.[330] Difficulties yet to overcome include the following: signal quality is dependent on high-quality 2D echocardiographic images; a region of interest needs to be defined manually by the user; and endocardial image dropout requires repetitive readjustments by the user to optimize the image using power settings, gain adjustments, and probe manipulation.

Three-dimensional echocardiographic cardiac output. 3D echocardiography may result in a major advance in minimally invasive CO monitoring. Calculations of 3D images require sequential acquisition of 2D echocardiographic data from multiple imaging planes. To date, image processing capacities allow only offline reconstruction and display of images.[331] In addition to some technical problems, costs are still too high for widespread use, and validation studies must be conducted to demon-

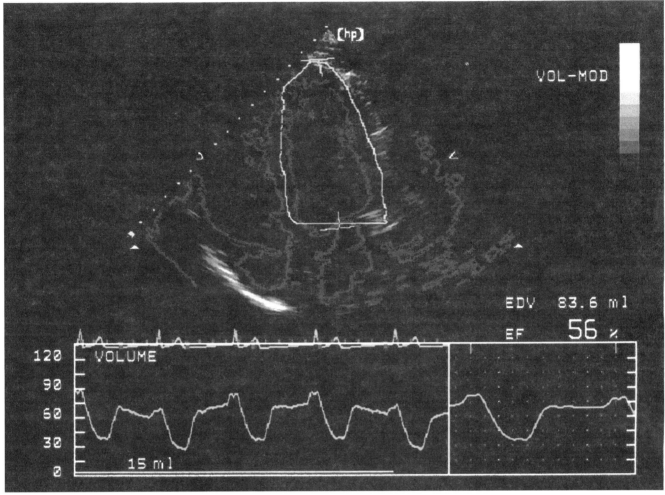

FIGURE 8-14 An example of automated border detection of the left ventricular area.

strate its accuracy in clinical use. Early results of 3D evaluation of the heart are promising, and advances in processor speed and echocardiographic technology should help overcome some of the problems this technology still encounters today.[332-334]

Transesophageal Echocardiography (TEE)

One of the major advances in cardiovascular monitoring has been the introduction of TEE. Echocardiography provides the anesthesiologist with a new dimension in the assessment of cardiovascular function. Prior to echocardiography, most of the information on cardiac function was indirect and derived from pressure and flow measurements. Echocardiography has added the ability not only to visualize cardiac structures but also to observe and quantify their function. Whether it will one day replace conventional hemodynamic monitoring techniques is, as yet, unknown, but it is certain that it has increased the knowledge and understanding of vascular patients' hemodynamic responses to anesthesia and surgery.

In echocardiography, the heart and great vessels are probed with ultrasound, which is sound above the human audible range. The ultrasound is sent into the thoracic cavity and is partially reflected by the cardiac structures. From these reflections,

information on distance, velocity, and density of objects within the chest is derived.

Imaging Techniques

M-MODE. The most basic current form of ultrasound imaging is M-mode echocardiography. In this mode, the density and position of all tissues in the path of a narrow ultrasound beam (i.e., along a single line) are displayed as a scroll on a video screen. The scrolling produces an updated, continuously changing time plot of the studied tissue section, several seconds in duration. Because this is a timed motion display (normal cardiac tissue is always in motion), it is called M-mode. Because only a limited part of the heart is being observed at any one time and because interpretation of the image requires considerable skill, M-mode is not currently used as a primary imaging technique. This mode is, however, useful for the precise timing of events within the cardiac cycle and is often used in combination with color-flow Doppler for the timing of abnormal flows (see later). Quantitative measurements of size, distance, and velocity are also easily performed on M-mode images without the need for sophisticated analysis equipment. Whenever a measurement includes a temporal component, the M-mode image is more advantageous than a 2D image because it is updated a thousand times each second. Thus, more subtle changes in motion or dimension can be appreciated.

2D-MODE. By rapid, repetitive scanning along many different radii within an area in the shape of a fan (sector), echocardiography generates a 2D image of a section of the heart. This image resembles an anatomic section and, thus, can be more easily interpreted. Information on structures and motion in the plane of a 2D scan is updated 30 to 60 times per second. This produces a "live" (real-time) image of the heart. Most modern TEE systems scan the heart using an electronically steered ultrasound beam (phased-array transducer), whereas

some older devices used a mechanically steered transducer for their 2D imaging capabilities. The Society of Cardiovascular Anesthesiologists and the American Society of Echocardiography have standardized the images that are routinely obtained by 2D TEE (Figure 8-15).[335] The reader is referred to texts devoted to this topic for further information.

Doppler Techniques

Doppler techniques are utilized to gather information on the velocity of red blood cells within the circulation. From the velocity data, information is derived on normal and abnormal

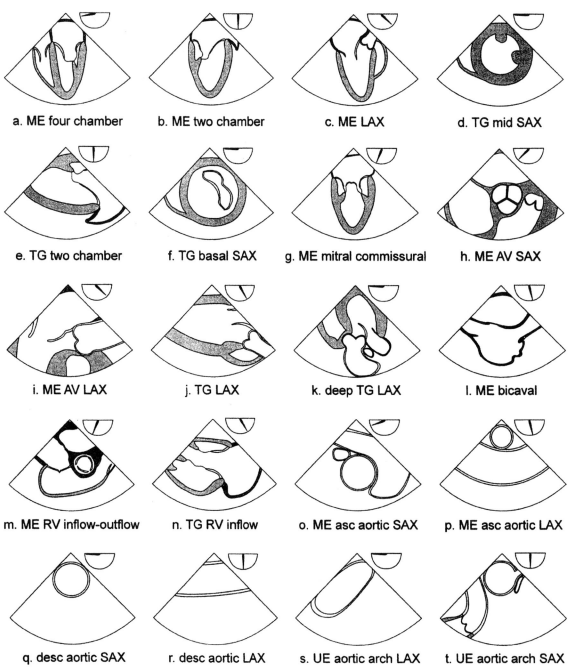

a. ME four chamber   b. ME two chamber   c. ME LAX   d. TG mid SAX

e. TG two chamber   f. TG basal SAX   g. ME mitral commissural   h. ME AV SAX

i. ME AV LAX   j. TG LAX   k. deep TG LAX   l. ME bicaval

m. ME RV inflow-outflow   n. TG RV inflow   o. ME asc aortic SAX   p. ME asc aortic LAX

q. desc aortic SAX   r. desc aortic LAX   s. UE aortic arch LAX   t. UE aortic arch SAX

FIGURE 8-15 The standard two-dimensional transesophageal echocardiography views described by the Society of Cardiovascular Anesthesiologists and the American Society of Echocardiography. (From Shanewise JS, Cheung AT, Aronson S, et al: *Anesth Analg* 89:870, 1999.)

flow patterns. The Doppler principle, as applied in echocardiography, states that the frequency of ultrasound reflected by a moving target (red blood cells) is different from the frequency of the emitted ultrasound. The magnitude and direction of the frequency shift are related to the velocity and direction of the moving target. The velocity of the target is calculated with the Doppler equation:

$$V = [C \times F_d] / [2F_0 \times \cos \theta]$$

where V is the flow velocity, C is a constant, F_d is the frequency shift, F_0 is the frequency of the emitted ultrasound, and θ is the angle between the ultrasound beam and the direction of blood flow.

PULSED-WAVE DOPPLER. In pulsed-wave Doppler, blood flow parameters are determined at precise locations within the heart by emitting repetitive short bursts of ultrasound at a specific frequency (pulse repetition frequency) and analyzing the frequency shift of the reflected echoes at an identical sampling frequency (f_s). A time delay between the emission of the ultrasound signal burst and the sampling of the reflected signal determines the depth at which the velocities are sampled. The delay is proportional to the distance between the transducer and the location of the velocity measurements.

When pulsed-wave Doppler is used in combination with 2D echocardiography, the sampling location or "sample volume" is displayed as a small marker on the 2D image. It can be positioned at any point along the Doppler beam by moving it up or down the Doppler cursor. On most devices, it is also possible to vary the width and height of the sample volume.

CONTINUOUS-WAVE DOPPLER. The continuous-wave Doppler technique uses continuous, rather than discrete, pulses of ultrasound waves. Continuous-wave probes have two transducers, one of which continuously emits ultrasound while the other continuously receives echoes. As a result, the region where flow dynamics are measured cannot be precisely localized. Blood flow velocity is, however, measured with great accuracy even at high flows. Continuous-wave Doppler is particularly useful for the evaluation of patients with valvular lesions and is also the preferred technique when attempting to derive hemodynamic information from Doppler signals.

COLOR-FLOW MAPPING. Color-flow Doppler ultrasound scanners display blood flow within the heart in colors and in real time while also imaging the tissues in two dimensions. In addition to showing the location, direction, and velocity of cardiac or intravascular blood flow, the images produced by these devices allow estimation of flow acceleration and differentiation of laminar and turbulent blood flow. Color-flow Doppler echocardiography is based on the principle of multigated pulsed-wave Doppler.[336] According to this principle, blood flow velocity is sampled at many locations, along many lines covering the entire imaging sector. At the same time, the sector is also scanned to generate a 2D image.

Color-flow Doppler imaging utilizes the three basic colors (red, green, and blue) used in standard color television. Each picture element (pixel) on the video monitor screen displays a particular combination of the colors red, blue, and green. A location in the heart where the scanner detects blood flow in a direction toward the transducer (the top of the image sector) is usually assigned the color red. At locations where flow away from the transducer is detected, the color blue is usually displayed. This color assignment (mapping) is completely arbitrary and determined by the user from the options provided by the ultrasound machine. In the most common color-flow mapping scheme, more rapid blood flow velocity (up to a limit) is exhibited as more intense color. The color green is added to either red or blue when flow velocities change by more than a preset value within a brief time interval ("flow variance"). Both rapidly accelerating laminar flow (change in flow speed) and turbulent flow (change in flow direction) satisfy the criteria for rapid changes in velocity and are, therefore, mapped in colors with added green. With the addition of green to red or blue, a whole range of intermediate colors including yellow, cyan, magenta, and white can be displayed. In areas where highly turbulent flows are detected, such as in regurgitant jets, a mosaic of all these colors is often noted.

Global Ventricular Function

SYSTOLIC FUNCTION. Before the introduction of TEE, hemodynamic parameters used to describe the overall cardiac performance were mainly assessed with invasive methods, such as the PAC. Unlike the PAC, TEE is a less invasive means of visualizing and assessing right and left ventricular function. Images are displayed in real time, on line, and allow a qualitative as well as a semiquantitative evaluation of the ventricular function and loading conditions.

The classic determinants of systolic ventricular function are preload, afterload, and contractility. A large number of echocardiographic measures of these determinants of ventricular function have been described in the literature. Data obtained from a comprehensive TEE examination, in combination with hemodynamic parameters, have enhanced the ability to assess the systolic function of the left ventricle.

PRELOAD. Preload can best be defined as the stretch of the muscle fibers at end-diastole with end-diastolic volume being the closest substitute.[337] In practice, preload is often estimated by measuring left ventricular filling pressures (PCWP or LVEDP). However, these have been shown to correlate poorly with end-diastolic volumes. Using TEE, left ventricular end-diastolic dimensions can be determined while providing a true estimate of the loading conditions of the heart. In 2D echocardiography, multiplane TEE probes allow visualization of multiple tomographic sections.

Standard guidelines have been promulgated to facilitate analysis and communication among practitioners. For that reason, ventricular preload is often assessed using the transgastric midleft ventricular short-axis view at the level of the midpapillary muscles. End-diastolic short-axis areas measured at this level correlated well with end-diastolic volumes simultaneously measured with standard techniques.[338] During surgery, a simple visual examination of the short-axis view at end-diastole is often sufficient for assessing loading conditions. Obliteration of the end-systolic area (the "kissing ventricle" sign) indicates severe hypovolemia. If quantitative information is required, the endocardial outline may be electronically delineated and the end-diastolic area calculated. It has been proposed that the end-diastolic area measured in this manner is a better index of preload than the PCWP.[339] Strong correlations between end-diastolic areas or end-diastolic volumes and cardiac index have been observed, but no significant correlation was found between PCWP and CO.[340] In clinical practice, however, it is best to measure both the end-diastolic volume and the left ventricular filling pressure because, together, they define the compliance of the left ventricle.

AFTERLOAD. Afterload is defined as the left ventricular wall stress during ejection.[341] Although afterload cannot be determined by echocardiography alone, the combination of ventricular dimensions with ventricular wall thickness and systolic arterial pressure may be used to measure end-systolic wall stress. Ventricular wall thickness is derived by calculating the distance between the epicardial and endocardial borders.[342] The formula to calculate wall stress was derived by Sandler and Dodge from the basic Laplace equation:

$$Wall\ stress = (1.33 \times P \times LVEDD)/[4WT\ (1 + WT/LVEDD)]$$

where P equals the systolic arterial pressure, WT represents wall thickness, LVEDD represents the end-diastolic cavity dimension, and 1.33 converts mmHg to dynes/cm^2.[343]

A simplified version of the wall stress equation is the following:

$$Wall\ stress = (P \times LVEDD)/WT$$

where P is systolic arterial pressure, LVEDD is left ventricular end-diastolic dimension, and WT is left ventricular wall thickness.

Wall stress is directly related to the shape of the ventricle. Diastolic dimensions are selected because it is assumed that peak systolic wall stress occurs during isovolumic ventricular contraction while the ventricle still possesses its diastolic anatomic configuration. Elevations in wall stress have been observed in patients with left ventricular enlargement related to systemic hypertension, aortic stenosis, or aortic regurgitation.[344] Wall stress provides a better index of afterload than SVR when forward SV is not equal to the total ventricular ejection such as in mitral regurgitation or in the presence of a ventricular septal defect. Whether the same is true in patients without such lesions is unclear. In one animal study, it was observed that, during pharmacologic interventions, SVR and wall stress did not correlate well and occasionally varied in opposite directions.[345] In patients undergoing carotid artery surgery, Smith et al studied wall stress under various anesthetic regimens.[346] They noted, during carotid cross-clamping, that patients receiving high concentrations of volatile agents, with phenylephrine to maintain BP, had significantly higher wall stress values than those receiving low concentrations of volatile agents without phenylephrine. The close association between wall stress and myocardial oxygen consumption should provide a strong impetus for future investigations on the importance of wall stress measurements during vascular surgery.

CONTRACTILITY. Indices of contractility are traditionally divided into isovolumic phase indices and ejection phase indices. Echocardiography has been utilized to estimate contractility with either type of index, although it is, by design, better suited for the evaluation of the ejection phase. Contractility, by definition, is independent of loading conditions. However, most of the indices used in common practice are dependent on loading conditions and heart rate. The use of indices that more specifically measure the intrinsic inotropic state of the heart,

such as the end-systolic pressure-volume relationship, has been promoted.

Isovolumic phase indices. The isovolumic phase indices, such as dP/dt, are obtained during the isovolumic phase of systole, prior to the opening of the aortic valve. Because of technical and anatomic limitations, TEE is not particularly well suited for the assessment of the isovolumic phase of the contraction. Some information on the isovolumic phase can, however, be gathered by measuring the length of the preejection period. The preejection period is the time between the onset of the QRS on ECG and the opening of the aortic valve on M-mode echocardiography. The usefulness and limitations of the preejection period as well as the other systolic time intervals have been extensively reviewed elsewhere.[347,348]

Another measurement that, to some extent, is related to the isovolumic phase of the contraction is the maximal acceleration of blood flow in the aorta.[349] Maximal blood flow acceleration occurs in the early part of the left ventricular ejection and can be measured by Doppler echocardiography. In the ascending aorta, using a transthoracic approach, it is determined by the placement of a Doppler transducer in the suprasternal notch and by aiming the ultrasound beam at the aortic valve. A variety of studies have demonstrated that maximum blood flow acceleration, sampled in this manner, provides information on left ventricular contractility.[350-352] However, even with multiplane TEE probes, it is not always feasible to obtain imaging planes suitable for this type of measurement.

Ejection phase indices. Using echocardiography, contractility has been most frequently estimated with ejection phase indices. A wide array of ejection phase indices have been described, but all require that end-diastolic and end-systolic dimensions be measured. With 2D echocardiography, multiple tomographic cuts can be obtained. End-diastolic and end-systolic endocardial areas can be delineated with the help of tracing software, and contractility may be estimated using the fractional area of contraction (FAC):

$$FAC = [LVEDA - LVESA]/LVEDA$$

where LVEDA is the left ventricular end-diastolic area and LVESA is the left ventricular end-systolic area.

More than one beat may need to be traced in order to account for beat-to-beat variation. Ventricular volumes can be calculated from 2D data using a variety of formulas such as Simpson's rule.[353] The ratio of SV to ventricular end-diastolic volume, the ejection fraction (EF), is then calculated using the standard formula:

$$EF = (LVEDV - LVESV)/LVEDV$$

where LVEDV is left ventricular end-diastolic volume and LVESV is left ventricular end-systolic volume.

It must be remembered, though, that ejection phase indices are highly dependent on preload and afterload and do not represent the intrinsic inotropic state of the heart. An EF of 55% to 60%, however, nearly always indicates normal ventricular contractility (except with severe mitral regurgitation).

Load-independent indices of ventricular function. The ability to assess the intrinsic inotropic state of the heart has been hampered by the load dependence of indices traditionally used to describe the ventricular performance of the heart. Suga and

Sagawa introduced a different approach that eliminates this load dependence.[354] Their method is a measure of ventricular performance based on the Frank-Starling relationship, displayed through the construction of pressure-volume loops at varying preload. The steepness of the slope of a curve connecting the end-systolic points on these pressure-volume loops at different levels of preload is described as the end-systolic elastance of the left ventricle (Figure 8-16). The ventricular elastance is considered to be a measure of the intrinsic inotropic state of the heart. In a somewhat less invasive approach, these volume measurements were estimated using TEE.[355-357] This index has never been widely used in clinical practice, mainly because of the complexity of the measurement.

DIASTOLIC FUNCTION. There is increasing awareness that left ventricular diastolic dysfunction plays a major role in the diseased heart. In some patients, the signs and symptoms of congestive heart failure are primarily due to diastolic dysfunction.[358-360] In these patients, various degrees of congestive heart failure are observed in the presence of normal or even increased left ventricular systolic function. In another study, diastolic left ventricular dysfunction was the earliest change noted after coronary occlusion, and it often preceded the development of abnormal systolic function.[361] The techniques most frequently utilized to assess diastolic function are radionuclide angiography and echocardiography.[362] TEE is particularly well suited for this type of examination because of the close proximity of the esophageal transducer to the left atrium and mitral valve.

Technique and interpretation. To assess diastolic function, the transesophageal transducer is positioned to obtain a four-chamber view of the heart. After valvular dysfunction has been excluded, the sample volume of the pulsed Doppler system is placed in the mitral inflow. The best location for the sample volume is in the center of the mitral flow, just slightly to the ventricular side of the mitral valve. Flow velocity measured with the sample volume in this location results in a typical flow

End-Systolic Pressure-Volume Relationship

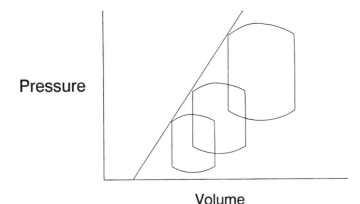

FIGURE 8-16 The end-systolic pressure volume relationship (elastance) of the left ventricle is a load-independent index of left ventricular contractility. It is measured by rapidly altering preload. The slope of the line connecting the end-systolic points of the resulting pressure-volume loops represents the elastance and is directly related to contractility.

Transmitral Doppler

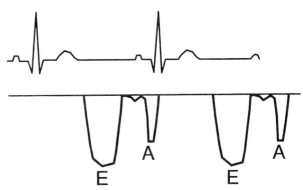

FIGURE 8-17 Pulsed-wave Doppler measurement at the level of the mitral valve. The E wave represents the passive filling of the left ventricle, the A wave corresponds to the atrial contraction in late diastole and follows the P wave on the ECG tracing.

velocity pattern (Figure 8-17). After opening of the mitral valve, the early inflow into the left ventricle is recognized as a large velocity peak (E wave). It is followed by a period of diastasis and a second, smaller velocity peak (A wave), representing the flow produced by the atrial contraction. Analysis of the diastolic inflow includes the analysis of the general velocity pattern (E/A peak ratio), measurement of peak E and A velocity, derivation of acceleration and deceleration for each peak, calculation of various time intervals, and integration of the total area, or parts of the area, under the velocity display. Generally, diastolic dysfunction is present when the height of the A wave exceeds that of the E wave.

In addition, pulmonary venous flow patterns are used to differentiate between more advanced stages of diastolic dysfunction. As diastolic function worsens, filling pressures may rise, increasing early transmitral diastolic pressures leading to an increased E velocity and pseudonormalization of the mitral inflow patterns. This condition may be unmasked by evaluating the pulmonary vein flow with pulsed-wave Doppler, where the normal pattern is altered.

The implications of assessing diastolic dysfunction intraoperatively are yet to be determined. A specific treatment for diastolic dysfunction is not yet available, and the therapeutic consequences of diagnosing diastolic dysfunction intraoperatively are limited. Diastolic function has been assessed intraoperatively by pulsed-wave Doppler echocardiography in only a few studies. In cardiac surgical patients, it was observed that some patients with normal mitral inflow patterns before cardiopulmonary bypass had signs of impaired ventricular filling after bypass.[363] In another study, Rinder et al reported that diastolic filling was significantly impaired 2 hours after cardiopulmonary bypass.[364] They noted a trend toward recovery by 4 hours and a return to baseline by 18 hours.

Intraoperative Application of Echocardiography

DIFFERENTIAL DIAGNOSIS. The use of intraoperative TEE has been beneficial in the differential diagnosis of hemodynamic disturbances. By viewing the heart in real time, TEE can guide the specific treatment of complicated hemodynamic situations. A fluid challenge may be indicated if a small left ventricular cavity is noted in the presence of systemic hypotension and a low or normal PCWP. A large left ventricular cavity with low ejection and systemic hypotension may present an indication for the administration of inotropic drugs.

EFFECTS OF INTERVENTIONS. Intraoperative echocardiography has also been utilized to assess the effects of surgical and anesthetic interventions on global left ventricular function in vascular surgery. It can be particularly useful in patients undergoing aortic surgery during aortic cross-clamping. Roizen et al observed marked reduction in FAC during aortic cross-clamping, while only minimal changes in CO were noted.[365] On the basis of this information, therapeutic maneuvers may be instituted to correct the abnormalities. Positional and respiratory maneuvers have also been shown to affect hemodynamic indices as assessed by TEE.[366,367]

PHARMACODYNAMICS. It is not surprising that one of the first studies describing the use of echocardiography in anesthetized patients was a pharmacodynamic study.[368] Indeed, echocardiography appears ideally suited to obtain information on the cardiovascular effects of drugs without the use of invasive monitoring or, alternatively, to complement the information provided by the conventional monitoring techniques. In patients scheduled for peripheral vascular surgery, Coriat et al, using TEE, compared ventricular function in patients during anesthetic inductions with thiopental or a flunitrazepam-fentanyl combination.[369] They noted that thiopental produced a marked impairment in ventricular function with a decrease in FAC and an increase in the end-systolic area (ESA). In another study of vascular patients, Reich et al confirmed that a neuromuscular blocker had little effect on ventricular function.[370]

THE DETECTION OF ISCHEMIA. Because the rate of left ventricular relaxation is an important determinant of early ventricular filling, it would be expected that impaired relaxation would result in impaired early ventricular filling. Ventricular relaxation is an energy-dependent process and one of the early signs of dysfunction related to myocardial ischemia. When myocardial ischemia is produced by transient occlusion of a coronary artery, as during angioplasty, the observation of a rapid reduction in E peak velocity is suggestive of impaired relaxation. In one study, diastolic left ventricular dysfunction was the earliest change noted after coronary occlusion and it often preceded the development of abnormal systolic function.[371] In another study, it was observed that acute ischemia not only altered early ventricular filling but also produced marked abnormalities in late ventricular filling.[372]

Regional wall motion abnormalities (RWMAs) have also been described as early signs of ischemia. They occur within seconds of inadequate blood flow or oxygen supply.[373] RWMA detected by TEE has been shown to be a more sensitive method of detecting myocardial ischemia in patients undergoing coronary artery bypass grafting than ST-segment changes.[374] Regional systolic function can be estimated by echocardiographic determination of wall thickening and wall motion during systole in both long- and short-axis views of the ventricle.[375,376]

Conclusions

A wide array of cardiovascular monitoring techniques is currently available to anesthesiologists caring for patients undergoing vascular surgery. Some, such as ECG and BP monitoring, are indispensable and will undoubtedly continue to be used. Other techniques will evolve over time as evidence is gathered. The increasing awareness that minimally invasive vascular surgical procedures can decrease perioperative risk and improve patients' outcome is also reflected in the newest trends in hemodynamic monitoring. Less invasive monitoring devices, such as TEE, have gained wider acceptance and their role continues to increase. Unfortunately, the increased cost associated with some of the less invasive techniques, such as continuous CO monitors, may slow their adoption in perioperative and critical care settings.

REFERENCES

1. Mangano DT: Perioperative cardiac morbidity, *Anesthesiology* 72:153, 1990.
2. http://www.asahq.org/practice/.
3. O'Kelly B, Browner WS, Massie B, et al: Ventricular arrhythmias in patients undergoing noncardiac surgery. The Study of Perioperative Ischemia Research Group, *JAMA* 268:217, 1992.
4. Atlee JL, Rusy BF: Ventricular conduction times and AV nodal conductivity during enflurane anesthesia in dogs, *Anesthesiology* 47:498, 1977.
5. Guler N, Kati I, Demirel CB, et al: The effects of volatile anesthetics on the Q-Tc interval, *J Cardiothorac Vasc Anesth* 15:188, 2001.
6. Kuenszberg E, Loeckinger A, Kleinsasser A, et al: Sevoflurane progressively prolongs the QT interval in unpremedicated female adults, *Eur J Anaesthesiol* 17:662, 2000.
7. Michaloudis D, Fraidakis O, Lefaki T, et al: Anaesthesia and the QT interval in humans. The effects of isoflurane and halothane, *Anaesthesia* 51:219, 1996.
8. London MJ, Hollenberg M, Wong MG, et al: Intraoperative myocardial ischemia: localization by continuous 12-lead electrocardiography, *Anesthesiology* 69:232, 1988.
9. Landesberg G, Mosseri M, Wolf Y, et al: Perioperative myocardial ischemia and infarction, *Anesthesiology* 96:264, 2002.
10. Mangano DT, Hollenberg M, Fegert G, et al: Perioperative myocardial ischemia in patients undergoing noncardiac surgery. I: Incidence and severity during the 4 day perioperative period. The Study of Perioperative Ischemia (SPI) Research Group, *J Am Coll Cardiol* 17:843, 1991.
11. Mangano DT, Wong MG, London MJ, et al: Perioperative myocardial ischemia in patients undergoing noncardiac surgery. II: Incidence and severity during the 1st week after surgery. The Study of Perioperative Ischemia (SPI) Research Group, *J Am Coll Cardiol* 17:851, 1991.
12. Kates RA, Zaidan JR, Kaplan JA: Esophageal lead for intraoperative electrocardiographic monitoring, *Anesth Analg* 61:781, 1982.
13. Mylera KC, Calkins JM, Carlson J, et al: ECG lead with the endotracheal tube, *Crit Care Med* 11:199, 1983.
14. Chatterjee K, Swan HJC, Ganz W, et al: Use of a balloon-tipped flotation electrode catheter for cardiac monitoring, *Am J Cardiol* 36:56, 1975.
15. Borello G: ECG artifacts simulating atrial flutter, *JAMA* 223:439, 1973.
16. Doss JD, McCabe CW, Weiss GK: Noise-free data during electrosurgical procedures, *Anesth Analg* 52:156, 1973.
17. Michelson E, Morganroth J, MacVough H: Postoperative arrhythmias after coronary artery and cardiac valvular surgery detected by long-term electrocardiographic monitoring, *Am Heart J* 97:442, 1979.
18. de Soyza N, Thenabadu P, Murphy M, et al: Ventricular arrhythmia before and after aortocoronary bypass surgery, *Int J Cardiol* 1:123, 1981.
19. Dewar M, Rosengarten M, Blundell P, et al: Perioperative Holter monitoring and computer analysis of dysrhythmias in cardiac surgery, *Chest* 87:593, 1985.
20. Raby KE, Brull SJ, Timimi F, et al: The effect of heart rate control on myocardial ischemia among high-risk patients after vascular surgery, *Anesth Analg* 88:477, 1999.

21. Romhilt DW, Bloomfield SS, Chai TC, et al: Unreliability of conventional electrocardiographic monitoring of arrhythmia detection in coronary care units, *Am J Cardiol* 31:457, 1973.

22. Holmberg S, Ryder L, Waldenstrom A: Efficiency of arrhythmia detection by nurses in a coronary care unit using a decentralized monitoring system, *Br Heart J* 39:1019, 1977.

23. Sheffield LT: Computer-aided electrocardiography, *J Am Coll Cardiol* 56:13, 1985.

24. Willems JL, Abreu-Lima C, Arnaud P, et al: The diagnostic performance of computer programs for the interpretation of electrocardiograms, *N Engl J Med* 325:1767, 1991.

25. Sekiguchi K, Kanda T, Osada M, et al: Comparative accuracy of automated computer analysis versus physicans in training in the interpretation of electrocardiograms, *J Med* 30:75, 1999.

26. Keats AS: Anesthesia mortality in perspective, *Anesth Analg* 71:113, 1990.

27. Pedersen T, Petersen P, Moller AM: Pulse oximetry for perioperative monitoring, *Cochrane Database Syst Rev* (2):CD002013, 2001

28. Moller JT, Pedersen T, Rasmussen LS, et al: Randomized evaluation of pulse oximetry in 20802 patients, I, *Anesthesiology* 78:436, 1993.

29. Moller JT, Johannessen NW, Espersen K, et al: Randomized evaluation of pulse oximetry in 20802 patients, II, *Anesthesiology* 78:445, 1993.

30. Tremper KK, Barker SJ: Pulse oximetry, *Anesthesiology* 70:98, 1989.

31. Reich DL, Timcenko A, Bodian CA, et al: Predictors of pulse oximetry failure, *Anesthesiology* 84:859, 1996.

32. Dripps RD, Eckenhoff JE, Vandam LD: *Introduction to anesthesia*, ed 7, Philadelphia, 1988, WB Saunders, 77.

33. Alpert BS: Cuff width and accuracy of measurement of blood pressure, *Blood Press Monit* 5:151, 2000.

34. Wallace CT, Baker JD, Alpert CC, et al: Comparison of blood pressure measurement by Doppler and by pulse oximetry techniques, *Anesth Analg* 66:1018, 1987.

35. Korotkoff NS: On the subject of methods of determining blood pressure, *Bull Imp Med Acad* 11:365, 1905.

36. Ramsey M: Noninvasive blood pressure monitoring methods and validation. In Gravenstein JS (ed): *Essential noninvasive monitoring in anesthesia*, New York, 1980, Grune & Stratton, 37.

37. Hutton P, Prys-Roberts C: The oscillotonometer in theory and practice, *Br J Anaesth* 54:581, 1982.

38. Ramsey M III: Noninvasive automatic determination of mean arterial pressure, *Med Biol Eng Comput* 17:11, 1979.

39. Borrow KM, Newburger JW: Noninvasive estimation of central aortic pressure using the oscillometric method for analyzing systemic artery pulsatile blood flow: comparative study of indirect systolic, diastolic, and mean brachial artery pressure with simultaneous direct ascending aortic pressure measurements, *Am Heart J* 103:879, 1982.

40. Friesen RH, Lichtor JL: Indirect measurement of blood pressure in neonates and infants utilizing an automatic noninvasive oscillometric monitor, *Anesth Analg* 60:742, 1981.

41. Peñaz J: *Photoelectric measurement of blood pressure volume and flow in the finger*, Digest, 10th International Conference of Medical Biological Engineers, 1973, 104.

42. Wesseling KH, van Bemmel R, van Dieren A, et al: Two methods for the assessment of hemodynamic parameters of epidemiology, *Acta Cardiol* 33:84, 1978.

43. Molhoek GP, Wesseling KH, Settels JJ, et al: Evaluation of the Peñaz servo-plethysmo-manometer for the continous, noninvasive measurement of finger blood pressure, *Basic Res Cardiol* 79:598, 1984.

44. Silke B, McAuley D: Accuracy and precision of blood pressure determination with the Finapres: an overview using re-sampling statistics, *J Hum Hypertens* 12:403, 1998.

45. Novak V, Novak P, Schondorf R: Accuracy of beat-to-beat noninvasive measurement of finger arterial pressure using the Finapres: a spectral analysis approach, *J Clin Monit* 10:118, 1994.

46. Gravenstein JS, Paulus DA, Feldman J, et al: Tissue hypoxia distal to a Peñaz finger blood pressure cuff, *J Clin Monit* 1:120, 1985.

47. Dorlas JC, Nijboer JA, Butijn T, et al: Effects of peripheral vasoconstriction on the blood pressure in the finger, measured continuously by a new noninvasive method (the FinapresR), *Anesthesiology* 62:342, 1985.

48. Kurki T, Smith NT, Head N: Noninvasive continuous blood pressure measurement from the finger: optimal measurement conditions and factors affecting reliability, *J Clin Monit* 3:6, 1987.

49. Hernandez A, Goldring D, Hartman AF: Measurement of blood pressure in infants and children by the Doppler ultrasound technique, *Pediatrics* 48:788, 1971.

50. Stegall HF, Kardon MB, Kemmerer WT: Indirect measurement of arterial blood pressure by Doppler ultrasonic sphygmomanometry, *J Appl Physiol* 25:793, 1968.

51. Sy WP: Ulnar nerve palsy possibly related to the use of an automatically cycled blood pressure cuff, *Anesth Analg* 60:687, 1981.

52. van Egmond J, Lenders JW, Weernink E, Thien T: Accuracy and reproducibility of 30 devices for self-measurement of arterial blood pressure, *Am J Hypertens* 6:873, 1993.

53. Boutros A, Albert S: Effect of the dynamic response of transducer-tubing system on accuracy of direct blood pressure measurement in patients, *Crit Care Med* 11:124, 1983.

54. Shinozaki T, Deane RS, Mazuzan JE: The dynamic responses of liquid-filled catheter systems for direct measurements of blood pressure, *Anesthesiology* 53:498, 1980.

55. Hunziker P: Accuracy and dynamic response of disposable pressure transducer-tubing systems, *Can J Anaesth* 34:409, 1987.

56. Abrams JH, Olson ML, Marino JA, Cerra FB: Use of a needle valve variable resistor to improve invasive blood pressure monitoring, *Crit Care Med* 12:978, 1984.

57. Gardner RM: Direct blood pressure measurement-dynamic response requirements, *Anesthesiology* 54:227, 1981.

58. Van Bergen FH, Weatherhead DS, Treloar AE, et al: Comparison of indirect and direct methods of measuring arterial blood pressure, *Circulation* 10:481, 1954.

59. Reich DL, Moskowitz DM, Kaplan JA: Hemodynamic monitoring. In Kaplan JA (ed): *Cardiac anesthesia*, ed 4, Philadelphia, 1999, WB Saunders, 321.

60. Szold A, Pizov R, Segal E, Perel A: The effect of tidal volume and intravascular volume state on systolic pressure variation in ventilated dogs, *Intensive Care Med* 15:368, 1989.

61. Rooke GA, Schwid HA, Shapira Y: The effect of graded hemorrhage and intravascular volume replacement on systolic pressure variation in humans during mechanical and spontaneous ventilation, *Anesth Analg* 80:925, 1995.

62. Mozersky DJ, Buckley CJ, Hagood C, et al: Ultrasonic evaluation of the palmar circulation, *Am J Surg* 126:810, 1973.

63. Allen EV: Thromboangiitis obliterans: methods of diagnosis of chronic occlusive arterial lesions distal to the wrist with illustrated cases, *Am J Med Sci* 178:237, 1929.

64. Cable DG, Mullany CJ, Schaff HV: The Allen test, *Ann Thorac Surg* 67:876, 1999.

65. Greenhow DE: Incorrect performance of Allen's test: ulnar artery flow erroneously presumed inadequate, *Anesthesiology* 37:356, 1972.

66. Brodsky JB: A simple method to determine patency of the ulnar artery intraoperatively prior to radial artery cannulation, *Anesthesiology* 42:626, 1975.

67. Nowak GS, Moorthy SS, McNiece WL: Use of pulse oximetry for assessment of collateral arterial flow, *Anesthesiology* 64:527, 1986 (letter).

68. Kumar P, Tendolkar AG, Reddy S: Preoperative assessment of hand circulation by means of Doppler ultrasonography and the modified Allen test, *J Thorac Cardiovasc Surg* 123:396, 2002.

69. Marshall AG, Erwin DC, Wyse RKH, et al: Percutaneous arterial cannulation in children, *Anesthesia* 39:27, 1984.

70. Slogoff S, Keats AS, Arlund C: On the safety of radial artery cannulation, *Anesthesiology* 59:42, 1983.

71. Mangano DT, Hickey RF: Ischemic injury following uncomplicated radial artery catheterization, *Anesth Analg* 58:55, 1979.

72. Jarvis MA, Jarvis CL, Jones PR, Spyt TJ: Reliability of Allen's test in selection of patients for radial artery harvest, *Ann Thorac Surg* 70:1362, 2000.

73. Ryan JF, Raines J, Dalton BC, et al: Arterial dynamics of radial artery cannulation, *Anesth Analg* 52:1015, 1973.

74. Barnes RW, Foster E, Jansen GA, et al: Safety of brachial artery catheters as monitors in the intensive care unit—prospective evaluation with the Doppler ultrasonic velocity detector, *Anesthesiology* 44:260, 1976.

75. Pascarelli EF, Bertrand CA: Comparison of blood pressures in the arms and legs, *N Engl J Med* 270:693, 1964.

76. Gurman GM, Kriemerman S: Cannulation of big arteries in critically ill patients, *Crit Care Med* 13:217, 1985.

77. Yacoub OF, Bacaling JH, Kelly M: Monitoring of axillary arterial pressure in a patient with Buerger's disease requiring clipping of an intracranial aneurysm, *Br J Anaesth* 59:1056, 1987.

78. Muralidhar K: Complication of femoral artery pressure monitoring, *J Cardiothorac Vasc Anesth* 12:128, 1998.

79. Johnstone RE, Greenhow DE: Catheterization of the dorsalis pedis artery, *Anesthesiology* 39:654, 1973.

80. Wada T, Yao H, Miyamoto T, et al: Prevention and detection of spinal cord injury during thoracic and thoracoabdominal aortic repairs, *Ann Thorac Surg* 72:80, 2001.

81. Griepp RB, Ergin MA, Galla JD, et al: Minimizing spinal cord injury during repair of descending thoracic and thoracoabdominal aneurysms: the Mount Sinai approach, *Semin Thorac Cardiovasc Surg* 10:25, 1998.

82. Safi HJ, Campbell MP, Miller CC, et al: Spinal cord protection in descending thoracic and thoracoabdominal aortic aneurysm repair, *Semin Thorac Cardiovasc Surg* 10:41, 1998.

83. Prian GW: New proximal approach works well in temporal artery catheterization, *JAMA* 235:2693, 1976.

84. Pierson DJ, Hudson LD: Monitoring hemodynamics in the critically ill, *Med Clin North Am* 67:1343, 1983.

85. Bedford RF, Wollman H: Complications of percutaneous radial artery cannulation: an objective prospective study in man, *Anesthesiology* 38:228, 1973.

86. Bedford RF: Radial arterial function following percutaneous cannulation with 18- and 20-gauge catheters, *Anesthesiology* 47:37, 1977.

87. Bedford RF: Wrist circumference predicts the risk of radial arterial occlusion after cannulation, *Anesthesiology* 48:377, 1978.

88. Jones RM, Hill AB, Nahrwold ML, Bolles RE: The effect of method of radial artery cannulation on postcannulation blood flow and thrombus formation, *Anesthesiology* 55:76, 1981.

89. Bedford RF, Ashford TP: Aspirin pretreatment prevents post-cannulation radial artery thrombosis, *Anesthesiology* 51:176, 1979.

90. Bedford RF: Removal of radial artery thrombi following percutaneous cannulation for monitoring, *Anesthesiology* 46:430, 1977.

91. Sfeir R, Khoury S, Khoury G, et al: Ischaemia of the hand after radial artery monitoring, *Cardiovasc Surg* 4:456, 1996.

92. Bedford RF, Wollman H: Complications of percutaneous radial artery cannulation: an objective prospective study in man, *Anesthesiology* 38:228, 1973.

93. Kim JM, Arakawa K, Bliss J: Arterial cannulation: factors in the development of occlusion, *Anesth Analg* 54:836, 1975.

94. Vender JS, Watts RD: Differential diagnosis of hand ischemia in the presence of an arterial cannula, *Anesth Analg* 61:465, 1982.

95. Chang C, Dughi J, Shitabata P, et al: Air embolism and the radial arterial line, *Crit Care Med* 16:141, 1988.

96. Lowenstein E, Little JW, Lo HH: Prevention of cerebral embolization from flushing radial artery cannulae, *N Engl J Med* 285:1414, 1971.

97. Freeark RJ, Baker WH: Arterial injuries. In Sabiston DC (ed): *Textbook of surgery*, Philadelphia, 1986, WB Saunders, 1902.

98. Thalhammer C, Kirchherr AS, Uhlich F, et al: Postcatheterization pseudoaneurysms and arteriovenous fistulas: repair with percutaneous implantation of endovascular covered stents, *Radiology* 214:127, 2000.

99. Criado E, Marston WA, Ligush J, et al: Endovascular repair of peripheral aneurysms, pseudoaneurysms, and arteriovenous fistulas, *Ann Vasc Surg* 11:256, 1997.

100. Stamm WE, Colella JJ, Anderson RL, et al: Indwelling arterial catheters as a source of nosocomial bacteremia, *N Engl J Med* 292:1099, 1975.

101. Band JD, Maki DG: Infection caused by arterial catheters used for hemodynamic monitoring, *Am J Med* 67:735, 1979.

102. Shinozaki T, Deane R, Mazuzan JE, et al: Bacterial contamination of arterial lines: a prospective study, *JAMA* 249:223, 1983.

103. Weinstein RA, Stamm WE, Kramer L: Pressure monitoring devices: overlooked sources of nosocomial infection, *JAMA* 236:936, 1976.

104. Hurst JW, Schlant RC: Examination of veins. In Hurst FW, Logue RB (eds): *The heart*, ed 4, New York, 1978, McGraw-Hill, 193.

105. Mark JB: Central venous pressure monitoring: clinical insights beyond the numbers, *J Cardiothorac Vasc Anesth* 5:163, 1991.

106. Mangano DT: Monitoring pulmonary arterial pressures in coronary artery disease, *Anesthesiology* 53:364, 1980.

107. Reich DL, Moskowitz DM, Kaplan JA: Hemodynamic monitoring. In Kaplan JA (ed): *Cardiac anesthesia*, ed 4, Philadelphia, 1999, WB Saunders, 321.

108. Neustein SM, Narang J, Bronheim D: Use of the color test for safer internal jugular vein cannulation, *Anesthesiology* 76:1062, 1992.

109. Denys BG, Uretsky BF, Reddy PS: Ultrasound-assisted cannulation of the internal jugular vein. A prospective comparison to the external landmark-guided technique, *Circulation* 87:1557, 1993.

110. Slama M, Novara A, Safavian A, et al: Improvement of internal jugular vein cannulation using an ultrasound-guided technique, *Intensive Care Med* 23:916, 1997.

111. Gordon AC, Saliken JC, Johns D, et al: US-guided puncture of the internal jugular vein: complications and anatomic considerations, *J Vasc Interv Radiol* 9:333, 1998.

112. Bennett J, Bromley P: Doppler ultrasound-guided vascular access needle in paediatric patients, *Paediatr Anaesth* 11:505, 2001.

113. Troianos CA, Jobes DR, Ellison N: Ultrasound-guided cannulation of the internal jugular vein. A prospective, randomized study, *Anesth Analg* 72:823, 1991.

114. Keenan SP: Use of ultrasound to place central lines, *J Crit Care* 17:126, 2002.

115. English IC, Frew RM, Pigott JF, et al: Percutaneous catheterization of the internal jugular vein, *Anaesthesia* 24:521, 1969.

116. Blitt CD, Wright WA, Petty WC, et al: Cardiovascular catheterization via the external jugular vein: a technique employing the J-wire, *JAMA* 229:817, 1974.

117. Defalque RJ: Subclavian venapuncture: a review, *Anesth Analg* 47:677, 1968.

118. Ruesch S, Walder B, Tramer MR: Complications of central venous catheters: internal jugular versus subclavian access—a systematic review, *Crit Care Med* 30:454, 2002.

119. Kellner GA, Smart JF: Percutaneous placement of catheters to monitor "central venous pressure," *Anesthesiology* 36:515, 1972.

120. Webre DR, Arens JF: Use of cephalic and basilic veins for introduction of cardiovascular catheters, *Anesthesiology* 38:389, 1973.

121. Burgess GE, Marino RJ, Peuler MJ: Effect of head position on the location of venous catheters inserted via the basilic vein, *Anesthesiology* 46:212, 1977.

122. Merrer J, De Jonghe B, Golliot F, et al: Complications of femoral and subclavian venous catheterization in critically ill patients: a randomized controlled trial, *JAMA* 286:700, 2001.

123. Goldstein AM, Weber JM, Sheridan RL: Femoral venous access is safe in burned children: an analysis of 224 catheters, *J Pediatr* 130:442, 1997.

124. Murr MM, Rosenquist MD, Lewis RW 2nd, et al: A prospective safety study of femoral vein versus nonfemoral vein catheterization in patients with burns, *J Burn Care Rehabil* 12:576, 1991.

125. Jobes DR, Schwartz AJ, Greenhow DE, et al: Safer jugular vein cannulation: recognition of arterial puncture, *Anesthesiology* 59:353, 1983.

126. Gobiel F, Couture P, Girard D, et al: Carotid artery–internal jugular fistula: another complication following pulmonary artery catheterization via the internal jugluar venous route, *Anesthesiology* 80:230, 1994.

127. Robinson R, Errett L: Arteriovenous fistula following percutaneous internal jugular vein cannulation: a report of carotid artery–to–internal jugular vein fistula, *J Cardiothorac Anesth* 2:488, 1988.

128. Cook TL, Deuker CW: Tension pneumothorax following internal jugular cannulation and general anesthesia, *Anesthesiology* 45:554, 1976.

129. Thomas CJ, Butler CS: Delayed pneumothorax and hydrothorax with central venous catheter migration, *Anaesthesia* 54:987, 1999.

130. Kurekci E, Kaye R, Koehler M: Chylothorax and chylopericardium: a complication of a central venous catheter, *J Pediatr* 132:1064, 1998.

131. Khalil DG, Parker FB, Mukherjee N, Webb WR: Thoracic duct injury: a complication of jugular vein catheterization, *JAMA* 221:908, 1972.

132. DiLello F, Werner P, Kleinman E, et al: Life-threatening chylothorax after left internal mammary dissection: therapeutic considerations, *Ann Thorac Surg* 44:660, 1987.

133. Teba L, Dedhia HV, Bowen R, Alexander JC: Chylothorax review, *Crit Care Med* 13:49, 1985.

134. Loeb T, Jean N, Estournet-Mathiaud B: Chylothorax complicating a subclavian puncture controlled by positive-pressure expiratory ventilation, *Ann Fr Anesth Reanim* 16:527, 1997.

135. Arditis J, Giala M, Anagnostidou A: Accidental puncture of the right lymphatic duct during pulmonary artery catherization, *Acta Anaesthesiol Scand* 32:67, 1988.

136. Darling JC, Newell SJ, Mohamdee O, et al: Central venous catheter tip in the right atrium: a risk factor for neonatal cardiac tamponade, *J Perinatol* 21:461, 2001.

137. Schummer W, Schummer C: Pericardial tamponade as a delayed complication of central venous catheterization, *Eur J Anaesthesiol* 18:780, 2001.

138. van Engelenburg KC, Festen C: Cardiac tamponade: a rare but life-threatening complication of central venous catheters in children, *J Pediatr Surg* 33:1822, 1998.

139. Vesely TM: Air embolism during insertion of central venous catheters, *J Vasc Interv Radiol* 12:1291, 2001.

140. Sing RF, Thomason MH, Heniford BT, et al: Venous air embolism from central venous catheterization: under-recognized or over-diagnosed? *Crit Care Med* 28:3377, 2000.

141. Heckmann JG, Lang CJ, Kindler K, et al: Neurologic manifestations of cerebral air embolism as a complication of central venous catheterization, *Crit Care Med* 28:1621, 2000.

142. Green HL, Nemir P Jr: Air embolism as a complication during parenteral alimentation, *Am J Surg* 121:614, 1971.

143. Smyth NPD, Rogers JB: Transvenous removal of catheter emboli from the heart and great veins by endoscopic forceps, *Ann Thorac Surg* 11:403, 1971.

144. Trentman TL, Rome JD, Messick JM Jr: Brachial plexus neuropathy following attempt at subclavian vein catheterization, *Reg Anesth* 21:163, 1996.

145. Hadeed HA, Braun TW: Paralysis of the hemidiaphragm as a complication of internal jugular vein cannulation: report of a case, *J Oral Maxillofac Surg* 46:409, 1988.

146. Burns S, Herbison GJ: Spinal accessory nerve injury as a complication of internal jugular vein cannulation, *Ann Intern Med* 125:700, 1996.

147. Parikh RD: Horner's syndrome: a complication of percutaneous catheterization of the internal jugular vein, *Anaesthesia* 27:327, 1972.

148. Swan HJC, Ganz W, Forrester JS, et al: Catheterization of the heart in man with the use of a flow-directed balloon-tipped catheter, *N Engl J Med* 283:447, 1970.

149. Lappas D, Lell WA, Gabel JC, et al: Indirect measurement of left atrial pressure in surgical patients—pulmonary capillary wedge and pulmonary artery diastolic pressures compared with left atrial pressure, *Anesthesiology* 38:394, 1973.

150. Raper R, Sibbald WJ: Misled by the wedge? *Chest* 89:427, 1986.

151. Nadeau S, Noble WH: Misinterpretation of pressure measurements from the pulmonary artery catheter, *Can Anaesth Soc J* 33:352, 1986.

152. Forrester J, Diamond G, Ganz W, et al: Right and left heart pressures in the acutely ill patient, *Clin Res* 18:306, 1970.

153. Lorzman J, Powers SR, Older T, et al: Correlation of pulmonary wedge and left atrial pressure: a study in the patient receiving positive end-expiratory pressure ventilation, *Arch Surg* 109:270, 1974.

154. Manjuran RS, Agarwal JB, Roy SB: Relationship of pulmonary artery diastolic and pulmonary artery wedge presssures in mitral stenosis, *Am Heart J* 89:207, 1975.

155. Hildick-Smith DJ, Walsh JT, Shapiro LM: Pulmonary capillary wedge pressure in mitral stenosis accurately reflects mean left atrial pressure but overestimates transmitral gradient, *Am J Cardiol* 85:512, A11, 2000.

156. Schmitt EA, Brantigan CO: Common artifacts of pulmonary artery pressures: recognition and interpretation. *J Clin Monit* 2:44, 1986.

157. Haggmark S, Hohner P, Ostman M, et al: Comparison of hemodynamic, electrocardiographic, mechanical, and metabolic indicators of intraoperative myocardial ischemia in vascular surgical patients with coronary artery disease, *Anesthesiology* 70:19, 1989.

158. Connors AF, Speroff T, Dawson NV, et al: The effectiveness of right heart catheterization in the initial care of critically ill patients, *JAMA* 276:889, 1996.

159. Dalen JE, Bone RC: Is it time to pull the pulmonary artery catheter? *JAMA* 276:916, 1996.

160. Guyatt G, Ontario Intensive Care Group: A randomised control trial of right heart catheterization in critically ill patients, *J Intensive Care Med* 6:91, 1991.

161. Gore JM, Goldberg RJ, Spodick DH, et al: A community-wide assessment of the use of pulmonary artery catheters in patients with acute myocardial infarctions, *Chest* 92:721, 1987.

162. Shoemaker WC, Appel PL, Kram HB, et al: Prospective trial of supra-normal values of survivors as therapeutic goals in high-risk surgical patients, *Chest* 94:1176, 1988.

163. Boyd O, Grounds RM, Bennett ED: A randomised clinical trial of the effect of deliberate perioperative increase of oxygen delivery on mortality in high-risk surgical patients, *JAMA* 270:2699, 1993.

164. Barone JE, Tucker JB, Rassias D, Corvo PR: Routine perioperative pulmonary artery catheterization has no effect on rate of complications in vascular surgery: a meta-analysis, *Am Surg* 67: 674, 2001.

165. Gnaegi A, Feihl F, Perret C: Intensive care physicians' insufficient knowledge of right-heart catheterization at the bedside: time to act? *Crit Care Med* 25:213, 1997.

166. Iberti TJ, Fischer EP, Leibowitz AB, et al: A multicenter study of physicians' knowledge of the pulmonary artery catheter. Pulmonary Artery Catheter Study Group, *JAMA* 264:2928, 1990.

167. Polanczyk CA, Rohde LE, Goldman L, et al: Right heart catheterization and cardiac complications in patients undergoing noncardiac surgery. JAMA 286: 309-314, 2001.

168. Sandham JD, Hall RD, Brant RF, et al: A randomized, controlled trial of the use of pulmonary artery-catheters in high-risk surgical patients. *N Eng J Med* 348: 5-14, 2003.

169. Shah KB, Rao TLK, Laughlin S, El-Etr AA: A review of pulmonary artery catheterization in 6245 patients, *Anesthesiology* 61:271, 1984.

170. Baldwin IC, Heland M: Incidence of cardiac dysrhythmias in patients during pulmonary artery catheter removal after cardiac surgery, *Heart Lung* 29:155, 2000.

171. Spring CL, Pozen RG, Rozanski JJ, et al: Advanced ventricular arrhythmias during bedside pulmonary artery catheterization, *Am J Med* 72:203, 1982.

172. Salmenpera M, Peltola K, Rosenberg P: Does prophylactic lidocaine control cardiac arrhythmias associated with pulmonary artery catheterization? *Anesthesiology* 56:210, 1982.

173. Shaw TJI: The Swan-Ganz pulmonary artery catheter. Incidence of complications with particular reference to ventricular dysrhythmias and their prevention, *Anaesthesia* 34:651, 1979.

174. Keusch DJ, Winters S, Thys DM: The patient's position influences the incidence of dysrhythmias during pulmonary artery catheterization, *Anesthesiology* 70:582, 1989.

175. Abernathy WS: Complete heart block caused by a Swan-Ganz catheter, *Chest* 65:349, 1974.

176. Thomson IR, Dalton BC, Lappas DG, et al: Right bundle-branch block and complete heart block caused by the Swan-Ganz catheter, *Anesthesiology* 51:359, 1979.

177. Bashour CA, Fitzpatrick D, Yared JP, Starr NJ: Transient complete heart block during pulmonary artery catheter removal, *Intensive Care Med* 26:483, 2000.

178. Sprung CL, Elser B, Schein RMH, et al: Risk of right bundle-branch block and complete heart block during pulmonary artery catheterization, *Crit Care Med* 17:1, 1989.

179. Morris D, Mulvihill D, Lew WYW: Risk of developing complete heart block during bedside pulmonary artery catheterization in patients with left bundle-branch block, *Arch Intern Med* 147:2005, 1987.

180. McDaniel DD, Stone JG, Faltas AN, et al: Catheter-induced pulmonary artery hemorrhage, *J Thoracic Cardiovasc Surg* 82:1, 1981.

181. Daccache G, Depoix JP, Provenchere S, et al: Pulmonary artery catheter during cardiac surgery: a rare but severe adverse effect, *J Cardiothorac Vasc Anesth* 12:125, 1998.

182. Neerukonda SK, Jantz RD: Pulmonary artery perforation caused by a flow-directed balloon-tipped catheter, *Chest* 103:1928, 1993.

183. Mullerworth MH, Angelopoulos P, Couyant MA, et al: Recognition and management of catheter-induced pulmonary artery rupture, *Ann Thorac Surg* 66:1242, 1998.

184. Shah KB, Rao TLK, Laughlin S, El-Etr AA: A review of pulmonary artery catheterization in 6,245 patients, *Anesthesiology* 61:271, 1984.

185. Dhamee MS, Pattison CZ: Pulmonary artery rupture during cardiopulmonary bypass, *J Cardiothoracic Anesth* 1:51, 1987.

186. Hannan AT, Brown M, Bigman O: Pulmonary artery catheter–induced hemorrhage, *Chest* 85:128, 1984.

187. Urschel JD, Myerowitz PD: Catheter-induced pulmonary artery rupture in the setting of cardiopulmonary bypass, *Ann Thorac Surg* 56:585, 1993.

188. Stein JM, Lisbon A: Pulmonary hemorrhage from pulmonary artery catheterization treated with endobronchial intubation, *Anesthesiology* 55:698, 1981.

189. Gourin A, Garzon AA: Operative treatment of massive hemoptysis, *Ann Thorac Surg* 18:52, 1974.

190. Klafta JM, Olson JP: Emergent lung separation for management of pulmonary artery rupture, *Anesthesiology* 87:1248, 1997.

191. Foote GA, Schabel SI, Hodges M: Pulmonary complications of the flow-directed balloon-tipped catheter, *N Engl J Med* 290:927, 1974.

192. Colbert S, O'Hanlon DM, Quill DS, et al: Swan-Ganz catheter—all in a knot, *Eur J Anaesthesiol* 14:518, 1997.

193. England MR, Murphy MC: A knotty problem, *J Cardiothorac Vasc Anesth* 11:682, 1997.

194. Mond HG, Clark DW, Nesbitt SJ, Schlant RC: A technique for unknotting an intracardiac flow-directed balloon catheter, *Chest* 67:731, 1975.

195. Tremblay N, Taillefer J, Hardy JF: Successful non-surgical extraction of a knotted pulmonary artery catheter trapped in the right ventricle, *Can J Anaesth* 39:293, 1992.

196. Tan C, Bristow PJ, Segal P, Bell RJ: A technique to remove knotted pulmonary artery catheters, *Anaesth Intensive Care* 25:160, 1997.

197. Lipp H, O'Donoghue K, Resnekov L: Intracardiac knotting of a flow-directed balloon catheter, *N Engl J Med* 284:220, 1971.

198. Boscoe MJ, deLange S: Damage to the tricuspid valve with a Swan-Ganz catheter, *Br Med J* 283:346, 1981.

199. Arnaout S, Diab K, Al-Kutoubi A, Jamaleddine G: Rupture of the chordae of the tricuspid valve after knotting of the pulmonary artery catheter, *Chest* 120:1742, 2001.

200. O'Toole JD, Wurtzbacher JJ, Wearner NE, Jain AC: Pulmonary valve injury and insufficiency during pulmonary-artery catheterization, *N Engl J Med* 301:1167, 1979.
201. Greene JF Jr, Fitzwater JE, Clemmer TP: Septic endocarditis and indwelling pulmonary artery catheters, *JAMA* 233:891, 1975.
202. Kim YL, Richman KA, Marshall BE: Thrombocytopenia associated with Swan-Ganz catheterization in patients, *Anesthesiology* 53:261, 1980.
203. Kim YL, Richman KA, Marshall BE: Thrombocytopenia associated with Swan-Ganz catheterization in patients, *Anesthesiology* 53:261, 1980.
204. Moberg PQ, Geary VM, Sheikh FM: Heparin-induced thrombocytopenia: a possible complication of heparin-coated pulmonary artery catheters, *J Cardiothorac Anesth* 4:226, 1990.
205. Mureebe L, Silver D: Heparin-induced thrombocytopenia: pathophysiology and management, *Vasc Endovasc Surg* 36:163, 2002.
206. King DJ, Kelton JG: Heparin-associated thrombocytopenia, *Ann Intern Med* 100:535, 1984.
207. Jain A, Shroff SG, Jnicki JS, et al: Relation between venous oxygen saturation and cardiac index. Nonlinearity and normalization for oxygen uptake and hemoglobin, *Chest* 99:1403, 1991.
208. Magilligan DJ, Teasdall R, Eisinminger R, Peterson E: Mixed venous saturation as a predictor of cardiac output in the postoperative cardiac surgical patient, *Ann Thorac Surg* 44:260, 1987.
209. Inomata S, Nishikawa T, Taguchi M: Continous monitoring of mixed venous oxygen saturation for detecting alterations in cardiac output after discontinuation of cardiopulmonary bypass, *Br J Anaesth* 72:11, 1994.
210. Boylan JF, Teasdale SJ: Con: perioperative continuous monitoring of mixed venous oxygen saturation should not be routine in high-risk cardiac surgery, *J Cardiothorac Anesth* 4:651, 1990.
211. O'Connor JP, Townsend GE: Pro: perioperative continuous monitoring of mixed oxygen saturation should be routine during high-risk cardiac surgery, *J Cardiothorac Anesth* 4:647, 1990.
212. Vedrinne C, Bastien O, De Varax R, et al: Predictive factors for usefulness of fiberoptic pulmonary artery catheter for continuous oxygen saturation in mixed venous blood monitoring in cardiac surgery, *Anesth Analg* 85:2, 1997.
213. Zaidan J, Freniere S: Use of a pacing pulmonary artery catheter during cardiac surgery, *Ann Thorac Surg* 35:633, 1983.
214. Mora CT, Seltzer JL, McNulty SE: Evaluation of a new design pulmonary artery catheter for intraoperative ventricular pacing, *J Cardiothorac Anesth* 2:303, 1988.
215. Trankina MF, White RD: Perioperative cardiac pacing using an atrioventricular pacing pulmonary artery catheter, *J Cardiothorac Anesth* 3:154, 1989.
216. Thys DM: Cardiac output, *Anesthesiol Clin North Am* 4:803, 1988.
217. Fegler G: Measurement of cardiac output in anesthetized animals by a thermodilution method, *Q J Exp Physiol* 39:153, 1954.
218. Branthwaite MA, Bradley RD: Measurement of cardiac output by thermal dilution in man, *J Appl Physiol* 24:434, 1968.
219. Forrester JS, Ganz W, Diamond G, et al: Thermodilution cardiac output determination with a single flow-directed catheter, *Am Heart J* 83:306, 1972.
220. Swan HJC, Ganz W, Forrester J, et al: Catheterization of the heart in man with use of a flow-directed balloon-tipped catheter, *N Engl J Med* 283:447, 1970.
221. Salgado CR, Galletti PM: In vitro evaluation of the thermodilution technique for the measurement of ventricular stroke volume and end-diastolic volume, *Cardiologia* 49:65, 1966.
222. Bilfinger TV, Lin CY, Anagnostopoulos CE: In vitro determination of accuracy of cardiac output measurements by thermal dilution, *J Surg Res* 33:409, 1982.
223. Levett JM, Replogle RL: Thermodilution cardiac output: a critical analysis and review of the literature, *J Surg Res* 27:392, 1979.
224. Goodyer AVN, Huvos A, Eckhardt WF, et al: Thermal dilution curves in the intact animal, *Circ Res* 7:432, 1959.
225. Pavek K, Lindquist O, Arfors KE: Validity of thermodilution method for measurement of cardiac output in pulmonary oedema, *Cardiovasc Res* 7:419, 1973.
226. Pelletier C: Cardiac output measurement by thermodilution, *Can J Surg* 22:347, 1979.
227. Runciman WB, Ilsley AH, Roberts JG: Thermodilution cardiac output—a systematic error, *Anaesth Intensive Care* 9:135, 1981.
228. Sorensen MB, Bille-Brahe NE, Engell HC: Cardiac output measurement by thermodilution, *Ann Surg* 183:67, 1976.
229. Weisel RD, Berger RL, Hechtman HB, et al: Measurement of cardiac output by thermodilution, *N Engl J Med* 292:682, 1975.
230. Wetzel RC, Latson TW: Major errors in thermodilution cardiac output measurement during rapid volume infusion, *Anesthesiology* 62:684, 1985.
231. Kahan F, Profeta J, Thys DM: High cardiac output measurements in a patient with congestive heart failure, *J Cardiothorac Anesth* 1:234, 1987.
232. Mackenzie JD, Haite NS, Rawles JM: Method of assessing the reproducibility of blood flow measurement: factors affecting the performance of thermodilution cardiac output computers, *Br Heart J* 55:14, 1986.
233. Hoel BL: Some aspects of the clinical use of thermodilution in measuring cardiac output, *Scand J Clin Lab Invest* 38:383, 1978.
234. Stetz CW, Miller RG, Kelly GE, et al: Reliability of the thermodilution method in the determination of cardiac output in clinical practice, *Am Rev Respir Dis* 126:1001, 1982.
235. Stevens JH, Raffin TA, Mihm FG, et al: Thermodilution cardiac output measurement: effects of the respiratory cycle on its reproducibility, *JAMA* 253:2240, 1985.
236. Pearl RG, Rosenthal MH, Nieson L, et al: Effect of injectate volume and temperature on thermodilution cardiac output determination, *Anesthesiology* 64:798, 1986.
237. Matthew EB, Vender JS: Comparison of cardiac output measured by different computers, *Crit Care Med* 15:989, 1987.
238. Nishikawa T, Dohi S: Slowing of heart rate during cardiac output measurement by thermodilution, *Anesthesiology* 57:538, 1982.
239. Harris AP, Miller CF, Beattie C, et al: The slowing of sinus rhythm during thermodilution cardiac output determination and the effect of altering injectate temperature, *Anesthesiology* 63:540, 1985.
240. Neto EP, Piriou V, Durand PG, et al: Comparison of the two semicontinuous cardiac output pulmonary artery catheters after valvular surgery, *Crit Care Med* 27:2694, 1999.
241. Jacquet L, Hanique G, Glorieux D, et al: Analysis of the accuracy of continuous thermodilution cardiac output measurement. Comparison with intermittent thermodilution and Fick cardiac output measurements, *Intensive Care Med* 22:1125, 1996.
242. Jakobsen CJ, Melsen NC, Andresen EB: Continuous cardiac output measurements in the perioperative period, *Acta Anaesthesiol Scand* 39:485, 1995.
243. Mihaljevic T, von Segesser LK, Tonz M, et al: Continuous thermodilution measurements of cardiac output: in-vitro and in-vivo evaluation, *Thorac Cardiovasc Surg* 42:32, 1994.
244. Hogue CW, Rosenbloom M, McCawley C, Lappas DG: Comparison of cardiac output measurements by continuous thermodilution with electromagnetometry in adult cardiac surgical patients, *J Cardiothorac Vasc Anesth* 8:631, 1994.
245. Zollner C, Polasek J, Kilger E, et al: Evaluation of a new continuous thermodilution cardiac output monitor in cardiac surgical patients: a prospective criterion standard study, *Crit Care Med* 27:293, 1999.
246. Medin DL, Brown DT, Wesley R: Validation of continuous thermodilution cardiac output in critically ill patients with analysis of systematic errors, *J Crit Care* 13:184, 1998.
247. Jurado RA: Measurement of cardiac output by the direct Fick method. In Litwak RS, Jurado RA: *Care of the cardiac surgical patient*, Norwalk, CT, 1982, Appleton-Century-Crofts, 495.
248. Huggins RA, Smith EL, Sinclair MA: Comparison between the cardiac output measured with a rotameter and output determined by the direct Fick method in open-chest dogs, *Am J Physiol* 160:183, 1950.
249. Seely RD, Gregg DE: A technique for measuring cardiac output directly by cannulation of the pulmonary artery, *Proc Soc Exp Biol Med* 73:269, 1950.
250. Seely RD, Nerlich WE, Gregg DE: Comparison of cardiac output determined by the Fick procedure and a direct method using the rotameter, *Circulation* 1:1261, 1950.
251. Cross KW, Groom AC, Mottram RF, et al: Cardiac output in the cat: a comparison between the Fick method and a radioactive indicator dilution method, *J Physiol (Lond)* 136:24P, 1957.
252. Doyle JT, Wilson JS, Lepine C, et al: An evaluation of the measurement of the cardiac output and of the so-called pulmonary blood volume by the dye dilution method, *J Lab Clin Med* 41:29, 1953.
253. Eliasch H, Lagerlof H, Bucht H, et al: Comparison of the dye dilution and the direct Fick methods for the measurement of cardiac output in man, *Scand J Clin Lab Invest* 7(Suppl 20):73, 1955.
254. Etsten B, Li TH: The determination of cardiac output by the dye dilution method: modifications, comparison with the Fick method, and application during anesthesia, *Anesthesiology* 15:217, 1954.
255. Hamilton WF, Riley RL, Attyah AM, et al:. Comparison of Fick and dye injection methods of measuring cardiac output in man, *Am J Physiol* 153:309, 1948.

256. Moore JW, Kinsman JM, Hamilton WF, et al:. Studies on the circulation. II. Cardiac output determinations: comparison of the injection method with the direct Fick procedure, *Am J Physiol* 89:331, 1929.

257. Howell CD, Horvath SM: Reproducibility of cardiac output measurements in the dog, *J Appl Physiol* 14:421, 1959.

258. Selzer A, Sudrann RB: Reliability of the determination of cardiac output in man by means of the Fick principle, *Circ Res* 6:485, 1958.

259. Thomasson B: Cardiac output in normal subjects under standard basal conditions; the repeatability of measurements by the Fick method, *Scand J Clin Lab Invest* 9:365,1957.

260. Wood EH, Bowers D, Shepherd JT, et al: O_2 content of mixed venous blood in man during various phases of the respiratory and cardiac output cycles in relation to possible errors in measurement of cardiac output by conventional applications of the Fick method, *J Appl Physiol* 215:605, 1968.

261. Grossman W (ed): Fick oxygen method. In *Cardiac Catheterization and angiography*, ed 3, Philadelphia, 1986, Lea & Febiger, 105.

262. Guyton AC: The Fick principle. In Guyton AC, Jones CE, Coleman TG: *Cardiac output and its regulation*, ed 2, Philadelphia, 1973, WB Saunders, 21.

263. Linton RA, Band DM, Haire KM: A new method of measuring cardiac output in man using lithium dilution, *Br J Anaesth* 71:262, 1993.

264. Kurita T, Morita K, Kato S, et al: Comparison of the accuracy of the lithium dilution technique with the thermodilution technique for measurement of cardiac output, *Br J Anaesth* 79:770, 1997.

265. Linton R, Band D, O'Brian T, et al: Lithium dilution cardiac output measurement: a comparison with thermodilution, *Crit Care Med* 25:1767, 1997.

266. Band DM, Linton RAF, O'Brian TK, et al: The shape of indicator dilution curves used for cardiac output measurement in man, *J Physiol (Lond)* 498:225, 1997.

267. Erlanger J, Hooker DR: An experimental study of blood pressure and of pulse-pressure in man, *Johns Hopkins Hosp Rep* 12:145, 1904.

268. Rodig G, Prasser C, Keyl C: Continuous cardiac output measurement: pulse contour analysis vs thermodilution technique in cardiac surgical patients, *Br J Anaesth* 82:525, 1999.

269. Buhre W, Weyland A, Kazmaier S, et al: Comparison of cardiac output assessed by pulse-contour analysis and thermodilution in patients undergoing minimally invasive direct coronary artery bypass grafting, *J Cardiothorac Vasc Anesth* 13:437, 1999.

270. Godje O, Friedl R, Hannekum A: Accuracy of beat-to-beat cardiac output monitoring by pulse contour analysis in hemodynamically unstable patients, *Med Sci Monit* 7:1344, 2001.

271. Linton NWF, Linton RAF: Estimation of changes in cardiac output from the arterial blood pressure waveform in the upper limb, *Br J Anaesth* 86:486, 2001.

272. Zollner C, Haller M, Weis M, et al: Beat-to-beat measurement of cardiac output by intravascular pulse contour analysis: a prospective criterion standard study in patients after cardiac surgery, *J Cardiothorac Vasc Anesth* 14:125, 2000.

273. Godje O, Hoke K, Lamm P, et al: Continuous, less invasive, hemodynamic monitoring in intensive care after cardiac surgery, *Thorac Cardiovasc Surg* 46:242, 1998.

274. Jansen JR, Schreuder JJ, Mulier JP, et al: A comparison of cardiac output derived from the arterial pressure wave against thermodilution in cardiac surgery patients, *Br J Anaesth* 87:212, 2001.

275. van Lieshout JJ, Wesseling KH: Continuous cardiac output by the pulse contour analysis? *Br J Anaesth* 86:467, 2001.

276. Gratz I, Kraidin J, Jacobi AG, et al: Continuous non invasive cardiac output as estimated from the pulse contour curve, *J Clin Monit* 8:20, 1992.

277. Kubicek WG, Karegis JN, Patterson RP, et al: Development and evaluation of an impedance cardiac output system, *Aerospace Med* 37:1208, 1966.

278. Cohen AJ, Arnaudov D, Zabeeda D, et al: Non invasive measurement of cardiac output during coronary artery bypass grafting, *Eur J Cardiothorac Surg* 14:64, 1998.

279. Shoemaker WC, Wo CC, Bishop MH, et al: Multicenter trial of a new thoracic electrical bioimpedance device for cardiac output estimation, *Crit Care Med* 22:1907, 1994.

280. Belardinelli R, Ciampani N, Costanini C: Comparison of impedance cardiography with thermodilution and direct Fick methods for noninvasive measurements of stroke volume and cardiac output during incremental exercise in patients with ischemic cardiomyopathy, *Am J Cardiol* 77:1293, 1996.

281. Spinale FG, Reines HD, Crawford FA Jr: Comparison of bioimpedance and thermodilution methods for determining cardiac output: experimental and clinical studies, *Ann Thorac Surg* 45:421, 1988.

282. Castor G, Molter G, Helms J, et al: Determination of cardiac output during positive end-expiratory pressure—noninvasive electrical bioimpedance compared with standard thermodilution, *Crit Care Med* 18:544, 1990.

283. Spinale FG, Smith AC, Crawford FA: Relationship of bioimpedance to thermodilution and echocardiographic measurements of cardiac function, *Crit Care Med* 18:414, 1990.

284. Fuller HD: The validity of cardiac output measurements by thoracic impedance: a meta-analysis, *Clin Invest Med* 15:103, 1992.

285. Barry BN, Mallick A, Bodenham AR, et al: Lack of agreement between bioimpedance and continuous thermodilution measurement of cardiac output in intensive care unit patients, *Crit Care* 1:71, 1997.

286. Young JD, McQuillan P: Comparison of thoracic electrical bioimpedance and thermodilution for the measurement of cardiac index in patients with severe sepsis, *Br J Anaesth* 70:58, 1993.

287. Clarke DE, Raffin TA: Thoracic electrical bioimpedance measurement of cardiac output—not ready for prime time, *Crit Care Med* 21:1111, 1993.

288. Sagemann WS, Amundsen DE: Thoracic electrical bioimpedance measurements of cardiac output in postaortocoronary bypass patients, *Crit Care Med* 21:1139, 1993.

289. Siegel LC, Shafer SL, Martinez GM, et al: Simultaneous measurements of cardiac output by thermodilution, esophageal Doppler, and electrical impedance in anesthetized patients, *J Cardiothorac Anesth* 2:590, 1988.

290. Shoemaker WC, Belzberg H, Wo C, et al: Multicenter study of noninvasive monitoring systems as alternatives to invasive monitoring of acutely ill emergency patients, *Chest* 114:1643, 1998.

291. Perrino AC Jr, Lippman A, Ariyan C, et al: Intraoperative cardiac output monitoring: comparison of impedance cardiography and thermodilution, *J Cardiothorac Vasc Anesth* 8:24, 1994.

292. Sageman WS, Riffenburgh RH, Spiess BD: Equivalence of bioimpedance and thermodilution in measuring cardiac index after cardiac surgery, *J Cardiothorac Vasc Anesth* 16:8, 2002.

293. Gotshall RW, Wood VC, Miles DS: Comparison of two impedance cardiographic techniques for measuring cardiac output in critically ill patients, *Crit Care Med* 17:806, 1989.

294. Jaffe MB: Partial CO_2 rebreathing cardiac output: operating principles of the NICOTM system, *J Clin Monit* 15:387, 1999.

295. Nilsson LB, Eldrup N, Berthelsen PG: Lack of agreement between thermodilution and carbon dioxide–rebreathing cardiac output, *Acta Anaesthesiol Scand* 45:680, 2001.

296. Arnold JH, Stenz RI, Grenier B, et al: Noninvasive determination of cardiac output in a model of acute lung injury, *Crit Care Med* 25:864, 1997.

297. Russell AE, Smith SA, West MJ, et al: Automated non invasive measurements of cardiac output by the carbon dioxide rebreathing method: comparisons with dye dilution and thermodilution, *Br Heart J* 63:195, 1990.

298. Arnold JH, Stenz RI, Thompson JE, Arnold LW: Noninvasive determination of cardiac output using single breath CO_2 analysis, *Crit Care Med* 24:1701, 1996.

299. Binder JC, Parkin WG: Non invasive cardiac output determination: comparison of a new partial-rebreathing technique with thermodilution, *Anaesth Intensive Care* 29:19, 2001.

300. van Heerden PV, Baker S, Lim SI, et al: Clinical evaluation of the non-invasive cardiac output (NICO) monitor in the intensive care unit, *Anaesth Intensive Care* 28:427, 2000.

301. Feigenbaum H, Popp RL, Wolfe SB, et al: Ultrasound measurements of the left ventricle: a correlative study with angiocardiography, *Ann Intern Med* 129:461, 1972.

302. Kronik G, Slany J, Moslacher H: Comparative value of eight M-mode echocardiographic formulas for determining left ventricular stroke volume, *Circulation* 60:1308, 1979.

303. Nosir YF, Fioretti PM, Vletter WB, et al: Accurate measurement of left ventricular ejection fraction by three-dimensional echocardiography. A comparison with radionuclide angiography, *Circulation* 94:460, 1996.

304. Katz WE, Gasior TA, Quinlan JJ, Gorscan J 3rd: Transgastric continuous wave Doppler to determine cardiac output, *Am J Cardiol* 71:853, 1993.

305. Darmon PL, Hillel Z, Mogtabar A, et al: Cardiac output by transesophageal echocardiography using continuous wave Doppler across the aortic valve, *Anesthesiology* 80:796, 1994.

306. Roewer N, Bednarz F, Schulte am Esch J: Continuous measurement of intracardiac and pulmonary blood flow velocities with transesophageal pulsed Doppler echocardiography: technique and initial clinical experience, *J Cardiothorac Anesth* 1:418, 1987.

307. Muhiudeen IA, Kuecherer HF, Lee E, et al: Intraoperative estimation of cardiac output by transesophageal pulsed Doppler echocardiography, *Anesthesiology* 74:9, 1991.

308. Pu M, Griffin BP, Vandervoort PM, et al: Intraoperative validation of mitral inflow determination by transesophageal echocardiography: comparison of single-plane, biplane and thermodilution techniques, *J Am Coll Cardiol* 26:1047, 1995.

309. Estagnasie P, Djedaini K, Mier L, et al: Measurement of cardiac output by transesophageal echocardiography in mechanically ventilated patients. Comparison with thermodilution, *Intensive Care Med* 23:753, 1997.

310. Perrino AC Jr, Harris SN, Luther MA: Intraoperative determination of cardiac output using multiplane transesophageal echocardiography: a comparison to thermodilution, *Anesthesiology* 89:350, 1998.

311. Dabaghi SF, Rokey R, Rivera J, et al: Comparison of echocardiographic assessment of cardiac hemodynamics in the intensive care unit with right-sided cardiac catheterization, *Am J Cardiol* 76:392, 1995.

312. Roewer N, Bednarz F, Dziadka A, et al: Intraoperative cardiac output determination from transmitral and pulmonary blood flow measurements using transesophageal pulsed Doppler, *J Cardiothorac Anesth* 1:418, 1987.

313. Savino JS, Trolanos CA, Aukburg S, et al: Measurement of pulmonary blood flow with two-dimensional echocardiography and Doppler echocardiography, *Anesthesiology* 75:445, 1991.

314. Miller WE, Richards KL, Crawford MH: Accuracy of mitral Doppler echocardiographic cardiac output determinations in adults, *Am Heart J* 119:905, 1990.

315. Maslow A, Communale M, Haering M, et al: Pulsed wave Doppler measurements of cardiac output from the right ventricular outflow tract, *Anesth Analg* 83:466, 1996.

316. Darmon P, Hillel Z, Mogtader A, et al: Cardiac output by transesophageal echocardiography using continous-wave Doppler across the aortic valve, *Anesthesiology* 80:796, 1994.

317. Hillel Z, Thys DM, Keene D, et al: A method to improve the accuracy of esophageal Doppler cardiac output determinations, *Anesthesiology* 71:A386, 1989.

318. Siegel LC, Shafer SL, Martinez GM, et al: Simultaneous measurements of cardiac output by thermodilution, esophageal Doppler, and electrical impedance on anesthetized patients, *J Cardiothorac Anesth* 2:590, 1989.

319. Muhiudeen IA, Kuecherer HF, Lee E, et al: Intraoperative estimation of cardiac output by transesophageal pulsed Doppler echocardiography, *Anesthesiology* 79:9, 1991.

320. Ryan T, Burwash I, Lu J, et al: The agreement between ventricular volumes and ejection fraction by transesophageal echocardiography or a combined radionuclear and thermodilution technique in patients after coronary artery surgery, *J Cardiothorac Vasc Anesth* 10:323, 1996.

321. Urbanowicz JH, Shaaban MJ, Cohen NH, et al: Comparison of transesophageal echocardiographic and scintigraphic estimates of left ventricular end-diastolic volume index and ejection fraction in patients following coronary artery bypass grafting, *Anesthesiology* 72:607, 1990.

322. Liu N, Darmon PL, Saada M, et al: Comparison between radionuclide ejection fraction and fractional area changes derived from transesophageal echocardiography using automated border detection, *Anesthesiology* 85:468, 1996.

323. Goens MB, Martin GR: Acoustic quantification: a new tool for diagnostic echocardiography, *Curr Opin Cardiol* 11:52, 1996.

324. Perez JE, Miller JG, Holland MR, et al: Ultrasonic tissue characterization: integrated backscatter imaging for detecting myocardial structural properties and on-line quantitation of cardiac function, *Am J Cardiac Imag* 8:106, 1994.

325. Gorcsan J III, Morita S, Mandarino WA, et al: Two-dimensional echocardiographic automated border detection accurately reflects changes in left ventricular volume, *J Am Soc Echocardiogr* 6:482, 1993.

326. Gorcsan J III, Denault A, Mandarino WA, Pinsky MR: Left ventricular pressure-volume relations with transesophageal echocardiographic automated border detection: comparison with conductance-catheter technique, *Am Heart J* 131:544, 1996.

327. Pinto FJ, Siegel LC, Chenzbraun A, Schnittger I: On-line estimation of cardiac output with a new automated border detection system using transesophageal echocardiography: a preliminary comparison with thermodilution, *J Cardiothorac Vasc Anesth* 8:625, 1994.

328. Tardif JC, Cao QL, Pandian NG, et al: Determination of cardiac output using acoustic quantification in critically ill patients, *Am J Cardiol* 74:810, 1994.

329. Morrissey RL, Siu SC, Guerrero JL, et al: Automated assessment of ventricular volume and function by echocardiography: validation of automated border detection, *J Am Soc Echocardiogr* 7:107, 1994.

330. Katz WE, Gasior TA, Reddy SCR, Gorscan J III: Utility and limitations of biplane transesophageal echocardiographic automated border detection for estimation of left ventricular stroke volume and cardiac output, *Am Heart J* 128:389, 1994.

331. Pandian NG, Roelandt J, Nanda NC, et al: Dynamic three-dimensional echocardiography: methods and clinical potential, *Echocardiography* 11:237, 1994.

332. Kuhl HP, Franke A, Janssens U, et al: Three-dimensional echocardiographic determination of left ventricular volumes and function by multiplane transesophageal transducer: dynamic in vitro validation and in vivo comparison with angiography and thermodilution, *J Am Soc Echocardiogr* 11:1113, 1998.

333. Lee D, Fuisz AR, Fan PH, et al: Real-time 3-dimensional echocardiographic evaluation of left ventricular volume: correlation with magnetic resonance imaging—a validation study, *J Am Soc Echocardiogr* 14:1001, 2001.

334. Panza JA: Real-time three-dimensional echocardiography: an overview, *Int J Card Imaging* 17:227, 2001.

335. Shanewise JS, Cheung AT, Aronson S, et al: ASE/SCA guidelines for performing a comprehensive intraoperative multiplane transesophageal echocardiography examination: recommendations of the American Society of Echocardiography Council for Intraoperative Echocardiography and the Society of Cardiovascular Anesthesiologists Task Force for Certification in Perioperative Transesophageal Echocardiography, *Anesth Analg* 89:870, 1999.

336. Kisslo J, Adams DB, Belkin RN: *Doppler color-flow imaging*, New York, 1988, Churchill Livingstone.

337. Braunwald E, Sonnenblick EH, Ross J Jr: Mechanisms of cardiac contraction and relaxation. In Braunwald E (ed): *Heart disease*, ed 4, Philadelphia, 1992, WB Saunders, 379.

338. Clements FM, Harpole D, Quill T, et al: Simultaneous measurements of cardiac volumes, areas and ejection fractions by transesophageal echocardiography and first-pass radionuclide angiography, *Anesthesiology* 69:A4, 1988.

339. Swenson JD, Bull D, Stringham J: Subjective assessment of left ventricular preload using transesophageal echocardiography: corresponding pulmonary artery occlusion pressures, *J Cardiothorac Vasc Anesth* 15:580, 2001.

340. Thys DM, Hillel Z, Goldman ME, et al: A comparison of hemodynamic indices by invasive monitoring and two-dimensional echocardiography, *Anesthesiology* 67:630, 1987.

341. Norton JM: Toward consistent definitions for preload and afterload, *Adv Physiol Educ* 25:53, 2001.

342. Reichek N, Wilson J, St John Sutton M, et al: Noninvasive determination of left ventricular end-systolic stress: validation of the method and initial application, *Circulation* 65:99, 1982.

343. Sandler H, Dodge HT: Left ventricular tension and stress in man, *Circ Res* 13:91, 1963.

344. Hartford M, Wilstand JCM, Wallentin I, et al: Left ventricular wall stress and systolic function in untreated primary hypertension, *Hypertension* 7:97, 1985.

345. Lang RL, Borow KM, Newman A, et al: Systemic vascular resistance: an unreliable index of afterload, *Circulation* 74:1114, 1986.

346. Smith JS, Roizen MF, Cahalan MK, et al: Does anesthesia technique make a difference? Augmentation of systolic blood pressure during carotid endarterectomy: effects of phenylephrine versus light anesthesia and isoflurane versus halothane on the incidence of myocardial ischemia, *Anesthesiology* 69:846, 1988.

347. Weissler AM: Systolic time intervals, *N Engl J Med* 296:321, 1977.

348. Lewis RP, Rittgers SE, Forester WF, et al: A critical review of the systolic time intervals, *Circulation* 56:146, 1977.

349. Noble MIM, Trenchard D, Guz A: Left ventricular ejection in conscious dogs: 1. Measurement and significance of the maximum acceleration of blood from the left ventricle, *Circ Res* 19:139, 1966.

350. Bennett ED, Else W, Miller GAH, et al: maximum acceleration of blood from the left ventricle in patients with ischaemic heart disease, *Clin Sci Mol Med* 46:49, 1974.

351. Mehta N, Bennett DE: Impaired left ventricular function in acute myocardial infarction assessed by Doppler measurement of ascending aortic blood velocity and maximum acceleration, *Am J Cardiol* 57:1052, 1986.

352. Sabbah HN, Khaja F, Brymer JF, et al: Noninvasive evaluation of left ventricular performance based on peak aortic blood acceleration measured with a continuous-wave Doppler velocity meter, *Circulation* 74:323, 1986.

353. Folland ED, Parisi AF, Moynihan PF, et al: Assessment of left ventricular ejection fraction and volumes by real-time, two-dimensional echocardiography, *Circulation* 60:760, 1979.

354. Suga H, Sagawa K: Determinants of instantaneous pressure in canine left ventricle: time and volume specification, *Circ Res* 46:256, 1980.

355. Gorcsan J, Denault A, Gaisor TA, et al: Rapid estimation of left ventricular contractility from end-systolic relations by echocardiographic automated border detection and femoral arterial pressure, *Anesthesiology* 81:553, 1994.

356. Gorcsan J 3rd: Load-independent indices of left ventricular function using automated border detection, *Echocardiography* 16:63, 1999.

357. Mandarino WA, Pinsky MR, Gorcsan J 3rd: Assessment of left ventricular contractile state by preload-adjusted maximal power using echocardiographic automated border detection, *J Am Coll Cardiol* 31:861, 1998.

358. Dodek A, Kassenbaum DG, Bristow JD: Pulmonary edema in coronary artery disease without cardiomegaly, *N Engl J Med* 25:1347, 1972.

359. Dougherty AM, Naccarelli GV, Gray EL, et al: Congestive heart failure with normal systolic function, *Am J Cardiol* 54:778, 1984.

360. Topol EJ, Traill TA, Fortuin NJ: Hypertensive hypertrophic cardiomyopathy of the elderly, *N Engl J Med* 312:277, 1985.

361. Labovitz AJ, Lewen MK, Kern M, et al: Evaluation of left ventricular systolic and diastolic dysfunction during transient myocardial ischemia produced by angioplasty, *J Am Coll Cardiol* 10:748, 1987.

362. Labovitz AJ, Pearson AC: Evaluation of left ventricular diastolic function: clinical relevance and recent Doppler echocardiographic insights, *Am Heart J* 114:836, 1987.

363. Thys DM, Hillel Z, Konstadt S, et al: *The intraoperative evaluation of left ventricular filling by esophageal Doppler echocardiography*, Proceedings of the 8th Annual Meeting, Society of Cardiovascular Anesthesiologists, Montreal, 1986, 80.

364. Rinder CS, Wheeler LR, Alpern WD: Pulsed Doppler assessment of diastolic function before and after cardiopulmonary bypass, *Anesthesiology* 69:A2, 1988.

365. Roizen M, Beaupre P, Alpert R, et al: Monitoring with two-dimensional transesophageal echocardiography. Comparison of myocardial function in patients undergoing supraceliac, suprarenal-infraceliac, or infrarenal aortic occlusion, *J Vasc Surg* 1:300, 1984.

366. Terai C, Venishi M, Sugimoto H, et al: Transesophageal echocardiographic dimensional analysis of four cardiac chambers during positive end-expiratory pressure, *Anesthesiology* 63:640, 1985.

367. Koolen J, Visser C, Wever E, et al: Transesophageal two-dimensional echocardiographic evaluation of biventricular dimension on function during positive end-expiratory pressure ventilation after coronary artery bypass grafting, *Am J Cardiol* 59:1047, 1987.

368. Barash P, Glanz S, Katz J, et al: Ventricular function in children during halothane anesthesia: an echocardiographic evaluation, *Anesthesiology* 49:79, 1978.

369. Coriat P, Pamela F, Evans J, et al: Left ventricular function monitored by transesophageal 2-D echocardiography during induction of anesthesia, *Anesthesiology* 65:A26, 1986.

370. Reich DL, Guffin AV, Thys DM, et al: Hemodynamic consequences of doxacurium in abdominal aortic surgery, *Anesth Analg* 70:S321, 1990.

371. Labovitz AJ, Lewen MK, Kern M, et al: Evaluation of left ventricular systolic and diastolic dysfunction during transient myocardial ischemia produced by angioplasty, *J Am Coll Cardiol* 10:748, 1987.

372. Bowman LK, Cleman MW, Cabin HS, et al: Dynamics of early and late left ventricular filling determined by Doppler two-dimensional echocardiography during percutaneous transluminal coronary angioplasty, *Am J Cardiol* 61:541, 1988.

373. Vatner SF: Correlation between acute reductions in myocardial blood flow and function in conscious dogs, *Circ Res* 47:201, 1980.

374. Comunale ME, Body SC, Ley C, et al: The concordance of intraoperative left ventricular wall-motion abnormalities and electrocardiographic S-T segment changes: association with outcome after coronary revascularization. Multicenter Study of Perioperative Ischemia (McSPI) Research Group, *Anesthesiology* 88:945, 1998.

375. Corda DM, Caruso LJ, Mangano DM: Myocardial ischemia detected by transesophageal echocardiography in a patient undergoing peripheral vascular surgery, *J Clin Anesth* 12:491, 2000.

376. Rouine-Rapp K, Ionescu P, Balea M, et al: Detection of intraoperative segmental wall-motion abnormalities by transesophageal echocardiography: the incremental value of additional cross sections in the transverse and longitudinal planes, *Anesth Analg* 83:1141, 1996.

Anesthetic Techniques for Major Vascular Surgery

9

Mark P. Yeager, MD
Kathleen H. Chaimberg, MD

THE era of modern vascular surgery began in the 1950s after many decades of intermittent progress. Developments in blood transfusion, anticoagulant drugs, and angiography were necessary antecedents to the widespread application of previously developed vascular surgical techniques.[1] In the half century since the first successful repair of an aortic aneurysm, surgery of the aorta and its branches has become commonplace, offering measurable survival and quality-of-life benefits for patients.[2] Anesthetic management of vascular surgical patients has undergone considerable evolution since the reports of early surgical series.[3] Anesthetic options were limited during the first decades of vascular surgery; patients were commonly managed with a light general anesthetic as a means to limit postoperative respiratory depression, to allow early tracheal extubation after surgery, and to minimize the hemodynamic consequences of aortic declamping. Regional anesthesia was not commonly used.

New techniques for the care of vascular surgical patients have been particularly prominent in the past 10 years. Aggressive preoperative evaluation has led to a clearer identification of patients at risk for postoperative cardiac morbidity, the single most important cause of death after major vascular surgery.[4] New methods to minimize cardiac morbidity after surgery include perioperative β-blockade, α_2-arenergic blocking agents, and thoracic epidural local anesthesia.[5-7] Further advances have occurred in the understanding of systemic responses to major vascular surgery, especially the neuroendocrine and inflammatory responses, their metabolic consequences, and their effects on organ function.[8-10] Effective new techniques for postoperative pain control have gained prominence. Finally, an emerging interest in outcomes research has provided important new perspectives on the many interventions that are commonly used to care for patients undergoing major vascular surgery.[11-13] New emphasis is placed on evaluating health-related quality-of-life measures and functional recovery with less emphasis placed on "intermediate" outcomes such as pain scales, pulmonary function, or transient organ dysfunction.

In the discussions that follow, comparisons are made between the physiologic effects and clinical outcomes that are induced by different anesthetic techniques, especially the documented differences between general anesthesia and regional anesthesia. These techniques have important physiologic differences, some of which may provide unique benefits for the vascular surgical population.

This chapter begins with a brief perspective on the profile of patients who present for major vascular surgery, followed by a review of new and important outcome data that have been published in the anesthesia literature and that are relevant to the care of vascular surgery patients. A discussion of organ-specific considerations and their anesthetic implications then precedes the final sections on the current status of endovascular surgical repairs and management issues related to regional anesthesia.

The Vascular Surgery Patient

Given the systemic nature of vascular disease, patients presenting for major vascular surgery are presumed to be at risk for coronary artery disease (CAD) (see Chapter 5). Cardiac events remain the most common complication following elective vascular procedures, and CAD is the most common cause of death in long-term follow-up of patients who undergo vascular surgery.[14-17] In a subset of 263 patients scheduled for elective abdominal aortic aneurysm (AAA) repair, 31% were found to have severe, correctable coronary lesions detected by routine preoperative angiography.[18] Notably, a substantial percentage of these patients were not suspected to have CAD by clinical criteria alone (Table 9-1). Thus, there is an unreliable relationship between the severity of patients' symptoms and coronary anatomy. In fact, coronary stenoses in the setting of vascular surgery should be viewed from a dynamic perspective, increasing a patient's vulnerability to ischemia or infarction when precipitated by anemia, hemodynamic instability, thrombosis, or plaque rupture.[19,20] When evaluating the cardiac status of a patient presenting for vascular surgery, an assessment of left ventricular function is important. Whatever the severity of CAD, decreased left ventricular function is associated with a worsened prognosis.[21] In addition, evidence of limited cardiac reserve may alter decisions regarding the appropriate level and type of monitoring as well as anesthetic technique (see Chapter 8).

Although some degree of cardiovascular disease is assumed to be present in almost all vascular surgery patients, the goal of preoperative evaluation should be to identify the patients at greatest risk for perioperative cardiac morbidity. This not only facilitates decision making regarding the timing and appropriateness of the planned procedure but also may direct interventions designed to attenuate risk.[14] One such intervention with a documented benefit for reducing cardiac complications in

Angiographic Classification of Coronary Artery Disease, According to Clinical Indications

| Finding | Clinical Coronary Disease | | | |
| | No Indication | | Suspected | |
	No.	%	No.	%
Normal coronary arteries	64	14	21	4
Mild-to-moderate CAD	218	49	99	18
Advanced but compensated CAD	97	22	192	34
Severe, correctable CAD	63	14	188	34
Severe, inoperable CAD	4	1	54	10

CAD, coronary artery disease.
Adapted from Hertzer NR, Beven EG, Young JR, et al: *Ann Surg* 199:223, 1984.

high-risk patients is the use of medications that block β-adrenergic receptors.[19,22,23] In a randomized, multicenter trial, Poldermans et al demonstrated a decreased incidence of nonfatal myocardial infarction and death from cardiac causes within 30 days of major vascular surgery in patients identified preoperatively as at high risk who were then treated with perioperative bisoprolol.[19] In a related study by the same investigators, patients undergoing vascular surgery who received β-blockers had a significantly reduced risk of cardiac death or myocardial infarction compared with those not taking such medication.[22] This finding was particularly notable given the fact that patients taking β-blockers had a considerably worse overall risk profile than those not taking them (see Chapters 2 and 6).

In addition to cardiovascular disease, patients presenting for vascular surgery have a high incidence of associated comorbidities including tobacco abuse with concomitant chronic obstructive pulmonary disease and diabetes mellitus with or without renal insufficiency. Given the progressive nature of most vascular pathology, many patients are also elderly. There is, in fact, evidence to suggest that the average age of the patient coming to surgery is increasing over time.[24] Maximum organ function declines progressively from about age 35, although the rate of decline varies depending upon the individuals and their lifestyle.[25] It is important to appreciate that a decline in organ function in elderly people may not be apparent during the preoperative evaluation and may be manifest only with the added stresses of the perioperative period. Numerous authors have reported worse outcomes following major surgery in the elderly population.[14,22,26-29]

There is some evidence to suggest that surgical mortality associated with many procedures, including aortic surgery, has declined over time.[24,30] Using a statewide database, Katz et al performed a mortality rate analysis on all patients with a primary diagnosis of AAA who underwent repair from 1980 to 1990 in Michigan.[24] Hospital mortality rates for nonruptured AAA decreased from 13.6% in 1980 to 5.6% in 1990 ($p \leq 0.001$). The authors noted that improvement in survival rates was associated with an overall increase in surgical volume and a decrease in the number of hospitals performing the surgery.[24] This finding is consistent with the growing body of evidence that suggests that operative mortality rates for select surgical procedures are inversely related to the number of such procedures performed at any given hospital per year.[31,32] That is, for certain diagnoses or procedures, lower mortality rates are seen at so-called high-volume hospitals than at low-volume hospitals. This effect has been specifically shown for elective AAA repair.[31,33] The question to address in the future then becomes whether or not patients identified as at high risk for major vascular surgery should be referred to specialized regional centers. Noninvasive stent graft techniques may further decrease the morbidity and mortality associated with elective AAA repair in the sickest patients. The apparent minimally invasive nature of this endovascular approach has expanded the inclusion criteria for elective AAA repair to patients who were once considered nonsurgical candidates on the basis of their comorbidities. Whether or not the endovascular technique will ultimately result in a decreased incidence of morbidity and mortality for the highest risk patients is unclear at this time.

Anesthetic Techniques for Vascular Surgery: Effects on Outcome

Because vascular surgery patients are at increased risk for perioperative morbidity, they have been aggressively studied to determine the impact of different anesthetic techniques on postoperative outcomes. Many early studies showed that a selected physiologic endpoint such as pain, pulmonary function, or cardiovascular performance could be altered or improved when one particular anesthetic technique was used and compared with another. The appropriate response to these findings was to examine the treatments to determine whether they offered unique clinical benefits unobtainable by any other anesthetic method and to measure the impact of those benefits on outcomes of patients' care. These studies are generally designed to test the impact of regional anesthetic and analgesic techniques on surgical outcomes compared with nonregional techniques. Although investigators have suggested potential benefits from the use of regional techniques for many decades, it was not until the introduction of microprocessor pump technology and the discovery of spinal opioid analgesia as an effective method to control postoperative pain that larger randomized clinical trials were conducted to evaluate the impact of anesthetic techniques on surgical outcomes.[34,35]

The majority of anesthetic "outcome" studies in the 1980s measured the effect of anesthetic techniques on clinical variables during the intra- and early postoperative periods. Studies reported, for example, significant differences in hemodynamic performance during abdominal aortic surgery with some suggestion that regional anesthetic techniques acted to sustain global cardiovascular performance better than a standardized general anesthetic.[36] These investigators documented, not surprisingly, that an epidural local anesthetic block extending into the high thoracic region resulted in lower systemic vascular resistance and higher cardiac outputs during the period of aortic cross-clamping when compared with a routine general anesthetic.[37] The unanswered question was whether these physiologic outcomes would actually minimize cardiac complications and whether or not they could be obtained by other interventions. A considerable body of literature also evolved demonstrating that certain anesthetic techniques, such as regional anesthesia and high-dose opioid anesthesia, could minimize the neural and endocrine responses to major surgery.[38]

Although some practitioners supported the use of regional techniques to minimize this stress response to surgery, it was not clear that limiting the stress response per se would favorably affect surgical recovery. Although these and other studies generally failed to demonstrate a correlation between these intermediate outcomes and measures of the effectiveness of health care, they helped to define an important question in anesthetic practice: "Does the choice of anesthetic technique affect patients' recovery after vascular surgery?"

Three randomized clinical trials have reported data on the impact of anesthetic technique on surgical outcomes in vascular surgical patients. Park et al completed a multicenter trial within the Department of Veterans Affairs Cooperative Study Program to test the influence of epidural anesthesia and postoperative epidural analgesia on the frequency of death and major complications after intra-abdominal surgery including abdominal aortic reconstruction.[39] The comparison control group received general anesthesia and parenteral opioid analgesia after surgery. With 15 participating centers, the study protocols for anesthetic management allowed for variations in local practice patterns, which is one of the study's important design features. The protocol included general anesthesia for all patients, utilizing thiopental and fentanyl during induction, succinylcholine or vecuronium for tracheal intubation, and nitrous oxide and isoflurane for anesthetic maintenance. Criteria for extubation at the end of the procedure included a negative inspiratory pressure greater than 20 cmH_2O and "stable cardiopulmonary status." Patients in the epidural group also received, in addition to general anesthesia, a lumbar or low thoracic epidural anesthetic using 0.5% bupivacaine with epinephrine to achieve a sensory level to T6. The epidural catheter was resupplied with a bolus of 5 to 10 mL of the same local anesthetic every 3 to 5 hours. Postoperative analgesia in the control group was provided by either intramuscular or intravenous opioid analgesia (including patient-controlled analgesia [PCA]), and patients in the epidural group received intermittent bolus injections of epidural morphine, 3 to 6 mg, every 12 to 24 hours or as a continuous infusion in some centers. The decision of whether or not to use invasive hemodynamic monitoring was not dictated by study protocol.

The results from this study showed no difference in the primary endpoints in the total population of 1021 patients (Table 9-2). However, in the subgroup of 374 patients undergoing abdominal aortic surgery, there were significant differences

in the number of patients with one or more primary endpoints (Table 9-3). This was true for major cardiovascular complications, especially new myocardial infarctions after surgery, and for total pulmonary complications, especially prolonged mechanical ventilation and pneumonia. In both the total study group and the subgroup of vascular surgical patients, postoperative pain control was significantly better in patients receiving regional analgesia, with less use of parenteral opioids (Table 9-4). There was also a decrease in the duration of mechanical ventilation in the patients receiving regional anesthesia and analgesia. Mortality and length of hospital stay were not significantly different between study groups in either the total population of patients or the subgroup of patients undergoing abdominal aortic surgery. These data document that, under the conditions of this study and during the time in which the study was conducted, there was a benefit to be achieved with the use of regional techniques because of better pain relief with less opioid use, a shorter duration of mechanical ventilation, and, in the abdominal aortic surgery subgroup, fewer total cardiopulmonary complications.

Some details of the Veterans Affairs study protocol are important. First, the study included only patients in American Society of Anesthesiologists (ASA) class III or IV undergoing major intra-abdominal surgery; thus, the investigators were interested in outcomes for relatively high-risk patients undergoing high-risk surgery. Second, patients were prospectively stratified by type of surgery, and all postrandomization measures of surgical difficulty were similar between the two study groups. Third, the study was conducted during a period of

---

TABLE 9-3

Primary and Secondary Endpoint Variables for 30 Days after Operation

Primary Endpoints	Abdominal Aortic Surgery		
	Group 1 GA	Group 2 RSGA	p Value
Total number	190	184	
Patients with one or more primary endpoints	70	40	<0.01
Deaths	5	4	0.96
Major cardiovascular complications	34	18	0.03
New myocardial infarction	15	5	0.05
Major pulmonary complications	55	26	<0.01

GA, general anesthesia; RSGA, regional supplemented general anesthesia.
Adapted from Park W, Thompson J, Lee K: *Ann Surg* 234:560, 2001.

TABLE 9-2

Primary and Secondary Endpoint Variables for 30 Days after Operation

Primary Endpoints	Group 1 GA	Group 2 RSGA	p Value
Total number	507	514	
Patients with one or more primary endpoints	111	91	0.11
Deaths	17	20	0.74
Major cardiovascular complications	57	44	0.18
Major pulmonary complications	73	51	0.06
Patients with one or more secondary endpoints	88	76	0.30

GA, general anesthesia; RSGA, regional supplemented general anesthesia.
Adapted from Park W, Thompson J, Lee K: *Ann Surg* 234:560, 2001.

TABLE 9-4

Ancillary Variables

Variable	Total Patients		
	Group 1 GA	Group 2 RSGA	p Value
Number of patients	507	514	
Postoperative pain scores (SD)			
Day 1	4.6 (2.5)	3.8 (2.6)	<0.01
Day 3	3.4 (2.3)	3.1 (2.2)	0.03
Day 7	2.4 (2.2)	2.1 (2.1)	0.03

GA, general anesthesia; RSGA, regional supplemented general anesthesia.
Adapted from Park W, Thompson J, Lee K: *Ann Surg* 234:560, 2001.

transition in opioid analgesia techniques; some patients received intramuscular opioid analgesia and some received intravenous PCA. Fourth, there was no study protocol directing perioperative hemodynamic management. Although many patients were managed with systemic arterial, central venous, and pulmonary artery catheters, there was no uniform approach to monitoring and management of cardiovascular performance. Although these data demonstrate a clinical benefit from the use of regional techniques during and after major vascular surgery under the study conditions noted, a similar study published at approximately the same time reported conflicting results.

Norris and Beattie and colleagues reported their results from a single-center study to test the hypothesis that regional anesthesia and/or analgesia could improve recovery from abdominal aortic surgery as assessed by length of hospital stay, resource utilization, and mortality.[40] This study is unique because it used a randomized, double-blind 2 × 2 factorial design to test the independent effects of epidural anesthesia versus general anesthesia and of epidural analgesia versus systemic opioid analgesia or combinations of both on indices of surgical outcome (Figure 9-1). The study is notable for several other design features. First, treatment interventions were

masked; this meant that some patients would receive epidural catheters that were infused only with a saline placebo. Nonepidural treatments (intravenous opioid analgesia) were also administered as masked injections of opioid analgesics. Second, patients were not randomly assigned until after the insertion of a T8-9 or T10-11 epidural catheter and after the catheter had been tested and documented to be functioning. Third, the study included well-developed protocols for management of hemodynamics, fluid administration, hemoglobin concentrations, and postoperative pain control. Fourth, all patients underwent continuous electrocardiographic monitoring for myocardial ischemia beginning the morning of or the night before surgery and, in addition, they all underwent intra-arterial and pulmonary artery catheterization for hemodynamic monitoring. Fifth, all patients were managed with a period of postoperative mechanical ventilation in the intensive care unit after receiving 250 μg of fentanyl and 5 mg of midazolam at the end of surgery. Finally, the study utilized hospital length of stay as its measure of "important health outcomes." Data collection was thorough and complete.

The study was initially powered to study 204 patients to detect a hypothesized 20% decrement in the expected hospital length of stay, or a 2.5-day decrease. The study was terminated after 168 patients had been enrolled on the advice of the Data Monitoring Committee because there was no suggestion of an improvement in surgical outcomes with the use of either regional anesthetic or analgesic techniques. This was true for both the intraoperative measurements (Table 9-5) and postoperative events (Table 9-6). Although patients who received epidural analgesia after surgery were extubated significantly earlier than control patients who did not receive this intervention, there was no suggestion that this earlier extubation had a favorable impact on pulmonary morbidity or other major outcomes after surgery. Similarly, there were no differences in direct medical costs. The results of this excellent study should focus attention on the importance of *perioperative* anesthetic management as a potential determinant of surgical outcomes because the number of adverse events recorded in this study for all groups was small and it seems likely that, in fact, these results were produced, at least in part, by the aggressive treatment protocols that were used during and after surgery. The

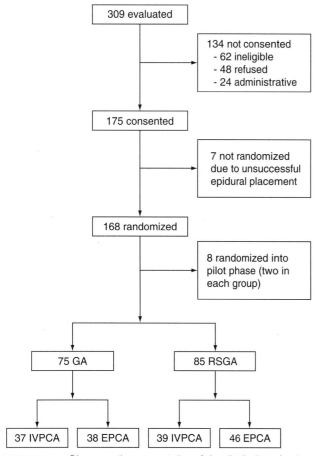

FIGURE 9-1 Diagrammatic representation of the distribution of patients. EPCA, epidural patient-controlled analgesia; GA, general anesthesia; IVPCA, intravenous patient-controlled analgesia; RSGA, regional supplemented general anesthesia. (From Norris E, Beattie C, Perler B, et al: *Anesthesiology* 95:1054, 2001.)

TABLE 9-5

Intraoperative Data by Anesthesia Treatment for Patients Surviving to Discharge

Observation	GA	RSGA	*p* Value
No. of patients	71	80	
Mean arterial blood pressure limits			
Maximum (mmHg)	111 (9.8)	113 (7.2)	0.402
Minimum (mmHg)	81 (9.8)	80 (6.5)	0.686
Fluids			
PRBCs (units)	2.0 (1.5)	2.0 (2.2)	0.179
Crystalloid (mL/hr)	1037 (272)	1045 (313)	0.406
Urine output (mL/hr)	99 (63)	101 (73)	0.391

Values are mean (SD).
GA, general anesthesia; PRBCs, packed red blood cells; RSGA, regional supplemented general anesthesia.
Adapted from Norris E, Beattie C, Perler B, et al: *Anesthesiology* 95:1054, 2001.

TABLE 9-6

Postoperative Data by Treatment Assignment for Patients Surviving to Discharge

Observation	GA-IVPCA	RSGA-IVPCA	GA-EPCA	RSGA-EPCA	p Value
No. of patients	35	36	36	44	
Hours to					
Extubation	19 (7)	19 (10)	16 (6)	13 (8)	0.010
ICU discharge	46 (9)	43 (29)	43 (29)	43 (17)	0.424
PCA discontinuation	81 (13)	78 (14)	78 (16)	79 (13)	0.523

Values are median ($SD_{resistant}$).

GA-IVPCA, general anesthesia and intravenous patient-controlled analgesia; RSGA-IVPCA, regional supplemented general anesthesia and intravenous patient-controlled analgesia; GA-EPCA, general anesthesia and epidural patient-controlled analgesia; RSGA-EPCA, regional supplemented general anesthesia and epidural patient-controlled analgesia; ICU, intensive care unit.

Adapted from Norris E, Beattie C, Perler B, et al: *Anesthesiology* 95:1054, 2001.

question posed in this study—"Does choice of anesthetic techniques per se influence postoperative outcomes?"—was answered by data showing that aggressive and sustained control of physiologic variables throughout the perioperative period keeps morbidity low independent of the anesthetic technique that is chosen. Interestingly, the length of hospital stay, based on a review of historical controls prior to the onset of the study, was 12.5 days. At the end of the study, however, the mean length of stay for all patients had decreased from 12.5 to 8.8 days because of (according to the authors) either increasing cost control measures, improved care with fewer complications, or both.

The third outcome study from which results have been reported was designed to test the effect of anesthetic technique on surgical outcomes in high-risk surgical patients.[41,42] The Multicenter Australian Study of Epidural Anesthesia and Analgesia in Major Surgery (MASTER trial) enrolled 915 patients randomly assigned (at 25 sites in six countries) to receive either regional anesthesia and analgesia or general anesthesia and opiate analgesia during and after "high-risk" surgical procedures including 170 abdominal aortic procedures. Because this was a multicenter study, the treatment protocols were not as tightly defined as they were in the study by Norris et al. The study was powered to measure a reduction in the postoperative complication rate (mortality plus major morbidity) from 50% to 40%. The results (Table 9-7) showed that the total morbidity and mortality rates were not significantly

different between the two groups. However, the incidence of respiratory failure was again significantly less in the group receiving regional anesthesia-analgesia and pain control was also better in this group on the first 3 postoperative days.

Overall, the results from these three large and well-planned studies suggest that the most successful approach for the minimization of morbidity and improvement of outcomes after major vascular surgery is one that uses aggressive, sustained, and goal-directed protocols to minimize the physiologic disruptions imposed by major vascular surgery. Aggressive and sustained protocols for management of hemodynamics, pain, pulmonary gas exchange, and mobilization after surgery appear to be the most effective intervention to improve results from vascular surgery.[40,43] This approach acknowledges the important concept that vascular surgical patients commonly present for surgery with minimal functional reserves, often arrive on the edge of decompensation, and are able to function only at rest. As a consequence of the minimal reserve of vascular surgery patients, the best perioperative care minimizes perturbations in global organ function. With these data as an introduction, the important effects of different anesthetic techniques on perioperative organ function including the cardiac, pulmonary, neuroendocrine-metabolic, and renal systems are reviewed.

Anesthetic Technique and Cardiovascular Function

Vascular surgery patients have a high incidence of accompanying cardiac disease that is the most common and significant cause of morbidity after vascular surgery. Hertzer et al found that only 8% of patients presenting for vascular surgery had normal coronary arteries; the remainder had varying degrees of CAD (see Table 9-1).[18] Although it is not practical to perform coronary angiography on every patient who presents for peripheral vascular surgery, these data clearly support a high level of suspicion and a low threshold for performance of noninvasive studies to determine perioperative cardiac risk. Guidelines regarding preoperative cardiovascular evaluations before noncardiac surgery have been published[44,45] (see Chapter 5). Because cardiac complications are such a significant determinant of perioperative morbidity, many studies have

TABLE 9-7

Postoperative Outcomes in the Master Trial

Endpoint	Control (n = 441)	Epidural (n = 447)	p Value*
Postoperative death	4.3	5.2	0.67
Respiratory failure	30.2	23.3	0.02
Cardiovascular event	24.0	25.7	0.61
Inflammation/sepsis	46.7	42.7	0.26
At least one morbid endpoint	60.5	56.6	0.26
Death or at least one morbid endpoint	60.7	57.1	0.29

Frequency of Endpoint (%)

*χ^2 test.
Adapted from Rigg J, Jamrozik K, Myles P, et al: *Lancet* 359:1276, 2002.

tested the effect of anesthetic techniques on cardiac performance and complications during and after vascular surgery. These studies must be evaluated carefully because they are a mix of many different trials.

Effects of Anesthetic Technique on Coronary Artery Blood Flow and Distribution

Intravenous anesthetics by themselves have little effect on the coronary vasculature; changes in coronary blood flow during intravenous anesthesia are primarily a function of sympathetic tone and local regulation of coronary vessel diameter. Inhaled anesthetics, particularly isoflurane, can have potent vasodilating effects on the coronary arteries, but this appears to be clinically significant only at relatively high concentrations and in individuals with "steal-prone" coronary anatomy.[46,47] Because neuraxial administration of local anesthetics can inhibit the sympathetic innervation of the heart, this approach has received extensive laboratory and clinical investigation as a possible means to improve coronary circulation. The size of an experimental myocardial infarction can be decreased with a thoracic epidural block. Epicardial ST-segment mapping in anesthetized dogs before and after induction of thoracic epidural block showed that ligation of the left anterior descending coronary artery resulted in measurable ST-segment elevations, which were significantly reduced by a local anesthetic thoracic block.[48] However, all of the beneficial effects of the epidural block could be minimized by restoration of heart rate and blood pressure to control values through phenylephrine infusions and pacing, suggesting that the beneficial effect was due to determinants of myocardial oxygen consumption and not to improvement in coronary blood flow distribution.

Klassen et al conducted a similar study, looking at intramyocardial blood flow distribution with labeled microspheres.[49] In this study, cervical epidural block significantly reduced indices of myocardial oxygen consumption and, following the occlusion of the left coronary artery, caused a favorable redistribution of epicardial-endocardial blood flow toward the at-risk myocardium in the endocardial region. Similar animal data were reported by Davis et al.[50] In humans with severe CAD, high thoracic administration of epidural local anesthetic (T1 to T6) can increase the angiographic diameter of diseased coronary arteries distal to stenotic segments.[51] These patients were all receiving maximum medical therapy, suggesting that, in fact, the sympathetic blockade provided by epidural local anesthetics could have effects that are additive to standard therapy. The same clinical effects have been sustained for months using epidural catheter implantation for infusion of local anesthetics in the treatment of unstable or inoperable angina.[52]

Anesthetic Technique and Determinants of Myocardial Oxygen Consumption

Most of the clinical data that compare the effects of different anesthetic techniques on myocardial oxygen consumption have compared regional anesthesia techniques with general anesthesia. Lunn et al randomly assigned patients undergoing abdominal surgery into two groups, who received a high-dose opiate general anesthetic or a light general anesthetic with lumbar epidural anesthesia.[37] The groups were then further randomly divided into those who received volume loading to maintain

pulmonary capillary wedge pressure 3 to 4 mmHg above baseline or to keep the pulmonary capillary wedge pressure at baseline. Hemodynamic stability was achieved in the epidural anesthesia group only by maintaining pulmonary capillary wedge pressure 3 to 4 mmHg above the baseline value during the intraoperative period (Table 9-8). The importance of maintaining circulatory volume has been shown by looking for myocardial wall motion abnormalities in patients with CAD before and after they received a lumbar epidural anesthetic. One study reported a worsening of preexisting myocardial wall motion abnormalities or new-onset wall motion abnormalities in previously normal segments in a large number of patients.[53] In this study the wall motion abnormalities were coincident with systemic hypotension that followed the onset of the epidural block that was achieved with a bolus injection of 2% lidocaine. Thirty minutes after the lidocaine injection, when the systemic diastolic pressure had decreased to approximately 50 mmHg, the increase in wall motion abnormalities was observed. These data clearly indicate that careful management of loading conditions on the heart during neuraxial blockade is critical for the vascular surgery patient.

There may be important differences with regard to hemodynamic stability between lumbar epidural anesthesia and thoracic epidural anesthesia. In theory, thoracic epidural anesthesia can have favorable effects on sympathetic outflow to the heart and on intramyocardial blood flow distribution as noted earlier. Lumbar epidural anesthesia, with peripheral vasodilatation, clearly lowers the peripheral vascular resistance as well as venous return to the heart. Although this may have a beneficial effect in terms of decreasing myocardial oxygen consumption, coronary perfusion can be severely compromised, as noted previously. In addition, the decrease in venous return to the heart induced by lumbar epidural anesthesia can significantly alter the baroreflex response to hypotension. This effect was clearly demonstrated in a study that tested the heart rate response to changes in blood pressure before and after the initiation of a lumbar epidural block.[54] Lumbar epidural

---

TABLE 9-8

Cardiovascular Responses to Aortic Occlusion during General and Epidural Anesthesia (mean ± SD)

Response by Group	Before Cross-Clamping	After Cross-Clamping Release
BP (mmHg)		
I (LEA + volume)	73 ± 8	74 ± 6
II (LEA)	78 ± 7	50 ± 7*
III (GA + volume)	100 ± 8*	87 ± 8*
IV (GA)	96 ± 9†	78 ± 9†
CO (L/min)		
I (LEA + volume)	4.1 ± 0.6	3.8 ± 0.6
II (LEA)	3.7 ± 0.7	3.4 ± 0.6
III (GA + volume)	3.6 ± 0.6	3.6 ± 0.7
IV (GA)	4.1 ± 0.5	3.6 ± 0.7

*$p < 0.05$ using Student's unpaired t-test when compared to group I values.

†$p < 0.05$ using Student's unpaired t-test when compared to group II values.

GA, general anesthesia; LEA, lumbar epidural anesthesia; volume, pulmonary capillary wedge pressure 3-4 mmHg above baseline.

Adapted from Lunn J, Dannemiller J, Stanley T: *Anesth Analg* 58:372, 1979.

anesthesia enhanced cardiac vagal tone associated with decreases in venous return. Although this could theoretically have a favorable effect on myocardial oxygen consumption, cardiac output could also be impaired with a potential for hemodynamic compromise.

The hemodynamic alterations induced by epidural local anesthetic blockade can be treated with a variety of vasoactive agents. Lundberg et al have studied this in patients undergoing abdominal aortic surgery.[55] Invasive hemodynamic measurements were made before surgery and then the effects of dopamine, phenylephrine, and dobutamine were all tested before and after the initiation of an epidural block. Dopamine, at approximately 4 μg/kg/min, restored hemodynamic indices to near-normal values. Phenylephrine restored the mean arterial pressure, although myocardial contractility, which was depressed with the onset of the block, was not improved with restoration of blood pressure. Dobutamine induced unacceptable increases in heart rate. All of these studies were performed in patients who were not receiving β-blocking agents. The onset of a thoracic epidural block in patients who *are* receiving β-blockers appears to have minimal impact on hemodynamics.[56] A group of patients were studied prior to coronary artery bypass graft surgery, all of whom were receiving β-blocking medications. The injection of 10 mL of 0.5% bupivacaine at the T7 to T9 interspace to achieve a T1 to T12 thoracic sensory block resulted in minimal changes in hemodynamics, although there was a modest decrease in the mean arterial pressure from 84 to 76 mmHg. The subsequent effect of general anesthesia was dependent primarily on the dose of fentanyl that was used to induce general anesthesia, with 35 μg/kg causing far more hemodynamic changes than 5 μg/kg. In patients who receive a spinal subarachnoid block with local anesthetics, hemodynamic changes can be minimized by using a very slow injection of medication and sustained positioning following injection (Figure 9-2).[57]

In summary, the effects of any anesthetic technique on myocardial oxygen consumption are a function of the degree of sympathetic blockade (level of epidural catheter placement, volume and concentration of local anesthetics used, use of β-blocking agents), the preanesthetic volume status of the patient and intravascular volume replacement therapy, concurrent vasoactive medication use, and the ongoing physiologic effects of surgery. The outcome data presented earlier suggest that either a general or a regional anesthetic technique, or both, can be used in patients with cardiac disease and that, in order to minimize cardiac complications, careful and ongoing cardiovascular monitoring and treatment are vital.

Anesthetic Technique and Clinical Cardiac Outcomes

Myocardial ischemia is the most significant risk factor for cardiac complications in the vascular surgical population. Continuous preoperative electrocardiographic monitoring detects an ischemic frequency of approximately 15% to 20% before vascular surgery, with 30% to 50% of patients demonstrating postoperative myocardial ischemia.[58] Allowing for the fact that different electrocardiographic monitoring systems may have slightly different sensitivities for detection of ischemia, it is unclear whether the new onset of myocardial

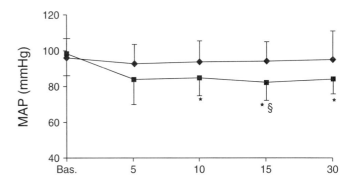

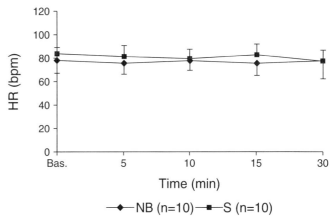

FIGURE 9-2 Changes in mean arterial blood pressure (MAP) and heart rate (HR) recorded before the block (Bas.) and at 5, 10, 15, and 30 minutes after anesthetic injection in patients receiving combined sciatic-femoral nerve block (group NB) and unilateral spinal anesthesia (group S). $*P < 0.05$ vs. Bas.; $\S P < 0.05$ vs. NB. (From Fanelli G, Casati A, Aldegheri G, et al: *Acta Anaesthesiol Scand* 42:80, 1998.)

wall motion abnormalities provides a more specific or sensitive detector of intraoperative myocardial ischemia.[59] Some studies have shown minimal concordance between electrocardiographic evidence of ischemia and ischemia detected by echocardiography.[60,61] Dodds et al studied the incidence of myocardial ischemia during abdominal aortic surgery using both Holter analysis and intermittent transesophageal echocardiographic assessments of the short-axis view of the myocardium.[61] Although intraoperative myocardial ischemia was commonly detected by both methods, there was little concordance between the two modalities (Figure 9-3). Perhaps just as important, hemodynamic measurements were a poor indicator of the onset of myocardial ischemia. There was no hemodynamic measurement that could reliably predict the onset of either electrocardiographic or echocardiographic ischemia. Similar data have been reported from other studies.[62]

Attention to postoperative pain is important. In one study of 100 abdominal aortic surgery patients, investigators tested the effect of intra- and postoperative epidural anesthesia and analgesia on the incidence of perioperative myocardial ischemia.[63] Epidural catheters were placed in the high lumbar or low thoracic region and loaded with 10 to 15 mL of 2% lidocaine with meperidine. All patients then received a general anesthetic,

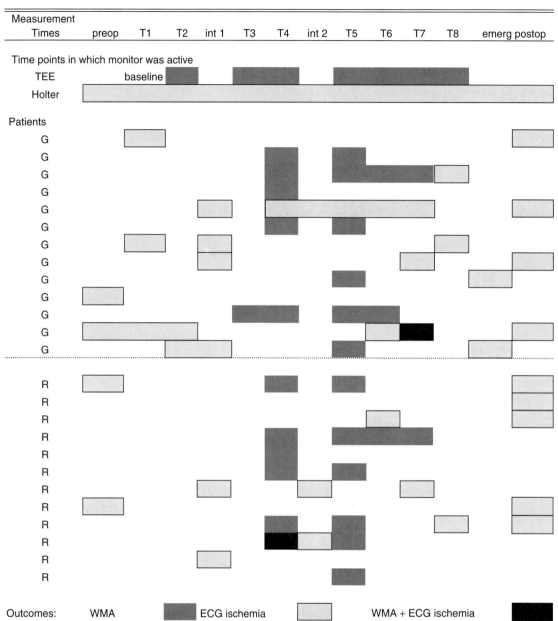

FIGURE 9-3 Temporal occurrence of wall motion abnormalities (WMA) and electrocardiographic (ECG) ischemia. G, general anesthesia; R, regional supplemented general anesthesia. Time points: preop, preoperative; int 1, interval between T2 and T3; int 2, interval between T4 and T5; emerg, 30 minutes after emergence; Postop, balance of 24-hour Holter recording; aortic cross-clamp placed between T3 and T4 and removed after T5. (From Dodds T, Burns A, DeRoo D, et al: *J Cardiothorac Vasc Anesth* 11:129, 1997.)

which included 20 to 30 µg of fentanyl during induction with supplemental doses of intravenous fentanyl in the nonepidural group. Low-dose dopamine was infused in all patients, and all patients received overnight mechanical ventilation. The incidence of ischemia was the same in both groups before, during, and immediately after surgery. However, on the morning of the second postoperative day, when the epidural catheters were removed in the treatment group, there was a marked increase in the number of ischemic events in this group, coincident with increases in heart rate and blood pressure (Table 9-9). Similar results were reported following peripheral vascular surgery

after patients left an intensive care environment when their epidural catheter or PCA opioid analgesia was discontinued.[58] An increase in the incidence of ischemic events has also been shown in the operating room during mesenteric traction coincident with decreases in systemic blood pressure.[63]

Important new clinical information has been published regarding the effect of β-blockade on cardiac outcomes in patients with known or suspected CAD who are undergoing major surgery. Mangano et al studied the effect of intraoperative and early postoperative β-blockade on survival of patients at risk for CAD who were undergoing noncardiac surgery.[64]

TABLE 9-9

Myocardial Ischemia as Detected by Holter Monitoring

Observation	Preoperative	Intraoperative	Day 1	Day 2
Number of events				
GA	6	21	17	26
Epidural	25	34	17	*60
	NS	NS	NS	*p = 0.03

GA, general anesthesia; NS, not significant.
Adapted from Garnett R, MacIntyre A, Lindsay P, et al: *Can J Anaesth* 43:769, 1996.

Patients who received β-blocking drugs during and for several days after surgery had fewer cardiac complications in the hospital and an improved survival rate for up to 2 years after surgery (Figure 9-4). Further investigations by this group showed that the beneficial effects of β-blockade were most likely due to prevention of perioperative myocardial ischemia.[65] Two hundred surgical patients, all at high risk for CAD, were studied during and after major surgery. All patients received general anesthesia and were randomly assigned to receive either atenolol or a placebo in the perioperative period. Ischemic episodes were significantly greater in the placebo-treated group and were associated with a higher mortality rate 2 years after surgery.[65] It is unclear at the moment exactly what aspect of β-blockade confers this apparent beneficial effect, whether it is control of heart rate, alterations of myocardial contractility, or some other effect that is yet to be identified.

The best available data do not support the use of any particular anesthetic technique as long as there is aggressive control of hemodynamics during and after surgery. In this situation, the incidence of myocardial complications appears to be the same with the effective use of either regional or general anesthesia followed by regional or systemic analgesia.

Anesthetic Technique and Perioperative Pulmonary Function

Impaired pulmonary function after major surgery is common. Age itself leads to predictable changes in pulmonary function including a decrease in motor power of the respiratory muscles, a decrease in elastic recoil of lung tissue, diminished compliance of the chest wall, and a decrease in the size in the intervertebral-rib spaces. These changes cause chronic small airway closure in elderly people and create the potential for clinically significant small airway closure after abdominal surgery when closing capacity often becomes greater than functional residual capacity, leading to decreases in arterial oxygenation. Surgery in the abdomen markedly decreases pulmonary function. Forced vital capacity may be reduced to 30% to 40% of preoperative values immediately after surgery and may take 7 to 10 days to return to preoperative values. Functional residual capacity is also reduced within 24 hours of surgery and takes several days to return toward normal. In addition, tidal volume, peak expiratory flow, and pulmonary compliance are all reduced after abdominal surgery.

The cause of these surgery-induced abnormalities is probably multifactorial, as documented by studies investigating the clinical effects of pain, diaphragmatic dysfunction, muscle spasm, and sedative drugs, all of which may adversely affect postoperative pulmonary function.[66,67] Ischemic reperfusion injury after lower extremity revascularization can also impair pulmonary function because of a circulating systemic inflammatory response that injures the pulmonary microcirculation.[68] As a direct consequence of all these events, postoperative pulmonary complications are common after vascular surgery. In a large retrospective review of more than 2500 abdominal surgeries, there was a 12% incidence of pulmonary complications after abdominal aortic surgery.[69] Other investigators have also documented a high incidence of pulmonary complications after abdominal aortic surgery with rates that vary between reporting institutions and depend upon the definitions used for pulmonary complications.[70]

Effect of Anesthetic Technique on Postoperative Lung Function

Although postoperative pulmonary complications are a comparatively uncommon cause of postoperative death, they increase hospital length of stay and resource utilization. Regional anesthetic techniques have been investigated for more than 50 years as a way to diminish the incidence of pulmonary complications in subgroups of high-risk surgical patients. Simpson et al, following the work of Cleland and Bromage, reported that thoracic epidural catheter analgesia after elective abdominal operations led to a decrease in the incidence of respiratory complications.[34] Their technique did not gain widespread acceptance at the time because of the practical difficulty of performing repeated injections of local anesthetic (an average of 18 to 20 injections over 2 to 3 days was required). Many years later, Rawal et al reported similar data on the effects of epidural morphine for postoperative analgesia after upper abdominal surgery in a double-blind study of 30 patients undergoing upper abdominal surgery for morbid obesity.[71] This study was noteworthy because it used a double-blind design to administer either intravenous or epidural morphine, with half of the patients receiving placebo intramuscular injections and half receiving placebo epidural catheter injections. Postoperatively, the peak expiratory flow rate was consistently higher in the group that received epidural morphine than in the group that

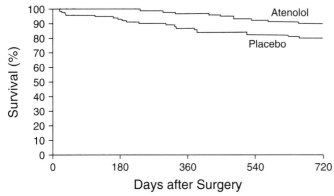

FIGURE 9-4 The rate of survival at 6 months (180 days) was 100% in the atenolol group and 92% in the placebo group (P < 0.001); at 1 year (360 days), the rates were 97% and 86%, respectively (P = 0.005), and at 2 years (720 days), 90% and 79% (P = 0.019). (From Mangano DT, Layug EL, Wallace A, et al: *N Engl J Med* 335:1713, 1996.)

received intramuscular morphine for pain relief. The peak expiratory flow also returned to normal several days earlier in the treatment group. Another important result of this study was that visual analog pain scales were virtually identical in the two groups, documenting that differences in pulmonary function may be present despite a similarity in reported pain perception.

The mechanism(s) by which regional analgesia improves postoperative pulmonary function was evaluated in vascular patients after abdominal aortic surgery by measuring abdominal excursion and transdiaphragmatic pressures.[72] On the first postoperative day, while patients were receiving systemic opiate analgesia as needed for pain, transdiaphragmatic pressure generated by diaphragmatic excursions was severely reduced, as was the abdominal contribution to tidal volume (Table 9-10). One hour after the epidural injection of 0.5% bupivacaine, both measures of diaphragmatic function were restored to normal or nearly normal in association with a significant improvement in the forced vital capacity. A similar study used intramuscular electrodes implanted on the costal and crural portions of the diaphragm during abdominal aortic surgery to assess muscle contractility after surgery.[73] On the first postoperative day, patients demonstrated an increase in respiratory rate and a decrease in tidal volume as well as a decrease in the contribution of diaphragmatic excursion to tidal volume that was accompanied by a diminution in diaphragmatic electrical activ-

TABLE 9-10

Sequential Changes in Respiratory Variables

Variable	Preoperatively (Control)	Postoperatively Prior to Epidural Injection	1 Hour after Epidural Injection
RR (c/min)	12.9	18.7‡	15.9†,¶
V_T(mL)	531	337‡	464¶
V_{AB}/V_T(%)	69.2	15.2‡	46.2‡,**
Pgas/Pes (%)	50.5	7.4‡	51.7**

RR, respiratory rate; V_T, tidal volume; V_{AB}/V_T, abdominal contribution to tidal volume; Pgas/Pes, change of gastric to esophageal pressure.
$*P < 0.05$; $†P < 0.01$; $‡P < 0.001$ vs. control; $§P < 0.05$; $¶P < 0.01$; $**P < 0.001$ vs. prior to epidural injection.
Adapted from Mankikian B, Cantineau J, Bertrand M, et al: Anesthesiology 68:379, 1988.

ity. Electromyograms of the diaphragm showed that, even when the patients were receiving systemic opioids as needed for analgesia, the subsequent injection of local anesthetics into a thoracic epidural catheter resulted in significant increases in diaphragmatic contraction and electromyogram activity (Figure 9-5). Abdominal aortic surgery, therefore, impairs diaphragmatic activity without impairing diaphragmatic contractility, presumably through a reflex arc that arises in the viscera, muscles, or chest wall and is mediated by phrenic, vagal, or

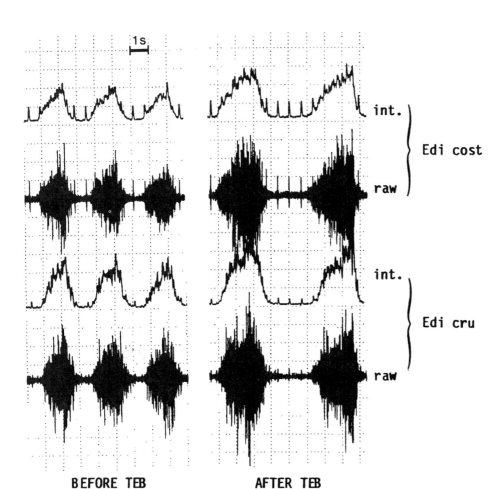

FIGURE 9-5 Effects of thoracic extradural block (TEB) on raw (raw) and integrated (int) electromyogram of costal (Edi cost) and crural (Edi cru) parts of the diaphragm after upper abdominal surgery, before and after TEB. The increase in diaphragmatic electromyogram is associated with a decrease in respiratory rate. (From Pansard J, Mankikian B, Bertrand M, et al: Anesthesiology 78:63, 1993.)

sympathetic pathways. Limiting the clinical effects of this reflex arc represents a relatively unique mechanism by which regional analgesia, compared with systemic opiate analgesia, can improve postoperative pulmonary function.

In order to test whether regional anesthetic techniques impair pulmonary mechanics in patients with severe lung disease, the effect of thoracic epidural bupivacaine (10 to 12 mL of 0.25%) on pulmonary function was evaluated in patients with severe chronic obstructive pulmonary disease (forced expiratory volume in 1 second [FEV_1] of 40% of predicted or less).[74] Thoracic epidural bupivacaine caused a modest increase in minute ventilation as a consequence of increased tidal volume, but no other significant changes in any measure of pulmonary function were observed. A similar study involving high thoracic epidural anesthesia (C4 to T8) using higher concentrations of bupivacaine (0.375%) in patients with chronic pulmonary disease prior to surgery found that high thoracic epidural anesthesia decreased FEV_1 modestly from 1.23 to 1.12 L with no other significant changes in pulmonary function noted.[75] These studies document that, even in patients with severe chronic lung disease, the use of neuraxial local anesthetic blockade with potential inhibition of pulmonary sympathetic fibers and/or paralysis of intercostal muscles does not significantly impair pulmonary function.

Anesthetic Technique and Postoperative Pulmonary Complications

Although significant improvements in pulmonary function have been repeatedly shown with the use of postoperative regional analgesia, these are "intermediate" outcome data that may not correlate with the incidence of postoperative pulmonary complications.[76,77] Studies that measure the potential impact of regional anesthetic and analgesic techniques on postoperative pulmonary complications have appeared in the literature with inconsistent results. Some researchers have suggested that the use of regional analgesic techniques can decrease the incidence of postoperative pulmonary complications in high-risk surgical patients.[77] These results are not uniformly supported by other studies. One possible explanation is that many patients in noncorroborative studies were relatively healthy compared with the high-risk patients studied in other investigations and, therefore, experienced a relatively low incidence of preoperative pulmonary dysfunction.[78,79]

A meta-analysis of the comparative effects of postoperative analgesic treatments on pulmonary outcomes found that epidural opioids decreased the risk of atelectasis after surgery and had a weak tendency to reduce the incidence of pulmonary infections and complications.[77] Epidural local anesthetics had a stronger effect and decreased the incidence of pulmonary infections and complications overall when compared with systemic opioids. These results are similar to those from another meta-analysis in which the investigators reported that the risk of pneumonia or respiratory depression was significantly reduced in a group of patients receiving any neuraxial medication (4871 patients) compared with patients who did not receive neuraxial medication (4688 patients).[80]

The use of routine mechanical ventilation in the first hours after abdominal aortic surgery has been reported by several investigators who noted very low rates of complications.[40,69]

This finding suggests that routine postoperative mechanical ventilation may be beneficial for patients having major vascular surgery. Pronovost et al evaluated the outcome after abdominal aortic surgery in the state of Maryland over a 2-year period to identify the characteristics of patients' management that were associated with adverse outcomes.[69] One of the findings of this study was that extubation of patients in the operating room was associated with a significant increase in resource use after surgery. After adjusting for patients' characteristics and hospital and surgeon volumes, the authors reported that extubation in the operating room was associated with significantly increased risk of reintubation and postoperative pulmonary complications. Although some studies have found no benefit from delayed endotracheal extubation after abdominal aortic surgery, a number of centers reporting excellent results after major vascular surgery all use postoperative mechanical ventilation for a brief period in an intensive care unit environment.[40,81,82]

Anesthetic Technique and the Neuroendocrine-Inflammatory Response to Surgery

With new technologies available to support cardiovascular, pulmonary, and renal functions, it has become increasingly clear that future advances in the care of surgical patients will require a greater understanding of the neuroendocrine, metabolic, and inflammatory consequences of traumatic injury. Clinical studies of the stress response have been conducted for well over a century with a recent upsurge in interest related to the availability of sophisticated techniques for testing cellular and molecular responses to injury. Some excellent reviews of this subject are available.[8,83] With specific reference to the vascular surgical population, three important effects of a systemic stress response arise during and after surgery: the effect of stress hormones on cardiovascular function and morbidity, a prolonged catabolic response that delays recovery because of muscle weakness and impaired immunity, and the initiation of a systemic inflammatory response. New data are available regarding interventions that can limit certain stress responses in vascular surgical patients using different anesthetic agents, β-blocking drugs, and α_2-adrenergic agonists.

Clinical investigations of the hormonal influences on cardiovascular responses to major surgery have been ongoing for at least two decades. Very high doses of opioids, for example, can temporarily limit the catecholamine and cortisol responses to coronary artery bypass surgery.[84] Fentanyl can actually decrease circulating levels of epinephrine and norepinephrine even after the onset of surgical trauma and may prevent the usual increase in cortisol (Table 9-11). These data were further developed as a clinical intervention for patients at risk for perioperative cardiovascular complications when researchers showed that intensive postoperative analgesia with systemic opioids could limit the incidence and duration of postoperative myocardial ischemia in coronary artery bypass patients.[85] The apparent site of action for fentanyl-induced inhibition of the pituitary-adrenal response to surgery is at the level of the hypothalamus or higher because it can be overcome by the administration of corticotropin-releasing factor.[86]

TABLE 9-11

Hormonal Responses to Fentanyl-Oxygen Anesthesia and Operation (Mean ± SD)

Compound	Control	Following Intubation	Surgical Stimulation
Epinephrine (pg/mL)	44 ± 12	33 ± 11	29* ± 11
Norepinephrine (pg/mL)	203 ± 27	198 ± 31	158† ± 19
Cortisol (mg/dL)	7.4 ± 0.7	7.2 ± 0.6	5.9* ± 0.5

*$P < 0.05$, †$P < 0.01$, utilizing analysis of variance when compared with control.
Adapted from Stanley T, Berman L, Green O, et al: *Anesthesiology* 53:250, 1980.

Similar stress-reducing effects can be observed during deep inhalation anesthesia, but both opioid and inhalation techniques have practical limitations on their postoperative use whereas regional techniques can be continued during recovery from surgery.[87] A single dose of 6 mg of epidural morphine, for example, was shown to decrease sympathetic nervous system activity and arterial blood pressure after abdominal aortic surgery.[88] In this double-blind study, in which no further epidural medications were administered, treatment and control patients both received the same general anesthetic and the same intravenous opioid analgesia after surgery. Both during and after the operation for up to 24 hours, the mean arterial pressure in the patients receiving epidural morphine was significantly lower than it was in the patients who received a placebo injection of epidural saline. This was coincident with reduced levels of plasma norepinephrine after (but not during) surgery. The diminution in the sympathetic response to surgery was associated with significantly better pain control, greater fluid requirements, and a reduction in the number of patients requiring antihypertensive therapy in the first 24 postoperative hours. These data suggest that one of the mechanisms by which adverse hyperdynamic events are initiated after vascular surgery involves afferent nociceptive signals from the site of surgical trauma ascending through the dorsal spinal cord. Limiting these signals appears to limit sympathetic nervous system activation as reflected by lowered circulating norepinephrine levels. The same results were not observed regarding adrenal release of epinephrine, which is a much more rapidly responding hormone.

A similar study investigated 24 abdominal aortic surgery patients; control patients received 50 to 100 µg/kg of fentanyl as part of a general anesthetic and treatment patients received a light general anesthetic and 2% lidocaine through a lumbar epidural catheter to achieve a T4 sensory level.[89] The investigators measured norepinephrine levels and hemodynamics before and for 10 minutes after placement of the aortic cross-clamp. They found that, in the group that received the high dose of fentanyl, there was a large increase in the norepinephrine levels 15 minutes prior to the placement of the clamp that was accompanied by an increase in epinephrine levels. In the treatment group that received lumbar epidural anesthesia, there was no change in norepinephrine or epinephrine levels before the placement of the clamp, with a modest increase after placement that was significantly less than in the control group. Epinephrine levels did not change in the treatment group. Despite these differences in circulating catecholamines, systemic vascular resistance rose in both groups by 10 minutes after placement of the clamp documenting that other factors, such as placement of the aortic cross-clamp per se, are more important in determining cardiovascular afterload during aortic surgery.

Another important consequence of adrenergic activation during vascular surgery is the effect on coagulation and fibrinolytic activity in the blood after surgery. Hypercoagulability is well described in the vascular surgical population characterized, in part, by an increase in plasma fibrinogen, increased platelet consumption and production, and impaired fibrinolysis with increases in plasminogen activator inhibitor (PAI).[90] These abnormalities often persist for a week or longer. Circulating hormonal response mediators alone appear to have little effect on coagulability. Using a model in which they infused a combination of epinephrine, cortisol, glucagon, angiotensin II, and vasopressin into healthy volunteers, researchers measured changes in plasma coagulability and plasminogen activation during and after a 24-hour infusion of these hormones.[91] Levels of hormones in the volunteer individuals were similar to those observed in postsurgical patients. Although there was a hormone-induced increase in the peripheral platelet count, other measures of coagulation including plasminogen activator, PAI, protein C, platelet function, and fibrinogen were unaffected by the hormone infusion. These data suggest, therefore, that the hypercoagulability that occurs after major surgery is not due solely to release into the circulation of stress hormones but probably involves interactions with inflammatory mediators released from injured tissue and from changes in endothelial cell function that occur as a consequence of trauma and ischemia-reperfusion injuries.

Coagulation changes after vascular surgery may be affected by anesthetic management. Under some circumstances, epidural anesthesia and postoperative epidural analgesia may improve fibrinolysis and decrease the occurrence of postoperative arterial thrombotic events after lower extremity revascularization.[90] Twenty-four hours after surgery, PAI levels were found to be higher in a general anesthesia group than in a regional anesthesia group, while fibrinogen levels were the same in both groups (probably reflecting the response of the liver to circulating cytokines that are released as the consequence of tissue trauma and are unaffected by anesthetic management). PAI levels correlated with the incidence of postoperative thrombotic events (cardiac or vascular graft occlusion), and both general anesthesia and preoperative PAI levels were predictive of postoperative arterial thrombotic complications. Increases in norepinephrine at the time of emergence from anesthesia also correlated with the requirement for a reoperation for graft occlusion, suggesting that control of norepinephrine levels during and immediately after surgery may be an important component of care for these patients.[92] Norepinephrine levels in this study were also correlated with postoperative pain scores. These results are similar to those reported from a mixed population of patients undergoing abdominal and lower extremity vascular surgical procedures.[93] In this study, regional anesthesia and postoperative regional analgesia were associated with fewer thrombotic events after surgery and with a decrease in hypercoagulability as assessed by thromboelastography.

The potential effect of clonidine on the sympathetic response to surgery was tested in a study that used preoperative and postoperative clonidine, sustained at therapeutic concentrations, in patients undergoing major abdominal surgery.[6] Catecholamine levels, especially norepinephrine, were significantly reduced with clonidine for up to 72 hours after surgery, resulting in a reduced frequency of postoperative hypertension. Interestingly, clonidine had no effect on circulating levels of interleukin-6, urine cortisol, or urine nitrogen excretion. The results of this study demonstrate that catecholamine levels can, in fact, be reduced with the use of clonidine, similar to what has been reported with the use of epidural anesthesia.

Metabolic responses to major trauma have received considerable attention lately because they limit recovery by prolonging hospitalization and the return to preoperative functional status. The use of aggressive regional anesthesia and postoperative analgesia after major abdominal surgery may help to limit the protein catabolism that normally occurs after surgery. Carli et al tested the effect of intraoperative epidural anesthesia and continued postoperative analgesia in patients undergoing major abdominal surgery.[94] In this study, nitrogen intake was carefully controlled using a standard diet and intravenous infusions for 6 days before surgery and for 2 days after surgery. Patients in a treatment group received epidural anesthesia during surgery with a T3 to S5 sensory block and postoperative analgesia with 0.25% bupivacaine to achieve a T8 to L5 sensory block for 48 hours. Sustained neuraxial blockade with epidural analgesia maintained and even increased the protein synthetic rate as determined by muscle biopsies 48 hours after surgery. In the control group receiving general anesthesia and opiate analgesia, muscle synthetic rate decreased significantly after surgery. These carefully obtained data demonstrate that aggressive epidural analgesia can minimize protein breakdown and help sustain protein synthesis after major surgery. Future investigations are needed to determine the clinical implications of this finding, especially because many patients in the treatment group had lower extremity neurosensory changes that limited postoperative mobilization.

Regional anesthesia-analgesia has also been reported to help control the inflammatory response to major surgery. The effect of epidural anesthesia and analgesia has been tested in combination with systemic glucocorticoid therapy and indomethacin.[95] Patients in the treatment group received a single dose of methylprednisolone 90 minutes before the induction of anesthesia with postoperative epidural analgesia using a combination of local anesthetic and morphine. Treatment improved postoperative pain and pulmonary function as reflected by peak expiratory flow and also lessened the systemic circulation of interleukin-6 and C-reactive protein after surgery. These investigators also measured collagen turnover and collagen accumulation in the wound and found no evidence that treatment with the single dose of glucocorticoid acted to impair wound healing, although delayed-type hypersensitivity was abolished in the treatment group. The same investigators have shown that this treatment regimen may result in less postoperative fatigue and earlier return of patients to their daily activities.[96]

Anesthetic Technique and Perioperative Renal Function

Acute postoperative renal failure is associated with markedly increased mortality rates in vascular surgical patients.[97] In addition, patients who undergo aortic surgery who have preoperative renal dysfunction are at greater risk for postoperative morbidity and diminished survival, perhaps because infrarenal abdominal aortic reconstruction, by itself, is associated with a decrease in glomerular filtration rate for up to 6 months after surgery.[98] Several investigators have shown that preoperative renal failure is a highly predictive indicator of an adverse event in the postoperative period and is associated with a reduction in survival rate after abdominal aortic surgery.[99-102] The data are less clear in patients undergoing peripheral vascular surgery. Two groups have reported survival rates for patients with preexisting renal failure following peripheral vascular surgery.[103,104] They found that 30-day mortality rates were significantly greater in patients with preexisting renal disease. The median survival was less than 2 years in patients with end-stage renal disease compared with more than 5 years in patients without end-stage renal disease. These results differ from those published by a third group who reported on a subset of patients with end-stage renal disease in a cohort of 622 infrainguinal bypass graft patients.[105] They found that 4-year survival, perioperative mortality, and graft patency rates were similar for patients with normal renal function and those with abnormal renal function. These results are reported from an institution that also reports the use of aggressive hemodynamic monitoring during and after surgery,[43] which may lend support for the use of pulmonary artery catheters in patients at risk for perioperative renal dysfunction.

Specific anesthetic techniques have been studied with regard to their effects on renal function and, in general, they appear to be minimal.[106] Intravenous anesthetics and inhalation anesthetics have relatively modest effects with small reductions in glomerular filtration rate and urine output, which can be largely overcome by preoperative hydration. Although these observed effects may be slightly less with regional anesthesia, the clinical significance of the difference is negligible. Direct anesthetic toxicity of inhaled agents, especially sevoflurane, does not appear to be of any clinical relevance.[107] Anesthesia is more likely to affect renal function through its indirect effects on hemodynamic responses to surgery, sympathetic nervous system activity, release of neurohumoral mediators, and the use of positive-pressure ventilation in patients who require general anesthesia. Mechanical ventilation alters urine volume and natriuresis because of baroreceptor alterations, antidiuretic hormone release, renin and angiotensin activation, and the effects of positive intrathoracic pressure. These effects are of minimal importance in a patient with normal cardiovascular function and normal preoperative renal function.

Although some data support the use of hemodynamic monitoring to maintain optimal volume loading, it seems clear that intraoperative urine output per se has no correlation with postoperative changes in renal function. This relationship was specifically studied in a group of 137 vascular surgery patients and no correlation was found between mean intraoperative urine output and postoperative changes in blood urea nitrogen or creatinine (Figure 9-6).[108] Placement of an aortic cross-clamp, even when below the renal arteries, can have a profound effect on renal blood flow and renal vascular resistance (Table 9-12).[109] Local neural reflexes associated with the placement of an aortic cross-clamp appear to be partly responsible for the changes in renal function that are observed during abdominal aortic surgery.

Other interventions to maintain renal function in the perioperative period have focused on the restoration of renal perfusion and glomerular filtration rate utilizing specific renal vasodilators. Dopamine clearly restores and supports hemodynamic performance in the presence of thoracic epidural anesthesia during abdominal aortic surgery,[55] but the increments in renal perfusion and glomerular filtration rate are modest.[55,110] During aortic cross-clamping, a dopamine infusion can produce significant increases in sodium and potassium clearance as well as urine output, although the long-term benefit, if any, of this intervention remains uncertain. Similar results have been reported for fenoldopam, a selective dopamine agonist.[111-113] When low-dose dopamine was randomly administered to patients following abdominal aortic surgery, there was no benefit in 24-hour creatinine clearance compared with a placebo.[110] Although the data are consistent with regard to the renal vascular effects of dopamine, the maintenance of intravascular volume and cardiac performance is probably more important.

Anesthetic Techniques for Endovascular Repair of the Abdominal Aorta

Parodi and colleagues described the first use of an endoluminal stent graft deployed through the femoral vessels for the management of AAAs.[114] Initial enthusiasm for the minimally invasive treatment encouraged widespread enrollment of patients in clinical trials to evaluate the technique's effectiveness. Since that time there has been a continuous evolution in device technology as well as in the indications for their use. In the early 1990s, endovascular grafts were deployed predominantly in patients who were deemed to be at prohibitively high risk to undergo a conventional open repair on the basis of their medical comorbidities.[115] As surgeons became more familiar with the technique and the design of the device and delivery systems improved, endovascular grafts were increasingly implanted in those who could be considered good surgical candidates. Similarly, the anesthetic technique of choice for these procedures has evolved in concert with surgical advances such that the early series of patients underwent general anesthesia almost exclusively, with later reports describing increasing numbers of patients who were managed with regional or local anesthesia with intravenous sedation (see Chapters 7 and 11).

Endoluminal Grafting Procedure

Understanding the anesthetic considerations for endoluminal grafting of aortic aneurysms is facilitated by a brief description of the procedure itself. The patient is prepared and draped as for an open procedure. Bilateral groin incisions are made, and access to either the femoral or iliac vessels is obtained. A large-bore sheath is then passed into the aorta over a guide wire. An arteriogram is performed to define precisely the anatomy of the aneurysm. The patient is systemically administered heparin, and the endovascular graft device, consisting of a delivery system, the prosthetic graft, and an attachment mechanism, is then advanced over the guide wire and carefully positioned by the use of an image intensifier and repeated injections of intra-arterial radio-opaque contrast material. The delivery system

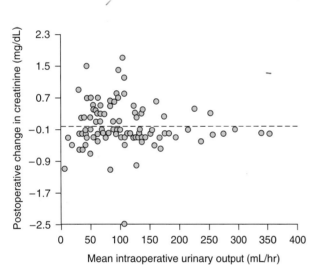

FIGURE 9-6 For 137 patients, no significant correlation ($r = 0.08$) existed between mean intraoperative urinary output and the greatest change in patient's creatinine level on postoperative day 1, 3, or 7. (From Alpert R, Roizen M, Hamilton W, et al: *Surgery* 95:707, 1984.)

TABLE 9-12

Renal Hemodynamic and Functional Changes Produced by Infrarenal Aortic Cross-Clamping and Declamping

Variable	Preclamp	Perclamp	Postclamp
Urinary output (mL/min)	4.45 ± 3.42	3.10 ± 1.58	3.03 ± 1.69
^{51}Cr EDTA clearance (mL/min)	90 ± 27	71 ± 18	71 ± 30
Renal blood flow (mL/min)	1,034 ± 254	622 ± 135[‡]	566 ± 226[‡]
Filtration fraction	0.22 ± 0.06	0.25 ± 0.06	0.27 ± 0.06
Renal vascular resistance (dyn · sec · cm^{-5})	7,901 ± 2,617	13,517 ± 4,144[*]	14,884 ± 6,124[†]

($X \pm SD$, $n = 12$).

Statistical difference from preclamp data: [*]$P < 0.05$, [†]$P < 0.01$, [‡]$P < 0.001$.

Adapted from Gamulin Z, Forster A, Morel D, et al: *Anesthesiology* 61:394, 1984.

is then withdrawn to expose the graft. The details of graft deployment are, to some extent, device specific and differ, in part, with respect to whether the stent is self-expanding or requires balloon expansion in order to affix the graft to the arterial wall. The majority of devices in current use for bifurcated grafts, when necessary, require that the iliac limb be deployed separately via the contralateral leg. After deployment, a completion arteriogram is performed to ensure exclusion of the aneurysm as well as to look for endoleaks. Endoleaks may be due either to incomplete adhesion of the graft to the arterial wall or to continued perfusion and expansion of the aneurysm sac by patent branch arteries. Detection of an endoleak intraoperatively may require further intervention, increasing both the length and complexity of the operation. There is currently considerable debate within the vascular community with regard to the prognostic significance and appropriate management of endoleaks that are discovered or that persist into the postoperative period.[115,116]

Perioperative Issues

Major issues of concern to the anesthesiologist include preparation for an emergent conversion to an open procedure, potentially accompanied by sudden and massive blood loss, the need for an immobile patient to facilitate precise radiographic positioning of the graft, and the significant potential for postoperative impairment of renal function. Conversion to an open procedure may be required at any time because of rupture or dissection of the aneurysm, disruption or trauma to the vasculature by the catheter delivery system, or malposition of the graft such that the renal or mesenteric vessels are occluded. Movement of the patient hinders the surgeon's ability to position the graft reliably for deployment. The surgeon may request that the patient's ventilation be suspended as even diaphragmatic excursion causes motion artifact and can interfere with accurate graft placement. This maneuver is facilitated either by having a patient awake enough to be cooperative or by controlling ventilation during general anesthesia with an endotracheal tube, as opposed to a laryngeal mask airway.

Patients are at risk for renal complications following endovascular AAA repair. The incidence of postoperative renal insufficiency, as defined by an increase in serum creatinine above baseline, was as high as 24% in one series, with no single factor being identified by multivariate analysis as significantly correlating with postoperative renal dysfunction.[117] The etiology is probably multifactorial.[117,118] Patients presenting for vascular surgery often have comorbidities that are associated with renal insufficiency (e.g., hypertension, diabetes). Initial screening and preoperative planning for an endovascular procedure are normally performed with computed tomography, which may be enhanced by a potentially nephrotoxic contrast agent. Intraoperatively, renal function may be further compromised by contrast angiography, thromboembolic events related to catheter manipulation within a diseased aorta, or graft occlusion of the renal arteries.

Anesthetic Techniques

A variety of anesthetic techniques for endovascular AAA repair have been reported in the literature, including local anesthesia with intravenous sedation, general anesthesia, combined spinal-epidural, combined epidural–general anesthesia, epidural, and continuous spinal.[118-124] The majority of these reports, however, are limited to case series or retrospective reviews and, therefore, there is little information available regarding the relative benefit of choosing one technique over another. Any attempt to understand the influence of anesthetic technique on outcome after endovascular AAA repair must consider the confounding variables of a surgical learning curve, device-specific complications, and variable populations of patients.

Baker et al retrospectively reviewed the records of 100 patients who underwent endovascular treatment of their aortic aneurysm over a 4-year period, from 1992 to 1996.[118] The authors noted that nearly half of the patients in this series had been refused conventional open treatment of their aneurysm on the basis of perioperative risk. Fifty patients underwent general anesthesia (N_2O, O_2, isoflurane, opioid, relaxant), 41 patients were managed with a combination of general anesthesia and thoracic epidural anesthesia, and 9 patients received lumbar epidural anesthesia with intravenous sedation. The technique employed was at the discretion of the anesthesiologist. Data regarding intraoperative use of invasive monitoring, mannitol, length of procedure, highest perioperative creatinine, and rates of conversion to an open procedure were collected. Main outcome measures included 30-day mortality, acute myocardial infarction or cardiac failure, postoperative respiratory dysfunction, acute renal failure, and the need for additional surgery. Of the 100 cases, there were 6 deaths at 30 days. Fourteen patients required an open repair (10 in the first 50 patients treated, 4 in the next 50). Thirty-seven patients experienced a major morbidity, of which respiratory dysfunction was the most common (16 patients). Mortality rate was increased in patients with a documented hemoglobin less than 8 mg/dL (22% vs. 5% in the nonanemic group) and in patients whose procedures took more than 4 hours (15% vs. 3% if it was < 4 hours). Although the authors outline the potential benefits of sympathetic blockade with the use of a thoracic or high lumbar epidural in these patients, no specific data are presented regarding outcome measures with respect to anesthetic technique.

Whether or not regional anesthesia confers a benefit in terms of reduced mortality and morbidity after major vascular surgery remains the subject of considerable debate. One potential advantage of the endovascular approach to aneurysm exclusion is that it expands the anesthetic options to include local anesthesia with conscious sedation. The feasibility of this technique was examined in an observational study over a 14-month period by Henretta et al.[119] Forty-seven patients underwent endovascular repair of infrarenal AAAs with local anesthesia supplemented by intravenous sedation. Thirty-three patients (70%) were classified as ASA III and 30% as ASA IV. Local anesthesia consisted of 10 to 20 mL of 1% lidocaine injected at each groin incision site. Intravenous sedation was described as a titration of midazolam and propofol. Conversion to general anesthesia was required in one patient to facilitate repair of an injured iliac artery. The average time to discharge was 2.13 days. There were no deaths and no cardiopulmonary morbidity reported in the 30-day perioperative period. The authors attributed this favorable outcome largely to the decreased physiologic stress associated with endovascular as opposed to open AAA repair. They argued further that their results testify to the safety of performing this procedure under local anesthesia. Whether that conclusion is supported by these data is limited by the fact that neither titration endpoints nor depth of sedation was defined. In fact, the authors noted that only one quarter of the patients were awake enough to be cooperative during the entire case. Further, three patients required an oral airway or "other airway protectant." It should be recognized that sedation represents a continuum. At the far end of the spectrum, the distinction between "deep" sedation and general anesthesia may be blurred.

In an initial attempt to compare two different anesthetic techniques, Cao et al reported on their experience with 119 patients who underwent elective endovascular AAA repair over an 18-month period ending in 1998.[123] The authors' intent was to evaluate whether epidural anesthesia was a feasible technique for this procedure and to compare it with general anesthesia in terms of mortality, morbidity, and technical outcome. Four patients (3%) required immediate conversion to an open repair and were excluded from the analysis. The first 15 patients represented the surgical learning curve for the specific device used during the study. These patients were offered only general anesthesia. The subsequent group of 100 patients underwent either lumbar epidural anesthesia with intravenous sedation or general endotracheal anesthesia (fentanyl, nitrous oxide, sevoflurane, vecuronium) based on the patient's or anesthesiologist's preference.

Data regarding intraoperative events (e.g., operating time, blood loss, amount of contrast material used) as well as perioperative variables (e.g., length of stay, incidence of complications) were collected and analyzed on the basis of intention to treat as well as by type of anesthesia actually received. In addition, the authors hypothesized that a patient with an epidural who was able to move on the operating table may compromise precise graft deployment. Therefore, the incidences of immediate graft-related endoleaks and technical complications were also compared between the two groups. Sixty-one patients (54%) underwent the procedure with epidural anesthesia; 54 patients (46%) had general anesthesia. There were no differences between the groups with respect to demographics or medical comorbidities. Fifteen percent of the patients in each group were classified as ASA IV. Conversion from epidural to general anesthesia was required in 3 of the 61 (5%) patients. Patients' intolerance and anxiety accounted for two cases, insufficient analgesia for the third. There were no differences between the groups with respect to any of the intraoperative variables examined. Technical success as measured by incidence of endoleak was not influenced by having a patient awake during the procedure. More patients who underwent general anesthesia were transferred to the intensive care unit (ICU) postoperatively, although this variable reached statistical significance only in the on-treatment univariate analysis. Further, it should be noted that transfer of a patient to the ICU was a decision left to the discretion of the nonblinded anesthesiologist. Although these data suggest that epidural anesthesia is a satisfactory technique for endovascular AAA repair, no definitive conclusion can be drawn from this nonrandomized study regarding any advantage over general anesthesia.

The significance of nonrandomization of patients to groups when comparing outcomes between anesthetic techniques is highlighted by a retrospective study by Bettex et al.[120] The authors analyzed 91 consecutive patients, both elective and emergent, undergoing endovascular AAA repair under local anesthesia, epidural anesthesia, or general anesthesia. Patients receiving either local or epidural anesthesia were also given midazolam and/or a continuous propofol infusion for sedation. Titration endpoints for sedation were not defined. Allocation to anesthesia type was dependent on site of surgical incision (local for femoral incisions, epidural or general anesthesia for iliac access) and anesthesiologist's preference. Main outcome measures included mortality, major cardiopulmonary morbidity, hemodynamic stability (as inferred from use of vasopressors), and ICU and hospital length of stay. There was a significant size disparity among the three groups; 63 patients (69%) had local-intravenous sedation, 8 (9%) epidural, and 20 (22%) had general anesthesia. No patient experienced a major cardiopulmonary complication, and the 30-day mortality rate was zero. The main finding as reported by the authors was reduced fluid balance and vasopressor requirement in the patients in the local anesthesia group. They concluded that local anesthesia confers an advantage over epidural or general anesthesia because of the hemodynamic stability it provides. On closer examination, however, 6 of the 20 patients included for analysis in the general anesthesia group (30%) represent conversions from local (5 patients) or epidural (1 patient). The majority (four of the six) required conversion because of surgical complications (i.e., bleeding). A further 35% of the general anesthesia group included the first seven patients entered into the cohort, who were considered the surgical learning curve and therefore not appropriate for local-regional anesthesia. A true comparison of local versus general anesthesia will necessitate a randomized trial.

A more important question to ask may be whether mortality and/or the incidence of major morbidity is decreased for patients who undergo endovascular AAA repair instead of a conventional, open repair. Within that framework, it would be advantageous to determine the relative contributions of patients' characteristics and anesthetic technique to outcome. One hypothesis might be that overall rates of mortality and morbidity are not different between the open and endovascular groups but that they are decreased in a subpopulation of older, sicker patients. If that were true, it would have important implications for counseling younger, healthier patients with regard to their surgical options given that the durability of endovascular repair is as yet undetermined and that it requires a lifetime of postoperative radiographic surveillance.[115,125] A further question to answer is whether there is a demonstrable benefit for any particular anesthetic technique within the subgroup of patients who are considered ineligible for conventional repair. Lastly, can a survival benefit be demonstrated for the sickest patients who have an endovascular procedure as opposed to those who have no intervention? Given the fact that the endovascular technique is one that is evolving and long-term follow-up data are not yet available, there is limited evidence from which to draw definitive conclusions regarding any of these questions.

A comparison of cardiac morbidity and mortality in patients undergoing endovascular versus open AAA repair was reported by de Virgilio et al.[126] The authors prospectively studied 83 patients who underwent endovascular AAA and compared their outcomes with those of 63 patients who underwent open repair during the same time period. Data for the open group were reviewed retrospectively. Cardiac risk factors for the two groups were defined using the Eagle criteria (age older than 70 years, diabetes, angina, history of congestive heart failure [CHF], Q wave on electrocardiography, and ventricular arrhythmia requiring therapy).[45] Adverse postoperative cardiac events were defined as Q-wave and non–Q-wave myocardial infarction, CHF, ventricular tachycardia, unstable angina, cardiac arrest, and cardiac death. Endovascular repairs were performed using general anesthesia in 79 patients (95%), local in 3 patients (4%), and epidural in 1 patient (1%). All patients in the open repair group had general anesthesia. Most patients in the endovascular group represented outside referrals for the technique because of either the patient's preference or a perceived increased risk for open repair by the referring physician. They were, as a group, significantly older than those undergoing open repair (73 vs. 68 years, $p = 0.003$); although there was otherwise no difference in risk factors. There was no significant difference between the groups with respect to number of adverse cardiac events (6% endovascular vs. 4% open). A higher mean number of risk factors was associated with an adverse cardiac event rate in both the endovascular and open groups. Within the endovascular but not the open group, patients who suffered an adverse cardiac event were significantly older (82 vs. 72 years, $p = 0.007$). There were six (4.1%) postoperative deaths, three each in the open and endovascular groups. The authors speculated in their discussion that the lack of decreased mortality and morbidity with the less invasive endovascular approach may, in part, be attributable to risk factors not captured by the preoperative criteria or to the "cardiac stress" of general anesthesia. Their approach now is to use local anesthesia for high-risk patients undergoing endovascular repair. Whether this practice change will affect the cardiac event rate remains to be studied.

Romero et al retrospectively reviewed data regarding adverse cardiac event rates following endovascular AAA repair during two consecutive time periods in order to examine the influence of surgical experience on outcome.[127] Adverse events were as defined for the preceding study. The patients were similar in age and number of risk factors across the two time periods. Although not statistically significant, the adverse cardiac event rate was 8.5% in the earlier operations and nearly twice as high (16.5%) in the later group. The authors noted that more patients in the later group underwent operations with local or regional anesthesia (23%) than those in the earlier cohort (1%). In contrast to the opinion expressed by the de Virgilio group, these authors raised the question of whether being awake under regional or local anesthesia is more stressful during this procedure than having general anesthesia.

A direct comparison of cardiac response and the incidence of adverse cardiac events during and after endovascular versus open AAA repair were reported by Cuypers et al.[128] Seventy-six patients considered fit for open repair and with aneurysms suitable for an endovascular approach were randomly assigned in a 3:1 ratio to endovascular (57 patients) or open (19 patients) procedures. Patients' demographics and cardiac risk factors were similar in the two groups. All patients underwent stan-

dardized general endotracheal anesthesia. Signs of myocardial ischemia, as defined by ST-segment changes on the electrocardiogram or new wall motion abnormalities on transesophageal echocardiography, were significantly less frequent in the endovascular group than in the open group. However, the incidence of combined clinical complications (including cardiac death, myocardial infarction, and CHF) did not differ between the two groups (5% after endovascular, 11% after open repair). A similar result was reported by May and colleagues from a prospective nonrandomized study of 303 patients who underwent elective AAA repair over a 4-year period.[129] Conventional open repair was performed in 195 patients; an endovascular approach was used in 108 patients. No difference was found between the perioperative mortality rates for open repair (5.6%) and endovascular repair (5.6%).

The significance of this result is further highlighted by the fact that 48 patients in the endovascular group (44%) were considered unsuitable candidates for conventional surgery on the basis of severe medical comorbidities. Given the advances in surgical technique and perioperative anesthetic management in the last decade, it may be appropriate to reconsider which factors truly indicate that a patient is at too high a risk to undergo open repair. In the patients who are deemed to be at prohibitively high risk to undergo conventional surgery using clinical criteria, there is growing evidence to suggest that their mortality rates following endovascular repair are significantly higher than those of patients who are considered good surgical candidates.[130-132] The risk of endovascular aneurysm repair, therefore, may exceed that of nonoperative management in the patients with the most significant medical comorbidities. To date, there has been no study comparing patients classified as ineligible for conventional surgery who undergo endovascular repair versus unfit patients who are observed without intervention. Using a mathematical model and data from the EUROSTAR group (EUROpean collaborators on Stent-graft Techniques for abdominal aortic Aneurysm Repair), Buth et al concluded that the life expectancy of patients at high surgical risk who are considered for endovascular AAA repair should be greater than 1 year before any realistic gain in life span would be realized.[132]

In summary, the indications for the endovascular stent-graft approach to AAA repair and the long-term durability of this procedure continue to be examined and redefined. In parallel, the optimal anesthetic technique has yet to be determined. Intraoperative goals include preparation for anticipated blood loss, control of patients' movement, and protection of renal function. In good surgical candidates, rates of mortality and morbidity are similar with endovascular and conventional surgical approaches. Future investigations should aim to determine the factors that will prospectively identify patients who are at high risk for a conventional open repair and who would receive the greatest benefit from the endovascular approach.

Complications of Regional Anesthesia

With the possible exception of cervical plexus blockade for carotid endarterectomy, neuraxial anesthesia by a subarachnoid or epidural block is the most common regional anesthetic method performed for major vascular surgery. Complications of neuraxial anesthesia may be attributable to a variety of factors including those related to patients' characteristics, to the technique itself, or to the injected drug. Complications range from transient and mild (e.g., urinary retention, localized back pain, hypotension) to permanent and disabling (i.e., adverse neurologic sequelae). One of the most feared complications of conduction anesthesia is the development of a spinal or epidural hematoma with subsequent spinal cord or nerve root compression resulting in permanent paralysis. Patients whose coagulation status has been altered by medication or their disease process are at risk for the development of spinal hematoma following neuraxial anesthesia. This complication is particularly relevant to the vascular surgical population, in whom perioperative anticoagulation is common. The specific agent used for anticoagulation (e.g., unfractionated versus low-molecular-weight heparin [LMWH]) has important implications for the relative risk of hematoma formation. In addition, increasing numbers of vascular patients are being treated preoperatively with platelet aggregation inhibitors. The safety of neuraxial anesthesia in the presence of these newer agents is not yet defined.

The actual incidence of neurologic dysfunction secondary to bleeding complications associated with neuraxial anesthesia is unknown, although it is rare. Cited estimates for the risk of spinal hematoma following conduction blockade are 1:150,000 after epidural and 1:220,000 after spinal anesthesia.[133] These estimates are based on a statistical analysis of 13 case series including more than 850,000 patients of whom only 3 developed a spinal hematoma. Information regarding specific risk factors, including use of anticoagulants, in these patients is unfortunately unavailable. In a comprehensive review of the literature between 1906 and 1994, Vandermeulen et al found 61 published cases of spinal hematoma associated with spinal ($n = 15$) or epidural ($n = 46$) anesthesia.[134] The use of anticoagulant drugs or the presence of a clotting disorder was identified in 42 (68%) of those cases. Twenty-five had received some form of heparin therapy (18 intravenous, 3 subcutaneous, and 4 low molecular weight). Notably, whether the heparin preceded or followed needle placement was not reported. An additional five patients were presumed to have received systemic heparinization as they were undergoing a major vascular procedure. In nearly half of the 61 cases, the puncture itself was described as difficult, traumatic, or bloody. In 45% of patients with an indwelling epidural catheter, the spinal hematoma occurred immediately after catheter removal, suggesting that this maneuver should be considered as traumatic as needle or catheter placement.

The issue of timing is an important one as several studies involving large numbers of patients have demonstrated that spinal or epidural anesthesia can be safely followed by systemic heparinization.[135-138] Rao and El-Etr prospectively studied more than 4000 patients scheduled for lower extremity vascular surgery under continuous spinal ($n = 847$) or epidural ($n = 3164$) anesthesia.[135] All patients were systemically given heparin approximately 60 minutes following catheter placement. Activated coagulation time was monitored and maintained at twice the baseline value. Postoperatively, patients received low-dose unfractionated heparin. Catheters were removed 24 hours after insertion and 1 hour prior to the next scheduled heparin

maintenance dose. No spinal hematomas were reported. Odoom and Sih described their experience with 950 patients undergoing reconstructive vascular surgery under combined general and epidural anesthesia.[137] In contrast to the Rao study, in addition to the intraoperative anticoagulation, all patients received preoperative oral anticoagulant therapy. Catheters were placed after the induction of general anesthesia and left in place for 48 hours postoperatively. None of the patients developed any neurologic sequelae. In a retrospective study of 912 vascular surgical patients undergoing a continuous epidural anesthetic, Baron et al reported no neurologic complications despite systemic anticoagulation given intraoperatively.[138] Common to these reports are careful selection of patients with exclusion of those who had preexisting coagulopathies, a minimum time interval of 1 hour between needle placement and administration of heparin, close monitoring of heparin effect, and an atraumatic technique with cancellation of surgery if blood is obtained through the needle or catheter.

Despite the large numbers of patients who have undergone regional anesthesia followed by heparinization without hematoma formation, the procedure is still not without risk. Ruff and Dougherty reported seven spinal hematomas in 342 patients (2%) who received heparin following a diagnostic lumbar puncture.[139] Initiation of heparin therapy within 1 hour of needle placement was a significant risk factor for spinal hematoma. Concomitant aspirin therapy and traumatic or bloody taps were also identified as risk factors.

In contrast to the relative safety of spinal-epidural anesthesia followed by unfractionated heparin when appropriate precautions are taken, there have now been more than 50 cases of spinal hematomas reported to the U.S. Food and Drug Administration (FDA) with the concurrent use of LMWH and neuraxial anesthesia or lumbar puncture. Because the events described to the FDA were reported voluntarily from a population of unknown size, the actual frequency of spinal hematomas in patients receiving LMWH while undergoing neuraxial anesthesia is impossible to determine. In fact, two large retrospective reviews have described the safe use of spinal or epidural anesthesia in conjunction with perioperative LMWH thromboprophylaxis.[140,141] It is important to note, however, that more than 90% of the patients in these studies received LMWH on a once-daily dosing schedule as was common in European practice. In 1993, when LMWH was approved for use in the United States 6 years after its introduction in Europe, the recommended dosing regimen was twice daily. Such dosing may provide a greater degree of anticoagulation and not result in the same nadir of heparin effect that would allow safe needle-catheter placement or removal.[141] Based largely on retrospective review of the initial cases reported to the FDA, the risk of hematoma formation is probably further increased by the following: use of indwelling epidural catheters (versus a single-shot epidural or spinal), the concurrent use of other medications known to affect hemostasis (nonsteroidal anti-inflammatory drugs, platelet inhibitors, oral anticoagulants), and traumatic or repeated attempts at epidural catheter placement or spinal puncture. To aid clinicians in their decision making regarding the use of regional anesthesia in the presence of LMWH, the American Society of Regional Anesthesia has published guidelines regarding the timing of needle or catheter placement or removal with respect to LMWH dosing.[142] Recommendations for management should a bloody tap occur are also included.

Antiplatelet agents are commonly prescribed for patients with atherosclerotic disease and recognized for their efficacy in reducing the incidence of cerebrovascular accidents and myocardial infarctions. Further, evidence has suggested that platelet aggregation inhibitors may confer a unique benefit, specifically in patients with peripheral arterial disease. Clopidogrel, a derivative of ticlopidine, has demonstrated an advantage over aspirin in preventing secondary thromboembolic events in patients with peripheral vascular disease.[143] Cilostazol, a platelet aggregation inhibitor with vasodilating activity, has been shown to increase the pain-free walking distance in patients with intermittent claudication.[144,145] Thus, an increasing number of patients presenting for vascular surgery can be expected to be receiving at least one antiplatelet agent.

Whether platelet inhibition contributes to the risk of spinal hematoma following neuraxial anesthesia is not entirely clear. Whereas the combined use of LMWH and platelet inhibitors is a recognized risk for hematoma formation, the use of antiplatelet drugs alone is not thought to represent an increased risk.[146] Horlocker et al prospectively studied 924 orthopedic surgical patients given spinal or epidural anesthesia.[147] Thirty-nine percent of the patients had been taking antiplatelet medications preoperatively, of which aspirin was the most common. No patient developed a spinal hematoma, and the occurrence of blood in the needle or catheter was not increased in the patients receiving antiplatelet therapy. Although the authors concluded that preoperative antiplatelet therapy does not increase the risk of spinal hematoma associated with regional anesthesia, it should be noted that their sample size may be considered too small to detect what is known to be a rare event. Caution is clearly warranted when considering a regional anesthetic for a patient taking multiple antiplatelet drugs or a platelet inhibitor concurrent with another medication known to affect hemostasis.[142,148]

When a patient undergoing major vascular surgery develops a neurologic deficit postoperatively, it is important to consider etiologies other than spinal hematoma secondary to a regional anesthetic. For example, the incidence of paraparesis-paraplegia secondary to spinal cord ischemia after thoracoabdominal aneurysm (TAA) resection has been as high as 16% in one large series.[149] The variable anatomy of the blood supply to the anterior spinal cord in the midthoracic region places this segment in jeopardy during aortic occlusion or as a consequence of hypotension. A variety of strategies have been proposed to protect the spinal cord during TAA repair, many of which focus on the maintenance of spinal cord perfusion pressure.[150] Aortic occlusion increases cerebrospinal fluid pressure and decreases distal aortic systolic pressure, resulting in reduced spinal cord perfusion (see Chapter 11).

Currently, one of the most widely studied and clinically utilized methods of spinal cord protection has been cerebrospinal fluid drainage (CSFD).[151] CSFD is thought to be beneficial by reducing CSF pressure, thereby promoting spinal cord blood flow. Attempts to validate this technique have been limited by nonrandomized studies with disparate aneurysm classifications

and the confounding use of other adjunctive protective strategies.[150] A randomized trial in which patients underwent Crawford type I or II TAA repair with a standardized surgical technique demonstrated a reduced incidence of paraparesis-paraplegia in the group who underwent CSFD (to maintain CSF pressure at or below 10 mmHg) as compared with control subjects (2.7% vs. 12.2%, $p = 0.03$). Future randomized studies are needed to confirm this finding as well as to define the optimal CSF pressure or spinal cord perfusion pressure. With regard to regional anesthesia, it is important to understand that injection of fluid (e.g., local anesthetic) into an epidural catheter raises the CSF pressure.[152] Bolus epidural injections should be avoided if possible during aortic clamping or whenever spinal cord perfusion pressure may be compromised.

Whatever the etiology, it is important to maintain a high index of suspicion for neurologic complications in the postoperative vascular patient who has had a regional anesthetic because the longer the interval between diagnosis of spinal hematoma and surgical decompression, the poorer the prognosis for recovery.[153] Neurologic monitoring in the patient receiving postoperative peridural analgesia is facilitated by using the lowest concentration of local anesthesia that provides pain relief with the least degree of motor blockade. Alternatively, a straight epidural narcotic technique can be employed. Early imaging with magnetic resonance is encouraged in any patient with an unexplained sensory or motor deficit.

Neurologic complications following regional anesthesia for vascular surgery are rare. However, increased risk is associated with heparinization within 1 hour of needle placement or catheter removal, the use of LMWH or multiple concurrent anticoagulants, and traumatic or repeated attempts at spinal injections or epidural catheter placement. The differential diagnosis of paraplegia after thoracoabdominal aortic surgery should include anterior spinal cord ischemia for which CSFD may decrease the risk. Finally, the decision to initiate a regional anesthetic in any given patient should be made only after a careful consideration of the risks and benefits for that particular patient.

REFERENCES

1. Dale W: The beginnings of vascular surgery, *Surgery* 76:849, 1974.
2. Dubost C, Allary M, Oeconomos N: Resection of an aneurysm of the abdominal aorta. Reestablishment of the continuity by a preserved human arterial graft, with result after five months, *Arch Surg* 62:405, 1951.
3. Seller A, Didier E: An anesthetic perspective on vascular surgery of the abdomen, *Surg Clin North Am* 45:881, 1965.
4. Sprung J, Abdelmalak B, Gottlieb A, et al: Analysis of risk factors for myocardial infarction and cardiac mortality after major vascular surgery, *Anesthesiology* 93:129, 2000.
5. Auerbach A, Goldman L: Beta-blockers and reduction of cardiac events in noncardiac surgery: scientific review, *JAMA* 287:1435, 2002.
6. Dorman T, Clarkson K, Rosenfeld B, et al: Effects of clonidine on prolonged postoperative sympathetic response, *Crit Care Med* 25:1147, 1997.
7. Meifsner A, Rolf N, Van Aken H: Thoracic epidural anesthesia and the patient with heart disease: benefits, risks, and controversies, *Anesth Analg* 85:517, 1997.
8. Weissman C: The metabolic response to stress: an overview and update, *Anesthesiology* 73:308, 1990.
9. Kehlet H: Manipulation of the metabolic response in clinical practice, *World J Surg* 24:690, 2000.
10. Breslow M: The role of stress hormones in perioperative myocardial ischemia, *Int Anesthesiol Clin* 30:81, 1992.

11. Liu S, Carpenter R, Neal J: Epidural anesthesia and analgesia—their role in postoperative outcome, *Anesthesiology* 82:1474, 1995.

12. Wu C, Fleisher L: Outcomes research in regional anesthesia and analgesia, *Anesth Analg* 91:1232, 2000.

13. Kehlet H, Holte K: Effect of postoperative analgesia on surgical outcome, *Br J Anaesth* 87:62, 2001.

14. Brady AR, Fowkes FG, Greenhalgh RM, et al: Risk factors for postoperative death following elective surgical repair of abdominal aortic aneurysm: results from the UK Small Aneurysm Trial, *Br J Surg* 87:742, 2000.

15. Mamode N, Scott RN, McLaughlin SC, et al: Perioperative myocardial infarction in peripheral vascular surgery, *Br Med J* 312:1396, 1996.

16. Blankensteijn JD, Lindenburg FP, Van Der Graaf Y, et al: Influence of study design on reported mortality and morbidity rates after abdominal aortic aneurysm repair, *Br J Surg* 85:1624, 1998.

17. Bry JD, Belkin M, O'Donnell TF: An assessment of the positive predictive value and cost-effectiveness of dipyridamole myocardial scintigraphy in patients undergoing vascular surgery, *J Vasc Surg* 19:112, 1994.

18. Hertzer NR, Beven EG, Young JR, et al: Coronary artery disease in peripheral vascular patients. A classification of 1000 coronary angiograms and results of surgical management, *Ann Surg* 199:223, 1984.

19. Poldermans D, Boersma E, Bax JJ, et al: The effect of bisoprolol on perioperative mortality and myocardial infarction in high-risk patients undergoing vascular surgery, *N Engl J Med* 341:1789, 1999.

20. Brown FG, Bolson EL, Dodge HT: Reflex constriction of significant coronary stenosis as a mechanism contributing to ischemic left ventricular dysfunction during isometric exercise, *Circulation* 70:18, 1974.

21. Mock MB, Ringquist I, Fisher LD, et al: Survival of medically treated patients in the coronary artery surgery study (CASS) registry, *Circulation* 66:562, 1982.

22. Boersma E, Poldermans D, Bax JJ, et al: Predictors of cardiac events after major vascular surgery: role of clinical characteristics, dobutamine echocardiography, and beta-blocker therapy, *JAMA* 285:1865, 2001.

23. Mangano DT, Layug EL, Wallace A, et al: Effect of atenolol on mortality and cardiovascular morbidity after noncardiac surgery, *N Engl J Med* 335:1713, 1996.

24. Katz DJ, Stanley JC, Zelenock GB: Operative mortality rates for intact and ruptured abdominal aortic aneurysms in Michigan: an eleven-year statewide experience, *J Vasc Surg* 19:804, 1994.

25. Williams ME: Clinical implications of aging physiology, *Am J Med* 76:1049, 1984.

26. Kazmers A, Perkins AJ, Jacobs LA: Outcomes after abdominal aortic aneurysm repair in those >80 years of age: recent Veterans Affairs experience, *Ann Vasc Surg* 12:106, 1998.

27. Fleisher LA, Eagle KA, Shaffer T, et al: Perioperative and long-term mortality rates after major vascular surgery: the relationship to preoperative testing in the Medicare population, *Anesth Analg* 89:849, 1999.

28. Sprung J, Abdelmalak B, Gottlieb A, et al: Analysis of risk factors for myocardial infarction and cardiac mortality after major vascular surgery, *Anesthesiology* 93:129, 2000.

29. Finlayson EV, Birkmeyer JD: Operative mortality with elective surgery in older adults, *Eff Clin Pract* 4:172, 2001.

30. Ghali WA, Ash AS, Hall RE, et al: Statewide quality improvement initiatives and mortality after cardiac surgery, *JAMA* 277:379, 1997.

31. Birkmeyer JD, Siewers AE, Finlayson EV, et al: Hospital volume and surgical mortality in the United States, *N Engl J Med* 346:1128, 2002.

32. Hannan EL, O'Donnell JF, Kilburn H, et al: Investigation of the relationship between volume and mortality for surgical procedures performed in New York State hospitals, *JAMA* 262:503, 1989.

33. Dudley R, Adams MD, Johansen KL, et al: Selective referral to high-volume hospitals: estimating potentially avoidable deaths, *JAMA* 283:1159, 2000.

34. Simpson B, Parkhouse J, Marshall R, et al: Extradural analgesia and the prevention of postoperative respiratory complications, *Br J Anaesth* 33:628, 1961.

35. Bromage P, Camporesi E, Chestnut D: Epidural narcotics for postoperative analgesia, *Anesth Analg* 59:473, 1980.

36. Reiz S, Peter T, Rais O: Hemodynamic and cardiometabolic effects of infrarenal aortic and common iliac artery declamping in man—an approach to optimal volume loading, *Acta Anaesthesiol Scand* 23:579, 1979.

37. Lunn J, Dannemiller J, Stanley T: Cardiovascular responses to clamping of the aorta during epidural and general anesthesia, *Anesth Analg* 58:372, 1979.

38. Kehlet H: The modifying effect of general and regional anesthesia on the endocrine-metabolic response to surgery, *Reg Anesth* 7(Suppl):S38, 1982.

39. Park W, Thompson J, Lee K: Effect of epidural anesthesia and analgesia on perioperative outcome, *Ann Surg* 234:560, 2001.

40. Norris E, Beattie C, Perler B, et al: Double-masked randomized trial comparing alternate combinations of intraoperative anesthesia and postoperative analgesia in abdominal aortic surgery, *Anesthesiology* 95:1054, 2001.

41. Rigg J, Jamrozik K, Myles P, et al: Design of the Multicenter Australian Study of Epidural Anesthesia and Analgesia in Major Surgery: the MASTER trial, *Control Clin Trials* 21:244, 2000.

42. Rigg J, Jamrozik K, Myles P, et al: Epidural anaesthesia and analgesia and outcome of major surgery: a randomised trial, *Lancet* 359:1276, 2002.

43. Bode R, Lewis K, Zarich S, et al: Cardiac outcome after peripheral vascular surgery—comparison of general and regional anesthesia, *Anesthesiology* 84:3, 1996.

44. Society of Cardiovascular Anesthesiologists: ACC/AHA guideline update for perioperative cardiovascular evaluation for noncardiac surgery—executive summary, *Anesth Analg* 94:1052, 2002.

45. Eagle K, Brundage B, Chaitman B: Guidelines for perioperative cardiovascular evaluation for noncardiac surgery. Report of the American College of Cardiology/American Heart Association Task Force on practice guidelines. Committee on perioperative cardiovascular evaluation for noncardiac surgery, *Circulation* 93:1278, 1996.

46. Slogoff S, Keats A, Dear W, et al: Steal-prone coronary anatomy and myocardial ischemia associated with four primary anesthetic agents in humans, *Anesth Analg* 72:22, 1991.

47. Pulley D, Kirvassilis G, Kelermenos N, et al: Regional and global myocardial circulatory and metabolic effects of isoflurane and halothane in patients with steal-prone coronary anatomy, *Anesthesiology* 75:756, 1991.

48. Vik-Mo H, Ottesen S, Renck H: Cardiac effects of thoracic epidural analgesia before and during acute coronary artery occlusion in open-chest dogs, *Scand J Clin Lab Invest* 38:737, 1978.

49. Klassen GA, Bramwell RS, Bromage PR, Zborowska-Sluis DT: Effect of acute sympathectomy by epidural anesthesia on the canine coronary circulation, *Anesthesiology* 52:8, 1980.

50. Davis RF, DeBoer LWV, Moroko PR: Thoracic epidural anesthesia reduces myocardial infarct size after coronary artery occlusion in dogs, *Anesth Analg* 65:711, 1986.

51. Blomberg S, Emanuelsson H, Kvist H, et al: Effects of thoracic epidural anesthesia on coronary arteries and arterioles in patients with coronary artery disease, *Anesthesiology* 73:840, 1990.

52. Blomberg S: Long-term home self-treatment with high thoracic epidural anesthesia in patients with severe coronary artery disease, *Anesth Analg* 79:413, 1994.

53. Saada M, Duval A, Bonnet F, et al: Abnormalities in myocardial segmental wall motion during lumbar epidural anesthesia, *Anesthesiology* 71:26, 1989.

54. Baron J, Decaux-Jacolot A, Edouard A, et al: Influence of venous return on baroreflex control of heart rate during lumbar epidural anesthesia in humans, *Anesthesiology* 64:188, 1986.

55. Lundberg J, Norgren L, Thomsen D, et al: Hemodynamic effects of dopamine during thoracic epidural analgesia in man, *Anesthesiology* 66:641, 1987.

56. Stenseth R, Berg E, Bejella L, et al: The influence of thoracic epidural analgesia alone and in combination with general anesthesia on cardiovascular function and myocardial metabolism in patients receiving β-adrenergic blockers, *Anesth Analg* 77:463, 1993.

57. Fanelli G, Casati A, Aldegheri G, et al: Cardiovascular effects of two different regional anaesthetic techniques for unilateral leg surgery, *Acta Anaesthesiol Scand* 42:80, 1998.

58. Christopherson R, Beattie C, Frank SM, et al: Perioperative morbidity in patients randomized to epidural or general anesthesia for lower extremity vascular surgery. Perioperative Ischemia Randomized Anesthesia Trial Study Group, *Anesthesiology* 79:422, 1993.

59. Slogoff S, Keats A, David Y, et al: Incidence of perioperative myocardial ischemia detected by different electrocardiographic systems, *Anesthesiology* 73:1074, 1990.

60. Ellis J, Shah M, Briller J, et al: A comparison of methods for the detection of myocardial ischemia during noncardiac surgery: automated ST-segment analysis systems, electrocardiography, and transesophageal echocardiography, *Anesth Analg* 75:764, 1992.

61. Dodds T, Burns A, DeRoo D, et al: Effects of anesthetic technique on myocardial wall motion abnormalities during abdominal aortic surgery, *J Cardiothorac Vasc Anesth* 11:129, 1997.

62. Urban M, Gordon M, Harris S, et al: Intraoperative hemodynamic changes are not good indicators of myocardial ischemia, *Anesth Analg* 76:942, 1993.

63. Garnett R, MacIntyre A, Lindsay P, et al: Perioperative ischaemia in aortic surgery: combined epidural/general anaesthesia and epidural analgesia vs general anaesthesia and iv analgesia, *Can J Anaesth* 43:769, 1996.

64. Mangano D, Layug E, Wallace A, et al: Effect of atenolol on mortality and cardiovascular morbidity after noncardiac surgery. Multicenter study of perioperative ischemia research group, *N Engl J Med* 335:1713, 1996.

65. Wallace A, Layug B, Tateo I, et al: Prophylactic atenolol reduces postoperative myocardial ischemia, *Anesthesiology* 88:7, 1998.

66. Simonneau G, Vivien A, Sartene R, et al: Diaphragm dysfunction induced by upper abdominal surgery. Role of postoperative pain, *Am Rev Respir Dis* 128:899, 1983.

67. Beydon L, Hassapopoulos J, Quera M, et al: Risk factors for oxygen desaturation during sleep, after abdominal surgery, *Br J Anaesth* 69:137, 1992.

68. Groeneveld A, Raijmakers P, Rauwerda J, et al: The inflammatory response to vascular surgery–associated ischaemia and reperfusion in man: effect on postoperative pulmonary function, *Eur J Vasc Endovasc Surg* 14:351, 1997.

69. Pronovost P, Jenckes M, Dorman T, et al: Organizational characteristics of intensive care units related to outcomes of abdominal aortic surgery, *JAMA* 281:1310, 1999.

70. Diehl J, Cali R, Hertzer N, et al: Complications of abdominal aortic reconstruction. An analysis of perioperative risk factors in 557 patients, *Ann Surg* 197:49, 1983.

71. Rawal N, Sjostrand U, Christoffersson E, et al: Comparison of intramuscular and epidural morphine for postoperative analgesia in the grossly obese: influence on postoperative ambulation and pulmonary function, *Anesth Analg* 63:583, 1984.

72. Mankikian B, Cantineau J, Bertrand M, et al: Improvement of diaphragmatic function by a thoracic extradural block after upper abdominal surgery, *Anesthesiology* 68:379, 1988.

73. Pansard J, Mankikian B, Bertrand M, et al: Effects of thoracic extradural block on diaphragmatic electrical activity and contractility after upper abdominal surgery, *Anesthesiology* 78:63, 1993.

74. Gruber E, Tschernko E, Kritzinger M, et al: The effects of thoracic epidural analgesia with bupivacaine 0.25% on ventilatory mechanics in patients with severe chronic obstructive pulmonary disease, *Anesth Analg* 92:1015, 2001.

75. Groeben H, Schäfer B, Pavlakovic G, et al: Lung function under high thoracic segmental epidural anesthesia with ropivacaine or bupivacaine in patients with severe obstructive pulmonary disease undergoing breast surgery, *Anesthesiology* 96:536, 2002.

76. Hendolin H, Lahtinen J, Länsimies E, et al: The effect of thoracic epidural analgesia on respiratory function after cholecystectomy, *Acta Anaesthesiol Scand* 31:645, 1987.

77. Ballantyne J, Carr D, deFerranti S, et al: The comparative effects of postoperative analgesic therapies on pulmonary outcome: cumulative meta-analyses of randomized, controlled trials, *Anesth Analg* 86:598, 1998.

78. Jayr C, Thomas H, Rey A, et al: Postoperative pulmonary complications, *Anesthesiology* 78:666, 1993.

79. Hjortsø NT, Neumann P, Frøsig F, et al: A controlled study on the effect of epidural analgesia with local anaesthetics and morphine on morbidity after abdominal surgery, *Acta Anaesthesiol Scand* 29:790, 1985.

80. Rodgers A, Walker N, Schug S, et al: Reduction of postoperative mortality and morbidity with epidural or spinal anaesthesia: results from overview of randomised trials, *Br Med J* 321:1, 2000.

81. Cohen J, Loewinger J, Hutin K, et al: The safety of immediate extubation after abdominal aortic surgery: a prospective, randomized trial, *Anesth Analg* 93:1546, 2001.

82. Boylan J, Katz J, Kavanagh B, et al: Epidural bupivacaine-morphine analgesia versus patient-controlled analgesia following abdominal aortic surgery, *Anesthesiology* 89:585, 1998.

83. Chrousos G, Gold P: The concepts of stress and stress system disorders. Overview of physical and behavioral homeostasis, *JAMA* 267:1244, 1992.

84. Stanley T, Berman L, Green O, et al: Plasma catecholamine and cortisol responses to fentanyl-oxygen anesthesia for coronary artery operations, *Anesthesiology* 53:250, 1980.

85. Mangano DT, Siliciano D, Hollenberg M, et al: Postoperative myocardial ischemia. Therapeutic trials using intensive analgesia following surgery. The Study of Perioperative Ischemia (SPI) Research Group, *Anesthesiology* 76:342, 1992.

86. Hall G, Lacoumenta S, Hart G, et al: Site of action of fentanyl in inhibiting the pituitary-adrenal response to surgery in man, *Br J Anaesth* 65:251, 1990.

87. Roizen M, Horrigan R, Frazer B: Anesthetic doses blocking adrenergic (stress) and cardiovascular responses to incision—MAC BAR, *Anesthesiology* 54:390, 1981.

88. Breslow M, Jordan D, Christopherson R, et al: Epidural morphine decreases postoperative hypertension by attenuating sympathetic nervous system hyperactivity, *JAMA* 261:3577, 1989.

89. Gold M, DeCrosta D, Rizzuto C, et al: The effect of lumbar epidural and general anesthesia on plasma catecholamines and hemodyamics during abdominal aortic aneurysm repair, *Anesth Analg* 78:225, 1994.

90. Rosenfeld B, Beattie C, Christopherson R, et al: The effects of different anesthetic regimens on fibrinolysis and the development of postoperative arterial thrombosis, *Anesthesiology* 79:435, 1993.

91. Rosenfeld B, Nguyen N, Sung I, et al: Neuroendocrine stress hormones do not recreate the postoperative hypercoagulable state, *Anesth Analg* 86:640, 1998.

92. Parker S, Breslow M, Frank S, et al: Catecholamine and cortisol responses to lower extremity revascularization: correlation with outcome variables, *Crit Care Med* 23:1954, 1995.

93. Tuman KJ, McCarthy RJ, March RJ, et al: Effects of epidural anesthesia and analgesia on coagulation and outcome after major vascular surgery, *Anesth Analg* 73:696, 1991.

94. Carli F, Phil M, Halliday D: Continuous epidural blockade arrests the postoperative decrease in muscle protein fractional synthetic rate in surgical patients, *Anesthesiology* 86:1033, 1997.

95. Schultze S, Andersen J, Overgaard H, et al: Effect of prednisolone on the systemic response and wound healing after colonic surgery, *Arch Surg* 132:129, 1997.

96. Schulze S, Moller W, Bang U, et al: Effect of combined prednisolone, epidural analgesia and indomethacin on pain, systemic response and convalescence after cholecystectomy, *Acta Chir Scand* 156:203, 1990.

97. Braams R, Vossen V, Lisman B, et al: Outcome in patients requiring renal replacement therapy after surgery for ruptured and non-ruptured aneurysm of the abdominal aorta, *Eur J Vasc Endovasc Surg* 18:323, 1999.

98. Awad R, Barham W, Taylor D, et al: The effect of infrarenal aortic reconstruction on glomerular filtration rate and effective renal plasma flow, *Eur J Vasc Surg* 6:362, 1992.

99. LeMaire S, Miller C 3rd, Conklin L, et al: A new predictive model for adverse outcomes after elective thoracoabdominal aortic aneurysm repair, *Ann Thorac Surg* 71:1233, 2001.

100. Moro H, Sugawara M, Shinonaga M, et al: The long-term survival rates of patients after repair of abdominal aortic aneurysms, *Surg Today* 28:1242, 1998.

101. Batt M, Staccini P, Pittaluga P, et al: Late survival after abdominal aortic aneurysm repair, *Eur J Vasc Endovasc Surg* 17:338, 1999.

102. Powell R, Roddy S, Meier G, et al: Effect of renal insufficiency on outcome following infrarenal aortic surgery, *Am J Surg* 174:126, 1997.

103. Gerrard DJ, Ray SA, Barrio EA, et al: Effect of chronic renal failure on mortality rate following arterial reconstruction, *Br J Surg* 89:70, 2002.

104. Redden DN, Marcus RJ, Owen WF Jr, et al: Long-term outcomes of revascularization for peripheral vascular disease in end-stage renal disease patients, *Am J Kidney Dis* 38:57, 2001.

105. Lantis J II, Conte M, Belkin M, et al: Infrainguinal bypass grafting in patients with end-stage renal disease: improving outcomes? *J Vasc Surg* 33:1171, 2001.

106. Burchardi H, Kaczmarczyk G: The effect of anaesthesia on renal function, *Eur J Anaesthesiol* 11:163, 1994.

107. Obata R, Bito H, Ohmura M, et al: The effects of prolonged low-flow sevoflurane anesthesia on renal and hepatic function, *Anesth Analg* 91:1262, 2000.

108. Alpert R, Roizen M, Hamilton W, et al: Intraoperative urinary output does not predict postoperative renal function in patients undergoing abdominal aortic revascularization, *Surgery* 95:707, 1984.

109. Gamulin Z, Forster A, Morel D, et al: Effects of infrarenal aortic cross-clamping on renal hemodynamics in humans, *Anesthesiology* 61:394, 1984.

110. De Lasson L, Hansen H, Juhl B, et al: A randomised, clinical study of the effect of low-dose dopamine on central and renal haemodynamics in infrarenal aortic surgery, *Eur J Vasc Endovasc Surg* 10:82, 1995.

111. Salem M, Crooke J, McLoughlin G, et al: The effect of dopamine on renal function during aortic cross clamping, *Ann R Coll Surg* 70:9, 1988.

112. Gilbert T, Hasnain J, Flinn W, et al: Fenoldopam infusion associated with preserving renal function after aortic cross-clamping for aneurysm repair, *J Cardiovasc Pharmacol* 6:31, 2001.

113. Halpenny M, Rushe C, Breen P, et al: The effects of fenoldopam on renal function in patients undergoing elective aortic surgery, *Eur J Anaesthesiol* 19:32, 2002.

114. Parodi JC, Palmaz JC, Barone hd: Transfemoral intraluminal graft implantation for abdominal aortic aneurysms, *Ann Vasc Surg* 5:491, 1991.

115. Ohki T, Veith FJ, Shaw P, et al: Increasing incidence of midterm and long-term complications after endovascular graft repair of abdominal aortic aneurysms: a note of caution based on a 9-year experience, *Ann Surg* 234:323, 2001.

116. Harris PL, Vallabhaneni SR, Desgranges P, et al: Incidence and risk factors of late rupture, conversion, and death after endovascular repair of infrarenal aortic aneurysms: the EUROSTAR experience, *J Vasc Surg* 32:739, 2000.

117. Carpenter JP, Fairman RM, Barker CF, et al: Endovascular AAA repair in patients with renal insufficiency: strategies for reducing adverse renal events, *Cardiovasc Surg* 9:559, 2001.

118. Baker AB, Lloyd G, Fraser TA, et al: Retrospective review of 100 cases of endoluminal aortic stent-graft surgery from an anesthetic perspective, *Anaesth Intensive Care* 25:378, 1997.

119. Henretta JP, Hodgson KJ, Mattos MA, et al: Feasibility of endovascular repair of abdominal aortic aneurysms with local anesthesia with intravenous sedation, *J Vasc Surg* 29:793, 1999.

120. Bettex DA, Lachat M, Pfammatter T, et al: To compare general, epidural and local anesthesia for endovascular aneurysm repair (EVAR), *Eur J Vasc Endovasc Surg* 21:179, 2001.

121. Greiff JM, Thompson MM, Langham BT: Anaesthetic implications of aortic stent surgery, *Br J Anaesth* 75:779, 1995.

122. Aadahl P, Lundbom J, Hatlinghus S, et al: Regional anesthesia for endovascular treatment of abdominal aortic aneurysms, *J Endovasc Surg* 4:56, 1997.

123. Cao P, Zannetti S, Parlani G, et al: Epidural anesthesia reduces length of hospitalization after endoluminal abdominal aortic aneurysm repair, *J Vasc Surg* 30:651, 1999.

124. Mathes DD, Kern JA: Continuous spinal anesthetic technique for endovascular aortic stent graft surgery, *J Clin Anesth* 12:487, 2000.

125. Carpenter JP, Baum RA, Barker CF, et al: Durability of benefits of endovascular versus conventional abdominal aortic aneurysm repair, *J Vasc Surg* 35:222, 2002.

126. de Virgilio C, Bui H, Donayre C, et al: Endovascular vs open abdominal aortic aneurysm repair: a comparison of cardiac morbidity and mortality, *Arch Surg* 134:947, 1999.

127. Romero L, de Virgilio C, Donayre C, et al: Trends in cardiac morbidity and mortality after endoluminal abdominal aortic aneurysm repair, *Arch Surg* 136:996, 2001.

128. Cuypers PW, Gardien M, Buth J, et al: Randomized study comparing cardiac response in endovascular and open abdominal aortic aneurysm repair, *Br J Surg* 88:1059, 2001.

129. May J, White GH, Yu W, et al: Concurrent comparison of endoluminal versus open repair in the treatment of abdominal aortic aneurysms: analysis of 303 patients by life table method, *J Vasc Surg* 27:213, 1998.

130. Laheij RJ, van Marrewijk CJ: Endovascular stenting of abdominal aortic aneurysm in patients unfit for elective open surgery, *Lancet* 356:832, 2000.

131. Riambau V, Laheij RJ, Garcia-Madrid C, et al: The association between co-morbidity and mortality after abdominal aortic aneurysm endografting in patients ineligible for elective open surgery, *Eur J Endovasc Surg* 22:265, 2001.

132. Buth J, van Marrewijk CJ, Harris PL, et al: Outcome of endovascular abdominal aortic aneurysm repair in patients with conditions considered unfit for an open procedure: a report on the EUROSTAR experience, *J Vasc Surg* 35:211, 2002.

133. Tryba M: Epidural regional anesthesia and low-molecular-weight heparin: Pro (German), *Anasthesiol Intensivmed Notfallmed Schmerzther* 28:179, 1993.

134. Vandermeulen EP, Van Aken H, Vermylen J: Anticoagulants and spinal-epidural anesthesia, *Anesth Analg* 79:1165, 1994.

135. Rao TL, El-Etr AA: Anticoagulation following placement of epidural and subarachnoid catheters: an evaluation of neurologic sequelae, *Anesthesiology* 55:618, 1981.

136. Ellison N, Jobes DR, Schwartz AJ: Implications of anticoagulant therapy, *Int Anesthesiol Clin* 20:121, 1982.

137. Odoom JA, Sih IL: Epidural analgesia and anticoagulant therapy: experience with 1000 cases of continuous epidurals, *Anaesthesia* 38:254, 1983.

138. Baron HC, LaRaja RD, Rossi G, et al: Continuous epidural analgesia in the heparinized vascular patient: a retrospective review of 912 patients, *J Vasc Surg* 6:144, 1987.

139. Ruff RL, Dougherty JH: Complications of lumbar puncture followed by anticoagulation, *Stroke* 12:879, 1981.

140. Bergqvist D, Lindblad B, Matzsch T: Low-molecular-weight heparin for thromboprophylaxis and epidural/spinal anesthesia: is there a risk? *Acta Anaesthesiol Scand* 36:605, 1992.

141. Horlocker TT, Heit JA: Low-molecular-weight heparin: biochemistry, pharmacology, perioperative prophylaxis regimens, and guidelines for regional anesthesia management, *Anesth Analg* 85:874, 1997.

142. ASRA: Recommendations for neuraxial anesthesia and anticoagulation, *http://www.asra.com/consensus/index.shtml*. Accessed October 2, 2001.

143. Gorelick PB, Born GV, D'Agostino RB: Therapeutic benefit. Aspirin revisited in light of the introduction of clopidogrel, *Stroke* 30:1716, 1999.

144. Strandness DE, Dalman RL, Panian S, et al: Effect of cilostazol in patients with intermittent claudication: a randomized, double-blind, placebo-controlled study, *Vasc Endovasc Surg* 36:83, 2002.

145. Regensteiner JG, Hiatt WR: Current medical therapies for patients with peripheral arterial disease: a critical review, *Am J Med* 112:49, 2002.

146. Urmey WF, Rowlingson J: Do antiplatelet agents contribute to the development of perioperative spinal hematoma? *Reg Anesth Pain Med* 23(Suppl 2):146, 1998.

147. Horlocker TT, Wedel DJ, Schroeder DR, et al: Preoperative antiplatelet therapy does not increase the risk of spinal hematoma associated with regional anesthesia, *Anesth Analg* 80:303, 1995.

148. Benzon HT, Wong HY, Siddiqui T, et al: Caution in performing epidural injections in patients on several antiplatelet drugs, *Anesthesiology* 91:1558, 1999.

149. Svensson LG, Crawford ES, Hess KR, et al: Experience with 1509 patients undergoing thoracoabdominal aortic operations, *J Vasc Surg* 17:357, 1993.

150. Ling E, Arellano R: Systematic overview of the evidence supporting the use of cerebrospinal fluid drainage in thoracoabdominal aneurysm surgery for the prevention of paraplegia, *Anesthesiology* 93:1115, 2000.

151. Heller LB, Chaney MM: Paraplegia immediately following removal of a cerebrospinal fluid drainage catheter in a patient after thoracoabdominal aortic aneurysm surgery, *Anesthesiology* 95:1285, 2001.

152. Hilt H, Gramm JH, Link J: Changes in intracranial pressure associated with extradural anaesthesia, *Br J Anaesth* 56:676, 1986.

153. Foo D, Rossier AB: Preoperative neurologic status in predicting surgical outcome of spinal epidural hematomas, *Surg Neurol* 15:389,

Anesthetic Considerations for Carotid Artery Surgery

Christopher J. O'Connor, MD

Kenneth J. Tuman, MD

THE intraoperative management of carotid endarterectomy (CEA) involves several critical goals: (1) prevention and prompt detection of cerebral and myocardial ischemia, (2) maintenance of hemodynamic stability, and (3) rapid recovery from anesthetic drug effects for prompt evaluation of neurologic function. Despite the relatively short duration of the procedure, the minimal amount of tissue destruction and blood loss, and modest anesthetic requirements, CEA can be associated with substantial intraoperative alterations in blood pressure and heart rate. These adverse hemodynamic events must be properly managed to reduce the risk of adverse neurologic and cardiovascular outcome.

Preoperative Considerations

Surgical Indications

Current indications for CEA are based upon prospective randomized trials in symptomatic and asymptomatic patients with carotid artery disease.[1,2] It is well accepted that symptomatic patients (previous transient ischemic attack, reversible ischemic neurologic deficit, or mild stroke within 6 months), with greater than 70% carotid artery stenosis (CAS), are candidates for CEA.[3] In addition, treatment of asymptomatic CAS of 60% or greater with aspirin and CEA reduces the 5-year risk of fatal and nonfatal strokes compared with aspirin alone (Table 10-1).[2]

Preoperative conditions other than angiographic anatomy have not consistently been identified as predictive of adverse outcome in CEA patients. A multicenter review of nearly 700 CEAs found that only angiographic characteristics (ipsilateral carotid occlusion, stenosis near the carotid siphon, or intraluminal thrombosis) and age older than 75 years were predictive of perioperative complications.[4] Another multivariate analysis was unable to identify any predictive association of age, gender, indication for surgery, bilaterality of CAS, hypertension, or smoking with adverse outcome after CEA.[5] In contrast, a larger multicenter study ($n = 1160$) identified several clinical predictors of adverse outcome (cerebrovascular accident [CVA], myocardial infarction [MI], or death) after CEA, including age older than 75 years, symptom status (ipsilateral symptoms versus asymptomatic or nonipsilateral symptoms), severe hypertension (diastolic blood pressure [BP] >110 mmHg), CEA prior to coronary artery bypass graft (CABG) surgery, history of angina, evidence of internal carotid artery thrombus, as well as internal CAS near the carotid siphon.[6] The presence of more than two factors was associated with a twofold increase in adverse events. Data from other series suggest that heart disease (a history of MI, angina, heart failure, or arrhythmia), diabetes, and stroke were significant risk factors for stroke or death within 30 days of CEA.[7]

Preoperative Assessment

Coexistent coronary artery disease (CAD) remains a major cause of morbidity and mortality after CEA, and assessment of the severity of CAD is an important aspect of evaluation before CEA (see Chapter 5). The decision to proceed with preoperative testing to assess cardiac risk should be based on the presence of clinical markers (major, intermediate, or minor predictors), functional capacity, and the surgical procedure–specific cardiac risk (see Table 5-1 in Chapter 5). CEA is typically considered an intermediate-risk procedure and specific preoperative cardiac testing is generally not indicated in this setting in the absence of major clinical predictors of increased cardiac risk (unstable coronary syndromes, such as acute MI [documented MI less than 7 days previously], recent MI [more than 7 days but less than 1 month before surgery], unstable or severe angina, evidence of a large ischemic burden by clinical symptoms or noninvasive testing, decompensated congestive heart failure, significant arrhythmias, or severe valvular disease) (see Table 5-2 in Chapter 5).

Patients with internal CAS often have associated impairment of cerebrovascular reactivity (CVR) and reduced ability to dilate intracerebral arterioles further in response to decreases in cerebral perfusion pressure. Use of transcranial Doppler (TCD) assessment of changes in middle cerebral artery blood

---

TABLE 10-1

Combined Results of Randomized Trials of Carotid Endarterectomy: NASCET, ECST, and VACS

	Risk Ratio	95% Confidence Interval
Stroke	0.56	0.42-0.75
Myocardial infarction	1.00	0.61-1.63
Death	0.75	0.53-1.07
Any event	0.67	0.54-0.83

Data from a comparison and meta-analysis of randomized trials of carotid endarterectomy (CEA) for symptomatic carotid stenosis demonstrate that CEA reduces the stroke rate, the risk of death, and the combined risk of stroke, myocardial infarction, and death combined compared with medical therapy alone. The risk of myocardial infarction was no different between surgical and medical treatment groups.

ECST, European Carotid Surgery Trial; NASCET, North American Symptomatic Carotid Endarterectomy Trial; VACS, Veterans Affairs Cooperative Study.

Data from Goldstein LB, McCrory DC, Landsman PB, et al: *Stroke* 25:1116, 1994.

flow velocity as a marker of CVR has been recommended for prediction of cerebral ischemic risk and to identify asymptomatic patients with CAS who are at greatest stroke risk.[8] Patients with impaired CVR to CO_2 demonstrated by TCD preoperatively have not been shown to have increased risk of cerebral ischemia during CEA, as assessed by somatosensory evoked potential (SSEP) recording.[9] Patients with residual cerebral ischemia after obstructive carotid artery lesions are removed or bypassed may have impaired CVR with an increased risk of stroke, and decreases in BP should be meticulously avoided in such patients.[10]

Although adequate preoperative BP control should logically be associated with decreased incidences of cardiac and neurologic morbidity, there are no conclusive prospective data to confirm that delaying CEA to achieve a certain level of preoperative BP actually reduces morbidity and no data to define how long a period of control might be required to realize such a potential benefit. What is known is that patients with poorly controlled hypertension frequently have labile intraoperative BP and are more likely to have both postoperative hypotension and hypertension. Although not strictly applicable to patients undergoing CEA, prospective data from 2069 CABG patients demonstrated that isolated preoperative systolic hypertension (BP > 140 mmHg) was associated with a 40% increase in the likelihood of cardiovascular morbidity after surgery.[11] Retrospective data indicate that hypertensive patients whose BP is pharmacologically controlled before CEA have a lower incidence of postoperative hypertension (and transient neurologic deficits) than patients with poorly controlled BP (≥170/95 mmHg).[12] Given the known alterations in cerebral blood flow autoregulation with chronic hypertension, BP reductions should be undertaken gradually and complete normalization of BP is probably not required and may even have detrimental effects.

The current American College of Cardiology/American Heart Association (ACC/AHA) guidelines define a systolic BP = 180 mmHg and diastolic BP =110 mmHg as stage 3 hypertension and recommend that patients with these values have BP controlled before surgery.[13] The guidelines indicate that an effective regimen can be achieved over several days to weeks with outpatient preoperative therapy and stress the importance of continuing antihypertensive therapy throughout the perioperative period.[13] It may be difficult to wait this interval of time for BP control when CEA is more urgent because the patient is neurologically symptomatic (e.g., preoperative transient ischemic attacks). BP control is especially critical for patients after CEA, in whom hypertension may exacerbate cerebral hyperperfusion in susceptible patients.

Intraoperative Considerations

The major goals of management for patients undergoing CEA are modulations of risks for myocardial and cerebral ischemia that are amenable to modification. Maintaining adequacy of cerebral perfusion, continual adjustment of cardiovascular parameters, and monitoring the patient appropriately to facilitate prompt intervention to reduce the risk of potential adverse neurologic or cardiovascular events are the essential elements of anesthetic management.

Cerebral Monitoring

A large number of methods are available for intraoperative neurologic monitoring, although no single method is infallible, in large part because of the heterogeneity of the causes of cerebral ischemia and the complex sequelae of cellular events along with the variable location of ischemic insults (i.e., lacunar versus cortical) (Table 10-2). The ideal method of monitoring cerebral perfusion during CEA remains controversial. Available techniques include xenon blood flow, TCD ultrasonography, cerebral oximetry, SSEP, electroencephalography (EEG), and continual clinical neurologic examination during regional anesthesia (RA). The latter two methods are the most commonly utilized and are probably better monitors of the adequacy of cerebral perfusion than carotid stump pressure alone.[14] Although reduced carotid stump pressure is generally associated with a greater risk of ischemic EEG changes, it is generally considered to be neither sufficiently sensitive nor specific to serve as a guide to selective carotid shunting, and it is difficult to define a critical pressure that does not result in an unacceptably high number of false positives or false negatives (Figure 10-1).[15,16] Combining stump pressure measurements with TCD monitoring also fails to improve specificity and positive predictive value.[17]

Neurologic testing during CEA in the awake patient with RA is generally accepted as a sensitive monitor of cerebral function and can reveal clinically significant cerebral ischemia even when sensitive EEG monitoring remains unchanged.[18-20] This situation can potentially occur when the ischemic insult is located within deeper brain structures and when preexisting electrophysiologic abnormalities make it difficult to identify superimposed new abnormalities.[21] Although processed EEG data are more "user friendly," sensitivity is reduced compared with multichannel analog EEG. For example, density spectral array analysis simplifies interpretation of EEG data, but it may not reliably detect mild analog EEG pattern changes of cerebral ischemia.[22] Compressed spectral array analyses of EEG data, especially decreases in the spectral edge frequency, are also less sensitive than the raw EEG data as a marker for ischemia.[23] One observational, noninterventional study collected EEG data during CEA without shunting and documented that 80% of immediate strokes after awakening from general anesthesia (GA) for CEA are associated with severe intraoperative EEG changes.[24] However, no data define how severe or how long intraoperative

---

TABLE 10-2

Intraoperative Monitors of Cerebral Perfusion

Neurologic assessment of awake patient
Assessment of cerebral blood flow
  Stump pressures
  ^{133}Xe washout
  Transcranial Doppler (middle cerebral artery flow)
Cerebral electrical activity
  Electroencephalography ± computer processing
  Somatosensory evoked potentials
Cerebral oxygenation
  Jugular venous oxygen saturation
  Cerebral oximetry

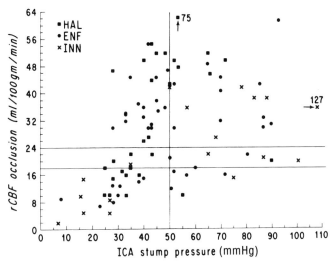

FIGURE 10-1 The poor correlation between stump pressures and radiolabeled xenon–determined cerebral blood flow (rCBF) is clearly demonstrated in this study of a large number of patients undergoing carotid endarterectomy. It is apparent from the figure that stump pressures below the "critical" value of 50 mmHg are frequently associated with adequate cerebral blood flow, and stump pressures considered "safe" (i.e., >50 mmHg) may be seen with low cerebral blood flow. HAL, halothane; ENF, enflurane; INN, isoflurane. (From McKay RD, Sundt TM, Michenfelder JD, et al: *Anesthesiology* 45:390, 1976.)

EEG changes must persist to be predictive of stroke after CEA, nor are there prospective data to define whether the EEG is decisively better than alternative methods of assessing the adequacy of cerebral perfusion.

TCD ultrasonography applied across the relatively thin temporal bone allows continuous measurement of blood flow velocity in the middle cerebral artery distribution and may be helpful in distinguishing between intraoperative hemodynamic versus embolic neurologic events (Figure 10-2).[25] Failure to obtain interpretable TCD signals occurs in 15% to 20% of cases because of temporal hyperostosis or other technical difficulties. Unfortunately, values for blood flow velocity and/or pulsatility index that correlate with critical cerebral blood flow reduction have not been identified. Patients with minimal changes in blood flow velocity during carotid clamping (with shunting) have been shown to have stroke rates similar to (or even slightly greater than) those when flow velocity is unchanged and shunts are not used.[26] TCD-detected embolization occurs in more than 90% of patients during CEA.[27] Emboli having TCD characteristics of air (occurring at shunt opening and during restoration of flow) are generally not associated with adverse clinical outcome. However, particulate emboli (>10) detected by TCD during carotid dissection correlate with significant deterioration in cognitive function after CEA, postoperative ischemic events, and new ischemic lesions on magnetic resonance images of the brain.[27,28] More careful surgical dissection of the artery and more meticulous attention to backbleeding and flushing to avoid embolization may be guided by acoustic evidence for embolism, although it is unknown whether such an approach alters outcome. TCD monitoring may also indicate which patients should have aggressive hemodynamic interventions and/or receive anticoagulation because cerebral embolic events and decreased cerebral blood flow velocity can be differentiated.

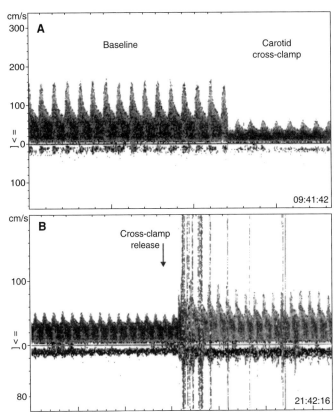

FIGURE 10-2 **A**, Transcranial Doppler (TCD) tracing of middle cerebral artery blood flow velocity before and after clamping of the internal carotid artery during a carotid endarterectomy. Although the velocities decreased with clamping, they decreased by only 30% of the preclamp mean value and thus represent competent collateral flow. In contrast, TCD velocities would have completely disappeared with inadequate collateral flow. **B**, Microemboli in the middle cerebral artery after carotid clamp release and restoration of cerebral blood flow. Embolic events appear as sharp spikes on the TCD recording and are common with reperfusion. (Adapted from Davis DA: Intraoperative transcranial Doppler monitoring in carotid endarterectomy. In Bailes JE, Spetzler RF [eds]: *Microsurgical carotid endarterectomy*, Philadelphia, 1996, Lippincott-Raven, Figures 6, 9; 89.)

Near-infrared spectroscopy (NIRS) can also be used to assess changes in cerebral blood flow by measuring regional cerebral oxygenation (rSo_2). NIRS assesses oxygenation of arterial, capillary, and venous hemoglobin and predominantly estimates venous oxygenation (i.e., venous blood makes up ~80% of cerebral blood volume).[29] Purported advantages of NIRS compared with EEG monitoring during CEA include ease of use, simplicity of displayed values, lower cost, and the noninvasive and portable nature of the device. Carotid artery clamping typically produces a significant decrease in ipsilateral rSo_2 values compared with preclamp and postclamp values in patients undergoing CEA.[30] Unfortunately, these changes are inconsistently related to reductions in cerebral flow and evoked potential amplitude during CEA.[31-34] Specific rSo_2 threshold values defining critical cerebral ischemia have yet to be definitively established. Samra et al noted that a 20% postclamp decrease in rSo_2 after carotid occlusion had a 66% false-positive rate but a 97.4% negative predictive value (i.e., if rSo_2 does not decrease, cerebral ischemia is unlikely, but a decrease does not always indicate ischemia).[35] In a comparison with TCD, Grubhofer et al also showed a significant negative predictive value (100%) but poor specificity and positive predictive value of rSo_2.[36] Using linear regression analysis to compare relative changes in mean TCD velocity and ΔrSo_2, they determined that a critical rSo_2 decrease after carotid clamping of 13% would have resulted in unnecessary shunting in 7 of their patients (Figure 10-3).[36]

These limitations of NIRS are related to (1) placement of the sensors on the scalp overlying the frontal lobes, whereas the area at greatest risk for ischemia during CEA is the parietal lobes supplied by the middle cerebral artery; (2) contamination by extracranial blood flow; (3) incorrect sensor placement; (4) major shifts of intracranial blood volume away from the frontal lobes (i.e., related to changes in CO_2 partial pressure); (5) the absence of "normal" absolute values because of a wide range of rSo_2 values reported in patients without neurologic changes during CEA; and (5) artifact from incomplete shielding of ambient light.[29,30,35] The inability to define a "biologic zero" is also a significant limitation, and the finding of an average rSo_2 value of 51% in dead subjects (compared with 68% in normal control subjects) invokes serious concerns regarding the validity of this monitoring technique.[29] Finally, the finding that the degree of change in rSo_2 values after CO_2 challenge varies significantly between two commercially available NIRS monitors—the INVOS 4100 (Somanetics, Troy, MI) and the NIRO 300 (Hamamatsu Photonics, Hamamatsu, Japan)—raises further questions regarding the validity and precise role of NIRS monitoring compared with other monitors of cerebral ischemia.[37]

Currently, no single method of intraoperative neurologic monitoring during CEA using selective shunting has been shown to improve postoperative neurologic outcome.[38] Moreover, the use of either routine or selective shunting remains controversial because available data remain inadequate to validate the efficacy of either surgical approach.[38]

Cerebral and Myocardial Ischemia

Hyperventilation has been proposed to redistribute blood flow from normal areas of the brain with preserved CO_2 reactivity to ischemic areas in which CO_2 reactivity has been lost, but controlled studies have not identified any benefit attributable to this "inverse steal" phenomenon.[39] Available data do not support reduction of arterial CO_2 pressure ($Paco_2$) as a routine intervention to reduce cerebral injury, and normocapnia seems to be most appropriate during CEA in most situations.

Cerebral ischemia during carotid clamping can be reduced with the use of a carotid shunt, although to optimize benefit the shunt must be functional within 2 to 4 minutes without dissection or embolization. Even functioning shunts do not guarantee adequacy of cerebral perfusion, and there are markedly variable flow rates for different types of shunts. For example, the flow through a long Inahara-Pruitt shunt is about half that through a Javid shunt under similar conditions.[40] Of course, hypotension and low cardiac output compound such flow discrepancies and may be associated with decreased cerebral perfusion despite shunt patency.

Most practitioners advocate maintenance of BP close to the preoperative level, but some recommend a BP of 10% to 20% above normal. The rationale for maintaining normal or mildly increased systemic BP during CEA is based upon three concerns: (1) the normally occurring reduction in cerebral perfusion pressure in boundary zones between principal vascular territories, (2) the increased vulnerability of these areas to declines in BP if intracranial occlusive disease or cerebral infarction is present, and (3) alteration of normal autoregulation in the presence of volatile anesthetics or chronic hypertension. Definite neurologic benefits of intraoperative "hypertension" have not been documented, although some concern has been raised about potential myocardial risks. Smith et al showed that transesophageal echocardiography (TEE)–diagnosed myocardial ischemia (identified as new segmental wall motion abnormalities [SWMAs]) occurs frequently during CEA when phenylephrine is administered to support BP with moderately deep levels of inhaled anesthesia.[41] These changes may be related to changes in ventricular loading conditions when a pure α_1-receptor agonist is administered in the presence of a volatile anesthetic with negative inotropic effects, resulting in altered regional wall motion and overdiagnosis of ischemia. Mutch et al found no evidence for Holter-monitored ischemia when phenylephrine was infused to support mean arterial pressure at 110% ± 10% of ward values during carotid artery clamping.[42] However, Holter-diagnosed myocardial ischemia that is prolonged and occurring during carotid artery clamping or within 2 hours following declamping is highly predictive of adverse cardiac complications.[43]

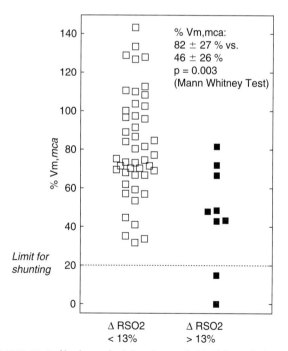

FIGURE 10-3 Number and relative changes in blood flow velocity versus baseline (%Vm,mca) in patients developing the calculated decrease in regional cerebral oxygenation (ΔRSo_2 >13%) indicated for shunting. The figure demonstrates that seven patients would have been "unnecessarily" shunted if only the criterion of a ΔRSo_2 >13% had been applied. (From Grubhofer G, Plöchl W, Skolka M, et al: *Anesth Analg* 91:1339, 2000.)

During CEA, myocardial ischemia can occur in close association with marked fluctuations in BP partially related to carotid baroreceptor deactivation (during clamping) and reactivation (after declamping).[43] Although intraoperative carotid sinus infiltration with local anesthetic has been recommended to reduce such hemodynamic fluctuation, this approach is associated with a greater frequency of intraoperative and postoperative hypertension.[44,45] The extent of surgical or pharmacologic denervation of the carotid sinus during CEA is probably an important determinant of postclamp hemodynamic responses. Perioperative hypertension has a multifactorial etiology, is dependent on the adequacy of preoperative BP control as well as the presence of peripheral vascular disease, and may be significantly affected by the choice of the anesthesia.[46] Hemodynamic instability with episodes of tachycardia and hypertension upon awakening or tracheal extubation after CEA is associated with myocardial ischemia.[42]

The appropriate temperature of the patient during CEA is unknown. Moderate hypothermia (34 to 35°C) has been shown to increase postoperative catecholamine levels and induce myocardial ischemia in susceptible vascular surgery patients with underlying CAD, whereas other data suggest a potential neuroprotective effect of moderate hypothermia in the setting of cerebral ischemia. Given the absence of any data regarding temperature management for patients undergoing CEA, a sensible approach is to minimize significant reductions in core temperature (i.e., maintain temperature > 35°C) while simultaneously avoiding the known deleterious cerebral effects of hyperthermia (temperature > 37.5°C). Thus, active warming is typically unnecessary during CEA.

Choice of Anesthesia

Debate over the choice of RA versus GA persists because of differing conclusions of various studies of risks and benefits (Figure 10-4).[47-50] The main advantage of RA is the ability to predict cerebral ischemia after carotid artery clamping, although various retrospective analyses have not been able to identify a clear difference in stroke or mortality rate between GA and RA.[51-56] Uncontrolled retrospective studies have suggested that carotid artery shunting is required less frequently with RA and that there is a lower incidence of postoperative hemodynamic instability as well as a shorter duration of postoperative hospital stay with RA.[46,51,57-59]

However, other retrospective analyses have found no difference in cardiovascular outcome or hospital stay after CEA regardless of anesthetic technique.[56,60] Interestingly, one prospective investigation found RA for CEA to be associated with a high incidence of tachycardia.[61] A retrospective review of GA versus RA for CEA found a greater incidence of ventricular arrhythmias with GA, but other adverse cardiac and neurologic events occurred with similar frequency with the two techniques.[62] Another retrospective analysis of more than 1000 CEAs (two thirds with cervical block) could not identify any difference in cardiac complication rates between GA and RA.[63] The latter retrospective study did, however, report a lower stroke rate after CEA with RA (1.3%) compared with GA (3.2%).[63] Most studies evaluating the influence of choice of anesthesia on MI after CEA are not prospective and have screened for MI on the basis of clinical symptoms only, so the question of whether there are differences in true rates of adverse cardiac outcome remains unresolved.[64] The Cochrane Collaboration has applied meta-analytic techniques to the prevailing literature through 2002 that examined outcome after CEA using RA versus GA.[65] This analysis included three randomized trials involving 143 patients and 17 nonrandomized studies involving approximately 5970 patients.[65] The methodologic quality of the randomized trials was assessed as questionable, and the absolute number of patients was not clearly defined in 9 of the 17 nonrandomized studies. Although these nonrandomized studies suggested a potential benefit of RA, there were insufficient data to draw conclusions from the randomized trials. Unfortunately, no carefully controlled randomized trial has been conducted to identify whether any definite cardiac or neurologic outcome difference exists with RA versus GA for CEA.

Opponents of RA for CEA are often concerned about its finite "failure rate," defined as need for conversion to GA. Failure may be reduced by supplemental infiltration with local anesthetic by the surgeon. A major factor in success of RA for CEA is gentle handling of tissues by the surgeon as well as appropriate and frequent communication with the patient during the procedure. Success of RA is also improved with infiltration of local anesthetic at the ramus and lower border of the mandible. Even with these qualifiers, RA is not ideal for patients with an expected long operative time or difficult vascular anatomy, especially a more cephalad carotid bifurcation or high carotid plaque requiring vigorous submandibular retraction (Table 10-3). In addition, unsatisfactory conditions may become manifest with RA in patients with short necks presenting difficulty in surgical exposure. Intraoperative mandibular nerve block can relieve discomfort associated with forceful or prolonged retraction on the mandible. Patients who become uncomfortable or restless may require airway intervention under physically awkward conditions, and the clinician must be ready to deal with this circumstance whenever embarking on RA for CEA. RA and GA are both acceptable options for CEA,

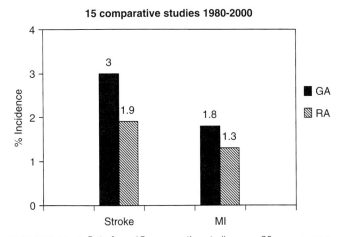

15 comparative studies 1980-2000

FIGURE 10-4 Data from 15 comparative studies over 20 years encompassing 9408 patients reveal that the pooled incidences of stroke and myocardial infarction (MI) are similar between patients undergoing carotid endarterectomy (CEA) using either regional anesthesia (RA) or general anesthesia (GA).

TABLE 10-3
Comparison of Regional and General Anesthesia for Carotid Endarterectomy

Technique	Advantages	Disadvantages
Regional	Less intraoperative hypotension	More intraoperative hypertension, higher catecholamine levels
	Technically simple block	Unfamiliarity for operative team
	Intubation not required	Awkward airway control if GA required
	Sensitive neurologic monitor	Sedation may obscure neurologic monitoring or falsely suggest ischemia
	Avoids postoperative somnolence seen with GA	Patient's discomfort if ischemia develops or if procedure is lengthy
	Shorter postoperative hospitalization, lower costs, possible ↓ cardiac complications	Sedation-induced ↑ Pco_2, ↓ Pao_2 may increase cerebral ischemia
	Provides postoperative analgesia	Need to convert to GA
General	Reliable airway control	Intubation/airway device required
	Secure control of Pco_2, Pao_2	More intraoperative hemodynamic changes
	Possible neuroprotective effects of anesthetics	Delayed emergence versus new neurologic event

GA, general anesthesia; Pco_2, arterial carbon dioxide tension; Po_2, arterial oxygen tension.

and the decision to use one or the other technique should depend on the combined desires and experience of the anesthesiologist and surgeon as well as the patient's preference. With regard to RA techniques, prospective, randomized comparisons of deep versus superficial cervical plexus block for CEA have found no significant differences in patients' satisfaction or intraoperative conditions, although deep cervical plexus block may prolong postoperative analgesia in the first 24 hours after CEA (Figure 10-5).[66,67]

Most anesthetic agents commonly used for induction and/or maintenance of GA decrease cerebral metabolism, although it is likely that any neuroprotective effect of anesthetics is more related to complex biochemical effects on ischemic brain tissue than simply to reduction of cerebral metabolism. Although isoflurane has been associated with fewer EEG changes during carotid clamping and with a lower critical regional cerebral blood flow compared with older volatile agents such as halothane or enflurane, retrospective comparison of these three anesthetics could not identify any difference in neurologic outcome or in cardiac outcome after CEA (Figure 10-6).[68-70] The cerebral vascular effects and impact of sevoflurane on brain energy metabolism appear similar to those of isoflurane, although return of consciousness and time to extubation after CEA may be shorter with sevoflurane and desflurane than isoflurane.[71-73] When compared with propofol for anesthesia for CEA, sevoflurane had a similar safety profile and demonstrated comparable recovery profiles.[74]

Hemodynamic stability during GA for CEA can be enhanced with moderate amounts of opioids such as fentanyl or its derivatives, although care must be exercised to avoid doses that compromise rapid emergence at the end of the procedure. Use of the ultrashort-acting opioid remifentanil may allow prompt awakening after GA and more effectively blunt the hypertensive response to intubation compared with fentanyl and sufentanil.[75-77] However, bradycardia and hypotension may be more intense with remifentanil anesthesia for CEA.[77] Judicious administration of β-adrenergic blockers is also useful to minimize surges in heart rate and BP during stressful intraoperative periods, and perioperative β-blockade may have beneficial effects on cardiac outcome. α_2-Receptor agonists are also useful to attenuate adverse hemodynamic responses during CEA (see Chapter 2).

Endovascular Surgery for Extracranial Revascularization

Endovascular treatment of extracranial carotid artery disease, including angioplasty and stenting, has emerged as an increasingly popular approach to the treatment of carotid disease. The success of angioplasty and stenting for coronary, renal, and iliac disease, along with the limitations and known complications of CEA, have led to an emerging interest in endovascular techniques as an alternative to surgery (Figure 10-7).[78] Percutaneous interventions for carotid angioplasty and stenting may be performed either by the femoral artery approach or (less commonly) by direct puncture of the common carotid artery. Sedation is usually sufficient for groin cannulation, with the patient awake during carotid balloon inflation. Anticholinergic agents (atropine or glycopyrrolate) are administered to attenuate the baroreceptor response during balloon dilation or stent deployment.[79] Particular vigilance to monitoring hemodynamic and neurologic status is required during these procedures, especially during balloon inflations and after sheath removal for the cervical approach. Control of hypertension is particularly important because it increases the risk of hematoma formation, a potentially catastrophic event, especially if residual anticoagulation is present. Maintenance of adequate perfusion pressure is particularly important to facilitate collateral blood flow during balloon dilation. Technical success rates of 98% have been reported.[80,81] Newer "brain protection devices" are being introduced that may reduce the risk of neurologic injury from distal embolization of plaque and low flow during the endovascular procedure. Two types are available: (1) balloon protection devices that remain inflated distal to the plaque during stenting and angioplasty and (2) filter protection devices located beyond the stent that theoretically capture atheromatous debris and plaque that are dislodged during balloon inflation and/or stent deployment (Figure 10-8).[80]

Although CEA is currently the "gold standard" therapy for CAS, experience with endovascular techniques suggests complication rates comparable to those with CEA, with carotid patency even after 6-year follow-up.[82] Because stroke, MI, and recurrent carotid stenosis can complicate both procedures, two multicenter, randomized, prospective trials have been initiated to compare the clinical efficacy of CEA versus endovascular therapy—The Carotid and Vertebral Artery Transluminal Angioplasty Study (CAVATAS) and the Carotid Revascularization Endarterectomy vs. Stent Trial (CREST). Preliminary 3-year follow-up of the CAVATAS study revealed insignificant differences in the risk of

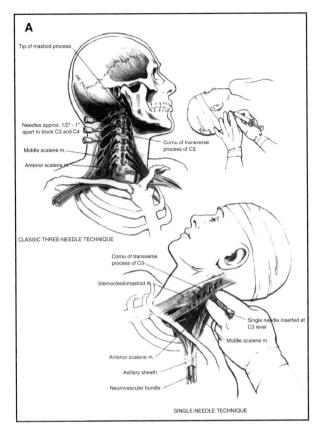

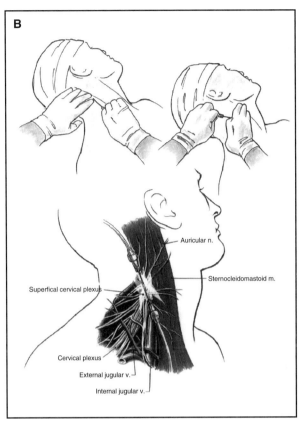

FIGURE 10-5 A, Deep cervical plexus block. Upper frame: The classic three-needle approach involves placing a skin wheal about 1 inch below the tip of the mastoid process and then inserting a 2-inch block needle in a slightly caudad fashion until the tip of the transverse process is reached, usually at a depth of about 1 inch. The other two needles are similarly inserted approximately ½ to 1 inch apart in a caudad direction to block C3 and C4. From 3 to 5 mL of solution is then injected after careful aspiration for cerebrospinal fluid and blood. Lower frame: The single-needle technique involves a position of the patient similar to that for the preceding technique with caudad localization of the C3 or C4 transverse process. A single injection of 8 to 10 mL of local anesthetic produces an adequate block because of the larger volume. **B,** Superficial cervical plexus block. This block provides anesthesia similar to that for the deep block but without muscle relaxation. The patient's head is raised to outline the sternocleidomastoid muscle. A skin wheal is raised along its posterior border midway between the origin on the clavicle and the insertion on the mastoid. A 2-inch 25-gauge needle is inserted, and 10 mL of local anesthetic is injected as the needle is advanced from 1 to 2 inches superiorly and inferiorly along the edge of the muscle. (Text and illustration from Katz Jordan: Section II. Neck. In: *Atlas of regional anesthesia*, ed 2, East Norwalk, CT, 1994, Appleton & Lange, 40-43.)

major stroke or death within the first 30 days between endovascular treatment and CEA (6.4% vs. 5.9%), nor were there differences in stroke rates after 3 years.[83] Cranial nerve injury and major neck hematoma occurred less frequently after endovascular treatment. Future analysis of these two randomized trials will provide further evaluation of the utility of endovascular stenting and angioplasty in the treatment of extracranial carotid disease.

Postoperative Considerations

Neurologic Injury

Table 10-4 lists common perioperative complications after CEA and typical incidence rates. Undoubtedly, neurologic injury is one of the complications that CEA is designed to prevent. Perioperative stroke after CEA has many causes, with more than half of surgical etiology (ischemia during carotid clamping, postoperative thrombosis and embolism) and the

remainder related to other factors such as reperfusion injury, intracranial hemorrhage, or other postoperative events. Embolization is the most common cause of strokes developing intraoperatively and is invariably associated with surgical events. It is estimated that only approximately 20% of strokes caused by intraoperative events are hemodynamic in origin (related to carotid clamping, intracranial occlusive disease, shunt problems). Nonetheless, hemodynamic strokes may follow a critical reduction in boundary zone perfusion secondary to intracranial occlusive disease or in areas around old cerebral infarcts, where apparently innocuous reductions in cerebral perfusion pressure may result in an adverse outcome. After CEA, strokes tend to be related to embolization and/or thrombosis, although intracerebral hemorrhage may also occur. Early thrombosis may be related to intimal injury and/or flap formation as well as enhanced platelet activation or deposition at the operative site.

Critical CBF and EEG Ischemia
N = 2,223 CEA

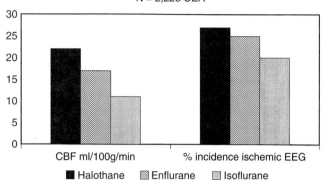

■ Halothane   ▨ Enflurane   ▨ Isoflurane

FIGURE 10-6 This figure from a retrospective analysis of 2223 carotid endarterectomies (CEAs) from single institution demonstrated that although isoflurane was associated with fewer electroencephalographic (EEG) changes during carotid clamping and a lower critical regional cerebral blood flow (CBF) compared with older volatile agents such as halothane or enflurane, retrospective comparison of these three anesthetics could not identify any difference in either neurologic outcome or cardiac outcome after CEA. (From Michenfelder JD, Sundt TM, Fode N, et al: *Anesthesiology* 67:336, 1987.)

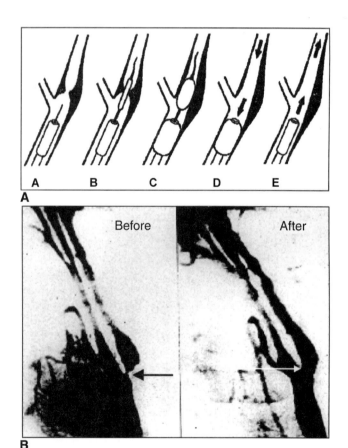

FIGURE 10-7 A, Endovascular repair of an internal carotid artery lesion involves placement of a double-balloon catheter (A) with positioning of the angioplasty balloon across the occluding lesion (B). After balloon dilation (C), blood is aspirated retrograde (D) to avoid embolization before reestablishing anterograde flow (E). **B,** Angiography of a carotid lesion shows the narrowing *before* angioplasty (*black arrow*) and the newly dilated lesion *after* balloon inflation (*white arrow*). (From Kachel R: *J Endovasc Surg* 3:22, 1996.)

TABLE 10-4

Perioperative Complications after Carotid Endarterectomy

Complication	Incidence (%)
Myocardial infarction	1-3
Stroke	3-4
Hypertension	28-58
Hypotension	8-10
Cranial nerve injury	10-16
Wound hematoma	3

Rockman et al reviewed 2024 CEAs over a 12-year period and observed that 63% of postoperative neurologic events were thromboembolic in nature and intraluminal thrombus was found in 83% of patients who underwent immediate surgical exploration.[84] Neurologic events occurring during CEA are not necessarily predictive of postoperative complications, which may explain the variable findings of studies examining the effects of intraoperative interventions on overall stroke incidence. Retrospective data from 835 consecutive CEAs revealed that 73% of new neurologic deficits were diagnosed in the operating room or the recovery room and 19% within 8 hours of surgery; the remaining patients experienced a deficit after 8 but less than 24 hours after surgery.[85] Thus, most patients manifest a new deficit soon after completion of the procedure, and diagnostic testing with Duplex ultrasonography or surgical reexploration can be immediately pursued.

Postoperative Hyperperfusion Syndrome

Postoperative hyperperfusion syndrome describes an abrupt increase in blood flow with loss of autoregulation in surgically reperfused brain. Patients with severe hypertension after CEA are at increased risk for developing this syndrome, which may arise with a spectrum of findings including headache, signs of transient cerebral ischemia, seizures, brain edema, and even intracerebral hemorrhage (Figure 10-9).[86] Middle cerebral artery blood flow has been shown to be pressure dependent in patients with post-CEA hyperperfusion (consistent with defective autoregulation), and systemic BP should be meticulously controlled in the immediate recovery period after CEA, especially when there was a large pressure gradient across a severe CAS preoperatively.[87]

Blood Pressure Lability

Before CEA, carotid sinus baroreceptors may reset secondary to proximal arterial occlusion. After CEA, the reset baroreceptor may sense sudden increases in BP, triggering subsequent baroreceptor-mediated hypotension. As noted previously, although anesthetizing the carotid sinus nerve can improve hemodynamic stability during CEA, this practice as well as surgical denervation of the carotid sinus compounds the risk of postoperative hypertension, especially in patients with significant preoperative hypertension.

Cranial Nerve and Carotid Body Dysfunction

Transient dysfunction of adjacent cranial nerves and their branches may occur despite gentle dissection and retraction during CEA. Injury to the superior laryngeal nerve can occur

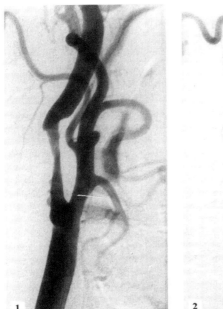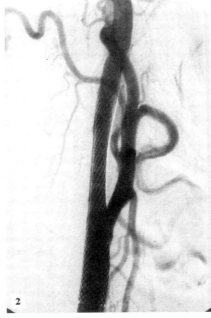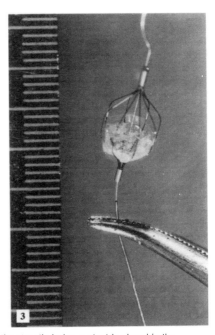

FIGURE 10-8 Carotid bulb stenosis is seen **(1)**. Following angioplasty of the stenotic lesion, a stent is placed in the previously stenotic vessel **(2)** under protection of a filter device **(3)**. After removal of the filter, yellowish material was found coating the surface of the filter. These filter devices may reduce the incidence of neurologic injury from distal embolization of plaque during the angioplasty and stenting procedure. (From Bonaldi G: *Neuroradiology* 44:164, 2002.)

and primarily results in mild relaxation of the ipsilateral vocal cord manifested by early fatigability of the voice and impairment of high-pitched phonation. Recurrent laryngeal nerve (RLN) dysfunction after CEA may result in paralysis of the ipsilateral vocal cord in the paramedian position, hoarseness, and impairment of the cough mechanism. If RLN injury occurs and contralateral CEA is planned, consideration should be given to postponing the subsequent operation until satisfactory RLN function returns, or at least precautions for postoperative airway management should be planned if operation cannot be delayed. Although bilateral CEA is known to result in carotid body dysfunction and increases in resting Paco$_2$, carotid body function can be

abnormal even after unilateral CEA, with impaired ventilatory response to mild hypoxemia.

Airway and Ventilation Problems

Upper airway obstruction after CEA is a rare but potentially fatal complication, which may occur not only because of hematoma formation but also more commonly because of tissue edema, secondary to venous and lymphatic congestion. This diffuse type of neck edema (lateral and retropharyngeal) may be associated with markedly edematous supraglottic mucosal folds. Although such edema has also been postulated to be the effect of tissue trauma with increased capillary permeability induced by release of vasoactive mediators, steroid

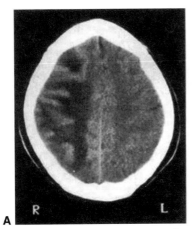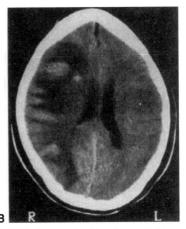

FIGURE 10-9 Hyperperfusion syndrome after carotid endarterectomy (CEA). **A,** noncontrast head computed tomography (CT) scan on postoperative day 5 reveals diffuse edema in the right frontal and parietal lobes. **B,** Midline shift from right-sided edema and a small hyperdense lesion in the right frontal lobe, representing a small cerebral hemorrhage, are evident in this scan. (From Breen JC, Caplan LR, DeWitt LD, et al: *Neurology* 46:175, 1996.)

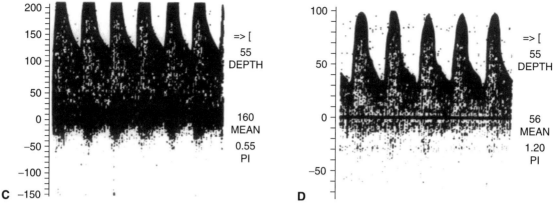

FIGURE 10-9 Cont'd. C, transcranial Doppler (TCD) recordings from a different patient with the hyperperfusion syndrome noted on postoperative day 1 after CEA. The mean velocity of 160 cm/sec was an increase of 400% over preoperative values and was accompanied by a severe unilateral headache. **D,** By postoperative day 2, the mean velocity (56 cm/sec) had returned to normal and the symptoms had resolved. (From Powers AD, Smith RR: *Neurosurgery* 26:56, 1990.)

administration immediately prior to CEA does not reduce edema formation.[88] The presence of supraglottic edema after CEA may make intubation and mask ventilation difficult.[89,90] Neck hematomas occur in 5% to 7% of patients, and the vast majority are typically diagnosed within 8 hours of surgery.[83,85] Nearly 80% of these patients eventually required reexploration for hematoma evacuation. Opening of the neck wound for

evacuation of the hematoma is thus not uniformly effective in this situation and may induce significant hypertension that may worsen further bleeding.

The most prudent approach to this problem is to return the patient to the operating room for controlled surgical exploration. Local anesthetic infiltration for evacuation of the hematoma is preferred over GA because the latter approach

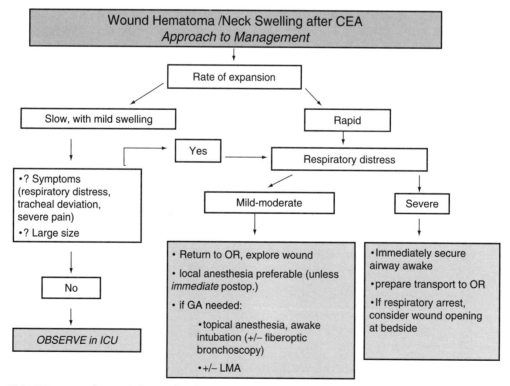

FIGURE 10-10 A suggested approach to the management of wound hematomas after carotid endarterectomies (CEAs) that are accompanied by neck swelling. Mild swelling with minimal symptoms may be conservatively managed with observation in an intensive care unit. The presence of respiratory symptoms, or a rapid increase in neck diameter, requires immediate reexploration in the operating room (OR) and securing of the airway while the patient is awake. Neck swelling immediately (<1 hour) after surgery may produce less glottic edema because of the short duration of bleeding, but cautious assessment of the airway is still advised before proceeding with general anesthesia (GA) for reexploration. Opening of the wound at the bedside should be reserved for acute respiratory arrest. ICU, intensive care unit; LAM, laryneal mask airway.

may induce airway obstruction and difficulty in intubation (Figure 10-10). In a series of 15 patients with a postoperative neck hematoma after CEA, no patient receiving local anesthesia sustained a complication.[90] In contrast, in seven patients administered GA, laryngoscopy was described as extremely difficult with obscured glottic structures and upper airway edema. Severe hypoxemia ensued in several patients, and two sustained severe neurologic and cardiac complications.[90] Awake intubation is thus strongly advised if respiratory distress develops or surgical exploration is required.

Phrenic nerve paresis is common after cervical plexus block. Although this normally has little clinical consequence (except for mildly increased $Paco_2$), it is a potentially more serious problem in some patients with severe pulmonary disease or with preexisting contralateral diaphragm dysfunction.

Fast-Track Recovery

Most patients undergoing CEA have historically been hospitalized for a few days, commonly with overnight observation in an intensive care unit (ICU) to treat BP and monitor for neurologic deficits or cervical swelling. As with other surgical procedures, fast-track recovery without routine ICU admission and with early home discharge is being applied to patients after CEA. The feasibility and safety of fast-tracking protocols have been examined, and the majority of patients do not require ICU admission and may be safely discharged home 1 to 2 days after CEA.[91] Acute postoperative neurologic events usually occur early in the postoperative course, which allows timely identification of patients who specifically require overnight ICU admission.[92]

REFERENCES

1. Moore WS, Barnett HJM, Beebe HG, et al: Guidelines for carotid endarterectomy. A multidisciplinary consensus statement from the Ad Hoc committee, American Heart Association, *Circulation* 91:566, 1995.
2. Executive Committee for the Asymptomatic Carotid Atherosclerosis Study: Endarterectomy for asymptomatic carotid stenosis, *JAMA* 273:1421, 1995.
3. Goldstein LB, Hasselblad V, Matchar DB, et al: Comparison and meta-analysis of randomized trials of carotid endarterectomy for symptomatic carotid stenosis, *Neurology* 45:1965, 1995.
4. Goldstein LB, McCrory DC, Landsman PB, et al: Multicenter review of preoperative risk factors for carotid endarterectomy in patients with ipsilateral symptoms, *Stroke* 25:1116, 1994.
5. Davies AH, Hayward JK, Currie I, et al: Risk prediction of outcome following carotid endarterectomy, *Cardiovasc Surg* 4:338, 1996.
6. McCrory DC, Goldstein LB, Samsa GP, et al: Predicting complications of carotid endarterectomy, *Stroke* 24:1285, 1993.
7. Kuhan G, Gardiner ED, Abidia AF, et al: Risk modelling study for carotid endarterectomy, *Br J Surg* 88:1590, 2001.
8. Gur AY, Bova I, Bornstein NM: Is impaired cerebral vasomotor reactivity a predictive factor of stroke in asymptomatic patients? *Stroke* 27:2188, 1996.
9. Thiel A, Zickmann B, Stertmann WA, et al: Cerebrovascular carbon dioxide reactivity in carotid artery disease, *Anesthesiology* 82:655, 1995.
10. Yonas H, Smith HA, Durham, SR, et al: Increased stroke risk predicted by compromised cerebral blood flow reactivity, *J Neurosurg* 79:483, 1993.
11. Aronson S, Boisvert D, Lapp W: Isolated systolic hypertension is associated with adverse outcomes from coronary artery bypass grafting surgery, *Anesth Analg* 94:1079, 2002.
12. Asiddao CB, Donegan JH, Witesell RC, et al: Factors associated with perioperative complications during carotid endarterectomy, *Anesth Analg* 61:631, 1982.
13. Eagle KA, Berger PB, Calkins H, et al: ACC/AHA Guideline Update for Perioperative Cardiovascular Evaluation for Noncardiac Surgery—Executive Summary, *Anesth Analg* 94:1052, 2002.
14. Whitley D, Cherry KJ: Predictive value of carotid artery stump pressures during carotid endarterectomy, *Neurosurg Clin North Am* 7:723, 1996.
15. Harada RN, Comerota AJ, Good GM, et al: Stump pressure, electroencephalographic changes, and the contralateral carotid artery: another look at selective shunting, *Am J Surg* 170:148, 1995.
16. McKay RD, Sundt TM, Michenfelder JD, et al: Internal carotid artery pressure and cerebral blood flow during carotid endarterectomy: modification by halothane, enflurane, and Innovar, *Anesthesiology* 45:390, 1976.
17. Cao P, Giordano G, Zannetti S, et al: Transcranial Doppler monitoring during carotid endarterectomy: is it appropriate for selecting patients in need of a shunt? *J Vasc Surg* 26:973, 1997.
18. Stoughton J, Nath R, Abbott W: Comparison of simultaneous electroencephalographic and mental status monitoring during carotid endarterectomy with regional anesthesia, *J Vasc Surg* 28:1014, 1998.
19. Lawrence PF, Alves JC, Jicha D, et al: Incidence, timing, and causes of cerebral ischemia during carotid endarterectomy with regional anesthesia, *J Vasc Surg* 27:329, 1998.
20. Pruitt J: 1009 consecutive carotid endarterectomies using local anesthesia, EEG, and selective shunting with Pruitt-Inahara carotid shunt, *Contemp Surg* 23:49, 1983.
21. Silbert BS, Kluger R, Cronin KD, et al: The processed electroencephalogram may not detect neurologic ischemia during carotid endarterectomy, *Anesthesiology* 70:356, 1989.
22. Kearse LA, Martin D, McPeck K, et al: Computer-derived density spectral array in detection of mild analog electroencephalographic ischemic pattern changes during carotid endarterectomy, *J Neurosurg* 78:884, 1993.
23. Hanowell LH, Soriano S, Bennett HL: EEG power changes are more sensitive than spectral edge frequency variation for detection of cerebral ischemia during carotid artery surgery: a prospective assessment of processed EEG monitoring, *J Cardiothorac Vasc Anesth* 6:292, 1992.
24. Redekop G, Ferguson G: Correlation of contralateral stenosis and intraoperative electroencephalogram change with risk of stroke during carotid endarterectomy, *Neurosurgery* 30:191, 1992.
25. Davis DA: Intraoperative transcranial Doppler monitoring in carotid endarterectomy. In Bailes JE, Spetzler RF (eds): *Microsurgical carotid endarterectomy*, Philadelphia, 1996, Lippincott-Raven, Figures 6 and 9, 89.
26. Halsey JH: Risks and benefits of shunting in carotid endarterectomy. The International Transcranial Doppler Collaborators, *Stroke* 23:1583, 1992.
27. Gaunt ME, Martin PJ, Smith JL, et al: Clinical relevance of intraoperative embolization detected by transcranial Doppler ultrasonography during carotid endarterectomy: a prospective study of 100 patients, *Br J Surg* 81:1435, 1994.
28. Ackerstaff RGA, Jansen C, Moll FL, et al: The significance of microemboli detection by means of transcranial Doppler ultrasonography monitoring in carotid endarterectomy, *J Vasc Surg* 21:963, 1995.
29. Schwarz G, Litscher G, Kleinert R, et al: Cerebral oximetry in dead subjects, *J Neurosurg Anesth* 8:189, 1996.
30. Samra SK, Dorje P, Zelenock GB, et al: Cerebral oximetry in patients undergoing carotid endarterectomy under regional anesthesia, *Stroke* 27:49, 1996.
31. Cho H, Nemoto EM, Yonas H, et al: Cerebral monitoring by means of oximetry and somatosensory evoked potentials during carotid endarterectomy, *J Neurosurg* 89:533, 1998.
32. Kuroda S, Houkin K, Abe H, et al: Near-infrared monitoring of cerebral oxygenation state during carotid endarterectomy, *Surg Neurol* 45:450, 1996.
33. Duffy CM, Manninen PH, Chan A, et al: Comparison of cerebral oximeter and evoked potential monitoring in carotid endarterectomy, *Can J Anaesth* 44:1077,. 1997.
34. Beese U, Langer H, Lang W, et al: Comparison of near-infrared spectroscopy and somatosensory evoked potentials for the detection of cerebral ischemia during carotid endarterectomy, *Stroke* 29:2032, 1998.
35. Samra SK, Dy EA, Welch K, et al: Evaluation of a cerebral oximeter as a monitor of cerebral ischemia during carotid endarterectomy, *Anesthesiology* 93:964, 2000.
36. Grubhofer G, Plöchl W, Skolka M, et al: Comparing Doppler ultrasonography and cerebral oximetry as indicators for shunting in carotid endarterectomy, *Anesth Analg* 91:1339, 2000.
37. Yoshitani K, Kawaguchi M, Tatsumi K, et al: A comparison of the INVOS 4100 and the NIRO 300 near-infrared spectrophotometers, *Anesth Analg* 94:586, 2002.
38. Bond R, Rekasem K, Counsell C, et al: Routine or selective shunting for carotid endarterectomy (and different methods of monitoring in selective shunting), *The Cochrane Library*, issue 2, Oxford, 2002, Update Software.

39. Michenfeder JD, Milde JH: Failure of prolonged hypocapnia, hypothermia, or hypertension to favorably alter acute stroke in primates, *Stroke* 8:87, 1977.

40. Grossi EA, Giangola G, Parish MA, et al: Differences of flow rates in carotid shunts: consequences in cerebral perfusion, *Ann Vasc Surg* 19:206, 1994.

41. Smith JS, Roizen MF, Cahalan MK, et al: Does anesthetic technique make a difference? Augmentation of systolic blood pressure during carotid endarterectomy: effects of phenylephrine versus light anesthesia and of isoflurane versus halothane on the incidence of myocardial ischemia, *Anesthesiology* 69:846, 1988.

42. Mutch WAC, White IWC, Donen N, et al: Haemodynamic instability and myocardial ischaemia during carotid endarterectomy: a comparison of propofol and isoflurane, *Can J Anaesth* 42:577, 1995.

43. Landesberg G, Erel J, Anner H, et al: Perioperative myocardial ischemia in carotid endarterectomy under cervical plexus block and prophylactic nitroglycerin infusion, *J Cardiothorac Vasc Anesth* 7:259, 1993.

44. Gottlieb A, Satariano-Hayden P, Schoenwald P, et al: The effects of carotid sinus nerve blockade on hemodynamic stability after carotid endarterectomy, *J Cardiothorac Vasc Anesth* 11:67, 1997.

45. Elliott BM, Collins GJ, Youkey JR, et al: Intraoperative local anesthetic injection of the carotid sinus nerve, *Am J Surg* 152:695, 1986.

46. Corson JD, Chang BB, Leopold PW, et al: Perioperative hypertension in patients undergoing carotid endarterectomy: shorter duration under regional block anesthesia, *Circulation* 75(Suppl I):1, 1986.

47. Shah DM, Darling RC, Chang BB, et al: Carotid endarterectomy in awake patients: its safety, acceptability, and outcome, *J Vasc Surg* 19:1015, 1994.

48. Sbarigia E, DarioVizza C, Antonini M, et al: Locoregional versus general anesthesia in carotid surgery: is there an impact on perioperative myocardial ischemia? Results of a prospective monocentric randomized trial, *J Vasc Surg* 30:131, 1999.

49. Takolander R, Bergqvist D, Hulthen UL, et al: Carotid artery surgery. Local versus general anesthesia as related to sympathetic activity and cardiovascular effects, *Eur J Vasc Surg* 4:265, 1990.

50. Magnadottir H, Lightdale N, Harbaugh RE: Clinical outcomes for patients at high risk who underwent carotid endarterectomy with regional anesthesia, *Neurosurgery* 45:786, 1999.

51. Papavasiliou AK, Magnadottir H, Gonda T, et al: Clinical outcomes after carotid endarterectomy: comparison of the use of regional and general anesthesia, *J Neurosurg* 92:291, 2000.

52. Gabelman CG, Gann DS, Ashworth CJ, et al: One hundred consecutive carotid reconstructions: local versus general anesthesia, *Am J Surg* 145:477, 1983.

53. Becquemin JP, Paris E, Valverde A, et al: Carotid surgery. Is regional anesthesia always appropriate? *J Cardiovasc Surg (Torino)* 32:592, 1991.

54. Rockman CB, Riles TS, Gold M, et al: A comparison of regional and general anesthesia in patients undergoing carotid endarterectomy, *J Vasc Surg* 24:946, 1996.

55. Allen BT, Anderson CB, Rubin BG, et al: Influence of anesthetic technique on perioperative complications after carotid endarterectomy, *J Vasc Surg* 19:834, 1994.

56. Palmer MA: Comparison of regional and general anesthesia for carotid endarterectomy, *Am J Surg* 157:329, 1989.

57. Forssell C, Takolander R, Bergqvist D, et al: Local versus general anaesthesia in carotid surgery: a prospective randomized study, *Eur J Vasc Surg* 3:503, 1989.

58. Corson JD, Chang BB, Shah DM, et al: The influence of anesthetic choice on carotid endarterectomy outcome, *Arch Surg* 122:807, 1987.

59. Muskett A, McGreevy J, Miller M: Detailed comparison of regional and general anesthesia for carotid endarterectomy, *Am J Surg* 152:691, 1986.

60. Sbarigia E, Speziale F, Colonna M, et al: The selection for shunting in patients with severe bilateral carotid lesions, *Eur J Vasc Surg* 7(Suppl A):3, 1993.

61. Davies MJ, Murrell GC, Cronin KD, et al: Carotid endarterectomy under cervical plexus block: a prospective clinical audit, *Anaesth Intensive Care* 18:219, 1990.

62. Ombrellaro MP, Freeman MB, Stevens SL, et al: Effect of anesthetic technique on cardiac morbidity following carotid artery surgery, *Am J Surg* 171:387, 1996.

63. Fiorani P, Sbarigia E, Speziale F, et al: General anaesthesia versus cervical block and perioperative complications in carotid artery surgery, *Eur J Vasc Endovasc Surg* 13:37, 1997.

64. Peitzman AB, Webster MW, Loubeau JM, et al: Carotid endarterectomy under regional (conductive) anesthesia, *Ann Surg* 196:59, 1982.

65. Tangkanakul C, Counsell C, Warlow C: Local versus general anaesthesia for carotid endarterectomy (Cochrane review), *The Cochrane Library*, issue 2, 2002.

66. Pandit JJ, Bree S, Dillon P: A comparison of superficial versus combined (superficial and deep) cervical plexus block for carotid endarterectomy: a prospective, randomized study, *Anesth Analg* 91:781, 2000.

67. Stoneham MD, Doyle A, Knighton J, et al: Prospective, randomized comparison of deep or superficial cervical plexus block for carotid endarterectomy, *Anesthesiology* 89:907, 1998.

68. Michenfelder JD, Sundt TM, Fode N, et al: Isoflurane when compared to enflurane and halothane decreases the frequency of cerebral ischemia during carotid endarterectomy, *Anesthesiology* 67:336, 1987.

69. Messick JM, Casement B, Sharbrough FW, et al: Correlation of regional cerebral blood flow (rCBF) with EEG changes during isoflurane anesthesia for carotid endarterectomy: critical rCBF, *Anesthesiology* 66:344, 1987.

70. Cucchiara RF, Sundt TM, Michenfelder JD: Myocardial infarction in carotid endarterectomy patients anesthetized with halothane, enflurane, or isoflurane, *Anesthesiology* 69:783, 1988.

71. Nakajima Y, Moriwaki G, Ikeda K, et al. The effects of sevoflurane on recovery of brain energy metabolism after cerebral ischemia in the rat: a comparison with isoflurane and halothane, *Anesth Analg* 85:593, 1997.

72. Summors AC, Gupta AK, Matta BF: Dynamic cerebral autoregulation during sevoflurane anesthesia: a comparison with isoflurane, *Anesth Analg* 88:341, 1999.

73. Umbrain V, Keeris J, D'Haese J, et al: Isoflurane, desflurane and sevoflurane for carotid endarterectomy, *Anaesthesia* 55:1052, 2000.

74. Godet G, Watremez C, El Kettani, C: A comparison of sevoflurane, target-controlled infusion propofol, and propofol/isoflurane anesthesia in patients undergoing carotid surgery: a quality of anesthesia and recovery profile, *Anesth Analg* 93:560, 2001.

75. Mouren S, De Winter G, Guerrero SP, et al: The continuous recording of blood pressure in patients undergoing carotid surgery under remifentanil versus sufentanil analgesia, *Anesth Analg* 93:1402, 2001.

76. Wilhelm W, Schlaich N, Harrer J, et al: Recovery and neurological examination after remifentanil-desflurane or fentanyl-desflurane anaesthesia for carotid artery surgery, *Br J Anaesth* 86:44, 2001.

77. Doyle PW, Coles JP, Leary TM, et al: A comparison of remifentanil and fentanyl in patients undergoing carotid endarterectomy, *Eur J Anaesthesiol* 18:13, 2001.

78. Chaloupka JC, Weigele JB, Mangla S, et al: Cerebrovascular angioplasty and stenting for the prevention of stroke, *Curr Neurol Neurosci Rep* 1:39, 2001.

79. Guimaraens L, Sola MT, Matali A, et al: Carotid angioplasty with cerebral protection and stenting: report of 164 patients (194 carotid percutaneous transluminal angioplasties), *Cerebrovasc Dis* 13:114, 2002.

80. Bonaldi G: Angioplasty and stenting of the cervical carotid bifurcation: report of a 4-year series, *Neuroradiology* 44:164, 2002.

81. Criado FJ, Lingelbach JM, Ledesma DF, et al: Carotid artery stenting in a vascular surgery practice, *J Vasc Surg* 35:430, 2002.

82. Kackel R: Results of balloon angioplasty in the carotid arteries, *J Endovasc Surg* 3:22, 1996.

83. CAVATAS Investigators: Endovascular versus surgical treatment in patients with carotid stenosis in the Carotid and Vertebral Artery Transluminal Angioplasty Study (CAVATAS): a randomized trial, *Lancet* 357:1729, 2001.

84. Rockman CB, Jacobowitz GR, Lamparello PJ, et al: Immediate reexploration for the perioperative neurologic event after carotid endarterectomy: is it worthwhile? *J Vasc Surg* 32:1062, 2000.

85. Sheehan MK, Baker WH, Littooy FN, et al: Timing of postcarotid complications: a guide to safe discharge planning, *J Vasc Surg* 34:13, 2001.

86. Breen JC, Caplan LR, DeWitt LD, et al: Brain edema after carotid surgery, *Neurology* 46:175, 1996.

87. Jorgensen LG, Schroeder TV: Defective cerebrovascular autoregulation after carotid endarterectomy, *Eur J Vasc Surg* 7:370, 1993.

88. Hughes R, McGuire G, Montanera W, et al: Upper airway edema after carotid endarterectomy: the effect of steroid administration, *Anesth Analg* 84:475, 1997.

89. O'Sullivan JC, Wells DG, Wells GR: Difficult airway management with neck swelling after carotid endarterectomy, *Anaesth Intensive Care* 14:460, 1986.

90. Kunkel JM, Gomez ER, Spebar MJ, et al: Wound hematomas after carotid endarterectomy, *Am J Surg* 148:844, 1984.

91. Kaufman JL, Frank D, Rhee SE, et al: Feasibility and safety of 1-day postoperative hospitalization for carotid endarterectomy, *Arch Surg* 131:751, 1996.

92. Geary KJ, Ouriel K, Geary JE, et al: Neurologic events following carotid endarterectomy: prediction of outcome, *Ann Vasc Surg* 7:76, 1993.

93. Katz J: Section II. Neck. In: *Atlas of Regional Anesthesia*, ed 2, East Norwalk, CT, 1994, Appleton & Lange, 40.

Surgery of the Thoracic and Abdominal Aorta

11

Michael J. Murray, MD, PhD
Timothy S. J. Shine, MD

VASCULAR disease is extremely prevalent in the United States, so much so that a large proportion of patients requiring anesthesia have vascular disease and, in many circumstances, are administered an anesthetic for a noncardiac vascular procedure. Vascular disease of the coronary arteries is present is most of these patients. The most complex cases involve patients with diffuse arteriosclerosis including disease of the aorta. Anesthesia for patients having aortic surgery is the focus of this chapter, excluding aortic endovascular stents, which are discussed in Chapter 7, and ascending aortic and arch aneurysm surgeries, which, because they are performed using cardiopulmonary bypass, are discussed in cardiac anesthesia textbooks. The evaluation of the aorta and the preoperative evaluation of patients having aortic surgical procedures are discussed in earlier chapters (Chapters 3 to 6).

Coarctation of the aorta, traumatic injury to the aorta, dissection, and atherosclerotic and aneurysmal disease of the aorta (predominantly the abdominal aorta) often require surgical repair and, therefore, are the main topics of this chapter (Table 11-1).

Background

History

In the second century AD, Galen recognized and described peripheral vascular aneurysms, and Vesalius described aneurysms of the thoracic aorta in the 16th century.[1] Over the centuries, there have been several attempts to prevent enlargement and rupture of aneurysms by ligation of the aneurysm at its base.[2] Most vascular specialists, however, consider the mid-20th century as the time point at which their specialty began. Carrel used homologous and heterologous arteries and veins to replace blood vessels in dogs, but in the early 20th century, nonbiologic impervious material was used to serve as passive vascular conduits, none of which were long-term solutions for replacing arteries or veins.[3] It was not until 1948, when Gross and colleagues used human arterial grafts to treat cardiovascular defects, that the modern era of vascular surgery (and anesthesia) began.[4] A wide variety of tissues and materials have been used as vascular grafts over the last century (Table 11-2).[1] Polyester (Dacron) grafts were first used and reported by DeBakey et al (Figure 11-1), and the bovine heterograft revolutionized the new field, as did the use of an endovascular stent by Parodi and colleagues.[5-7] As surgeons developed the tools to replace larger and lengthier segments of endogenous vessels, the need arose to anesthetize and manage patients who were undergoing aortic surgical procedures and who had extensive cardiovascular disease.

Definitions

A *coarctation* is a congenital narrowing of the thoracic aorta at the level of the ligamentum arteriosum caused by a shelf-like thickening on the posterior lateral wall of the aorta (Figure 11-2). The lesion is found most commonly in males (ratio 2:1). Twenty percent of patients with Turner's syndrome and X-O karyotype have coarctation. Eighty-five percent of patients with a coarctation have a bicuspid aortic valve. The most common complications associated with coarctation are hypertension (proximal to the coarctation), cardiac failure related to the increased left ventricular afterload, aortic valvular disease, rupture of the aorta, endarteritis, and cerebral aneurysm rupture. The last is most likely due to defects in the vessel wall within the circle of Willis and the proximal hypertension that is a hallmark of coarctation.

Aortic injury related to trauma can result in an incomplete laceration or a complete *transection* of the aorta, usually caused by extensive blunt chest trauma as might occur in a fall from an elevated platform or from a severe deceleration injury as happens in a motor vehicle crash when an unbelted driver's torso slams forward against the steering wheel. Eighty percent of these injuries occur in close proximity to the aortic isthmus just distal to the left subclavian artery at the level of the ligamentum arteriosum. Complete rupture of the aorta with exsanguination is the most feared complication, but less severe trauma can lead to dissection, pseudoaneurysm formation, and other complications.

An aortic *dissection* involves a tear of the aortic endothelium that allows the pulsatile force of the aortic blood pressure to be transmitted through the tear, dilating and tearing the aortic media in a longitudinal fashion. More than 50 years ago, DeBakey classified dissections as type I, II, and III (Figure 11-3). Type I dissections involve the ascending aorta and extend into the arch and distal aorta, type II dissections involve only the ascending aorta, and type III dissections affect the aorta distal to the left subclavian artery.

The Stanford classification system divides dissections into type A and type B (Figure 11-4). Type A dissections involve the ascending aorta, independent of the entry site, and type B dissections involve the descending aorta, distal to the left subclavian artery.

Unfortunately, neither the DeBakey nor the Stanford classification scheme works for all dissections. It is often easiest to classify the dissections as either proximal or distal. Dissections are acute if the diagnosis is made within 14 days of onset of symptoms and chronic if diagnosed after this time period. Dissections, in and of themselves, may rupture, may lead to

TABLE 11-1
Diseases of the Aorta That May Require Surgery

Aneurysms
- Pseudoaneurysm
- True aneurysm
  - Congenital (Marfans)
  - Degenerative (cystic medial degeneration)
  - Infectious (mycotic)
  - Inflammatory (Takayasu's arteritis)

Atherosclerosis

Coarctation
- Adulthood
- Childhood

Dissection
- Proximal (DeBakey I, II; Type A)
- Distal (DeBakey III; Type B)

Traumatic injury to the aorta
- Blunt
  - Acute
  - Chronic
- Penetrating

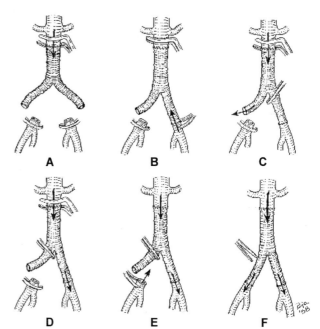

FIGURE 11-1 Technical application of bifurcation Dacron graft for replacement following resection of aneurysm or occlusive disease of abdominal aorta. **A,** Following completion of aortic anastomosis, the proximal occluding clamp on the aorta is released for a few seconds to permit flushing of atheromatous debris or accumulated clot formation. **B,** Following completion of the left iliac anastomosis, the occluding clamp on this vessel is released, permitting retrograde blood flow into the graft and thus flushing it of accumulated clot. **C,** An occluding clamp is applied to the left iliac limb of the graft just distal to the bifurcation, and the occluding clamp on the aorta is momentarily released to flush out thoroughly any accumulated clots. **D,** The occluding clamp on the left iliac limb of the graft is removed and applied to the right iliac limb, and the aortic occluding clamp is slowly and intermittently released over a period of several minutes, permitting restoration of circulation through the graft and into the left iliac artery. **E,** Distal occluding clamp on right iliac artery is temporarily released to permit retrograde flushing of any accumulated clots before performing anastomosis. **F,** After completing anastomosis to the right iliac artery, the distal occluding clamp is removed first and the proximal clamp is then slowly and intermittently released, permitting restoration of circulation to the right iliac artery. (From DeBakey ME, Cooley DA, Crawford ES, et al: *Am Surg* 24:862, 1958.)

aneurysm formation (true aneurysm vs. pseudoaneurysm), or may precipitate multiple organ system failure if the dissection obliterates or compromises the arterial blood supply to vital organs.

Atherosclerosis is the most common vascular disease that can lead to *aneurysm* formation in a significant number of patients. An aortic aneurysm is diagnosed when the diameter of the aorta exceeds 3.0 cm (Figure 11-5).

Incidence

The incidence of almost every kind of aortic disease, with the exception of syphilitic aortitis, has been steadily increasing, predominantly because of the incidental detection of more disease by the increasing use of ultrasonography and radiographic

TABLE 11-2
History of Vascular Grafts

Author	Type of Graft
Carrel et al, 1906	Homologous and heterologous artery and vein transplant in dogs
Goyanes, 1906	First autologous vein transplant in man
Tuffier, 1915	Paraffin-lined silver tubes
Blakemore, 1942	Vitallium tubes
Hufnagel, 1947	Polished methyl methacrylate tubes
Gross et al, 1948	Arterial allografts
Donovan, 1949	Polyethylene tubes
Voorhees, 1952	Vinyon-N®
Egdahl, 1955	Siliconized rubber
Edwards and Tapp, 1955	Crimped nylon
Edwards, 1957	Polytetrafluoroethylene
DeBakey, 1960	Polyester (Dacron®)
Rosenberg, 1966	Bovine heterograft
Sparks, 1968	Dacron-supported autogenous fibrous tubes
Soyer et al, 1972	Expanded polytetrafluoroethylene
Dardik, 1975	Human umbilical cord vein
Parodi, 1991	Stented endograft

From Kempczinski RF: vascular conduits; an overview. In Rutherford RB (ed): *Vascular Surgery*, ed 5, Philadelphia, 2000, WB Saunders, 527.

techniques. The "incidence" of coarctation is reported as 1 per 1550 patients based on autopsies; the premorbid diagnosis is more commonly and readily made today with improvements in health care and imaging techniques.[8] The incidence of traumatic injury to the aorta varies with the incidence of blunt and penetrating injury to the thorax and abdomen and, therefore, appears to be increasing.[9] In the United States, about 2000 new cases of aortic dissection are reported annually. The incidence of dissection of the aorta, based on an autopsy study, is reported as 3.2 per 100,000 of both sexes.[10]

In one study from the Mayo Clinic, there was a threefold increase in the incidence of abdominal aortic aneurysm (AAA) from 12.2 per 100,000 to 36.2 per 100,000 from 1950 to 1980.[11] This was most likely due to improved diagnostic techniques. However, in a second study from the same institution, more aneurysms of all sizes were discovered between 1970 and 1980 than in the previous two decades, which suggests a true increase in the incidence of aneurysmal disease independent of

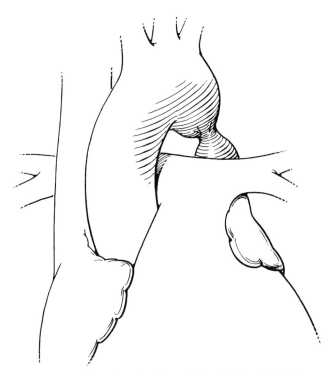

FIGURE 11-2 The aortic arch with coarctation at the level of the ligamentum arteriosum, the remnant of the ductus arteriosus.

any diagnostic improvements.[12] The increase is mostly likely due to the increasing longevity of the population, along with the effects of environmental factors that predispose patients to aneurysmal disease.

The incidence in men (older than 65) increases to a peak of 5.9% at age 80.[13] More than 10,000 deaths occur annually in the United Kingdom from aneurysmal disease, and aneurysm rupture is now the 13th most common cause of death in the Western world.[14] In the United States, a population-based screening study suggested that the combined effects of aging and comorbid conditions have increased the incidence of AAA to as high as 9% in patients older than 65 years, and ruptured AAAs account for at least 15,000 deaths annually.[15] Smoking is associated with AAA; given the prevalence of smoking, it is not surprising that as the population ages, the incidence and prevalence of AAA increase.[16]

Diagnosis

Aneurysms are most cost-effectively diagnosed by ultrasonography, but angiographic techniques are often used for patients with atherosclerotic and obliterative disease of the distal aorta and iliac arteries (see Chapters 3 and 4).[17] Aneurysms of the aorta are diagnosed when the aortic lumen is found to be greater than 3.0 cm (see Figure 11-5). The risk of rupture increases exponentially when the aneurysm is greater than

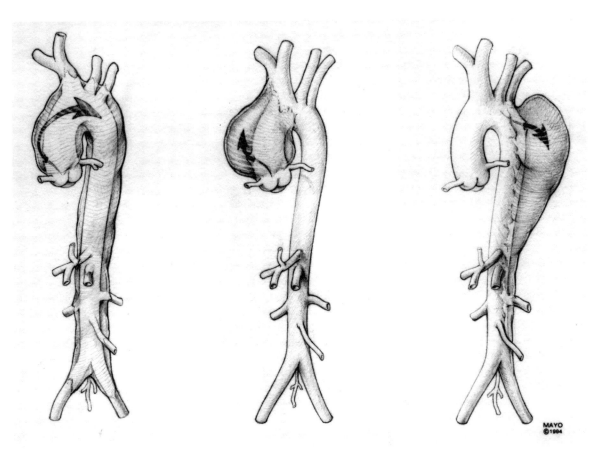

FIGURE 11-3 Types of aortic dissections. Type I: ascending aorta extending into the arch. Type II: ascending aorta only. Type III: descending aorta distal to the left subclavian artery.

STANFORD TYPE A   **STANFORD TYPE B**

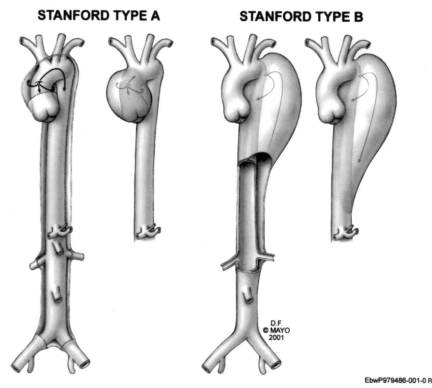

EbwP979486-001-0 R

FIGURE 11-4 The Stanford classification of aneurysms divides dissections into those involving the ascending aorta (type A) and those affecting the distal aorta (type B).

5.0 cm or if there is a superimposed inflammatory lesion. False aneurysms or *pseudoaneuryms* of the aorta are diagnosed when the aortic lumen is not dilated beyond normal (3.0 cm), yet the aorta itself is dilated to greater than 3.0 cm. The diagnosis of coarctation is most commonly suspected when during a routine physical examination increased blood pressure is found, but only in the upper extremities. Coarctation is more often found in young patients and confirmed through additional clinical and imaging tests.

Traumatic injury to the aorta is diagnosed when clinicians, on the basis of the history and physical examination, suspect aortic injury and confirm their impression with imaging studies. Angiography is still the "gold standard," but, increasingly, spiral or helical computed tomographic (CT) aortography is being used to diagnose and evaluate both blunt and penetrating aortic injury.[9]

Aortic dissections occur most commonly in the fifth to seventh decade of life and, as with almost all aortic disease, occur most commonly in men (2:1 to 3:1 ratio). The diagnosis should be considered in any patient with an acute onset of chest pain, especially if the pain penetrates to the back and radiates to the abdomen. A chest radiograph may help, but the diagnosis can be confirmed with an echocardiogram or an intravenous contrast CT aortogram. An angiogram remains the definitive imaging study.

Pathophysiology

Coarctation of the aorta occurs at the level of the ligamentum arteriosum, which is thought to play a role in the development of the coarctation. The exact mechanism is unknown, but current thinking is that oxygen-sensitive tissue from the ductus

arteriosus is incorporated into the aortic wall. After birth, as oxygen-rich blood perfuses the aorta, this tissue contracts, eventually becoming a permanent stricture. Most coarctations are immediately distal to the site of the ligamentum, with a minority being proximal or preductal.

Traumatic rupture of the thoracic aorta often occurs at the same site, at the ligamentum arteriosum, because of the anchoring effect of the ductal remnant on the aorta. During a motor vehicle crash, if the driver slams forward into the steering wheel (a common scenario for this type of injury), the thoracic contents jolt forward, with the ligamentum arteriosum tethering the aorta. A shear force is created that disrupts the integrity of the aorta. Penetrating wounds (gunshot, knife) are the most common traumatic injuries to the abdominal aorta.

In 95% of patients, aortic dissection occurs when a tear develops in the aortic wall. The exact cause is unknown but is probably multifactorial. Cystic medial necrosis is no longer thought to be one of those factors. Hypertension and an intrinsic defect of the aortic wall no doubt both play a role. The tear is usually horizontal, extending through the intima and into the media, which allows blood to eject through the tear. As the pulsating blood further dissects the media, a second or false lumen is created as the tear extends distally. The tear most commonly occurs proximally, secondary to the combination of hydraulic and mechanical forces that occur closer to the heart. Sixty-five percent of dissections occur in the ascending aorta, 20% in the descending aorta, 10% in the arch, and 5% more distally.[18]

Observational studies show that genetics, and endothelial and environmental factors, influence the development of aneurysmal and atherosclerotic disease (Figure 11-6). For example, men are five times more likely than women to have aortic aneurysmal

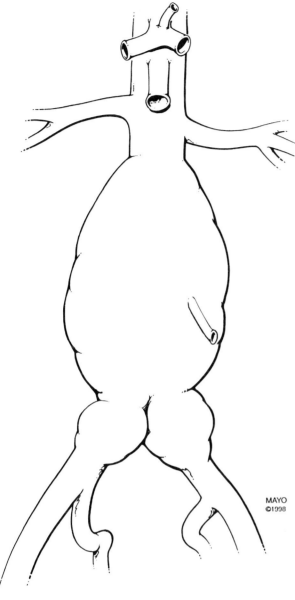

FIGURE 11-5 An infrarenal aortic aneurysm.

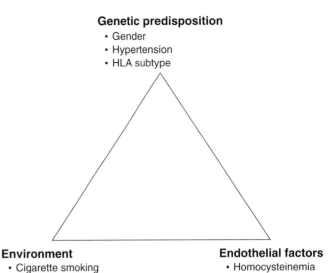

Genetic predisposition
- Gender
- Hypertension
- HLA subtype

Environment
- Cigarette smoking

Endothelial factors
- Homocysteinemia

FIGURE 11-6 Pathophysiology of aneurysm is multifactorial. HLA, human leukocyte antigen.

disease, and, similarly, men are 1.8 times more likely to have their aneurysm treated surgically.[19] Interestingly, women who have their aneurysm treated surgically have a 1.4 times greater risk of death than men who have elective aneurysm repair.[20]

Genetic factors that influence the development of AAAs include the methylene tetrahydrofolate reductase genotype, which correlates with levels of homocysteine. In patients with hyperhomocysteinemia, aortic aneurysms are larger. Homocysteine is believed to play a role because it induces serine elastase through activation of matrix metalloproteinase (MMP).[21] Serine elastase destroys elastin, one of the two important structural proteins in the wall of the aorta. Further support for this concept comes from the observation that MMP-2 production is increased in the wall of aortic aneurysms, and there is a relationship between the amount of MMP-9 expression and aortic diameter.[22,23] Unfortunately, lowering homocysteine levels does not decrease the mortality from atherosclerosis.[24]

Another enzyme that might destroy elastin is cysteine proteinase, which is overexpressed at sites of elastin damage. Cystatin C, expressed in vascular smooth muscle cells (VSMCs), is an inhibitor of cysteine proteinase. Any injury to VSMCs would, therefore, decrease inhibition of cysteine proteinase, leading to elastolysis.[25]

The destruction of VSMCs may be one of the critical events leading to the development of aneurysmal disease. Approximately 5% of aortic aneurysms are thought to be inflammatory, developing through a mechanism similar to that which causes Takayasu's arteritis, but the remaining 95% of aneurysms are also thought to have an inflammatory component. Macrophages and lymphocytes are often found on histopathologic examination of the aneurysm wall. These inflammatory cells destroy VSMCs that release an MMP inhibitor and a cystatin C inhibitor. With the loss of MMP and cystatin C inhibition, levels of serine elastase and cysteine proteinases (enzymes that can destroy elastin) are increased. Cigarette smoking is thought to affect aneurysm formation through increased production of these elastolytic enzymes. Current smokers are six to seven times more likely to have aneurysmal disease than nonsmokers. Ex-smokers are three times more likely to have AAAs than nonsmokers. The duration of smoking is thought to play an important role.[26] Elastase enzymatically destroys elastin, leaving collagen as the remaining structural protein in the aortic wall.[27] Although there is not a consistent relationship between aortic aneurysms and hypertension, there is an independent association between pulse pressure and aortic aneurysms.[28] Increased pulse pressure over time damages the collagen remaining in the aortic wall, resulting in aneurysm formation.

Prognosis

Observational data on the natural history of coarctation indicate that the median age of death is approximately 31 years, with complications of the coarctation accounting for 76% of the deaths.[29] Patients younger than 31 years die of aortic rupture, bacterial endocarditis, or intracranial hemorrhage; of those who die of intracranial hemorrhage, approximately one third die secondary to rupture of a cerebral aneurysm. Patients older than 31 years die from complications of congestive heart failure. Even if the coarctation is resected and repaired surgically or dilated with an intraluminal balloon, the long-term mortality is relatively high and, in one study, reported to be 12% at a mean duration of 9 years postoperatively.[30] In this study, the mortality was due to the same causes as observed in autopsy studies of untreated aortic aneurysm, for example, congestive heart failure, aortic rupture, and subarachnoid hemorrhage. But in the latter study, myocardial infarction accounted for a significant number of deaths. Some of the mortality is thought to be secondary to the effects of hypertension that exists in these patients, hypertension that is not necessarily corrected with repair of the coarctation (Table 11-3). Operative repair modifies the natural history of coarctation but, unfortunately, does not eliminate the associated morbidity and mortality.[31]

The prognosis of traumatic injury to the aorta has been determined from observational studies. Galli and colleagues reported their results for 42 patients who had traumatic injury of the thoracic aorta.[32] Of the 42 patients, 21 had immediate surgery, with the remaining 21 patients treated "conservatively" with cardiopulmonary resuscitation, hemodynamic stabilization with fluid administration, and induced hypotension. Among the 21 patients treated aggressively, the operative mortality was 19% (4 patients), with 3 of the 17 patients who survived having complications; 1 was paraplegic, 1 had paraparesis, and 1 had acute renal failure. In the conservatively managed group of patients, the aorta was evaluated by CT scan or magnetic resonance imaging every 3 to 5 days for 3 weeks and, thereafter, the patients were observed every 3 to 4 months. Eleven patients required surgery at approximately 7 months, with 10 of the patients under close monitoring still asymptomatic several months to years later.

Outcome is probably related not just to how the injury occurred, the extent of damage, and whether conservative (observational) therapy or a surgical procedure is undertaken but also to the hospital at which the operation is performed. Patients fare better if managed in a system or a hospital that has a large experience caring for patients requiring emergency vascular surgery.[33,34]

Approximately 21% of patients with aortic dissections die acutely before ever reaching a hospital or health care facility.[35] For patients admitted to a hospital for a proximal aortic dissection, the mortality is high—approximately 1.3% per hour, averaging 25% over the first 24 hours, 70% over 7 days, and 80% over 2 weeks.[36-38] If left untreated, half of the remaining patients succumb from their disease within 1 year.[35] Patients with acute distal aortic dissections can be medically managed because the survival rate of 75% is the same for both medical and surgical management.[39]

The prognosis for patients with AAAs has been extensively studied.[40-42] In a retrospective analysis of patients from Olmsted County (Minnesota) evaluated at the Mayo Clinic, the cumulative risk of rupture was 6% at 5 years after diagnosis and 8% after 10 years. However, the risk was different depending on the size of the aneurysm. For the 130 patients with an aneurysm less than 5 cm, the risk was 0%; and for the 46 patients with an aneurysm greater than 5 cm, the risk was 25%.[40]

For thoracic aneurysms, data also from the Mayo Clinic suggest different pathogenesis and outcome. Whereas men were five times more likely to have AAAs, women constituted 57% of the group who had thoracoabdominal aortic aneurysms (TAAAs) and tended to be older than patients diagnosed with AAAs, with an overall incidence of 10.4 per 100,000 persons years. The chances of rupture were 20% over 5 years, with 76% of the ruptures occurring in women.[41] On the basis of these observations, investigators in the United Kingdom studied 1090 patients with AAAs with a diameter of 4.0 to 5.5 cm and assigned them to one of two groups—early elective surgery or periodic surveillance with ultrasonography. Surgery was offered to the latter patients if the aneurysm grew to be greater than 5.5 cm or expanded more than 1.0 cm per year. There was no difference in outcome between the two groups. In the control group, the rupture rate was 1.6% per year; women had a fourfold risk of rupture, and if a woman's aneurysm ruptured, it was more likely to be fatal (Figure 11-7).[42]

TABLE 11-3

Risk Factors for Complications Following Repair of Coarctation of the Aorta

Complication	Prevalence, %	Proportion of Deaths, %	Risk Factors
Coronary artery disease	5-23	25-66	Duration of preoperative hypertension
Hypertension	25-75	–	Postoperative hypertension
			Age at repair
			Recoarctation
			Duration of follow-up
			Severe aortic regurgitation
Cerebrovascular accident	3	0–12	Preoperative and postoperative hypertension
			Preexisting Berry aneurysm
			Age at operation
Heart failure	NA	9–35	Hypertension
			Aortic valve disease
			Coronary artery disease
Recoarctation	3.1-10.8	–	Repair in infancy
			Subclavian flap aortoplasty
			Balloon angioplasty

From Jenkins NP, Ward C: *QJM* 92:365, 1999.

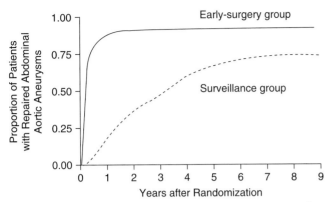

FIGURE 11-7 Kaplan-Meier estimates of the cumulative proportion of patients who underwent surgery for aneurysm repair, according to treatment group assignment. Data were not censored at the time of death. (From The United Kingdom Small Aneurysm Trial Participants: *N Engl J Med* 346:1445, 2002.)

In another study from the United Kingdom, the Multicenter Aneurysm Screening Study (MASS), patients (67,800 men 64 to 74 years of age) were routinely screened for AAAs at four centers. There were 47 fewer deaths in those assigned to the screening group who were then treated surgically if an aneurysm was found, versus a control group. Unfortunately, women were not included in this population-based study.[43]

Similar results were found in a somewhat larger study in the United States.[44] In the Aneurysm Detection and Management (ADM) Veterans Affairs Cooperative Study, 50- to 80-year-old patients with a 4.0- to 5.4-cm aneurysm, 99% of whom were men, were assigned at random to one of two groups. A total of 569 patients had immediate surgical repair, and 567 were assigned to a surveillance group.[44] All patients were seen every 6 months for the duration of the study; patients in the surveillance group had ultrasonography or CT scanning at these visits to monitor the size of the aneurysm. In this study, similarly to the United Kingdom study, patients in the surveillance group had surgical resection of the aneurysm with a graft interposition (similar surgical management to the early surgical repair group) when the aneurysm had expanded to be at least 5.5 cm or grew by 0.7 cm in the preceding 6 months. The immediate surgical repair group had an operative mortality rate of 2.7% (in contrast to the data reported by Pronovost and colleagues for the state of Maryland, with an operative mortality of 5.0% to 7.3%[45]). The mortality from any cause, the primary endpoint for the ADM study, was not different between groups. The authors concluded that early surgical intervention for aneurysms less than 5.5 cm, even when operative mortality was low, did not improve long-term survival.[44]

Management
Surgical Management

Changes in the management of aortic disease are no different from what has been observed in other cardiovascular disciplines in that less invasive techniques are increasingly being used to manage these patients, with associated decreases in morbidity, mortality, and cost, and improvements in patients' satisfaction and outcome. For coarctation of the aorta, resection of the aorta with patch angioplasty has long been the standard

of care, but balloon aortoplasty has been increasingly used over the last two decades. Balloon dilatation is not without complications and, unfortunately, recurrence of the coarctation and development of chronic hypertension are relatively high. However, even patients who have their coarctation repaired with an open surgical intervention have a high incidence of persistent hypertension, especially if the coarctation is repaired at an older age.[46]

Management of traumatic aortic rupture has not changed appreciably in that some patients are managed conservatively; on the basis of the extent of injury, the hemodynamic status, and bleeding complications, however, open surgical repair remains the treatment of choice.[47]

Patients with aortic dissection are commonly treated medically if they have a type III, type B, or a distal dissection and surgically with an interpositional aortic graft for type I or II, type A, or proximal aortic dissection. Increasingly, however, dissections are being treated with endovascular aortic stents with good results, but long-term observational studies are still ongoing.

Proximal aortic dissections require a surgical procedure unless serious comorbid conditions would make surgical intervention futile. A concomitant stroke is a relative contraindication because of the perioperative need for anticoagulation, which would greatly increase the risk for intracerebral bleeding, both because of the anticoagulation and because open surgical repair requires aortic cross-clamping, which significantly raises proximal aortic pressure. Surgical repair of a distal aneurysm is indicated if blood is leaking from the aneurysm, if there is ongoing dissection with intractable pain, or if the mechanical effects of the dissection occlude flow to a limb or organ.[48]

For patients with aneurysmal disease, as mentioned previously, the aneurysms are observed and monitored periodically if they are less than 5.5 cm, and surgery is recommended for aneurysms greater than 5.5 cm.[49] Depending on where the neck of the aneurysm is and the proximity to other blood vessels, descending thoracic aortic aneurysms can be managed with endovascular stents rather than an open surgical procedure. Whereas previous data have not justified open surgical procedures for aneurysms less than 5.5 cm, the size at which consideration should be given to placement of an endovascular stent for an aortic aneurysm has not yet been determined. Presumably, with an even lower mortality rate associated with an aneurysm compared with the 2.7% reported in the ADM, an endovascular stent may be warranted in patients with smaller aneurysms.[44]

The TAAA is the aneurysm of the aorta that is most difficult to manage surgically for a variety of reasons. Given the extent of the incision, the length of aorta to be resected, and the multiple organs that are affected by the ischemic cross-clamp time, alternative approaches are continually being evaluated. Some surgeons are advocating a combined open and endovascular stent approach to TAAAs as a means of decreasing the morbidity and mortality associated with this disease entity.[50]

Anesthetic Management

GLOBAL CONSIDERATIONS. Patients with vascular disease, especially aortic disease, often have comorbid conditions.[51] Many either currently smoke or are former smokers, leading to the development not only of vascular disease but of pulmonary disease as well. Many have coronary artery disease, and many have hypertension. It would not be unusual for 90% of patients to have all three comorbid conditions. In addition, diabetes is prevalent; approximately 10% of patients presenting for surgical repair of an aneurysm have diabetes, which further complicates the intraoperative management of these patients.

The anesthesiologist should ascertain the extent of all these disease processes during the preoperative period and optimize, as much as possible, the patient's preoperative health status. For example, many of these patients have angiography, and a significant number have preexisting renal disease. A bolus of intravascular contrast material given for imaging purposes in the days preceding an operation increases the risk of perioperative renal dysfunction, a risk that is magnified if the patient has an aortic surgical procedure. Prophylactic measures should be instituted prior to angiography if appropriate, and renal status should be restored to "baseline" status before surgery. Many patients are current or past smokers, a large proportion of whom have chronic obstructive pulmonary disease (COPD). Any intervention that results in cessation of smoking is of benefit to the patients who currently smoke. Treating pulmonary problems preoperatively to improve lung reserve and status should also improve overall morbidity and mortality.

When assessing comorbid conditions as part of the perioperative management of such patients, the anesthetic plan should include interventions that minimize additional complications and improve outcome. In addition, during the preoperative period, the imaging studies should be reviewed, and the case should be discussed with the vascular surgeon. Only by doing so can the anesthesiologist appreciate the extent of the vascular disease and the fact that perhaps not all the vascular abnormal-

ities will be corrected with the planned surgical intervention. For example, some arch aneurysms and TAAAs are repaired in stages. In the first operation, the proximal portion of the aneurysm is repaired, with the graft sutured proximally and then inserted into the distal aneurysm as an "elephant trunk" (Figure 11-8); the patient then returns to the operating room several weeks later for repair of the distal portion of the aneurysm.[52] Furthermore, if the incision will involve the thorax, discussion with the surgeon is necessary to ascertain whether or not a double-lumen endotracheal tube (ETT) is required. The use of a double-lumen ETT is relatively indicated, as the majority of anesthesiologists and surgeons find them to be beneficial. In this circumstance, patients undergoing TAAA resection develop facial and upper airway edema. The use of a bronchial blocker is more appropriately indicated in this circumstance because changing to a single-lumen ETT from a double-lumen ETT at the end of the surgical procedure can be difficult.

MONITORING

Cardiac ischemia. Because these patients have a high incidence of vascular disease, monitoring for cardiac ischemia is critical, often including electrocardiography, pulmonary artery occlusion pressure (PAOP) monitoring, and transesophageal echocardiography (TEE). Because most ischemia (approximately 97%) occurs inferolaterally, leads II and V_5 of the electrocardiogram (ECG) should be monitored. If the surgical field obviates monitoring V_5, lead II is monitored continuously (which can detect 90% to 95% of myocardial ischemia).

In addition to monitoring of the ECG, many of these patients have a pulmonary artery catheter (PAC) placed. An increase of 4 mmHg or more in the PAOP is a very sensitive but not very

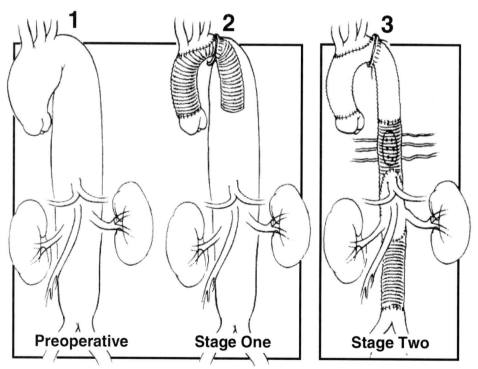

FIGURE 11-8 1, Preoperative aortic aneurysm. **2,** First stage of elephant trunk repair. **3,** Completed second stage of elephant trunk repair. (From Safi HJ, Miller CC III, Iliopoulos DC, et al: *Ann Surg* 226:599, 1997.)

specific monitor of cardiac ischemia. The role of the PAC in monitoring patients undergoing anesthesia is increasingly controversial, but most anesthesiologists continue to use PACs to monitor patients undergoing operations on the aorta.[53-55]

Finally, TEE is often used to monitor the effects of aortic cross-clamping and the associated increase in afterload on the left ventricle. It is also an excellent monitor of myocardial ischemia but, unfortunately, requires constant monitoring to detect regional wall motion abnormalities. If TEE is going to be used as a continuous monitor of ischemia, what most commonly occurs is that the TEE is performed shortly after induction and intubation, completing a baseline examination of the heart; if the aneurysm involves the thoracic aorta, the aorta can also be scanned. Immediately after the aorta is cross-clamped, the TEE scan is again repeated to assess the effects of the increase in afterload on the left ventricle. After the cross-clamp is removed and the patient's intravascular volume restored, the TEE examination can be repeated, especially if there is any hemodynamic instability. The purpose of this repeated examination is to check for left ventricular global dysfunction, as might be expected to occur if the patient was acidotic; regional wall motion abnormalities if the patient did indeed have myocardial ischemia; or a hyperdynamic heart with small chambers if the patient was hypotensive and had inadequate intravascular volume.

Temperature. Core temperature must be monitored for a variety of reasons. In 1984, Crawford and Sade published a report of three children who developed paraplegia following a simple aortic coarctation repair.[56] All three children had hyperthermia, and the authors speculated that the hyperthermia contributed to an increase in the metabolic rate for oxygen within the spinal cord, which became ischemic during the procedure. Following this publication, the safe ischemic time was decreased because of the increased metabolic rate of the cord.

Conversely, hypothermia might protect the spinal cord by extending the safe ischemic time (Figure 11-9), although hypothermia is also associated with an increase in coagulopathy, which in one series led to an 8% incidence of disseminated intravascular coagulation and an associated mortality rate of

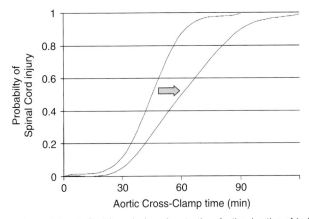

FIGURE 11-9 Goal for spinal cord protection. As the duration of ischemia increases, the likelihood of spinal cord injury increases. Hypothermia should protect the spinal cord by shifting the curve to the right and extending the safe ischemic time.

75%.[51] Therefore, patients should be maintained with a core temperature of 35 to 37°C when undergoing aortic surgical procedures, a temperature that is most commonly achieved by maintaining room temperature and through the use of forced-air warming blankets.[57] Depending on the type of surgical exposure required for the procedure, however, the amount of body surface that can be covered with an air blanket is often limited. Furthermore, if the aorta is going to be cross-clamped, the lower extremities should not be warmed for the same reason speculated upon earlier—the warmed extremities would have a higher metabolic rate, one that could not be supported during the aortic cross-clamping. Under these circumstances then, although upper and lower body warming blankets are placed, carefully avoiding the surgical site, the lower body warming device is not used until after the aortic cross-clamp is removed.

In order to monitor temperature, a nasopharyngeal probe works relatively well, although if a PAC is in place it can be used to monitor the core temperature. Bladder temperatures can be used as an assessment of core temperature, but during aortic cross-clamping, because of the low urine output, they are not very accurate.

Intravascular arterial catheters. Patients undergoing aortic surgical procedures with cross-clamping of the aorta require an indwelling arterial catheter for continuous measurement of blood pressure and for withdrawal of blood samples. In the upper extremities, an arterial catheter in the right radial artery is often used because blood flow to the left subclavian can occasionally be altered by a very proximal aortic cross-clamp, rendering blood pressure measured by a left-sided radial arterial catheter inaccurate. In addition to a proximal arterial catheter, if the thoracic or thoracoabdominal aorta is to be cross-clamped, many clinicians place a distal arterial catheter in either the femoral artery or the dorsalis pedis artery. Femoral arterial catheters can be difficult to place because many patients have had an arteriogram, and a hematoma in the groin can make placement of an arterial cannula difficult. Furthermore, if a bypass of the aorta is to be used, the left groin is not available for arterial pressure monitoring as it is reserved for a left atrial-to-iliac or atrial-to-femoral artery bypass using a centrifugal blood pump.[58] The advantage of having an arterial catheter under these circumstances is that if a left atrial-to-distal shunt is used, the perfusionist can monitor distal perfusion pressure and balance proximal and distal arterial pressures using the values from the arterial cannulas in the upper and lower extremities.

Intravascular central venous catheters. In addition to an intravascular arterial cannula, patients require placement of a central catheter both for volume administration and to measure intravascular filling pressures. It is not uncommon for aneurysms to rupture on induction of anesthesia and for patients with traumatic injury and dissections to be in hemorrhagic shock. Large-bore venous access needs to be achieved as quickly as possible upon entering the operating room, balancing this need with the placement of monitors and induction of anesthesia.

Because these patients have a high incidence of cardiac disease, a right atrial or central venous pressure monitoring catheter does not give as accurate information as a PAC with utilization of PAOP to monitor the left-sided filling pressures.[59] At many institutions, PACs are routinely inserted into patients undergoing aortic surgical procedures, but there are exceptions.[60] When inserting the PAC, a variety of techniques can be used to gain access to the central circulation, including double sticking the right internal jugular vein. However, if a large-bore intravenous catheter can be placed peripherally, a quadruple-lumen catheter can be inserted into the internal jugular or subclavian vein that would allow placement of a PAC, along with providing an indwelling cannula to monitor right atrial pressure, a large-bore venous access, and two other catheters for infusion of vasoactive medications.

Evoked potentials. A number of institutions find evoked potential monitoring helpful. One of the most feared complications of aortic surgery is the development of paraplegia secondary to inadequate perfusion of the anterior spinal artery (ASA), resulting in loss of motor neurons in the anterior portion of the spinal cord and rendering the patient paraplegic. Patients have motor evoked potential (and occasionally somatosensory evoked potential) monitors placed preoperatively. If the evoked potentials change in either latency or amplitude after the aorta is cross-clamped, the surgeon may move the aortic cross-clamps to allow greater perfusion of intercostal arteries and improved spinal cord blood flow. If repositioning of the clamps does not restore the evoked potentials, the surgeon may cancel the procedure.

When using motor evoked potential monitors, a certain degree of muscle activity must be allowed and, therefore, the compound motor action potential (CMAP) is monitored with infusion of neuromuscular blocking agents to maintain the CMAPs at approximately 10% of the baseline amplitude. Sensitivity and specificity of motor evoked potentials are not known, but currently this is the only monitoring technique available to assess spinal cord function intraoperatively. When evoked potential monitoring is used, the anesthetic should be adjusted carefully, and the use of benzodiazepines should be avoided if possible. In some circumstances, if the evoked potentials are lost, an increase in the proximal aortic pressure to improve perfusion through the vertebral arteries and the vessels that coalesce to form the ASA occasionally restores them to normal.[61]

The exact role of evoked potential monitors in aortic surgery is yet to be determined, but, as stated previously, physicians at several centers believe they are beneficial and use them routinely.

Transesophageal echocardiography. Increasingly, a number of centers use TEE in all their cardiovascular procedures and, depending upon the extent of the patient's coronary artery and vascular disease and the anticipated aortic surgery, TEE is often used.[62] It can be used not only to define the extent of the aortic disease, with respect to calcification, disruption, and so forth, but also to monitor for myocardial ischemia and for the effects of aortic cross-clamping on the left ventricle. If regional wall motion abnormalities develop in response to the aortic cross-clamping, the proximal pressure needs to be decreased (using a vasodilator such as sodium nitroprusside or nitroglycerin) until the regional wall motion abnormalities resolve.

Intraoperative Management
Anesthetic management of patients with aortic disease is challenging for a variety of reasons. Coarctations are commonly resected in children, often young children.

Traumatic rupture of the aorta can occur at any age, but because of the factors that contribute to motor vehicle crashes, these patients may be intoxicated and frequently have multiple other traumatic injuries.

Patients with dissections or aneurysms often have multiple comorbid conditions that present their own anesthetic challenges and frequently have diffuse vascular disease that can compromise blood flow to the heart, kidneys, brain, and so on. The heart is the organ most likely to become ischemic during the surgical procedure. Multiple complications can occur, but morbidity and mortality correlate with preoperative risk factors and with whether or not the patient has evidence of myocardial ischemia prior to surgery (Figure 11-10).

In addition to providing the usual standard of care that any patient undergoing an anesthetic should have, the anesthesiologist must give special care to maintaining core temperature (avoiding hyperthermia and hypothermia), stable hemodynamics, and an adequate myocardial oxygen supply-demand ratio and avoiding hypertension, hypotension, tachycardia, and high pulse pressure. This is important in all patients but especially in patients with dissection or large aneurysms because a high pulse pressure with tachycardia can create shear forces that further dissect or rupture the aorta. These hemodynamic goals can be achieved by titrating a combination of hypnotic and opioid agents and a short-acting β-blocker (such as esmolol) and vasodilators (sodium nitroprusside, nitroglycerin) to attenuate adverse hemodynamic responses to intubation, cross-clamping the aorta, and releasing the cross-clamp. Clinical experience suggests that maintenance of stable hemodynamics throughout the perioperative period decreases the likelihood of aortic rupture.[63]

TYPE OF ANESTHETIC. Patients having a surgical procedure on the aorta, unless it is an endovascular stent procedure, require general anesthesia. There are some reports of patients having AAAs repaired under a pure regional anesthetic technique, and others using a thoracic epidural with intubation,

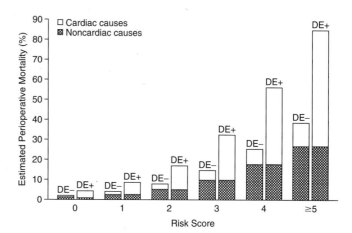

FIGURE 11-10 Estimate of the perioperative risk of death from noncardiac and cardiac causes. The risk score was determined by the number of risk factors present; risk factors included chronic pulmonary disease, angina, myocardial infarction, diabetes mellitus, heart failure, stroke, and renal failure. Patients with a negative result on dobutamine echocardiography (DE−) were considered not to have stress-induced ischemia, and those with a positive result (DE+) were considered to have stress-induced ischemia. (From Kertai MD, Bowersma E, Poldermans D: *N Engl J Med* 347:1112, 2002.)

ventilation, and sedation for patients with a TAAA.[64,65] The question is not whether these procedures should be performed with general versus regional anesthesia but whether regional anesthesia has a role in managing these patients intraoperatively and postoperatively (see Chapter 9).

Numerous articles have appeared over the last several decades outlining the benefits of epidural anesthesia and analgesia in managing patients with aortic disease, although demonstrating the benefits of regional anesthesia in this population of patients is difficult.[66-70] As Sitzman and his colleagues commented, "Although much literature has been published suggesting benefits of thoracic epidural anesthesia and analgesia on the cardiac, respiratory, and immune systems as well as on the surgical stress response, most currently published studies lack the power to provide definitive answers to the question, 'Does intraoperative use of epidural local anesthetics improve outcome?' "[71] Unfortunately, despite these many studies, most are simply not powered to answer the question of whether epidural anesthesia provides documented clinical utility. Having said that, however, most clinicians do use epidurals during the perioperative period. Some of the difficulties with using epidurals have to do with the use of local anesthetics in patients who become hypotensive after removal of the cross-clamp for a procedure in which the aorta is cross-clamped. Under those circumstances, the sympathectomy induced by local anesthetics can compound the difficulty of treating the accompanying hypotension. Another issue has to do with placement of an epidural in a patient who is going to receive heparin or some form of anticoagulation during the intraoperative period. This question has been addressed in several studies, and even though several hundred patients have been enrolled in such studies, the size of the studies does not allow an answer to the question of what happens to the incidence of epidural hematoma when heparin is given to these patients.[72,73] Presumably it is increased, but it is not known by how much.

The incidence of neurologic complications is typically reported as 1 in 20,000, but Lund, in a review of 150,000 patients who had epidural blockade, could find no incidence of an epidural hematoma resulting in a neurologic deficit.[74] However, if the incidence of epidural hematoma is 1 in 20,000, and if the incidence increased to 1 in 10,000, a 100% increase

in the incidence of epidural hematoma, in patients who were heparinized, although the incidence does double, the risk is so small that the potential benefits may outweigh the risks.[67-69]

When epidurals are placed, they are inserted at the level at which benefit is most likely to accrue. For example, patients undergoing abdominal laparotomy benefit most from a lumbar or low thoracic epidural, whereas patients undergoing a thoracotomy for resection of a coarctation or a descending thoracic aneurysm benefit most from a thoracic epidural. In these circumstances, the common practice is to administer an opioid along with a dilute concentration of a local anesthetic such as 0.05% or 0.075% bupivacaine or ropivacaine. Concentrations higher than this lead to intraoperative hypotension and, during the postoperative period, make it difficult for patients to ambulate because of the motor weakness associated with the higher concentration of local anesthetic. Increasingly in the United States, the practice is to have patients undergoing these major vascular procedures out of bed within 24 hours and with ambulation beginning soon thereafter. An epidural can improve the hemodynamic response, improve outcome by decreasing pulmonary complications, and attenuate the sequelae of ineffectively managed pain in patients undergoing aortic surgery, with a risk-benefit ratio that is acceptable. In this practice, the authors are of the opinion that epidurals provide so much benefit that when regional lumbar epidural cooling has been used in patients who receive heparin intraoperatively, two epidurals and an intrathecal catheter are placed because the benefits outweigh the risks, even in patients with several catheters within the epidural space.[75]

AIRWAY. Another major issue to be addressed when managing patients having aortic surgery has to do with the airway. Whereas the management of patients undergoing surgery on the abdominal aorta involves concerns no different from those for any other patient requiring oral intubation, if the surgery is to be performed on the thoracic aorta or on the thoracoabdominal aorta, a plan must be formulated for managing the airway during the perioperative period.

Surgical exposure of the descending thoracic aorta is often achieved using one-lung anesthesia (Table 11-4).[76] To achieve this goal, a left-sided, double-lumen ETT is commonly recommended because of the difficulty of placing a right-sided ETT without compromising the right upper lobe. However, large aneurysms

TABLE 11-4

Summary of Lung Isolation Devices and Recommendations for Placement

Device	Indication	Tube Size
Left-sided DLT	Majority of elective left or right thoracic surgical procedures	Can be determined by measurements of the tracheal width from chest radiograph
Right-sided DLT	Left bronchus-distorted anatomy Left pneumonectomy	
Univent® blockers	Selective lobar blockade Difficult airways	
WEB blockers	Critically ill intubated patient who requires lung isolation Selective lobar blockade Nasotracheal intubation	Standard endotracheal tube at least 8.0 mm ID
Fogarty occlusion catheter	Critically ill intubated patient who requires lung isolation Small bronchus Nasotracheal intubation	Standard endotracheal tube at least 6.0 mm ID

ID, inside diameter; DLT, double-lumen tube; WEB, wire-guided endobronchial blocker.
From Campos JH: *Anesthesiology* 97:1295, 2002.

can obstruct the left main bronchus and make it difficult or impossible to insert a left-sided endobronchial tube.[77] In such situations, a right-sided double-lumen tube would be used and carefully placed so as not to occlude the right upper lobe takeoff from the right mainstem bronchus (Figure 11-11).

One-lung anesthesia can also be accomplished using a single-lumen ETT with an endobronchial blocker either manufactured within the wall of the ETT (Univent tube) or inserted through the lumen of a single-lumen ETT. A Fogarty catheter or a wire-guided endobronchial tube (Figure 11-12) can be used in this manner. All these techniques require the use of a fiberoptic bronchoscope for placement and positioning of the tubes or catheters. The advantage of a single-lumen tube with a bronchial blocker is that there is no requirement to exchange the double-lumen tube for a single-lumen tube at the end of the operation. This exchange involves the risk of losing the airway while performing the tracheal tube exchange in a patient who has airway edema from the proximal hypertension and third spacing of fluid that occurs during proximal aortic cross-clamping. It is not uncommon for patients to have a 10- to 15-L positive fluid balance at the end of an operation that is primarily confined to the upper extremities and head and neck. Should the anesthesia team's assessment of the airway at the end of the operation indicate that changing a double-lumen for a single-lumen tube would present difficulties because of

edema and swelling in the glottic area, ventilation in the intensive care unit can be maintained with the double-lumen tube, deflating the bronchial cuff and withdrawing the double-lumen tube into the trachea. This situation could be avoided by using a bronchial blocker intraoperatively to manage the airway.

Oxygenation during one-lung anesthesia is maintained by adjusting respiratory rate and minute volume using arterial blood gases and pulse oximetry and positive end-expiratory pressure. Continuous positive airway pressure to the collapsed lung may be used to improve oxygenation if saturations fall below 88% to 90%.

AORTIC CROSS-CLAMPING. A number of sequelae occur with cross-clamping of the aorta (Figure 11-13). Mean arterial pressure above the cross-clamp increases up to 40% of baseline after cross-clamping the aorta because of an increase in afterload from the mechanical effect of the cross-clamp and from the effects of catecholamines, renin, and angiotensin. Although myocardial contractility may initially increase, cardiac output and global ventricular function deteriorate during cross-clamping and can be best evaluated using TEE. Mean arterial pressure decreases by up to 80% below the cross-clamp.[78-80] These hemodynamic changes result in increased intracranial pressure related to proximal hypertension and obstruction of cerebrospinal fluid (CSF) outflow. Renal blood flow and urine output are decreased, as is perfusion of the liver and all tissues below the cross-clamp,

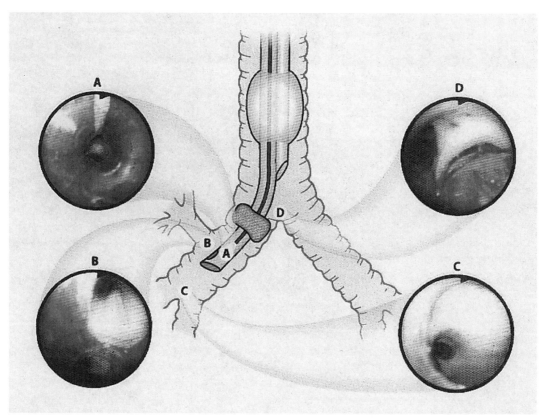

FIGURE 11-11 Fiberoptic bronchoscopic examination for a right-sided double-lumen tube. **A,** White line marker when the bronchoscope is passed through the endobronchial lumen. **B,** Slot of the endobronchial lumen properly aligned within the entrance of the right upper bronchus. **C,** Part of the bronchus intermedius when the bronchoscope is advanced through the distal portion of the endobronchial lumen. **D,** Edge of the endobronchial cuff around the entrance of the right mainstem bronchus when the bronchoscope is passed through the tracheal lumen. (From Campos JH: *Anesthesiology* 97:1295, 2002.)

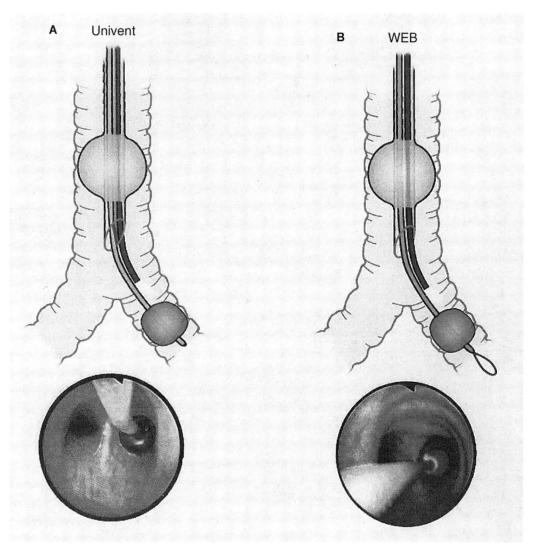

FIGURE 11-12 A, Univent bronchial blocker; the optimal position of the Univent in the left mainstem bronchus. **B,** Wire-guided endobronchial blocker (WEB); the optimal position of the WEB blocker in the left mainstem bronchus. (From Campos JH: *Anesthesiology* 97:1295, 2002.)

resulting in lactic acid production and metabolic acidosis. In an effort to improve renal function during and after cross-clamping, mannitol and low-dose dopamine are often administered prior to cross-clamping. Unfortunately, dopamine has not been found to be efficacious in controlling blood pressure and renal blood flow.[81] A relatively new dopamine-1 agonist, fenoldopam, has been found to lower blood pressure, maintain renal blood flow and urine output, and decrease the incidence of renal failure in patients undergoing aortic surgery.[82,83]

The surgical team can use bypass techniques and shunts to reduce proximal hypertension, improve distal perfusion, and preserve organ function in the vascular beds distal to the aortic cross-clamp. Before unclamping the aorta, fluid resuscitation should be started, replacing blood loss with salvaged blood or transfusion of packed red blood cells; metabolic acidosis should be corrected with sodium bicarbonate, and inotropic support should be ready and available.

Management of TAAAs and that of AAAs are similar; however, the hemodynamic instability is easier to control and treat in most patients following open repair of an AAA. Although it is generally true that the more distally the cross-clamp is placed, the less hemodynamic change and the fewer effects on the heart, cross-clamping the aorta at any site produces profound hemodynamic changes with effects on the heart and organs both above and below the cross-clamp.[62] Interestingly, patients with aneurysms are likely to have more profound hemodynamic changes upon aortic cross-clamping than patients who have obstructive disease, most often of the distal aorta, the iliac arteries, and the proximal femoral arteries (Leriche's syndrome).[84] This is thought to be due to the fact that patients with occlusive disease have more periaortic collateral vessels and, therefore, can withstand the placement of the cross-clamp with less hemodynamic compromise.[85]

With placement of the cross-clamp, a significant change occurs in the proximal blood pressure, as already noted. As was also mentioned, cardiac output can increase initially but deteriorates over time. This is most likely because of a redistribution of blood flow with collapse of the venous circulation distal to the cross-clamp and augmentation of flow above the cross-clamp.[86] Filling pressures increase immediately after placement

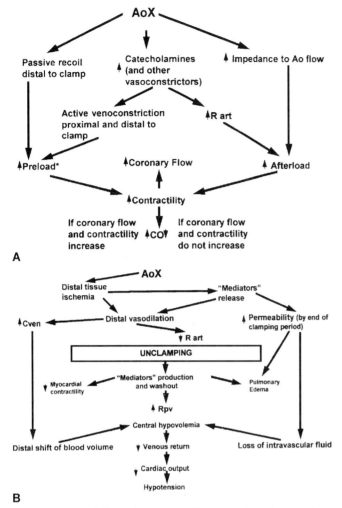

A

B

FIGURE 11-13 A, Systemic hemodynamic response to aortic cross-clamping. Preload does not necessarily increase. If, during infrarenal aortic cross-clamping, blood volume shifts into the splanchnic vasculature, preload does not increase. **B,** Systemic hemodynamic response to aortic unclamping. Ao, aortic; AoX, aortic cross-clamping; Cven, venous capacitance; Rart, arterial resistance; Rpv, pulmonary vascular resistance; $\uparrow$ and $\downarrow$, increase and decrease, respectively. *Different patterns are possible. (From Gelman S: *Anesthesiology* 82:1026, 1995.)

of the cross-clamp, which can lead to the increase in cardiac output. The deterioration in cardiac output is due to an adverse oxygen supply-demand ratio. The left ventricle can become overdistended because of the increased afterload. This often leads to myocardial ischemia. The anesthesiologist treating such patients must optimize myocardial oxygen supply-demand ratios. Although the surgeon can place a shunt or insert a bypass around the aorta to be cross-clamped, many surgeons do not because it has not been shown to be of benefit.[87] Furthermore, independent of whether a shunt or bypass is placed and independent of the use of vasodilators, such as sodium nitroprusside to control the hemodynamic response to cross-clamping, the vascular beds above the cross-clamp are at risk for the development of hypoperfusion, ischemia, and organ dysfunction. This may seem surprising because of the increase in flow above the cross-clamp, but studies in animals have demonstrated evidence of depletion of high-energy phosphate storage

in both myocardial and skeletal muscle above the cross-clamp.[88] Shunts develop during aortic cross-clamping, certainly distal to the cross-clamp but probably above the cross-clamp as well. Flow through shunts within skeletal, myocardial, and other organ beds proximal to the cross-clamp increases with no increase in nutritive blood flow.[89]

When treating the proximal hypertension that develops after placement of the cross-clamp on the aorta, many clinicians use a vasodilator such as sodium nitroprusside.[87] Additional literature reports that arterial vasodilators such as sodium nitroprusside work better than venodilators such as nitroglycerin.[90] Controlling the proximal hypertension that develops following cross-clamping is important in protecting the heart and tissues proximal to the aortic cross-clamp. Conversely, treating the hemodynamic sequelae that develop after removal of the aortic cross-clamp is equally important. Following release of the cross-clamp, a prolonged period of profound hypotension can occur. This hypotension is thought to be secondary to several factors and is most likely multifactorial. During placement of the aortic cross-clamp, blood pools in the periphery, and following removal of the cross-clamp, central hypovolemia is manifested. Furthermore, a number of cytokines produced in the organ beds distal to the cross-clamp are released. As these vasodilators wash into the central circulation following removal of the cross-clamp, systemic vasodilation is a consequence, with a decrease in total systemic vascular resistance and development of profound hypotension.

A third mechanism for the hypotension that is seen after aortic cross-clamping is the anoxia that develops. Anoxia per se in the peripheral vascular bed distal to the cross-clamp relaxes smooth muscles. As blood flow is restored in the distal circulation, the smooth muscle relaxation is manifested by a decrease in systemic vascular resistance and hypotension.

Treatment of the hypovolemia that develops following release of aortic cross-clamping focuses on several factors. Volume resuscitation must be initiated at once and often prior to removal of the aortic cross-clamp.[91] In this circumstance, interestingly, the fluid requirements for patients with aneurysmal disease versus aortic occlusive disease are often greater, and some patients require twice as much fluid following replacement of an aneurysm as opposed to tube grafting the aorta for aortic occlusive disease.[91]

Acidosis is also noted after removal of the aortic cross-clamp, but no evidence exists that correcting the metabolic acidosis with bicarbonate improves outcome.[92] However, in common practice, most clinicians administer 1 to 2, 50-mEq ampules of sodium bicarbonate prior to releasing the aortic cross-clamp, independent of any evidence-based medicine to suggest that such a practice has any benefit. At a minimum, it does improve the acidosis that develops during cross-clamping and, as long as perfusion (primarily with volume resuscitation) and ventilation are maintained, the accompanying increase in carbon dioxide production should not have any adverse physiologic consequences.

In addition to the volume resuscitation and use of bicarbonate, many clinicians add a vasoconstrictor and sometimes an inotrope. Many patients do not respond to vasoconstrictors because during the aortic cross-clamping, as already noted, the smooth muscle in the peripheral circulation may be relaxed and initially unresponsive to the use of any vasopressor. Furthermore, following aortic cross-clamping, a large amount of cate-cholamines is released. These excess catecholamines, over a relatively short period of time, can lead to downregulation of the adrenergic receptors in the periphery with an attenuated response of the peripheral vasculature to exogenous vasoconstrictors such as phenylephrine and norepinephrine. However, clinical practice often dictates that if volume resuscitation is proving inadequate, one or two amps of bicarbonate and a vasoconstrictor such as phenylephrine should be used, either as a bolus or as a continuous infusion. Because the hypotension is usually transient, lasting one to several minutes, most clinicians elect to use a bolus of a vasoconstrictor if it is used at all.

If during the aortic cross-clamping decreased myocardial function occurs—because of myocardial ischemia or the release of myocardial depressant factors—the dysfunction should be assessed with TEE as previously mentioned.[62] Following assessment, an inotrope such as dobutamine or epinephrine can be used. The advantage of using epinephrine in this circumstance is that because of its α and β properties, it can augment myocardial contractility at the same time that it augments peripheral vascular tone. Unfortunately, in this circumstance, the vasculature proximal to the cross-clamp is more likely to respond to adrenergic stimulation as opposed to the circulation distal to the area perfused by the aorta that was cross-clamped.

The main reason for controlling these hemodynamic sequelae of cross-clamping and unclamping has to do with attenuating the profound organ dysfunction that frequently develops after aortic surgery. In a review of more than 1500 patients undergoing thoracoabdominal aortic operations, Crawford and colleagues at Baylor College of Medicine noted that cardiac complications, neurologic complications, renal failure, and gastrointestinal ischemia were manifest in 7% to 18% of patients.[93] As noted previously, the incidence of cardiac dysfunction is not as great as it once was, primarily because many of these patients undergo extensive preoperative cardiac assessment and lesions are treated preoperatively when found (Chapter 5).

Even so, it cannot be emphasized enough that it is imperative for anesthesiologists managing these patients to optimize myocardial oxygen supply-demand ratios. The ratio can be improved by the judicious use of vasodilators and by the use of drugs that decrease heart rate and contractility such as β-adrenergic blocking agents. Esmolol is often used because of its short half-life, which is an extremely important feature when, later in the surgical procedure following removal of the cross-clamp from the aorta, hypotension is a problem. Furthermore, because a significant number of these patients have pulmonary disease, if airway obstruction manifests itself, because of esmolol's sufficiently short half-life, its pulmonary sequelae should be relatively short lived.

Pulmonary complications are common following aortic surgery, not because of reactive airway disease but because of several factors, including the extent of the surgical wound, especially if the incision extends into the thorax, and the effects of ileus that are common with repair of AAAs and TAAAs.[94] In their assessment of respiratory failure following operations on the TAAA, Svensson and colleagues found that 8% had pulmonary complications that required prolonged ventilatory sup-

port leading to tracheostomy.[95] Although the premorbid conditions of the patients, including a history of smoking and COPD, were important, other factors that were associated with respiratory failure included multiple organ dysfunction syndrome, coagulopathy, and reoperation. The independent predictors of respiratory failure in their study were a history of COPD, a history of smoking, and cardiac and renal complications.

Visceral ischemia is also common following surgery secondary to hypoperfusion of the abdominal vasculature during aortic cross-clamping, whether that cross-clamp is placed in the chest or in the supraceliac position within the abdomen.[96] Although ischemic colitis is common and these patients are at increased risk for gastrointestinal bleeding, of greater concern is the development of postoperative renal failure.[97] Initially after cross-clamping, a large amount of renin is released with conversion to angiotensin, but this release is insufficient to maintain renal blood flow during and following aortic cross-clamping.[98] Therefore, the incidence of renal dysfunction in patients following aortic surgery is high and independent of whether the cross-clamp was placed in the infrarenal or suprarenal position (see Chapter 14).

NEUROLOGIC COMPLICATIONS. Of all the complications associated with aortic surgery, the most feared and most devastating are the neurologic complications. Cerebrovascular accidents (CVAs) are major sequelae of surgical repair of aortic arch aneurysms, especially if the patient is undergoing a surgical repair for Takayasu's arteritis.[99,100] CVAs following dismissal from the hospital are also fairly common, even for patients undergoing AAA repair, but this is most likely secondary to the fact that patients with aortic disease have extensive systemic vascular disease, which would manifest itself as organ dysfunction occurring because of pathology in the arterial tree in those organs.[101] Shine and colleagues have reported that the incidence of CVAs in the immediate postoperative period in patients undergoing TAAAs is 7.6%.[102] In the series of patients they studied, most of those CVAs involved the left hemisphere, implicating placement of the proximal aortic cross-clamp.

Although stroke is an unfortunate complication of aortic surgery, even more feared is the development of a spinal cord infarction manifested by postoperative paraplegia. This can occur even with endovascular repair of AAA but most commonly occurs with AAA repair (Figure 11-14) and most likely has to do with the anatomy of the arterial blood supply of the spinal cord (Figure 11-15).[103]

The blood supply to the ASA, the artery that supplies nutrient blood flow to the anterior motor neurons, is formed from two branches of the vertebral artery, which coalesce to form the ASA that runs in the midline and the anterior aspect of the spinal cord all the way to the conus of the cord. The ASA has several feeder arteries that supply additional blood throughout its course.[104] Of the arteries that supply the cord, the most important is the so-called artery of Adamkiewicz, the arteria medullaris magna anterior. All these medullary feeding arteries arise from radicular arteries, which in turn are offshoots of lumbar arteries that derive from intercostal arteries from the aorta. Paraplegia develops in patients with coarctation because of the anatomy of the aorta, the intercostal arteries, and the distal spinal cord, which contains the motor neurons that innervate the lower extremities (Figure 11-16).[105] Any time the aorta is cross-clamped in its

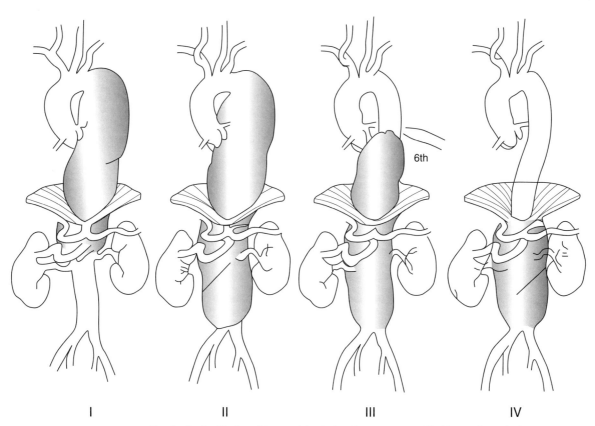

FIGURE 11-14 Crawford's classification of thoracoabdominal aortic aneurysms and incidence of paraplegia.

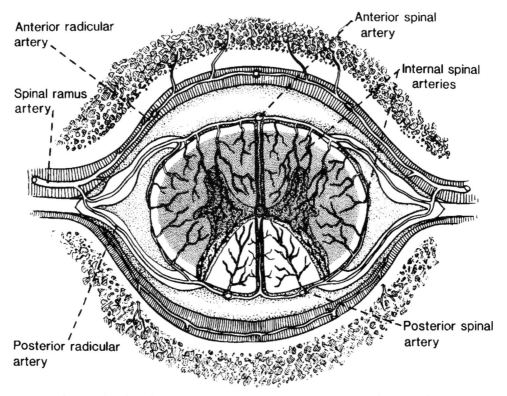

FIGURE 11-15 Cross section of the distal thoracic cord with blood supply. (From Whitley D, Gloviczki P: Spinal cord ischemia associated with high aortic clamping: methods of protection. In Sidawy AN, Sumpio BE, DePalma RG, Armonk NY [eds]: *The basic science of vascular disease*, Armonk, NY, 1997, Futura Publishing Company, 797.)

two that have the most promise, CSF drainage and hypothermia, currently demand the most attention.

In 1960, Miyamoto and colleagues attempted CSF drainage in patients undergoing coarctation repair to minimize the incidence of spinal cord injury.[107] Two years later, Blaisdell and Cooley demonstrated in dogs that drainage of CSF augmented spinal cord perfusion pressure.[108] Although CSF drainage has often been considered controversial, a number of case reports demonstrate its benefit.[109-114] Importantly, Safi and colleagues, in a series of patients undergoing TAAA, demonstrated in a prospective, randomized, controlled trial the benefit of CSF drainage. By keeping CSF pressure low, spinal cord perfusion pressure is augmented.[115] This would underscore the importance not only of draining CSF but also of maintaining proximal aortic pressure.[114] It is the authors' practice in patients undergoing TAAA repair to drain CSF fluid.

Of equal interest is the role of hypothermia in protecting the spinal cord. More than 50 years have elapsed since Beattie and colleagues commented upon the importance of hypothermia in protecting the spinal cord during surgery on the aorta.[116] This finding has been demonstrated in animals as well.[117] Unfortunately, hypothermia is associated with a number of infectious complications, severe coagulopathies, and prolonged recovery from anesthesia.[118,119] However, Marsala et al developed a technique in which the spinal cord itself was cooled without the use of systemic hypothermia.[120] This led Davison and his colleagues at Massachusetts General Hospital to use epidural cooling during TAAA repair.[121] Davison and colleagues continue to use regional spinal cord cooling, but De Ruyter and his colleagues at the Mayo Clinic have been unable to duplicate their findings.[122] Given the fact that others have found a benefit of moderate hypothermia in protecting the central nervous system, there is no doubt a role for hypothermia in protecting the cord, but the best way to use this technique in managing patients with TAAAs is yet to be found.[123]

Conclusion

Managing patients undergoing open aortic surgical procedures is one of the greatest challenges an anesthesiologist faces, but if they are managed correctly, the anesthesiologist's care can have a huge impact on their outcome.

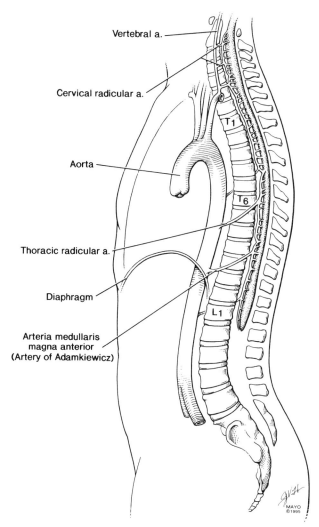

FIGURE 11-16 Cross section of a human torso showing the origin of the anterior spinal artery (ASA) from cervical radicular arteries. The ASA, through its course to the conus, receives additional blood from medullary arteries that derive from intercostals off the aorta. The majority of these arteries arise from the thoracic aorta. Any time the thoracic aorta is cross-clamped, the spinal cord is at risk of ischemia leading to the development of paraplegia postoperatively.

thoracic distribution, the distal spinal cord is at risk of hypoperfusion. Even patients undergoing AAA surgery are at risk of developing paraplegia if the artery of Adamkiewicz comes off lower than normal.[106] Placement of a left atrial-to-distal aortic bypass with retrograde perfusion, presumably of the ASA through intercostal and radicular arteries, does not necessarily prevent paraplegia. This may be because ischemia not only is secondary to the ischemia that occurs during cross-clamping but also may be related to intraoperative thromboembolic events that might develop. It might result if the intercostal arteries supplying the critical blood flow to the ASA are not reimplanted, or it may be related to the anatomy of the ASA itself.[104] The ASA proximal to the junction of the artery of Adamkiewicz is 67% of the size of the artery distal to the junction. Therefore, if flow through a distal bypass is marginal, it may not be enough to perfuse the entire ASA in a retrograde fashion.

Many attempts have been made to minimize the incidence of paraplegia, but all of them have met with limited success. The

REFERENCES

1. Kempczinski RF: Vascular conduits: an overview. In: Rutherford RB (ed): *Vascular surgery*, ed 5, Philadelphia, 2000, WB Saunders, 527.
2. Dale AW: The beginnings of vascular surgery, Surgery 76:849, 1974.
3. Carrel A, Guthrie CG: Uniterminal and biterminal venous transplantations, *Surg Gynecol Obstet* 2:266, 1906.
4. Gross RE, Hurwitt ES, Bill AH Jr, et al: Preliminary observations on the use of human arterial grafts in the treatment of certain cardiovascular defects, *N Engl J Med* 239:578, 1948.
5. DeBakey ME, Cooley DA, Crawford ES, et al: Clinical application of a new flexible knitted Dacron arterial substitute, *Am Surg* 24:862, 1958.
6. Rosenberg N, Gaughran ERL, Henderson J, et al: The use of segmental arterial implants prepared by enzymatic modification of heterologous blood vessels, *Surg Forum* 6:242, 1955.
7. Parodi JC, Palmaz JC, Barone HD: Transfemoral intraluminal graft implantation for abdominal aortic aneurysms, *Ann Vasc Surg* 5:491, 1991.
8. Blackford LM: Coarctation of the aorta, *Arch Intern Med* 41:702, 1928.
9. Degiannis E, Boffard K: Critical decisions in trauma of the thoracic aorta, *Injury* 33:317, 2002.

10. Svensjo S, Bengtsson H, Bergqvist D: Thoracic and thoracoabdominal aortic aneurysm and dissection: an investigation based on autopsy, *Br J Surg* 83:68, 1996.
11. Melton LJ III, Bickerstaff LK, Hollier LH, et al: Changing incidence of abdominal aortic aneurysms: a population-based study, *Am J Epidemiol* 120:379, 1984.
12. Bickerstaff LK, Hollier LH, Van Peenen HJ, et al: Abdominal aortic aneurysms: the changing natural history, *J Vasc Surg* 1:6, 1984.
13. Bengtsson H, Bergqvist D, Sternby NH: Increasing prevalence of abdominal aortic aneurysms: a necropsy study, *Eur J Surg* 158:19, 1992.
14. Thompson MM, Bell PRF: ABC of arterial and venous disease. Arterial aneurysms, *Br Med J* 320:1193, 2000.
15. Alcorn HG, Wolfson SK Jr, Sutton-Tyrrell K, et al: Risk factors for abdominal aortic aneurysms in older adults enrolled in the Cardiovascular Health Study, *Arterioscler Thromb Vasc Biol* 16:963, 1996.
16. MacSweeney STR, Ellis M, Worrell PC, et al: Smoking and growth rate of small abdominal aortic aneurysms, *Lancet* 344:651, 1994.
17. Greenhalgh RM, Powell JT: Screening men for aortic aneurysm. A national population screening service will be cost effective, *Br Med J* 325:1123, 2002.
18. Crawford ES: The diagnosis and management of aortic dissection, *JAMA* 264:2537, 1990.
19. Kuivaniemi H, Tromp G, Prockop DJ: Genetic causes of aortic aneurysms. Unlearning at least part of what the textbooks say, *J Clin Invest* 88:1441, 1991.
20. Katz DJ, Stanley JC, Zelenock GB: Gender differences in abdominal aortic aneurysm prevalence, treatment, and outcome, *J Vasc Surg* 25:561, 1997.
21. Brunelli T, Prisco D, Fedi S, et al: High prevalence of mild hyperhomocysteinemia in patients with abdominal aortic aneurysm, *J Vasc Surg* 32:531, 2000.
22. Davis V, Persidskaia R, Baca-Regen L, et al: Matrix metalloproteinase-2 production and its binding to the matrix are increased in abdominal aortic aneurysms, *Arterioscler Thromb Vasc Biol* 18:1625, 1998.
23. McMillan WD, Tamarina NA, Cipollone M, et al: Size matters: the relationship between MMP-9 expression and aortic diameter, *Circulation* 96:2228, 1997.
24. Hung J, Beilby JP, Knuiman MW, Divitini M: Folate and vitamin B-12 and risk of fatal cardiovascular disease: cohort study from Busselton, Western Australia, *BMJ* 326:131, 2003.
25. Shi GP, Sukhova GK, Grubb A, et al: Cystatin C deficiency in human atherosclerosis and aortic aneurysms, *J Clin Invest* 104:1191, 1999.
26. Wilmink TB, Quick CR, Day NE: The association between cigarette smoking and abdominal aortic aneurysms, *J Vasc Surg* 30:1099, 1999.
27. Shah PK: Inflammation, metalloproteinases, and increased proteolysis: an emerging pathophysiological paradigm in aortic aneurysm, *Circulation* 96:2115, 1997.
28. Naydeck BL, Sutton-Tyrrell K, Schiller KD, et al: Prevalence and risk factors for abdominal aortic aneurysms in older adults with and without isolated systolic hypertension, *Am J Cardiol* 83:759, 1999.
29. Reifenstein GH, Levine SA, Gross RE: Coarctation of the aorta: a review of 104 autopsied cases of the "adult-type," 2 years of age or older, *Am Heart J* 33:146, 1947.
30. Maron BJ, O'Neal-Humphries J, Rowe RD, Mellitis ED: Prognosis of surgically corrected coarctation of the aorta: a 20-year post operative appraisal, *Circulation* 47:119, 1973.
31. Clarkson PM, Nicholson MR, Barratt-Boyes BG, et al: Results after repair of coarctation of the aorta beyond infancy: a 10-to-28 year follow-up with particular reference to late systemic hypertension, *Am J Cardiol* 51:1481, 1983.
32. Galli R, Pacini D, Di Bartolomeo R, et al: Surgical indications and timing of repair of traumatic ruptures of the thoracic aorta, *Ann Thorac Surg* 65:461, 1998.
33. Cernaianu AC, Cilley JH Jr, Baldino WA, et al: Determinants of outcome in lesions of the thoracic aorta in patients with multiorgan system trauma, *Chest* 101:331, 1992.
34. Campbell B, Chester J: Emergency vascular surgery. Patients need to travel for specialist treatment, *BMJ* 324:1167, 2002.
35. Meszaros I, Morocz J, Szlavi J, et al: Epidemiology and clinicopathology of aortic dissection, *Chest* 117:1271, 2000.
36. Hirst AE Jr, Johns VJ Jr, Kime SW Jr: Dissecting aneurysms of the aorta: a review of 505 cases, *Medicine (Baltimore)* 37:217, 1958.
37. Archer AG, Choyke PL, Zeman RK, et al: Aortic dissection following coronary artery bypass surgery: diagnosis by CT, *Cardiovasc Intervent Radiol* 9:142, 1986.
38. Pitt MP, Bonser RS: The natural history of thoracic aortic aneurysm disease: an overview, *J Card Surg* 12:270, 1997.
39. Chirillo F, Marchiori MC, Andriolo L, et al: Outcome of 290 patients with aortic dissection: a 12-year multicenter experience, *Eur Heart J* 11:311, 1990.
40. Nevitt MP, Ballard DJ, Hallett JW Jr: Prognosis of abdominal aortic aneurysms. A population-based study, *N Engl J Med* 321:1009, 1989.
41. Clouse WD, Hallett JW Jr, Schaff HV, et al: Improved prognosis of thoracic aortic aneurysms. A population-based study, *JAMA* 280:1926, 1998.
42. The United Kingdom Small Aneurysm Trial Participants: Long-term outcomes of immediate repair compared with surveillance of small abdominal aortic aneurysms, *N Engl J Med* 346:1445, 2002.
43. Muticentre Aneurysm Screening Study Group: Multicentre aneurysm screening study (MASS): cost-effectiveness analysis of screening for abdominal aortic aneurysms based on four year results from randomized controlled trial, *BMJ* 325:1135, 2002.
44. Lederle FA, Wilson SE, Johnson GR, et al: Immediate repair compared with surveillance of small abdominal aortic aneurysms, *N Engl J Med* 346:1437, 2002.
45. Pronovost PJ, Jenckes MW, Dorman T, et al: Organizational characteristics of intensive care units related to outcomes of abdominal aortic surgery, *JAMA* 281:1310, 1999.
46. Sakopoulos AG, Hahn TL, Turrentine M, Brown JW: Recurrent aortic coarctation: is surgical repair still the gold standard? *J Thorac Cardiovasc Surg* 116:560, 1998.
47. von Oppell UO, Dunne TT, De Groot MK, Zilla P: Traumatic aortic rupture: twenty-year metaanalysis of mortality and risk of paraplegia, *Ann Thorac Surg* 58:585, 1994.
48. Khan IA, Nair CK: Clinical, diagnostic, and management perspectives of aortic dissection, *Chest* 122:311, 2002.
49. Hallett JW Jr: Management of abdominal aortic aneurysms, *Mayo Clin Proc* 75:395, 2000.
50. Morrissey NJ, Hollier LH: Anatomic exposures in thoracoabdominal aortic surgery, *Semin Vasc Surg* 13:283, 2000.
51. Murray MJ, Bower TC, Oliver WC, et al: Effects of cerebrospinal fluid drainage in patients undergoing thoracic and thoracoabdominal aortic surgery, *J Cardiothorac Vasc Anesth* 7:266, 1993.
52. Safi HJ, Miller CC III, Iliopoulos DC, et al: Staged repair of extensive aortic aneurysm: improved neurologic outcome, *Ann Surg* 226:599, 1997.
53. Dalen JE, Bone RC: Is it time to pull the pulmonary artery catheter? *JAMA* 276:916, 1996.
54. Vincent J-L, Dhainaut J-F, Perret C, Suter P: Is the pulmonary artery catheter misused? A European view, *Crit Care Med* 26:1283, 1998.
55. Vender JS: Resolved: a pulmonary artery catheter should be used in the management of the critically ill patient, *J Cardiothorac Vasc Anesth* 12:9, 1998.
56. Crawford FA Jr, Sade RM: Spinal cord injury associated with hyperthermia during aortic coarctation repair, *J Cardiothorac Vasc Anesth* 87:616, 1984.
57. Stoneham M, Howell S, Neill F: Heat loss during induction of anaesthesia for elective aortic surgery, *Anaesthesia* 55:79, 2000.
58. Safi HJ: Role of the BioMedicus pump and distal aortic perfusion in thoracoabdominal aortic aneurysm repair, *Artif Organs* 20:694, 1996.
59. Drazner MH, Hamilton MA, Fonarow G, et al: Relationship between right and left-sided filling pressures in 1000 patients with advanced heart failure, *J Heart Lung Transplant* 18:1126, 1999.
60. Romagnoli A, Cooper JR Jr: Anesthesia for aortic operations, *Cleve Clin Q* 48:147, 1981.
61. Grundy BL, Nash CL Jr, Brown RH: Arterial pressure manipulation alters spinal cord function during correction of scoliosis, *Anesthesiology* 54:249, 1981.
62. Roizen MF, Beaupre PN, Alpert RA, et al: Monitoring with two-dimensional transesophageal echocardiography. Comparison of myocardial function in patients undergoing supraceliac, suprarenal-infraceliac, or infrarenal aortic occlusion, *J Vasc Surg* 1:300, 1984.
63. Wang CH, Cheng KW, Jawan B, Lee JH: Anesthesia for patients with aortic aneurysm for non-aneurysmal surgery—a retrospective study, *Acta Anaesthesiol Sin* 38:3, 2000.
64. McGregor WE, Koler AJ, Labat GC, et al: Awake aortic aneurysm repair in patients with severe pulmonary disease, *Am J Surg* 178:121, 1999.
65. Bonnet F, Touboul C, Picard AM, et al: Neuroleptanesthesia versus thoracic epidural anesthesia for abdominal aortic surgery, *Ann Vasc Surg* 3:214, 1989.
66. Bunt TJ, Manczuk M, Varley K: Continuous epidural anesthesia for aortic surgery: thoughts on peer review and safety, *Surgery* 101:706, 1987.
67. Houweling PL, Ionescu TI, Leguit P, et al: Comparison of the cardiovascular effects of intravenous, epidural and intrathecal sufentanil analgesia as a supplement to general anaesthesia for abdominal aortic aneurysm surgery, *Eur J Anaesthesiol* 10:403, 1993.

68. Gold MS, DeCrosta D, Rizzuto C, et al: The effect of lumbar epidural and general anesthesia on plasma catecholamines and hemodynamics during abdominal aortic aneurysm repair, *Anesth Analg* 78:225, 1994.
69. Norman JG, Fink GW: The effects of epidural anesthesia on the neuroendocrine response to major surgical stress: a randomized prospective trial, *Am Surg* 63:75, 1997.
70. Oyen LJ, Murray MJ, John D, et al: A pilot study of epidural analgesia and anesthesia and cardiac morbidity following abdominal vascular operations, *Crit Care Med* 29:A182, 2001.
71. Sitzman BT, Watson D, Schug SA: Combined general and epidural anesthesia for abdominal aortic aneurysm surgery, *Tech Reg Anesth Pain Manage* 4:91, 2000.
72. Cunningham FO, Egan JM, Inahara T: Continuous epidural anesthesia in abdominal vascular surgery. A review of 100 consecutive cases, *Am J Surg* 139:624, 1980.
73. Baron HC, LaRaja RD, Rossi G, Atkinson D: Continuous epidural analgesia in the heparinized vascular surgical patient: a retrospective review of 912 patients, *J Vasc Surg* 6:144, 1987.
74. Lund PC: *Peridural analgesia and anesthesia*, Springfield, IL, 1966, Charles C Thomas.
75. De Ruyter ML, Torres NE, Harrison BA, et al: Regional lumbar epidural cooling (RELEC) for spinal cord protection in patients undergoing TAAA repair, *Anesthesiology* 89:A314, 1998.
76. Campos JH: Current techniques for perioperative lung isolation in adults, *Anesthesiology* 97:1295, 2002.
77. Mora C, Chuma R, Kiichi Y, et al: The anesthetic management of patient with a thoracic aortic aneurysm that caused compression of the left mainstem bronchus and the right pulmonary artery, *J Cardiothorac Vasc Anesth* 7:579, 1993.
78. Shine T, Nugent M: Sodium nitroprusside decreases spinal cord perfusion pressure during thoracic aortic cross-clamping in the dog, *J Cardiothorac Anesth* 4:185, 1990.
79. Gelman S. Reves JG, Fowler K, et al: Regional blood flow during cross-clamping of the thoracic aorta and infusion of sodium nitroprusside, *J Thorac Cardiovasc Surg* 85:287, 1983.
80. Gelman S: The pathophysiology of aortic cross-clamping and unclamping, *Anesthesiology* 82:1026, 1995.
81. Kellum JA, Decker MJ: Use of dopamine in acute renal failure: a meta-analysis, *Crit Care Med* 29:1526, 2001.
82. Gilbert TB, Hasnain JU, Flinn WR, et al: Fenoldopam infusion associated with preserving renal function after aortic cross-clamping for aneurysm repair, *J Cardiovasc Pharmacol Ther* 6:31, 2001.
83. Halpenny M, Rushe C, Breen P, et al: The effects of fenoldopam on renal function in patients undergoing elective aortic surgery, *Eur J Anaesthesiol* 19:32, 2002.
84. Meloche R, Pottecher T, Audet J, et al: Haemodynamic changes due to clamping of the abdominal aorta, *Can Anaesth Soc J* 24:20, 1977.
85. Johnston WE, Balestrieri FJ, Plonk G, et al: The influence of periaortic collateral vessels on the intraoperative hemodynamic effects of acute aortic occlusion in patients with aorto-occlusive disease or abdominal aortic aneurysm, *Anesthesiology* 66:386, 1987.
86. Gelman S, Khazaeli MD, Orr R, Henderson T: Blood volume redistribution during cross-clamping of the descending aorta, *Anesth Analg* 78:219, 1994.
87. Crawford ES, Walker HS III, Saleh SA, Normann NA: Graft replacement of aneurysm in descending thoracic aorta: results without bypass or shunting, *Surgery* 89:73, 1981.
88. Balschi JA, Henderson T, Bradley EL, Gelman S: Effects of crossclamping the descending aorta on the high-energy phosphates of myocardium and skeletal muscle. A phosphorus 31-nuclear magnetic resonance study, *J Thorac Cardiovasc Surg* 106:346, 1993.
89. Gelman S, Patel K. Bishop SP, et al: Renal and splanchnic circulation during infrarenal aortic cross-clamping, *Arch Surg* 119:1394, 1984.
90. Van Hemelrijck J, Waets P, Van Aken H, et al: Blood pressure management during aortic surgery: urapidil compared to isosorbide dinitrate, *J Cardiothorac Vasc Anesth* 7:273, 1993.
91. Walker PM, Johnston KW: When does limb blood flow increase after aortoiliac bypass grafting? *Arch Surg* 115:912, 1980.
92. Baue AE, McClerkin WW: A study of shock: acidosis and the declamping phenomenon, *Ann Surg* 161:41, 1965.
93. Svensson LG, Crawford ES, Hess KR, et al: Experience with 1509 patients undergoing thoracoabdominal aortic operations, *J Vasc Surg* 17:357, 1993.
94. Spargo PM, Crosse MM: Anaesthetic problems in cross-clamping of the thoracic aorta, *Ann R Coll Surg Engl* 70:64, 1988.
95. Svensson LG, Hess KR, Coselli JS, et al: A prospective study of respiratory failure after high-risk surgery on the thoracoabdominal aorta, *J Vasc Surg* 14:271, 1991.
96. Jonung T, Ribbe E, Norgren L, et al: Visceral ischemia following aortic surgery, *Vasa* 20:125, 1991.
97. Svensson LG, Coselli JS, Safi HJ, et al: Appraisal of adjuncts to prevent acute renal failure after surgery on the thoracic or thoracoabdominal aorta, *J Vasc Surg* 10:230, 1989.
98. Grindlinger GA, Vegas AM, Williams GH, et al: Independence of renin production and hypertension in abdominal aortic aneurysmectomy, *Am J Surg* 141:472, 1981.
99. Kazui T, Washiyama N, Bashar M, et al: Improved results of atherosclerotic arch aneurysm operations with a refined technique, *J Thorac Cardiovasc Surg* 121:491, 2001.
100. Giordano JM: Surgical treatment of Takayasu's arteritis, *Int J Cardiol* 75:S123, 2000.
101. Plate G, Hollier LH, O'Brien PC, et al: Late cerebrovascular accidents after repair of abdominal aortic aneurysms, *Acta Chir Scand* 154:25, 1988.
102. Shine TS, Stapelfeldt WH, De Ruyter ML, et al: Incidence of stroke following thoracoabdominal aortic aneurysm (TAAA) repair, *Anesthesiology* 96:A248, 2002.
103. Gravereaux EC, Faries PL, Burks JA, et al: Risk of spinal cord ischemia after endograft repair of thoracic aortic aneurysms, *J Vasc Surg* 34:997, 2001.
104. Zhang T, Harstad L, Parisi JE, Murray MJ: The size of the anterior spinal artery in relation to the arteria medullaris magna anterior in humans, *Clin Anat* 8:347, 1995.
105. Brewer LA, Fosburg RG, Mulder GA, Verska JJ: Spinal cord complications following surgery for coarctation of the aorta. A study of 66 cases, *J Thorac Cardiovasc Surg* 64:368, 1972.
106. Rosenthal D: Spinal cord ischemia after abdominal aortic operation: is it preventable? *J Vasc Surg* 30:391, 1999.
107. Miyamoto K, Veno A, Wada T, Kimoto S: A new and simple method of preventing spinal cord damage following temporary occlusion of the thoracic aorta by draining the cerebrospinal fluid, *J Cardiovasc Surg* 16:188, 1960.
108. Blaisdell FW, Cooley DA: The mechanism of paraplegia after temporary thoracic aortic occlusion and its relationship to spinal fluid pressure, *Surgery* 51:351, 1962.
109. Nugent M: Pro: cerebrospinal fluid drainage prevents paraplegia, *J Cardiothorac Vasc Anesth* 6:366, 1992.
110. Wallace L: Con: cerebrospinal fluid drainage does not protect the spinal cord during thoracoabdominal aortic reconstruction surgery, *J Cardiothorac Vasc* Anesth 16:650, 2002.
111. Afifi S: Pro: cerebrospinal fluid drainage protects the spinal cord during thoracoabdominal aortic reconstruction surgery, *J Cardiothorac Vasc Anesth* 16:643, 2002.
112. Heller L, Chaney M: Paraplegia immediately following removal of a cerebrospinal fluid drainage catheter in a patient after thoracoabdominal aortic aneurysm surgery, *Anesthesiology* 95:1285, 2001.
113. Garutti I, Fernández C, Bardina A, et al: Reversal of paraplegia via cerebrospinal fluid drainage after abdominal aortic surgery, *J Cardiothorac Vasc Anesth* 16:471, 2002.
114. Weiss SJ, Hogan MS, McGarvey ML, et al: Successful treatment of delayed onset paraplegia after suprarenal abdominal aortic aneurysm repair, *Anesthesiology* 97:504, 2002.
115. Safi HJ, Bartoli S, Hess KR, et al: Neurologic deficit in patients at high risk with thoracoabdominal aortic aneurysms: the role of cerebral spinal fluid drainage and distal aortic perfusion, *J Vasc Surg* 20:434, 1994.
116. Beattie EJ Jr, Adovasio D, Keshishian JM, Blades B: Refrigeration in experimental surgery of the aorta, *Surg Gynecol Obstet* 96:711, 1953.
117. Rokkas CK, Sundaresan S, Shuman TA, et al: Profound systemic hypothermia protects the spinal cord in a primate model of spinal cord ischemia, *J Thorac Cardiovasc Surg* 106:1024, 1993.
118. Sessler DI: Mild perioperative hypothermia, *N Engl J Med* 336:1730, 1997.
119. Lenhardt R, Marker E, Goll V, et al: Mild intraoperative hypothermia prolongs postanesthetic recovery, *Anesthesiology* 87:1318, 1997.
120. Marsala M, Vanicky I, Galik J, et al: Panmyelic epidural cooling protects against ischemic spinal cord damage, *J Surg Res* 55:21, 1993.
121. Davison JK, Cambria RP, Vierra DJ, et al: Epidural cooling for regional spinal cord hypothermia during thoracoabdominal aneurysm repair, *J Vasc Surg* 20:304, 1994.
122. De Ruyter ML, Torres NE, Harrison BA, et al: Regional lumbar epidural cooling (RELEC) for spinal cord protection in patients undergoing TAAA repair, *Anesthesiology* 89:314A, 1998.
123. Marion DW, Penrod LE, Kelsey SF, et al: Treatment of traumatic brain injury with moderate hypothermia, *N Engl J Med* 336:540, 1997.

Anesthesia for Patients with Diseases of Peripheral Arteries and Veins

12

Christine Lallos, MD
Arnold J. Berry, MD, MPH

PATIENTS with peripheral venous or arterial disease raise important questions for the anesthesiologist. Because the population of patients with peripheral vascular disease is generally composed of older patients with multiple medical problems and limited physical reserves, much of the challenge in caring for these individuals revolves around the complexity and severity of their coexisting illnesses. Once the patient's medical conditions are defined and optimized, the anesthesiologist must select from among several anesthetic and postoperative pain management techniques. Determining which technique is likely to result in the "best outcome" continues to be controversial. Endovascular stent placement and other minimally invasive procedures are being utilized more frequently to treat peripheral vascular disease, and these present new challenges to anesthesiologists. This chapter explores these controversies and presents the pertinent data to help clinicians make informed decisions.

Epidemiology of Peripheral Vascular Disease

Because peripheral vascular disease occurs most commonly in elderly patients, its prevalence is likely to increase as the population ages. Data from the National Hospital Discharge Survey, covering patients discharged from nonfederal hospitals in the United States, demonstrated that from 1985 to 1987 there were more than 228,000 males and 183,000 females diagnosed with peripheral arterial occlusive disease.[1] The majority were older than 65 years, and the rate was 60% greater in men than women. As these data represent only hospitalized patients, the true prevalence of the disease is likely to be greater. According to epidemiologic studies, up to 5% of men and 2.5% of women older than 60 have symptoms of arterial insufficiency.[2] Although up to 70% of patients report no change in their symptoms up to 10 years after diagnosis, 20% to 30% have progression of their disease requiring intervention.[2] A small, but significant, proportion (10%) require amputation.[2,3] The reported prevalence of peripheral vascular disease is also dependent upon the method used to detect arterial insufficiency. If diagnosis is based upon an ankle/brachial index (ABI) of less than 0.9, up to 10% of the population aged 55 to 77 years meet diagnostic criteria (see Chapter 1).[2]

The Census Bureau has made estimates of the growth and aging of the population of the United States. In 2000, there were 34.8 million individuals older than 65 years and 4.3 mil-

lion older than 85 in the United States; in 2010, these figures are projected to increase to 39.7 million and 5.8 million, respectively.[4] These data indicate that if the rate of peripheral vascular disease does not change, the prevalence of this disease in the United States will significantly increase.

Arterial Disease

Diseases of the peripheral vasculature encompass a broad spectrum of pathophysiologic processes. Atherosclerosis is the most common etiology necessitating surgical intervention on the arteries of the lower extremities. Other processes that can lead to surgical intervention include aneurysmal dilation, fibromuscular disease, embolic phenomena, and traumatic injury.

Atherosclerotic occlusive disease is a progressive disease in which atheromatous plaques gradually obliterate the lumen of arteries and reduce perfusion of distal tissues.[5,6] The disease process begins in childhood, and the rapidity of its progression depends on numerous factors including concomitant hypertension, genetic predisposition, hyperlipidemia, smoking, diabetes, and gender. Initially, a fatty streak forms within the intimal layer of the arterial wall. A fibrous plaque then develops within the intima of the artery. Over time, the plaque enlarges and matures into a more complex lesion with increased lipid deposition, internal hemorrhage, and calcium deposition. There is new work indicating that inflammatory processes play an important role in atherosclerosis with interactions among endothelial cells, monocytes, T cells, platelets, and chemokines.[5]

When the atherosclerotic plaque enlarges enough to reduce blood flow below a critical level, symptoms of ischemia are noted. Ischemic changes may become acute if internal hemorrhage occurs within the plaque and results in sudden arterial occlusion. If the degenerative process includes the medial layer of the arterial wall, aneurysmal dilation can result.

Subsets of Patients with Arterial Insufficiency

ACUTE ISCHEMIA. The sudden cessation of blood supply to an extremity may be caused by embolism, thrombosis, trauma, intense vasospasm, or iatrogenic interventions. Most emboli originate from the heart with the following etiologies: atrial or ventricular thrombus, diseased or prosthetic cardiac valves, bacterial endocarditis, left atrial myxoma, or paradoxical embolus from a venous source. Emboli can also arise from ulcerated plaques in the central circulation (e.g., aortic aneurysms), tumors, or even invasive cannulas placed during catheterization of a vessel. When dislodged, arterial emboli most often migrate

This manuscript is partially based on a chapter in the first edition by Jane D. Lowdon, MD and Ira J. Isaacson, MD.

219

to the bifurcation of the common femoral artery, followed in frequency by the iliac, popliteal, and brachial arteries, respectively.[7]

Thrombosis is another major cause of acute arterial insufficiency. Acute occlusion of the artery may occur with hemorrhage and enlargement of a preexisting plaque or with trauma resulting in compression or intimal dissection. Less frequent causes of acute thrombosis include thromboangiitis obliterans, collagen vascular disease, hypercoagulable states, and intra-arterial injections of thrombogenic substances.

With the acute onset of ischemia, pain is the first symptom. Patients may describe a burning paresthesia progressing from the distal to proximal aspects of the limb, and this sensation may eventually progress to complete anesthesia. Early signs of ischemia include absent pulses, a cool extremity, pallor, cyanosis, slow capillary refill, and decreased sensation. With progressive ischemia, paralysis, muscle tenderness, and necrosis are seen. This constellation of symptoms and signs is commonly known as the *five Ps* of acute ischemia: pain, paresthesia, pallor, pulselessness, and paralysis.[3,8]

Once suspected, acute ischemia must be rapidly evaluated because irreversible injury to muscle can occur within 4 to 6 hours of arterial occlusion.[7] Classification of the level of acute ischemia is of importance because it determines the appropriate intervention. To permit a standardized nomenclature for ischemic conditions, the Society of Vascular Surgeons has developed a classification scheme (Table 12-1).[3,8] Diagnostic techniques such as Doppler, arteriography, or magnetic resonance angiography may be required for localization of the acute obstruction. The goals of therapy are survival of the patient and limb viability. When limb viability is acutely threatened, the patient may have to proceed directly to the operating room without the aid of diagnostic tests.

Emergency surgical procedures limit the time available to treat the patient's coexisting diseases. Reperfusion injury following revascularization compounds the many problems facing the clinician. Initial laboratory evaluation should include a hematocrit, platelet count, serum electrolytes, and coagulation studies. Lactate and creatine phosphokinase (CPK) levels may be of additional value. A preoperative electrocardiogram (ECG) is needed, but a more complete cardiac evaluation by a cardiologist is often unobtainable because of the emergent nature of the procedure. In the case of embolic causes, an echocardiogram is indicated to determine whether there is a cardiac source of the emboli, but this diagnostic test should not postpone surgical treatment to save an extremity. If there is laboratory evidence of rhabdomyolysis (elevated CPK, myoglobin, potassium, and lactate with metabolic acidosis), intraoperative use of mannitol and maintenance of good urine output are indicated to prevent acute renal injury. Serum potassium concentration should be closely monitored, and hyperkalemia from muscle necrosis should be aggressively treated. When there are no contraindications, systemic anticoagulation with heparin may be initiated to limit clot formation and minimize recurrent embolization.[3] Other therapies include analgesics to minimize pain, oxygen therapy to maximize oxygen delivery to the ischemic tissue, and treatment of decompensated heart disease, such as congestive heart failure or arrhythmias. Limb perfusion may be improved by avoidance of cold environments, treatment of hypotension, and limiting external pressure on the extremity.

The therapeutic options that exist for acute limb ischemia include alleviation of symptoms, heparin anticoagulation, intra-arterial thrombolytics, endovascular repair, traditional open surgical revascularization procedures, and amputation. With the advance of thrombolytics and endovascular techniques, many patients may first undergo a trial of catheter-directed thrombolytic therapy or percutaneous mechanical thrombectomy in an attempt to reperfuse the extremity and to avoid traditional operative interventions.[3,9,10] These therapies usually require an interventional radiologist, vascular surgeon, and well-equipped angiography suite or operating room. Thrombolytic drugs (streptokinase, tissue plasminogen activator, or urokinase) are generally used in patients with a viable extremity and are administered through a catheter directed into the affected artery.[2] During the arteriogram, a decision is made by the surgeon and interventional radiologist whether the lesion is amenable to thrombolytic therapy. One advantage of thrombolytic therapy is that it produces a slow reperfusion of the ischemic tissues, which may avoid some of the complications associated with the acute reperfusion that occurs with traditional open techniques.[11] Local anesthesia with monitored anesthesia care can usually be employed, obviating general anesthesia. The contraindications to thrombolysis are listed in Table 12-2 (see Chapter 4).[3]

Catheter-directed thrombolytic therapy is successful in 50% to 80% of patients.[12] Complications include fatal local hemor-

---

TABLE 12-1

Clinical Categories of Acute Limb Ischemia

Category	Description/Prognosis	Findings		Doppler Signals	
		Sensory Loss	Muscle Weakness	Arterial	Venous
I. Viable	Not immediately threatened	None	None	Audible	Audible
II. Threatened;					
a. Marginally	Salvageable if promptly treated	Minimal (toes) or none	None	(Often) inaudible	Audible
b. Immediately	Salvageable with immediate revascularization	More than toes, associated with rest pain	Mild, moderate	(Usually) inaudible	Audible
III. Irreversible*	Major tissue loss or permanent nerve damage inevitable	Profound, anesthetic	Profound, paralysis (rigor)e	Inaudible	Inaudible

*When presenting early, the differentiation between class IIb and III acute limb ischemia may be difficult.
From Trans-Atlantic Inter-Society Concensus: *J Vasc Surg* 31: S143, 2000.

TABLE 12-2

Contraindications to Thrombolysis

Absolute contraindications
1. Established cerebrovascular event (excluding TIA within previous 2 months)
2. Active bleeding diathesis
3. Recent gastrointestinal bleeding (within previous 10 days)
4. Neurosurgery (intracranial, spinal) within previous 3 months
5. Intracranial trauma within previous 3 months

Relative contraindications
1. Cardiopulmonary resuscitation within previous 10 days
2. Major nonvascular surgery or trauma within previous 10 days
3. Uncontrolled hypertension (systolic > 180 mmHg or diastolic > 110 mmHg)
4. Puncture of noncompressible vessel
5. Intracranial tumor
6. Recent eye surgery

Minor contraindications
1. Hepatic failure, particularly those with coagulopathy
2. Bacterial endocarditis
3. Pregnancy
4. Diabetic hemorrhagic retinopathy

TIA, transient ischemic attack.
From Trans-Atlantic Inter-Society Concensus: *J Vasc Surg* 31: S152, 2000.

rhage or intracerebral hemorrhage (1%), nonfatal stroke (1%), and hemorrhage requiring blood transfusion or surgical intervention (5%).[12] Other associated complications include pseudoaneurysm, renal failure, retroperitoneal hemorrhage, and gastrointestinal bleeding.[2] After acute thrombolytic therapy, some patients may require surgical revascularization to provide long-term vessel patency.

With the advancement of endovascular technology, percutaneous mechanical thrombectomy and percutaneous aspiration thrombectomy may be alternatives to open procedures. These techniques may be of benefit to patients who are considered at high risk for an operative procedure (see Chapter 7).[13]

Indications for surgical revascularization include situations that are immediately limb threatening (category IIb or III in Table 12-1).[3] In up to 30% of cases, there may be inadequate return of flow after operative embolectomy or thrombectomy. An intraoperative angiogram often reveals a distal thrombus. In this situation, intra-arterial thrombolytics may be utilized or traditional surgical revascularization is performed. In the case of a nonviable extremity, primary amputation is necessary. Acute lower extremity ischemia continues to be associated with significant mortality and a high rate of limb loss, with 10% to 20% of complications secondary to preexisting cardiac disease.[12,14,15]

CHRONIC ISCHEMIA OF THE LOWER EXTREMITIES. Atherosclerotic occlusive disease is a progressive disorder, but its manifestations may remain silent or asymptomatic for a number of years. When muscle oxygen demand exceeds blood supply, the patient may note intermittent claudication. Claudication is characterized by pain, cramping, or fatigue in muscles, brought on by exercise and relieved by rest.[3] The anatomic site of the obstruction can be accurately predicted by the symptoms. For example, calf pain is typically caused by superficial femoral artery occlusion, thigh and calf pain by iliofemoral occlusion, and hip and buttock pain by aortoiliac occlusion.

For most patients, the symptoms of claudication remain stable over several years and may improve with exercise and medical therapy when there is the development of collateral flow. The clinical progress of intermittent claudication can vary and may consist of improvement or stabilization, progression not requiring intervention, or progression requiring surgical intervention, angioplasty, or amputation. Jelnes et al analyzed the outcome of patients with intermittent claudication and noted that 25% of patients had progression of their disease, the majority within the first year of diagnosis.[16] In another series, 79% of patients with intermittent claudication remained stable or improved over a mean follow-up time of 2.5 years.[17] Of the patients with worsening symptoms, 5.8% underwent arterial reconstruction and an equal number suffered gangrene and amputation. The risk of amputation was greatest in patients with diabetes mellitus.[2,3]

As the arterial occlusion worsens, the patient's symptoms progress from intermittent claudication to pain at rest and may result in critical limb ischemia. Critical limb ischemia defines patients who, because of the arterial insufficiency, have experienced skin breakdown (ulcers or gangrene) or pain at rest.[3] Patients with critical ischemia report severe burning pain, which awakens them from sleep and which is relieved by dependent positioning. Infection may develop in areas of ischemic necrosis and can progress to cellulitis, osteomyelitis, or sepsis.[17]

Evaluation of anatomic obstruction begins with the physical examination. Noninvasive tests include segmental blood pressure measurements with plethysmographic tracings. The ankle-brachial index (ABI) correlates with the patient's symptoms and is derived by dividing the ankle systolic blood pressure, obtained with the Doppler technique, by the brachial systolic blood pressure. Normal, healthy patients have an ABI greater than 1.0, claudicants have a value of 0.6, and critical limb ischemia occurs with a value less than 0.5.[18] In diabetic patients, however, the ABI can give a false-negative result because of the incompressibility of distal vessels. For these patients, measurement of toe systolic pressure index (TSPI) is performed.[2] Normally, the TSPI should be greater than 0.6. Absolute pressures are measured, and when there is a pressure differential greater than 30 mmHg, impaired healing of distal ulcers is likely.

Modification of risk factors, including hypertension, smoking, glucose, and lipid levels, is initially emphasized for patients with claudication. Exercise therapy has been shown to minimize disease progression and increase pain-free walking distance.[3] Smoking cessation should be encouraged. Smokers have a fourfold increased risk of developing peripheral arterial disease and a greater chance of disease progression, myocardial infarction, stroke, limb loss, and death.[19,20] Diabetes is a well-known risk factor, and intensive glycemic control has been found to provide significant reduction in diabetic endpoints and myocardial infarction. The Trans-Atlantic InterSociety Consensus (TASC) recommendations are fasting blood glucose less than 120 mg/dL, postprandial glucose less than 180 mg/dL, and hemoglobin A_{1c} less than 7.0%.[3] Management of hyperlipidemia should have a goal of low-density lipoprotein less than 125 mg/dL with initial use of diet modification and the addition of medications if needed.[3]

Arteriography is used in the evaluation of arterial occlusive disease to delineate and define its extent (Figure 12-1). The hemodynamic significance of an arterial stenosis is determined by a combination of the location and flow velocity across the stenosis.[3] The use of radiologic contrast agents is routine for angiography, and patients should be assessed for allergies to contrast agents and iodine. The presence of allergies indicates the need to avoid use of these agents and/or to employ measures to prevent allergic reactions (premedication with corticosteroids and H_1 and H_2 blockers). Baseline renal function should also be noted because it may be worsened by contrast agents. To help minimize renal impairment with arteriography, prehydration with saline and/or the use of N-acetylcysteine may be indicated. Finally, there has been an association between arteriographic procedures and metabolic acidosis in patients taking the oral hypoglycemic agent metformin. It is now recommended that metformin be withheld for 48 hours prior to intravenous contrast agents.[21] Advances in intravascular imaging techniques such as intravascular ultrasonography and angioscopy may obviate the need for use of contrast agents.[21]

Historically, surgical intervention has been the mainstay for treatment of severe arterial obstruction; however, percutaneous transluminal angioplasty (PTA) is emerging as an alternative. The many advantages to the patient of PTA over traditional surgery include the avoidance of general anesthesia, rapid recovery, relatively low treatment cost, and decreased hospital stay.[3,22] Although PTA has been utilized to relieve obstructions in the aorta and in vessels as distal as the tibial artery, it is best utilized to relieve obstructions caused by localized, stenotic lesions and short, segmental occlusions of the superficial femoral artery. The TASC group recommends the use of endovascular procedures for type A or single, short, segmental stenoses and classical surgical intervention for complete occlusion of the common or superficial femoral arteries, popliteal artery, or the proximal trifurcation (see Tables 12-3 and 12-4 for TASC classifications).[3] Lesions of intermediate classification may be treated on the basis of the judgment of the surgeon (see Chapters 3, 4, and 7).[3]

The success of PTA is predicted by several independent variables: an indication of intermittent claudication versus limb salvage, arterial stenosis versus occlusion, a non-diabetic patient, a single stenotic area for dilatation, and good distal runoff. Success is defined by both subjective criteria (progressive improvement in symptoms and signs from ulceration or gangrene to rest pain, to intermittent claudication, and then to an asymptomatic state) and objective criteria (ABI increase of 0.10). The success rate in one large, prospective study was initially 88.6% but decreased to 48.2% at 5 years.[23] Twenty-five percent of patients underwent vascular surgery after failed PTA. Matsi and Manninen performed a prospective analysis of 410 percutaneous transluminal angioplasties of the lower extremities.[24] In this series, the total complication rate was 10% and the rate of major complications requiring intervention was 5%.

To help maintain vessel patency after PTA, stents can be placed in the dilated vessel.[21] In general, there are two types of stents, balloon-expandable and self-expanding. When the stent is deployed, a completion angiogram is performed to assess patency.

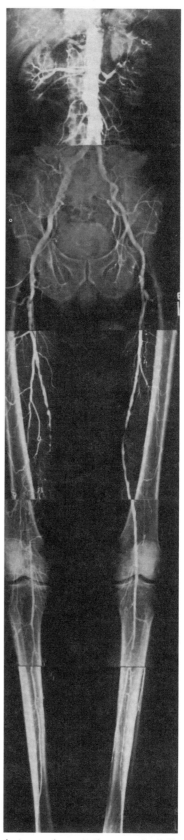

FIGURE 12-1 Aortogram demonstrating generalized atherosclerotic plaque disease with a tightly stenotic left renal artery and totally occluded superficial arteries bilaterally. (From Smith RB, Perdue GD: Diseases of the Peripheral arteries and veins. In Hurst JW, Schlant RC, Rackley CE, et al (eds): *The Heart*, McGraw-Hill, New York, 1990.)

TABLE 12-3

Morphologic Stratification of Femoropopliteal Lesions

TASC type A iliac lesions:
1. Single stenosis <3 cm of the CIA or EIA (unilateral/bilateral)

TASC type B iliac lesions:
2. Single stenosis 3-10 cm in length, not involving the distal popliteal artery
3. Heavily calcified stenosis up to 3 cm in length
4. Multiple lesions, each less than 3 cm (stenoses or occlusions)
5. Single or multiple lesions in the absence of continuous tibial runoff to improve inflow for distal surgical bypass

TASC type C femoropopliteal lesions:
6. Single stenosis or occlusion longer than 5 cm
7. Multiple stenoses or occlusions, each 3-5 cm, with or without heavy calcification

TASC type D femoropopliteal lesions
8. Complete common femoral artery or superficial femoral artery occlusions or complete popliteal and proximal trifurcation occlusions.

CIA, common iliac artery; EIA, external iliac artery; TASC, Trans-Atlantic Inter-Society Consensus.
From Trans-Atlantic Inter-Society Consensus: *J Vasc Surg* 31: S235, 2000.

Complications of PTA range from technical difficulties such as inability to pass a catheter through the stenoses (3.8%) to severe hemorrhage, arterial dissection or distal emboli producing extremity ischemia, and formation of a false aneurysm or arteriovenous fistula.[23] Such events usually require emergent surgical intervention and, therefore, consultation with an anesthesiologist.

Anesthesiologists may be asked to be present during PTA, especially when the patient is anxious or is at high risk for complications. Vigilance and an appropriate degree of monitoring are necessary. Many of these procedures can be performed under monitored anesthesia care. The surgeon or interventional radiologist performing the procedure injects a local anesthetic at the skin site, and parenteral analgesics and hypnotic agents are administered for the patient's comfort. Local anesthetic toxicity and anaphylactoid reactions to dye are risks in this setting.[21,23]

TABLE 12-4

Morphologic Stratification of Infrapopliteal Lesions

TASC type A infrapopliteal lesions:
1. Single stenoses shorter than 1 cm in the tibial or peroneal vessels

TASC type B infrapopliteal lesions:
2. Multiple focal stenoses of the tibial or peroneal vessel, each less than 1 cm in length
3. One or two focal stenoses, each less than 1 cm long, at the tibial trifurcation
4. Short tibial or peroneal stenosis in conjunction with femoropopliteal PTA

TASC type C infrapopliteal lesions:
5. Stenoses 1-4 cm in length of the tibial or peroneal vessels
6. Occlusions 1-2 cm in length of the tibial or peroneal vessels
7. Extensive stenoses of the tibial trifurcation

TASC type D infraopopliteal lesions:
8. Tibial or peroneal occlusions longer than 2 cm
9. Diffusely diseased tibial or peroneal vessels

PTA, percutaneous transluminal angioplasty; TASC, Trans-Atlantic Inter-Society Concensus.
From Trans-Atlantic Inter-Society Consensus: *J Vasc Surg* 31: S236, 2000.

If surgical intervention is chosen for relief of occlusive disease distal to the inguinal ligament, the femoral popliteal bypass graft and autogenous saphenous graft are the surgical procedure and conduits of choice. In this procedure, the saphenous vein is exposed and removed. Once the branches are ligated, the vein is reversed, reimplanted, and anastomosed to the arteries.[25] The graft patency rate with this approach was reported as 75% to 80% at 5 years, and the limb salvage rate was 90%.[26] When a suitable saphenous vein is not available for use for infrainguinal revascularization, a vein may be taken from the patient's arm.[27] When arm veins are used, the primary patency and limb salvage rates at 1 year were 80% and 90%, respectively, in one series.[27]

If an in situ saphenous vein graft is used, the vein remains in its bed. Valves in the vein are excised with microscissors or a valvulotome to allow free retrograde arterial flow. The proximal saphenous vein is anastomosed to the femoral artery and the distal vein to the distal artery. The in situ graft allows the use of small distal veins to revascularize smaller distal arteries. Because the vein is not completely excised from its bed, the graft tends to have fewer problems with twisting or kinking compared with reversed autogenous grafts.[28] The in situ graft patency rate at 5 years is about 80%, with limb salvage rates of 84% to 90%.[29] When no suitable veins are available, other graft materials such as human umbilical vein, Dacron, and polytetrafluoroethylene (Gore-Tex) have been used. Long-term patency rates with prosthetic grafts are not as high as those with autogenous vein grafts.

If the patient has disabling claudication related to aortic occlusive disease but is an unsuitable candidate for abdominal aortic reconstructive surgery, an extra-anatomic bypass may be performed for revascularization. Axillofemoral, axillo-bifemoral, and femorofemoral grafts are reserved for patients with comorbid illnesses that leave them at very high risk for perioperative morbidity and mortality. Compared with abdominal aortic reconstructive surgery, extra-anatomic bypasses appear to represent a less stressful procedure with lower mortality rates and minimal postoperative complications.[30]

Anesthetic Management for Lower Extremity Procedures

Preoperative Evaluation

When the decision to intervene with surgery is reached, each patient deserves a thorough preoperative evaluation to define the extent of concurrent diseases and to evaluate whether the patient is in optimal condition to undergo surgery. Emergent, limb-saving procedures may preclude extensive preoperative evaluation and treatment. For patients undergoing distal revascularization procedures, the long-term survival rate is low and reflects both patients' advanced age and concomitant disease processes. In a large study of men undergoing femorodistal bypass grafts in Veterans Affairs hospitals, the 30-day mortality rate was 2.1%.[31] Survival probability was 88% at 1 year and 63% at 5 years. The limb salvage rates at 1 and 5 years were 87% and 74% for femoropopliteal bypass grafts and 77% and 63% for tibial bypass grafts.

CARDIAC DISEASE. The major cause of perioperative and late postoperative mortality in patients with peripheral vascular disease is related to atherosclerotic heart disease.[32] Weitz et al noted that 28% of patients with peripheral vascular disease also have coronary disease.[2] All-cause mortality was two to three times greater than in age-matched control subjects. In another study, patients having infrainguinal peripheral vascular surgery had a 3.5 times greater risk of fatal and nonfatal myocardial infarction than those undergoing abdominal aortic aneurysm repair (21% vs. 6%).[33] Therefore, each patient must be evaluated to determine the extent of cardiac disease (see Chapters 2, 5, and 6).

Angiography. Hertzer et al utilized coronary angiography in 1000 patients with peripheral vascular disease (cerebrovascular, aortic aneurysmal, or lower extremity occlusive disease) to determine the prevalence of coronary artery disease (CAD).[32] Of the patients with lower extremity ischemia (*n* = 381), only 10% had normal coronary arteries. Mild-to-moderate CAD was found in 33% of patients; advanced, but compensated, CAD in 29%; severe, correctable CAD in 21%; and severe, inoperable disease in 7%. The degree of CAD was not consistently predicted by the commonly used screening tests, such as history, physical examination, and ECG. Severe, correctable CAD was found in 19% of patients with no history of angina and in 19% of patients with normal ECGs. Of the patients with lower extremity occlusive disease, 18% underwent coronary artery bypass grafting (CABG) on the basis of angiographic findings. The overall mortality rate for CABG was 5.3%, and it was 1.8% for lower extremity revascularization in the patients with peripheral vascular disease who had had the following procedures: aortoiliofemoral (0% mortality), extra-anatomic (3.3%), profundoplasty (2.7%), and femoropopliteal or distal arterial bypass (4.5%).[32]

Risk indices. Indices based on clinical factors have been proposed to identify patients with increased risk for perioperative adverse cardiac events after noncardiac surgery.[34,35] Clinical factors such as high-risk (major vascular) or emergency surgery, history of CAD or prior myocardial infarction, congestive heart failure, and type I diabetes mellitus are included in most indices. The American College of Cardiology (ACC) and the American Heart Association (AHA) have published guidelines for the perioperative cardiovascular evaluation and treatment of patients undergoing noncardiac surgery.[36] The algorithms are based on clinical predictors, the patient's functional capacity, and the risk associated with the operative procedure. Peripheral vascular surgical procedures are included in the high-risk category of this classification (see Chapter 5).

Stress testing. Although there is a small subset of patients with peripheral vascular disease who have no clinical symptoms, signs, or risk factors for CAD, the majority of patients require further diagnostic evaluation and risk stratification. Treadmill exercise testing with electrocardiographic monitoring is commonly utilized as an initial test for CAD.[36] For patients requiring peripheral vascular surgery, this test predicts only advanced CAD, and patients with severe claudication are often reluctant or unable to exercise adequately to obtain meaningful treadmill testing.[37] From 64% to 79% of patients with intermittent claudication were unable to complete the protocol for treadmill testing, whereas testing was halted in 8% to 10% of these patients because of ECG changes.[38]

Other noninvasive tests, independent of the patient's ability to exercise, may be used to evaluate cardiac function and diagnose CAD. These include 24-hour Holter monitoring, myocardial perfusion scintigraphy or dipyridamole-thallium imaging, and dobutamine stress echocardiography (see Chapter 5).

During dipyridamole-thallium imaging, intravenous dipyridamole pharmacologically causes maximal coronary vasodilation and induces a state that resembles that produced by exercise. Injection of thallium allows imaging of regional myocardial blood flow. Thallium is taken up into perfused myocardium, and decreased or absent blood flow is reflected as decreased thallium uptake. The heart is imaged again several hours later. If thallium uptake is noted in areas not previously visualized, a phenomenon known as reperfusion or redistribution, that zone of myocardium is considered ischemic and at risk for infarction during periods of stress such as major vascular surgery.[39] An area of myocardium without thallium uptake on either scan is nonfunctioning and represents scarring from previous myocardial infarction (see Chapter 5).

Dipyridamole-thallium imaging has been validated as accurate in the stratification of cardiac risk in patients undergoing peripheral vascular surgery and as a better predictor of risk than exercise testing.[40-42] From early reports, the positive predictive value of the thallium test was 4% to 20% depending on the patients who were studied.[36] Eagle et al demonstrated that the specificity of dipyridamole-thallium imaging was improved when patients also had a clinical predictor of CAD (Q wave on ECG, history of ventricular ectopic activity, diabetes mellitus, advanced age, or angina).[43] The negative predictive value of a normal scan is approximately 99%, and, therefore, patients without thallium redistribution are at low risk for postoperative ischemic events.[36] There are reports, however, of mortality from CAD in patients undergoing noncardiac surgery who had normal dipyridamole-thallium scans.[44] The patients with thallium redistribution should be considered for coronary angiography and possibly myocardial revascularization by percutaneous coronary balloon angioplasty or coronary artery bypass prior to their planned peripheral vascular procedure.[41]

Dobutamine stress echocardiography (DSE) is another test that can be utilized to identify patients with significant CAD.[45] The test is performed in the following manner. After performing baseline transthoracic echocardiography, an infusion of dobutamine is administered in a stepwise fashion to accelerate the heart rate to 85% of age-predicted maximum while the patient is monitored for angina or ECG changes of ischemia. If necessary, atropine may be added to reach the target heart rate. Repeated echocardiography is then performed, and a positive test is defined as the presence of a new regional wall motion abnormality, a finding that is indicative of impaired coronary flow to the area. A review of published studies indicates that the positive predictive value of DSE ranged from 7% to 25% for postoperative myocardial infarction or death and the negative predictive value ranged from 93% to 100%.[36] The degree of impairment and the number of affected myocardial wall segments are also considered important predictors.[46] Many clinicians prefer using DSE over dipyridamole-thallium imaging for cardiac risk stratification because comprehensive echocardiography provides additional information that may be useful in the clinical management of the patient (i.e., left and right ventricular function, the presence of valvular abnormalities, and estimates of pulmonary arterial pressure).

Following the ACC/AHA guideline for risk stratification, patients with positive noninvasive screening tests are candidates for cardiac catheterization to assess for significant coronary artery stenosis.[36] When coronary angiography demonstrates significant CAD, the clinician must decide on the best treatment option. Possibilities include cancellation of any elective surgical procedure or institution of medical therapy, CABG, or percutaneous transluminal coronary angioplasty followed by the peripheral revascularization procedure.

Prior CABG. There is some evidence to suggest that for patients with significant CAD undergoing high-risk noncardiac surgery, CABG lowers the risk of a perioperative myocardial event. The Coronary Artery Surgery Study (CASS) maintained a large registry of patients (n = 24,959 from 1974 to 1979) to help assess cardiac morbidity after noncardiac surgery.[47] Within this database, 3368 patients with CAD had a CABG or were medically treated and subsequently had at least one noncardiac surgery. In the subgroup of 314 patients having vascular surgery, CABG significantly reduced the risk of death (2.4% to 1.1%) and perioperative myocardial infarction (8.5% to 0.6%) compared with medical therapy. These data also suggest that the protective effect of CABG persisted for at least 6 years.

Several other studies support the benefits for coronary revascularization prior to high-risk surgery. An observational study of Medicare beneficiaries who underwent elective infrainguinal or abdominal aortic reconstructive surgery demonstrated that stress testing, with or without CABG, was associated with improved survival after aortic surgery but not infrainguinal surgery.[48] It is of interest that stress testing alone was associated with decreased long-term mortality in patients having infrainguinal vascular surgery. This result suggests that patients who were tested may have been at decreased risk. Other studies by Hertzer, Crawford, and Nielsen and their colleagues indicated that patients who have undergone myocardial revascularization have a perioperative mortality rate comparable to that of those without CAD after noncardiac surgery.[31,49,50]

For appropriate assessment of the rates of adverse outcomes after vascular surgery in patients who have previously undergone CABG, the risk of cardiac catheterization and CABG must be included. In considering this problem in patients undergoing abdominal aortic reconstructive surgery, Fleisher et al used a decision tree model consisting of risk estimates taken from published studies.[51] Sensitivity analyses indicated that the specific institutional complication rate associated with CABG and with vascular surgery performed without preoperative intervention determines the optimal strategy for treatment. These data are from patients undergoing abdominal aortic reconstructive surgery, and the conclusion for patients having lower extremity revascularization may differ (see Chapter 5).

Myocardial revascularization may improve survival for subsequent noncardiac surgery and be in the best interest of the patient's long-term welfare. The indications for and timing of coronary revascularization must be balanced against the urgency of the vascular surgical procedure, the complication rate associated with CABG at the specific institution, and the possibility of other treatment options. When there is severe limb ischemia, the need for rapid intervention to preserve the limb would preclude CABG.

Perioperative β-blockade. Several investigators have demonstrated the benefits of perioperative β-blockers for preventing adverse cardiac events in patients with CAD having high-risk surgical procedures.[46,52-55] Mangano et al studied 200 patients at risk for CAD who were having noncardiac surgery.[53] The use of atenolol preoperatively and in the postoperative period reduced morbidity and mortality from cardiac events for up to 2 years. Wallace et al performed a randomized, placebo-controlled trial evaluating the use of perioperative atenolol in 220 patients at high risk for cardiac ischemia who were undergoing noncardiac surgery.[54] They concluded that atenolol, 5 to 10 mg intravenously, begun 30 minutes prior to the induction of anesthesia and continued for 1 week postoperatively, decreased the incidence of postoperative myocardial ischemia 30% to 50%. There was no increased risk of bronchospasm, hypotension, severe bradycardia, or arrhythmia in the atenolol-treated group.

In a randomized, multicenter trial, Poldermans et al demonstrated that administration of a β-blocker, bisoprolol, to high-risk patients (positive DSE) undergoing major vascular surgery reduced the perioperative incidence of death from cardiac events and nonfatal myocardial infarction.[52] Patients with extensive left ventricular wall motion abnormalities, asthma, and evidence of left main or severe three-vessel CAD were excluded from this study. The data from these investigations suggest that perioperative use of β-blockers is warranted in most patients with CAD to prevent postoperative cardiac morbidity (see Chapters 2 and 6).

An interesting multicenter, randomized study by Boersma and colleagues assessed the role of clinical predictors, DSE, and β-blocker therapy in patients with CAD having abdominal aortic or infrainguinal vascular surgery.[46] Multivariate analysis identified five clinical factors (prior cerebrovascular accident, congestive heart failure, prior myocardial infarction, current stable angina or prior angina, and age ≥70 years) that were associated with a greater risk of adverse outcomes (cardiac death or nonfatal myocardial infarction) within 30 days of vascular surgery. In the 83% of patients with fewer than three of these risk factors, perioperative β-blockade significantly reduced the rate of cardiac complications (2.3% to 0.8%) and DSE findings did not provide additional prognostic information. For the 17% of patients with three or more clinical risk factors, DSE was useful in risk stratification. In the subgroup with no new wall motion abnormalities on DSE (11% of all patients), β-blockade reduced the rate of cardiac events from 5.8% to 2.0%. When there were one to four new wall motion abnormalities on DSE (4% of all patients), β-blockade was associated with a decrease from 33% to 2.8%, and in the subgroup with five or more new wall motion abnormalities (2% of all patients), β-blockade resulted in no improvement in outcome (33% vs. 36%). If these data can be confirmed by other investigators, it appears that the five clinical predictors would be useful in deciding which patients should undergo DSE. The results of the DSE would then determine the need for coronary arteriography and myocardial revascularization prior to elective vascular surgery.

Use of β-blockade in high-risk patients is, therefore, an alternative strategy for patients considered at high risk for CAD when there is insufficient time for risk stratification and more definitive therapy such as myocardial revascularization. Further research must be performed to determine whether any particular β-blocking agent is superior to others, whether β-blockers can be safely administered to patients with significant bronchospastic lung disease or left ventricular dysfunction, and the appropriate duration of pre- and postoperative treatment with β-blockers.

Prior percutaneous transluminal coronary angioplasty.

Preoperative percutaneous transluminal coronary angioplasty (PTCA) with or without stent placement may be considered for some patients with documented critical coronary artery stenosis. Although there have been no randomized controlled trials of PTCA to reduce the risk for adverse cardiac outcomes after noncardiac surgery, there have been several small retrospective evaluations and one larger observational study that used a control group.[56-58] Posner et al compared the rate of cardiac events within 30 days after noncardiac surgery in patients who were without known CAD, those with CAD not having PTCA, and those who had undergone preoperative PTCA.[56] Although patients with PTCA had their risk of postoperative angina and congestive heart failure reduced by 50%, there were no differences in the rates of myocardial infarction or death. When PTCA was performed within 90 days of surgery, there was no risk reduction compared with patients with untreated CAD. Other studies provide only limited data on the benefit of PTCA prior to noncardiac surgery. Therefore, the ACC/AHA Task Force could not recommend prophylactic PTCA prior to noncardiac surgery but indicated that their general guidelines for PTCA be followed.[36]

Several case reports have indicated the risk of bleeding complications in patients having surgery within several days of PTCA and stent placement when antithrombotic agents were used to prevent thrombosis at the site of the coronary stent.[59,60] In a series of 40 patients having PTCA with stent placement within 6 weeks of noncardiac surgery, there were 7 myocardial infarctions, 11 patients with major bleeding, and 8 deaths.[60] The 8 deaths, all with myocardial infarctions, and 8 of the 11 bleeding episodes occurred among patients having surgery within 14 days of PTCA with stent placement. Therefore, there is an increased risk of thrombosis at the site of coronary stent placement when antiplatelet regimens are held before surgery and a risk of severe bleeding when the antiplatelet drugs are administered. The authors recommend postponing elective noncardiac surgery for at least 2 to 4 weeks after PTCA and stent placement so that the antiplatelet medications can be safely stopped.[60] If the surgery is performed more than 8 weeks after PTCA, there is an increased risk of restenosis at the angioplasty site, which may be associated with an increased risk of an adverse cardiac event in the perioperative period. Therefore, timing of surgery after PTCA should be based on balancing these risks.

For patients having PTCA months or years prior to presenting for vascular surgery, cardiac risk stratification must consider whether the previous procedure continues to confer protection against myocardial ischemic events. Unfortunately, there are not adequate data to support any recommendations in this regard. For patients who have been active and asymptomatic since a PTCA more than 8 to 12 months previously, it is likely that the affected area of myocardium remains revascularized.[36] In symptomatic patients or those with limited exercise ability, cardiac risk stratification should take place.

OTHER DISEASES. In addition to CAD, patients with peripheral vascular disease commonly have coexisting disease processes such as hypertension, chronic obstructive pulmonary disease, renal disease, and diabetes mellitus. Each pathophysiologic process requires attention and may influence the anesthetic plan (see Chapters 2 and 6).

Hypertension is present in 40% to 60% of patients with peripheral vascular disease.[16] Long-standing, untreated hypertension causes pathologic deterioration in all arterial beds. End-organ changes in the cerebral, myocardial, and renal vasculature are important and leave these patients more susceptible to cerebrovascular events, myocardial ischemia, congestive heart failure, and renal insufficiency. In the nonsurgical setting, antihypertensive therapy improves survival and lowers mortality. In the perioperative period, hypertension alone may affect outcome, especially when the systolic blood pressure is greater than 180 mmHg and the diastolic greater than 110 mmHg (stage 3 and 4 hypertension).[61,62] Although hypertension may serve as a marker for CAD, it is included as a "minor" clinical factor in the ACC/AHA guidelines for assessing cardiovascular risk.[36] Left ventricular hypertrophy is likely with long-standing hypertension and, if diastolic dysfunction is present, may produce congestive heart failure with excessive intravascular volume.

Prior to elective surgery, systemic arterial hypertension should be reasonably well controlled. Preoperative antihypertensive medications should be continued through the day of surgery. Patients treated with angiotensin II inhibitors may have more episodes of intraoperative hypotension than those receiving other antihypertensive agents.[63] Acute withdrawal of β-blockers or clonidine may be associated with rebound hypertension or tachycardia. Use of intraoperative β-blockers is associated with reductions in blood pressure fluctuation and risk of perioperative myocardial ischemia.[64] Most clinicians recommend that in the intraoperative period, blood pressure should remain within 20% to 30% of preoperative values with the proper use of vasoactive agents. With prolonged hypertension producing end-organ changes, the lower limit for blood pressure autoregulation may be shifted upward, requiring blood pressure to be maintained at higher levels during the perioperative period.[65]

Cigarette smoking is associated with the development and acceleration of atherosclerotic disease. Analysis of data from more than 5209 persons in the Framingham study demonstrated a threefold increased risk for peripheral vascular disease in smokers compared with nonsmokers.[19,66,67] In the 36-year follow-up analysis, tobacco use was found to be an independent risk factor for the development of intermittent claudication.[66] The quantity of tobacco use (number of cigarettes per day) directly correlated with the severity of peripheral vascular disease and was associated with the progression to critical ischemia, failure of revascularization, limb amputation, and death.[20,66] Cessation of smoking has several advantages. It has been shown to reduce symptoms, limit disease progression, and improve graft patency.[3,68] Smoking cessation for more than 8 weeks preoperatively significantly reduces the risk of postoperative pulmonary complications.[69] Other preoperative benefits include a reduction in carboxyhemoglobin concentration and improved mucociliary clearance of tracheal secretions.[70]

Chronic obstructive pulmonary disease (COPD), from long-term smoking or from other pathophysiology, is present in a significant proportion of patients with peripheral vascular disease. Patients with COPD deserve preoperative evaluation to define the degree of pulmonary dysfunction as well as to optimize respiratory function.[71] A history of respiratory failure and mechanical ventilation or findings of right ventricular failure would dictate thorough preoperative assessment or even a change in the surgical procedure. Although not all patients require preoperative pulmonary function tests (PFTs), the findings provide information on the degree and type of pulmonary impairment and the possibility of any reversible component. If the forced expired volume in 1 second (FEV_1) is less than 1 L or if the maximum breathing capacity (MBC) is less than 50% of predicted, the patient is at high risk for postoperative respiratory sequelae.[72] In addition, patients with a ratio of FEV_1 to forced vital capacity (FVC) less than 65% and an FVC less than 70% of predicted may be at increased risk for postoperative respiratory complications.[73] A preoperative radiograph of the chest and arterial blood gas with the patient breathing room air may be useful in defining the extent of the pulmonary disease.

Preoperative preparation of patients with COPD includes several possible interventions. Patients should be taught the value of deep breathing, coughing, and incentive spirometry for their pre- and postoperative benefits. Assessment of nutritional status is important in the preoperative period because malnutrition is associated with poor immunologic and respiratory function. Another critical preoperative intervention is the maximization of pharmacologic therapy. The patient may benefit from the proper administration of aerosols (β-agonists and/or anticholinergics) and a short course of corticosteroids. Antibiotics may also be indicated to treat a preexisting pulmonary or bronchial infection.

The intraoperative management of patients with peripheral vascular disease who have concomitant COPD raises several issues including the "best" type of anesthesia. Inherent in the choice of anesthesia is the method of postoperative pain control. Postoperative analgesia is critically important in patients with significant pulmonary disease, with the goals being minimal respiratory depression and maximal respiratory function. Patients may benefit from direct arterial pressure monitoring to obtain baseline measurements of arterial blood gases as well as intraoperative arterial partial pressures of oxygen and carbon dioxide.

Diabetes mellitus is associated with the development of atherosclerosis and peripheral vascular disease.[3,66] The incidence of diabetes mellitus in patients with peripheral vascular disease ranges from 8% to 12%.[74] In the Framingham study, the risk for the development of peripheral vascular disease was two times greater in diabetic men and three times greater in diabetic women than in nondiabetic controls.[75] Individuals with diabetes were more likely to have distal vessel disease and a higher rate of amputation and complications.

Diabetes mellitus has significant implications with regard to preoperative assessment. CAD and silent myocardial ischemia are more prevalent, as are cardiomyopathy and congestive heart failure. Diabetic nephropathy is a frequent finding in long-standing type 1 diabetes. Nephropathy with chronic renal insufficiency has significant implications for the perioperative period, such as altered drug pharmacokinetics, hyperkalemia,

and the potential of worsening renal function with hypotension, hypovolemia, or nephrotoxic agents.

Diabetic neuropathy affects perioperative anesthetic management in several ways. Diabetic patients with autonomic neuropathy may have delayed gastric emptying and impaired esophageal and intestinal motility.[76] Because of the increased risk of aspiration, the preoperative administration of an H_2-receptor blocker and metoclopramide may be indicated. Cardiac manifestations of diabetic autonomic dysfunction include orthostatic hypotension, resting tachycardia, and decreased beat-to-beat variation in heart rate during deep breathing. These changes may be associated with more pronounced intraoperative hemodynamic fluctuations and cardiac complications.[77] Peripheral neuropathy may produce numb distal extremities, reducing the need for analgesics in the perioperative period.

Hyperglycemia can result from the metabolic stress of surgery. Although intraoperative hypoglycemia from aggressive insulin treatment can result in grave neurologic consequences, hyperglycemia may cause profound metabolic disturbances, such as ketoacidosis, hyperosmolar coma, electrolyte disturbances, and osmotic diuresis.

Postoperative outcome for patients with diabetes is improved when tight glycemic control (less than 120 mg/dL) is instituted.[3,75] Numerous regimens have been suggested for the control of serum glucose during the perioperative period. Untreated glucose levels vary with each patient, depending on the severity of disease, the stress of surgery, and even the type of anesthesia. Therefore, each patient's insulin regimen should be tailored to the individual needs. A traditional method of perioperative glucose control is to give from one fourth to one half of the usual daily intermediate-acting insulin dose subcutaneously prior to surgery. As an alternative, a continuous infusion of regular insulin at low doses along with supplemental intravenous dextrose may produce better glycemic control and can be continued into the postoperative period.[78] In one protocol, intravenous fluid containing 5% dextrose is administered at 100 mL/hr along with an infusion of insulin (0.5 to 1.0 units/hr) by infusion pump.[78] Blood glucose is checked every 1 to 2 hours and the insulin infusion appropriately adjusted. When the patient begins eating, the intravenous dextrose and insulin infusions can be discontinued and appropriate subcutaneous dosing of insulin restarted.

Medications—Anticoagulant, Antiplatelet, and Thrombolytic Agents

Anticoagulation therapy is frequently employed for patients with peripheral vascular disease to minimize disease progression, decrease the risk of cerebral or cardiac events, prevent graft occlusion, and, in the acute setting, to reopen an acutely thrombosed vessel or graft. Intraoperatively and postoperatively, patients may receive dextran to increase the rate of arterial patency.[79] For long-term protection, warfarin or aspirin plus dipyridamole may be administered.[79] It is important for the anesthesiologist to understand the implications of these medications for the perioperative care of this population (Table 12-5).

Because the majority of morbidity and mortality in the perioperative period for patients undergoing vascular surgery is due to thromboembolic and cardiac events, TASC has recommended the routine use of antithrombotic medications.[3] Aspirin, 80 to 325 mg/day, has been shown to decrease cardiovascular morbidity and mortality and is the primary drug recommended for the perioperative period.[3,79] Aspirin therapy may modify the natural history of chronic arterial insufficiency and prevent death and disability from stroke and myocardial infarction.[2,3] Bleeding time is often used to monitor aspirin's effect on platelets, but the results of this test can be unreliable. Aspirin is usually continued up until the time of surgery. Dipyridamole may be added because it may modify the natural history of atherosclerosis and decrease risk of cardiac events.[3] On the basis of a decision analysis, Neilipovitz et al demonstrated that aspirin should be continued preoperatively in patients undergoing infrainguinal peripheral vascular surgery because it increased life expectancy and decreased mortality despite increasing the rate of hemorrhagic complications.[80] Therefore, when considering the use of neuraxial anesthesia, anesthesiologists should be aware that some patients may be receiving aspirin at the time of operation.

If aspirin is contraindicated, clopidogrel or ticlopidine can be utilized. These medications have been shown to minimize the risk of death and morbidity from stroke and myocardial infarction in patients with peripheral vascular disease.[74,79] The manufacturers recommend that these drugs be withheld for 7 days prior to surgery to permit normalization of platelet function.

Pentoxifylline alters red blood cell morphology, decreases platelet aggregation, and improves the distance that patients with peripheral vascular disease can walk.[2] Data are insufficient to recommend that pentoxifylline be continued perioperatively. Cilostazol, a type 3 phosphodiesterase inhibitor with antiplatelet and vasodilating properties, can be used for the treatment of intermittent claudication.[79]

Unfractionated heparin is routinely administered during peripheral vascular surgery before occlusion of arterial inflow. In addition, some patients may present to the operating room already receiving intravenous heparin to prevent embolization or vascular thrombosis. Close monitoring of the activated partial thromboplastin time (aPTT) and anti-Xa level is indicated

TABLE 12-5
Medications Affecting Coagulation

Drug	Mechanism of Action	Metabolism	Half-Life	Monitoring	Reversal
A. Antiplatelets					
Clopidogrel (Plavix)	Platelet inhibitor	Hepatic	10 d	Bleeding time	Stop 7 d preoperatively Administer platelets
Ticlopidine (Ticlid)	Platelet inhibitor	Hepatic	10 d	Bleeding time	Stop 7 d preoperatively Administer platelets
Aspirin	Platelet inhibitor	Hepatic	10 d	Bleeding time	Stop 7-10 d preoperatively Administer platelets
B. IIb/IIIa inhibitors					
Abciximab (ReoPro)	IIb/IIIa receptor	Plasma protease	>48 hr	Bleeding time	nl BT in 12 hr Administer platelets
Eptifibatide (Integrelin)	IIb/IIIa receptor	Renal	2-4 hr	Bleeding time	BT nl 4 hr after stopping Platelet infusion not effective
Tirofiban (Aggrastat)	IIb/IIIa receptor	Renal (30%-60%) Biliary (40%-70%)	2-4 hr	Bleeding time ACT a PTT	BT nl 4 hr after stopping Platelet infusion not effective
C. Thrombolytics					
Streptokinase	Thrombolytic	Unknown	25 min	PT/aPTT	36-48 hr for fibrinogen level to normalize cryoprecipitate
Anistreplase	Thrombolytic	Unknown	5 min	PT/aPTT	Cryoprecipitate
Alteplase	Thrombolytic	Hepatic	88 min	PT/aTT	Cryoprecipitate
Reteplase	Thrombolytic	Renal, hepatic	15 min	PT/aPTT	Cryoprecipitate
Urokinase	Thrombolytic	Hepatic	24-48 hr	PT/aPTT	Cryoprecipitate
D. Indirect thrombin inhibitor					
Heparin	Binds antithrombin III	Renal	90 min	aPTT	Hold 6 hr preoperatively Fresh frozen plasma protamine
Warfarin (Coumadin)	Vitamin K–dependent factor inhibition	Hepatic	40 hr	PT	Hold 10 mg IV vitamin K (effective in 3 hr) Fresh frozen plasma for immediate effect
E. Low-molecular-weight heparins					
Enoxaparin (Lovenox)	Anti-Xa greater than antithrombin	Renal	4 hr	Anti-Xa	Protamine effective only for reversing anti-IIa portion
Dalteparin (Fragmin)	Anti-Xa greater than anti-thrombin	Renal	3 hr	Anti-Xa	Protamine effective only for reversing anti-IIa portion
F. Low-molecular-weight heparinoid					
Danaparoid (Orgaran)	Anti-Xa	Renal elimination, unchanged	24 hr	Anti Xa	Plasma exchange (protamine not effective)
G. Direct thrombin inhibitor					
Hirudin	Direct thrombin inhibitor	Hydrolysis with renal elimination	1.3 hr, 2 days if on hemodialysis	aPTT	

ACT, activated clotting time; aPTT, activated partial thromboplastin time; BT, bleeding time; nl, normal; PT, prothrombin time.

to minimize bleeding complications associated with long-term heparin use. If reversal of anticoagulation is indicated, the heparin infusion can be terminated for at least 6 hours or its effect reversed with titration of protamine or administration of fresh frozen plasma.[81-83] The half-life of heparin may be prolonged in patients with severe hepatic failure and end-stage renal disease.[83]

Long-term heparin administration may be associated with thrombocytopenia, and, therefore, the platelet count should be measured in this setting.[84,85] There are two types of heparin-induced thrombocytopenia (HIT). In type I HIT, there is a decreased platelet count 2 to15 days after initiation of heparin therapy caused by the direct action of heparin producing platelet aggregation.[86] This type of HIT is usually of little clinical significance and generally improves without discontinuation of the heparin. HIT type II, produced by immunoglobulin G antibodies directed against a complex of platelet factor 4 and heparin, generally occurs 2 to 5 days after initiation of unfractionated heparin in less than 1% of patients, and there is a lower incidence with low-molecular-weight heparin (LMWH).[81] Type II HIT results in a rapid decline in platelet count to less than 100,000 or to below 50% of baseline and may be associated with arterial or venous thrombosis.[86] If type II HIT is suspected on a clinical basis, treatment should not be delayed for laboratory confirmation. Serum can be sent for HIT-immunoglobulin assay or antigen assay such as platelet factor 4–heparin enzyme-linked immunosorbent assay. Therapy for HIT includes discontinuation of all heparin including heparin flushes of intravascular catheters and removal of all heparin-coated intravascular devices. With significant thromboses or if the original need for anticoagulation continues to exist, lepirudin, argatroban, and danaparoid can be used for anticoagulation.[86] Lepirudin is highly immunogenic and must be closely monitored with aPTT levels.[86] Its half-life may exceed 2 days for patients with renal failure. Argatroban has a half-life of only 40 to 50 minutes and is excreted normally in patients with renal failure, but the dose should be reduced in those with hepatic failure. Anticoagulation with argatroban is monitored with aPTT. Danaparoid can also be used for anticoagulation in HIT. It is administered subcutaneously and has a half-life of 25 hours that is prolonged in renal failure.[86] Anticoagulation after danaparoid cannot be reversed with protamine, and plasma exchange is the only method that can be used to clear the drug.[86]

Heparin resistance is the inability to achieve therapeutic anticoagulation despite appropriate dosing. It results from diminished antithrombin III levels, often from prolonged heparin infusion, and can be treated with administration of fresh frozen plasma or antithrombin III concentrate. In the presence of heparin resistance, it is more accurate to determine the level of anticoagulation with anti-Xa levels (target 0.3 to 0.7 U/mL) as opposed to aPTT.[86]

LMWHs such as enoxaparin or dalteparin are derived from heparin.[83] The benefits of LMWHs over unfractionated heparin include subcutaneous administration with less frequency as well as predictable clearance and an anticoagulant effect based on body weight.[83,86] The initial indication for their use was deep venous thrombosis prophylaxis, but enoxaparin is also approved by the Food and Drug Administration to treat deep

venous thrombosis, pulmonary embolism, unstable angina, and atrial fibrillation and to prevent thrombosis on prosthetic heart valves.[86] The anticoagulation effect of LMWHs cannot be assessed using the aPTT because they have their primary effect on factor Xa levels. Anti-Xa levels are assessed clinically and take about 1 hour to obtain from the laboratory. Protamine has an inconsistent effect on the neutralization of LMWH.

Warfarin is the most commonly used orally administered anticoagulant. Its main mechanism of action is inhibition of vitamin K–dependent clotting factors. Warfarin may be administered postoperatively to maintain graft patency or to prevent deep venous thrombosis.[3,79,86] The degree of anticoagulation is monitored using the prothrombin time (PT) with the goal of increasing the international normalized ratio (INR) to 2.0 to 3.0 for full-dose anticoagulation or 1.5 to 2.0 for low-dose anticoagulation. Stopping warfarin for approximately 5 days usually results in return of the PT to a normal level. More rapid reversal of warfarin-induced anticoagulation can be achieved with administration of fresh frozen plasma or vitamin K.[81,86]

Fibrinolytic agents such as streptokinase, urokinase, anistreplase, alteplase, and reteplase are used to treat acute arterial thrombosis or embolic occlusions.[82] Intra-arterial thrombolytic therapy can be utilized alone or in combination with angioplasty and stent placement.[3,79] The recent administration of thrombolytics is associated with an increased risk of hemorrhage in the perioperative setting. The thrombolytic agent should be stopped and antifibrinolytic therapy such as aprotinin should be considered.[82] Cryoprecipitate, fresh frozen plasma, and platelets may also be indicated.

Platelets play a central role in thrombus formation. Because the platelet glycoprotein IIb/IIIa receptor plays a key role in platelet adhesion, IIb/IIIa inhibitors may be administered to maintain vascular patency after coronary angioplasty, cerebral interventions, and peripheral vascular angioplasty and stent placement.[87] The most commonly used intravenous agents include abciximab, eptifibatide, and tirofiban.[87] Bleeding time can be used to monitor the antiplatelet activity; however, this is often unreliable. Glycoprotein IIb/IIIa antagonists prolong the activated coagulation time, but because the test is also affected by other factors, it may not be the best method for monitoring anticoagulation. Tests of platelet aggregation may be useful, and the development of more accurate methods is under investigation.[87] To reduce bleeding complications, platelet transfusions benefit patients receiving abciximab but are not effective in patients who have received eptifibatide or tirofiban. Reversal of antiplatelet effects requires abciximab to be discontinued for 12 hours, but only 4 to 6 hours are required for eptifibatide and tirofiban.

NEURAXIAL ANESTHESIA AND AGENTS AFFECTING HEMOSTASIS. Although neuraxial anesthesia and postoperative analgesia are advocated by many practitioners for lower extremity vascular surgical procedures, the risk of spinal or epidural hematoma formation must be considered in patients receiving anticoagulants, thrombolytics, and antiplatelet agents. The American Society of Regional Anesthesia has published a series of consensus statements on neuraxial anesthesia and anticoagulation that suggest strategies for evaluating the use of neuraxial blockade when anticoagulants are utilized.[88-92] Subsequently, Horlocker published a review that also addressed the use of neuraxial anesthesia in patients receiving these agents.[93]

Spinal hematomas have been reported after both spinal and epidural anesthesia in patients receiving anticoagulants or antiplatelet drugs, but in the majority of cases patients had a clotting abnormality or there was difficulty with needle placement.[93] The risk of spinal hematoma must always be balanced against the benefit of neuraxial anesthesia along with a consideration of the effects of the specific anticoagulants or antiplatelet agents that have been or are to be administered.

The following are some general recommendations regarding neuraxial blockade in the setting of anticoagulation. Because this is a complex but important issue, clinicians should consult current recommendations as new information becomes available.[93] Use of aspirin or nonsteroidal anti-inflammatory drugs is not a contraindication for use of neuraxial anesthesia, but the risks associated with ticlopidine, clopidogrel, and platelet IIb/IIIa inhibitors are unknown. If intraoperative heparinization (unfractionated heparin) will not take place until at least 1 hour after needle placement and if there is no preexisting coagulopathy or thrombocytopenia, neuraxial anesthesia may be used. When heparin is given while an epidural catheter is in place or is continued postoperatively, the aPTT should be followed. The catheter should not be removed until several hours after stopping the heparin and normalization of the aPTT. The situation related to use of LMWH is more complex, and use of neuraxial anesthesia may not be appropriate depending on the timing of the LMWH and the dose administered. For patients started on warfarin after surgery, the PT should be monitored, and an existing neuraxial catheter should not be removed until the INR is less than 1.5. Neuraxial block is not recommended when fibrinolytics have been administered.

There are numerous reports of hemorrhage following either epidural or subdural puncture in anticoagulated patients or patients with coagulopathy.[94-96] When symptoms occur, the spinal or epidural hematoma must be diagnosed and swiftly treated with appropriate surgical exploration. Although some patients may recover complete neurologic function, many others suffer permanent deficits including paraplegia or quadriplegia with respiratory failure and death.[94,97,98]

Monitoring Considerations

The choice of monitoring during peripheral arterial revascularization is determined by the extent of concurrent disease, especially cardiac, pulmonary, or renal disease. Although certain procedures such as aortic reconstructive surgery or CABG may dictate an aggressive approach to invasive hemodynamic monitoring, surgical procedures to revascularize an extremity may not require invasive monitors. Peripheral vascular (nonaortic) procedures generally are not associated with major fluid shifts, blood loss, or hemodynamic derangements, and the surgical physiologic trespass is not as great as with cardiac or aortic procedures. The clinician should, therefore, choose invasive monitors on the basis of the patient's constellation of disease states and factors associated with the specific surgical procedure.

Regardless of the type of anesthesia, there are certain recommended minimal standards for monitoring.[99] Continuous dual-channel ECG monitoring with automated ST-segment analysis using a modified V_5 lead and lead II is suggested for detection of myocardial ischemia. Respirations are monitored with a precordial stethoscope or with an esophageal stethoscope during general anesthesia. Pulse oximetry, to assess oxygenation continuously, and end-tidal carbon dioxide measurements, to assess ventilation during general anesthesia, are considered standard care.[99] Insertion of a urinary bladder catheter is usually recommended because the procedures may be of long duration, there is the potential for blood loss, and urine output reflects adequate renal perfusion.

Monitoring of temperature and maintenance of normothermia are mandatory, especially during general anesthesia.[100] In a randomized trial of patients with high risk for CAD undergoing major surgical procedures, mild hypothermia (35.4°C) was associated with a two times greater risk for an adverse cardiac event compared with that of patients who were actively warmed (36.7°C) during general or regional anesthesia.

Accurate monitoring of blood pressure is critical because intraoperative hemodynamic changes are likely to be exaggerated in older individuals with hypertension and atherosclerotic, noncompliant vessels. Sphygmomanometer or automated oscillometric blood pressure measurement may be accurate, but direct intra-arterial monitoring and sampling may be desirable and indicated in patients with hypertension, diabetes mellitus, or significant pulmonary disease or in cases expected to have major blood loss. The benefits of arterial cannulation must be weighed against the risks of distal ischemia and embolism. Percutaneous radial artery catheterization may be difficult because of generalized atherosclerotic disease.

In this group of patients with a high incidence of CAD, the clinician must be especially attentive to ECG abnormalities such as arrhythmias and ST-segment changes that may reflect ischemia. The most sensitive monitor of myocardial ischemia may be transesophageal echocardiography (TEE). In many instances, TEE detects myocardial segmental wall motion abnormalities well before the ECG changes and is more sensitive than the pulmonary artery catheter (PAC) in detecting ischemia.[101-103] Although TEE is a valuable monitor, the technology requires costly equipment, trained personnel, and, usually, general anesthesia for the patient.[104]

The PAC, although less sensitive than TEE in detecting myocardial ischemia, yields far more information than the ECG alone. Ischemia can be detected as an increase in pulmonary artery pressures or as a change in the morphology of the pulmonary capillary wedge tracing. The appearance of a V wave in the pulmonary capillary wedge tracing reflects mitral regurgitation caused by either intrinsic valvular disease or papillary muscle ischemia.[105] A PAC also allows the measurement of cardiac output and mixed venous oxygen saturation as well as the assessment of interventions made in an effort to optimize hemodynamics. Although there are theoretical advantages associated with PAC monitoring during vascular surgery, the benefit is not supported in several outcome studies.[106-109] Prospective randomized studies in patients undergoing abdominal aortic reconstructive surgery or other vascular surgery failed to demonstrate improved morbidity or mortality associated with PAC monitoring.[106,107,109] In an observational study of 4059 patients (221 with PAC) undergoing noncardiac surgery (17% underwent vascular surgery), there was no difference in complication rates associated with use of PAC monitoring.[108] Therefore, these data demonstrate that routine PAC monitoring in vascular surgical patients is not associated with an improved outcome.

Choice of Anesthesia

The choice of anesthetic technique for patients undergoing major vascular surgery raises numerous questions and controversies. There are certain procedures in which one type of anesthetic (general anesthesia, regional anesthesia, or monitored anesthetic care with infiltration of local anesthetic and intravenous sedation) is preferred or most advantageous. For example, patients undergoing embolectomy with a balloon catheter for acute femoral artery thrombosis usually fare well with local anesthesia administered by the surgeon, accompanied by parenteral sedation and analgesia. If simple embolectomy is unsuccessful, the patient may require a more extensive surgical procedure under regional or general anesthesia. On the other end of the spectrum, there are procedures that almost always require general anesthesia. For example, grafts originating from the aortic arch for relief of upper extremity ischemia require general anesthesia, as do most extrathoracic upper extremity bypasses.

Patients undergoing emergency limb revascularization procedures frequently require general anesthesia. If the viability of an extremity is jeopardized, the patient may be fully anticoagulated with heparin on arrival to the operating room and regional anesthesia is thus contraindicated. When an extremity has been profoundly ischemic, with rigidity and edema, severe metabolic derangements such as myoglobinuria, rhabdomyolysis, metabolic acidosis, hyperkalemia, and azotemia may occur during and after the revascularization procedure.[110] In this setting, invasive hemodynamic monitors are strongly recommended, with attention to volume, acid-base status, electrolytes, and urine output.

Debate continues about whether neuraxial blockade or general anesthesia constitutes the better choice of anesthesia for elective lower extremity revascularization. The most commonly used types of neuraxial blockade include continuous epidural anesthesia-analgesia and subarachnoid block consisting of either single-shot or continuous spinal anesthesia. For procedures of longer duration, neuraxial blockade may be combined with a light general anesthetic. There are many possible advantages to neuraxial blockade compared with general anesthesia for patients undergoing lower extremity revascularization procedures. Potential benefits include hemodynamic stability, reduced blood loss, improved distal arterial blood flow from the accompanying sympathectomy, and an opportunity to provide continuing postoperative analgesia. Although early investigations comparing regional versus general anesthesia focused on intermediate variables such as changes in intraoperative blood pressure, more recent studies have assessed outcomes such as mortality and major morbidity rates. In addition, as new anesthetic agents and monitors have been introduced into clinical practice, general anesthesia may be associated with fewer complications, possibly making older studies less pertinent to current practice.[111] Finally, in some reports, the study design did not permit the reader to determine whether an improved outcome was attributable to the choice of

intraoperative anesthetic or type of postoperative pain management (see Chapter 9).

The prospective, randomized study of Yeager and colleagues was one of the first to demonstrate the beneficial effects of epidural anesthesia and postoperative analgesia in high-risk patients undergoing intra-abdominal, intrathoracic, or major vascular surgery.[112] When light general anesthesia was combined with epidural analgesia, there were decreases in mortality (0% versus 16%) and the incidence of postoperative complications, cardiovascular failure, and major infections compared with rates in patients having general anesthesia with postoperative parenteral narcotics. Because of the significant differences in the major outcomes, the trial was terminated after only 53 patients.

The results of subsequent studies comparing anesthetic techniques in patients undergoing peripheral vascular surgery have been less dramatic and have conflicted. Tuman and coworkers randomly assigned 80 patients undergoing major vascular surgery of either the abdominal aorta or the lower extremities to receive either general anesthesia combined with epidural anesthesia (GEN-EPI) and analgesia or general anesthesia with postoperative narcotics (GEN).[113] Although there were no deaths in either group, the rates of infectious and overall postoperative complications were decreased in the GEN-EPI patients. Regression analysis demonstrated that preoperative congestive heart failure and GEN were associated with cardiovascular complications. Patients in the GEN-EPI group were less hypercoagulable and had fewer thrombotic complications, including arterial graft thromboses. In a study by Christopherson et al, 100 patients having elective vascular reconstructive surgery of a lower extremity were randomly assigned to receive either epidural anesthesia for surgery with postoperative epidural analgesia (fentanyl) or general anesthesia with postoperative patient-controlled morphine analgesia.[114] Although there were no differences in cardiac complications, the main outcome of the study, patients receiving epidural anesthesia and analgesia had a decreased rate of regrafting and embolectomy. Unfortunately, this study did not report on surgical factors that may have been responsible for graft occlusion. In a companion publication, the investigators demonstrated that the increased rate of thrombotic events in the patients receiving general anesthesia and postoperative narcotics was associated with impaired fibrinolysis and an increased concentration of plasminogen activator inhibitor-1.[115]

The previous studies suggest that neuraxial anesthesia and analgesia may be preferable to general anesthesia because the regional technique was not associated with a hypercoagulable state and postoperative graft failure. Choice of anesthetic and postoperative analgesia technique was not clearly associated with improvement in other outcome measures. In a larger study, 423 patients undergoing femoral-to-distal artery bypass surgery were randomly assigned to general, epidural, or spinal anesthesia, and all received parenteral narcotics for postoperative analgesia.[116] There were no differences in mortality, cardiovascular morbidity, or length of stay between the groups of patients. Additional data collected from the same patients indicated no differences in graft patency or amputation.[117] This finding would suggest that when parenteral opioids are used for postoperative analgesia, there is no best type of anesthesia for lower extremity revascularization surgery. Because long-term graft patency depends on several factors including the conduit material, adequacy of arterial inflow and outflow, and technical quality of the anastomoses, there are conditions outside the control of the anesthesiologist that may have a greater effect on the overall success of the surgical procedure.

Other studies have also examined whether neuraxial anesthesia and analgesia are associated with improved outcome after major surgical procedures. A large meta-analysis of data from randomized studies available before January 1, 1997 compared outcome for patients receiving either general or regional anesthesia for all types of surgical procedures.[118] Although overall mortality was reduced by about one third in patients receiving neuraxial blockade, there was no significant difference in mortality in the subgroup having vascular surgery. A multicenter trial randomly assigned 920 patients with one of nine significant comorbid states to receive either epidural-general anesthesia with postoperative epidural analgesia or general anesthesia with postoperative parenteral narcotics.[119] All patients underwent major abdominal surgery, and the primary study endpoint was death at 30 days or major postoperative morbidity. There was no difference in 30-day mortality between groups, but the rate of respiratory failure was less and there was better pain relief during the first three postoperative days in the epidural group. To assess whether there are improved outcomes from either intraoperative neuraxial block or postoperative epidural analgesia, a prospective randomized study (consisting of the four possible combinations with general anesthesia and postoperative patient-controlled analgesia) was conducted in 168 patients undergoing surgery of the abdominal aorta.[120] There were no differences between the groups in any of the major outcome measures (length of hospital stay and direct medical costs) or secondary outcomes (rates of death, myocardial infarction, myocardial ischemia, reoperation, pneumonia, and renal failure). From the studies involving patients undergoing vascular surgery as well as other well-conducted trials involving patients having other major surgical procedures, the data demonstrate that neuraxial block is not associated with a decreased mortality rate. In some studies, patients may be more comfortable when epidural postoperative analgesia is administered, but their overall postoperative course does not appear to be improved.

The cardiovascular changes characteristic of neuraxial anesthesia are not necessarily desirable for all patients. When the subarachnoid or epidural block is established, the resulting sympathectomy can cause significant hemodynamic derangements such as hypotension and bradycardia, especially in patients with untreated systemic arterial hypertension or hypovolemia.[121] Perioperative intravascular fluid shifts may lead to hemodynamic lability and its associated risks during regional anesthesia. If neuraxial block is utilized, adequate hydration with crystalloid or colloid solutions should be ensured and vasoconstrictors administered in a timely manner to prevent significant hypotension.

Femoral Pseudoaneurysm

A pseudoaneurysm, or false aneurysm, is an arterial dilatation produced by a disruption of the arterial wall and most commonly results from trauma or iatrogenic injury such as following an arterial puncture for vascular intervention. Because larger diameter devices are more commonly used for percutaneous vascular procedures and postprocedure anticoagulation is utilized after vascular stent placement, the incidence of femoral pseudoaneurysms appears to be increasing. Pseudoaneuryms most commonly develop at the bifurcation of the superficial and deep femoral artery where external compression is less effective in providing hemostasis.

A pseudoaneurysm arises as a painful mass, and when it continues to expand, it is at significant risk for rupture. Small, stable pseudoaneurysms may be observed, but larger pseudoaneurysms should be repaired. Diagnosis is best made with duplex ultrasonography. Nonoperative treatment modalities include ultrasound-guided compression and percutaneous ultrasound-guided thrombin injection, but these are most effective with smaller pseudoaneurysms.[122,123] Surgical treatment consists of evacuation of hematoma and repair of the arterial defect or puncture. Satisfactory anesthesia for this surgical procedure can often be accomplished using infiltration of local anesthetic combined with intravenous sedation and analgesia. With large pseudoaneurysms, especially when there is an extensive hematoma compressing the femoral nerve, or in obese patients, infiltration of local anesthetic is likely to be inadequate. Under these circumstances, neuraxial or general anesthesia is usually preferable. Hypovolemia may exist if there has been significant blood loss around the femoral artery or into the retroperitoneum. In addition, intraoperative blood loss may be quite large if the surgeon has difficulty controlling the artery and identifying the arterial puncture site or when the patient continues to receive anticoagulants or antiplatelet agents. Therefore, a large-bore intravenous catheter should be placed so that fluids can be rapidly administered.

Venous Disease of the Lower Extremities

There are several diseases involving the veins of the lower extremities that may require surgical treatment. These include the acute and chronic sequelae of venous insufficiency and thrombosis.

Venous Thrombosis

Acute thrombosis of deep veins in the legs or pelvis may occur when there is stasis of blood flow, injury to the vessel wall, and hypercoagulability. Patients who are not ambulating in the postoperative period, with venous stasis in the lower extremities, and who are hypercoagulable are at increased risk for deep vein thrombosis (DVT). Some patients have no symptoms of DVT whereas others report pain and/or swelling of the leg. In some unfortunate circumstances, pulmonary embolus (PE) may be the initial presentation of DVT.

The clinical signs of DVT are inconsistent but may include swollen and edematous muscle tissue or tenderness to palpation. When DVT is suspected, diagnostic testing should be performed. Although ascending contrast phlebography had been the standard test for lower extremity DVT, venous duplex imaging is now utilized as the initial screening test because of its simplicity and accuracy. Magnetic resonance venography is another diagnostic modality that has a sensitivity comparable to that of phlebography, but its use may be limited by cost, availability, and metal implants.

If thrombophlebitis remains untreated, the clot may undergo spontaneous lysis. If clot lysis is incomplete, significant valvular injury and incompetence may occur and result in chronic venous hypertension. The most serious complication of DVT is PE with its associated morbidity and mortality.

Treatment for DVT includes bed rest and anticoagulation with intravenous heparin followed by LMWH or oral warfarin. Thrombolytic therapy with drugs such as recombinant tissue plasminogen activator may be useful in acute DVT to preserve venous valvular function.[124] Patients with iliofemoral DVT are not likely to respond to systemic thrombolytic therapy and may be treated with delivery of the thrombolytic agent directly into the clot using a catheter-directed approach.

If medical therapy fails, venous thrombectomy may be attempted, especially when an iliofemoral clot threatens limb viability. For these procedures, general anesthesia with positive end-expiratory pressure may reduce the risk of pulmonary embolism during thrombectomy. Blood should be available for transfusion because there may be a large blood loss. The operating room should be prepared for fluoroscopy because intraoperative phlebography may be required.

Surgical interruption of the inferior vena cava may be indicated in some circumstances such as recurrent PE in the presence of adequate anticoagulation. There are several methods of vena cava interruption, but percutaneous insertion of an inferior vena cava filter is currently the most desirable choice. These filters can be percutaneously placed while the patient receives monitored anesthesia care with local anesthetic infiltrated by the surgeon and intravenous sedation provided by the anesthesiologist. Close monitoring is particularly desirable in the patient with DVT and recurrent PE whose cardiopulmonary status is unstable. PE is often associated with hypoxemia and tachypnea and, therefore, minimally invasive procedures are better tolerated. A vena cava filter may be inserted through either the femoral or jugular vein. When the jugular vein is utilized, the filter and deployment device must be passed through the right atrium and may result in air embolus or may induce arrhythmias.

Chronic Venous Insufficiency

Chronic venous insufficiency (CVI) can produce symptoms ranging from aching and swelling to dilatation of superficial veins and skin changes of the lower extremity. Signs of CVI include telangiectasia, varicose veins, lipodermatosclerosis, and skin ulceration. CVI, produced by venous hypertension resulting from structural or functional abnormalities of veins, has a high prevalence in Western countries and a significant socioeconomic impact. The incidence of varicose veins was 2.6% per year and 1.9% per year in women and men, respectively, in the Framingham study.[125] The prevalence of venous ulcers appears to be less than 1%.

Venous hypertension results from venous obstruction, reflux, or a combination of the two. Most commonly, CVI results in varicose veins, which result from abnormal distensibility of connective tissue in the vein wall. Varicosities frequently occur at the saphenofemoral and saphenopopliteal junctions and in the perforating venous systems. The varicosities may be primary, from dilatation without previous thrombosis, or secondary from incompetent valves produced after DVT and recanalization. Chronic obstruction and reflux may lead to abnormal microcirculation in the skin that may produce skin changes, eczema, and ulceration. Coagulation abnormalities including impaired fibrinolysis with an increase in plasminogen activator-1 have also been associated with CVI.[126]

To permit uniformity in the diagnosis and treatment of CVI, the CEAP classification was proposed in the consensus report of the American Venous Forum in 1994. The classification is based on *c*linical signs (asymptomatic to active ulceration), *e*tiologic classification (congenital, primary, secondary), *a*natomic distribution (superficial, deep, or perforator), and *p*athophysiologic dysfunction (reflux or obstruction, alone or in combination).[127] History and physical examination are not sufficient to define the extent and location of the venous pathology.[128] Although ascending phlebography had been the mainstay for diagnosing patency and anatomy of veins, newer technology such as duplex scanning has become the preferred initial noninvasive test.

Many patients with CVI can be treated nonoperatively. Initial therapy is often external compression with elastic stockings and periods of intermittent sequential pneumatic compression. Because edema contributes to the impaired microcirculation, external limb compression with bed rest and leg elevation, along with antibiotics to treat associated cellulitis, may be sufficient to speed ulcer healing. Sclerotherapy may be effective for some forms of CVI.[129]

When the nonoperative therapies fail, surgical correction of CVI may be directed at superficial, perforating, or deep veins. Treatment for superficial venous insufficiency includes stripping of the upper and/or lower portions of the greater saphenous vein, saphenous vein ligation, and/or stab avulsion of varicosities. These procedures involve several short incisions that can be infiltrated with local anesthetic to increase the patient's comfort postoperatively. Some surgeons pull a gauze soaked in bupivacaine with epinephrine through the saphenous tunnel as the vein is stripped to provide analgesia and vasoconstriction. Perforating vein ligation may be added to the surgical procedure. Subfascial endoscopic perforator surgery is a technique that is used for perforating vein ligation and involves creation of a subfascial working space with a balloon dissection device. Direct repair of an incompetent femoral vein valve or deep venous reconstruction may be used in some patients. These reconstruction procedures generally require that the patients receive heparin anticoagulation intraoperatively and warfarin after surgery.

The choice of anesthetic for lower extremity venous surgery needs to be based on the specific procedure to be performed, the use of anticoagulants, and the postoperative disposition of the patient. Regional anesthesia or monitored anesthesia care with sedation may be adequate for some procedures and general anesthesia may be preferred for the remainder.

Upper Extremity Ischemia

Chronic upper extremity ischemia usually results from obstruction of a proximal vessel, such as the brachiocephalic, subclavian, or axillary artery. Because extensive collateral circulation usually exists, gradual arterial occlusion may be well tolerated. Ischemia may produce symptoms in the hand or arm, such as pain or early fatigue with exercise. Another presentation of obstruction is the subclavian steal syndrome. If the vessels of the circle of Willis remain patent while the subclavian or innominate artery is obstructed, the direction of blood flow in the vertebral artery may reverse and may compromise the vertebrobasilar circulation of the brain. Symptoms include bilateral visual disturbances (blurred vision or total blindness) or manifestations of brainstem ischemia including dysarthria, dysphagia, perioral numbness, and weakness or paresthesias of all extremities.

The causes of upper extremity ischemia are numerous and are noted in Table 12-6. In contrast to lower extremity ischemia, upper extremity ischemia is most often the result of nonatherosclerotic disease, often occurring in the palmar or digital arteries or smaller vessels. Large artery disease makes up less than 10% of upper extremity ischemia. The diagnosis and anatomy of obstructive lesions can be determined with segmental pressure measurements, duplex ultrasonography, arteriography, computed tomography with intravenous contrast administration, and magnetic resonance angiography.

For occlusive disease of the proximal branches of the aortic arch, some lesions can be treated with PTA and stenting. The preferred surgical intervention is an extrathoracic bypass graft, performed as follows: axillary to axillary, carotid to subclavian, subclavian to subclavian, or a combination of these procedures.[131] If an extrathoracic bypass is not feasible, a transthoracic procedure may be required so that a prosthetic graft may be anastomosed to the aortic arch.

A common cause of upper extremity ischemia in young adults is thoracic outlet compression syndrome in which the subclavian artery is compressed by one of several mechanisms such as a cervical or anomalous first rib. An aneurysm may form at the site of compression and emboli to distal arteries in the extremity may be the presenting symptom. When conservative management of thoracic outlet syndrome fails, surgical decompression can be accomplished by a transaxillary or a supraclavicular approach under general anesthesia. Surgical complications include pneumothorax and brachial plexus, long thoracic, or phrenic nerve injury.

Other conditions that require surgical intervention are emboli, aneurysms, or stenosis of the brachial or more distal arteries. Roddy and colleagues have reported on a series of patients with brachial artery reconstruction using bypass conduits of autogenous vein (greater saphenous or arm vein) or polytetrafluoroethylene.[132] The majority of the patients were women (55%) and smoked (73%). The most common presenting symptom was exertional arm pain.

The choice of anesthetic for upper extremity vascular surgical procedures should be based on the surgical site or sites, the duration of the procedure, and any coexisting diseases. Localized procedures may be performed under brachial plexus block. A continuous regional technique offers the advantage of providing postoperative analgesia. Indwelling brachial plexus catheters can be inserted utilizing the interscalene, infraclavicular, and axillary approaches, but the placement site must be based upon the location of the surgical procedure. Sympathectomy and vasodilatation associated with upper extremity blocks may be beneficial, but postoperative analgesia may mask ischemic limb pain associated with inadequate perfusion resulting from a complication of the vascular surgery.

TABLE 12-6
Etiology of Upper Extremity Ischemia

Emboli
Arteriosclerosis
Thoracic outlet syndrome
Trauma
Systemic disease
  Scleroderma
  Uremia
  Thromboangiitis obliterans
  Systemic lupus erythematosus
  Giant cell arteritis
  Dermatomyositis
  Malignancy
  Cryoglobulinemia
  Myeloma

From Stewart MT: Assessment of peripheral vascular disease. In Hurst JW, Schlant RC, Rackley CE, et al (eds): *The Heart*, McGraw-Hill, 1990, New York, 368.

REFERENCES

1. Guillum RF: Peripheral arterial occlusive disease of the extremities in the United States: hospitalization and mortality, *Am Heart J* 120:1414, 1990.
2. Weitz JI, Byrne J, Clagett P, et al: Diagnosis and treatment of chronic arterial insufficiency of the lower extremities: a critical review, *Circulation* 94:3026, 1996.
3. Trans-Atlantic Inter-Society Concensus: Management of peripheral arterial disease, *J Vasc Surg* 31:S1, 2000.
4. *Projections of the total resident population by 5-year age groups, and sex with special age categories*, Washington, DC, 2000, Population Projections Program U. S. Census Bureau.
5. Ross R: Atherosclerosis—an inflammatory disease, *N Engl J Med* 340:115, 1999.
6. Braunwald E: Shattuck Lecture—cardiovascular medicine at the turn of the millennium: triumphs, concerns, and opportunities, *N Engl J Med* 337:1360, 1997.
7. Perdue GD, Smith RB: Atheromatous microemboli, *Ann Surg* 169:954, 1969.
8. Rutherford RB, Baker JD, Ernst C, et al: Recommended standards for reports dealing with lower extremity ischemia: revised version, *J Vasc Surg* 26:517, 1997.
9. Ouriel K, Veith J, Sasahara AA, and the Thrombolysis or Peripheral Arterial Surgery (TOPAS) Investigators: A comparison of recombinant urokinase with vascular surgery as initial treatment of acute arterial occlusion of the legs, *N Engl J Med* 338:1105, 1998.
10. Diffin DC, Kandarpa K: Assessment of peripheral intra-arterial thrombolysis versus surgical revascularization in acute lower-limb ischemia: a review of limb-salvage and mortality statistics, *J Vasc Interv Radiol* 7:57, 1996.
11. Beyersdorf R, Matheis G, Kruger S, et al: Avoiding reperfusion injury after limb revascularization: experimental observations and recommendations for clinical application, *J Vasc Surg* 9:757, 1989.
12. Golledge J: Lower limb arterial disease, *Lancet* 350:1459, 1997.
13. Nilsson L, Albrechtssen U, Jonung T, et al: Surgical treatment versus thrombolysis in acute arterial occlusion: a randomized controlled study, *Eur J Vasc Surg* 6:189, 1992.
14. Aune S, Trippestad A: Operative mortality and long-term survival of patients operated on for acute lower extremity ischemia, *Eur J Vasc Endovasc Surg* 15:143, 1998.
15. Braithwaite BD, Davies B, Birch PA, et al: Management of acute leg ischemia, *Br J Surg* 85:217, 1998.
16. Jelnes R, Gaardsting O, Hougaard JK, et al: Fate in intermittent claudication: outcome and risk factors, *Br Med J* 293:1137, 1986.
17. Imparato AM, Kim G, Davidson T, Crowley JC: Intermittent claudication: its natural course, *Surgery* 78:795, 1975.
18. Yao S: Hemodynamic studies in peripheral arterial disease, *Br J Surg* 57:761, 1970.
19. Kannel W, McGee DL: Update on some epidemiological features of intermittent claudication, *J Am Geriatr Soc* 33:13, 1985.
20. Smith I, Franks PJ, Greenhalgh RM, et al: The influence of smoking cessation and hypertriglyceridemia on the progression of peripheral arterial

disease and the onset of critical ischemia, *Eur J Vasc Endovasc Surg* 11:402, 1996.

21. Weiss VJ, Lumsden AB: Minimally invasive vascular surgery. In Morris PJ, Wood WC (eds): *Oxford textbook of surgery*, ed 2, New York, 2000, Oxford University Press, 937.

22. Krajcer A, Howell MH: Update on endovascular treatment of peripheral vascular disease: new tools, techniques, and indications, *Texas Heart Inst J* 27:369, 2000.

23. Johnston K, Rae M, Hogg-Johnson S: 5-Year results of a prospective study of percutaneous transluminal angioplasty, *Ann Surg* 206:403, 1987.

24. Matsi PJ, Manninen HI: Complications of lower-limb percutaneous transluminal angioplasty. A prospective analysis of 410 procedures on 295 consecutive patients, *Cardiovasc Intervent Radiol* 21:361, 1998.

25. Smith R, Fulenwider J: Reversed autogenous vein graft for lower extremity occlusive disease. In Ernst CB, Stanley JC (eds): *Current therapy in vascular surgery*, Toronto, 1987, BC Decker, 206.

26. Taylor LM, Edwards JM, Porter JM: Present status of reversed vein bypass grafting: five-year results of a modern series, *J Vasc Surg* 11:193, 1990.

27. Faries PL, Arora S, Pomposelli FB, et al: The use of arm vein in lower-extremity revascularization: results of 520 procedures performed in eight years, *J Vasc Surg* 31:50, 2000.

28. Leather R, Shah D, Buchbinder D: Further experience with the saphenous vein used in-situ for arterial bypass, *Am J Surg* 142:506, 1981.

29. Donaldson MC, Mannick JA, Whittemore AD: Femoral-distal bypass with in situ greater saphenous vein: long-term results using the Mills valvulatome, *Ann Surg* 213:457, 1991.

30. Bunt T: Aortic reconstruction vs extra-anatomic bypass and angioplasty, *Arch Surg* 121:1166, 1986.

31. Feinglass J, Pearce WH, Martin GJ, et al: Postoperative and amputation-free survival outcomes after femorodistal bypass grafting surgery: findings from the Department of Veterans Affairs National Surgical Quality Improvement Program, *J Vasc Surg* 34:283, 2001.

32. Hertzer N, Beven E, Youns J: Coronary artery disease in peripheral vascular patients, *Ann Surg* 199:223, 1984

33. Krupski WC, Littooy EP, Reilly LM, et al: Comparison of cardiac morbidity rates between aortic and infrainguinal operations. Two-year followup, *J Vasc Surg* 18:609, 1993.

34. Goldman L, Caldera DL, Nussbaum SR, et al: Multifactorial index of cardiac risk in noncardiac surgical procedures, *N Engl J Med* 297:845, 1977.

35. Lee TH, Marcantonio ER, Mangione CM, et al: Derivation and prospective validation of a simple index for prediction of cardiac risk of major noncardiac surgery, *Circulation* 100:1043, 1999.

36. Eagle KA, Berger PB, Calkins H, et al: ACC/AHA guideline update for the perioperative cardiovascular evaluation for noncardiac surgery. A report of the American College of Cardiology/American Heart Association Task Force on Practice Guidelines (Committee to Update the 1996 Guidelines on Perioperative Cardiovascular Evaluation for Noncardiac Surgery), 2002. American College of Cardiology Web site. Available at: http://www.acc.org/clinical/guidelines/perio/dirIndex.htm.

37. von Knorring J, Lapanfalo M: Prediction of perioperative cardiac complications by electrocardiographic monitoring during treadmill exercise testing before peripheral vascular surgery, *Surgery* 99:610, 1986.

38. Kovamees A, Brundin T: Continuous electrocardiography recording at examination of walking capacity in patients with intermittent claudication, *J Cardiovasc Surg* 17:509, 1976.

39. Brewster D, Okada R, Strauss H: Selection of patients for preoperative coronary angiography: use of dipyridamole-stress-thallium myocardial imaging, *J Vasc Surg* 2:504, 1985.

40. Jain K, Patil K, Doctor U, Peck S: Preoperative cardiac screening before peripheral vascular operations, *Am Surg* 51:77, 1985.

41. Boucher C, Brewster D, Darling R: Determination of cardiac risk by dipyridamole-thallium imaging before peripheral vascular surgery, *N Engl J Med* 312:389, 1985.

42. Leppo J, Plaja J, Gionet M: Noninvasive evaluation of cardiac risk before elective vascular surgery, *J Am Coll Cardiol* 9:269, 1987.

43. Eagle KA, Coley CM, Newell JB, et al: Combining clinical and thallium data optimizes preoperative assessment of cardiac risk before major vascular surgery, *Ann Intern Med* 110:859, 1989.

44. Chin WL, Go R, Lenehan S, et al: Failure of dipyridamole-thallium myocardial imaging to detect severe coronary disease, *Cleve Clin J Med* 56:587, 1989.

45. Davila-Roman VG, Waggoner AD, Sicard GA, et al: Dobutamine stress echocardiography predicts surgical outcome in patients with an aortic aneurysm and peripheral vascular disease, *J Am Coll Cardiol* 21:957, 1993.

46. Boersma E, Poldermans D, Bax JJ, et al: Predictors of cardiac events after major vascular surgery: role of clinical characteristics, dobutamine echocardiography, and β-blocker therapy, *JAMA* 285:1865, 2001.

47. Eagle KA, Rihal CS, Micket MC, et al: Cardiac risk of noncardiac surgery: influence of coronary disease and type of surgery in 3368 operations, *Circulation* 96:1882, 1997.

48. Fleisher LA, Eagle KA, Shaffer T, et al: Perioperative and long-term mortality rates after major vascular surgery: the relationship to preoperative testing in the Medicare population, *Anesth Analg* 89:849, 1999.

49. Crawford ES, Morris GC, Howell JF, et al: Operative risk in patients with previous coronary artery bypass, *Ann Thorac Surg* 26:215, 1978.

50. Nielsen JL, Page CP, Mann C, et al: Risk of major elective operation after myocardial revascularization, *Am J Surg* 164:423, 1992.

51. Fleisher LA, Skolnick ED, Holroyd KJ, et al: Coronary artery revascularization before abdominal aortic aneurysm surgery: a decision analytic approach, *Anesth Analg* 74:661, 1994.

52. Poldermans D, Boersma E, Bax JJ, et al: The effect of bisoprolol on the perioperative mortality and myocardial infarction in high-risk patients undergoing vascular surgery, *N Engl J Med* 341:1789, 1999.

53. Mangano DT, Layug EL, Wallace A, et al: The effect of atenolol on the mortality and cardiovascular morbidity after noncardiac surgery, *N Engl J Med* 335:1713, 1996.

54. Wallace A, Layug B, Tateo I, et al: Prophylactic atenolol reduced postoperative myocardial ischemia, *Anesthesiology* 88:7, 1998.

55. Urban MK, Markowitz SM, Gordon MA, et al: Postoperative prophylactic administration of β-adrenergic blockers in patients at risk for myocardial ischemia, *Anesth Analg* 90:1257, 2000.

56. Posner KL, Van Norman GA, Chan V: Adverse cardiac outcomes after noncardiac surgery in patients with prior percutaneous transluminal coronary angioplasty, *Anesth Analg* 89:553, 1999.

57. Allen JR, Helling TS, Hartzier GO: Operative procedures not involving the heart after percutaneous transluminal coronary angioplasty, *Surg Gynecol Obstet* 173:285, 1991.

58. Gottlieb A, Banoub M, Sprung J, et al: Perioperative cardiovascular morbidity in patients with coronary artery disease undergoing vascular surgery after percutaneous transluminal coronary angioplasty, *Cardiothorac Vasc Anesth* 12:501, 1998.

59. Vicenzi MN, Ribitsch D, Luha O, et al: Coronary artery stenting before noncardiac surgery: more threat than safety? *Anesthesiology* 94:367, 2001.

60. Kaluza GL, Joseph J, Lee JR, et al: Catastrophic outcomes of noncardiac surgery soon after coronary stenting, *J Am Coll Cardiol* 35:1288, 2000.

61. Goldman L, Caldedra DL: Risks of general anesthesia and elective operation in the hypertensive patient, *Anesthesiology* 50:285, 1979.

62. Stone JG, Foex P, Sear JW, et al: Risk of myocardial ischaemia during anaesthesia in treated and untreated hypertensive patients, *Br J Anaesth* 61:675, 1988.

63. Brabant SM, Bertrand M, Eyraud D, et al: The hemodynamic effects of anesthetic induction in vascular surgical patients chronically treated with angiotensin II receptor antagonists, *Anesth Analg* 89:1388, 1999.

64. Magnusson J, Thulin T, Werner O, et al: Haemodynamic effects of pretreatment with metoprolol in hypertensive patients undergoing surgery, *Br J Anaesth* 58:251, 1986.

65. Farnett L, Mulrow C, Linn W, et al: The J-curve phenomenon and the treatment of hypertension: is there a point beyond which pressure reduction is dangerous? *JAMA* 265:489, 1991.

66. Muribito JM, D'Agostino RB, Silbershatz H, Wilson WF: Intermittent claudication: a risk profile from the Framingham Heart Study, *Circulation* 96:44, 1997.

67. Kannel W, Shurleff D: The Framingham Study: cigarettes and the development of intermittent claudication, *Geriatrics* 28:61, 1973.

68. Krupski W: The peripheral vascular consequences of smoking, *Ann Vasc Surg* 5:291, 1992.

69. Doyle R: Assessing and modifying the risk of postoperative pulmonary complications, *Chest* 115:77S, 1999.

70. Warner MA, Offord KP, Warner ME, et al: Role of perioperative cessation of smoking and other factors in postoperative pulmonary complications: a blinded prospective study of coronary artery bypass patients, *Mayo Clin Proc* 64:609, 1989.

71. Smetana GW: Preoperative pulmonary evaluation, *N Engl J Med* 340:937, 1999.

72. Tisi GM: Preoperative identification and evaluation of the patient with lung disease, *Med Clin North Am* 71:399, 1987.

73. Gass CD, Olsen GN: Preoperative pulmonary function testing to predict postoperative morbidity and mortality, *Chest* 89:127, 1986.

74. Haitt W: Medical treatment of peripheral arterial disease and claudication, *N Engl J Med* 344:1608, 2001.

75. Akbari CM, Lo Gerfo FW: Diabetes and peripheral vascular disease, *J Vasc Surg* 30:373, 1999.

76. Wright RA, Clemente R, Wathen R: Diabetic gastroparesis: an abnormality of gastric emptying of solids, *Am J Med Sci* 289:240, 1985.

77. Burgos LUG, Bert TJ, Asiddao C, et al: Increased intraoperative cardiovascular morbidity in diabetics with autonomic neuropathy, *Anesthesiology* 70:591, 1989.

78. Hirsh IB, Magill JOB, Cryer EG, et al: Perioperative management of surgical patients with diabetes mellitus, *Anesthesiology* 74:346, 1991.

79. Jackson MR, Clagett GP: Antithrombotic therapy in peripheral arterial occlusive disease, *Chest* 119:283S, 2001.

80. Neilipovitz DT, Bryson GL, Nichol G: The effect of perioperative aspirin therapy in peripheral vascular surgery: a decision analysis, *Anesth Analg* 93:573, 2001.

81. Martin R: Perioperative use of anticoagulants and thrombolytics. Perioperative approach to the anticoagulated patient, *Anesth Clin North Am* 17:813, 1999.

82. Fitch JCK, Hines R: Perioperative use of anticoagulants and thrombolytics. Thrombolytic therapy, *Anesth Clin North Am* 17:787, 1999.

83. Akhtar S, Brull S: Perioperative use of anticoagulation and thrombolytics. Intraoperative use of anticoagulants and antithrombotics. Heparin and beyond, *Anesth Clin North Am* 17:831, 1999.

84. Lindhoff-Last E, Eichler P, Stein M, et al: A prospective study on the incidence and clinical relevance of heparin-induced antibodies in patients after vascular surgery, *Thromb Res* 97:387, 2000.

85. Warkentin TE, Kelton JG: Temporal aspects of heparin-induced thrombocytopenia, *N Engl J Med* 344:1286, 2001.

86. Abu-Hajiir M, Mazzeo AJ: Perioperative use of anticoagulants and thrombolytics. The pharmacology of antithrombotic and antiplatelet agents, *Anesth Clin North Am* 17:479, 1999.

87. Kam PCA, Egan MK: Platelet glycoprotein IIb/IIIa antagonists, *Anesthesiology* 96:1237, 2002.

88. Liu SS, Mulroy MG: Neuraxial anesthesia and analgesia in the presence of standard heparin, *Reg Anesth Pain Med* 23:157, 1998.

89. Horlocker TT, Wedel DJ: Neuraxial block and low-molecular-weight heparin: balancing perioperative analgesia and thromboprophylaxis, *Reg Anesth Pain Med* 23:1641998.

90. Enneking KF, Benzon HT: Oral anticoagulants and regional anesthesia: a perspective, *Reg Anesth Pain Med* 23:140, 1998.

91. Rosenquist RW, Brown DL: Neuraxial bleeding: fibrinolytics/thrombolytics, *Reg Anesth Pain Med* 23:152, 1998.

92. Urmey WF, Rowlingson JC: Do antiplatelet agents contribute to the development of perioperative spinal hematoma? *Reg Anesth Pain Med* 23:146, 1998.

93. Horlocker TT: Regional anesthesia and anticoagulation: are the benefits worth the risks? In Chaney MA (ed): *Regional anesthesia for cardiothoracic surgery*, Philadelphia, 2002, Lippincott, Williams & Wilkins, 139.

94. Edelson R, Chenik N, Posner J: Spinal subdural hematomas complicating lumbar puncture. Occurrence in thrombocytopenic patients, *Arch Neurol* 31:134, 1974.

95. Messer H, Forshan V, Brust J, Hughes J: Transient paraplegia from hematoma after lumbar puncture. A consequence of anticoagulant therapy, *JAMA* 235:529, 1976.

96. DeAngelis J: Hazards of subdural and epidural anesthesia during anticoagulant therapy: case report and review, *Anesth Analg* 51:676, 1972.

97. Costabile G, Husag L, Probst C: Spinal epidural hematoma, *Surg Neurol* 21:489, 1984.

98. Bamford C: Spinal epidural hematoma due to heparin, *Arch Neurol* 85:693, 1978.

99. American Society of Anesthesiologists: Standards for basic anesthetic monitoring, 1998. Can be obtained at the American Society of Anesthesiologists web site: http://www.asahq.org/Standards/02.html#2.

100. Frank SM, Fleisher LA, Breslow MJ, et al: Perioperative maintenance of normothermia reduces the incidence of morbid cardiac events: a randomized trial, *JAMA* 277:1127, 1997.

101. Smith J, Cahalan M, Benefiel P: Intraoperative detection of myocardial ischemia in high-risk patients: electrocardiography versus two-dimensional transesophageal echocardiography, *Circulation* 72:1015, 1985.

102. Thys D, Hillel Z, Goldman M: A comparison of hemodynamic indices derived by invasive monitoring and two-dimensional echocardiography, *Anesthesiology* 67:630, 1987.

103. Kalman P, Wellwood M, Weisel R: Cardiac dysfunction during abdominal aortic operation: the limitations of pulmonary wedge pressures, *J Vasc Surg* 3:773, 1986.

104. Shanewise, JS, Cheung AT, Aronson S, et al: ASE/SCA guidelines for performing a comprehensive intraoperative multiplane transesophageal echocardiography examination: recommendations of the American Society of Echocardiography Council for Intraoperative Echocardiography and the Society of Cardiovascular Anesthesiologists Task Force for Certification in Perioperative Transesophageal Echocardiography, *Anesth Analg* 89:870, 1999.

105. Haskell R, French W: Accuracy of left atrial and pulmonary artery wedge pressure in pure mitral regurgitation in predicting left ventricular end-diastolic pressure, *Am J Cardiol* 61:136, 1988.

106. Valentine RJ, Duke ML, Inman MH, et al: Effectiveness of pulmonary artery catheters in aortic surgery: a randomized trial, *J Vasc Surg* 27:203, 1998.

107. Bender JS, Smith-Meek MA, Jones CE: Routine pulmonary artery catheterization does not reduce morbidity and mortality of elective vascular surgery: results of a prospective, randomized trial, *Ann Surg* 226:229, 1997.

108. Polanczyk CA, Rohde LE, Goldman L, et al: Right heart catheterization and cardiac complications in patients undergoing noncardiac surgery: an observational study, *JAMA* 286:309, 2001.

109. Isaacson I, Lowdon JD, Berry AJ, et al: The value of pulmonary artery and central venous monitoring in patients undergoing abdominal aortic reconstructive surgery: a comparative study of two selected, randomized groups, *J Vasc Surg* 12:754, 1990.

110. Haimovici H: Myopathic-nephrotic-metabolic syndrome associated with massive acute arterial occlusions, *J Cardiovasc Surg* 14:589, 1973.

111. Kohn L, Corrigan J, Donaldson M: *To err is human: building a safer health system.* Washington, DC, 1999, National Academy Press.

112. Yeager MP, Glass DD, Neff RK, Brinck-Johnsen T: Epidural anesthesia and analgesia in high-risk surgical patients, *Anesthesiology* 56:729, 1987.

113. Tuman KJ, McCarthy RJ, March RJ, et al: Effects of epidural anesthesia and analgesia on coagulation and outcome after major vascular surgery, *Anesth Analg* 73:696, 1991.

114. Christopherson R, Beattie C, Frank S, et al: Perioperative morbidity in patients randomized to epidural or general anesthesia for lower extremity vascular surgery, *Anesthesiology* 79:422, 1993.

115. Rosenfeld B, Beattie C, Christopherson R, et al: The effects of different anesthetic regimens on fibrinolysis and the development of postoperative arterial thrombosis, *Anesthesiology* 79:435, 1993.

116. Bode R, Lewis K, Zarich S, et al: Cardiac outcome after peripheral vascular surgery: comparison of general and regional anesthesia, *Anesthesiology* 84:3, 1996.

117. Pierce E, Pomposelli F, Stanley G, et al: Anesthesia type does not influence early graft patency or limb salvage rates of lower extremity arterial bypass, *J Vasc Surg* 25:226, 1997.

118. Rodgers A, Walker N, Schug S, et al: Reduction of postoperative mortality and morbidity with epidural or spinal anaesthesia: results from overview of randomised trials, *BMJ* 321:1493, 2000.

119. Rigg JRA, Jamrozik K, Myles PS, et al: Epidural anaesthesia and analgesia and outcome of major surgery: a randomised trial, *Lancet* 359:1276, 2002.

120. Norris EJ, Beattie C, Perler BA, et al: Double-masked randomized trial comparing alternate combinations of intraoperative anesthesia and postoperative analgesia in abdominal aortic surgery, *Anesthesiology* 95:1054, 2001.

121. Dagnino J, Prys-Roberts C: Studies of anaesthesia in relation to hypertension. VI: Cardiovascular responses to extradural blockade of treated and untreated hypertensive patients, *Br J Anaesth* 56:1065, 1984.

122. Hertz SM, Brener BJ: Ultrasound-guided pseudoaneurysm compression: efficacy after coronary stenting and angioplasty, *J Vasc Surg* 26:913, 1997.

123. Kang SS, Labropoulos N, Mansour MA, Baker WH: Percutaneous ultrasound guided thrombin injection: a new method for treating postcatheterization femoral pseudoaneurysms, *J Vasc Surg* 27:1032, 1998.

124. Comerota AJ, Aldridge SA: Thrombolytic therapy for acute deep vein thrombosis, *Semin Vasc Surg* 5:76, 1992.

125. Brand FN, Dannenberg AL, Abbott RD, et al: The epidemiology of varicose veins: the Framingham study, *Am J Prev Med* 4:96, 1988.

126. Margolis DJ, Kruithof EK, Barnard M, et al: Fibrinolytic abnormalities in two different cutaneous manifestations of venous disease, *J Am Acad Dermatol* 34:204, 1996.

127. Kistner RL, Eklof B, Masuda EM: Diagnosis of chronic venous disease of the lower extremities: the "CEAP" classification, *Mayo Clinic Proc* 71:338, 1996.

128. Nicolaides AN: Investigation of chronic venous insufficiency: a consensus statement, *Circulation* 102:e126, 2000.

129. Baccaglini U: Consensus conference on sclerotherapy, *Int Angiol* 14:239, 1995.

130. Stewart MT: Assessment of peripheral vascular disease. In Hurst JW, Schlant RC, Rackley CE, et al (eds): *The heart*, McGraw-Hill, 1990, New York, 368.

131. AbuRahma AF, Robinson PA, Jennings TG: Carotid-subclavian bypass grafting with polytetrafluoroethylene grafts for symptomatic subclavian artery stenosis or occlusion: a 20-year experience, *J Vasc Surg* 32:411, 2000.

132. Roddy SP, Darling RC, Chang BB, et al: Brachial artery reconstruction for occlusive disease: a 12-year experience, *J Vasc Surg* 33:802, 2001.

Liver Transplantation

13

Yoogoo Kang, MD
Mathai Kurien, MD

END-STAGE liver disease (ESLD) is the ninth leading cause of death in the United States with a mortality rate of 10 per 100,000 population.[1] Medical treatment of ESLD, however, has been ineffective in most cases. For example, survival after fulminant hepatic failure with medical treatment alone is 5% to 20%; mortality of patients with chronic liver disease is 60% to 80% when variceal bleeding occurs; and treatment of neoplasms is generally ineffective.

Liver transplantation was considered "what was exactly needed for patients with ESLD" and pioneered by Dr. Thomas Starzl with the first successful orthotopic liver transplantation in a 3-year-old boy with biliary atresia in 1963.[2] During the first two decades, pioneers of liver transplantation, led by Starzl of Denver and Sir Roy Calne of Cambridge, experienced great difficulties with surgical technique, immunosuppression, and infection control. The number of procedures performed was relatively few, and their success rate was low. It is important to note, however, that physicians and scientists of the 1960s laid the foundation of modern liver transplantation.

Major changes were seen in the early 1980s. Cyclosporine was a breakthrough in immunosuppression, and the National Institutes of Health Consensus Development Conference statement in 1983 promoted the use of orthotopic liver transplantation as clinically effective therapy for patients with ESLD, paving the way for a large increase in the number of centers and procedures.[3,4] Furthermore, surgical technique became simpler with the introduction of venovenous bypass. Anesthesiologists and intensivists took a scientific approach to perioperative medical management. The next evolution was seen in the late 1980s. Tacrolimus was shown to be a superior immunosuppressant, University of Wisconsin solution was introduced to extend the safe cold ischemia time to 24 hours, and the piggyback technique became popular among well-trained surgeons.[5-7] Liver transplantation flourished in the following 10 years; in the year 2000, 4954 liver transplantations were performed in 122 centers in the United States with 1- and 3-year survival rates of 80% and 70%, respectively.[8] In addition to saving many patients with ESLD, liver transplantation has allowed physicians and scientists to understand the pathogenesis of many types of congenital as well as acquired diseases. The number of liver transplantation candidates has ballooned to more than 17,000 patients, but, unfortunately, more than 1700 patients died in 1999 while waiting for organs. The acute shortage of donor organs led to the development of reduced-size and living-related liver transplantation in the late 1990s.

In this chapter, pathophysiology of liver disease, surgical approaches, and anesthetic management of liver transplantation are described.

Anatomy of the Liver

The liver develops as a diverticulum from the primitive gut as early as the eighth day of gestation, and the diverticulum splits into the cranial pars hepatica and caudal pars cystica. The pars hepatica forms the hepatic parenchyma, hepatic ducts, and proximal common bile duct; the pars cystica forms the gallbladder and cystic duct. At the 12th week of gestation, bile begins to flow.

The liver, weighing 1200 to 1500 g in adults, lies in the right upper quadrant of the abdominal cavity and is attached to the diaphragm by the falciform ligament. Traditionally, the liver is divided into the right and left lobes in reference to the location of the falciform ligament. Couinaud, however, divided the liver into the right and left hemiliver using Cantlie's line, which extends from the inferior vena cava (IVC) to the gallbladder. Each hemiliver is further divided into four segments, each containing a pedicle of portal vessels, bile ducts, and hepatic vessels. The left hemiliver is composed of the traditional left lobe along with the caudate and quadrate lobes. Liver resections based on these segmental definitions are right hepatectomy (segments 4 to 8), right lobectomy (segments 5 to 8), left hepatectomy (segments 1 to 4), and left lobectomy (segments 1 to 3) (Figure 13-1).[9]

The liver has a dual blood supply—arterial supply from the hepatic artery, a branch of the celiac axis, and venous supply from the portal vein formed by the union of the splenic and superior mesenteric vein. The total hepatic blood flow is approximately 100 mL/100 g/min, or 25% of cardiac output. The hepatic artery supplies approximately 25% to 30% of hepatic blood flow and 45% to 50% of oxygen, and the portal vein supplies 70% to 75% of hepatic blood flow and 50% to 55% of oxygen. The venous drainage is through the right, middle, and left hepatic veins that merge into the IVC. Hepatic blood flow is primarily regulated by local metabolic demand with an inverse relationship between portal venous and hepatic arterial flow; an increase in hepatic adenosine level triggered by reduced portal venous flow increases hepatic arterial blood flow.[10,11] In addition, the arterial sphincter tone and the contraction state of the sinusoidal endothelial cells influence relative flow between the portal vein and the hepatic artery.[12,13] In contrast to healthy subjects, patients with ESLD cannot tolerate a disruption of arterial blood supply because of their reduced portal venous flow.[14]

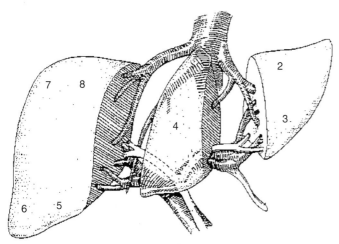

FIGURE 13-1 Segments of the liver. (From Ghobrial RM, Amersi F, Busuttil RW: *Clin Liver Dis* 4:553, 2000.

Diminished hepatic arterial flow in a transplanted liver results in bile duct ischemia, indicating a significant role of arterial blood in the perfusion of the biliary tree.[15]

The liver is innervated by the left and right vagi, the right phrenic nerve, and fibers from the T7-T10 sympathetic ganglia. The hepatic artery is innervated mainly by sympathetic fibers, and unmyelinated sympathetic fibers innervate individual hepatocytes. The bile ducts are innervated by both sympathetic and parasympathetic fibers. The role of hepatic innervation is unclear, as denervation of the transplanted liver does not affect its function.[16,17]

Bile flows from the bile canaliculi to ductules, intrahepatic bile ducts, the right and left hepatic bile ducts, and finally to the common hepatic duct. The union of the common hepatic duct and cystic duct forms the common bile duct, which drains bile into the duodenum. Hepatic lymph forms in the space between the sinusoid and the hepatocyte (space of Disse) and flows to lymph nodes in the hilum and IVC. The transdiaphragmatic lymphatic flow is the cause of pleural effusions in the presence of large ascites.

Hepatocytes are polyhedral, with a central spherical nucleus, and are arranged in one-cell-thick plates with endothelium-lined sinusoids on both sides. Each hepatocyte cell membrane has three distinct membrane domains. The sinusoidal membrane is adjacent to the sinusoidal endothelium and has numerous microvilli abutting into the space of Disse. Fenestrae within the sinusoidal endothelium without a basement membrane permit intimate contact between sinusoidal blood and the hepatocytes to allow the passage of big molecules including lipoproteins. The space of Disse contains phagocytic Kupffer cells that participate in the hepatic inflammatory process. The Ito cells, also known as stellate cells, are high in fat content and are the major site of vitamin A storage. Activation of stellate cells results in their transformation into a myelofibroblast-like state and subsequent hepatic fibrosis and cirrhosis. Reticulin fibers in the space of Disse support the sinusoidal framework. Weakening of these supporting fibers results in rupture of sinusoidal walls and formation of blood-filled cysts known as peliosis hepatis, a forerunner of cirrhosis. The apical membrane circumscribes the canaliculus, the earliest component of the

biliary system. Tight junction complexes between adjacent hepatocytes separate the sinusoidal space from the bile canaliculus. The lateral hepatic membrane is found between adjacent hepatocytes.

The functional unit of the liver is the acinus. As proposed by Rapaport and modified by Matsumoto and Kawakami, terminal portal veins communicate with terminal hepatic venules with sinusoids bridging the gap between the two vessels.[18] Conceptually, this can be visualized as a wheel with the central hepatic vein being the hub and four to six portal triads representing the rim (Figure 13-2). The acinus is bulb shaped, and the classical lobule is composed of several wedge-shaped portions called primary lobules that have cylindrical (sickle-shaped) isobars. In this model, the margins of the shaded zones represent planes of equal blood pressure (isobars), oxygen content, or other characteristics. Periportal tissue (zone 1) receives blood higher in oxygen content than pericentral or perivenular tissue (zone 3). As a result, the hepatocytes in the perivenular zone are more vulnerable to ischemic damage and nutrient depletion. Oxidative and reductive functions are predominantly performed by hepatocytes of the periportal zone and glucuronidation by those of the pericentral zone, although hepatocytes of the two different zones are functionally integrated.[19] The unique structure of the liver acinus is well suited for bidirectional transfer of nutrients. The low pressure in the portal venous system allows blood to flow slowly through the sinusoids. Hepatic arterial blood flows mainly to the terminal bile canaliculi, although it augments sinusoidal flow to give a gentle pulsatility. In patients with cirrhosis, the sinusoids acquire features of systemic capillaries; the space of Disse widens with collagen deposition, endothelial fenestrations become smaller and fewer, and hepatic microvilli efface. All these changes reduce transport across the sinusoidal walls and result in hepatic dysfunction. Further, widespread fibrosis and scarring reduce the number and size of the small portal and hepatic veins and increase intrahepatic vascular resistance to develop portal hypertension.[20] Sluggish blood flow in the altered vascular architecture promotes thrombosis, causing further cell necrosis and fibrosis.[21]

Physiology of the Liver

The liver has three major functions—metabolism, bile production and secretion, and filtration of harmful substances.

Carbohydrate Metabolism

Glucose is the primary nutrient for the brain, erythrocytes, muscle, and the renal cortex. The principal role of the liver is to provide the body with normal glucose levels under the regulation of insulin, glucagon, growth hormone, and catecholamines.[22] In response to a high glucose level, the liver converts glucose into glycogen (glycogenesis) and utilizes glucose for the synthesis of fatty acids. The healthy liver has a 2-day storage of glycogen and maintains euglycemia by triggering gluconeogenesis and glycogenolysis during starvation. The liver is able to produce 240 g of glucose per day through gluconeogenesis, twice the daily needs of the brain, retina, and red blood cells.

Matsumoto and Kawakami   ## Rappaport

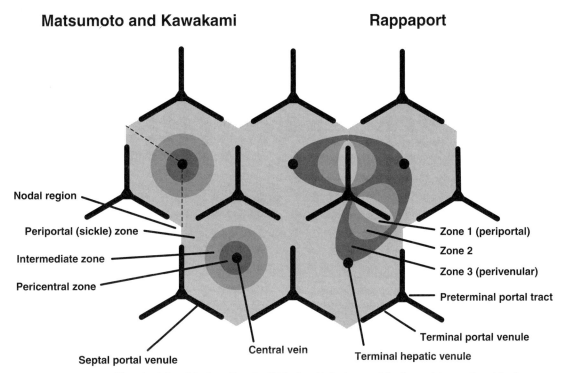

Nodal region

Periportal (sickle) zone

Intermediate zone

Pericentral zone

Zone 1 (periportal)

Zone 2

Zone 3 (perivenular)

Preterminal portal tract

Terminal portal venule

Septal portal venule

Central vein

Terminal hepatic venule

FIGURE 13-2 Microcirculation of the liver. (From Ian R. Wanless IR: Anatomy and developmental anomalies of the liver. In Feldman M [ed]: *Sleisenger & Fordtran's gastrointestinal and liver disease*, ed 6, Philadelphia, 1998, WB Saunders, 1059.)

Cirrhotic patients are frequently hyperglycemic, although their insulin level is elevated.[23,24] This insulin resistance is caused by multiple mechanisms. Cirrhotic patients have an increased basal metabolic rate and preferentially use fatty acids as an energy source. Reduced glucose uptake and storage in the muscle and liver lead to hyperglycemia. Other contributing factors are increased serum fatty acids, which inhibit glucose uptake by muscle, altered second-messenger activity after insulin binding to its receptors, an increased concentration of serum cytokines associated with elevated levels of endotoxins, and increased levels of glucagon and catecholamines.

Protein and Amino Acid Metabolism

The liver is the major organ for protein synthesis, and albumin is the most important protein product. Albumin is the major contributor to plasma oncotic pressure, and hypoalbuminemia results in peripheral edema, ascites, and pleural effusions. It also binds and transports bilirubin, hormones, fatty acids, and other substances. Hypoalbuminemia is commonly caused by decreased hepatic synthetic function, although it can be seen in patients with enlarged volume of distribution, reduced level of amino acid precursors, and losses into urine, peritoneum, and pleural cavity.[25] The low serum oncotic pressure stimulates hepatic albumin synthesis in healthy subjects, although synthesis is impaired in patients with cirrhosis.[26] The liver synthesizes all coagulation factors (except von Willebrand factor) and proteins C and S. Factors II, VII, IX, and X undergo a post-translational vitamin K–dependent modification involving γ-carboxylation of specific glutamic acid residues in the liver.[27]

The liver is the primary site of interconversion of amino acids. Anabolic processes synthesize proteins from amino acids, and catabolic processes convert amino acids either to keto acids by transamination or to keto acids and ammonia by oxidative deamination. Ammonia, in turn, is converted to urea by the Krebs-Henseleit cycle. In patients with liver disease, derangement of both anabolic and catabolic processes results in decreased production of blood urea nitrogen and accumulation of ammonia, a contributing factor in the development of hepatic encephalopathy. The liver produces acute phase reactants, such as α-fetoprotein, ceruloplasmin, fibrinogen, transferrin, complement, and ferritin. They are expressed during acute and chronic systemic inflammation, and their activation is mediated by interleukin-6, tumor necrosis factor, interferon-γ, and glucocorticoids.

Lipid Metabolism

The liver takes up fatty acids and cholesterol from the diet and peripheral tissues to produce and release lipoprotein complexes into circulation. Fatty acids released from adipocytes are bound to serum albumin and transported to the liver for synthesis of phospholipids and triglycerides.[28] The liver produces fatty acids from small molecular weight precursors, and cholesterol synthesis is regulated by the rate-limiting enzyme 3-hydroxyl-3-methylglutaryl coenzyme A reductase (HMG-CoA reductase). Lipids are exported from the liver by very low density lipoprotein particles that are the major carriers of plasma triglycerides during nonabsorptive states.[29] Lipids may be temporarily stored in the liver as fat droplets or as cholesteryl esters in the case of cholesterol and directly excreted into bile or metabolized into bile acids. The liver is the major site for sterol excretion and the site of production of bile acids.

Various abnormalities in lipid metabolism are common in liver disease. Hypertriglyceridemia (250 to 500 mg/dL) is the most common presentation and may be caused by decreased synthesis of lipoproteins, decreased hepatic clearance of lipoprotein complexes, or reentry of biliary content into the serum. Alcoholic liver injury results in increased fatty acid synthesis and steatosis.[30] Paradoxically, an increased high-density lipoprotein 3 (HDL3) level has been noted with moderate alcohol consumption, which may explain the reduced risk of atherosclerosis in these patients.[31] Patients with cholestatic liver diseases have elevated total serum cholesterol and triglycerides because the bile is rich in cholesterol, phospholipids, and lecithin.

Detoxification and Hormone Alteration

The liver eliminates drugs by two types of reactions. The phase 1 reactions include oxidation, reduction, hydroxylation, sulfoxidation, deamination, dealkylation, and methylation of reactive substances. These reactions involve systems such as cytochrome P-450 and typically occur in the periportal area of the liver. The phase 2 reactions that transform lipophilic agents into more water-soluble compounds take place in the pericentral area. In patients with liver disease, hepatic drug clearance is usually reduced owing to the enlarged volume of distribution and decreased hepatic metabolism. As a result, a large initial dose followed by small, titrated maintenance doses of medications is required to achieve the desired pharmacologic effects. Several hormones are deactivated or altered in the liver. Those deactivated include insulin, glucagon, steroid hormones, aldosterone, thyroxine, and triiodothyronine. The liver converts testosterone into androsterone and estrogen into estrone and estriol. Abnormal levels of estrogen and testosterone in patients with liver disease lead to testicular atrophy, loss of pubic and axillary hair, spider angioma, and gynecomastia.

Excretory Functions

The liver removes various substances from the body, and bile formation is one of the most important excretory functions. When membranes of old erythrocytes rupture, the released hemoglobin is taken up by the reticuloendothelial cells and is split into heme and globin. Heme is converted to biliverdin, which, in turn, is reduced to free bilirubin and released into the plasma. The free bilirubin–albumin complex is taken up by the hepatocytes. Bilirubin primarily conjugates with glucuronic acid and is actively transported into the bile. A small portion of conjugated bilirubin returns to the plasma directly from the sinusoids or indirectly by absorption from the bile ducts and lymphatics. Bilirubin is converted into urobilinogen by the intestinal bacterial flora. Some urobilinogen is reabsorbed through the intestinal mucosa and is reexcreted into the intestine. Bile acids, which enhance absorption of vitamin K, are also excreted into the bile by the liver.

Filtration Function

The liver, located between the splanchnic and systemic venous systems, acts as a vascular filter. Kupffer cells phagocytose immune complexes, endotoxins, and bacteria in the portal venous blood and process antigens for presentation to immunocompetent cells. The liver also removes activated clotting elements from the circulation to prevent excessive coagulation or fibrinolysis.

Hepatocyte Regeneration and Apoptosis

The liver undergoes rapid regeneration through proliferation of hepatocytes to maintain the critical mass necessary for normal liver function.[32] For example, the newly transplanted hemiliver from a living-related donor regenerates to about 85% of its original whole liver size in 7 to 14 days. The major hepatic growth factors are epidermal growth factor and the hepatocyte growth factor.[33,34] It is interesting that administration of the epidermal or hepatocyte growth factor to normal rats does not cause hepatocyte replication. This negative response suggests that liver regeneration involves a two-step process: the initial signal generated by an acute increase in metabolic demand associated with the loss of hepatocytes triggers a set of early response genes that prime hepatocytes to respond to various growth factors. In apoptosis or programmed cell death, aging hepatocytes are removed and new cells produced in a continuous manner.[35] Although it is unclear, Fas/Apo 1 antigen may play a major role in the removal of senescent hepatocytes.[36]

Pathophysiology of Liver Cirrhosis

Liver cirrhosis, defined as progressive fibrosis and the formation of regenerative nodules, is the final common pathway in which hepatocytes are replaced by connective tissue after various repetitive insults. The amount of remaining functional hepatic mass and the degree of architectural distortion determine the functional state of the liver. Portal hypertension is inevitable in advanced cirrhosis and leads to ascites, variceal bleeding, encephalopathy, and spontaneous bacterial peritonitis. The severity of cirrhosis is frequently classified by the Child-Pugh score (Table 13-1), and a score greater than 6 suggests a short life expectancy.

Central Nervous System

Hepatic encephalopathy is a reversible neuropsychiatric condition of both acute and chronic liver failure. In chronic liver disease, hepatic encephalopathy develops in 28% of patients within 10 years of compensated cirrhosis and is associated with spontaneously developed or surgically created portosystemic shunting.[37] The degree of encephalopathy is stratified by a coma scale: grade 1, subtle confusion; grade 2, somnolence; grade 3, unconsciousness with response to pain stimulation; and grade 4, deep coma. Clinically, asterixis, flapping tremor,

TABLE 13-1

The Child-Pugh Score

Presentation	Points		
	1	2	3
Albumin (g/dL)	>3.5	2.8-3.5	<2.8
Prothrombin time			
Seconds prolonged	<4	4-6	>6
INR	<1.7	1.7-2.3	>2.3
Bilirubin (mg/dL)			
Hepatocellular disease	<2	2-3	>3
Cholestatic disease	<4	4-10	>10
Ascites	Absent	Mild-moderate	Tense
Encephalopathy	None	Grade 1-2	Grade 3-4

Class A, 5-6 points; B, 7-9 points; C, 10-15 points; INR, international normalized ratio.

and fetor hepaticus (musty, sweet breath odor) are confirmatory of hepatic encephalopathy.

Neurotransmitter dysfunction is thought to be central in the pathogenesis of hepatic encephalopathy.[38] Chronic liver failure appears to alter expression of several gene codings for various neurotransmitter proteins in the brain. Decreased expression of the glutamate transporter GLT-1 increases extracellular brain glutamate. Increased expression occurs in some receptors: monoamine oxidase increases degradation of monoamine transmitters, the peripheral-type benzodiazepine receptor increases inhibitory neurosteroids, and neuronal nitric oxide synthase increases nitric oxide production. Ammonia, although its plasma level is not closely related to the severity of encephalopathy, is still considered as the major contributing factor. Ammonia and manganese, normally removed by the liver, accumulate in the brain of patients with portosystemic shunting and are known to alter the expression of peripheral-type benzodiazepine receptor and neuronal nitric oxide synthase in exposed cells.[39]

Magnetic resonance spectroscopy reveals brain edema and increased brain glutamine-glutamate with reductions in choline and myoinositol in the frontal and parietal lobes. Histological findings include swelling and glycogen deposition in astrocytes.[40] These changes in the brain coincide with impairment in visuopractic capacity, visual scanning, and perceptual-motor speed on neuropsychiatric testing.[41] Subclinical hepatic encephalopathy can be detected by having patients perform a simple timed connect-the-numbers test.

Treatment of hepatic encephalopathy is based on an ammonia-lowering strategy with protein restriction, oral nonabsorbable antibiotics, and lactulose. Neomycin reduces the plasma ammonia level by destroying intestinal bacteria, producing urease. Although it is mostly nonabsorbable, gastrointestinal absorption of a small quantity of neomycin may cause nephrotoxicity and ototoxicity. Metronidazole (800 mg/day) is an alternative to neomycin, although its adverse effects limit its use to a week at a time. Lactulose is a substrate for gut bacteria and reduces the formation of ammonia by lowering intestinal pH. Lactitol, a more palatable agent causing less nausea and bloating, is an alternative to lactulose. Although the combination of neomycin and lactulose is beneficial, an increase in stool pH indicates the eradication of disaccharide-metabolizing intestinal bacteria and the need to discontinue the antibiotic. Oral or parenteral ornithine aspartate, a substrate for the conversion of ammonia to urea and glutamine, has effects similar to those of lactulose with fewer adverse effects. Zinc supplementation is not particularly useful, and flumazenil appeared to be beneficial in limited studies.[42,43] In patients with severe encephalopathy, the molecular absorbent recycling system (MARS) may be utilized to remove small and middle molecular weight water-soluble substances.[44] The system appears to increase blood pressure and systemic vascular resistance, possibly by removing nitric oxide.

In fulminant hepatic failure, progressive hepatic coma is accompanied by a gradual increase in cerebral blood flow and intracranial hypertension. Subsequently, vasogenic cerebral edema and severe intracranial hypertension develop, and approximately 30% to 50% of patients die of brain herniation.[45] Intracranial pressure monitoring using a Ladd epidural sensor is useful in detecting intracranial hypertension, monitoring the therapeutic effects, and identifying patients who would survive after transplantation without neurologic damage.[46] Noninvasive neurologic assessment includes transcranial Doppler to measure cerebral blood flow velocity, determination of cerebral metabolic rate for oxygen by calculating the oxygen content difference between arterial and jugular venous blood, evoked potentials, and serial computed tomography (CT) scans.[47,48] Treatment includes osmotic and loop diuretics, barbiturate-induced coma, and hypothermia. The definitive treatment is usually transplantation.

Pulmonary System

Hypoxemia of varying severity is present in 45% to 69% of patients with significant liver disease.[49] The common causes are pleural effusions, impaired diffusion capacity, arteriovenous shunting, atelectasis caused by ascites or diaphragmatic dysfunction, aspiration secondary to encephalopathy, and muscular weakness.[50] Ventilation-perfusion mismatch, pulmonary vasodilation, and infection also contribute to hypoxemia. Mild forms of hypoxemia are most common, although moderate-to-severe hypoxemia may be found in patients with advanced liver disease complicated by acute respiratory distress syndrome (ARDS), infection, and multiple organ failure.

Severe hypoxemia that occurs in a subset of patients with liver disease was first described by Fluckiger in 1884 and subsequently confirmed by others.[51] The hepatopulmonary syndrome consists of a triad of liver dysfunction, severe hypoxemia (arterial oxygen pressure < 70 mmHg in room air), and pulmonary vasodilation and is characterized by dyspnea, cyanosis, clubbing of the digits, exercise desaturation, and orthodeoxia.[52] Other concomitant clinical signs are markedly increased alveolar-arterial oxygen gradient, portal hypertension, and vascular abnormality such as spider angioma and pulmonary vasodilation. The pulmonary vascular dilatation (from 8 to 15 μ to 15 to 100 μ) at the precapillary level is believed to be the main pathology of the hepatopulmonary syndrome.[53] The pulmonary vasodilation decreases erythrocyte transit time and impairs diffusion of oxygen to the erythrocytes at the center of the bloodstream. As a result, oxygenation is impaired as ventilation-perfusion mismatching and the alveolar-arterial gradient increase. Contrary to the findings in other pulmonary diseases, oxygenation improves dramatically with high fraction of inspired oxygen (F_IO_2); a high alveolar concentration of oxygen overcomes the diffusion barrier and oxygenates the erythrocytes in the center of the bloodstream.

The pathophysiology of the pulmonary vasodilation is complex. Reversal of hypoxia by liver transplantation in many patients implies that functional changes in pulmonary vasculature are the primary cause.[54] Various humoral vasodilators have been implicated in causing the pulmonary vasodilation, namely glucagon, histamine, serotonin, calcitonin-related peptides, vasoactive intestinal polypeptides, atrial natriuretic peptide, substance P, and arachidonic acid metabolites.[55-62] Glucagon, however, does not appear to be a major contributing substance because somatostatin, an inhibitor of glucagon release, does not reverse pulmonary vasodilation.[63] Arachidonic acid metabolites do not appear to play a significant role, although long-term aspirin therapy improves cyanosis and dyspnea of patients with this syndrome.[64]

There is increasing evidence that nitric oxide may be the prime mediator of these vasodilatory changes. It has been shown that increased levels of exhaled nitrites and nitrates, the end products of nitric oxide metabolism, rapidly decrease after liver transplantation as the oxygenation improves.[65] In a cirrhotic rat model, the reduced contractile response of isolated pulmonary arterial rings to phenylephrine was normalized when animals were pretreated with L-NOArg, a nitric oxide synthase inhibitor.[66] In a case report of a patient with the hepatopulmonary syndrome, administration of methylene blue, a nitric oxide synthase inhibitor, reversed hypoxemia and increased systemic arterial pressure.[67]

The hepatopulmonary syndrome is best diagnosed by perfusion scanning with technetium 99–labeled macroaggregated albumin or contrast echocardiography, and more selectively by pulmonary angiography. Embolotherapy, in which sclerosing material is selectively injected into the areas of dilation, may benefit patients with large discrete pulmonary vascular dilatations. In general, the hepatopulmonary syndrome can be reversed by liver transplantation, although patients with severe hepatopulmonary syndrome (alveolar-arterial gradient > 300 mmHg in 100% oxygen) may have a prolonged postoperative course with a mortality rate of up to 30%.[68,69]

Noncardiogenic pulmonary edema occurs in 37% to 79% of patients with advanced liver disease, particularly in those with fulminant hepatic failure. Although its mechanism is unclear, sepsis and neurogenic mechanisms appear to be prime causes. The presence of this complication is ominous: Matuschak and Shaw reported that all 29 patients who developed noncardiogenic pulmonary edema died before liver transplantation.[70] In contrast, a rapid reversal of ARDS after liver transplantation has been reported.[71] Pulmonary edema caused by fluid overload responds to diuretics and has a benign course.

Pleural effusions are found on chest radiographs in about 10% of patients.[72] They are usually right sided (66%) but may be bilateral (17%) or unilateral (17%). Described as hepatic hydrothorax in the absence of primary pulmonary or cardiac disease, this transudate accumulation is caused by the unidirectional passage of fluid through diaphragmatic defects into the pleural space. Diagnostic thoracentesis is necessary to confirm the transudative nature and to exclude infection, malignancy, or embolic disease. Optimal ascites control may prevent symptomatic pleural effusions, and transjugular intrahepatic portosystemic shunt (TIPS) is effective in treating refractory hydrothorax in 84% of patients.[73]

Cardiovascular System

The presence of hyperkinetic circulation with a markedly increased cardiac output and decreased systemic vascular resistance was first described by Kowalski and Abelmann in the early 1950s.[74] Several hypotheses have been proposed to explain this phenomenon, including an overactive sympathetic nervous system, inadequate clearance of vasoactive substances by the diseased liver, the presence of arteriovenous shunts, nitric oxide–induced vasodilation, and relative hypoxia in peripheral tissues.[75-78]

Although cardiac output is frequently two to three times normal, impaired systolic and diastolic function, together with attenuated cardiac responsiveness to stimuli, suggest that cardiomyopathy is present in cirrhotics (cirrhotic cardiomyopathy).[79,80] Caramelo et al noted a 50% decrease in cardiac output with volume expansion in a CCl_4-induced cirrhotic rat model.[81] In another rat model, the chronotropic response to a β-agonist, isoproterenol, was attenuated compared with that in control animals.[82] Cardiac response to physical exercise is blunted in patients with cirrhosis as indicated by alterations in preejection period, isometric contraction time, and the ratio of preejection period to left ventricular ejection time.[83] In addition, abnormalities in myocardial diastolic indices suggest noncompliant ventricles.[84] Histologically, myocardial fibrosis, mild subendocardial edema, and vacuolation of myocyte nucleus and cytoplasm are observed.

Several mechanisms are proposed for the development of cirrhotic cardiomyopathy. It appears that the β-receptor system, the main stimulant of the ventricle, is dysfunctional. In humans, lymphocyte β-receptor density, which reflects cardiac β-receptor status, is reduced in patients with severe ascites, and the β-receptor density of cardiomyocyte sarcolemmal plasma membrane is reduced in cirrhotic rats.[85,86] Further, the β-receptor signal transduction pathway is impaired at several levels, including membrane content and function of the stimulatory G proteins, coupling of the receptor-ligand complex, and activity of the adenyl cyclase enzyme itself.[86,87] Although cardiac contractile impairment may result from muscarinic M_2-receptor overactivity, the receptor density and binding affinity are unchanged, suggesting normal parasympathetic function. Overall muscarinic function may even be depressed as a compensatory response to the impaired β-adrenergic system.[88]

Biophysical and biochemical changes in plasma membrane are also seen in cirrhosis.[89] The membrane fluidity, the ability of lipid and protein moieties in the plasma membrane to move in various directions, is vital for many receptors to function properly. In a cirrhotic rat model, an increase in the membrane cholesterol content decreases membrane fluidity, and restoration of membrane fluidity normalizes isoproterenol-stimulated adenyl cyclase activity. The abnormal plasma membrane also reduces the outward K^+ currents, which prolongs the action potential and QT interval.[90] This prolongation is commonly observed in cirrhotics and correlates with the Child-Pugh score.[91]

Increased serum catecholamine levels, a result of desensitization and downregulation of β-receptors, may lead to myocardial dysfunction in the presence of α-mediated coronary vasoconstriction. In addition, overproduction of nitric oxide in cirrhosis inhibits β-receptor–stimulated cyclic adenosine monophosphate release to cause myocardial dysfunction and vasodilation.[92-94]

Endocarditis is three times more common in patients with liver disease because of translocation of intestinal bacteria through the intestinal wall, portosystemic collaterals, and reduced immune response.[95] The reported incidence of pericardial effusions in cirrhotics is approximately 32% to 63% and correlates with the degree of liver failure.[96,97] The effusions are usually small but may require drainage if they affect cardiac function.

Pulmonary hypertension associated with portal hypertension was first described in 1951.[98] Pulmonary hypertension defined as a mean pulmonary artery pressure greater than 25 mmHg and pulmonary vascular resistance greater than 120 dyne/sec/cm^{-5} is more common in patients with liver disease with a prevalence of 0.25% to 0.73%.[99,100] Pulmonary artery pressure is a function of pulmonary venous pressure, pulmonary vascular resistance, and cardiac output [Ppa = Ppv + (PVR × Q)]. Therefore, pulmonary hypertension is likely to develop in patients with liver disease because of their poor left ventricular compliance, increased pulmonary vascular resistance, and increased pulmonary blood flow from portosystemic shunting.

Pulmonary venous pressure is dependent on left ventricular function. In cirrhosis, impaired systolic and diastolic function decreases left ventricular compliance and increases pulmonary venous congestion and pulmonary capillary pressure. This, in turn, provokes peribronchial edema, which decreases lung compliance. Subsequently, ventilation-perfusion mismatching results in alveolar hypoxia, which further increases pulmonary vascular resistance and pulmonary artery pressure.[101,102] Naeije and colleagues demonstrated an increase in pulmonary vascular resistance in cirrhotic patients, although there was no evidence of any humoral vasoconstrictor involvement.[103] The combination of a high cardiac output and additional inflow from portopulmonary shunts increases the overall blood flow to the lungs and contributes to pulmonary hypertension. Based on this premise, surgical portosystemic shunting may increase the risk of developing pulmonary hypertension, although Hadengue et al reported that pulmonary hypertension was delayed in those with a surgical portosystemic shunt, and the degree of portal hypertension had no bearing on the presence of pulmonary hypertension.[104,105]

The diagnosis of pulmonary hypertension is difficult to establish in patients with liver disease owing to its nonspecific symptoms and limited physical activity of patients. Hence, it is not uncommon to observe pulmonary hypertension during preparation for liver transplantation in the operating room. Echocardiography is the most commonly used screening test for pulmonary hypertension. The presence of an enlarged right ventricle with paradoxical septal motion and significant tricuspid regurgitation are common findings. Pulmonary artery pressure can be estimated by measuring flow velocity in the pulmonary artery and right heart catheterization confirms the diagnosis.

The presence of pulmonary hypertension is a significant risk factor for liver transplantation with extremely high perioperative mortality.[106,107] It is generally agreed that patients with mild-to-moderate pulmonary hypertension may tolerate liver transplantation as long as right ventricular function is normal. However, the risk of liver transplantation in patients with severe pulmonary hypertension (mean pulmonary artery pressure > 35 mmHg) or mild-to-moderate pulmonary hypertension with right ventricular dysfunction is prohibitively high because volume shifts and myocardial depression associated with reperfusion precipitate acute right heart failure. Its treatment has been a dilemma for clinicians. Pulmonary hypertension associated with liver disease does not appear to respond to vasodilators. Preoperative trial of various vasodilators including nitric oxide did not reduce pulmonary arterial pressure,[108] and calcium channel blockers are generally ineffective. Long-term intravenous administration of epoprostenol was reported to reduce pulmonary hypertension.[109] Sildenafil and bosentan appear to be beneficial for patients with pulmonary hypertension, but additional clinical trials are required. The prognosis of

pulmonary hypertension is unclear; pulmonary hypertension is corrected in some patients after liver transplantation.

Coronary artery disease was believed to be relatively uncommon in patients with cirrhosis because of generalized vasodilation and elevated levels of high-density lipoprotein and estrogen. In addition, autopsy findings showed relatively less atherosclerotic changes and myocardial infarction. However, more recent studies show that coronary artery disease is not uncommon, and moderate-to-severe coronary artery disease is found in approximately 27% of patients who undergo coronary artery catheterization as a part of liver transplantation work-up.[110] The presence of coronary artery disease appears to have remarkable clinical significance. For example, Plotkin et al reported a mortality rate of 50% and morbidity rate of 81% among 32 liver transplantation recipients with known coronary artery disease.[111] This high morbidity and mortality may stem from the postoperative hypercoagulable state, poor cardiac reserve, which cannot handle fluid shifts and electrolyte imbalance during surgery, and normalizing vascular resistance after surgery.[112]

Identifying patients with significant coronary artery disease is a difficult task because symptoms of ischemic heart disease may not be recognizable in patients with limited physical activity. It appears that dobutamine stress echocardiography is the most reliable screening test with its high sensitivity and specificity.[113] Further, dobutamine-induced tachycardia may mimic intraoperative cardiac events. For patients with a positive dobutamine stress test, coronary angiography is recommended to identify the degree and type of obstruction. It is generally agreed that coronary artery disease should be aggressively treated using medications and percutaneous intervention. Coronary artery bypass grafting may be limited to patients with relatively well-preserved hepatic function, and liver transplantation is performed only after a thorough evaluation and counseling about cardiac risk.

Portal hypertension is a common circulatory change in patients with liver disease and is caused by increased intrahepatic vascular resistance and increased splanchnic blood flow. Intrahepatic vascular resistance is increased because of architecturally distorted hepatic tissues and increased intrahepatic vascular tone. Endothelin-1, a powerful vasoconstrictor produced by the sinusoidal endothelial cells, increases intrahepatic vascular resistance and activates stellate cells. It increases as cirrhosis progresses.[114-116] Normally, vasodilatory compounds, such as nitric oxide, counterbalance the increased intrahepatic vascular resistance induced by endothelin. In liver cirrhosis, however, nitric oxide production is inhibited by caveolin-1, a hepatic membrane protein that binds with endothelial nitric oxide synthase.

Renal System

Approximately 10% of hospitalized patients with cirrhosis and ascites develop the hepatorenal syndrome. It is a clinical condition that occurs in patients with chronic, advanced liver disease and portal hypertension and is characterized by impaired renal function with markedly abnormal arterial circulation.[117] The primary contributing factor for the hepatorenal syndrome is nitric oxide–induced vasodilation of the splanchnic vascular bed to cause systemic arterial underfilling.[118] Activation of baroreceptor-mediated sympathetic and renin-angiotensin systems constricts all vascular beds including the renal vasculature.[119] The initial prostaglandin-mediated compensatory renal vasodilation is followed by renal arterial vasoconstriction and renal hypoperfusion. A striking feature of the hepatorenal syndrome is the lack of any histologic change and its reversibility; the affected kidney resumes its function after successful liver transplantation. The renal failure may be rapid or insidious and results in sodium and water retention and dilutional hyponatremia. Because the hepatorenal syndrome is a functional renal failure, the urine is similar to that found in prerenal azotemia: oliguria, low urinary sodium, and increased urine osmolality and urine-to-plasma osmolality ratio.

The major criteria for the diagnosis of the hepatorenal syndrome are (1) advanced hepatic disease and portal hypertension; (2) low glomerular filtration rate (serum creatinine > 1.5 mg/dL or creatinine clearance < 40 mL/min); (3) absence of nephrotoxic drug use, shock, systemic infection, or recent fluid losses; (4) lack of sustained improvement after diuretic withdrawal and volume resuscitation with 1.5 L of normal saline; (5) proteinuria (<500 mg/dL); and (6) no ultrasound evidence of urinary obstruction or parenchymal disease. Minor criteria include oliguria (<500 mL/day), urinary sodium less than 10 mEq/L, urinary osmolality greater than plasma osmolality, urinary red blood cells less than 50 per high-power field, and serum sodium less than 130 mEq /L. It is noteworthy that conventional renal function tests, such as blood urea nitrogen and creatinine levels, overestimate renal function in patients with liver failure; malnutrition and muscle wasting contribute to low creatinine level, and liver dysfunction impairs urea synthesis.

The hepatorenal syndrome is treated with the administration of vasopressin-1 agonists such as terlipressin, TIPS, and, most reliably, liver transplantation. One uncontrolled trial using terlipressin with albumin for a median duration of 26 days (range 8 to 68 days) showed improvement in serum sodium as well as a decrease in creatinine level below 2 mg/dL.[120] Hemodialysis is a temporary measure and its efficacy is not reliable. The only primary preventive measure showing some promise is the administration of albumin along with antibiotics as soon as the presence of spontaneous bacterial peritonitis is diagnosed, possibly by preventing hypovolemia and subsequent activation of vasoconstrictor systems.

Coagulation System

Liver disease results in impairment of all phases of hemostasis, including coagulation, fibrinolysis, and their inhibitory processes. Thrombocytopenia is found in 30% to 64% of cirrhotic patients.[121] The platelet count is rarely below 30,000 to 40,000/mm^3 and spontaneous bleeding is uncommon. Thrombocytopenia is primarily caused by splenomegaly associated with portal hypertension, which pools up to 90% of platelets in the spleen. However, the degree of thrombocytopenia does not closely correlate with the size of the spleen. Impaired hepatic synthesis of thrombopoietin also leads to thrombocytopenia. Thrombopoietin is involved in the maturation and formation of platelets, and its return to normal coincides with a gradual increase in platelet count by the fifth day after liver transplantation.[122] Other contributing factors are increased destruction of platelets by immune mechanisms,

excessive activation of coagulation, direct bone marrow suppression by toxins such as ethanol, and folate deficiency. Additionally, platelet dysfunction is common as demonstrated by impaired platelet aggregation to adenosine diphosphate, collagen, and thrombin.[123]

The liver produces all coagulation factors except for von Willebrand factor. Therefore, plasma levels of clotting factors are directly related to the severity of liver disease, and prothrombin time (PT) is considered one of the most sensitive hepatic synthetic function tests. Plasma fibrinogen, an acute phase reactant, is typically normal or increased in chronic liver disease. A reduction in fibrinogen may indicate either greatly reduced hepatic reserve or significant ascites with extravascular loss. Markedly prolonged thrombin time indicates the presence of dysfibrinogenemia in some patients. Dysfibrinogenemia is characterized by an excessive number of sialic acid residues in the fibrinogen molecule and abnormal polymerization of fibrin monomers, and its clinical significance is unclear.

Patients with liver disease have a tendency to develop fibrinolysis owing to decreased hepatic clearance of plasminogen activators, especially tissue plasminogen activator (tPA), and reduced production of α_2-antiplasmin and thrombin-activatable fibrinolysis inhibitors.[124] Elevated levels of D-dimers and fibrin degradation products, together with low fibrinogen and plasminogen levels, have been found in ascitic fluid, indicating that absorption of ascitic fluid may contribute to the hyperfibrinolysis.

On the other hand, excessive activation of coagulation is common in liver disease owing to inadequate hepatic clearance of activated coagulation factors, reduced level of coagulation inhibitors, and enlarged vascular beds. The hypercoagulable state may lead to localized or disseminated intravascular coagulation, particularly in the presence of sepsis, trauma, or major surgery. The diagnosis is based on the presence of a known triggering factor, the progressive worsening of coagulation, and thrombocytopenia. In cholestatic liver diseases (primary biliary cirrhosis and sclerosing cholangitis), the hypercoagulable state may be caused by nonspecific activation of protein synthesis.

Other Complications

ASCITES. Development of ascites is the natural progression of cirrhosis, and the 2-year survival after ascites formation is approximately 50%. It is caused by renal sodium and water retention to compensate for renal hypoperfusion associated with systemic vasodilation. The initial management of ascites is dietary sodium restriction to 2000 mg/day (equivalent to 88 mmol/day) and diuretic therapy to accelerate sodium excretion. Spironolactone, a diuretic with an antialdosterone effect, is commonly used, as these patients have a high aldosterone level. Fluid restriction is usually added only when the serum sodium level falls to less than 120 mmol/L. Diuretic-resistant ascites is treated with paracentesis with or without concurrent plasma expansion with albumin.[125] TIPS can dramatically reduce portal pressure and may make ascites diuretic sensitive. This procedure, however, is associated with complications similar to those of portosystemic shunting, such as hepatic encephalopathy and hepatic and renal failure. Peritoneovenous shunts (LeVeen and Denver shunt) are seldom used because of frequent complications, such as shunt occlusion, infection, sepsis, vena caval thrombosis, and peritoneal fibrosis.

VARICEAL BLEEDING. Variceal bleeding is a potentially fatal complication that occurs with a 10-year cumulative probability of 25% in established cirrhosis. Varices, portosystemic communications, develop as the transhepatic pressure gradient (the difference between portal venous pressure and hepatic venous pressure) exceeds 12 mmHg. Variceal bleeding usually occurs at the distal esophagus, and an endoscopic investigation of esophageal varices is warranted in all patients with cirrhosis to avoid massive variceal bleeding.

Nonselective β-blockers and nitrates are commonly used to prevent variceal bleeding. Nonselective β-blockers (propranolol and nadolol) reduce portal blood flow by allowing unopposed α splanchnic arterial vasoconstriction. In higher doses, reductions in cardiac output and blood pressure decrease portal inflow. The dose is titrated to achieve the heart rate of 55 to 60 beats/min or a 25% reduction from the baseline value.[126] Nitrates decrease portal pressure by systemic vasodilation, postsinusoidal venodilation, and reduction of cardiac output. Variceal ligation is an alternative to drug therapy because it does not require constant hemodynamic monitoring to evaluate efficacy of drug therapy. However, at least one study has failed to show any advantage of the variceal ligation over propranolol.[127]

Variceal bleeding is aggressively treated by fluid resuscitation and prevention of complications such as aspiration pneumonia, electrolyte imbalance, and spontaneous bacterial peritonitis. Analogs of vasopressin (0.2 to 0.4 units/min in a 70-kg patient) are frequently administered during active bleeding to constrict mesenteric arterioles and decrease portal inflow. Triglycyl lysine vasopressin (Glypressin) slowly metabolizes to active vasopressin. It has a long duration of action, does not stimulate plasminogen activator, and has less cardiac toxicity.[128] Octreotide acetate, a synthetic long-acting analog of somatostatin, is the drug most commonly used to reduce portal flow; it acts by inhibiting the release of vasodilator hormones, such as glucagon and vasoactive intestinal polypeptides.[129]

Balloon tamponade is commonly used to control active variceal bleeding unresponsive to pitressin infusion, although its effectiveness is controversial.[130] Sclerotherapy is effective in preventing bleeding from varices before or after the control of active bleeding. It involves endoscopically injecting sclerosing agents (ethanolamine oleate or sodium morrhuate) into the varices. When a patient experiences variceal bleeding, the chance of rebleeding is high, and a shunting procedure (TIPS or surgical portosystemic shunt) or liver transplantation is considered.

SPONTANEOUS BACTERIAL PERITONITIS. Spontaneous bacterial peritonitis is a bacterial infection of ascitic fluid that occurs in the absence of a surgically treatable source of infection. It is seen in approximately 20% of hospitalized patients with cirrhosis, and members of the intestinal flora (*Escherichia coli* and *Klebsiella*) are the most common pathogens. Its clinical presentation includes abdominal pain, fever, and encephalopathy. Early antibiotic therapy, using the third-generation cephalosporins for 5 days, reduced mortality to about 20% to 30% from 80% in the 1970s. Failure to respond to antibiotics should suggest intestinal perforation or secondary peritonitis.

Artificial Hepatic Support

Although liver transplantation is the treatment of choice for patients with ESLD, several modes of temporary or permanent hepatic support have undergone clinical trials with limited success. Hepatic support is based on the fact that clinical effects of hepatic failure are caused by accumulation of toxins normally cleared by the liver (*toxin hypothesis*) and the loss of hepatocytes beyond the critical mass to meet the metabolic demand (*critical mass hypothesis*). In addition, injured hepatocytes contribute to amplification of liver injury by generating toxic substances or altering cell-to-cell interactions. The role of artificial hepatic support includes the removal of toxins, protein synthesis, and the reversal of inflammatory processes in the failing organ.

Nonbiologic Hepatic Support

HEMODIALYSIS. Hemodialysis has been utilized for the reversal of encephalopathy in liver disease. It was reported to improve hepatic encephalopathy by removing middle molecules in the range of 400 to 2000 daltons, although the results have not been consistent.[131] It does not appear to improve survival and may interfere with circulatory stability and fluid and electrolyte balance.

HEMOFILTRATION. Hemofiltration removes convective solutes by utilizing a permeable membrane to avoid any large volume and electrolyte shifts.[132] There is no dialysis fluid, and the ultrafiltrate is replaced by substitution fluid. This technique is more efficient than hemodialysis in the removal of middle molecules including vasoactive immunoglobulins such as interleukin-6 (IL-6), IL-1, tumor necrosis factor α, platelet-activating factor, C1q, C3a, and C5a.

HEMODIAFILTRATION. Hemodiafiltration combines the advantages of both convection (removal of larger molecules, 2000 to 3000 daltons) and diffusion (smaller molecules, up to 400 daltons). Yoshiba et al reported a survival rate of 85% in acute hepatic failure. Its adverse effects include activation of complement and coagulation and release of vasoactive compounds.[133]

HEMODIABSORPTION. Hemodiabsorption (the BioLogic-DT system) combines charcoal and a cation exchanger. Blood is dialyzed across the parallel-plate dialyzer with a cellulose membrane coated with sorbent. The sorbent contains powdered charcoal, sodium, and a cation exchange resin. No survival benefits have been demonstrated.

PLASMAPHERESIS. Plasmapheresis is considered a bridge to transplantation, although it has been moderately successful at best. Multiple studies have demonstrated its beneficial effects on systemic and cerebral hemodynamic variables, possibly through partial removal of neuroinhibitory plasma factors.[134,135] It has also been effective in sustaining life in a small group of patients while recovering from hepatic failure.

Biologic Hepatic Support

XENOGENEIC AND ALLOGENEIC EXTRACORPOREAL SUPPORTS. Xenogeneic and allogeneic extracorporeal supports have been investigated for decades, although no long-term survival has been noted. Further, endothelial antigens in the perfused liver react with antibodies in the recipient to activate the complement and coagulation systems. Eiseman et al described the first experience of heterologous liver perfusion in the treatment of liver failure in 1965.[136] They demonstrated bile flow, galactose elimination, and ammonia clearance in a pig liver extracorporeally perfused with human blood. Extracorporeal perfusion using human livers was reported in three patients with acute liver failure in 1993.[137] Two patients showed neurologic improvement as well as lower serum bilirubin and ammonia levels and subsequently underwent successful liver transplantation.

HYBRID HEPATIC SUPPORT. Hybrid hepatic support utilizes biologic tissue for synthetic and biotransformation functions and nonbiologic materials for toxin removal. Patients are connected to a dialysis circuit, and blood is passed through a metabolic circuit with a gel-type cellulose membrane, followed by a biologic circuit containing liver homogenate, liver slices, or freeze-dried granules. Three systems are available for clinical trials—Sussman's extracorporeal liver assist device (ELAD), Demetriou's bioartificial liver (BAL), and Gerlach's hybrid liver support system.[138-140]

HEPATOCYTE TRANSPLANTATION. Hepatocyte transplantation is performed on the basis of the principle that the injection of an adequate mass of hepatocytes into a patient with hepatic failure has the potential to provide normal liver function as long as the hepatocytes have access to plasma without rejection. A difficulty with this technique is that at least a third of the normal number of hepatocytes (3×10^{10}) is necessary to achieve a long-term benefit of hepatocyte transplantation. Encapsulation of hepatocytes in the semipermeable membrane that protects hepatocytes from immune reaction and mechanical trauma has a potential short-term benefit.[141,142]

XENOTRANSPLANTATION. Xenotransplantation, or the use of animal livers in lieu of human organs, has several advantages over allograft transplantation. It addresses the growing shortage of human organs, avoids recurrence of certain human diseases (eg, hepatitis B or C), and offers a means of gene delivery. The main limitation of xenotransplantation of the liver is the severe immunologic response.[143] Whole-organ xenotransplantation leads to either hyperacute rejection, in which antibodies binding to these cells trigger complement activation, or acute vascular rejection. Cellular rejection mediated by natural killer T cells also plays a role. Hepatocyte transplantation with xenogeneic cells involves similar challenges, including primary nonfunction, failure of neovascularization, and inability to survive in a hostile microenvironment. Other hurdles to xenotransplantation are the differences in physiology of nonhuman organs. For example, human thrombin and protein C are incompatible with porcine thrombomodulin, leading to a thrombotic state. In addition, there is the possibility of spreading a new infectious agent from the graft to the recipient.

Indications and Evaluation for Hepatic Transplantation

Indications

Patients with ESLD, in whom the morbidity and mortality from medical management are judged to be greater than those of liver transplantation, are candidates for transplantation. An expected 1-year survival of less than 90% with medical man-

agement alone is usually considered an indication for liver transplantation. The common diseases requiring liver transplantation are listed in Table 13-2. Chronic hepatocellular disease includes viral hepatitis, alcoholic liver disease, autoimmune disease, and cryptogenic cirrhosis. The presence of recurrent encephalopathy, recurrent spontaneous bacterial peritonitis, diuretic-resistant ascites, refractory variceal bleeding, muscular wasting, and hepatic osteodystrophy are additional reasons for urgency of liver transplantation in this group of patients. There are some controversies regarding transplantation in patients with hepatitis C because immunosuppression accelerates the replication of hepatitis C virus in the grafted liver, and interferon treatment does not eradicate the virus. The disease, however, runs a benign course in most patients; the short-term graft survival is acceptable, approximately 25% of patients develop chronic hepatitis, and progressive disease is seen in only 8% of patients. Liver transplantation in patients with hepatitis B virus is less controversial. The perioperative use of hepatitis B immunoglobulin (HBIg) and lamivudine has been successful in preventing recurrent infection in the allograft. Hepatitis B infection is, however, a premalignant condition, and surveillance for hepatocellular carcinoma is advisable.

TABLE 13-2

Indications and Contraindications for Liver Transplantation

Indications

Fulminant hepatic failure
  Viral hepatitis: A, B, C, D
  Chemical-induced hepatitis (e.g., mushrooms, gold, disulfiram, acetaminophen, quinidine, halothane, Wilson's disease)
Chronic liver disease
  Hepatocellular disease (viral, chemical, alcohol, autoimmune, Wilson's, congenital hepatic fibrosis)
  Cholestatic disease (primary biliary cirrhosis, sclerosing cholangitis, drug-induced)
  Vascular disease (Budd-Chiari syndrome, veno-occlusive disease)
  Neoplasms
    Hepatocellular carcinoma
    Hepatic metastasis (carcinoid)
  Inborn errors of metabolism
    Hemophilia (A, B), protein C deficiency, Crigler-Najjar syndrome
    Hyperoxaluria (I), urea cycle enzyme deficiency
    Hypercholesterolemia (type II), cystic fibrosis
    α_1-Antitrypsin deficiency, tyrosinemia, Niemann-Pick disease
    Glycogen storage disease (I, IV), protoporphyria

Contraindications

Extrahepatic malignancy
Cholangiocarcinoma
Hemangiosarcoma
HIV seropositivity
Active sepsis
Active alcohol or drug abuse
Advanced cardiopulmonary disease
Severe fulminant hepatic failure (ICP > 50 mmHg or CPP < 40 mmHg)
Inability to comply with immunosuppressive protocol
Severe hypoxia (Pa_{O_2}<50 mmHg) unresponsive to 100% oxygen
Technical difficulty associated with anatomic abnormalities

HIV, human immunodeficiency virus; Pa_{O_2}= arterial partial pressure of oxygen.

Chronic cholestatic diseases include primary biliary cirrhosis and slerosing cholangitis. Intractable pruritus, progressive osteodystrophy, xanthomatous neuropathy, and recurrent bacterial cholangitis are additional indications for liver transplantation.

Metabolic liver diseases necessitating transplantation include Wilson's disease, hemochromatosis, α_1-antitrypsin deficiency, hemophilia (A and B), glycogen storage diseases, Crigler-Najjar syndrome, hyperoxaluria, urea cycle enzyme deficiency, protein C deficiency, protoporphyria, and amyloidosis, to name a few.

Hepatic transplantation is contraindicated when either associated diseases or patients' conditions may not improve outcome after liver transplantation. These situations include malignancy with poor prognosis, active bacterial and viral infection, severe cardiopulmonary dysfunction, and anticipated technical difficulties. The recurrence rate of cholangiocarcinoma and hemangiosarcoma is very high, and liver transplantation does not prolong life. A majority of patients with human immunodeficiency virus (HIV) develop acquired immunodeficiency syndrome (AIDS) rapidly after liver transplantation and die of AIDS.[144] Active infection or sepsis must be treated before transplantation. Spontaneous bacterial peritonitis is a relative contraindication as a 5-day course of treatment is usually sufficient to ensure peritoneal sterility. Active alcoholism is a contraindication, although demonstrable abstinence for 6 months is considered acceptable. The presence of multiple organ dysfunction is a relative contraindication for liver transplantation as the 2-year survival is approximately 25%.[8]

Poor prognostic indicators of fulminant hepatic failure are progressive hepatic failure for 7 to 14 days, grade 3 to 4 encephalopathy, intracranial hypertension, cerebral swelling, severe coagulopathy, rapid shrinkage of the liver, metabolic acidosis, hemodynamic instability, and sepsis. Indications and contraindications for liver transplantation, however, have evolved in the past 40 years, and further modifications are expected to occur.

Pretransplantation Evaluation

Upon referral of a patient to the transplantation center, hepatologists, surgeons, anesthesiologists, and intensivists perform the pretransplantation evaluation. Consultations can be obtained to investigate specific issues, such as cardiac or psychosocial evaluation. All clinical and laboratory data are reviewed at the liver transplantation candidate conference for discussion of the hepatic disease, its complications, and extrahepatic organ function. When the patient is placed on the active candidate list, the United Network for Organ Sharing (UNOS) is notified. The UNOS network's transplantation centers are under contract with the Human Resources and Services Administration of the U.S. Department of Health and Human Services.[8] The mission statement of the nonprofit organization is "to advance organ availability and transplantation by uniting and supporting its communities for the benefit of patients through education, technology and policy development." It maintains the national database of organ transplantation and facilitates distribution of all organs and tissues for transplantation.

According to the policy adopted in 2002, patients with acute liver failure with a life expectancy of less than 7 days (fulminant hepatic failure, primary graft nonfunction, hepatic artery thrombosis, and decompensated Wilson's disease) are placed on the highest priority list. Donor livers are allocated to patients with chronic liver disease on the basis of the medical end-stage liver disease (MELD) score in adults and pediatric end-stage liver disease (PELD) score in children. The MELD and PELD scores evaluate the degree of liver disease by using the following laboratory values.

$$\text{MELD score} = 10 \times [0.957 \times \log_e(\text{creatinine, mg/dL}) + 0.378 \times \\ \log_e(\text{bilirubin, mg/dL}) + 1.120 \times \log_e(\text{INR}) + 0.643]$$

$$\text{PELD score} = 10 \times [0.480 \times \log_e(\text{bilirubin, mg/dL}) + 1.857 \times \log_e(\text{INR}) \\ + 0.687 \times \log_e(\text{albumin, g/dL}) + [0.436 \text{ when the child is younger than 1} \\ \text{year or } 0.667 \text{ when the child has growth failure } (<2 \text{ SD})]$$

In the MELD score system, the maximum serum creatinine value is considered 4.0 mg/dL. In the event of a tied score, the patient with a longer waiting period receives the higher priority. The priority scores are adjusted every 3 months to allow fair distribution of donor livers.

Organ Donor Procurement and Preservation of the Donor Liver

In the liver donor, aside from standard tests, serum levels of aspartate aminotransferase, alanine aminotransferase, amylase, bilirubin, and glucose are reviewed. A normal level of serum transaminase is considered ideal, although a donor with a gradual restoration from an increased level is acceptable. Antigens for viral hepatitis and antibodies for HIV should be negative.

Several liver procurement techniques (modified, rapid, super-rapid) are available to meet the needs of various donor conditions. In general, the liver is separated from the diaphragm by severing the falciform, round, and left triangular ligaments (Figure 13-3).[145] The gallbladder is opened and the gastrohepatic ligament is transected. The common bile duct is divided close to the duodenum, and the gastroduodenal and right gastric arteries are divided distally. The splenic and superior mesenteric veins are exposed, and the aorta is stripped off serosa and encircled proximal to its bifurcation. The donor is then administered heparin, and cannulas are inserted into the distal abdominal aorta and the splenic vein. The aorta is cross-clamped above the celiac axis, and cold preservative solution is rapidly infused through the aortic and splenic cannulas while the liver is decompressed through an opening in the suprahepatic IVC. When the liver is cooled and devoid of blood, the left gastric and splenic arteries and the splenic and superior mesenteric veins are ligated and transected. The celiac axis is divided at its junction with the aorta with the Carrell patch. The suprarenal, infrahepatic IVC is divided, and the liver is removed en bloc with a piece of diaphragm containing the suprahepatic IVC.

Donor Organ Preservation

The liver is preserved by the simple hypothermic preservation technique using University of Wisconsin solution, which mimics the intracellular electrolyte composition with a high potassium content (120 mmol/L). The solution contains several substances to protect hepatocytes, lactobionate and raffinose to prevent cell swelling, hydroxyethyl starch to increase oncotic pressure, allopurinol and glutathione to reduce oxygen free rad-

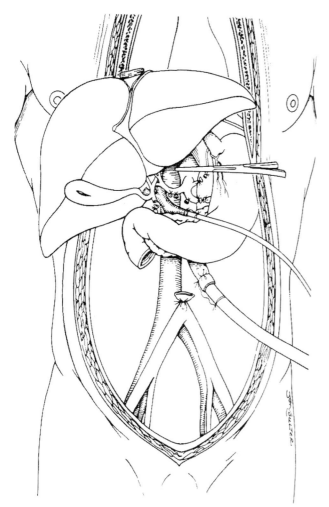

FIGURE 13-3 Procurement of the donor liver. (From Kang YG, Kormos RL, Casavilla A: Organ procurement from donors with brain death. In Grande C [ed]: *Textbook of trauma anesthesia and critical care*, St Louis, 1993, Mosby, 1020.)

ical formation, and adenosine to promote adenosine triphosphate production. This technique extends the safe organ preservation period up to 24 hours, a significant advantage over earlier preservation using Collins solution. However, a prolonged cold ischemia can be associated with more pronounced cytokine release and major histocompatibility complex class II antigen expression, leading to an increased inflammatory response on reperfusion.[146]

Surgical Aspects of Liver Transplantation

Orthotopic Liver Transplantation

In orthotopic liver transplantation (OLT), the engrafted liver is placed anatomically in the right upper quadrant after removing the diseased liver (Figure 13-4). The procedure is divided into three stages—stage 1 (dissection stage), stage 2 (anhepatic stage), and stage 3 (neohepatic stage) for convenience of description. The first stage (dissection stage) begins with skin incision and ends with the skeletonization of the diseased liver. Although the second stage (anhepatic stage) may vary depending on the technique used, it begins with occlusion of the IVC, portal vein, and hepatic artery for hepatectomy and ends with

anastomoses of the supra- and infrahepatic IVC and portal vein. The third stage (neohepatic stage) begins with reperfusion of the grafted liver by sequential unclamping of the infrahepatic IVC, portal vein, and suprahepatic IVC. Reperfusion is followed by hepatic arterial and biliary reconstruction and closure of the abdomen.

OLT WITH SIMPLE VENOUS CROSS-CLAMPING. After an inverted Y-shaped bilateral subcostal skin incision, the hepatic hilum is dissected to isolate the hepatic artery, portal vein, and common bile duct. The liver is then mobilized by severing the falciform, round, and left triangular ligaments and other supporting structures.[147] It is removed together with the retrohepatic IVC after cross-clamping the supra- and infrahepatic IVC, hepatic artery, and portal vein. After surgical hemostasis of the retrohepatic area, the donor liver is placed in the right upper quadrant, and sequential vascular anastomoses of the suprahepatic IVC, infrahepatic IVC, and portal veins are performed. During the infrahepatic IVC anastomosis, the liver allograft is flushed with 1000 mL of lactated Ringer's or 5% albumin solution through a cannula in the portal vein. This flush technique allows preservative solution, metabolites, and air in the donor liver to drain through the incompletely anastomosed infrahepatic IVC. In addition, a second flush technique is used in some centers by allowing 300 to 500 mL of blood to escape through the incompletely anastomosed portal vein by unclamping the infrahepatic IVC (backbleeding technique). When the portal vein of the recipient is less than optimal, the superior or inferior mesenteric vein, collateral vein, or venous graft may be used for portal blood supply.

The liver is reperfused by sequential unclamping of the infrahepatic IVC, portal vein, and suprahepatic IVC. After hemostasis, an end-to-end hepatic arterial anastomosis is commonly performed. However, when the size and anatomy of the hepatic arteries are less than optimal, an arterial graft is made between the infrarenal aorta of the recipient and the hepatic

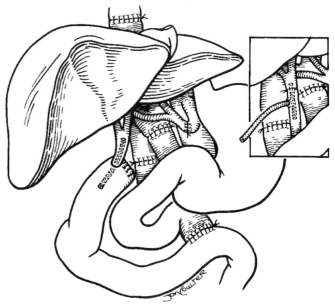

FIGURE 13-4 Orthotopic liver transplantation. (From Starzl TE, Demetris AJ: *Liver transplantation: a 31-year perspective*, Chicago, 1990, Year Book Medical.)

artery of the graft while a side clamp is applied to the aorta. After further hemostasis, choledochocholedochostomy is performed with or without a T-tube, and its patency can be confirmed by an operative cholangiogram. Choledochojejunostomy using a Roux-en-Y loop is performed when the bile ducts are diseased or mismatched in size. The abdomen is closed after the absence of foreign bodies in the peritoneal cavity is confirmed. For patients with a large graft or swollen intestine, the abdomen is closed using plastic mesh.

A major disadvantage of this traditional technique is that it interrupts venous return from the infrahepatic IVC and portal vein. As a result, it decreases cardiac output as much as 40%, exacerbates portal hypertension that causes bleeding and intestinal congestion and swelling, and leads to renal venous congestion, oliguria, and hematuria.

OLT WITH VENOVENOUS BYPASS. This technique was developed in 1983 to avoid reduction of venous return associated with the cross-clamping technique by diverting blood from the IVC and portal vein to the axillary vein using a centripetal magnetic pump (Figure 13-5).[148] Once the hepatic hilum is dissected, cannulas are inserted into the left superficial femoral vein (7 mm) and portal vein (9 mm) for outflow from the patient and into the left axillary vein (7 mm) for venous inflow. The cannula site and size can be modified depending on the preference of the surgical team or anatomic variations. The cannulas and heparin-bonded tubings are flushed with heparin solution (2000 U/L) to avoid thrombosis during preparation. Systemic heparinization is avoided because of preexisting coagulopathy and the use of heparin-bonded tubings. The bypass run begins by unclamping all cannulas while the pump speed is gradually increased to achieve the maximal flow rate. Hepatectomy and anastomoses of the suprahepatic and infrahepatic IVC are performed when full bypass is achieved. The portal cannula is removed during portal venous anastomosis resulting in partial

bypass and reduced venous return. Bypass is terminated after the engrafted liver is reperfused, and cannulas are removed.

Advantages of venovenous bypass are (1) well-preserved cardiac output because of uninterrupted venous return from the viscera and lower extremities; (2) effective decompression of the portal system that decreases bleeding and intestinal congestion; (3) avoidance of renal congestion, oliguria, and hematuria; and (4) simplified anhepatic stage allowing meticulous hepatectomy and vascular anastomoses. Potential acute complications of this technique are inadequate venous return caused by kinked tubing, too high or low bypass pump speed, or reduced preload. Thromboembolism may occur when preexisting mural thrombi are embolized or when the bypass flow rate is low (<1 L/min). Air embolism can also occur if air is permitted to enter the bypass circuit through lacerated blood vessels or cannula connection sites. Long-term complications are neurovascular injury, thrombosis, infection, lymphocele, and seroma at the cannulation sites.

THE FEMORAL VENOARTERIAL BYPASS TECHNIQUE. To maintain circulatory physiology, femoral venous blood is shunted to the femoral artery to decompress the venous system of the lower extremities.[149] This historical technique is no longer used because it does not effectively decompress the portal system and delivers desaturated blood to the systemic circulation.

PIGGYBACK OLT. Piggyback OLT was originally designed for patients with significant cardiovascular disease, portacaval shunt, superior vena caval syndrome, or small donor livers (Figure 13-6).[7] In this technique, the diseased liver is removed without the retrohepatic portion of the IVC by peeling the diseased liver off the IVC after cross-clamping the hepatic veins. Therefore, systemic venous return can be preserved through the intact IVC during the anhepatic stage. For hepatic venous drainage, vascular anastomoses are made between the reconstructed ostia of the recipient (combination of the left and

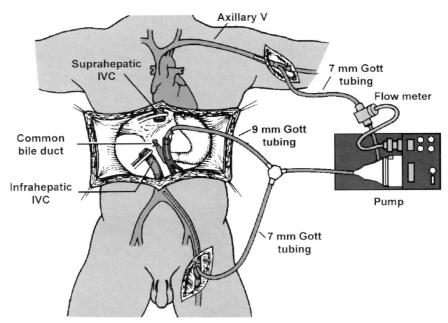

FIGURE 13-5 Venovenous bypass. IVC, inferior vena cava. (From Shaw BW Jr, Starzl TE, Iwatsuki S, et al: An overview of orthotopic transplantation of the liver. In Flye MW [ed]: *Principles of organ transplantation*, Philadelphia, 1989, WB Saunders, 359.)

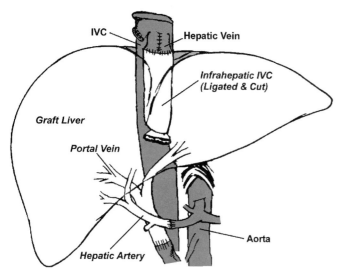

FIGURE 13-6 Piggyback orthotopic liver transplantation. IVC, inferior vena cava. (From Tzakis A, Todo S, Starzl TE: *Ann Surg* 210:649, 1989.)

middle hepatic veins) and the suprahepatic IVC of the graft. The portal veins of the recipient and the graft are anastomosed for portal blood supply, and the infrahepatic IVC of the graft is ligated. Hepatic arterial anastomosis and biliary reconstruction are similar to those described earlier.

Conceptually, this is a simple technique. Hepatectomy in the presence of portal hypertension, however, can be very difficult, and hypotension is not uncommon from inadvertent compression and partial clamping of the IVC during hepatectomy and cross-clamping of the portal vein during portal anastomosis. In some centers, portal venous blood is returned to the systemic circulation by portal-axillary venovenous bypass or temporary portacaval shunt.

Heterotopic (Auxiliary) Liver Transplantation

In this technique, the relatively small liver allograft is placed in the right lower paravertebral gutter without removing the diseased liver (Figure 13-7).[150] The hepatic artery and portal vein are anastomosed to adjacent vessels, and hepatic venous blood is drained into the IVC. This procedure is relatively simple as it avoids hepatectomy and manipulation of major vessels. It is well tolerated by recipients because the anhepatic stage is avoided, and the native liver absorbs metabolites and preservative solution from the relatively small graft. The engrafted liver, however, atrophies rapidly because portal inflow is from the iliac vein with insufficient insulin content. This technique, therefore, is reserved for patients with potentially reversible liver disease (eg, fulminant hepatic failure) or those with an extremely high surgical risk.

Specific Type of Liver Transplantation

Transplantation of cadaveric whole liver was the mainstay of liver transplantation for the first three decades. However, a rapid increase in the recipient pool with a relatively fixed number of donor organs necessitated finding alternative donor sources, using a portion of the liver from either a cadaveric or living-related donor.

REDUCED-SIZE LIVER TRANSPLANTATION. Large cadaveric donor livers can be reduced in size to meet the need of children or small recipients. In children, the most commonly used grafts are segments 2 and 3 (left lateral segment) or segments 2 to 4 (left lobe) (see Figure 13-1). The extended right lobe (segments 4 to 8) is rarely used in children because of the size discrepancy. The unused portion of the liver is discarded. This technique was associated with increased graft-related complications, such as hepatic abscess, primary nonfunction, hepatic artery thrombosis, biliary tract complications, and excessive bleeding.[151] One report, however, suggested that survival and complications are comparable to those of full-size graft transplantation.[152]

CADAVERIC SPLIT-LIVER TRANSPLANTATION. Cadaveric split-liver transplantation is the logical progression from reduced-size liver transplantation. An adult cadaveric organ is divided into two functioning allografts to increase the total number of available organs: segments 2 and 3 (the left lateral segment) for children and segments 4 to 8 (the extended right lobe) for adults. Two methods are commonly used for preparation of the donor liver. In the ex vivo split, the organ is divided in the operating room after removal from the cadaver. This potentially lengthy procedure may result in a long warm ischemia time and increase the incidence of hepatic artery thrombosis and biliary tract injury.[153] The in vivo split was developed to minimize donor ischemia. In this technique, the division of the graft is performed in the donor in a fashion similar to the adult-to-pediatric living-related technique. Using this method, Rogers et al achieved a 6-month graft survival rate of 85.7% with significantly low complications.[154]

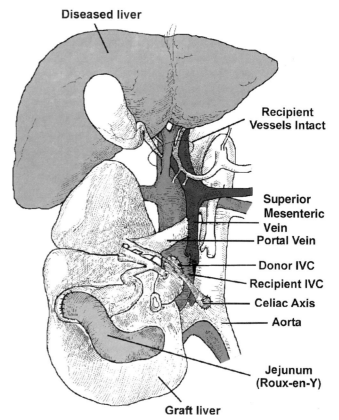

FIGURE 13-7 Heterotopic liver transplantation. IVC, inferior vena cava. (From Starzl TE: Clinical auxiliary transplantation. In Starzl TE, Putnam CW [eds]: *Experience in hepatic transplantation*, Philadelphia, 1969, WB Saunders, 503.)

ADULT-TO-PEDIATRIC LIVING-RELATED DONOR TRANSPLANTATION. Since the use of the left lateral segment of an adult living donor by Raia et al in 1988, more than 1000 adult-to-pediatric living-related liver transplantations have been performed with a survival rate equal to or better than those with cadaveric whole-organ transplantation.[155,156] The advantage of living-related liver transplantation is that it allows proper selection of a donor with adequate hepatic function and histocompatibility. However, the minimal hepatic mass necessary for full functional recovery is not completely known, and, more significantly, donor mortality has been reported.

ADULT-TO-ADULT LIVING-RELATED DONOR TRANSPLANTATION. The first successful adult-to-adult living-related liver transplantation using the left lobe was reported in 1994 by Hashikura et al.[157] The left lobe graft is commonly used in Asia. In the United States, however, the right lobe is preferred because of the large metabolic demand of the recipient.[158] Over the past several years, the number of transplantations has dramatically increased, with more than 500 procedures in 2001. It is noteworthy that the graft undergoes remarkable regeneration: the graft size increased from a mean of 862 to 1614 mL over 7 days in a series of patients.[159] This technique has enlarged the donor pool significantly, although death of donors has been a major concern.[160] Therefore, an extensive donor evaluation process is mandatory to minimize complications (Table 13-3).

Preparation for Liver Transplantation

An immediate preoperative consultation takes place when a donor organ is identified. The patient is reevaluated to identify any significant changes during the waiting period. Anesthetic and postoperative management and their risks are explained to the patient one more time. In general, premedication is withheld in most cases because of potential encephalopathy and hypovolemia, and narcotics (e.g., fentanyl, 1 to 5 µg/kg) are commonly administered intravenously (IV) in the operating room.

Necessary medications and anesthesia equipment are listed in Table 13-4. A device that delivers fluids and blood rapidly on demand is considered standard equipment (e.g., the Rapid Infusion System of Haemonetics, Braintree, MA or FMS2000 fluid warming system of Belmont Instrument Corp., Billerica, MA).[161-163] An autotransfusion system is helpful in minimizing the need for bank blood.[164,165] A system that monitors coagulation, either conventional coagulation profile or Thrombelastograph (Haemoscope Corporation, Niles, IL), is essential in monitoring and management of coagulation.[166,167] In general, 20 units each of cross-matched packed red blood cells (PRBCs) and fresh frozen plasma (FFP) are available at all times, and 10 units of each are prepared in the operating room. Platelets (10 to 20 units) should be available on demand.

Circumferential identification tags around the wrists or ankles are removed to avoid the compartment syndrome. Both arms are placed on padded arm boards in an abducted position; excessive abduction should be avoided to prevent plexus stretch injury. The extremities are protected with foam paddings to avoid pressure injuries.

Noninvasive monitoring is similar to that for patients undergoing major surgery. For invasive monitoring, two intra-arterial catheters (20 gauge in the right radial artery and 18 gauge in the

TABLE 13-3

Evaluation for Living-Related Liver Transplantation

Phase 1 (Recipient and Donor)

Recipient
  Age, ≤65 years
  Absence of major contraindications
    Obesity (>130% ideal body weight)
    Advanced cardiopulmonary disease
    Psychosocial instability
  Financial clearance
Donor
  Age, 18-60 years
  Identical or compatible blood type
  Absence of previous major abdominal surgery
  Absence of major medical problems
  Demonstrable, significant, long-term relationship with recipient
  Normal laboratory test results: liver function tests, serum electrolytes, and complete blood cell count, negative hepatitis B surface antigen, negative hepatitis B core antibody, and negative hepatitis C antibody

Phase 2 (Donor)

Complete medical history and physical examination
Laboratory tests
  Serum ferritin, iron, transferrin, and ceruloplasmin
  α_1-Antitrypsin level and phenotype
  Rapid plasmin reagin
  Cytomegalovirus antibody (IgG), Epstein-Barr virus antibody (IgG)
  Antinuclear antibody
  Human immunodeficiency virus antibody
  Substance abuse screening
  Urinalysis
  Hemoglobin oxygen saturation
Chest radiography
Electrocardiography
MRI of liver, biliary system, and hepatic vasculature
Surgical consultation
Anesthesiology consultation

Phase 3 (Donor)

Further tests or consultations
ERCP, hepatic angiography
Liver biopsy, stress echocardiography, etc.
ECRP, endoscopic retrograde cholangiopancreatography; IgG, immunoglobulin G; MRI, magnetic resonance imaging.

Modified from Trotter JF, Wachs M, Everson GT, et al: *N Engl J Med* 346:1079, 2002.

right femoral artery) are recommended. Femoral arterial pressure monitoring is preferred because it reflects central blood pressure more accurately in the presence of low systemic vascular resistance, particularly after reperfusion.[168] Radial arterial pressure monitoring is useful when the aorta is partially or completely clamped during aorta-to-hepatic artery anastomosis. A pulmonary artery catheter is inserted through the right internal jugular vein to monitor intracardiac pressures, cardiac output, and core temperature. Carotid artery puncture should be assiduously avoided because of the presence of coagulopathy. An oximetric-type pulmonary artery catheter provides additional information on mixed venous hemoglobin oxygen saturation ($S\bar{v}o_2$). The right ventricular ejection fraction-type pulmonary catheter monitors right ventricular ejection fraction and right ventricular end-diastolic volume. Central venous pressure and pulmonary capillary wedge

TABLE 13-4
Equipment and Medications

Equipment

Anesthesia machine
Volume ventilator (for ARDS and pulmonary edema)
Mass spectrometer or capnograph
Multiple-channel vital sign monitor
Pulse oximeter
Cardiac output computer (oximetry or right ventricular ejection fraction)
Warming blanket
Thrombelastograph
Rapid infusion device
Autotransfusion system
Drug infusion pumps
Defibrillator

Medications

Induction agents
  Thiopental (500 mg)
  Etomidate (30 mg)
Intravenous agents
  Midazolam (4 mg)
  Lorazepam (4 mg)
  Fentanyl (2000 μg of 50 μg/mL, 40 mL)
Inhalation agents
  Isoflurane
Muscle relaxants
  Succinylcholine (100 mg)
  Rocuronium (50 mg)
  Pancuronium (10 mg)
Other drugs
  Atropine: 0.4 mg
  Calcium chloride: 1000 mg (100 mg/mL) × 200
  $NaHCO_3$: 40 mEq × 10
  Tromethamine (THAM): 500 mL × 3
  Ephedrine: 50 mg (5 mg/mL) × 1
  Epinephrine: 40 μg (4 μg/mL) × 1
  Epinephrine: 400 μg (40 μg/mL) × 1
  ε-Aminocaproic acid (EACA): 1000 mg (250 mg/mL) × 1
  Protamine: 50 mg (10 mg/mL) × 1
  Insulin: available in the refrigerator
  Potent vasoactive infusions: as needed

ARDS, acute respiratory distress syndrome.

pressure are not as sensitive as right ventricular end-diastolic volume in estimating preload, particularly during the anhepatic stage.[169] Two large-bore intravenous catheters (8.5 or 9F) are secured, typically in the right antecubital and left internal jugular veins. When the antecubital vein is unavailable, two catheters may be placed in the same internal jugular vein. Catheter patency is confirmed by noting an infusion pressure of less than 300 mmHg during fluid infusion at 400 mL/min through the catheter. Sterile technique should be followed during catheterization, and antiseptic ointment (neomycin or bacitracin) is applied at the skin puncture site. Transesophageal echocardiography (TEE) may also be used to monitor myocardial contractility and ventricular end-diastolic volume, wall motion abnormality, air or thromboembolism, intrapulmonary shunting, and patency of the reconstructed major veins.[170,171] A naso- or orogastric tube is placed with copious lubrication to avoid nasal or esophageal variceal bleeding.

Multiple sets of measurements of arterial blood gas tensions and pH, electrolytes, ionized calcium, glucose, lactate, and pos-

sibly ionized magnesium are performed during surgery. Typical test times areas follows: before and after induction of anesthesia, every hour during the dissection stage; 5 minutes after the onset of the anhepatic stage; every 30 minutes during the anhepatic stage; 15 minutes before reperfusion; 5 minutes and 30 minutes after reperfusion; and every hour thereafter. Coagulation monitoring is performed by either conventional coagulation profile (PT, activated partial thromboplastin time [aPTT], fibrinogen level, and platelet count) or thromboelastography (TEG) at the following times: before induction of anesthesia; every hour during the dissection stage; 15 minutes and 60 minutes after the onset of the anhepatic stage; 15 minutes before reperfusion; 5, 30, and 90 minutes after reperfusion; and every hour thereafter. The authors prefer TEG and platelet count to conventional coagulation monitoring because they reliably and rapidly reflect blood coagulability.[172] Before reperfusion, the TEG of untreated blood is compared with that of blood treated with ε-aminocaproic acid (EACA) to identify the presence of fibrinolysis. After reperfusion, TEGs of untreated blood, EACA-treated blood, and protamine sulfate–treated blood are compared to identify the presence of fibrinolysis and heparin effect, respectively.

Anesthesia Management

A rapid-sequence induction is preferred because of uncertain gastric emptying. Anesthesia can be induced with sodium thiopental (4 mg/kg), etomidate (300 to 500 μg/kg), propofol (2 mg/kg), or ketamine (2 mg/kg). Fentanyl (2 to 5 μg/kg) is frequently added. Succinylcholine (1 to 2 mg/kg) is commonly used to facilitate intratracheal intubation, and rocuronium (0.7 mg/kg) may be used when the patient is hyperkalemic. Dental injury may occur during intratracheal intubation because periodontal disease is not uncommon.

Anesthesia is maintained using volatile inhalation agents and narcotics. Isoflurane is the preferred inhalation agent because of less myocardial depression and biotransformation. Nitrous oxide is usually avoided because it distends the bowel and increases the size of any entrained air. Lorazepam (1 to 4 mg) may be added for amnesia. For neuromuscular blockade, pancuronium bromide, vecuronium bromide, rocuronium, or atracurium is commonly used.

Antibiotics and immunosuppressants administered during surgery may vary from center to center. One example is as follows. Ceftriaxone (Rocephin, 1 g, IV) is given on induction of anesthesia and every 6 hours thereafter. For patients allergic to cephalosporin and penicillin, clindamycin (600 mg, IV) and aztreonam (1 g, IV) are administered on induction of anesthesia and every 6 hours thereafter. Methylprednisolone (Solu-Medrol) is given on induction of anesthesia (100 mg, IV) and before reperfusion (200 mg, IV). Tacrolimus administration begins in the immediate postoperative period.

Physiologic Homeostasis During Liver Transplantation

Liver transplantation imposes a great deal of physiologic stress upon patients, and maintenance of physiologic homeostasis is essential to a successful outcome.

Cardiovascular Homeostasis

The goal of hemodynamic management is to maintain the hyperdynamic state, characteristic of ESLD.

THE DISSECTION STAGE. Hemodynamic instability represented by hypotension is typically caused by hypovolemia associated with drainage of ascites, rapid third-space fluid loss, surgical bleeding, and inadvertent compression of the major vessels (IVC, portal vein, hepatic veins, and aorta) (Figure 13-8). Intravascular volume is usually replenished by administration of a combination of PRBCs and FFP (typically PRBC, FFP, and Plasma-Lyte A, 200:300:250 mL) using a rapid infusion device. Calcium-containing fluids are not used in the rapid infusion device to prevent clot formation in the reservoir. This mixture has a hematocrit of 26 to 28 vol% and coagulation factor levels of 30% to 50% of normal. A low hematocrit is chosen to minimize the RBC wastage and to optimize the microcirculation. Continuous infusion of FFP is necessary to compensate for the loss of coagulation elements (procoagulants, prolysins, and their inhibitors) by surgical bleeding, and excessive activation of coagulation. In patients with blood loss of less than one blood volume, additional colloids (albumin or FFP) and crystalloids may be required to compensate for the third-space fluid loss. Close communication with the surgical team and the blood bank is essential to identify the cause of hemodynamic instability and to ensure an adequate supply of blood products. Intraoperative autotransfusion is shown to be effective and safe during liver transplantation. Its use may be considered when the RBC requirement is more than 10 units.

Increased central venous pressures may be seen in patients with volume overload, ascites, and pleural or pericardial effusions. Drainage of ascites and effusions may decrease intrathoracic and central venous pressures and improve cardiac performance. Thoracentesis and pericardiocentesis may be performed after the abdomen is opened to minimize the risk of injury to the thoracoabdominal organs.

Unexpected pulmonary hypertension may be observed in some patients. Because of the high mortality rate in patients with pulmonary hypertension, right ventricular function should be assessed by intraoperative TEE, and the pulmonary vascular response to various vasodilators (e.g., diltiazem, nitroglycerin, epoprostenol) may be evaluated. Liver transplantation may continue when pulmonary hypertension is mild to moderate and right ventricular function is within the normal range. In such cases, right ventricular function is supported by maintaining optimal preload and coronary perfusion pressure and avoiding myocardial depressants. The need for inotropes should also be anticipated upon reperfusion of patients with pulmonary hypertension. Dopamine or epinephrine is preferred when low cardiac output is accompanied by hypotension, and dobutamine may be used when patients are normotensive.

Complications of massive blood transfusion (hypothermia, ionic hypocalcemia, ionic hypomagnesemia, hyperkalemia, and acidosis) may develop at this stage and should be aggressively treated.

THE ANHEPATIC STAGE. Hemodynamic changes that occur during the anhepatic stage are caused primarily by interruption of venous return from the IVC and portal vein. Cross-clamping of the IVC and portal vein reduces venous return by up to 40%, resulting in low cardiac output, hypotension, and compensatory tachycardia (Figure 13-9).[173] Calculated systemic vascular resistance is frequently increased, although its interpretation should include the recognition that a large portion of the venous system is also excluded from the circulation. It is noteworthy that cross-clamping of the IVC and the portal vein decreases the central blood volume while it progressively increases total intravascular blood volume as blood is sequestered in the vascular bed of the kidneys, gastrointestinal and pelvic organs, and lower extremities. The prolonged low-output state, portal hypertension, and renal venous congestion may lead to acidosis, intestinal swelling, and hematuria. The low-output state

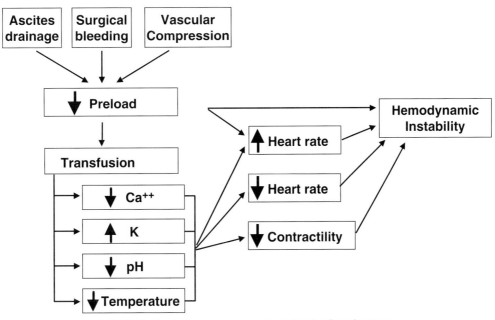

FIGURE 13-8 Hemodynamic changes during the dissection stage.

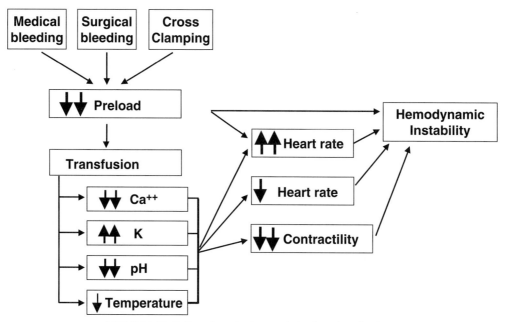

FIGURE 13-9 Hemodynamic changes during the anhepatic stage.

can be alleviated by administration of fluid or a vasopressor (dopamine or dobutamine, 2 to 5 μg/kg/min).

Venovenous bypass is a more physiologic technique than the simple cross-clamping technique as it returns venous blood from the portal and IVC system.[148] It is generally agreed that hemodynamic change is minimal when the bypass flow rate is greater than 25% of baseline cardiac output. Both the anesthesia and surgical teams, however, should be prepared for potential acute complications of venovenous bypass. Bleeding or air embolism may result from venous laceration during cannulation or improperly secured cannulas. Entry of a small volume of air (up to 50 mL) into the bypass pump does not cause immediate systemic air embolism because it is trapped in the cone-shaped pump head by centrifugal force. Thromboembolism may be caused by the migration of preexisting thrombi or those developed during bypass with a reduced bypass flow rate (<1000 mL/min), particularly in hypercoagulable conditions (eg, Budd-Chiari syndrome, neoplasms, and congenital protein C deficiency). The bypass flow rate is affected by several factors. Improper positioning of an intravascular cannula tip may not adequately drain blood, and the surgical team should correct the problem. A low pump speed reduces venous return, and a high pump speed collapses the venous wall and decreases the bypass flow. The perfusionist, therefore, should adjust the pump speed to maximize the bypass flow. In addition, hypovolemia decreases the bypass flow, which should be corrected by the anesthesia team. Most important, bypass may have to be terminated unexpectedly when serious complications occur. The anesthesiologist, therefore, should be prepared for unexpected cross-clamping of the IVC and portal vein at all times. After completion of the IVC anastomosis, the portal cannula is removed to facilitate the portal venous anastomosis, resulting in partial bypass. Low bypass flow and low cardiac output during this period can be improved by the administration of fluids or vasopressors, but full correction of central hypovolemia is avoided to prevent fluid overload on reperfusion.

In the original description of the piggyback technique, adequate venous return is maintained through the intact IVC and portal vein using portoaxillary venovenous bypass.[7] However, inadvertent compression of the IVC is inevitable and may decrease venous return and cardiac output. Furthermore, significant hemodynamic change may occur depending on technical modifications. When an end-to-side anastomosis is made between the suprahepatic IVC of the donor liver to the IVC of the recipient, side clamping of the IVC significantly reduces venous return. Reduced venous return also occurs during portal anastomosis; portal venous return is maintained in the portoaxillary bypass or temporary portosystemic shunt technique, but it is impaired in the portal cross-clamping technique. Hence, close communication with the surgical team is mandatory to prepare for technique-specific hemodynamic changes, and the surgical and anesthetic plan should be flexible enough not to derange circulatory homeostasis.

Typically, about 1000 mL of crystalloids or albumin is flushed through the portal vein and drained through the incompletely anastomosed IVC to remove preservative solution, metabolites, and air from the allograft. In addition, approximately 500 mL of blood may be allowed to escape through the incompletely anastomosed portal vein by partial unclamping of the IVC (back-bleeding technique). In this case, blood should be administered simultaneously to avoid hypovolemia.

Other factors that affect circulation during the anhepatic stage are similar to those of the dissection stage, although lactic acidosis, citrate intoxication, hypomagnesemia, hyperkalemia, and coagulopathy are more pronounced. At the end of the anhepatic stage, all biochemical variables are normalized to prepare for reperfusion.

THE NEOHEPATIC STAGE. Significant hemodynamic changes occur on reperfusion of the grafted liver (Figure 13-10). Unclamping of the infrahepatic IVC and portal vein results in transient hypovolemia and hypotension owing to acute sequestration of the blood in the engrafted liver. Unclamping of the

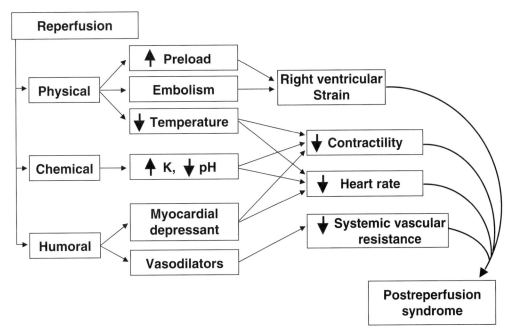

FIGURE 13-10 Hemodynamic changes on reperfusion of the graft liver.

suprahepatic IVC increases preload by mobilization of blood sequestered in the lower extremities and splanchnic circulation. This is followed by severe hemodynamic changes, the so-called postreperfusion syndrome.[174] The postreperfusion syndrome, which occurs in approximately 30% of patients, is characterized by abrupt hypotension (below 70% of the baseline value) that develops within 5 minutes of reperfusion and lasts for more than 1 minute. Other associated hemodynamic changes are bradycardia, high central venous pressure and pulmonary capillary wedge pressure, low systemic vascular resistance, conduction defects, and possible myocardial depression. The postreperfusion syndrome appears to be caused by a combination of several factors. An acute increase in preload from mobilization of blood formerly sequestered in the viscera and lower extremities may result in right ventricular strain. An acute decrease in blood temperature (1 to 2°C) by systemic entry of the cold preservation solution may decrease cardiac conduction and contractility. Other physical factors are air embolism and thromboembolism that may cause right ventricular outflow tract obstruction and right ventricular strain.[170,175] Chemical factors are acute hyperkalemia and acidosis. Systemic entry of hyperkalemic preservation solution increases serum potassium level (up to 12 mmol/L), causing severe conduction defects and bradycardia.[176] Return of the acidic blood from the viscera and lower extremities increases base deficit by 5 to 10 mmol/L. In addition, endogenous vasodilators or myocardial depressants (e.g., vasoactive intestinal polypeptide, nitric oxide, and eicosanoid) released from the allograft or congested viscera may decrease systemic vascular resistance and impair myocardial function.

Several measures may be taken to prevent the postreperfusion syndrome, although they are not always successful. At the end of the anhepatic stage, blood volume is adjusted to avoid reperfusion hypervolemia, and ionic hypocalcemia, hyperkalemia, and metabolic acidosis are corrected. Administration of $CaCl_2$ (20 mg/kg), $NaHCO_3$ (1 mmol/kg), regular insulin (10 units), 50% dextrose (1 mL/kg), and epinephrine (5 to 10 μg) is recommended by some centers.[170] When the postreperfusion syndrome develops, hypotension and bradycardia are treated with small doses of epinephrine (10-μg increments) to support contractility, heart rate, and vasomotor tone, followed by dopamine or epinephrine infusion, if necessary (Figure 13-11). Symptomatic hyperkalemia (tall, peaked T wave and widening QRS complex with bradycardia) is treated by administration of $CaCl_2$ (15 mg/kg) and $NaHCO_3$ (0.5 to 1 mmol/kg). Arrhythmias are treated in a standard fashion. When pulmonary edema develops, positive end-expiratory pressure (PEEP) is applied and inotropes may be given. Patients who develop intracardiac or pulmonary embolism are supported by inotropes. When severe fluid overloading is a concern, phlebotomy may be considered.

The postreperfusion syndrome dissipates gradually over the next 5 to 15 minutes, although low systemic vascular resistance and hypotension with a high cardiac output may persist for several hours. When hypotension is suspected to cause tissue and myocardial ischemia, it may be treated with ephedrine, dopamine, or epinephrine. Overzealous administration of fluids may result in hepatic congestion, and norepinephrine may interfere with hepatic blood flow by hepatic arterial vasoconstriction. Octreotide, by its effects on vasoactive intestinal polypeptides, increases splanchnic vasomotor tone and systemic blood pressure, although its effects on the hepatic circulation are unclear.[177] Hemodynamic changes that occur during hepatic arterial and biliary reconstruction are relatively minor, except for intermittent fluctuation of the preload associated with continuous third-space fluid loss and compression of the liver and great vessels.

Pulmonary Homeostasis

Gas exchange is satisfactorily maintained in most patients. Minute volume is gradually decreased during the anhepatic stage to match the reduced oxygen consumption and carbon

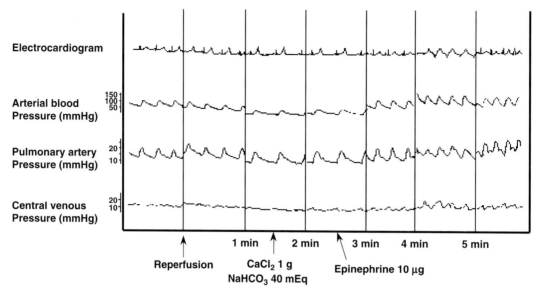

Electrocardiogram

Arterial blood
Pressure (mmHg)
150
100
50

Pulmonary artery
Pressure (mmHg)
20
10

Central venous
Pressure (mmHg)
20
10

1 min   2 min   3 min   4 min   5 min

Reperfusion   CaCl₂ 1 g   Epinephrine 10 µg
NaHCO₃ 40 mEq

FIGURE 13-11 The postreperfusion syndrome and its treatment. (From Kang YG, Gelman S: Liver transplantation. In Gelman S [ed]: *Anesthesia and organ transplantation*, Philadelphia, 1987, WB Saunders, 167.)

dioxide production and is increased during the neohepatic stage. Alveolar recruitment maneuvers are performed intermittently to avoid atelectasis caused by pleural effusions, cephalad traction of the rib cage, and compression of the diaphragm. Intermittent endotracheal suctioning, using a catheter or bronchoscope, may be required to remove secretions. Drainage of pleural effusions and ascites decreases intrathoracic pressure and improves oxygenation within 2 hours. Thoracentesis is performed after the abdominal cavity is entered to avoid potential injury to the thoracoabdominal organs.

Patients with preoperative ARDS may require an increased F_IO_2 and increased levels of PEEP to ensure adequate gas exchange. A volume ventilator may be necessary to overcome high airway pressure. Frank pulmonary edema may develop, particularly after reperfusion, from fluid overload or increased pulmonary capillary permeability. In such cases, patients are ventilated with a high level of F_IO_2 and PEEP while the underlying cause is treated. Closure of the abdominal cavity may interfere with ventilation by increasing intrathoracic and airway pressures. Primary closure with mesh or secondary closure may be necessary.

Coagulation

Intraoperative changes in coagulation are summarized in Table 13-5. Surgical bleeding is common owing to numerous collateral vessels associated with portal hypertension, difficulty in dissection of the diseased liver, preexisting coagulopathy, and pathologic changes in coagulation. The average blood loss in adults is 10 to 15 units each of PRBCs and FFP, although blood loss may reach more than 100 units each.

During the dissection stage, dilutional coagulopathy develops as bleeding reduces coagulation factors and platelets (Figure 13-12). Fibrinolysis may develop in patients with hepatocellular disease owing to a low level of inhibitors of fibrinolysis and impaired hepatic clearance of tPA.[178] Excessive activation of coagulation, evidenced by a gradual increase in thrombin-antithrombin complex, develops at the end of the dis-

TABLE 13-5

Intraoperative Changes in Coagulation

	Dissection Stage	Anhepatic Stage	Neohepatic Stage	
			Early	Late
Preexisting coagulopathy	++	+ +	++	+
Dilution	+++	+++	++	+
Hypocalcemia	+	+++	++	+
Hypothermia	+	++	+++	+
Fibrinolysis	+	++	++++	–
Excessive coagulation	+	++	++++	–
Heparin effect	–	+*	++	–

*In patients with venovenous bypass with heparin in the priming solution.

section stage.[179] Management of coagulation begins with normalization of physiologic variables because ionic hypocalcemia, hypothermia, and acidosis impair coagulation.[180] It is followed by continuous infusion of coagulation factor–rich blood (RBC, FFP, Plasma-Lyte A or normal saline, 1 unit, 1 unit, and 250 mL, respectively) to maintain coagulation factor levels above the critical level (30% to 50% of normal). Infusion of the coagulation factor–rich blood appears to be necessary in most patients because coagulation factors are continuously lost by surgical bleeding and, more importantly, by excessive activation of coagulation.

Specific blood components may be administered on the basis of the coagulation profile or TEG. The authors prefer to use TEG and platelet count to overcome shortcomings of the coagulation profile.[172] The conventional coagulation profile (PT, aPTT, fibrinogen) has several drawbacks to use during liver transplantation. PT is a sensitive hepatic function test and is prolonged in most patients undergoing liver transplantation. Administration of FFP to correct PT may not be possible or desirable in the course of surgery. The aPTT follows a time course similar to that of PT, and its correction may not be practical. It is a sensitive test for heparin effect, and its prolongation indicates the presence of heparin released from the grafted

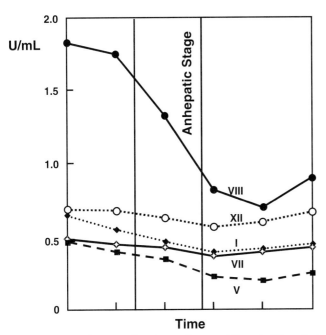

FIGURE 13-12 Intraoperative change in coagulation of 100 patients. (Modified from Lewis JH, Bontempo FA, Awad SA, et al: *Hepatology* 9:710, 1989.)

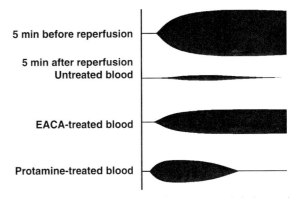

FIGURE 13-13 Effects of pharmacologic agents on pathologic coagulation. EACA, E-aminocaproic acid. (From Kang YG: Monitoring and treatment of coagulation. In Winter PM, Kang YG [eds]: *Hepatic transplantation: anesthetic and perioperative management*, New York, 1986, Praeger, 168.)

liver. Fibrinogen level is frequently maintained within the acceptable range, although severe hypofibrinogenemia may indicate either active fibrinolysis or excessive activation of coagulation. The level of fibrin(ogen) degradation products is usually elevated in most patients because of excessive activation of coagulation and reabsorption of defibrinated blood from the abdominal cavity and does not have any immediate clinical significance. Further, coagulation profile results may not be available in a timely manner.

TEG has several advantages over the conventional coagulation profile.[181] It rapidly and reliably measures blood coagulability, and an accurate differential diagnosis for replacement therapy and pharmacologic therapy can be made by comparing the TEG of untreated blood with that of blood treated with various blood components or pharmacologic agents (e.g., protamine sulfate, heparinase, EACA) (Figure 13-13).[182] In general, 8 to 10 units of platelets are administered for a small maximum amplitude (MA < 40 mm). Platelet administration, in addition to increasing MA, improves reaction time (r) and clot formation rate (α) because the coagulation cascade leading to fibrin formation occurs on the surface of platelets. Its administration, however, is withheld during the anhepatic stage to avoid potential thrombosis and during massive blood transfusion (>150 mL/min) to minimize wastage. Two units of FFP may be administered when the reaction time is prolonged even after platelet administration (r > 12 minutes). Cryoprecipitate (6 units) containing factors I and VIII may be infused to treat residual effects of fibrinolysis because plasmin selectively destroys factors I, V, and VIII. In addition, it may be used for patients with severe hypofibrinogenemia (< 100 mg/dL).

Pathologic coagulation superimposes on dilutional coagulopathy during the anhepatic stage. The heparin effect is seen as prolonged aPTT and reaction time on TEG at the onset of the venovenous bypass, as a small dose of heparin (2000 to 5000

units) in the bypass cannula enters the systemic circulation. This heparin effect dissipates over the next 30 to 60 minutes. The effects of the absence of the hepatic synthetic and clearance functions begin to develop during this stage. The absence of hepatic clearance of tPA promotes fibrinolysis in approximately 30% of patients.[182] A similar effect on activated coagulation factors results in excessive activation of coagulation evidenced by progressive increases in thrombin-antithrombin complex and fibrin(ogen) degradation products.[179] Severe fibrinolysis (fibrinolysis time < 60 minutes) may be treated by the administration of a single, small dose of EACA (250 to 500 mg).[182] Administration of a large or repeated dose of EACA is not recommended to avoid potential thromboembolism.[183]

The postreperfusion syndrome affects coagulation at the onset of the neohepatic stage. A typical coagulation profile shows prolonged PT, aPTT, reptilase time, and thrombin time. Generalized decreases in coagulation factors (I, V, VII, and VIII) and platelets are accompanied by a sharp increase in tPA level, a shortened euglobulin lysis time, and moderate increases in fibrin(ogen) degradation products and thrombin-antithrombin complex. Fibrinolysis is observed in up to 80% of patients and is severe in about 40%.[182] Fibrinolysis is caused by a 20-fold increase in tPA released from the allograft and congested viscera, which overwhelms the activity of the plasminogen activator inhibitor.[184,185] There are ample supports for the theory that fibrinolysis is primary in origin: a relatively steady level of antithrombin; only moderate levels of fibrin(ogen) degradation products and D-dimers; selective decreases in factors I, V, and VIII; and no known microthrombi formation.[178,186,187] Fibrinolysis resolves over the next 120 minutes after reperfusion.

Early treatment of fibrinolysis using a single, small dose of EACA (250 to 500 mg) is recommended to reduce delayed oozing and to minimize the loss of factors I, V, and VIII.[188] When oozing persists, additional FFP or cryoprecipitate may be administered to replenish factors I, V, and VIII. The heparin effect occurs in about 30% of patients, as heparin is released from the allograft. It dissipates over the next 60 to 90 minutes, but a small dose of protamine sulfate (25 to 50 mg) may be given in severe cases. In addition, blood coagulability is impaired by reperfusion hypothermia, acidosis, and ionic hypocalcemia. In contrast, excessive activation of coagulation leading to fatal intracardiac or pulmonary embolism may occur in some patients.[183] This complication appears to be associated with massive transfusion, release of a large quantity of tissue thromboplastin from the less-than-optimal allograft, impaired tissue perfusion, and, possibly, antifibrinolytic therapy. Coagulopathy improves gradually after reperfusion. Generalized oozing, however, may occur even in the presence of acceptable coagulation profiles and TEG, possibly by delayed bleeding caused by the loss of poorly formed clot or by the residual effects of reperfusion fibrinolysis.

Several other pharmacologic agents are reported to improve coagulation. Aprotinin (2,000,000 KIU followed by 500,000 KIU/hr), a nonspecific inhibitor of plasminogen and serine protease, reduces blood loss by inhibition of fibrinolysis as well as inhibition of excessive activation of coagulation.[189-191] Its clinical use, however, has declined; clinical reports do not show significant reduction of blood loss, and fibrinolysis can be more efficiently treated with EACA or tranexamic acid.[182,192-194] Desmopressin acetate, a synthetic analog of 8-arginine vasopressin, increases the endothelial release of factor VIII, von Willebrand factor, and plasminogen. Its beneficial effect has been demonstrated in vitro and in patients with liver disease. Doses of 0.3 µg/kg may be used to improve coagulation.[195] Conjugated estrogen was reported to improve coagulation and reduce blood loss, although its clinical use has not been widely accepted.[196]

Electrolyte and Acid-Base Homeostasis

CALCIUM METABOLISM. Ionic hypocalcemia, caused by chelation of serum calcium with citrate in the banked blood, invariably occurs in patients with hepatic dysfunction and begins to appear during the dissection stage.[197] Severe ionic hypocalcemia occurs during the anhepatic stage. The serum ionized calcium level is inversely related to serum citrate level, as the absence of hepatic metabolism of citrate increases the serum citrate level close to that in the banked blood. Significant hypocalcemia (Ca^{2+} < 0.55 mmol/L) is associated with a prolonged QT interval and decreases in cardiac index, stroke work index, and blood pressure. Therefore, ionized calcium concentration is monitored hourly or more frequently, and $CaCl_2$ (15 mg/kg) or calcium gluconate (30 mg/kg) is administered to maintain its normal level.[198] Ionic hypocalcemia gradually improves as the engrafted liver begins to metabolize citrate, unless the speed of transfusion exceeds the metabolic function of the liver.

POTASSIUM METABOLISM. Hypokalemia is not uncommon in patients with liver disease because of poor dietary intake of potassium and its loss through chronic diuretic therapy and diarrhea. Severe hypokalemia (< 2.5 mmol/L) is treated with potassium chloride to increase its level to greater than 3.0 mmol/L. Moderate hypokalemia (< 3.5 mmol/L) is untreated because it is well tolerated by patients and self-corrected by blood transfusion. In addition, progressive hyperkalemia inevitably occurs during massive transfusion and on reperfusion of the grafted liver.

Hyperkalemia is a serious concern because it decreases myocardial conduction and contractility, particularly in the presence of acidosis and hypocalcemia. Progressive hyperkalemia (up to 6 to 7 mmol/L) may occur in patients with renal dysfunction or requiring massive blood transfusion. Mild hyperkalemia (> 4.5 mmol/L) is treated with insulin (10 units)

and glucose (12.5 g).[199] For moderate-to-severe hyperkalemia (> 5.5 mmol/L), in addition to insulin therapy, transfusion of washed PRBCs using an autotransfusion system should be considered.[200]

Reperfusion hyperkalemia is caused by potassium influx from the preservative solution and hepatocytes, and its systemic effects and treatment have been described. The acute hyperkalemia returns to normal range within 5 to 10 minutes by redistribution. The potassium level gradually returns to the baseline value, as the RBCs and the engrafted liver take up excess potassium. Hypokalemia (< 3.5 mmol/L), which occurs toward the end of the procedure, is treated using KCl infusion (20-mmol increments).

SODIUM METABOLISM. Hyponatremia (< 130 mmol/L) is a common occurrence in patients with liver disease, particularly those with fluid retention, ascites, diuretic therapy, and a restricted sodium diet. Serum sodium level gradually increases toward normal during surgery with administration of FFP and balanced salt solution. The intraoperative concern is that patients with a rapid increase in serum sodium level (>10 mmol/L) have a higher chance of developing central pontine myelinolysis, neurologic damage caused by the destruction of the myelin sheath in the pons.[201] Therefore, the preoperative serum sodium level is increased to greater than 130 mmol/L, if possible, and a rapid increase in sodium is prevented by administration of low-sodium–containing crystalloids during surgery. In addition, tromethamine (THAM) is the preferred drug for treatment of metabolic acidosis because it does not contain sodium. Hypernatremia may be seen in some patients who receive a large dose of $NaHCO_3$ preoperatively. It is gradually normalized by administration of blood products and balanced electrolyte solution.

IONIC HYPOMAGNESEMIA. A clinical investigation revealed that serum ionized magnesium level has an inverse relationship with serum citrate level, as magnesium ion chelates with serum citrate in banked blood (Figure 13-14).[202] Although the clinical significance of ionic hypomagnesemia during liver transplantation is unclear, $MgSO_4$ (1 to 4 g) may be administered to minimize potential cardiac irritability and myocardial depression.

METABOLIC ACIDOSIS. Metabolic acidosis begins to appear during the dissection and anhepatic stages because of impaired hepatic metabolism of acid load from the banked blood and the peripheral tissues. Base deficit and lactate level increase further (approximately 5 mmol/L) on reperfusion owing to acid load from the graft and congested viscera and lower extremities. It gradually improves as hepatic function is restored and tissue perfusion improves during the neohepatic stage. Persistent lactic acidosis (>15 mmol/L) appears to be associated with graft dysfunction.[203]

Metabolic acidosis is aggressively corrected by administration of $NaHCO_3$ to maintain base deficit levels less than 5 mmol/L because acidosis leads to myocardial depression, inadequate cellular respiration, and decreased sensitivity to catecholamines. As described earlier, THAM is preferred in hyponatremic or hypernatremic conditions to avoid central pontine myelinolysis: 150 mL of 0.3 molar THAM is equivalent to 50 mmol of $NaHCO_3$. Alternatively, dichloroacetate (40 mg/kg every 4 hours) appears to reduce lactate production by stimulating pyruvate oxidation.[204]

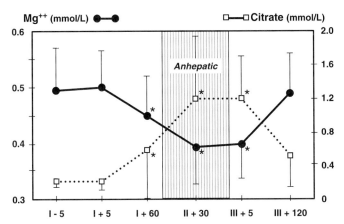

FIGURE 13-14 Intraoperative changes in serum ionized magnesium level during liver transplantation. (From Scott VL, De Wolf AM, Kang Y, et al: *Liver Transpl Surg* 2:343, 1996.)

METABOLIC ALKALOSIS. Metabolic alkalosis may develop during the neohepatic stage, and this was believed to be associated with the dose of $NaHCO_3$ administered and citrate metabolism generating bicarbonate. However, it has been shown that the degree of metabolic alkalosis is unrelated to citrate and $NaHCO_3$ load and may be associated with residual hyperaldosteronism.[205]

Metabolic Homeostasis

Body temperature may gradually decrease to 34°C during the dissection stage because of exposure of the abdominal contents to the cold environment, vasodilatation, and lack of shivering. Hypothermia continues during the anhepatic stage as energy production decreases further. An abrupt decrease in core temperature (1 to 2°C) occurs on reperfusion as cold preservative solution enters the systemic circulation. The temperature increases during the neohepatic stage, and the surgery ends with a body temperature of approximately 35 to 36°C. Hypothermia is difficult to avoid, although increasing room temperature, application of warming blankets, and use of a heat exchanger in the venovenous bypass system may be beneficial.

The blood glucose level is relatively well maintained (100 to 200 mg/dL) with blood transfusion, as the banked blood contains glucose (approximately 200 mg/dL). A gradual decrease in glycogenolysis reduces the blood glucose level during the dissection and anhepatic stages. In patients with fulminant hepatic failure or severe hepatocellular disease, the blood glucose level may decrease precipitously, and glucose supplementation is necessary. Hyperglycemia (up to 300 mg/dL) occurs on reperfusion as glucose is released from the engrafted liver.[206] Insulin does not appear to be effective in treating the reperfusion hyperglycemia because glucose reuptake requires restoration of hepatic function. The insulin concentration is relatively steady during surgery, and the glucagon concentration increases after reperfusion. Blood glucose level usually returns to normal within 12 to 24 hours. Persistent hyperglycemia caused by impaired hepatic glucose reuptake and hormonal imbalance is an early sign of poor graft function.[207]

Renal Homeostasis

Urine output is well preserved in most patients when intravascular volume is optimized. Oliguria or anuria, however, may persist in patients with the hepatorenal syndrome or with underlying renal disease. The presence of oliguria and hematuria during the anhepatic stage of the simple cross-clamping technique was described earlier. Urine output increases during the neohepatic stage from restoration of renal function and excretion of excess fluids. Various agents have been tried to protect or improve renal function. The role of dopamine is controversial, dopexamine appears to be beneficial, and triple drug therapy (dopamine [2 to 3 µg/kg/min], mannitol [250 mg/kg], and furosemide) improves urine output but not renal function.[208-211] When fluid overload or severe electrolyte imbalance is a concern, intraoperative venovenous ultrafiltration or hemodialysis may be utilized.

Conclusion of Surgery

The restoration of hepatic function is evident in about 2 hours after reperfusion: levels of citrate and lactate decrease, glucose level returns toward normal, coagulopathy improves, and bile production begins. Persistent citrate intoxication, acidosis, hyperglycemia, coagulopathy, and pale-colored bile are poor prognostic signs.

Recently, tracheal extubation in the operating room has been successful in several centers when the patient meets strict guidelines.[212] However, most patients are still transported to the ICU with invasive monitoring and ventilatory support. Upon arrival to the ICU, the ventilator setting is reported to the respiratory therapist, the lungs are auscultated, and vital signs are displayed on the ICU monitor. Detailed intraoperative information is reported to the ICU physician and nursing staff.

Postoperative Complications

Postoperative complications are outlined in Table 13-6.

Hepatic Complications
PRIMARY NONFUNCTION. Primary nonfunction is defined as graft failure occurring within 90 days after liver transplantation

TABLE 13-6
Postoperative Complications

Hepatic complications
  Allograft-related complications
  Primary nonfunction
  Acute rejection
Vascular complications
  Hepatic arterial stenosis
  Hepatic arterial thrombosis
  Vena caval stenosis or thrombosis
  Portal stenosis or thrombosis
Biliary complications
Abdominal complications
Extrahepatic complications
  Pulmonary complications
  Neurologic complications
  Renal complications
  Infectious complications

in the absence of either rejection or technical factors, such as hepatic arterial thrombosis.[213] This complication occurs in up to 10% of patients and is frequently caused by hepatic dysfunction of the donor liver and prolonged cold ischemia (>18 hours). The patient develops progressive multiorgan failure including encephalopathy, coagulopathy, minimal bile production, and oliguria. Supportive therapy may be helpful until the liver resumes its function, although urgent retransplantation may be the only solution in many patients.

ACUTE REJECTION. Worsening liver function in the second week after liver transplantation without technical complications suggests acute cellular rejection. Biopsy findings are inflammation of the intrahepatic endothelium and bile duct and a mononuclear cell infiltration with eosinophilia.[214] It is commonly treated by steroid (bolus followed by a gradual tapering) and increased immunosuppression. Steroid-resistant rejection is treated with monoclonal antibody, OKT3.

VASCULAR COMPLICATIONS

Hepatic arterial stenosis. Hepatic arterial stenosis occurs in approximately 5% of cases. It is suspected when an ultrasound examination shows increased focal arterial flow velocities and it is confirmed by angiography. In the immediate postoperative period, direct repair or reconstruction using an infrarenal arterial conduit is usually successful. Stenosis occurring several weeks after transplantation is treated with percutaneous hepatic arterial angioplasty, which has a success rate of greater than 90% in achieving long-term patency.[215]

Hepatic arterial thrombosis. Hepatic arterial thrombosis occurs in 2% to 12% of recipients, and its occurrence is four times more common in children. The grafted liver lacks collaterals and is often unable to survive dearterialization. The common presentations are biliary tract breakdown, recurrent bacteremia, hepatic abscess, and, occasionally, massive hepatic necrosis.[216] This complication may be caused by several contributing factors, such as anastomotic stenosis, intimal dissection, atherosclerotic celiac axis, hypotension, overtransfusion of PRBCs (hematocrit > 44 vol%) and coagulation factors, and deficiency of coagulation inhibitors (protein C, protein S, and antithrombin III).[217,218] It is diagnosed by angiography and treated by urgent thrombectomy and interposition of an arterial graft. Supportive management includes drainage of abscess and bilomas and control of intra-abdominal sepsis using antibiotics. Urgent retransplantation is necessary when the preceding measures do not restore hepatic circulation.

Vena caval stenosis and thrombosis. Vena caval stenosis and thrombosis occur in 1% to 2% of patients. In traditional liver transplantation, outflow obstruction is managed by balloon angioplasty with or without metallic wall stent placement.[219] In the piggyback technique, it is treated with an end-to-side anastomosis between the donor infrahepatic IVC and the recipient retrohepatic IVC.[220]

Portal venous stenosis and thrombosis. Portal venous stenosis and thrombosis are relatively uncommon in the adult population and arise with graft dysfunction, massive ascites formation, and hemodynamic instability. These complications are corrected by an urgent reconstruction of the portal vein or construction of a superior mesenteric venous graft to the liver together with a ligation of large collaterals that may reduce the portal flow.

BILIARY COMPLICATIONS. Biliary complications, more common in children, have an overall incidence of 8% to 15%, and the difficulty in their early recognition leads to high morbidity and mortality.[221] Most complications occur within the first 3 months, although bile leak may occur in the first 4 weeks. Diagnosis is made by liver function tests (serum bilirubin, γ-glutamyltransferase, and alkaline phosphatase) and imaging techniques. Bile leaks usually occur at the anastomotic site, although they may be from the T-tube site or aberrant ducts. Leaks are treated by percutaneous or endoscopic drainage of bile collections. In the case of Roux-en-Y choledochojejunostomy, surgical reconstruction is required. It is critical to evaluate patency of the hepatic artery to rule out bile duct ischemia. Biliary obstruction also occurs at the anastomotic site, and balloon dilatation with a stent is often successful. A conversion of a choledochocholedochostomy to a Roux-en-Y anastomosis may be required in some patients.

ABDOMINAL COMPLICATIONS

Intra-abdominal bleeding. Intra-abdominal bleeding occurs in about 7% to 15% of patients and requires exploration in about half the cases.[222] Gastrointestinal bleeding may develop from ulcers, viral enteritis, varices, and the afferent Roux-en-Y loop. Variceal bleeding is usually associated with portal vein thrombosis and requires urgent ultrasound or angiographic evaluation. Bleeding from the Roux-en-Y limb occurs 1 week after surgery and is usually self-limited. Bleeding can also be caused by persistent thrombocytopenia associated with splenic sequestration, drug toxicity, heparin-induced thrombocytopenia, and immunologic reaction.[223]

Intestinal perforation. Intestinal perforation is caused by serosal injury to the intestines, usually in patients with technically difficult hepatectomy, prolonged portal venous clamping, and massive blood transfusion.[224] Intestinal perforation is frequently complicated by fungal infection. Intestinal perforation or leakage is treated by urgent surgery and antifungal therapy.

Extrahepatic Complications

PULMONARY COMPLICATIONS. Most patients require mechanical ventilation only a few days after transplantation. Prolonged ventilatory support, however, is required in some patients with atelectasis, pleural effusions, and central nervous system depression. Intraoperative cross-clamping of the IVC occasionally results in right phrenic nerve crush injury and diaphragmatic paralysis in the immediate postoperative period.[225] ARDS may develop in patients with intra-abdominal infection, pancreatitis, hepatic necrosis, acute cellular rejection, and, occasionally, with OKT3 treatment.[226] Bronchoalveolar lavage and bacterial culture are frequently performed to rule out pulmonary infection from any other pulmonary pathology. Preexisting pulmonary hypertension may persist postoperatively and is controlled by epoprostenol or nitroglycerin.

NEUROLOGIC COMPLICATIONS. Neurologic complications occur in 12% to 20% of patients, mostly in the first week after transplantation.[227] These are more common in adults and arise as mental status changes ranging from dysphasia to frank coma. Dysfunction of the central nervous system is commonly caused by medications, such as cyclosporine, tacrolimus, H_2 blockers, acyclovir, and antibiotics such as imipenem. Nonconvulsive seizures may occur, and an electroencephalogram is performed for patients with unexplained mentation changes. Intracranial hemorrhage and watershed infarcts are ruled out by computed tomography scans. Hyponatremia and hypomagnesemia can also delay awakening. Central pontine myelinolysis may develop several days after transplantation, and recovery is often slow and incomplete.[228] Hepatic encephalopathy may be present for several days after transplantation in patients with persistent portosystemic shunting. Meningitis should be ruled out when the mental status change is accompanied by fever. Disseminated aspergillosis is a devastating complication in a patient with multiple brain infarcts and fever. Peripheral neuropathy arising as weakness or "failure to awaken" is usually myopathic in nature and more common in patients with preoperative severe liver disease, poor graft function, and high steroid doses and uremia; it is confirmed by electromyography and muscle biopsy.

RENAL DYSFUNCTION. Renal dysfunction is usually transient and is commonly associated with intraoperative hypovolemia and hypotension, allograft dysfunction, and nephrotoxicity of cyclosporine and tacrolimus.[229] Oliguria is an early sign of renal dysfunction and is managed by restoring intravascular volume and renal perfusion pressure. Patients with the preoperative hepatorenal syndrome have a tendency to develop postoperative renal dysfunction.[230] Hepatorenal syndrome may persist after transplantation, and recovery depends on its preoperative severity and allograft function. In some patients, addition of vasoconstrictive immunosuppressants (cyclosporine and tacrolimus) may lead to acute tubular necrosis. In general, renal function returns to the normal range in most patients, and approximately 10% of patients require temporary dialysis.[229] Long-term prognosis is reasonably good, although hypertension, diabetes, and chronic nephropathy induced by steroids and the calcineurin inhibitors may result in chronic renal failure.

INFECTIOUS COMPLICATIONS. More than half of the postoperative infections are bacterial in origin.[231] These infections typically occur in the first 2 weeks, when blood level of immunosuppressants is high. The most common sites of infection are the liver, biliary tract, peritoneal cavity, and pulmonary system.[232] The common organisms in the abdomen are aerobic gram-positive organisms (streptococci and staphylococci) and gram-negative bacilli (*E. coli*, *Enterobacter* species, and *Pseudomonas*). In the lung, *Pseudomonas* infection is most common.

Approximately 20% of infections are caused by fungus, with *Candida* species accounting for more than 80% of all fungal infections. The risk factors are high steroid dosage, broadspectrum antibiotic usage, and prolonged surgical time. *Candida* infection is treated with amphotericin or fluconazole. *Aspergillus* accounts for 15% of all fungal infections and is associated with high mortality. A high-dose liposomal amphotericin followed by prolonged itraconazole is the treatment of choice.

Viral infections are seen 2 to 3 months after transplantation, with cytomegalovirus and herpes simplex accounting for the bulk of these infections. Epstein-Barr virus is not usually seen until about 6 months after transplantation but is an important cause of lymphoproliferative disease. *Pneumocystis* pneumonia, an opportunistic infection, responds to trimethoprimsulfamethoxazole.

LATE METABOLIC COMPLICATIONS. These include diabetes, hyperlipidemia, weight gain, and hypertension. Diabetes is induced by steroids, cyclosporine, and tacrolimus and may respond to oral hypoglycemic agents or insulin. Hyperlipidemia is associated with diabetes, obesity, steroids, and immunosuppressive drugs and is treated by diet and exercise. Hypertension is seen in as many as 85% of patients after transplantation. The use of steroids, cyclosporine, and, to a lesser extent, tacrolimus is the most likely cause. Cyclosporine is a potent stimulant of endothelin and decreases prostaglandin E_2 production as well as nitric oxide–mediated vasodilation. Hypomagnesemia has been implicated as the cause of the hypertension in some cases. The presence of chronic renal insufficiency and hyperkalemia in most transplant recipients limits the choice of antihypertensives to β-blockers and calcium channel blockers.

Immunosuppression

Although better understanding of rejection and introduction of newer drugs allow transplant recipients to survive with a relatively low incidence of rejection, immunosuppression is still the major obstacle of liver transplantation. The principal goal of immunosuppression is the use of a combination of drugs to achieve satisfactory rejection control while reducing their side effects.

Corticosteroids

Corticosteroids have been present in virtually all immunosuppressive regimens to date. They act through intracellular receptors in multiple ways and are effective in preventing and treating acute rejection. In acute rejection, corticosteroids are administered in a short course of 3 to 5 days. Their side effects are osteoporosis, diabetes, hypertension, dyslipidemias, and enhanced viral replication. Therefore, serious attempts are made to eliminate the long-term use of steroids, and this is often possible about a year after transplantation.[233]

Calcineurin Inhibitors (Cyclosporine and Tacrolimus)

All calcineurin inhibitors bind to a family of intracellular proteins known as immunophilins. The drug-immunophilin complex competitively binds to calcineurin to inhibit the phosphatase activity of calcineurin. This, in turn, prevents dephosphorylation and translocation of the nuclear factor of activated T cells (NF-AT). NF-AT binds to the promoter region of a variety of genes involved in T cell activation, which interferes with the activity of IL-2, IL-3, IL-4, IL-5, and interferon-γ. The side effects of cyclosporine and tacrolimus are similar and include renal dysfunction, tremor, hypertension, and headache. Cyclosporine is associated with hirsutism and gingival hyperplasia and tacrolimus with a higher incidence of diabetes and gastrointestinal symptoms. This group of drugs, along with steroids, forms the basis of the various immunosuppressive protocols and is used for induction and maintenance.

Mycophenolate Mofetil

This drug is a potent noncompetitive inhibitor of inosine monophosphate dehydrogenase, which interferes with guanine nucleotide synthesis and DNA replication. Because lymphocytes depend on this pathway for purine synthesis, this drug results in a selective inhibition of lymphocyte proliferation. Mycophenolate mofetil is useful in both acute and chronic rejection and is used as an adjunct to cyclosporine- and tacrolimus-based protocols to reduce rejection as well as to facilitate a reduction in their dosages.[234] Common side effects are bone marrow suppression, nausea, diarrhea, and abdominal pain and usually subside with a reduction in dosage.

Antilymphocyte Agents

POLYCLONAL ANTILYMPHOCYTE/ANTITHYMOCYTE GLOBULIN. A horse or rabbit that has been immunized with human lymphocytes or thymocytes produces antilymphocyte globulin (ALG) or antithymocyte globulin (ATG), respectively. The administration of ALG/ATG blocks various lymphocyte receptors to deplete peripheral blood lymphocytes rapidly. Their side effects are allergic reactions, fever, serum sickness, and lymphoproliferative disease. The indication for ALG/ATG is renal dysfunction early in the induction phase.

OKT3. This monoclonal antibody targets specific epitopes expressed on the cell surface. OKT3 is directed against the CD3 molecular complex expressed on mature T cells. Although OKT3 is not superior to steroids and calcineurin inhibitors, it is effective in steroid-resistant graft rejection. Common side effects are fever, diarrhea, nausea, myalgia, and an increased risk of lymphoproliferative disease.

ANTI–IL-2 RECEPTOR MONOCLONAL ANTIBODIES. Both rat and mouse antibodies to IL-2 receptors are effective in preventing acute rejection in liver transplantation. The major limitation is the rapid development of neutralizing antibodies against the xenogeneic immunoglobulin. New chimeric monoclonal antibodies in which the murine variable region is fused to human immunoglobulin constant region domains are less immunogenic and have longer half-lives in serum. These agents decrease the incidence of acute cellular rejection, and their combination with the delayed introduction of low-dose cyclosporine or tacrolimus reduces rejection as well as renal dysfunction.

Retransplantation of the Liver

Approximately 15% of all patients require retransplantation of the liver. Early retransplantation is performed within several days after the primary transplantation to rescue patients from primary nonfunction (graft factor), secondary nonfunction (host factor) associated with poor hepatic perfusion, acute rejection, and technical failure (vascular thrombosis). Hepatic necrosis is the common pathway and results in progressive, severe encephalopathy, ARDS, lactic acidosis, coagulopathy, hypoglycemia, and significant circulatory instability. Although infrequent, hepatectomy with portacaval shunt may be performed to protect the patient from the ill effects of the necrotizing liver on extrahepatic organ functions. In such a case, retransplantation should be performed as soon as the donor organ is available. The surgical procedure itself is relatively simple because surgical dissection has already been made and adhesions have not yet formed. Anesthetic management of these patients is similar to that of patients undergoing the primary transplantation.

Late retransplantation is performed for patients with chronic rejection, vascular complications, and recurrence of the original disease. The physical condition of the patient may have improved, but complications of immunosuppression (hypertension, renal insufficiency) may be present. Adhesions and steroid-induced tissue fragility frequently complicate late retransplantation. Anesthetic management is similar to that of primary liver transplantation, but large blood loss is anticipated.

Pediatric Liver Transplantation

Survival after pediatric liver transplantation is somewhat better than that of adults: 1-year survival of 90% and 5- to 8-year survival of 60% to 80%.[235,236] The most common indication is congenital biliary atresia. Circulatory changes are less significant than those of adults, although hypoxia is more common because of pulmonary shunting. Restrictive pulmonary disease, portal hypertension, hypoglycemia, renal insufficiency, electrolyte imbalance, and anemia from chronic bleeding may all be present.

A rapid-sequence IV induction is preferred; however, a mask induction is chosen in patients in whom it is difficult to obtain IV access.[237] All large-bore intravenous catheters are placed in the upper extremities after induction of anesthesia. Central venous pressure is usually monitored, and pulmonary arterial catheterization is rarely indicated. Blood pressure is monitored using a femoral intra-arterial catheter. It appears that children tolerate cross-clamping of the IVC and portal vein reasonably well without significant hemodynamic changes, possibly by compliant vasomotor tone. Venovenous bypass is rarely used in children under 20 kg, as low bypass flows may cause thrombosis. Coagulation changes that occur during liver transplantation are not as severe as those of adults, and this may be associated with more prevalent cholestatic diseases in children.[238] Blood loss is more significant in patients with biliary atresia because of technical difficulty associated with previous biliary surgery. Maintenance of body temperature is difficult as the large surface area promotes heat loss. The long-term effects of immunosuppressive drugs are similar to those in adults. Children, however, rarely require dialysis or renal transplantation after transplantation.[238] Long-term studies in children and adolescents have shown that successful liver transplantation promotes nutritional rehabilitation and normal growth and development.[240] More significantly, children undergoing transplantation before significant growth or developmental retardation are expected to achieve normal psychosocial development.[241]

Anesthetic Management After Liver Transplantation

Early Postoperative Period

All types of surgical procedures may be necessary in the early postoperative period. In the first 2 months after transplantation, surgical procedures are performed to treat complications of transplantation, such as exploratory laparotomy for abdominal bleeding or reconstruction of the biliary system and hepatic blood supply. Some degree of hepatic dysfunction may still be present, and ventilatory and circulatory support and invasive monitoring may be required. Regional anesthesia is not recommended because of potential bleeding and infectious complications. Rapid-sequence induction or awake intubation is performed using sodium thiopental, propofol, or etomidate, and anesthesia is maintained with volatile inhalation agents and narcotics. The dose of muscle relaxants is titrated for early extubation and recovery.

Late Postoperative Period

Patients may return to the operating room at any time for biliary reconstruction, replacement of a hip joint, or almost any other procedure. Liver function and drug metabolism are usually within the normal range, and anesthetic management differs little from that of other patients. Side effects of immunosuppressants (hypertension and renal insufficiency) and drug interaction should be considered. The activity of cyclosporine is enhanced by cytochrome P-450 inhibitors (ketoconazole and cimetidine) and reduced by cytochrome P-450 inducers (phenobarbital, phenytoin, and rifampin). Cyclosporine prolongs sleep time of pentobarbital and potentiates the analgesic effects of fentanyl but does not alter the median effective dose of either halothane or enflurane in animals. Regional anesthesia is an acceptable choice.

Summary

Liver transplantation, one of the most stressful procedures for patients with multiple organ dysfunction, is a challenge to all anesthesiologists. It is remarkable that anesthesiologists have been the major contributors to the progress of liver transplantation and successful outcome of many patients. It cannot be overemphasized, however, that a thorough understanding of pathophysiology and close communication and cooperation of hepatologists, surgeons, anesthesiologists, intensivists, and other health care workers are vital to the successful outcome and further progress in this field.

REFERENCES

1. U.S. Department of Commerce Bureau of the Census. *Statistical abstract of the United States: national data book*, Washington, DC, 1990, 79.
2. Starzl TE, Marchioro TL, von Kaulla KN, et al: Homotransplantation of the liver in humans, *Surg Gynecol Obstet* 117:659, 1963.
3. Starzl TE, Demetris AJ, Van Thiel DH: Liver transplantation (first of two parts), *N Engl J Med* 321:1014, 1989.
4. National Institute of Health Consensus Development Conference Statement: Liver transplantation, *Hepatology* 4:107S, 1984.
5. Starzl TE, Todo S, Fung J, et al: FK 506 for liver, kidney, and pancreas transplantation, *Lancet* 2:1000, 1989.
6. Jamieson NV, Sundberg R, Lindell S, et al: Preservation of the canine liver for 24-48 hours using simple cold storage with UW solution, *Transplantation* 46:517, 1988.
7. Tzakis A, Todo S, Starzl TE: Orthotopic liver transplantation with preservation of the inferior vena cava, *Ann Surg* 210:649, 1989.
8. *www.UNOS.net*
9. Bismuth H: Surgical anatomy and anatomical surgery of the liver, *World J Surg* 6:3, 1982.
10. Lautt WW, Legare DJ, d'Almeida MS: Adenosine as a putative regulator of hepatic arterial flow (the buffer response), *Am J Physiol* 248:H331, 1985.
11. Gelman S, Ernst E: Role of pH, pCO_2, and O_2 content of portal blood in hepatic circulatory autoregulation, *Am J Physiol* 233:E255, 1977.
12. McCluskey RS, Reilly FD: Hepatic microvasculature: dynamic structure and its regulation, *Semin Liver Dis* 13:1, 1993.
13. Lautt WW: Relationship between hepatic blood flow and overall metabolism: the hepatic arterial buffer response, *Fed Proc* 42:1662, 1983.
14. Brittain RS, Marchioro TL, Hermann G, et al: Accidental hepatic artery ligation in humans, *Am J Surg* 107.822, 1964.
15. Hesselink J, Slooff MJ, Schuur KH, et al: Consequences of hepatic artery pathology after orthotopic liver transplantation, *Transplant Proc* 19:2476, 1987.
16. Kjaer M, Jurlander J, Keiding S, et al: No reinnervation of hepatic sympathetic nerves after liver transplantation in human subjects, *J Hepatol* 20:97, 1994.
17. Lindfeldt J, Balkan B, Vandijk G, et al: Influence of peri-arterial hepatic denervation on the glycemic response to exercise in rats, *J Auton Nerv Syst* 44:45, 1993.
18. Wanless IR: Physioanatomic considerations. In Schiff L, Schiff ER (eds): *Diseases of the liver*, ed 8, Philadelphia, 1998, JB Lippincott, 3.
19. Lamers WH, Hilberts A, Furt E, et al: Hepatic enzymic zonation: a reevaluation of the concept of the liver acinus, *Hepatology* 10:72, 1989.
20. Popper H: Pathologic aspects of cirrhosis, *Am J Pathol* 87:228, 1977.
21. Wanless I, Wong F, Blendis L, et al: Hepatic and portal vein thrombosis in cirrhosis: possible role in development of parenchymal extinction and portal hypertension, *Hepatology* 21:1238, 1995.
22. Pilkis SJ, Granner DK: Molecular physiology of the regulation of hepatic gluconeogenesis and glycolysis, *Annu Rev Physiol* 54:885, 1992.
23. Nolte W, Hartmann H, Ramadori G: Glucose metabolism and liver cirrhosis, *Exp Clin Endocrinol Diabetes* 103:63, 1995.
24. Petrides A, DeFronzo RA: Glucose metabolism in cirrhosis: a review with some perspectives for the future, *Diabetes Metab Rev* 5:691, 1989.
25. Rothschild MA, Oratz M, Schreiber SS: Serum albumin, *Hepatology* 8:385, 1988.
26. Pierrangelo A, Panduro A, Chowdhury JR, et al: Albumin gene expression is downregulated by albumin or macromolecule infusion in the rat, *J Clin Invest* 89:1755, 1992.
27. Suttie JW: Vitamin K-dependent carboxylase, *Annu Rev Biochem* 54:459, 1985.
28. Yeaman S: Hormone sensitive lipase—a multipurpose enzyme in lipid metabolism, *Biochim Biophys Acta* 1052:128, 1990.
29. Gibbons GF: Assembly and secretion of hepatic very-low-density lipoprotein, *Biochem J* 268:1, 1990.
30. Lieber CS: Biochemical factors in alcoholic liver disease, *Semin Liver Dis* 13:136, 1993.
31. Chait A, Brunzell JD: Acquired hyperlipidemia (secondary dyslipoproteinemias), *Endocrinol Metab Clin North Am* 19:259, 1990.
32. Steer CJ: Liver regeneration, *FASEB J* 9:1396, 1995.
33. Michalopoulos GK: Liver regeneration: molecular mechanisms of growth control, *FASEB J* 4:176, 1990.
34. Fausto N, Laird AD, Webber EM: Liver regeneration. 2. Role of growth factors and cytokines in hepatic regeneration, *FASEB J* 9:1527, 1995.
35. Ellis RE, Yuan JY, Horvitz HR: Mechanisms and functions of cell death, *Annu Rev Cell Biol* 7:663, 1991.
36. Ogasawara J, Watanabe-Fukunaga R, Adachi M, et al: Lethal effect of the anti-Fas antibody in mice, *Nature* 364:806, 1993.
37. Gines P, Quintero E, Arroyo V, et al: Compensated cirrhosis: natural history and prognostic factors, *Hepatology* 7:122, 1987.
38. Butterworth RF: Neurotransmitter dysfunction in hepatic encephalopathy: new approaches and new findings, *Metab Brain Dis* 16:55, 2001.
39. Warskulat U, Kreuels S, Muller HW, et al: Identification of osmosensitive and ammonia-regulated genes in rat astrocytes by Northern blotting and differential display reverse transcriptase–polymerase chain reaction, *J Hepatol* 35:358, 2001.
40. Cordoba J, Alonso J, Rovira A, et al: The development of low-grade cerebral edema in cirrhosis is supported by the evolution of ^{1}H-magnetic resonance abnormalities after liver transplantation, *J Hepatol* 33:1370, 2001.
41. Tarter RE, Hegedus AM, Van Thiel DH, et al: Nonalcoholic cirrhosis associated with neuropsychological dysfunction in the absence of overt evidence of hepatic encephalopathy, *Gastroenterology* 86:1421, 1984.
42. Riggio O, Ariosto F, Merli M, et al: Short-term oral zinc supplementation does not improve chronic hepatic encephalopathy. Results of a double-blind crossover trial, *Dig Dis Sci* 36:1204, 1991.
43. Barbaro G, Di Lorenzo G, Soldini M, et al: Flumazenil for hepatic encephalopathy grade III and IVa in patients with cirrhosis: an Italian multicenter double blind, placebo-controlled, crossover study, *Hepatology* 28:374, 1998.
44. Sorkine P, Ben Abraham R, Szold O, et al: Role of the molecular adsorbent recycling system (MARS) in the treatment of patients with acute exacerbation of chronic liver failure, *Crit Care Med* 29:1332, 2001.

45. Ware AJ, D'Agostino AN, Combes B: Cerebral edema: a major complication of massive hepatic necrosis, *Gastroenterology* 61:877, 1971.

46. Lidorsky SD, Bass NM, Prager MC, et al: Intracranial pressure monitoring in liver transplantation for fulminant hepatic failure, *Hepatology* 16:1, 1992.

47. Aggarwal S, Kang YG, DeWolf A, et al: Transcranial Doppler: monitoring of cerebral blood flow velocity during liver transplantation, *Transplant Proc* 25:1799, 1993.

48. Aggarwal S, Kramer D, Yonas H, et al: Cerebral hemodynamic and metabolic changes in fulminant hepatic failure: a retrospective study, *Hepatology* 19:80, 1994.

49. Krowka MJ, Cortese DA: Pulmonary aspects of chronic liver disease and liver transplantation, *Mayo Clin Proc* 60:407, 1985.

50. Hourani LM, Bellamy PE, Tashkin DP, et al: Pulmonary dysfunction in advanced liver disease: frequent occurrence of an abnormal diffusing capacity, *Am J Med* 90:693, 1991.

51. Fluckiger M: Vorkommen von trommelschlagel-formigen fingerendphalangen ohne chronische Veranderungeng an den lungen oder am Herzen, *Wien Med Wochenschr* 34:1457, 1884.

52. Castro M, Krowka MJ: Hepatopulmonary syndrome, *Clin Chest Med* 17:35, 1996.

53. Genovesi MG, Tierney DF, Taplin GA: An intravenous radionuclide method to evaluate hypoxemia caused by abnormal alveolar vessels, *Am Rev Respir Dis* 114:59, 1976.

54. Lange PA, Stoller JK: The hepatopulmonary syndrome: effect of liver transplantation, *Clin Chest Med* 17:115, 1996.

55. Pak JM, Lee SS: Glucagon in portal hypertension, *J Hepatol* 20:825, 1994.

56. Farrell DJ, Hines JE, Walls AF, et al: Intrahepatic mast cells in chronic liver diseases, *Hepatology* 22:1175, 1995.

57. Lebrec D: Portal hypertension: serotonin and pathogenesis, *Cardiovasc Drug Ther* 4(Suppl 1):33, 1990.

58. Bendtsen F, Schifter S, Henriksen JH: Increased circulating calcitonin gene–related peptide (CGRP) in cirrhosis, *J Hepatol* 12:118, 1991.

59. Lee SS, Huang M, Ma Z, et al: Vasoactive intestinal peptide in cirrhotic rats: hemodynamic effects and mesenteric arterial receptor characteristics, *Hepatology* 23:1174, 1996.

60. Laffi G, Barletta G, La Villa G, et al: Altered cardiovascular responsiveness to active tilting in nonalcoholic cirrhosis, *Gastroenterology* 113:891, 1997.

61. Fernandez-Rodriguez CM, Prieto J, Quiroga J, et al: Plasma levels of substance P in liver cirrhosis: relationship to the activation of vasopressor systems and urinary sodium excretion, *Hepatology* 21:35, 1995.

62. Ohara N, Voelkel NF, Chang SW: Tissue eicosanoids and vascular permeability in rats with chronic biliary obstruction, *Hepatology* 18:111, 1993.

63. Soderman C, Juhlin-Dannfelt A, Lagerstrand L, et al: Ventilation-perfusion relationships and central hemodynamics in patients with cirrhosis. Effect of a somatostatin analogue, *J Hepatol* 21:52, 1994.

64. Song JY, Choi JY, Ko JT, et al: Long-term aspirin therapy for hepatopulmonary syndrome, *Pediatrics* 97:917, 1996.

65. Cremona G, Higgenbottam TW, Mayoral V, et al: Elevated exhaled nitric oxide in patients with hepatopulmonary syndrome, *Eur Respir J* 8:1883, 1995.

66. Chabot F, Mestiri H, Sabry S, et al: Role of NO in the pulmonary artery hyporeactivity to phenylephrine in experimental biliary cirrhosis, *Eur Respir J* 9:560, 1996.

67. Rolla G, Bucca C, Brussino L: Methylene blue in the HPS, *N Engl J Med* 331:1089, 1994 (letter).

68. Krowka MJ, Porayko MK, Plevak DJ, et al: Hepatopulmonary syndrome with progressive hypoxemia as an indication for liver transplantation: case reports and literature review, *Mayo Clin Proc* 72:44, 1997.

69. Scott VL, Dodson SF, Kang Y: The hepatopulmonary syndrome, *Surg Clin North Am* 79:23, 1999.

70. Matuschak GM, Shaw BW: Adult respiratory distress syndrome associated with acute liver allograft rejection: resolution following hepatic transplantation, *Crit Care Med* 15:878, 1987.

71. Doyle HR, Marino IR, Miro A, et al: Adult respiratory distress syndrome secondary to endstage liver disease—successful outcome following liver transplantation, *Transplantation* 55:292, 1993.

72. Alberts WM, Salem AJ, Solomon DA, et al: Hepatic hydrothorax—cause and management, *Arch Intern Med* 151:2383, 1991.

73. Siegerstetter V, Deibert P, Ochs A, et al: Treatment of refractory hepatic hydrothorax with transjugular intrahepatic portosystemic shunt: long-term results in 40 patients, *Eur J Gastroenterol Hepatol* 13:529, 2001.

74. Kolawski HJ, Abelmann WH: The cardiac output at rest in Laennec's cirrhosis, *J Clin Invest* 32:1025, 1953.

75. Benoit JN, Barrowman JA, Harper SL, et al: Role of humoral factors in the intestinal hyperemia associated with chronic portal hypertension, *Am J Physiol* 247:G486, 1984.

76. Yokoyama I, Todo S, Miyata T, et al: Endotoxemia and human liver transplantation, *Transplant Proc* 21:3833, 1989.

77. Kalb TH, Walter M, Mayer M, et al: Intra-allograft production and systemic release of tumor necrosis factor-alpha: detection upon reperfusion, *Transplant Proc* 25:1817, 1993.

78. D'Souza MG, Plevak DJ, Kvols L, et al: Elevated neuropeptide levels decrease during liver transplant, *Transplant Proc* 25:1805, 1993.

79. Darsee JR, Heymsfield SB, Miklozek CL, et al: Cirrhotic cardiomyopathy: the hyperdynamic unloaded-failing heart, Circulation 60(Suppl 2): 38, 1979 (abstract).

80. Lee SS: Cardiac abnormalities in liver cirrhosis, *West J Med* 151:530, 1989.

81. Caramelo C, Fernandes-Munoz D, Santos JC, et al: Effect of volume expansion on hemodynamics, capillary permeability and renal function in conscious cirrhotic rats, *Hepatology* 6:129, 1986.

82. Lee SS, Marty J, Mantz J, et al: Desensitization of myocardial beta-adrenergic receptors in cirrhotic rats, *Hepatology* 12:481, 1990.

83. Bernardi M, Rubboli A, Trevisani F, et al: Reduced cardiovascular responsiveness to exercise-induced sympathoadrenergic stimulation in patients with cirrhosis, *J Hepatol* 12:207, 1991.

84. Finucci G, Desideri A, Sacerdoti D, et al: Left ventricular diastolic function in liver cirrhosis, *Scand J Gastroenterol* 31:279, 1996.

85. Gerbes A, Remien J, Jungst D, et al: Evidence for downregulation of beta-adrenoceptors in cirrhotic patients with severe ascites, *Lancet* 1:1409, 1986.

86. Liu H, Lee SS: Cardiopulmonary dysfunction in cirrhosis, *J Gastroenterol Hepatol* 14:600, 1999.

87. Ma Z, Miyamoto A, Lee SS: Role of altered beta-adrenoceptor signal transduction in the pathogenesis of cirrhotic cardiomyopathy in rats, *Gastroenterology* 110:1191, 1996.

88. Jaue DN, Ma, Z, Lee SS: Cardiac muscarinic receptor function in rats with cirrhotic cardiomyopathy, *Hepatology* 25:1361, 1997.

89. Le Grimellec C, Friedlander G, Yandouzi EH, et al: Membrane fluidity and transport properties in epithelia, *Kidney Int* 42:825, 1992.

90. Ward CA, Ma Z, Lee SS, et al: Potassium currents in atrial and ventricular myocytes from a rat model of cirrhosis, *Am J Physiol* 273:G537, 1997.

91. Bernardi M, Calandra S, Colantoni A, et al: Q-T interval prolongation in cirrhosis: prevalence, relationship with severity and etiology of disease and possible pathogenetic factors, *Hepatology* 27:28, 1998.

92. Hare JM, Colucci WS: Role of nitric oxide in the regulation of myocardial function, *Prog Cardiovasc Dis* 38:155, 1995.

93. Chung MK, Gulick TS, Rotondo RE, et al: Mechanism of cytokine inhibition of beta-adrenergic agonist stimulation of cyclic AMP in rat cardiac myocytes. Impairment of signal transduction, *Circ Res* 67:753, 1990.

94. Bomzon A, Blendis LM: The nitric oxide hypothesis and the hyperdynamic circulation in cirrhosis, *Hepatology* 20:1343, 1994.

95. Snyder N, Atterbury CE, Correia JP, et al: Increased concurrence of cirrhosis and bacterial endocarditis, *Gastroenterology* 73:1107, 1977.

96. Shah A, Variyam E: Pericardial effusion and left ventricular dysfunction associated with ascites secondary to hepatic cirrhosis, *Arch Intern Med* 148:585, 1988.

97. Kinney E: Pericardial effusion associated with ascites, *Arch Intern Med* 148:1879, 1988.

98. Mantz FA, Craige E: Portal axis thrombosis with spontaneous portocaval shunt and resulting cor pulmonale, *Arch Pathol* 52:91, 1951.

99. Lebrec D, Capron J-P: Pulmonary hypertension complicating portal hypertension, *Am Rev Respir Dis* 120:849, 1979.

100. McDonnell DJ, Toye PA, Hutchins GM: Primary pulmonary hypertension and cirrhosis: are they related? *Am Rev Respir Dis* 127:437, 1983.

101. Hoff JC, Agarawal JB, Gardiner AJS, et al: Distribution of airway resistance with developing pulmonary edema in dogs, *J Appl Physiol* 32:20, 1972.

102. Iliff LD, Greene RE, Hughes JMB: Effect of interstitial edema on distribution of ventilation and perfusion in isolated lung, *J Appl Physiol* 33:462, 1972.

103. Naeije RL, Melot C, Hallemans R, et al: Pulmonary hemodynamics in liver cirrhosis, *Semin Respir Med* 7:164, 1985.

104. Senior RM, Britton RC, Turino GM, et al: Pulmonary hypertension associated with cirrhosis of the liver and with portocaval shunts, *Circulation* 378:88, 1968.

105. Hadengue A, Benhayoun MK, Lebrec D, et al: Pulmonary hypertension complicating portal hypertension: prevalence and relation to splanchnic hemodynamics, *Gastroenterology* 100:520, 1991.

106. De Wolf AM, Gasior T, Kang Y: Pulmonary hypertension in a patient undergoing liver transplantation, *Transplant Proc* 23:2000, 1991.

107. Krowka MJ, Plevak DJ, Findlay JY, et al: Pulmonary hemodynamics and perioperative cardiopulmonary-related mortality in patients with portopulmonary hypertension undergoing liver transplantation, *Liver Transpl* 6:443, 2000.

108. De Wolf AM, Scott V, Bjerke R, et al: Hemodynamic effects of inhaled nitric oxide in four patients with severe liver disease and pulmonary hypertension, *Liver Transpl Surg* 3:594, 1997.

109. Kuo PC, Johnson LB, Plotkin JS, et al: Continuous infusion of epoprostenol for the treatment of portopulmonary hypertension, *Transplantation* 63:604, 1997.

110. Carey WD, Dumor JA, Pimentel RR, et al: The prevalence of coronary artery disease in liver transplant candidates over age 50, *Transplantation* 59:859, 1995.

111. Plotkin JS, Scott VL, Pinna A, et al: Morbidity and mortality in patients with coronary artery disease undergoing orthotopic liver transplantation, *Liver Transpl Surg* 2:426, 1996.

112. Keeffe BG, Valantine H, Keeffe EB: Direction and treatment of coronary artery disease in liver transplantation candidates, *Liver Transpl Surg* 7:755, 2001.

113. Plotkin JS, Benite RM, Kuo PC, et al: Dobutamine stress echocardiography for preoperative cardiac risk stratification in patients undergoing orthotopic liver transplantation, *Liver Transpl Surg* 4:253, 1998.

114. Kojima H, Sakurai M, Kuriyama S, et al: Endothelin-1 plays a major role in portal hypertension of biliary cirrhotic rats through endothelin receptor subtype B together with subtype A in vivo, *J Hepatol* 34:805, 2002.

115. Gandhi CR, Kang Y, DeWolf A, et al: Altered endothelin homeostasis in patients undergoing liver transplantation, *Liver Transpl Surg* 2:362, 1996.

116. Shah V, Cao S, Hendrickson H, et al: Regulation of hepatic eNOS by caveolin and calmodulin after bile duct ligation in rats, *Am J Physiol* 280:G1209, 2001.

117. Arroyo V, Gines A, Gerbes A, et al: Definition and diagnostic criteria of refractory ascites and hepatorenal syndrome in cirrhosis, *Hepatology* 23:164, 1996.

118. Martin PY, Gines P, Schrier RW: Role of nitric oxide as mediator of hemodynamic abnormalities and sodium and water retention in cirrhosis, *N Engl J Med* 339:553, 1998.

119. Guevara M, Gines P, Fernandez-Esparrach G, et al: Reversal of hepatorenal syndrome by prolonged administration of ornipressin and plasma volume expansion, *Hepatology* 27:35, 1998.

120. Mulkay JP, Louis H, Donckier V, et al: Long-term terlipressin administration improves renal function in patients with cirrhosis with type 1 hepatorenal syndrome: a pilot study, *Acta Gastroenterol Belg* 64:15, 2001.

121. Lechner K, Niessner H, Thaler E: Coagulation abnormalities in liver disease, *Semin Thromb Hemost* 4:40, 1977.

122. Kawasaki T, Takeshita A, Souda K, et al: Serum thrombopoietin levels in patients with chronic hepatitis and liver cirrhosis, *Am J Gastroenterol* 94:1918, 1999.

123. Rubin MH, Weston MJ, Langley MH, et al: Platelet function in chronic liver disease; relationship to disease severity, *Dig Dis Sci* 24:197, 1979.

124. Van Thiel DH, George M, Fareed J: Low levels of thrombin activatable fibrinolysis inhibitor (TAFI) in patients with chronic liver disease, *Thromb Haemost* 85:667, 2001.

125. Runyon BA: Treatment of patients with cirrhosis and ascites, *Semin Liver Dis* 17:249, 1997.

126. D'Amico G, Pagliaro L, Bosch J: The treatment of portal hypertension: a meta-analytic review, *Hepatology* 22:332, 1995.

127. Stanley AJ, Forrest EH, Lui HF, et al: Band ligation versus propranolol or isosorbide dinitrate in the primary prophylaxis of variceal hemorrhage: preliminary results of a randomized controlled trial, *Gut* 42(Suppl 1):A19, 1998 (abstract).

128. Vosmik J, Jedlicka K, Mulder J, et al: Action of the triglycyl hormonogen of vasopressin (Glypressin) in patients with liver cirrhosis and bleeding esophageal varices, *Gastroenterology* 72:605, 1977.

129. Bosch J, Kravetz D, Rodes J: Effects of somatostatin on hepatic and systemic hemodynamics in patients with cirrhosis of the liver. Comparison with vasopressin, *Gastroenterology* 80:518, 1981.

130. Chojkier M, Conn HO: Esophageal tamponade in the treatment of bleeding varices, *Dig Dis Sci* 25:267, 1980.

131. Oules R, Asaba H, Neuhauser M, et al: The removal of uremic small and middle molecules and free amino acids by carbon hemoperfusion, *Trans Am Soc Artif Intern Organs* 23:583, 1977.

132. Davenport A, Will EJ, Davison AM: Continuous vs intermittent forms of hemofiltration and/or dialysis in the management of acute renal failure in patients with defective cerebral autoregulation at risk of cerebral edema, *Contrib Nephrol* 93:225, 1991.

133. Yoshiba M, Inoue K, Sekiyama K, et al: Favorable effect of new artificial liver support on survival of patients with fulminant hepatic failure, *Artif Organs* 20:1169, 1996.

134. Winikoff S, Glassman MS, Spivak W: Plasmapheresis in a patient with fulminant hepatic failure awaiting hepatic transplantation, *J Pediatr* 107:547, 1985.

135. Kondrup J, Almdal T, Vilstrup H, et al: High-volume plasma exchange in fulminant hepatic failure, *Int J Artif Organs* 15:669, 1992.

136. Eiseman B, Liem DS, Raffucci F: Heterologous liver perfusion in treatment of hepatic failure, *Ann Surg* 162:329, 1965.

137. Fox IJ, Langnas AN, Fristoe LW, et al: Successful application of extracorporeal liver perfusion: a technology whose time has come, *Am J Gastroenterol* 88:1876, 1993.

138. Sussman NL, Chong MG, Koussayer T, et al: Reversal of fulminant hepatic failure using an extracorporeal liver assist device, *Hepatology* 16:60, 1992.

139. Rozga J, Holzman MD, Ro MS: Development of a hybrid bioartificial liver, *Ann Surg* 17:258, 1993.

140. Gerlach JC: Long-term liver cell cultures in bioreactors and possible application for liver support, *Cell Biol Toxicol* 13:349, 1997.

141. Soriano HE, Wood RP, Kang DC, et al: Hepatocellular transplantation in children with fulminant liver failure, *Hepatology* 26:A239, 1997 (abstract).

142. Bilir BM, Guenette D, Ostrowska A, et al: Percutaneous hepatocyte transplantation in liver failure, *Hepatology* 26:A252, 1997 (abstract).

143. Starzl TE, Fung J, Tzakis A, et al: Baboon-to-human liver transplantation, *Lancet* 341:65, 1993.

144. Tzakis AG, Cooper MH, Drummer JS, et al: Transplantation in HIV-positive patients, *Transplantation* 49:354, 1990.

145. Kang YG, Kormos RL, Casavilla A: Organ procurement from donors with brain death. In Grande C (ed): *Textbook of trauma anesthesia and critical care*, St Louis, 1993, Mosby, 1013.

146. Howard TK, Klintmalm GB, Corer JB, et al: The influence of preservation injury or rejection in hepatic transplant recipients, *Transplantation* 49:103, 1990.

147. Starzl TE: The recipient operation in man. In Starzl TE, Putnam CW (eds): *Experience in hepatic transplantation*, Philadelphia, 1969, WB Saunders, 112.

148. Shaw BW, Martin DJ, Marquez JM, et al: Venous bypass in clinical liver transplantation, *Ann Surg* 4:524, 1984.

149. Wheeldon DR, Gill RD: Partial cardiopulmonary bypass. In Cale RY (ed): *Liver transplantation. The Cambridge/King's College Hospital experience*, New York, 1983, Grune & Stratton, 145.

150. Fortner JG, Kinne DW, Shiu MH, et al: Clinical liver heterotopic (auxiliary) transplantation, *Surgery* 74:739, 1973.

151. Broelsch CE, Edmond JC, Thisticwaite JR, et al: Liver transplantation including the concept of reduced size liver transplants in children, *Ann Surg* 208:410, 1988 (abstract).

152. Houssin D, Soubrane O, Boillot O, et al: Orthotopic liver transplantation with a reduced size graft: an ideal compromise in pediatrics? *Surgery* 111:532, 1992.

153. Howard TK, Klintmalm GB, Corer JB, et al: The influence of preservation injury or rejection in hepatic transplant recipients, *Transplantation* 49:103, 1990.

154. Rogers X, Malago M, Gawad K, et al: In situ splitting of cadaveric livers: the ultimate expansion of the donor pool, *Ann Surg* 224:331, 1996.

155. Raia S, Nery JR, Mies S: Liver transplantation from live donors, *Lancet* 2:497, 1988.

156. Strong RW, Lynch SV, Ong TN, et al: Successful liver transplantation from a living donor to her son, *N Engl J Med* 322:1505, 1990.

157. Hashikura Y, Makuuchi M, Kawasaki S, et al: Successful living-related partial liver transplantation to an adult patient, *Lancet* 43:1233, 1994.

158. Wachs ME, Bak TE, Karrer FM, et al: Adult living donor liver transplantation using a right hepatic lobe, *Transplantation* 66:1313, 1998.

159. Marcos A, Fisher RA, Ham JM, et al: Liver regeneration and function in donor and recipient after right lobe adult-to-adult living donor transplantation, *Transplantation* 69:1375, 2000.

160. Malago M, Rogiers X, Burdelski M, et al: Living-related liver transplantation: 36 cases at the University of Hamburg, *Transplant Proc* 26:3620, 1994.

161. Sassano JJ: The rapid infusion system. In Winter PM, Kang YG (eds): *Hepatic transplantation, anesthetic and perioperative management*, Philadelphia, 1986, Praeger, 120.

162. Dunham CM, Belzberg H, Lyles R, et al: The rapid infusion system: a superior method for the resuscitation of hypovolemic trauma patients, *Resuscitation* 21:207, 1991.

163. Elia E, Kang Y: Rapid infusion devices for hemorrhagic cardiothoracic trauma, *Semin Cardiothorac Vasc Anesth* 6:105, 2002.

164. Dzik WH, Jenkins R: Use of intraoperative blood salvage during orthotopic liver transplantation, *Arch Surg* 120:946, 1985.

165. Kang Y, Aggarwal S, Virji M, et al: Clinical evaluation of autotransfusion during liver transplantation, *Anesth Analg* 72:94, 1991.

166. Kang YG: Monitoring and treatment of coagulation. In Winter PM, Kang YG (eds): *Hepatic transplantation, anesthetic and perioperative management*, Philadelphia, 1986, Praeger, 151.

167. Kang Y: Transfusion based on clinical coagulation monitoring does reduce hemorrhage during liver transplantation, *Liver Transpl Surg* 3:655, 1997.

168. Begliomini B, DeWolf A, Snyder J, et al: Is radial arterial pressure monitoring accurate during liver transplantation? *Eur J Anaesthesiol Relat Spec* 2:13, 1990 (abstract).

169. DeWolf AM, Begliomini B, Gasior RA, et al: Right ventricular function during orthotopic liver transplantation, *Anesth Analg* 76:562, 1993.

170. Ellis JE, Lichtor JL, Feinstein SB, et al: Right heart dysfunction, pulmonary embolism, and paradoxical embolization during liver transplantation. A transesophageal two-dimensional echocardiographic study, *Anesth Analg* 68:777, 1989.

171. De Wolf AM, Scott V, Kang Y, et al: Hepatic venous outflow obstruction during hepatic resection diagnosed by transesophageal echocardiography, *Anesthesiology* 80:1398, 1994.

172. Kang Y: Thromboelastography in liver transplantation, *Semin Thromb Haemost* 21(Suppl 4):34, 1995.

173. Pappas G, Palmer WM, Martineau GL, et al: Hemodynamic changes in clinical orthotopic liver transplantation, *Surg Forum* 22:335, 1971.

174. Aggarwal S, Kang Y, Freeman JA, et al: Postreperfusion syndrome: hypotension after reperfusion of the transplanted liver, *J Crit Care* 8:154, 1993.

175. Suriani RJ, Cutrone A, Feierman D, et al: Intraoperative transesophageal echocardiography during liver transplantation, *J Cardiothorac Vasc Anesth* 10:699, 1996.

176. Martin D: Fluid and electrolyte balance during liver transplantation. In Winter PM, Kang YG (eds): *Hepatic transplantation, anesthetic and perioperative management*, Philadelphia, 1986, Praeger, 33.

177. Cottam S, Potter D, Ginsburg R, et al: Effects of somatostatin on systemic and mesenteric hemodynamics during orthotopic liver transplantation, *Transplant Proc* 23:1959, 1991.

178. Lewis JH, Bontempo FA, Awad Sa, et al: Liver transplantation: intraoperative changes in coagulation factors in 100 first transplants, *Hepatology* 9:710, 1989.

179. Kratzer MAA, Dieterich J, Denecke H, et al: Hemostatic variables and blood loss during orthotopic human liver transplantation, *Transplant Proc* 23:1906, 1991.

180. Rohrer MJ, Natale AM: Effect of hypothermia on the coagulation cascade, *Crit Care Med* 20:1402, 1992.

181. Kang YG, Martin DJ, Marquez J, et al: Intraoperative changes in blood coagulation and thromboelastographic monitoring in liver transplantation, *Anesth Analg* 64:888, 1985.

182. Kang YG, Lewis JH, Navalgund A, et al: Epsilon-aminocaproic acid for treatment of fibrinolysis during liver transplantation, *Anesthesiology* 66:766, 1987.

183. Gologorsky E, De Wolf AM, Scott V, et al: Intracardiac thrombus formation and pulmonary thromboembolism immediately after graft reperfusion in 7 patients undergoing liver transplantation, *Liver Transpl* 7:783, 2001.

184. Virji MA, Aggarwal S, Kang Y: Alterations in plasminogen activator and plasminogen activator inhibitor levels during liver transplantation, *Transplant Proc* 21:3540, 1989.

185. Porte RJ, Bontempo FA, Knott EAR, et al: Systemic effects of tissue plasminogen activator–associated fibrinolysis and its relation to thrombin generation in orthotopic liver transplantation, *Transplantation* 47:978, 1989.

186. Lewis JH, Bontempo FA, Ragni MV, et al: Antithrombin III during liver transplantation, *Transplant Proc* 21:3543, 1989.

187. Hutchison DE, Genton E, Porter KA, et al: Platelet changes following clinical and experimental hepatic homotransplantation, *Arch Surg* 97:27, 1968.

188. Kang Y, Carranza JA, Chung CJ: A low-dose EACA during liver transplantation, *Liver Transpl Surg* 3:C-46, 1997 (abstract).

189. Neuhaus P, Bechstein WO, Lefebre B, et al: Effect of aprotinin on intraoperative bleeding and fibrinolysis in liver transplantation, *Lancet* 2:924, 1989.

190. Mallett SV, Cox D, Burroughs AK, et al: Aprotinin and reduction of blood loss and transfusion requirements in orthotopic liver transplantation, *Lancet* 336:886, 1990 (letter).

191. Hunt BJ, Cottam S, Segal H, et al: Inhibition by aprotinin of tPA-mediated fibrinolysis during orthotopic liver transplantation, *Lancet* 336:381, 1990.

192. Groh J, Welte M, Azad SC, et al: Does aprotinin really reduce blood loss in orthotopic liver transplantation? *Semin Thromb Hemost* 19:306, 1993.

193. Ickx B, Pradier O, DeGroote F, et al: Effect of two different dosages of aprotinin on perioperative blood loss during liver transplantation, *Semin Thromb Hemost* 19:300, 1993.

194. Boylan JF, Klinck JR, Sandler AN, et al: Tranexamic acid reduces blood loss, transfusion requirements, and coagulation factor use in primary orthotopic liver transplantation, *Anesthesiology* 85:1043, 1996.

195. Kang Y, Scott V, DeWolf A, et al: In vitro effects of DDAVP during liver transplantation, *Transplant Proc* 25:1821, 1993.

196. Frenette L, Cox J, McArdle P, et al: Conjugated estrogen reduces transfusion and coagulation factor requirements in orthotopic liver transplantation, *Anesth Analg* 86:1183, 1998.

197. Marquez J, Martin D, Kang YG, et al: Cardiovascular depression secondary to citrate intoxication during hepatic transplantation in man, *Anesthesiology* 65:457, 1986.

198. Martin TJ, Kang Y, Robertson KM, et al: Ionization and hemodynamic effects of calcium chloride and calcium gluconate in the absence of hepatic function, *Anesthesiology* 73:62, 1990.

199. DeWolf A, Frenette L, Kang Y, et al: Insulin decreases the serum potassium concentration during the anhepatic stage of liver transplantation, *Anesthesiology* 78:677, 1993.

200. Ellis R, Beeston JT, Witherington SS, et al: Liver transplantation: effect of washing bank blood on intraoperative control of hyperkalemia, *Transplant Proc* 19(Suppl 3):73, 1987.

201. Videira R, Kang YG, Martinez J, et al: A rapid increase in sodium is associated with CPM after liver transplantation, *Anesthesiology* 75:A222, 1991 (abstract).

202. Scott VL, De Wolf AM, Kang Y, et al: Ionized hypomagnesemia in patients undergoing orthotopic liver transplantation: a complication of citrate intoxication, *Liver Transpl Surg* 2:343, 1996.

203. Begliomini B, DeWolf A, Freeman J, et al: Intraoperative lactate levels can predict graft function after liver transplantation, Anesthesiology 71:A72, 1989 (abstract).

204. Shangraw RE, Robinson ST: Oxygen metabolism during liver transplantation: the effect of dichloroacetate, *Anesth Analg* 85:746, 1997.

205. Fortunato FL Jr, Kang Y, Aggarwal S, et al: Acid-base state during and after orthotopic liver transplantation, *Transplant Proc* 19(Suppl 3):59, 1987.

206. DeWolf AM, Kang YG, Todo S, et al: Glucose metabolism during liver transplantation in dogs, *Anesth Anal* 66:76, 1987.

207. Mallett S, Kang Y, Borland LM, et al: Prognostic significance of reperfusion hyperglycemia during liver transplantation, *Anesth Analg* 68:182, 1989.

208. Polson RJ, Park GR, Lindop MJ, et al: The prevention of renal impairment in patients undergoing orthotopic liver grafting by infusion of low-dose dopamine, *Anaesthesia* 42:15, 1987.

209. Swygert TH, Roberts LC, Valek TR, et al: Effect of intraoperative low-dose dopamine on renal function in liver transplant recipients, *Anesthesiology* 75:571, 1991.

210. Gray PA, Bodenham AR, Park GR: A comparison of dopexamine and dopamine to prevent renal impairment in patients undergoing orthotopic liver transplantation, *Anaesthesia* 46:638, 1991.

211. Planinsic RM, Kang Y, DeWolf AM, et al: Dopamine, furosemide and mannitol infusions and changes in serum creatinines after liver transplantation, *Liver Transpl Surg* 3:10, 1997.

212. Mandell MS, Lockrem J, Kelley SD: Immediate tracheal extubation after liver transplantation: experience of two transplant centers, *Anesth Analg* 84:249, 1997.

213. Bzeizi KI, Jalan R, Plevris JN, et al: Primary graft dysfunction after liver transplantation: from pathogenesis to prevention, *Liver Transpl Surg* 3:137, 1997.

214. Wiesner RH: Is hepatic histology the true gold standard in diagnosing acute hepatic allograft rejection? *Liver Transpl Surg* 2:165, 1996 (editorial).

215. Orons PD, Zajko AB, Bron KM, et al: Hepatic artery angioplasty after liver transplantation: experience in 21 allografts, *J Vasc Interv Radiol* 6:523, 1995.

216. Tzakis AG, Gordon RD, Shaw BW, et al: Clinical presentation of hepatic artery thrombosis after liver transplantation in the cyclosporine era, *Transplantation* 40:667, 1985.

217. Mazzaferro V, Esquivel CO, Makowka L, et al: Hepatic artery thrombosis after pediatric liver transplantation—a medical or surgical event? *Transplantation* 47:971, 1989.

218. Harper PL, Edgar PF, Luddington R, et al: Protein C deficiency and portal thrombosis in liver transplantation in children, *Lancet* 2:924, 1988.

219. Simo G, Echenagusia A, Camunez F, et al: Stenosis of the inferior vena cava after liver transplantation: treatment with Gianturco expandable metallic stents, *Cardiovasc Intervent Radiol* 18:212, 1993.

220. Stieber AS, Gordon RD, Bassi N: A simple solution to a technical complication in piggy back liver transplantation, *Transplantation* 64,654, 1997.

221. O'Connor TP, Lewis WD, Jenkins RL: Biliary tract complications after liver transplantation, *Arch Surg* 130:312, 1995.

222. Ozaki CF, Katz SM, Monsour HP, et al: Surgical complications of liver transplantation, *Surg Clin North Am* 74:1155, 1994.

223. Richards EM, Alexander GJ, Calne RY, et al: Thrombocytopenia following liver transplantation is associated with platelet consumption and thrombin generation, *Br J Haematol* 98:315, 1997.

224. Shaked A, Vargas J, Csete ME, et al: Diagnosis and treatment of bowel perforation following pediatric orthotopic liver transplantation, *Arch Surg* 128:994, 1993.

225. McAlister VC, Grant DR, Roy A, et al: Right phrenic nerve injury in orthotopic liver transplantation, *Transplantation* 55:826, 1993.

226. Stein KL, Ladowski J, Kormos R, et al: The cardiopulmonary response to OKT3 in orthotopic cardiac transplant recipients, *Chest* 95:817, 1989.

227. Singh N, Yu VL, Gayowski T: Central nervous system lesions in adult liver transplant recipients: clinical review with implications for management, *Medicine (Baltimore)* 73:110, 1994.

228. Winnock S, Janvier G, Parmentier F, et al: Pontine myelinolysis following liver transplantation: a report of two cases, *Transplant Int* 6:26, 1993.

229. McCaulley J, Van Thiel D, Starzl TE, et al: Acute and chronic renal failure after liver transplantation, *Nephron* 55:121, 1990.

230. Gonwa TA, Klintmalm GB, Levy M, et al: Impact of pretransplant renal function on survival after liver transplantation, *Transplantation* 59:361, 1995.

231. Singh N, Gayowski T, Wagener M, et al: Infectious complications in liver transplant recipients on tacrolimus, *Transplantation* 58:774, 1994.

232. George DL, Arnow PM, Fox AS, et al: Bacterial infection as a complication of liver transplantation: epidemiology and risk factors, *Respir Infect Dis* 13:387, 1991.

233. Everson G, Trouillot T, Wachs M, et al: Early steroid withdrawal in liver transplant is safe and beneficial, *Liver Transpl Surg* 5(Suppl 1):S48, 1999.

234. Fisher RA, Ham JM, Marcos A, et al: A prospective randomized trial of mycophenolate mofetil with neoral or tacrolimus after orthotopic liver transplantation, *Transplantation* l66:1616, 1998.

235. Cacciarelli TV, Esquivel CO, Moore DH, et al: Factors affecting survival after orthotopic liver transplantation in infants, *Transplantation* 64:242, 1997.

236. Andrews W, Sommerauer J, Roden J, et al: 10 years of pediatric liver transplantation, *J Pediatr Surg* 31:619, 1996.

237. Borland LM, Roule M, Cook DR: Anesthesia for pediatric orthotopic liver transplantation, *Anesth Analg* 64:117, 1985.

238. Kang Y, Borland LM, Picone J, et al: Intraoperative coagulation changes in children undergoing liver transplantation, *Anesthesiology* 71:44, 1989.

239. Ellis D, Avner E, Starzl TE: Renal failure in children with hepatic failure undergoing liver transplantation, *J Pediatr* 108:393, 1986.

240. Codoner-Franch P, Bernard O, Alvarez F: Long-term follow-up of growth in height after successful liver transplantation, *J Pediatr* 124:368, 1994.

241. Beath SV, Brook GD, Kelly DA, et al: Successful liver transplantation in babies under 1 year, *BMJ* 307:825, 1993.

Renal Transplantation and Renal Protection During Vascular Surgical Procedures

14

Claudia Crawford, MD
Perry Bechtle, DO
Michael J. Murray, MD, PhD

Renal Protection During Vascular Surgical Procedures

Patients with vascular disease who undergo vascular operations have a high risk of developing organ dysfunction, particularly kidney dysfunction. This risk is due not only to the disease that precipitated the operation, but also to comorbid conditions that many of these patients have. Even in patients without renal disease, most vascular surgical procedures carry a moderate-to-high risk of causing renal dysfunction, a risk that has not changed appreciably in many decades.

The incidence of renal failure requiring postoperative dialysis is as high as 5% in patients who undergo surgical procedures involving the aorta, even when the operation involves only the infrarenal aorta, and the incidence may be even higher in patients with preoperative renal dysfunction.[1] A study that examined complication rates of repair of Crawford type II thoracoabdominal aortic aneurysms (TAAAs) found that 15.9% of patients developed renal failure; patients with preoperative renal insufficiency had an increased risk of postoperative renal failure (odds ratio, 2.8). After cardiac operations, the incidence of renal failure requiring therapy was 1.1% in a study by Chertow et al; these researchers also found that the mortality rate was 64% in patients with and 4.3% in those without renal failure.[2]

In patients undergoing elective abdominal aortic aneurysm repair, Dardik et al found mortality rates of 11.8% in patients with perioperative renal failure versus 3.4% in patients without perioperative renal dysfunction.[3] Of patients whose kidneys were infused with a cold perfusate (79% of cases) during repair of a TAAA that involved a suprarenal aortic cross-clamp, acute renal failure developed in 11.5%, with 2.7% of patients requiring hemodialysis.[4] Patients who developed renal failure had a significantly increased mortality rate compared with those who did not develop renal failure (odds ratio, 9.2). Coselli et al reported a 5.9% rate of renal failure requiring hemodialysis in 1773 patients who underwent TAAA repair, one third of whom received a left atrial–to–iliac artery bypass (see Chapter 11).[5]

Endovascular aortic surgery is increasingly being used for patients deemed too sick for conventional open aortic surgery, although such cases may involve further procedures to treat leaks and malposition of the stent. Because endovascular procedures involve manipulation of atheromatous aortas, they are associated with renal risks. In one study of 164 patients who had undergone endovascular repair of abdominal aortic aneurysms, 9 of the 149 patients (6.2%) with normal preoperative renal function developed significant renal impairment postoperatively; 4 patients (2.8%) died, 2 perioperatively.[6] The mortality rate for patients with preoperative renal impairment was 27%. In another study in 50 subjects, the frequency of renal embolic events was 18%, and such events were correlated with the volume of aneurysm neck atheroma.[7]

Anatomy and Physiology of the Kidney

Because the kidneys are vulnerable to damage preoperatively from intravenously administered contrast imaging drugs, intraoperatively from hypoperfusion during aortic cross-clamping and embolization during manipulation of the aorta, and postoperatively as the result of hypoperfusion, anemia, hypotension, hypovolemia, or other causes, the kidneys need to be protected in any patient undergoing vascular surgical procedures. A review of renal anatomy (Fig. 14–1) and physiology allows the clinician to identify the pharmacologic agents and procedures that have the greatest positive and greatest negative impacts on the kidney and to ascertain potential strategies to protect the kidney.

The main functions of the kidneys are filtration, reabsorption, and secretion. To achieve these goals, the kidneys receive more blood flow for their size than any other organ in the body. They receive approximately 25% of the cardiac output, which is delivered to the kidneys through the renal arteries. The renal arteries enter the kidneys through the hilum, giving off interlobar arteries that pass between the medullary pyramids. At the junction of the medulla and the cortex, these arteries branch to form the arcuate arteries, which in turn branch off into cortical radial arteries (formerly called interlobular arteries). Branches of these arteries lead to afferent arterioles, which enter Bowman's capsule and form a capillary cluster called a glomerulus (Fig. 14–2). Bowman's capsule is an expansion of the proximal closed end of the renal tubule, which forms a cup around the glomerulus where renal filtration occurs. A glomerular filtration rate (GFR) of approximately 125 mL/minute (180 L/day) is achieved via hydrostatic pressure through the permeable capillaries. Changes in blood pressure, as well as variations in the constriction and dilation of the afferent and efferent arterioles, lead to alterations in the amount of filtration.

Bowman's capsule leads to the renal tubule, which coils to form the proximal convoluted tubule leading to the descending loop of Henle, the ascending loop of Henle, and the distal convoluted tubule leading to the collecting duct (Fig. 14–3). Multiple distal convoluted tubules merge in the renal cortex to form the collecting duct, which passes into the renal medulla. Multiple collecting ducts meet at the calyces, which join to form the renal pelvis leading to the ureter. The distal convoluted tubule contacts the afferent arteriole near the glomerulus,

271

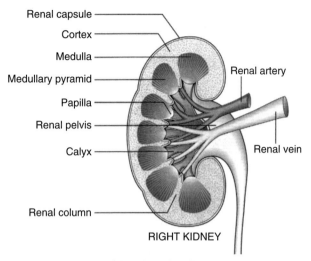

FIGURE 14-1 Anatomy of the kidney. (From Field MJ, Pollock CA, Harris DC: *The Renal System.* Philadelphia, 2001, Churchill Livingstone)

and the tubular cells and the arteriole form the juxtaglomerular apparatus (JGA), the site of renin release. The efferent arteriole leaves the glomerulus and forms a network called the *peritubular capillary system*, which surrounds the tubular system to participate in the exchange of fluids and solutes. The JGA includes the macula densa, a prominent cell plaque in the thick ascending limb (which acts as the substrate for the functional connection between the distal tubular fluid composition, afferent arterial tone, and renin release), the terminal portion of the afferent arteriole (with renin-producing cells), the initial portion of the efferent arteriole, and the extraglomerular mesangium.[8] This site, which is the main site for the regulation of renin secretion, allows the composition of the distal urine to influence the tone in the glomerular arterioles, resulting in a change in glomerular blood flow and GFR, known as *tubuloglomerular feedback.*

The cortical nephrons receive most of their blood flow from the renal arteries, maximizing the amount of blood filtered. Their corpuscles are near the surface of the kidney, and their loops of

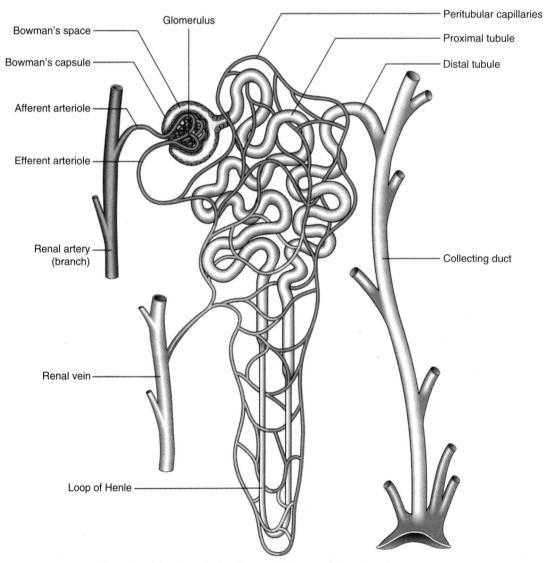

FIGURE 14-2 Formation of the glomerulus by afferent and efferent arterioles. (From Field MJ, Pollock CA, Harris DC: *The Renal System.* Philadelphia, 2001, Churchill Livingstone)

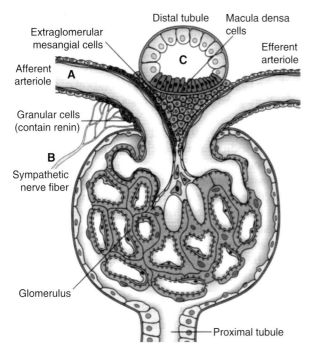

Extraglomerular mesangial cells

Afferent arteriole

Granular cells (contain renin)

Sympathetic nerve fiber

Glomerulus

Distal tubule   Macula densa cells

Efferent arteriole

Proximal tubule

FIGURE 14-3 Reabsorption of solute from the descending and ascending limbs of the loop of Henle. (From Field MJ, Pollock CA, Harris DC: *The Renal System.* Philadelphia, 2001, Churchill Livingstone)

Henle are relatively short. Most do not reach the medulla. A second population of nephrons, the juxtamedullary nephrons (which comprise approximately 20% of the total nephron population), have corpuscles close to the renal medulla, and their loops extend deep into the medulla. They are more involved in concentrating the urine. Although both sets of nephrons empty into common collecting tubules, their effluent is different.

Urine formation begins when hydrostatic pressure causes water and solutes to move from the glomeruli into the tubular system. Changes in the diameters of the afferent and efferent arterioles affect the hydrostatic pressure within the glomerulus and control the filtration rate. If the afferent arteriole is constricted, blood flow into the glomerulus is reduced, and pressure within the capillary bed is decreased. If the efferent arteriole is constricted, the volume of blood leaving the glomerulus is decreased, and the hydrostatic pressure is increased. Thus, different degrees of constriction and dilation at these sites can control filtration pressure and rate, a process called *autoregulation*, which, under normal conditions, protects the subunits of the kidneys from extremes of high or low blood pressure.

Filtrate passes from the glomerulus into the low-pressure proximal convoluted tubule. Water is actively reabsorbed through the tubule, but most transfer of water from the proximal tubule occurs passively by osmosis, leaving higher concentrations of the remaining substances within the tubule. Other substances, such as glucose, amino acids, small proteins, uric acid, lactic acid, phosphate, and sodium are actively reabsorbed into the blood from the filtrate in the proximal tubule. As the positively charged sodium ions are transported, negative ions such as chloride, bicarbonate, and phosphate accompany them (passive transport). As the solutes are transported, more water is osmotically pulled into the capillaries as well, reducing the amount of fluid in the proximal tubule.

A countercurrent mechanism is set up around the loops of the juxtamedullary nephrons. The fluid in the descending loop of Henle becomes hypertonic, as described earlier. As the solute moves into the ascending limb, it continues to be reabsorbed, but the tubules are impermeable to water. In the thick ascending limb, chloride ions are actively reabsorbed, and sodium molecules passively follow. Because water cannot follow, the ascending loop fluid is relatively hypotonic, and the interstitial fluid surrounding it becomes hypertonic. This fluid also surrounds the descending loop and reenters it by diffusion, making it more hypertonic. Thus, the fluid in the descending loop is hypertonic and that in the ascending loop is hypotonic. The interstitial fluid surrounding the medullary loops has the greatest concentration at the tips of the loops and is less concentrated as it approaches the renal cortex. The vessel loop surrounding the tubules—the vasa recta formed from the efferent arteriole—gradually takes in sodium and chloride by diffusion as it flows down the proximal loops and releases it back into the interstitium as it flows through the distal loops, so that little sodium chloride actually leaves the renal medulla.

When tubular fluid reaches the distal convoluted tubule, it is relatively dilute. The cells of the tubule are impermeable to water unless acted upon by antidiuretic hormone (ADH) in response to signals by osmoreceptors in the hypothalamus. In the absence of ADH, dilute urine will be transported to the renal pelvis. In the presence of ADH, the tubules become permeable, and water leaves the duct by osmosis as the collecting tubule passes through the hypertonic interstitial fluid in the renal medulla. Thus, in the presence of ADH, the urine becomes concentrated.

In addition, the kidneys excrete uric acid and urea, as well as actively secreting other substances into the urine. Some organic compounds, including antibiotics, histamine, phenobarbital, and others, are secreted. Hydrogen ions are actively secreted in large quantities, particularly in the proximal segment. Potassium ions are actively reabsorbed in the proximal tubule. Furthermore, active reabsorption of sodium ions out of the distal collecting ducts leaves a negative charge within the ducts; therefore, potassium ions pass back into the tubules to the more negative side.

While much of the cardiac output is diverted to the kidneys to allow them to filter large volumes of blood, most of the blood flow goes to the cortex; relatively little goes to the medulla, thus preserving the osmotic gradient and minimizing the risk of diluting the concentration.[9] In addition, the area of the thick ascending limb that is responsible for actively reabsorbing sodium consumes a large amount of oxygen, which is the main determinant of the medullary oxygen requirement. The P_{O_2} in the medulla is 10 mmHg to 20 mmHg, which is lower than the P_{O_2} in the cortex, which is about 50 mmHg.[10] Because of the low P_{O_2} in the medulla and the relatively low blood flow, this area becomes a watershed area. Thus, a delicate balance must be maintained between oxygen utilization and delivery.

During ischemia, intracellular adenosine triphosphate is broken down and depleted. Phospholipases are activated that release arachidonic acid stored in phospholipids in the cell membrane. There is loss of the epithelial brush border, destruction of tight junctions, and activation of cytokines. Cells die and slough into the lumen, obstructing the flow of filtrate. Commonly, this begins with a loss of concentrating ability, followed by oliguria and anuria.[11]

MODULATION OF RENAL BLOOD FLOW. Many agents can affect renal blood flow. Because oxygen demand in the medulla is regulated by the rate of active reabsorption in the thick ascending limb of the loop of Henle, factors that decrease the rate of delivery of filtrate to that area will decrease oxygen demand. Thus, constriction of the afferent limb in the glomerulus (eg, by angiotensin) or dilation of the efferent limb (eg, by prostaglandin E_2), as well as inhibition of active transport by loop diuretic drugs (which can increase the Po_2 from 16 mmHg to 35 mmHg), can favorably affect oxygen balance.[12]

Control of sodium and fluid balance is achieved through sensors of intravascular volume located in the atria, carotid arteries, and kidneys (in the JGA). Pressure in the atria can lead to release of atrial natriuretic peptide (ANP) and ADH. The carotid sinus modulates sympathetic nervous system activity and ADH secretion. Changes in the JGA affect the renin-angiotensin-aldosterone system.

HORMONAL INFLUENCES ON THE KIDNEY

Renin-angiotensin-aldosterone. Renin is secreted from the granular cells within the JGA, leading to release of angiotensin I, which is converted to angiotensin II, a potent vasoconstrictor. Angiotensin II also stimulates release of aldosterone from the adrenal glands, enhancing sodium reabsorption at the distal nephron.

Antidiuretic hormone is released from the posterior pituitary gland, primarily in response to stimulation of osmoreceptors in the anterior hypothalamus. Antidiuretic hormone is almost undetectable at levels of plasma osmolality less than 280 mOsm/kg and increases almost linearly at higher levels. Nonosmotic controls also exist, responding to changes in blood volume, left atrial pressure, catecholamines, angiotensin II, ANP, nausea, pain, and drugs.[8]

Atrial natriuretic peptide. Released in response to atrial distention, ANP causes arterial vasodilation and increased urinary sodium and water excretion. It can also modulate afferent arteriolar dilation and efferent constriction to increase GFR.

HYDROSTATIC FACTORS AFFECTING THE KIDNEYS. Low-pressure receptors are located in the atria. High-pressure arterial baroreceptors are present in the aortic arch, the carotid sinus, and the afferent arteriole. These receptors act by changing sympathetic outflow to the afferent and efferent arterioles. In addition, the low-pressure venous baroreceptors directly inhibit proximal tubular sodium transport, cause arteriolar and venous dilation, and inhibit renin secretion.[8]

INTRARENAL FACTORS AFFECTING THE KIDNEYS. Various intrarenal factors also affect vasodilation and sodium excretion. Prostaglandin E_2 inhibits sodium transport in the thick ascending limb and the collecting duct and also mediates the natriuretic response to pressure. Prostaglandin E_2 also relaxes mesangial cells, whereas thromboxane A_2 constricts them. Prostaglandin I_2 may mediate baroreceptor-induced changes in renin secretion. Nitric oxide mediates the vasodilating effect of bradykinin, and endothelium-derived nitric oxide modulates the GFR and renal sodium excretion.

Laboratory Evaluation of Renal Function

BLOOD UREA NITROGEN. Although multiple tests of renal function exist, none is ideally suited for evaluation during surgical procedures. The most commonly obtained blood tests are measurements of blood urea nitrogen (BUN) and serum creatinine levels. The BUN represents protein catabolism, the product of which (ammonia) is converted to urea by the liver. Thus, the BUN level can be elevated by high dietary protein intake, decreased GFR, metabolism of blood (as during a gastrointestinal bleed), and accelerated catabolism (eg, trauma or sepsis). Catabolic drugs (eg, corticosteroids) may elevate the BUN level. Liver failure, as well as starvation, may decrease the BUN level. In addition, although nitrogen is freely filtered at the glomerulus, it is variably reabsorbed by the renal tubules, particularly during dehydration. Measuring the BUN level is therefore an imprecise test of renal function.

CREATININE. Serum creatinine is produced through the conversion of creatine, a product of muscle metabolism. Creatinine is filtered from blood in the glomerulus but is not resorbed. The serum level of creatinine is normally constant in a given individual. Because the serum creatinine level is dependent on muscle mass, a muscular person would have a higher serum creatinine level than would an asthenic individual. Creatinine levels are generally higher in men than in women and generally higher in younger than in elderly persons. In an individual, an increase of serum creatinine of 0.5 mg/dL over 24 hours is compatible with a diagnosis of acute renal failure. After acute changes in the GFR, serum creatinine requires 48 to 72 hours to equilibrate. In the absence of flow to the kidneys, serum creatinine increases by 1 to 3 mg/dL per day.[12] The GFR decreases with age (approximately 5% per decade after 20 years of age). However, because increases in age are accompanied by decreasing muscle mass, creatinine tends to remain constant.

In a patient with changes in the GFR, a twofold increase in serum creatinine reflects a 50% reduction in the GFR. The GFR can be estimated by the following formula for creatinine clearance, which takes age and muscle mass into consideration; for women, the result of this equation is multiplied by 0.85 to compensate for their smaller muscle mass.

$$\text{GFR} = [(140 - \text{age}) \times \text{lean body weight}] \div (72 \times \text{plasma creatinine})$$

Normally, the BUN-to-creatinine ratio is between 10:1 and 20:1. Because BUN is affected by low tubular flow rates but serum creatinine is not, higher ratios are found in patients with decreased renal perfusion. In these cases, volume depletion should be suspected, as it should be with renal artery obstruction or diseases associated with low intravascular volume (prerenal azotemia). The ratio can also change with elevation of levels of other factors that increase the BUN level (eg, increased dietary protein, gastrointestinal bleeding). Creatinine clearance measurements involve 24-hour urine collections (or 2-hour collections through a catheter).[13] An ideal estimate of GFR would be based on measurements of a substance that is freely filtered and excreted only by glomerular filtration. One such substance is insulin. However, because measuring insulin clearance is inconvenient, creatinine is used to estimate the GFR using the following equation

$$C_x = (U_x) \times (V/P_x)$$

where C_x is clearance of substance x, U_x is urine concentration of substance x, P_x is plasma concentration of x, and V is urine volume. The V is derived because, if a substance is freely filtered across the capillary wall and excreted only by glomerular filtration, its rate of filtration is equal to its rate of urinary excretion. Thus, the following formula is used[8]:

$$GFR \times P_x = U_x \times V$$

URINE ANALYSES. Urinalysis, urine culture, urine sodium concentration, and fractional excretion of sodium are laboratory tests that can be performed to give insights into kidney function or dysfunction. A urinalysis gives information about urine pH, specific gravity, and the presence of blood, glucose, ketones, protein, bilirubin, and sediments such as crystals, cells, bacteria, or casts. Specific gravity reflects the ability of the kidneys to concentrate urine. The presence of glucose, ketones, red or white blood cells, bacteria, or casts invites further investigation. When glucose levels are normal, the nephron reabsorbs all the glucose that is filtered, and spilling of glucose into the urine indicates possible hyperglycemia. Protein in the urine may indicate glomerulonephritis, and the presence of red blood cells indicates a need for investigation for bleeding abnormalities. White blood cells are associated with infection. Diseased nephrons produce tubular casts. The presence of crystals may indicate metabolic abnormalities.

Tests of urinary sodium concentration and fractional excretion of sodium can be used to differentiate prerenal from renal causes of oliguria. Normally, in cases of hypovolemia, the kidneys effectively conserve water and sodium. With prerenal causes of oliguria, urine sodium concentration is usually less than 20 mEq/L. A urine sodium concentration greater than 40 mEq/L is indicative of a renal cause of oliguria. The fractional excretion of sodium compares the urine-to-plasma ratio of sodium to the urine-to-plasma ratio of creatinine $\times$ 100. Urinary fractional excretion of sodium of less than 1% indicates prerenal azotemia; a level of more than 2% points to ischemic or nephrotoxic acute renal failure.[8]

None of these tests is readily available during surgical procedures; thus, despite its inaccuracies, measurement of urine output is the method most commonly used for assessing renal function. Other methods that examine intravascular volume and pressure status can give a better estimate of organ perfusion than urine output.

Challenges to the Kidneys in Patients Undergoing Aortic Surgery

PATIENT FACTORS. Patients with vascular disease who require major vascular operations often have preexisting hypertension, cardiac disease, or diabetes or baseline renal insufficiency. Hypertension, cardiac disease, and diabetes are also risk factors for the development of chronic renal disease, which may be subclinical in daily life but becomes evident when the kidneys are subjected to the multiple insults involved in major vascular operations.

USE OF CONTRAST AGENTS. The injection of a contrast agent represents the first in a series of insults to the kidneys as a patient proceeds through diagnosis and work-up, the operation itself, and the postoperative course. Radiocontrast-induced nephropathy develops in approximately 10% to 20% of patients after administration of iodine-based dye.[14] The kidneys are particularly susceptible to contrast damage because they receive a high fraction of the cardiac output. Because solutes are absorbed and concentrated in the kidneys, exposure to toxins is increased. The effects of contrast agents on the kidneys may last several days or weeks. Typically, the serum creatinine level increases (peaking within 3 to 4 days) as creatinine clearance decreases and oliguria occurs.

Radiologic contrast agents aggravate outer medullary hypoxia by enhancing metabolic activity and oxygen consumption through osmotic diuresis and increased salt delivery to the distal nephron, increasing the workload of active salt reabsorption. Relative hypoxia occurs despite the fact that regional blood flow and oxygen supply actually increase.[15] Marked outer medullary vasodilation is accompanied by prominent cortical vasoconstriction.[16]

Patients arriving for aortic operations have usually had recent angiography and are dehydrated from diuresis caused by the contrast dye. They are then allowed no liquid or food for prolonged periods and frequently receive bowel-cleansing regimens before coming to the operating room. These patients are then susceptible to further morbidity during the operation.

Some patients are at particularly high risk of developing renal impairment, particularly those with preexisting renal disease such as diabetics with nephropathy. Because patients with preexisting kidney damage already have fewer nephrons, toxins are concentrated into smaller amounts of renal tissue, increasing exposure. Furthermore, patients with type II diabetes who are taking metformin may develop fatal lactic acidosis after injection of contrast media.

Preprocedural and postprocedural hydration to offset dehydration from contrast-induced diuresis has been shown to be effective in preventing nephropathy.[14] Volume expansion and facilitation of rapid flow through the kidneys by means of diuretic agents such as ANP, loop diuretics, and mannitol are also important. The use of other drugs, such as calcium channel-blocking agents, theophylline, or dopamine, may provide benefit as well. The authors recommend using low-osmolar nonionic contrast media in the smallest possible dose. Unfortunately, the cost of nonionic contrast agents is higher than that of ionic agents, although the substitution might be viewed as inexpensive, considering the cost of prolonged hospitalizations to treat the consequences of nephropathy. Avoidance of repeat studies that involve contrast injection within short time intervals and, whenever possible, allowing time for the kidneys to fully recover before subjecting them to further insults can reduce the risk of worsening failure with subsequent operations.

Interventions found to attenuate radiocontrast nephropathy include adequate intravascular filling, cardiac output, and renal perfusion pressure, as well as the avoidance of hypoxemia, marked anemia, and nephrotoxins.[17] The use of fenoldopam mesylate, a dopamine-1 receptor agonist that augments renal plasma flow, has shown promise in reducing the rate of contrast-induced nephropathy.[18]

CROSS-CLAMP. Placement of an aortic cross-clamp may interfere with the blood supply to the kidneys, and when the cross-clamp is removed, the ischemic kidneys are flooded with debris and byproducts of anaerobic metabolism from the hypoperfused areas distal to the cross-clamp. Achieving adequate oxygen delivery by maximizing cardiac output is a key factor in preventing renal damage due to ischemia. This process begins before placement of the aortic cross-clamp. If the kidneys become ischemic and are treated after they become oxygen deprived, the chances of recovery are much lower than if they are prevented from becoming ischemic in the first place. Thus, adequate cardiac output and reasonable oxygen-carrying capacity must be maintained throughout the operation. The length of cross-clamp time significantly affects tissue ischemia. The incidence of renal failure is as high as 6.3% in patients undergoing resections of descending thoracic aneurysms with clamp times of 46 to 60 minutes.[19] The experience of the surgeon in clamp placement can affect outcome as well. More experienced surgeons have better outcomes than do those with little experience, and individual surgeons have improved outcomes as they gain additional experience.[20,21]

The degree of ischemia depends on whether the cross-clamp is placed in a suprarenal or an infrarenal position. Whereas thoracic aorta cross-clamping is associated with an 85% to 94% decrease in renal blood flow, infrarenal clamping, which is associated with an increase in renal vascular resistance, can lead to a 30% decrease in blood flow.[22,23] With suprarenal clamping, adequate cardiac output is the key to perfusion through collateral vessels. Volume management remains important in the period after removal of the cross-clamp, during which vasodilation, lactate, and free radicals are present.

Placement of the cross-clamp taxes the heart as well as the organs distal to the clamp. The initial effect is a large increase in afterload, which causes an elevation in systemic vascular resistance and increases filling pressures of the heart.[24] Gelman et al demonstrated in a dog model that cross-clamping the aorta at the level of the diaphragm was associated with increased flow to organs and tissues proximal to that level.[25] In contrast, clamping at a suprarenal level did not significantly alter the blood volume in any area studied (brain, left and right ventricles, lungs, deltoid muscles, liver, and intestines). Blood flow to the area above the cross-clamp increased, while flow below it decreased. This phenomenon changed, however, with the level of the cross-clamp. When the clamp was below the celiac trunk, there was little increase in preload, presumably because of increased blood volume entering the splanchnic circulation. Cross-clamping above the celiac trunk was associated with a more significant increase in preload because of redistribution of blood flow and cardiac output to the organs above the clamp.

As demonstrated by Roizen et al using transesophageal echocardiography (TEE), cardiac output is decreased in the presence of a cross-clamp.[26] Gelman et al showed that the decrease could be caused by decreased oxygen consumption (increased mixed venous content) and not necessarily by deterioration of myocardial performance.[27] These authors also demonstrated a 40% decrease in ejection fraction with suprarenal clamping.[27] Effects on the kidney from this clamping are both direct (decreased flow past the clamp) and compensatory (increased systemic epinephrine and norepinephrine concentrations, leading to arteriolar constriction and further decreasing flow to the kidneys). Even an infrarenal cross-clamp can thus result in increased vascular resistance and a 30% decrease in renal blood flow.[28]

Depending on the level of the clamp, the surgeon may decide to perfuse the aorta distal to the cross-clamp, which has the advantage of helping to decrease hypertension proximal to the cross-clamp and thereby decreasing workload on the cardiovascular system. A second advantage is an increase in perfusion below the cross-clamp, potentially avoiding ischemia to the spinal cord and other organs distal to the clamp (Table 14–1).

Means of perfusion retrograde from distal to the cross-clamp include the following:

1. *Shunting between the proximal and distal aorta.* The most common type is the Gott shunt.
2. *Femoral vein to femoral artery bypass, utilizing an extracorporeal oxygenator and pump.* The disadvantage is that it requires heparinization.
3. *Atriofemoral pump.* Left atrial oxygenated blood is passed to the femoral artery via a pump. The rate can be controlled. Proximal hypertension can be controlled. Blood can be passed through heparin-bonded tubing, and systemic heparinization is not required. Compared with a cross-clamp-only group, patients undergoing this technique for repair of a TAAA had improved outcomes with regard to hospital mortality rates, need for postoperative dialysis, and paraplegia and paraparesis.[29]
4. *Selective organ perfusion used along with retrograde perfusion.* To perfuse the celiac trunk, the superior mesenteric artery, and both renal arteries, Jacobs et al used four 9F Pruitt catheters connected as an octopus to the extracorporeal circulation, administering at least 60 mL of fluid per hour through each catheter.[30] Svensson et al studied renal artery perfusion with cold Ringer's lactate solution in patients undergoing TAAA repairs.[31] Although no benefit was seen in a normal population, patients with preexisting renal dysfunction or renal artery occlusive disease had a significant reduction in the rate of acute renal failure. The investigators recommended using renal perfusion in such patients or in those for whom more than 45 minutes of cross-clamp time is anticipated. In another study, 30 patients undergoing Crawford II TAAA repair with left heart bypass had renal artery perfusion with either cold Ringer's lactate

TABLE 14-1

Advantanges and Disadvantages of Distal Perfusion Techniques

Advantages	Disadvantages
Control of proximal hypertension	Air emboli or embolic stroke
Reduction of visceral and renal ischemia	Increased operative time
Prevention of acidosis and declamping shock	Potential for excess hemorrhage with anticoagulation
Ability to rapidly warm patients	Shunt dislodgement.
Access for rapid volume infusion	
? Reduced incidence of paraplegia	

(at 4°C) or normothermic blood from the bypass circuit. One patient in the blood group experienced renal failure requiring hemodialysis. Ten patients (63%) in the blood-perfusion group and three patients (21%) in the cold-crystalloid-perfusion group had acute renal dysfunction.[32]

It is important to have a means of monitoring perfusion below the cross-clamp, particularly when the clamp is high on the aorta. Many practitioners use a femoral artery catheter to monitor below the clamp in addition to a radial artery catheter (right radial, if the clamp is proximal to the left subclavian artery or is likely to impede flow).

Cross-clamping may also result in the circulation of embolizing thrombotic material from the aorta, either to the kidneys and viscera or to the periphery, as a consequence of placement or removal of the clamp or any manipulation of the aorta. Furthermore, unclamping the aorta is associated with recirculation of acidotic and lactate-rich blood, followed by vasodilation, hypotension, and myocardial depression. Unclamping the aorta is also associated with prolonged decreases in renal blood flow and GFR, probably due to sympathetic stimulation and activation of the renin-angiotensin system during cross-clamping. Oyama et al measured blood flow in Macaque monkeys before and after hemorrhagic shock, after aortic cross-clamping and resuscitation, and following release of the cross-clamp and stabilization.[22] Total abdominal flow decreased with hemorrhage and then fell further with cross-clamping. Release of the cross-clamp produced profound acidosis, which was treated with sodium bicarbonate. After stabilization, kidney flow remained at 49% of baseline, although intestinal flow was 320% of baseline.

Prevention and Treatment of Renal Failure

The most important strategy for protecting the kidneys during aortic operations is to ensure delivery of adequate blood volume and oxygen to the tissues to balance supply and demand. Strategies for decreasing oxygen consumption and delivering optimal amounts of oxygen-carrying blood to the kidneys, coupled with strategies for minimizing oxygen uptake, need to be considered in order to minimize ischemic damage.

SUPRANORMAL HEMODYNAMIC VALUES. Shoemaker and various colleagues have looked at the intriguing concept of supranormal hemodynamic values. Although most of these studies were conducted with trauma patients, the following points should be noted. Patient outcome is better if hemodynamic values are optimized early (before organ failure) rather than late (after onset of organ failure). In a study of trauma patients who were randomly allocated to treatment aimed at normal values versus optimal values (cardiac index > 4.5 L/min/m², ratio of transcutaneous oxygen tension to F_IO_2 > 200, oxygen delivery index > 600 mL/min/m², and oxygen consumption index > 170 mL/min/m²), patients who reached optimal values (either in the optimal group or spontaneously among the control group) fared better. The investigators concluded that patients who can achieve optimal hemodynamic values are more likely to survive than those who cannot.[33,34] Although many patients undergoing major vascular operations might not be able to achieve or tolerate supranormal conditions, the concept of optimizing hemodynamic values before the onset of organ failure is worth considering.

MONITORING. Intraoperatively, urine output of 0.5 mL/kg/h is usually considered adequate. However, urine output cannot be relied upon as an indicator of adequate renal perfusion. Adequate urine output is not a guarantee that the kidneys are functioning normally and may occur when the patient is in high-output failure, is undergoing cold diuresis, or has received diuretics.

Oliguria may or may not portend problems with the kidneys and can have various causes. Prerenal oliguria can indicate decreased renal blood flow due to hypovolemia or obstruction of blood flow to the kidneys (eg, renal artery stenosis). Oliguria may indicate cellular dysfunction associated with ischemia or nephrotoxins. It may also be caused by postrenal obstruction at the level of the ureters, the prostate, or the urethra due to tumor or blood clots or simply a kink in the Foley catheter. Any of these conditions, as well as high-output renal failure, can occur during vascular operations. Thus, urine output is a nonspecific indicator, despite its major role in monitoring renal function during surgical procedures.

Close monitoring of intravascular volume status is paramount to maintaining adequate flow to the kidneys. Many authors advocate the use of a pulmonary artery catheter (PAC) for this purpose. Arguments for the use of a PAC rather than monitoring of central venous pressure (CVP) have been made for years. Mangano demonstrated good correlation between CVP and pulmonary artery occlusion pressure in patients with ejection fractions greater than 50% and poor correlation in patients with ejection fractions less than 40%.[35] More recently, Sandham et al randomly allocated 1994 patients (American Society of Anesthesiologists class III or IV) undergoing major abdominal, thoracic, vascular, or orthopedic operations to the use of PAC versus no PAC.[36] More than 50% of the patients were class III patients undergoing major vascular operations. Outcomes addressed included in-hospital mortality, 6- and 12-month mortality, and in-hospital morbidity. The investigators found no differences in median length of stay. The in-hospital mortality rate was 7.7% for the standard-care group and 7.8% for the PAC group. No difference was found between the two groups in mortality or morbidity rates, except an increase in pulmonary emboli in the PAC group. Postoperative renal insufficiency was 9.8% in the standard-care group and 7.4% in the PAC group ($P = 0.07$).

Transesophageal echocardiography (TEE), which is frequently used to help describe the extent and hemodynamics of a TAAA, represents another monitoring option. TEE has been shown to be as effective as a PAC in assessing volume status and is thus a valuable tool. Even with abdominal aneurysms, TEE is useful for assessing wall motion abnormalities in marginal status hearts when the cross-clamp is placed. The TEE can guide fluid therapy in such patients as well. In addition, TEE has been used (with angiography) to guide placement of endovascular stent grafts.[37]

PHARMACOLOGIC INTERVENTION. Many classes of drugs are potentially effective in preventing renal injury during major vascular operations because of their effects on various parts of the nephron, on delivery of oxygenated blood to the kidney, or on medullary oxygen utilization. Some are routinely used; others are still in the trial stage.

Diuretics. Diuretics have been used for many years with the aim of keeping the kidneys functioning and maintaining urine production when perfusion pressure to the kidneys is mechanically blocked by an aortic cross-clamp. However, maintenance of urine production in the presence of a cross-clamp is no guarantee that the kidneys are functioning well. In addition, diuretics may dehydrate patients, further aggravating the delivery of oxygen to the kidneys. Thus, it is critical that adequate cardiac output be maintained when these drugs are being used. In fact, such agents can give a false sense of security involving the kidneys, and the worry is that volume support may be less aggressive if active urine production is seen.

By improving intravascular volume, mannitol does succeed in delivering more blood to the kidneys and may indeed protect them. In addition, mannitol decreases blood viscosity, which may also diminish renin release.[38] However, the increase in urine output resulting from the use of mannitol can lead to depletion of intravascular volume and worsening renal function. In addition, by initially increasing intravascular volume, it can place an additional burden on a marginal status heart, which is already facing the increased workload imposed by the cross-clamp. A small group of 28 patients studied for the effects of mannitol on renal impairment after infrarenal aortic aneurysm repair received either mannitol (0.3 g/kg) or a saline bolus before cross-clamping.[39] Although there were no significant differences in postoperative BUN level, serum creatinine concentration, or creatinine clearance between the groups, the mannitol group had lower mean levels of urinary albumin and *N*-acetyl-glucosaminidase postoperatively, indicating a reduced level of subclinical glomerular and renal tubular damage. Of note, however, one patient in the control group developed fatal postoperative renal failure, and two patients in the mannitol group succumbed to perioperative myocardial infarction. Since mannitol can increase intravascular volume, it is possible that it played a role in this instance. Thus, although the use of mannitol may be indicated, consideration must be given to maintaining intravascular volume and the ability of the heart to handle the initial increased volume load.

Furosemide may act to decrease oxygen utilization in the renal medulla. Rat kidney studies by Brezis et al demonstrated that the use of furosemide, which inhibits reabsorptive transport in the medullary thick ascending limb, increased medullary Po_2 from 16 ± 4 mmHg to 35 ± 4 mmHg without altering cortical Po_2.[40] Medullary flow was also markedly reduced by the use of furosemide ($-28\% \pm 6\%$), indicating that the effect was directly due to decreased tubular oxygen consumption. Similar effects were found with the use of the loop diuretics ethacrynic acid and bumetanide.

Any benefit accorded by the use of furosemide should be accompanied by adequate hydration. Weinstein et al studied patients who had preexisting renal insufficiency and were at high risk of developing renal failure after receiving radiocontrast agents.[41] Study patients received furosemide (mean dose of 110 mg) and a control group received a mean dose of 3 L of intravenously administered fluids. Serum creatinine levels deteriorated significantly in the group receiving furosemide, whereas no change occurred in the patients receiving fluids. Adequate hydration is of paramount importance in preventing renal damage in patients receiving contrast agents.

Dopamine. Dopamine is commonly used during major vascular operations to maintain perfusion and urine output, the primary indicator of adequate volume delivery. Dopamine stimulates D_1- and D_2-type receptors. The postsynaptic D_1 receptor increases adenylate cyclase activity and intracellular cyclic adenosine monophosphate. The presynaptic D_2 receptor may indirectly cause dilation by inhibiting norepinephrine release. A biphasic blood-pressure effect occurs with increasing doses of dopamine. At 1 and 2 µg/kg/min, the mean blood pressure decreases through a decrease in diastolic blood pressure, whereas at levels above 7.5 µg/kg/min, mean blood pressure increases through an increase in systolic blood pressure. At 3 µg/kg/min, a maximum effective renal plasma flow occurs.[42]

The natriuretic effect of dopamine is seen throughout the dose ranges. At 1 µg/kg/min to 5 µg/kg/min, sodium excretion is doubled, and above 7.5 µg/kg/min, sodium clearance is further increased, even as renal plasma flow decreases. Dopamine natriuresis occurs independent of effective renal plasma flow and GFR. The effect is abolished by specific D_1-receptor antagonists.[42] In renal tubular cells, dopamine inhibits Na^+, $K^{(+)}$-ATPase, causing decreased sodium reabsorption and impairment of tubuloglomerular feedback.[43]

The role of dopamine is controversial. Although it increases urine flow, it does not necessarily improve outcome. The use of dopamine may improve flow to the splanchnic beds, which also are at risk for injury during major vascular operations, but some studies show that splanchnic ischemia worsens in pigs receiving renal-dose dopamine.[44] One prospective, randomized, double-blind clinical study looked at liver transplant patients receiving renal-dose dopamine (3 µg/kg/min) for 48 hours.[45] No benefits were seen in postoperative urine output, GFR, or need for dialysis.

Heyman et al demonstrated, in anesthetized rats, that dopamine given at 10 µg/kg/min had no effect on cortical flow but increased outer medullary flow by $35\% \pm 5\%$ while not significantly altering the medullary Po_2.[46] This flow is higher than that with the traditional renal-dose dopamine (1–3 µg/kg/min). Studies of renal-dose dopamine in healthy animals and volunteers revealed that, although dopamine causes diuresis and natriuresis, as well as some vasodilation, it is not without risk due to its catecholamine and neuroendocrine effects.[43] The investigators concluded that the routine use of prophylactic renal-dose dopamine in surgical patients should not be recommended.

Baldwin et al studied patients after major vascular operations (elective infrarenal abdominal aortic aneurysm or aorto-bifemoral grafting) who had adequate hydration and were randomly allocated to receive 3 µg/kg/min of dopamine or a saline infusion.[47] None of the measured parameters (creatinine levels, plasma urea levels, creatinine clearance at 24 hours, and urine volumes) showed significant differences between the groups, although urine volumes were slightly higher in the dopamine group. The lack of difference between the groups led the authors to suggest that generous fluid replacement alone was as effective as fluid combined with low-dose dopamine. Thus, although renal-dose dopamine is widely given to patients undergoing major vascular operations, there is no compelling evidence supporting this use.

Fenoldopam mesylate is a selective agonist of D_1 receptors that has been studied for a possible role in the prevention of renal failure. It causes relaxation of smooth muscle, vasodilation, and inhibition of tubular reabsorption of sodium in the kidney (thus inhibiting oxygen utilization and decreases in Po_2). Because it lacks D_2 effects, fenoldopam has no α- or β-adrenergic effects, and its use may avoid some of the negative effects found with dopamine.[48] Tumlin et al compared fenoldopam with normal saline in patients receiving radiocontrast agents, which induces intense vasoconstriction in the already hypoxic renal medulla.[49] A total of 51 patients with chronic renal insufficiency received either 0.5 normal saline or 0.5 normal saline with 0.1 μg/kg/min of fenoldopam, beginning at least 1 hour before administration of the contrast dye. Renal plasma flow improved from baseline in the fenoldopam group (+15.8%) but not in the group receiving saline alone. The incidence of nephropathy at 48 hours was 21% for the fenoldopam group versus 41% for the saline group (among diabetic patients, the incidence was 33% vs 64%). The peak serum creatinine level after 72 hours was 2.8 mg/dL in the fenoldopam group versus 3.6 mg/dL in the saline group. The investigators concluded that fenoldopam is a promising prophylactic agent for use in patients with radiocontrast-induced nephropathy. In still another study, patients undergoing infrarenal cross-clamping for aortic operations received an infusion of either fenoldopam at 0.1 μg/kg/min or placebo.[50] The infusions were started before surgical incision and continued until after the cross-clamp was removed. Multiple tests of renal function were performed. The use of fenoldopam was not associated with hemodynamic instability. Creatinine clearance remained stable in the fenoldopam group but decreased significantly in the placebo group (with the decrease persisting for at least 8 hours after release of the cross-clamp). On the first postoperative day, plasma creatinine concentration was increased with placebo but not with fenoldopam. This study included only 28 patients but supported the hypothesis that fenoldopam has a renoprotective effect during and after infrarenal aortic cross-clamping. However, fenoldopam does increase heart rate, which may limit its efficacy as a sole agent.

Another dopamine analog being studied is ibopamine, an agonist at D_1 and D_2 receptors that may be useful in retarding progressive renal failure. However, ibopamine has been shown to increase mortality in a study of its use in patients with heart failure.[51]

Vasodilators

Nitroglycerin. Management of the increase in blood pressure and afterload due to cross-clamping often includes the administration of vasodilators, which aid with afterload and preload issues proximal to the clamp. The use of nitroglycerin can help improve coronary flow, enabling the heart to tolerate the increased workload.[52] However, the improvement may not be enough to counteract the increased oxygen demand. Although the use of nitroglycerin helps control the increases in blood pressure above the clamp, it also causes vasodilation and lowering of blood pressure below the clamp, risking not only ischemia of the organs distal to the clamp, but also decreasing perfusion pressure to the spinal cord.

Thus, nitroglycerin infusion can help dilate the vascular beds to allow volume loading before placement of the cross-clamp and can help control blood pressure and preload when the aorta is cross-clamped. It then provides vascular dilation for fluid loading during the cross-clamp period. The nitroglycerin infusion should be stopped before the cross-clamp is removed. The use of nitroglycerin should be limited in patients at high risk for developing spinal cord ischemia, however, because it causes increased cerebrospinal fluid pressure and decreased spinal cord perfusion pressure.[38]

Sodium Nitroprusside. The use of sodium nitroprusside decreases perfusion pressure distally as well as proximally to the cross-clamp, thereby worsening the risk of ischemia in underperfused areas. Gregoretti et al used a dog model to demonstrate that sodium nitroprusside increased cardiac output and blood flow above the aortic occlusion but decreased blood flow and oxygen consumption below the occlusion.[53] Cernaianu et al also showed, in a dog model, that the use of sodium nitroprusside increases cerebrospinal fluid pressure, decreases spinal cord perfusion pressure, and increases ischemia.[54]

The actual shunting of blood due to cross-clamping is complex. In addition to increases in preload and afterload, an increase in mixed venous oxygen content is found, which is contrary to the expectation that inadequate cardiac output would lead to increased extraction and decreased mixed venous oxygen. The increase in mixed venous oxygen content does not necessarily imply adequacy of tissue perfusion, however. This phenomenon may reflect a decrease in uptake by the total body that is attributable to a decrease in the perfused mass of tissues and to increased arteriovenous shunting, which is not associated with nutritive flow to the tissues.[27]

Angiotensin-Converting Enzyme Inhibitors. The renin-angiotensin-aldosterone system causes an increase in renal vascular resistance and sodium resorption during cross-clamping that can last for hours after unclamping.[55] In an animal model comparing pretreatment with an angiotensin-converting enzyme inhibitor with controls, the use of an angiotensin-converting enzyme inhibitor was associated with lower values of renal blood flow during cross-clamping and higher values immediately after unclamping.[56] In another study, Licker et al looked at a small group of 22 patients undergoing aortic operations with infrarenal cross-clamping who received 50 μg/kg of enalapril versus saline before cross-clamping.[57] These patients had significantly better renal plasma flow and, on the first postoperative day, had significantly higher creatinine clearance when compared with the control group.

Nonsteroidal anti-inflammatory drugs. The use of nonsteroidal anti-inflammatory drugs has long been known to predispose patients to increased risks of developing acute or chronic renal disease. Agmon and Brezis demonstrated in 1993 that, in volume-expanded rats, the use of indomethacin caused a significant decrease in outer medullary blood flow.[58] More recently, the effects of the cyclooxygenase-2 antagonist nabumetone were studied in rat kidneys. The authors hypothesized that the cyclooxygenase-1 enzyme was physiologically important for prostaglandin synthesis in the normal kidney. Both nabumetone and its active metabolite reduced renal parenchymal prostaglandin E_2 to the same extent as did indomethacin. The kidneys of rats who had received oral nabumetone showed reduced GFR, filtration fraction, and urine volume. Hypoxic outer medullary tubular damage was seen when the kidneys were removed. However, the use of nabumetone showed no significant alteration in renal microcirculation in vivo when compared with controls, whereas the use of indomethacin, a nonselective cyclooxygenase inhibitor, did show significant changes.[59] In a study by Feldman et al, patients receiving intravenously administered ketorolac for 5 days did not show any increased incidence of acute renal failure when compared with patients receiving only opioids.[60]

Antioxidants. Oxygen free radicals are a product of metabolism in hypoxic conditions, inspiring research into the effects of antioxidants on hemodynamics after unclamping of the aorta. Wijnen et al specifically studied renal outcomes in patients undergoing infrarenal aortic aneurysm repair and treated with a multi-antioxidant regimen.[61] The ischemic injury resulted in albuminuria and impairment of renal function. The patients received standard treatment or standard treatment plus the antioxidants allopurinol, vitamin E, vitamin C, N-acetylcysteine, and mannitol. The albumin-to-creatinine ratio and 24-hour urine creatinine clearance were studied. Although the two groups showed no difference in the albumin-to-creatinine ratio, there was a significantly higher creatinine clearance in the antioxidant group at day 2.

Other pharmaceutical manipulations to counteract oxygen free radicals are under investigation. For example, superoxide dismutase, irbesartan (an angiotensin-II receptor antagonist), prostaglandin E_1, amlodipine (a calcium channel-blocking agent), and hydrochlorothiazide and hydralazine are being studied. Brosnan et al found that in rats, the use of irbesartan, amlodipine, and hydrochlorothiazide and hydralazine produced similar decreases in blood pressure, but irbesartan caused a greater reduction in superoxides.[62]

Natriuretic peptides. The natriuretic peptides regulate circulatory volume and promote renal sodium excretion by renal effects that increase renal flow in the glomerulus and increase GFR while decreasing release of renin. They also promote vasodilation through vascular smooth muscle by binding receptors that stimulate cyclic guanosine monophosphate (cGMP) synthesis. These peptides antagonize the effects of renin-angiotensin-aldosterone system activation, sympathetic nervous system activation, and endothelin.[63]

Atrial natriuretic peptide is normally released from the atrial cells after atrial distention. It appears both to have arterial vasodilating properties and to increase urinary sodium and water excretion in the renal tubules. It also mediates afferent arteriolar dilation and efferent constriction, thereby increasing GFR, inhibits renin and aldosterone at the level of the JGA, and inhibits ADH. Thus, ANP can significantly influence intravascular volume. Human ANP has been demonstrated to decrease peripheral vascular resistance, suppress the renin-angiotensin-aldosterone system, and exert a strong diuretic effect in patients undergoing cardiopulmonary bypass. Levels of ANP are increased in the circulation of patients with acute renal failure. The levels return to normal following renal transplantation but not after hemodialysis.[64]

Atrial natriuretic peptide has been studied in a number of situations involving the kidney. Its efficacy has been investigated in cases of radiocontrast-induced nephropathy. One study showed that the intravenous administration of anaritide (ANP 4-28) did not improve the incidence of nephropathy in a population of patients with preexisting stable chronic renal insufficiency when started at several dose regimens, 30 minutes before to 30 minutes after administration of radiocontrast agents.[65]

Other peptides, such as urodilatin, brain natriuretic peptide, and C-type natriuretic peptide, have been identified in various tissues. In view of their biologic effects, therapeutic efficacy might be anticipated for this class of drugs in cases of acute renal failure or congestive heart failure. A number of studies have investigated their efficacy in renal failure.[66]

Urodilatin is a natriuretic peptide isolated from human urine. It is processed from the same precursor as anaritide but is a 32-amino-acid peptide, whereas anaritide has 28 peptides. Urodilatin is synthesized in the tubular cells of the kidney and secreted into the lumens of the distal or collecting tubules to help regulate sodium and water resorption.[67]

Brain natriuretic peptide has been studied both as a treatment and as a marker for congestive heart failure. In people with suspected heart disease, a normal brain natriuretic peptide value indicates a low risk of cardiac impairment, whereas a consistently elevated plasma level of brain natriuretic peptide after myocardial infarction is associated with a distinctly poor prognosis. The cardiovascular and renal effects of anaritide and brain natriuretic peptide have great potential for patients with hypertension and conditions associated with volume overload. Limitations include the lack of an oral form of the drug.[68]

C-type natriuretic peptide is produced in vascular endothelial cells and acts as an endothelium-derived relaxing peptide. Infusions of C-type natriuretic peptide in volunteers have shown that it exerts significant diuretic, natriuretic, kaliuretic, and chloruretic actions, with increases in creatinine clearance. It also causes significant hypotension, with an accompanying increase in heart rate. Plasma aldosterone levels decreased significantly after administration of C-type natriuretic peptide.[69] Levels of C-type natriuretic peptide have been shown to be elevated in patients undergoing hemodialysis when compared with patients with normal renal function.[69]

Nitric oxide may play a role in protecting against renal failure. In a rat model, manipulating nitric oxide with a pan-nitric oxide-synthase inhibitor and then subjecting the rats to 60 minutes of infrarenal cross-clamping was associated with significantly worse renal failure when compared with controls.[70]

Renal Replacement Therapy

The most familiar type of renal replacement therapy is intermittent hemodialysis. Hemodialysis involves the movement of solutes diffusing along concentration gradients in an extracorporeal dialyzer. A semipermeable membrane separates the patient's blood from the moving dialysate, which flows away with the transported solutes. The toxins removed are usually the products of normal metabolism, which are typically found in urine. Excess fluid is removed through a hydrostatic pressure gradient across the membrane during dialysis treatment. Patients with renal failure undergo several hours of dialysis 3 days per week.

Bellomo et al compared dialysis modes in patients with acute renal failure who were in an intensive care unit.[71] They found in this population that there was better control of azotemia and hyperphosphatemia and increased nutritional intake in the patients undergoing acute continuous hemofiltration when compared with conventional dialytic therapy. The acute fluid shifts associated with conventional hemodialysis can have detrimental effects on organ perfusion in already unstable patients.

Continuous renal replacement therapy was developed to meet the needs of patients who developed acute renal failure or who were already on chronic dialysis but who were too unstable to undergo hemodialysis. Continuous renal replacement therapy can be used to address a patient's volume overload, as well as for solute removal. Patients receiving multiple intravenously administered medications and parenteral nutrition may have better hemodynamic status and improved cardiac and pulmonary function if continuous renal replacement therapy is used for fluid management.[72] In many intensive care units, continuous hemofiltration is used not only for blood purification, but also for treating certain drug intoxications and severe cardiac failure, controlling volume during and after cardiopulmonary bypass, and decreasing toxicity from chemotherapy.[73]

Although some continuous renal replacement therapy requires arterial and venous cannulation, several types use venous-to-venous flow, requiring large-bore double- or triple-lumen dialysis catheters. Access should be obtained through a large vessel, and scrupulously aseptic technique must be used. Because the venous-to-venous flow units are a low-pressure system, they require a pump.

Patients undergoing procedures with major fluid shifts have occasionally been treated intraoperatively with hemofiltration. Hemofiltration is often used during coronary artery bypass operations and has been used in patients with renal failure who are undergoing aortic aneurysm repair and in liver transplant recipients.[74,75]

Anesthetic Strategies

If patients have had injection of iodine-based contrast media, they should be given adequate recovery time—several days to 2 weeks—for their renal status to return to baseline. Patients should be hydrated generously. The administration of nonsteroidal anti-inflammatory drugs should be stopped before surgery.

Induction of anesthesia should be achieved in the customary fashion. Most induction agents have little effect on kidney function. However, in patients with existing renal disease, the hemodynamic effects may be altered because of decreased protein binding. Neuromuscular blocking agents should be chosen with the caveat that, if a patient has known renal disease, succinylcholine should not be used if the potassium concentration is elevated. Likewise, drugs that depend on renal excretion, such as pancuronium, should be used cautiously and should be carefully monitored if the patient is to be extubated at the end of the procedure.

Monitors for measuring volume status and assessing adequacy of hydration should be placed. A monitoring method other than urine output is recommended. PAC, CVP, or TEE may be used to ensure adequate hydration. Blood pressure should be manipulated with vasoactive infusions during aortic cross-clamping, but it is necessary to ensure that the patient is well hydrated. Retrograde perfusion should be used in patients at high risk for developing spinal cord ischemia.

Vasodilators and fluid loading should be used and should be stopped before the aortic cross-clamp is unclamped. Removal of the cross-clamp in increments by the surgeon may allow for gradual reintroduction of acidotic blood into the systemic circulation. Hypotension should be managed with inotropic agents or small doses of α_1-agonists to maintain vital organ perfusion.

The volatile anesthetic agents decrease renal flow because of vasodilation and, in the case of halothane, decrease cardiac output. Because halothane is associated with myocardial depression, it should probably not be used in situations in which the cardiac workload will be further increased by cross-clamping of the aorta. Some anesthetics have been shown to have deleterious effects on renal function. Metabolic products of methoxyflurane include fluoride ions, which can lead to vasopressin-resistant, high-output renal failure. Enflurane also has fluoride as a product of metabolism. Concentrations rise very slowly, and renal damage is unlikely, but it should not be used in patients with renal disease or in those at risk for developing renal dysfunction. Isoflurane is minimally metabolized to trifluoroacetic acid. The levels rise very slowly, and the risk of developing nephrotoxicity is extremely low from this agent. Desflurane is not associated with any nephrotoxic effects. It undergoes minimal metabolism, and fluoride levels are essentially unchanged by its use. Because of their low risk of causing renal damage, isoflurane and desflurane are good choices in patients undergoing major vascular operations. Sevoflurane metabolites include fluoride ions, and its use has been associated with impaired renal tubule function. In addition, degradation by soda lime can produce a product called compound A, which may also cause nephrotoxicity.

Placement of an epidural catheter before surgery should be considered. Although there is some concern about heparinization of patients who have epidural catheters in place, several studies have shown no instances of epidural hematomas in patients undergoing aortic operations. Baron et al found no significant benefit to using epidural versus general anesthesia for abdominal aortic surgery.[76] However, Yeager et al concluded that epidural anesthesia and postoperative analgesia exerted a significant beneficial effect on operative outcome in high-risk surgical patients.[77] If epidural anesthesia is used, it might be advisable to avoid administering the local anesthetic through the epidural catheter until the postoperative period, when the period of hypotension and decreased renal perfusion after removal of the cross-clamp has ended. Epidural opioids and local anesthetics are valuable in the emergent and extubation phases following the operation.

Positive pressure, positive end-expiratory pressure, and continuous positive airway pressure can all elevate mean intrathoracic pressure, decrease venous return to the heart, and decrease cardiac output, which in turn will decrease renal flow. These parameters should be optimized.

Whereas mild hypothermia may help reduce ischemic organ damage, generalized hypothermia can lead to multiple complications, including vasoconstriction from cold, elevated blood pressure, and increased myocardial oxygen consumption. In addition, hypothermia can lead to ventricular arrhythmias. It can also lead to disseminated intravascular coagulation, seriously complicating already challenging cases. Patients should be kept at normal or slightly below normal body temperature with fluid warmers, heating of the room, and warm air blankets. Warm air blankets should be used only above the level of the cross-clamp, as they can worsen ischemia in nonperfused areas and have been known to cause thermal burns in areas where there is minimal blood flow to carry away the accumulated heat.

The use of diuretics during cross-clamping may be of benefit but can be detrimental in patients with insufficient intravascular volume. The use of fenoldopam may significantly reduce renal morbidity associated with aortic operations. The primary issue for renal protection during major vascular operations is maintaining adequate volume replacement and maximizing renal flow. The authors therefore make the following recommendations: (1) allow sufficient time for renal recovery after an angiographic dye load, and (2) ensure adequate intraoperative hydration and renal perfusion by monitoring appropriately; using shunts, bypasses, or cold renal perfusion, if appropriate (as determined in consultation with the surgeon); maximizing renal flow during and after cross-clamping; and using diuretic agents while compensating for increased urine output.

Kidney Transplantation

In the United States, end-stage renal disease (ESRD) results from three major diseases, diabetes, hypertension, and glomerulonephritis, which affect nearly one-half million people. With more than 275,000 people dependent on dialysis, the annual cost is $19.35 billion. In 2000, 14,311 kidney transplants were performed, 62% from cadavers, 28% from living related donors, and 10% from living unrelated donors. With more effective organ preservation and immunosuppression, 1- and 10-year graft survival rates are 78% and 34.5% for cadaver transplants and 98% and 78% for living donor transplants, respectively.[78] Although numerous donor and recipient factors responsible for graft survival are largely out of the control of the anesthesiologist, the thoughtful evaluation and management of patients undergoing kidney transplantation are important in limiting the perioperative morbidity in these patients with severe systemic illness and optimally promoting graft function during the crucial first few hours after reperfusion of the organ.[79]

Surgical Principles of Kidney Transplantation

The technique of kidney transplantation typically proceeds with a right lower quadrant incision, exposure of the iliac vessels, and formation of a pocket in the iliac fossa. Venous anastomosis of the renal vein with the iliac vein is usually accomplished first, followed by arterial anastomosis of the donor renal artery with the hypogastric or iliac artery of the recipient. Reperfusion of the kidney is accomplished by unclamping of the proximal and distal venous clamps followed by the arterial clamp.[80] During the latter part of the vascular anastomoses, mannitol and furosemide are often given to promote diuresis, and, at some centers, a calcium channel-blocking agent may be injected into the renal artery. The urinary tract is then reestablished by a variety of means, depending on the condition of the bladder and ureter, but often by ureter-to-bladder anastomosis or renal pelvis-to-ureter anastomosis.

Renal Protection of the Donor Kidney

Continued function of a donor kidney is achieved by optimal management of donors and effective preservation, cooling, transport, and storage of the donor kidney, followed by timely reperfusion in combination with induction and long-term maintenance immunosuppression.

Kidney donors may be living related, living unrelated, heartbeating cadaver, or non-heart-beating cadaver donors. The techniques of harvest and preservation are according to institution-specific protocols, but the goal of each is to have adequate volume status, metabolic and hemodynamic stability, and established diuresis prior to harvest. Pharmacologic agents that may be given during this time include dopamine, mannitol, furosemide, calcium channel-blocking agents, steroids, and heparin. Once the donor kidney is removed, minimizing warm ischemic time is critical (often to less than a few minutes) by rapid flushing and cooling. A beneficial effect of cooling is significant reduction in metabolic activity, which is 5% at 5°C and is exemplified by satisfactory cold preservation of organs in excess of 24 hours and demonstration that 30 minutes of warm ischemic time is more damaging than an additional 24 hours of cold storage.[81,82] In the case of cadaver organs, a cold preserving solution such as the University of Wisconsin solution is flushed or continuously perfused into the organ. These preserving solutions contain a variety of buffers, electrolytes, and metabolic substances, such as glucose, amino acids, and adenosine, as well as osmotically active impermeable molecules that limit ischemia-related cellular edema.

Preoperative Evaluation of the Renal Transplant Recipient

The patient presenting for renal transplantation often has a considerable past medical history and is on a variety of therapeutic regimens aimed at controlling the morbidity associated with this serious chronic condition. Although the patient has likely been through a pretransplant evaluation, it is important to take a timely but thorough system-by-system approach to evaluating the patient; the perspectives of the transplant nephrologist and the anesthesiologist are quite different, and, typically, a significant period of time may have passed since the nephrologist's evaluation was completed. The underlying disease and therapeutic interventions, such as dialysis, can have profound short-term metabolic and hemodynamic effects that must be identified and quantified, and appropriate strategies must be instituted to safely navigate the patient through a major surgical procedure. An additional pressure in this critical preoperative period is the fact that time is of the essence. Increased cold ischemic time has recently been confirmed as the single and most important avoidable risk factor for graft failure,[79] and it is quite likely that the surgical team will enlist the anesthesiologist in promoting a timely course to the operating room.

ETIOLOGY OF END-STAGE RENAL DISEASE AND TYPE OF RENAL REPLACEMENT THERAPY. Diabetes remains the leading cause of ESRD, with hypertension and glomerulonephritis as other common causes. The etiology and treatment of ESRD are the key starting point for the evaluation of the renal-transplant recipient. Conditions severe enough to destroy the kidneys highlight the severity of the cause, and a search for etiology-related comorbidities must be sought because these comorbidities will likely be more common and more severe than in other patients. For example, in the patient with ESRD secondary to diabetes, the anesthesiologist should seek to identify symptoms suggestive of silent ischemia, autonomic neuropathy or gastroparesis, and occult infection.

Hemodialysis removes solutes and accomplishes fluid removal by diffusion across a semipermeable membrane in an extracorporeal circuit via a large venous access port or arteriovenous fistula. Patients usually have scheduled hemodialysis three times weekly and are heparinized at these sessions. Factors to consider preoperatively include timing since the last dialysis; presence, function, and protection of arteriovenous fistulas; volume status; heparin effect if the patient is dialyzed on the day of the impending operation; difficulty with peripheral or central vascular access due to repeated interventions; and electrolyte and acid-base status. Patients are often quite informative about their predialysis and postdialysis weight, fluid intake since last dialysis, and daily urine output, which are valuable clues to the patient's preinduction volume status. Preoperative dialysis is preferable in all patients to improve electrolyte disturbances, make volume management easier, and hopefully avoid early postoperative dialysis (and associated heparinization).

Peritoneal dialysis provides for solute and fluid removal by instilling dialysate fluid through a tunneled catheter into the abdomen and removing the fluid after a prescribed dwell time. Peritoneal dialysis has certain advantages, particularly with regard to patient quality of life, but these are tempered by the risk of peritonitis and pleural effusion, which are common in these patients.[83] Although the peritoneal cavity is not entered during a heterotopic renal transplant, it is important to ensure that the dialysate has been removed before proceeding to the operating room.

Noting the fact that a patient has had a previous renal transplant is important because it may affect the immunosuppressive regimen to be administered intraoperatively and may affect the complexity and length of the operation. The incidence of significant hypertension and coronary artery disease in the post-transplant population is very high.[84]

An increasing number of patients, particularly living-donor recipients, have yet to be started on renal replacement therapy despite their having significant uremic manifestations. Clues to subclinical volume overload, congestive heart failure, and pulmonary edema are important to elicit in these patients.

CARDIOVASCULAR DISEASE. Cardiovascular disease is an important cause, and result, of ESRD; both diabetes and hypertension, as leading causes of ESRD, are potent independent risk factors for perioperative cardiovascular complications.[85] The leading cause of graft failure after renal transplantation is death from a cardiovascular cause of a patient with a functioning graft.[78] It follows, then, that all patients with significant risk factors, particularly those with diabetes, should undergo a cardiac evaluation; even younger diabetic patients should have a cardiac evaluation if other traditional risk factors (ie, smoking or family history of diabetes) are present. Institutional protocol typically includes an electrocardiogram, an echocardiogram, and a dobutamine stress echocardiogram as part of the initial evaluation of potential transplant recipients.

PULMONARY AND AIRWAY EVALUATION. Other than being particularly mindful of the potential for patients to have effusions related to peritoneal dialysis or occult pulmonary infection, anesthesiologists need not undertake any extraordinary pulmonary investigations outside of normal practice. The airway

examination should address the presence of poor dentition, which may need to be addressed by the post-transplant medical team, as well as the possibility of limited temporomandibular or atlanto-occipital extension secondary to connective-tissue changes in diabetic patients.[86]

METABOLIC, ENDOCRINE, AND HEMATOLOGIC EVALUATION. Metabolic derangements are common, and their interaction and management are beyond the scope of this section but include hyperkalemia, hyperchloremia, hyponatremia, decreased bicarbonate and buffering capacity, chronic metabolic acidosis, secondary hyperparathyroidism, qualitative platelet disorder, and chronic anemia. Blood-gas and other laboratory evaluations should be completed in the immediate preoperative setting, after dialysis has been completed, to ensure that these abnormalities are managed appropriately during the dynamic perioperative period.

Attention to detail during the immediate preoperative examination, chart review, and preparation are of critical importance in achieving the best possible operative course. These factors include small details such as specifically noting deviations from the patient's normal antihypertensive and diabetes management, the antirejection (immunosuppressive induction) medication that has been given and the required intraoperative doses, and antibiotic orders. Specific to cadaveric renal transplantation is the need to confirm that tissue typing, if used at the institution, has been completed prior to proceeding to the operating room.

Intraoperative Management

Intraoperative management for renal transplantation is guided first and foremost by the comorbidities revealed during the preoperative evaluation, with four key points kept in mind: (1) carefully managing volume and hemodynamic status to maximize blood flow to the new graft, (2) avoiding the use of all medications and situations known to cause renal impairment, (3) ensuring prompt and accurate administration of immunosuppressive drugs (induction therapy), and (4) facilitating a smooth transition into the postoperative phase following recovery in the postanesthesia care unit, particularly in cases with suspected delayed early graft function.

Premedication with midazolam in divided doses is appropriate. Aspiration prophylaxis may be given at this time. Factors that make these patients potentially susceptible to pulmonary aspiration include autonomic dysfunction with delayed gastric emptying, recent peritoneal dialysis with residual dialysate, and recent ingestion of a meal in some cases when the preoperative notice has been short.

INDUCTION. Anesthetic induction should be guided by cardiovascular, hemodynamic, metabolic, and airway concerns. At this institution, induction with propofol or thiopental followed by succinylcholine with cricoid pressure until the airway is secured is the normal practice. In patients with acutely elevated potassium levels and the need to rapidly secure the airway, rocuronium may be used, with the realization that its duration of action may be unpredictable and possibly quite prolonged in the patient with ESRD. The metabolic characteristics of cisatracurium, relying on nonspecific ester hydrolysis and Hoffman elimination, make it the nondepolarizing neuromuscular-blocking agent of choice in renal transplantation and most general surgical cases in patients with ESRD.[87]

MONITORING. Standard noninvasive monitors must be placed to avoid artifact caused by or injury to existing arteriovenous shunts, which are so common in these patients; therefore, all patients are asked about the location of current functioning and previously placed nonfunctioning or poorly functioning shunts. Care must be taken to not place blood pressure cuffs on an extremity that has a shunt; the use of pulse oximetry on these extremities should also be avoided. Consistent with the theme of letting the preoperative evaluation guide the anesthetic technique, invasive monitoring of these patients is individualized within the following framework: nearly every patient should have a multiport CVP catheter placed to guide fluid replacement both intraoperatively and in the immediate post-transplant period. Placement of an arterial catheter is not required in most cases unless the preoperative evaluation reveals the potential for surgical technical difficulty or the patient's cardiovascular or pulmonary history suggests labile blood pressure, coronary ischemia, valvular disease, or the need for blood gas analysis. In all cases, the arterial catheter is removed in the postanesthesia care unit and direct pressure is held at the site in an effort to minimize the potential for injury because the vessel may be needed in the future for a shunt. Although not common in renal transplant practice, the use of PAC or TEE data to guide the intraoperative management in patients with untreated discrete or diffuse coronary artery disease, congestive heart failure, cardiomyopathies, or valvular lesions is certainly justified based on standard indications for these valuable monitors.[85,88] The need for immunosuppression mandates strict aseptic technique and proper sterile dressing of all invasive lines.

ANESTHETIC MAINTENANCE. Although the protocol calls for a balanced anesthetic technique of isoflurane, air, and oxygen and the use of fentanyl in moderate doses of 5 µg/kg to 10 µg/kg over several hours, it is the endpoints that matter most, and many techniques are appropriate. Importantly, avoiding the use of enflurane and sevoflurane because of their potential renal effects caused by fluoride and compound A, respectively, is prudent.

Intraoperative hemodynamic management is aimed at providing adequate blood pressure, intravascular volume, hemoglobin, and oxygenation following reperfusion of the graft. To this end, a variety of factors should be considered during the maintenance phase of the anesthetic procedure. Adequate intravascular volume improves allograft function,[89] and hydration with a potassium-free crystalloid solution with the addition of albumin, if necessary, to maintain the CVP at or above 8 mmHg to 10 mmHg is the typical therapeutic goal. Because of routine preoperative dialysis, this usually requires sequential fluid boluses. Blood loss during kidney transplantation is usually low (< 500 mL); however, because the patient may have preexisting anemia, transfusion with packed red blood cells may be necessary and is usually discussed with the surgeon or nephrologist preoperatively to sort out issues related to cytomegalovirus transmission and HLA sensitization. In some cases, such as the use of expanded-criteria (marginal) donors or long cold ischemic time, the anesthesiologist and the surgeon may agree upon an aggressive hydration regimen that will place a premium on the anesthesiologist's ability to detect subtle signs of overhydration prior to the onset of frank pulmonary edema. Some of these signs may be increasing

pulmonary artery pressures, rales, gallop, worsening oxygenation, and prominent jugular venous distention.

The surgical technique of heterotopic renal transplantation typically involves clamping and grafting of the iliac vessels. As in any vascular or orthopedic case involving limb ischemia, attention to the surgical field is important to avoid periods of hypotension associated with unanticipated reperfusion of the limb and of the graft. In the period preceding reperfusion, electrolytes, glucose level, and hemoglobin may need to be rechecked. At this institution, mannitol (25 g) and furosemide (100 mg) are administered intravenously during the vascular anastomoses, and some surgeons inject a calcium channel-blocking agent (verapamil 10 mg) directly into the renal artery following reperfusion. Of these interventions, the use of mannitol and calcium channel-blocking agents has been shown to decrease the incidence of acute tubular necrosis and early graft dysfunction.[90,91] Each of these surgical maneuvers and drug interventions, and certainly their combination, can lead to hypotension. For this reason, the use of long-acting antihypertensive agents is avoided in most circumstances; instead, early hypertension is managed by increasing anesthetic depth, using a short-acting antihypertensive agent (esmolol or nitroglycerine), or a combination of the two techniques. Renal-dose dopamine may be employed during the procedure to promote diuresis, although the benefit has not been unequivocally demonstrated.

Minutes before reperfusion, the volatile agent should be decreased and the intravascular volume reassessed. A systolic blood pressure of at least 120 mmHg is usually achieved following reperfusion; in all cases, systemic blood pressure should be maintained above 90 mmHg.[92] If the use of additional agents is required for adequate perfusion, low-dose dopamine (less than 5 µg/kg/min) or ephedrine in 5 to 10 mg doses is usually effective.

Management in the Postanesthesia Care Unit

Early postoperative care is straightforward and is often performed with early involvement of the transplant nephrologist. Occasionally, slow emergence to an alert state, which is presumed to be related to prolonged clearance of drugs, may be seen, but emergence should proceed steadily nevertheless. If not, an early metabolic work-up should begin without delay. Pain control is rarely problematic and is accomplished by intermittent bolus or patient-controlled analgesia. (The use of nonsteroidal anti-inflammatory drugs and meperidine should be avoided.) Hypertension may be significant and precipitous with emergence and is controlled by a variety of intravenously administered agents, including the β-adrenergic receptor-blocking agents, labetalol or esmolol, or vasodilating agents such as hydralazine. Unlike the use of short-acting antihypertensive agents in the period preceding graft reperfusion, the use of longer acting antihypertensive agents is appropriate postoperatively. Diabetes management may be complicated at this time due to earlier administration of high-dose corticosteroids and usually necessitates frequent measurements of blood glucose and, occasionally, therapy with insulin infusion.

Providing optimum conditions for diuresis and responding to early diuresis, or lack thereof, *and* communicating the clinician's efforts and concerns to the nephrologist, the surgeon, or both, are important aspects of the early postoperative period. Intravascular volume must be maintained at normal to high-normal levels to optimize conditions for graft function. Replacement of intravascular volume in accordance with urine output usually proceeds according to a set protocol with frequent assessment of volume status by monitoring of the CVP and clinical means. Particularly in the case of high urine output, serum potassium and sodium concentrations should be monitored, and adjustments should be made in the replacement fluid. In the event of postoperative oliguria, euvolemia must be ensured by maintaining the CVP at or above 8, and the urinary catheter must be checked for proper function and should be irrigated if necessary; after both of these interventions have taken place, a strategy for determining the cause of the oliguria should begin. The common reason for the early lack of function of the kidney in the euvolemic recipient is acute tubular necrosis, which should improve with time and meticulous care by the transplant team. The likelihood of other causes of oliguria in any particular patient must be considered because failure to quickly address mechanical or surgical causes of oliguria may lead to permanent loss of graft function in some cases. Surgical bleeding, vascular disruption or thrombosis, hematoma, urinary disruption, leak, or stenosis are among the possibilities.

Conclusion

Renal dysfunction is common in patients with vascular disease who are undergoing surgical procedures. Anesthesiologists must be familiar with renal physiology, with the pharmacology of drugs used throughout the perioperative period, with the surgical techniques used to correct vascular disease, and with the anesthetic principles that optimize outcome.

A subset of patients with ESRD will undergo renal transplantation. Anesthesiologists must likewise be familiar with the preoperative, intraoperative, and postoperative care of these patients.

REFERENCES

1. McCombs P, Roberts B: Acute renal failure following resection of abdominal aortic aneurysm, *Surg Gynecol Obstet* 148:175, 1979.
2. Chertow GM, Levy EM, Hammermeister KE, et al: Independent association between acute renal failure and mortality following cardiac surgery, *Am J Med* 104:343, 1998.
3. Dardik A, Lin J, Gordon T, et al: Results of elective abdominal aortic aneurysm repair in the 1990s: a population-based analysis of 2335 cases, *J Vasc Surg* 30:985, 1999.
4. Kashyap V, Cambria R, Davison J, et al: Renal failure after thoracoabdominal aortic surgery, *J Vasc Surg* 26:949; discussion 955, 1997.
5. Coselli JS, Conklin LD, LeMaire SA: Thoracoabdominal aortic aneurysm repair: review and update of current strategies, *Ann Thorac Surg* 74:S1881; discussion S1892, 2002.
6. Walker SR, Yusuf SW, Wenham PW, Hopkinson BR: Renal complications following endovascular repair of abdominal aortic aneurysms, *J Endovasc Surg* 5:318, 1998.
7. Harris JR, Fan CM, Geller SC, et al: Renal perfusion defects after endovascular repair of abdominal aortic aneurysms, *J Vasc Interv Radiol* 14:329, 2003.
8. Anger MS, Senkfor SI, Berl T: Water and sodium metabolism: control of water excretion. In Massry SG, Glassock RJ (eds): *Massry & Glassock's Textbook of Nephrology*, ed 4. Philadelphia, 2001, Lippincott Williams & Wilkins, 248.
9. Brezis M, Rosen S. Hypoxia of the renal medulla: its implications for disease, *N Engl J Med* 332:647, 1995.
10. Brezis M, Heyman SN, Epstein FH: Determinants of intrarenal oxygenation. II. Hemodynamic effects, *Am J Physiol* 267:F1063, 1994.
11. Lieberthal W, Koh JS, Levine JS: Necrosis and apoptosis in acute renal failure, *Semin Nephrol* 18:505, 1998.
12. Kassirer JP: Clinical evaluation of kidney function-glomerular function, *N Engl J Med* 285:385, 1971.
13. Sladen RN, Endo E, Harrison T: Two-hour versus 22-hour creatinine clearance in critically ill patients, *Anesthesiology* 67:1013, 1987.
14. Stone G, Tumlin J, Madyoon H, et al: Design and rationale of CONTRAST: a prospective, randomized placebo-controlled trial of fenoldopam mesylate for the prevention of radiocontrast nephropathy, *Rev Cardiovasc Med* 2:S31, 2001.
15. Heyman SN, Reichman J, Brezis M: Pathophysiology of radiocontrast nephropathy: a role for medullary hypoxia, *Invest Radiol* 34:685, 1999.
16. Heyman S, Goldfarb M, Carmeli F, et al: Effect of contrast agents on intrarenal nitric oxide and NO synthase activity, *Exp Nephrol* 6:557, 1998.
17. Ronco C, Bellomo R: Prevention of acute renal failure in the critically ill, *Nephron Clin Pract* 93:C13, 2003.
18. Madyoon H: Clinical experience with the use of fenoldopam for prevention of radiocontrast nephropathy in high-risk patients, *Rev Cardiovasc Med* 2:S26, 2001.
19. Livesay JJ, Cooley DA, Ventemiglia RA, et al: Surgical experience in descending thoracic aneurysmectomy with and without adjuncts to avoid ischemia, *Ann Thorac Surg* 39:37, 1985.
20. Forbes TL, De Rose G, Harris KA: A CUSUM analysis of ruptured abdominal aortic aneurysm repair, *Ann Vasc Surg* 16:527, 2002.
21. Batt M, Staccini P, Pittaluga P, et al: Late survival after abdominal aortic aneurysm repair, *Eur J Vasc Endovasc Surg* 17:338, 1999.
22. Oyama M, McNamara JJ, Suehiro GT, et al: The effects of thoracic aortic cross-clamping and declamping on visceral organ blood flow, *Ann Surg* 197:459, 1983.
23. Gamulin Z, Forster A, Morel D, et al: Effects of infrarenal aortic cross-clamping on renal hemodynamics in humans, *Anesthesiology* 61:394, 1984.
24. Roberts AJ, Nora JD, Hughes WA, et al: Cardiac and renal responses to cross-clamping of the descending thoracic aorta, *J Thorac Cardiovasc Surg* 86:732, 1983.
25. Gelman S, Khazaeli MB, Orr R, et al: Blood volume redistribution during cross-clamping of the descending aorta, *Anesth Analg* 78:219, 1994.
26. Roizen MF, Beaupre PN, Alpert RA, et al: Monitoring with two-dimensional transesophageal echocardiography: comparison of myocardial function in patients undergoing supraceliac, suprarenal-infraceliac, or infrarenal aortic occlusion, *J Vasc Surg* 1:300, 1984.
27. Gelman S, McDowell H, Varner PD, et al: The reason for cardiac output reduction after aortic cross-clamping, *Am J Surg* 155:578, 1988.
28. Gelman S: The pathophysiology of aortic cross-clamping and unclamping, *Anesthesiology* 82:1026, 1995.
29. Schepens MA, Vermeulen FE, Morshuis WJ, et al: Impact of left heart bypass on the results of thoracoabdominal aortic aneurysm repair, *Ann Thorac Surg* 67:1963; discussion 1979, 1999.
30. Jacobs MJ, de Mol BA, Legemate DA, et al: Retrograde aortic and selective organ perfusion during thoracoabdominal aortic aneurysm repair, *Eur J Vasc Endovasc Surg* 14:360, 1997.
31. Svensson LG, Crawford ES, Hess KR, et al: Thoracoabdominal aortic aneurysms associated with celiac, superior mesenteric, and renal artery occlusive disease: methods and analysis of results in 271 patients, *J Vasc Surg* 16:378; discussion 389, 1992.
32. Koksoy C, LeMaire SA, Curling PE, et al: Renal perfusion during thoracoabdominal aortic operations: cold crystalloid is superior to normothermic blood, *Ann Thorac Surg* 73:730, 2002.
33. Kern JW, Shoemaker WC: Meta-analysis of hemodynamic optimization in high-risk patients, *Crit Care Med* 30:1686, 2002.
34. Velmahos GC, Demetriades D, Shoemaker WC, et al: Endpoints of resuscitation of critically injured patients: normal or supranormal? A prospective randomized trial, *Ann Surg* 232:409, 2000.
35. Mangano DT: Monitoring pulmonary arterial pressure in coronary artery disease, *Anesthesiology* 53:364, 1980.
36. Sandham JD, Hull RD, Brant RF, et al: A randomized, controlled trial of the use of pulmonary artery catheters in high-risk surgical patients, *N Engl J Med* 348:5, 2003.
37. Gonzalez-Fajardo JA, Gutierrez V, San Roman JA, et al: Utility of intraoperative transesophageal echocardiography during endovascular stent-graft repair of acute thoracic aortic dissection, *Ann Vasc Surg* 16:297, 2002.
38. Simpson JI: *Anesthesia for Aortic Surgery.* Newton, Mass, 1997, Butterworth Heinemann.

39. Nicholson ML, Baker DM, Hopkinson BR, et al: Randomized controlled trial of the effect of mannitol on renal reperfusion injury during aortic aneurysm surgery, *Br J Surg* 83:1230, 1996.

40. Brezis M, Agmon Y, Epstein FH: Determinants of intrarenal oxygenation. I. Effects of diuretics, *Am J Physiol* 267:F1059, 1994.

41. Weinstein JM, Heyman S, Brezis M: Potential deleterious effect of furosemide in radiocontrast nephropathy, *Nephron* 62:413, 1992.

42. Olsen NV: Effects of dopamine on renal haemodynamics tubular function and sodium excretion in normal humans, *Dan Med Bull* 45:282, 1998.

43. Perdue PW, Balser JR, Lipsett PA, Breslow MJ: "Renal dose" dopamine in surgical patients: dogma or science? *Ann Surg* 227:470, 1998.

44. Segal JM, Phang PT, Walley KR: Low-dose dopamine hastens onset of gut ischemia in a porcine model of hemorrhagic shock, *J Appl Physiol* 73:1159, 1992.

45. Swygert TH, Roberts LC, Valek TR, et al: Effect of intraoperative low-dose dopamine on renal function in liver transplant recipients, *Anesthesiology* 75:571, 1991.

46. Heyman SN, Kaminski N, Brezis M: Dopamine increases renal medullary blood flow without improving regional hypoxia, *Exp Nephrol* 3:331, 1995.

47. Baldwin L, Henderson A, Hickman P: Effect of postoperative low-dose dopamine on renal function after elective major vascular surgery, *Ann Intern Med* 120:744, 1994.

48. Shorten GD: Fenoldopam: potential clinical applications in heart surgery, *Rev Esp Anestesiol Reanim* 48:487, 2001.

49. Tumlin JA, Wang A, Murray PT, et al: Fenoldopam mesylate blocks reductions in renal plasma flow after radiocontrast dye infusion: a pilot trial in the prevention of contrast nephropathy, *Am Heart J* 143:894, 2002.

50. Halpenny M, Rushe C, Breen P, et al: The effects of fenoldopam on renal function in patients undergoing elective aortic surgery, *Eur J Anaesthesiol* 19:32, 2002.

51. Doggrell SA: The therapeutic potential of dopamine modulators on the cardiovascular and renal systems, *Expert Opin Investig Drugs* 11:631, 2002.

52. Hummel BW, Raess DH, Gewertz BL, et al: Effect of nitroglycerin and aortic occlusion on myocardial blood flow, *Surgery* 92:159, 1982.

53. Gregoretti S, Gelman S, Henderson T, Bradley EL: Hemodynamics and oxygen uptake below and above aortic occlusion during crossclamping of the thoracic aorta and sodium nitroprusside infusion, *J Thorac Cardiovasc Surg* 100:830, 1990.

54. Cernaianu AC, Olah A, Cilley JH Jr, et al: Effect of sodium nitroprusside on paraplegia during cross-clamping of the thoracic aorta, *Ann Thorac Surg* 56:1035; discussion 1038, 1993.

55. Berkowitz HD, Shetty S: Renin release and renal cortical ischemia following aortic cross-clamping, *Arch Surg* 109:612, 1974.

56. Joob AW, Dunn C, Miller E, et al: Effect of left atrial to left femoral artery bypass and renin-angiotensin system blockade on renal blood flow and function during and after thoracic aortic occlusion, *J Vasc Surg* 5:329, 1987.

57. Licker M, Bednarkiewicz M, Neidhart P, et al: Preoperative inhibition of angiotensin-converting enzyme improves systemic and renal haemodynamic changes during aortic abdominal surgery, *Br J Anaesth* 76:632, 1996.

58. Agmon Y, Brezis M: Effects of nonsteroidal anti-inflammatory drugs upon intrarenal blood flow: selective medullary hypoperfusion, *Exp Nephrol* 1:357, 1993.

59. Reichman J, Cohen S, Goldfarb M, et al: Renal effects of nabumetone, a COX-2 antagonist: impairment of function in isolated perfused rat kidneys contrasts with preserved renal function in vivo, *Exp Nephrol* 9:387, 2001.

60. Feldman HI, Kinman JL, Berlin JA, et al: Parenteral ketorolac: the risk for acute renal failure, *Ann Intern Med* 126:193, 1997.

61. Wijnen MH, Vader HL, Van Den Wall Bake AW, et al: Can renal dysfunction after infra-renal aortic aneurysm repair be modified by multi-antioxidant supplementation? *J Cardiovasc Surg (Torino)* 43:483, 2002.

62. Brosnan MJ, Hamilton CA, Graham D, et al: Irbesartan lowers superoxide levels and increases nitric oxide bioavailability in blood vessels from spontaneously hypertensive stroke-prone rats, *J Hypertens* 20:281, 2002.

63. Conn PM: Natriuretic peptides in health and disease. In Sampson W, Levin E (eds): *Contemporary Endocrinology.* Totowa, NJ, 1997, Humana Press, 337.

64. Vesely DL: Natriuretic peptides and acute renal failure, *Am J Physiol Renal Physiol* 285:F167, 2003.

65. Kurnik BR, Allgren RL, Genter FC, et al: Prospective study of atrial natriuretic peptide for the prevention of radiocontrast-induced nephropathy, *Am J Kidney Dis* 31:674, 1998.

66. Michels P, Tarnow J: Natriuretic peptides: physiological, pathophysiological and clinical aspects, *Anasthesiol Intensivmed Notfallmed Schmerzther* 36:406, 2001.

67. Forssmann W, Meyer M, Forssmann K: The renal urodilatin system: clinical implications, *Cardiovasc Res* 51:450, 2001.

68. Stagnella G: Practical implications of current natriuretic peptide research, *J Renin-Angiotensin-Aldosterone System* 1:304, 2000.

69. Igaki T, Itoh H, Suga S, et al: C-type natriuretic peptide in chronic renal failure and its action in humans, *Kidney Int Suppl* 55:S144, 1996.

70. Pararajasingam R, Weight SC, Bell PR, et al: Prevention of renal impairment following aortic cross-clamping by manipulation of the endogenous renal nitric oxide response, *Eur J Vasc Endovasc Surg* 19:396, 2000.

71. Bellomo R, Mansfield D, Rumble S, et al: Acute renal failure in critical illness: conventional dialysis versus acute continuous hemodiafiltration, *ASAIO J* 38:M654, 1992.

72. Manns M, Sigler MH, Teehan BP: Continuous renal replacement therapies: an update, *Am J Kidney Dis* 32:185, 1998.

73. Ronco C, Bellomo R, Kellum J: Continuous renal replacement therapy, *Adv Renal Replace Ther* 9:229, 2002.

74. Sugawara Y, Sato O, Miyata T, et al: Continuous hemodiafiltration during aortic arch aneurysm repair in chronic renal failure patient, *Panminerva Med* 40:63, 1998.

75. Blackwell MM, Chavin KD, Sistino JJ: Perioperative perfusion strategies for optimal fluid management in liver transplant recipients with renal insufficiency, *Perfusion* 18:55, 2003.

76. Baron JF, Bertrand M, Barre E, et al: Combined epidural and general anesthesia versus general anesthesia for abdominal aortic surgery, *Anesthesiology* 75:611, 1991.

77. Yeager MP, Glass DD, Neff RK, et al: Epidural anesthesia and analgesia in high-risk surgical patients, *Anesthesiology* 66:729, 1987.

78. Annual Data Report United States Renal Data System, Vol. 2003. USRDS Coordinating Center, 2002.

79. Roodnat JI, Mulder PG, Van Riemsdijk IC, et al: Ischemia times and donor serum creatinine in relation to renal graft failure, *Transplantation* 75:799, 2003.

80. Lee HM: Surgical techniques of renal transplantation. In Morris PJ (ed): *Kidney Transplantation: Principles and Practice.* Philadelphia, 1994, WB Saunders, 128.

81. Harvey RB: Effect of temperature on isolated dog kidney, *Am J Physiol* 197:181, 1959.

82. Sacks SA, Petritsch PH, Kaufman JJ: Canine kidney preservation using a new perfusate, *Lancet* 1:1024, 1973.

83. Maiorca R, Cantaluppi A, Cancarini GC, et al: Prospective controlled trial of a Y-connector and disinfectant to prevent peritonitis in continuous ambulatory peritoneal dialysis, *Lancet* 2:642, 1983.

84. Massy ZA: Cardiovascular risk factors in kidney transplantation, *Curr Opin Urol* 11:139, 2001.

85. Eagle KA, Berger PB, Calkins H, et al: ACC/AHA Guideline Update for Perioperative Cardiovascular Evaluation for Noncardiac Surgery-Executive Summary: a report of the American College of Cardiology/American Heart Association Task Force on Practice Guidelines (Committee to Update the 1996 Guidelines on Perioperative Cardiovascular Evaluation for Noncardiac Surgery), *Anesth Analg* 94:1052, 2002.

86. Reissell E, Orko R, Maunuksela EL, Lindgren L: Predictability of difficult laryngoscopy in patients with long-term diabetes mellitus, *Anaesthesia* 45:1024, 1990.

87. Atherton DP, Hunter JM: Clinical pharmacokinetics of the newer neuromuscular blocking drug, *Clin Pharmacokinet* 36:169, 1999.

88. Practice guidelines for perioperative transesophageal echocardiography. A report by the American Society of Anesthesiologists and the Society of Cardiovascular Anesthesiologists Task Force on Transesophageal Echocardiography, *Anesthesiology* 84:986, 1996.

89. Lauzurica R, Teixido J, Serra A, et al: Hydration and mannitol reduce the need for dialysis in cadaveric kidney transplant recipients treated with CyA, *Transplant Proc* 24:46, 1992.

90. Richards KF, Belnap LP, Rees WV, et al: Mannitol reduces ATN in cadaveric allografts, *Transplant Proc* 21:1228, 1989.

91. Palmer BF, Davidson I, Sagalowsky A, et al: Improved outcome of cadaveric renal transplantation due to calcium channel blockers, *Transplantation* 52:640, 1991.

92. Barry JM: Technical aspects of renal transplantation. In Norman DJ, Turka LA (eds): *Primer on Transplantation.* Mt Laurel, NJ, 2001, American Society of Transplantation.

Hematologic Considerations in Vascular Surgery

15

Christopher A. Troianos, MD

Colleen Walker, DO

Normal Hemostasis

Hemostasis is a tripartite function depending on vascular integrity, adequate number and function of platelets, and a normal coagulation mechanism.[1] Bleeding occurs because of a defect in one or more of these individual elements. Vascular integrity is disrupted during any surgical procedure. Patients undergoing vascular surgery are particularly at risk because venous and arterial vessels are opened and have the potential for major bleeding. Restoration of hemostasis is dependent on surgical ligation of the bleeding site on the vessel, as well as the normal hemostatic mechanisms, in restoring vascular integrity. Blood clots in response to an insult to vascular integrity in two stages, termed primary and secondary hemostasis. The importance of these mechanisms can perhaps best be appreciated by the fact that the majority of blood vessels are less than 1 mm in diameter and that in vessels of this caliber, platelets and coagulation factors play the major role in securing (primary) hemostasis. The hemostatic mechanisms include a vascular reaction, formation of a platelet plug, and activation of the coagulation cascade (secondary hemostasis) to produce a firm fibrin clot.[2] However, these mechanisms alone are not sufficient to restore vascular integrity if a large defect develops, in which case surgical ligation is required.

Platelets are important because of their role in several phases of hemostasis. Platelets have been termed the firefighters of hemostasis because they respond first when a vessel is damaged. von Willebrand factor (vWF) released from endothelial injury combines with the platelet surface glycoprotein Ib to increase the affinity of platelets for the exposed collagen and for other platelets. The platelets release adenosine diphosphate (ADP) and thromboxane A_2, causing further platelet release and aggregation. Platelet adhesion is the affinity of platelets for nonplatelet surfaces, and platelet aggregation is the affinity of platelets for one another. This initial involvement results in the formation of a platelet plug in the area of the damaged endothelium. Thromboxane A_2 causes the injured vessel to constrict and exposes the IIb/IIIa platelet surface glycoprotein, stimulating platelet aggregation through cross-linked fibrin and factor XIII. Formation of a fibrin network within the platelet provides stabilization within the clot to prevent its dissolution. The final action of platelets is clot retraction, caused by the platelet protein thrombosthenin.

Secondary hemostasis involves activation of the coagulation cascade, as indicated in Figure 15-1.[3] The intrinsic coagulation system utilizes factors XII, XI, IX, and VIII, and the extrinsic pathway utilizes the VIIa tissue factor complex. Factor X is activated by the end product of either the intrinsic or extrinsic system to initiate the final common pathway converting prothrombin to thrombin. Thrombin converts fibrinogen to fibrin and activates factors V and VIII, which further increase thrombin production. The minimum levels of coagulation factors and platelets necessary for effective hemostasis are listed in Table 15-1. A primary hemostatic defect can often be differentiated from a secondary hemostatic defect by bedside evaluation. Platelet defects are usually manifested by petechiae, ecchymoses, and mucosal bleeding, whereas secondary (coagulation factor) defects are manifested by large hematomas or hemarthroses.

Fibrinolysis is the body's mechanism for keeping the clotting mechanism localized to the area of bleeding. This mechanism, also called the plasminogen system, results in the dissolution of the fibrin network that forms the fibrin-based clot. It is made up of enzymes, inhibitors, and activators that are closely related to the enzymes, inhibitors, and activators involved in coagulation. Fibrinolysis is important both for restoring vascular patency and in preventing widespread coagulation. The system is activated by tissue plasminogen activator (tPA), which binds to fibrin and activates the fibrin-bound plasminogen to plasmin. If released systemically, plasmin, in turn, digests a number of coagulation factors including fibrinogen and factors V and VIII. The therapeutic use of the fibrinolytic pathway and the pathologic syndrome associated with excessive fibrinolysis are discussed later.

Laboratory Evaluation

Evaluation of hemostasis begins with a properly taken history and physical examination. Rarely is a preexisting bleeding disorder first manifest intraoperatively in a patient with a negative history.[4] Specific questions regarding bleeding tendency or excessive bleeding associated with previous surgery may suggest further laboratory evaluation. With respect to any history of bleeding episodes, their frequency and severity, as well as the apparent cause, should be ascertained. Equally important is the need to obtain a record of all medications that the patient is taking. Family history of bleeding tendency should also be sought as a part of the preoperative evaluation. Physical examination should focus on the presence of petechiae and ecchymoses, with the former suggesting a platelet or vascular defect and the latter more likely a coagulation factor defect.

Laboratory tests, in addition to serving as a screening tool, help delineate the specific hemostatic defect. For screening purposes, determinations of the prothrombin time (PT), activated

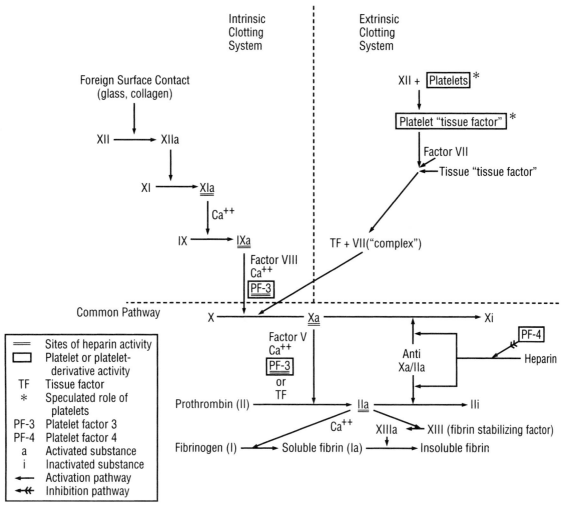

FIGURE 15-1 The coagulation cascade with special emphasis on the sites of platelet and heparin activity. (From Barrer MJ, Ellison N: *Anesthesiology* 46:202, 1977.)

partial thromboplastin time (aPTT), platelet count, fibrinogen level, and bleeding time are needed. In the operating room, an activated coagulation time (ACT) may be added to the list of baseline screening tests (Table 15-2). If all of these screening tests are normal and the patient has a negative history and physical examination, it may be reasonable to assume that any intraoperative bleeding disorder is not due to a preexisting defect.

The PT is dependent on the function of both the intrinsic and extrinsic pathways, and the aPTT is dependent on the function of the intrinsic and common pathways (see Figure 15-1). These pathways localize the specific defect by screening tests and direct further testing if necessary. For example, a patient with a prolonged PT but normal aPTT most likely has a factor VII defect. A patient with a normal PT but prolonged aPTT has a defect among factors VIII, IX, XI, and XII. A patient with prolonged PT and aPTT has factor deficiencies in both the intrinsic and extrinsic systems, the common pathway, or all three. A less common etiology is the presence of a circulatory inhibitor of a clotting factor protein without a clotting factor deficiency, such as a lupus anticoagulant or factor VIII inhibitor. Mixing the patient's blood with normal plasma 1:1 corrects a prolonged aPTT related to factor deficiency. A prolonged aPTT is not corrected with 1:1 mixing if a circulatory inhibitor is present.

Congenital Bleeding Disorders

Congenital bleeding disorders are usually due to the absence or decreased presence of a single coagulation factor. The most common of these disorders are hemophilia A (classic hemophilia, factor VIII deficiency), hemophilia B (Christmas disease, factor IX deficiency), plasma thromboplastin antecedent (factor XI) deficiency, and von Willebrand's disease.

Hemophilia A is probably the most common hereditary disease, with an incidence of 1 per 10,000 live births, and is due to a sex-linked autosomal recessive trait. The disease results in a prolongation of the aPTT with a normal PT. Perioperative management is aimed at increasing factor VIII activity to near normal preoperatively and maintaining levels at 30% or greater intraoperatively and for the duration of postoperative wound healing. This convalescent period can range up to 10 days, depending on the magnitude of the surgical procedure (Table 15-3).[5] Cryoprecipitate and factor VIII concentrate are the blood products available for treatment of the coagulopathy related to hemophilia A. The determinants of the dose necessary for correction are listed in Table 15-4.

Hemophilia B is due to an autosomal recessive trait, and in this disease the aPTT is also prolonged. A factor IX concentrate

TABLE 15-1

Minimum Levels of Coagulation Factors and Platelets Necessary for Effective Hemostasis—Distribution, Half-Life, and Dosing

	Minimal Level for Surgical Hemostasis (% of Normal)	Apparent Volume of Distribution (× Plasma Volume)	In Vivo Half-Life (h)	Therapeutic Agent	Dose (Per kg Body Weight)	
					Initial	Maintenance
Factor						
I	50-100	2-5	72-144	Cryoprecipitate	Ppt from 100 mL	Ppt from 14 to 20 mL, qd
II	20-40	1.5-2	72-120	Plasma	10-15 mL	5-10 mL, qd
V	5-20	?	12-36	Fresh or frozen plasma	10-15 mL	10 mL, qd
VII	10-20	2-4	4-6	Plasma	5-10 mL	5 mL, qd
VIII	30	1-1.5	10-18	Cryoprecipitate	Ppt from 70	Ppt from 35 mL, bid
Von Willebrand	30			Plasma	10 mL	10 mL, q2-3d
IX	20-25	2-5	18-36	Plasma or II,VII, IX, X concentrate	60 mL variable	7 mL, qd
X	10-20	1-2	24-60	Plasma	15 mL	10 mL, qd
XI	20-30	1-1.33	40-80	Plasma	10 mL	5 mL, qd
XII	0	?	?50-70	Plasma	5 mL	5 mL, qd
XIII	1-3	?	?72-120	Plasma	2-3 mL	None
Platelets	50,000- 100,000/mm^3			Platelet concentrate	1-2 U per desired 10,000 increment in count	

Adapted from Ellison N: Coagulation evaluation and management. In Ream AK, Fogdall RP (eds): *Acute cardiovascular management*, Philadelphia, 1982, JB Lippincott, 773.

is available, but because it is a pooled product, it is associated with a high risk of hepatitis as well as the potential to initiate disseminated intravascular coagulation (DIC) because of the presence of activated products. Factor IX concentrate is also used in patients with factor VIII deficiency who have developed inhibitors.

von Willebrand's disease results from decreased activity of the protein factor VIII:vonWillebrand factor (VIII:vWF), which plays an important role in both platelet function and factor VIII activity. The disease is classified according to the etiology of the defect. Type 1 involves a quantitative defect of factor VIII:vWF; type 2, a qualitative defect; and type 3, a defect in the synthesis of factor VIII. The disease is inherited as either an autosomal dominant (types 1 and 2) or, rarely, an autosomal recessive trait (type 3). The disease results in defective platelet aggregation, manifested by a prolonged bleeding time, and decreased levels of factor VIII, manifested by a prolonged aPTT. Desmopressin acetate is effective in increasing endogenous release of VIII:vWF, which may also be provided through the administration of cryoprecipitate. Desmopressin acetate administered the evening prior to surgery and the day of surgery is an effective way to neutralize the defective platelet aggregation and to increase levels of factor VIII, respectively.[5]

Factor XI deficiency is an autosomal recessive coagulation disorder with a predilection for certain ethnic groups, especially Ashkenazi Jews. The risk of bleeding does not correlate with factor XI levels. Fresh frozen plasma (FFP) is the treatment of choice. Factor XIII deficiency is an autosomal recessive bleeding disorder manifested by a deficiency of fibrin-stabilizing factor and a normal aPTT. The plasma clot of a patient with factor XIII deficiency is soluble in 5 molar urea,

TABLE 15-2

Baseline Screening Tests of Hemostasis

Activated coagulation time (ACT)	Can be done in operating room; observe for clot retraction and lysis
Fibrinogen level	Depressed in DIC
Prothrombin time (PT)	Prolonged in liver disease, vitamin K deficiency, warfarin (Coumadin) anticoagulation, DIC
Partial thromboplastin time (aPTT)	Prolonged in factors V, VIII deficiency (massive transfusion), the hemophilias, or the presence of heparin
Platelet count	Major cause of bleeding related to platelets is a decrease in number; thus, platelet count is first step in elevation; decreased in DIC (secondary fibrinolysis), but not primary fibrinolysis
Bleeding time	Most widely accepted clinical test of platelet function; the other cause of bleeding due to platelets

DIC, disseminated intravascular coagulation.

TABLE 15-3

Recommended Factor VIII Levels and Duration of Treatment for Surgical Procedure or Bleeding Condition

Factor VIII Level (U/mL)	Treatment	
	Frequency (hr)	Duration (days)
Hemarthrosis 0.30	Every 12	1
Dental (minor) 0.30	Every 12	1
Dental (extraction) 0.30	Every 8	1-1
All surgery 0.50	Every 8	2-10

From Ellison N, Silberstein LE: Hemostasis in the perioperative period. In Stoelting RK, Barash PG, Gallagher TJ (eds): *Advances in anesthesia*, vol 3, Chicago, 1986, Year Book Medical Publishers, 67.

TABLE 15-4

Determinants of Dose of Blood Component Used to Correct a Hemostatic Defect(s)

Patient's size
Initial level of deficient factor
Potency of preparation
Hemostatic level required
Magnitude of operation
Half-life of the factor
Redistribution
Metabolic rate

and this observation facilitates the diagnosis. Small volumes of FFP are used for treatment.

Acquired Bleeding Disorders

Unlike the congenital disorders, which are usually due to deficiencies of a single coagulation factor, the acquired bleeding disorders are commonly multifactorial. The most common acquired bleeding disorders include vitamin K deficiency, anticoagulants, liver disease, platelet dysfunction, DIC, massive blood transfusion, and inadequate surgical hemostasis.

Vitamin K is required for the production of factors II, VII, IX, and X (the prothrombin complex) and acts by enzymatically adding a γ-carboxyl group to the precursors of these factors.[2] This process occurs in the liver and, therefore, requires adequate liver function as well as adequate vitamin K absorption from the gastrointestinal tract. Without γ-carboxylation, these factors are produced in a dysfunctional state and are unable to bind calcium, a cofactor in the coagulation process. Causes of vitamin K deficiency include malabsorption; "intestinal sterilization syndrome" (elimination of intestinal flora, a major source of vitamin K, through antibiotic therapy); warfarin (Coumadin) therapy, which inhibits the action of vitamin K; and (rarely) a true dietary deficiency. Laboratory studies initially reveal a prolonged PT with a normal aPTT because factor VII is the most sensitive to vitamin K deficiency. As the vita-

min K deficiency becomes greater, factors II, IX, and X become affected and then the aPTT is also prolonged (Figure 15-2). Treatment depends on the urgency of correction, as the administration of parenteral vitamin K requires 3 to 6 hours or longer to neutralize the Coumadin effect, depending on the level of inhibition achieved and the adequacy of liver function. FFP can correct the coagulopathy immediately but carries the risk of homologous blood transfusion and should, therefore, be reserved for treatment of patients who are actively bleeding or undergoing emergency surgery.

Patients scheduled for vascular surgery are frequently treated with anticoagulants preoperatively; Coumadin and heparin are additional causes of acquired bleeding disorders. Coumadin interferes with coagulation by inhibiting the production of the prothrombin complex, resulting in the clinical picture of vitamin K deficiency just described. Heparin inhibits the action of factors IIa (thrombin), IXa, Xa, and XIa, also called the serine proteases, by the binding of heparin to a polypeptide, antithrombin III (AT-III). Heparin bound to AT-III produces a conformational change in AT-III, markedly enhancing the inhibitory effects of AT-III on the serine proteases. Small doses of heparin initially inhibit factor IXa, thus prolonging both the PT and aPTT (see Figure 15-2).

Liver disease can also lead to defects in coagulation by mechanisms other than vitamin K deficiency, such as malabsorption because of lack of bile salts. Factors not dependent upon vitamin K, but produced in the liver, are fibrinogen (I), V, and XI. These may also be decreased in patients with liver disease. Portal hypertension secondary to liver disease may also lead to bleeding from esophageal varices and to hypersplenism resulting in excessive sequestration of platelets and thrombocytopenia.

Platelet Defects

Platelet dysfunction can be qualitative or quantitative. Because the most common cause of bleeding related to platelet deficiency is one of number, a platelet count is the first step in the evaluation. Thrombocytopenia is generally defined as a platelet count less than 150,000/mm³. Thrombocytopenic

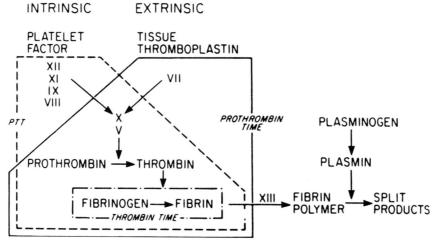

FIGURE 15-2 The coagulation mechanism. The diagram outlines the factors involved in the in vitro determination of prothrombin time, partial thromboplastin time (PTT), and thrombin time. (From Neerhout RC: *Pediatr Clin North Am* 16: 681, 1969.)

patients have a higher prevalence of bleeding and greater transfusion requirements. An acute decrease in platelet count of 30% or more is independently associated with increased mortality.[6] A decreased platelet count can be due to decreased production of platelets, increased destruction, or excessive sequestration. Decreased production can occur during chemotherapy, and increased destruction can be idiopathic, related to certain disease states (human immunodeficiency virus [HIV], marrow infiltration by tumor), or drug induced. Anemia and leukopenia often accompany decreased platelet production. Medications associated with platelet destruction include heparin, quinine, quinidine, thiazide diuretics, and medications derived from sulfa.[7] Hypersplenism causes excessive platelet sequestration but usually leads to only a modest decrease in the platelet count.

Idiopathic thrombocytopenic purpura (ITP) is an autoimmune disease mediated by immunoglobulin G (IgG) antibodies, which bind to platelets and lead to their destruction. Patients with acute ITP rarely present for elective vascular surgery. Chronic ITP is treated with steroids, splenectomy, or immunosuppression (for refractory cases). Appropriate anesthetic considerations are undertaken to include perioperative stress steroid coverage. Thrombotic thrombocytopenic purpura (TTP) is a systemic disorder manifested by platelet aggregation of unknown etiology in the microcirculation. Thrombocytopenia is associated with hemolytic anemia, neurologic deficits, fever, and renal insufficiency. Treatment usually includes plasma exchange and steroid therapy; platelet transfusion is relatively contraindicated because of the risk of further clinical deterioration.

Heparin-induced thrombocytopenia (HIT) is a manifestation of IgG antibodies to the heparin–platelet factor 4 complex, causing hypercoagulation and thrombocytopenia. Two percent of patients treated with standard (unfractionated) heparin develop HIT; the risk is lower with low-molecular-weight heparin (LMWH). The syndrome typically develops over 5 to 7 days in patients with no previous exposure to heparin and within 48 hours in those with previous exposure. Hypercoagulation may be manifested as venous or arterial thrombosis and thrombocytopenia in the range 50,000 to 100,000 platelets/mm[3] The diagnosis is suspected when the platelet count decreases after heparin exposure by any route (intravenous, subcutaneous, flush as necessary [prn], coated catheters), and confirmed by platelet aggregometry or enzyme-linked immunosorbent assay for heparin–platelet factor 4 complexes. Treatment includes discontinuing heparin therapy and administering inhibitors of platelet aggregation (hirudin, danaparoid), provided there is no active bleeding. Treatment should be considered in all other patients because there is a risk of thrombosis (arterial and venous) in 30% to 75% of patients with HIT.[8] Venous thrombosis is more prevalent in HIT patients receiving heparin for venous thromboembolism, whereas arterial thrombosis occurs more often in HIT patients receiving heparin for arterial disease.[8] LMWH is not an alternative treatment option for these patients.

DIC is relatively rare in the patient who presents for elective vascular surgery but may occur during emergent vascular surgery. DIC is a secondary condition that occurs in response to a serious underlying disease (infected vascular graft) or after massive fluid replacement in a patient who has suffered a catastrophic vascular event (ruptured aneurysm). The release of tissue factor initiates the coagulation cascade. Bleeding occurs because of factor deficiency and thrombocytopenia related to the formation of fibrin within the circulation and by secondary fibrinolysis. This digestion of fibrinogen and fibrin results in increased fibrin split products in the circulation that possess anticoagulant properties of their own. Laboratory findings reveal thrombocytopenia, prolonged PT and aPTT, decreased fibrinogen levels, and the presence of fibrin split products. Definitive treatment involves correcting the underlying problem that led to DIC. However, in cases of active bleeding and depletion of platelets or coagulation factors, the administration of platelets and coagulation factors is indicated in addition to treating the underlying problem. The use of heparin in this setting is controversial and is rarely indicated in the surgical patient.

Massive blood transfusion may be required for the patient with a large hemorrhage, as in a ruptured aortic aneurysm. The hemostatic defect introduced with massive transfusion is dilutional, the most important defect being dilutional thrombocytopenia. Dilution of clotting factors, especially the labile factors V and VIII, may also play a minor role in the acquired hemostatic defects. Treatment involves administration of platelets and FFP. The dilutional effects on the stable coagulation factors may be decreased by the administration of whole blood instead of packed red blood cells.

Acquired qualitative platelet disorders are more prevalent than hereditary disorders and usually predispose patients to less bleeding. Medications associated with platelet dysfunction include the nonsteroidal anti-inflammatory drugs (NSAIDs), antihistamines, tricyclic antidepressants, dextran, aminoglycosides, protamine, certain local anesthetics, and α-adrenergic antagonists.[2,7] Aspirin causes permanent impairment of platelet function through a covalent bond that persists throughout the life of the platelet. It is for this reason that aspirin therapy is discontinued 7 to 10 days before surgery to avoid the increased bleeding potential related to platelet dysfunction. Ticlopidine inhibits platelet aggregation by inhibiting ADP-induced platelet-fibrinogen binding and subsequent platelet-platelet interaction for the life of the platelet.

Other causes of platelet dysfunction include uremia and chronic liver disease. Uremia is treated with dialysis and desmopressin (DDAVP) administered intravenously at 0.3 μg/kg. Inherited platelet disorders are rare. Bernard-Soulier syndrome is an autosomal recessive disorder characterized by moderate thrombocytopenia, large platelets on microscopy, and increased bleeding time. Platelets lack glycoprotein Ib and therefore cannot bind vWF. Glanzmann's thrombasthenia is also an autosomal recessive disorder but is associated with a normal platelet count. The defect is a paucity of IIb-IIIa complexes, and patients bleed because of impaired ability of fibrinogen to cross-link platelets.

Finally, loss of vascular integrity induced during every surgical procedure is another acquired defect of hemostasis that must be considered. Inadequate surgical hemostasis may lead to prolonged postoperative bleeding not correctable by administration of coagulation products but requiring surgical correction.

Hypercoagulable States and Venous Thrombosis

There is a balance in normal hemostasis between clot formation and thrombolysis. Derangements may produce excessive hemorrhage or thrombosis. Thrombotic disorders become evident with a history of repeated thromboembolic events, unexpected thrombosis, thrombosis in the presence of anticoagulation, and perioperative thrombosis in the vascular surgical patient who has had a good surgical repair resulting in good blood flow through the repaired vessel.[9] Table 15-5 is a list of conditions that are associated with or may lead to thrombotic events. Most commonly, patients who present with thrombosis have one or more of these associated conditions. Less commonly, there exists a hereditary disorder that predisposes the patient to thrombosis. However, these patients may also have one of the predisposing conditions listed in Table 15-5.

Clot formation is limited by the fibrinolytic system and by three plasma proteins—AT-III, protein C, and protein S. Reduced levels of these three proteins predispose patients to excessive thrombosis.[10] In addition, disorders of the fibrinolytic system, dysfibrinogenemias, and the lupus anticoagulant have been associated with an increased risk of thrombosis.[11-13]

The risk of intravascular thrombus formation is further increased in the surgical patient when the vascular endothelium is damaged. Thrombus may result from obvious injury such as trauma or surgery or from more subtle forms of injury such as hypertension or vascular distention. Exposure of the subendothelium promotes adhesion of platelets, release of vasoactive substances, and activation of the coagulation cascade. Whether a thrombus develops at this point depends on a number of factors. These include characteristics of blood flow and velocity, including diameter of the vessel, presence and concentration of coagulation factors, presence of coagulation inhibitors, age

TABLE 15-5

Clinical Conditions Associated with Thrombosis

Trauma
Postoperative state, especially after orthopedic or other leg procedures
Advanced age
Previous history of thrombosis
Immobilization
Paralysis
Obesity
Malignancy
Pregnancy
Estrogen or contraceptive therapy
Infusion of prothrombin concentrates
Myeloproliferative disorders
Nephrotic syndrome
Diabetes
Congestive heart failure
Smoking
Vasculitis
Heparin-induced thrombocytopenia
Homocystinemia
Polycythemia
Leukemia
Sickle cell disease
Hyperlipidemia
Thrombotic thrombocytopenic purpura

of the patient, and activation of the fibrinolytic system. Venous thrombi tend to be red in color because they are formed in vessels with sluggish blood flow, resulting in a red cell–fibrin thrombus; arterial thrombi, which are formed under high-flow and shear conditions, tend to be white in color because they are platelet rich in composition, with few red blood cells in their matrix; thus, the names "red" and "white" thrombi.[9] Composition of the thrombus may be important in guiding therapy, that is, antiplatelet versus anticoagulant drugs.

For each surface, there is a critical velocity below which stasis becomes a significant factor in thrombosis and above which velocities provide adequate shearing forces to overcome the deposition of platelets and fibrin.[14] Any deviation from normal laminar flow may lead to turbulence and to platelet aggregation. Whether this aggregation leads to thrombosis depends not only on those physical factors but also on the presence or absence of coagulation factors and inhibitors. The intact endothelial surface is rich in fibrinolytic activity. As this surface becomes disrupted, however, the fibrinolytic activity is overcome and thrombosis may develop. If a hypercoagulable state is superimposed, thrombosis is even more likely and may, in fact, involve a greater extent of the vessel.

Antithrombin III Deficiency

AT-III is the primary inhibitor of thrombin (II_a) and other serine proteases in the coagulation cascade. The incidence of AT-III deficiency has been reported to be as high as 1 in 2000.[15] Congenital AT-III deficiency is acquired as an autosomal dominant trait. Variations in this disease can result in qualitative as well as quantitative deficiencies of AT-III.[16] Patients with AT-III deficiency present with spontaneous thrombosis (36%), thrombosis during pregnancy or immediately after delivery (28%), and postoperatively (13%).[10] Acquired AT-III deficiency may occur in patients with the nephrotic syndrome (enhanced protein elimination), liver disease (decreased production), and DIC (increased consumption).

AT-III exerts its effect through an arginine group that covalently binds to the clotting factors through their serine group. In the absence of heparin, AT-III is a slow inhibitor of the serine proteases. In the presence of heparin, however, the arginine group is more accessible through a conformational change induced by heparin, and binding to clotting factors is enhanced. When heparin is present as a cofactor, AT-III is approximately 50 times more effective as an inhibitor of coagulation. In the absence of AT-III, heparin is ineffective as an anticoagulant.

Treatment of patients with AT-III deficiency who present with thrombosis involves the administration of heparin to patients with a mild deficiency. If the deficiency is severe, levels of AT-III need to be increased through the administration of FFP or AT-III concentrates, where available.

Protein C Deficiency

Protein C is a vitamin K–dependent glycoprotein that proteolytically degrades the activated forms of factors V and VIII and inhibits factor Va activity on the platelet surface while inhibiting binding of factor Xa to the platelet surface. Protein C also has an effect on fibrinolysis by decreasing tPA inhibitor activity, permitting tPA to activate plasminogen to plasmin unchecked.[10]

Clinical manifestations of protein C deficiency in heterozygotes include venous thrombosis and warfarin-induced skin necrosis; purpura fulminans neonatalis is manifested in homozygotes. Massive and fatal neonatal thrombosis has been reported in homozygous protein C neonates, in whom plasma levels of protein C were virtually absent.[17]

Acquired protein C deficiency can occur in DIC, liver disease, acute respiratory distress syndrome, and following surgery.[18] Because it is a vitamin K–dependent protein, administration of Coumadin increases protein C deficiency. Treatment of acute thrombosis involves intravenous heparin administration, and chronic therapy is maintained with Coumadin. Coumadin in larger doses decreases protein C levels faster than decreasing factor X levels, thereby increasing the risk of thrombosis. For this reason, either intravenous heparin is administered or smaller doses of Coumadin are used during initiation of Coumadin therapy for chronic anticoagulation.[18] Danazol, an anabolic steroid, has been suggested as a treatment for protein C deficiency.[19] Danazol's mechanism of action involves increasing the synthesis of vitamin K–dependent proteins.

Protein S Deficiency

Protein S is a cofactor for the anticoagulant effects of activated protein C. Although it does not have anticoagulant effects of its own, protein S markedly enhances the inhibitory effect of protein C on factor Va and is required for the binding of activated protein C to platelets. Because protein S is a vitamin K–dependent cofactor, deficiency of protein S may be acquired in patients treated with Coumadin and in patients with liver disease. Protein S deficiency can also occur in DIC, nephrotic syndrome, pregnancy, after an acute thrombotic event, and with systemic lupus erythematosus.[18]

The usual clinical manifestation is venous thrombosis, although arterial thrombosis has also been reported in a patient with protein S deficiency.[20] Treatment includes intravenous heparin initially, followed by oral anticoagulants for chronic control of thromboses.

Defects in Fibrinolysis

Thrombosis can also develop in patients with defects in fibrinolysis. These result from impaired synthesis or release of plasminogen activator, the presence of excess inhibitors of plasminogen activator, the administration of ε-aminocaproic acid (EACA), or a functionally abnormal fibrinogen molecule.[12,21,22]

Venous Thrombosis

Venous thrombosis is a problem that occurs in approximately 30% of general surgery cases and is of particular concern for the patient undergoing lower extremity revascularization.[14] It may be associated with significant morbidity with the development of the post-thrombotic syndrome and can be fatal if it results in pulmonary embolism. Surgical intervention may be necessary in patients who have failed medical therapy or those patients who have a contraindication to anticoagulant therapy (Table 15-6).[23,24] If the venous thrombosis is extensive or involves large veins, surgical removal may be required. Rarely, a patient presents for surgical removal of a pulmonary embolus if there is a contraindication to anticoagulant therapy in the presence of repeated or massive pulmonary embolization.

TABLE 15-6
Relative Contraindications to Anticoagulant Therapy

Bleeding diathesis (exception may be consumptive coagulopathies)
Ulcerative lesions of the gastrointestinal, genitourinary (especially prostate), or respiratory tract
Recent central nervous system or eye surgery
Severe hypertension
Recent cerebral hemorrhage
Subactive bacterial endocarditis or pericarditis
Uncooperative patient or inadequate laboratory control
Pregnancy, first trimester and near term (applies only to Coumadin)[23]

Adapted from Ellison N, Ominsky AJ: *Anesthesiology* 39:328, 1973.

The process of venous thrombosis begins with damage to the endothelial lining of the vessel wall. This damage leads to a vascular and platelet reaction resulting in stasis and the initiation of coagulation. The process may be acute or chronic and may occur in visceral veins as well as in the veins of the extremities. It is termed *thrombophlebitis* when it is associated with an inflammatory process producing symptoms of pain, tenderness, and erythema. The majority of patients, however, lack any clinical manifestation of their disease.

Pulmonary embolism can be a fatal complication of venous thrombosis. The deep veins of the lower extremity are the source of 90% of pulmonary emboli. Patients with pulmonary embolism present with an acute onset of dyspnea and tachycardia. If it is a large embolus, associated signs and symptoms may include chest pain, hypotension, central venous distention, and the manifestations of hypoxia. Diagnosis may be made with a "mismatch" of pulmonary ventilation and perfusion scanning as well as with pulmonary angiography.

Anticoagulant Therapy

Patients treated with anticoagulants present interesting dilemmas to the anesthesiologist. One consideration is the initiation of invasive monitoring for an anticoagulated patient. The unintentional placement of a large-bore catheter in the carotid artery of a patient with a coagulopathy during attempted internal jugular vein cannulation can lead to hematoma formation and airway compression.[25] Ultrasound-guided cannulation of the internal jugular vein reduces the incidence of carotid artery puncture but the incidence is not zero.[26] Another approach is to neutralize the anticoagulant effect and then place all the necessary invasive cannulas. If therapeutic prophylactic anticoagulation is required, heparin therapy can be reinstituted after the successful placement of all vascular cannulas. This approach introduces the potential risk of extending an established thrombus when the anticoagulant is neutralized. Another approach would be to initiate invasive monitoring while maintaining anticoagulation and reverse the heparin only if complications arise, such as carotid puncture during attempted internal jugular cannulation or repeated unsuccessful attempts leading to hematoma formation at the cannulation site.

Even greater controversy surrounds the question of performing intraspinal techniques on patients who are anticoagulated. Most anesthesiologists would avoid intraspinal techniques in patients whose blood is anticoagulated and consider abnormalities in blood clotting a contraindication to performing these techniques.[27] Odoom and Sih, however, reported a series of 1000 epidural blocks performed on patients who were receiving anticoagulants preoperatively and without any side effects that could be related to epidural hematoma formation.[28] Perioperative considerations for patients treated with various classes of anticoagulant therapies are discussed next.

Heparin

Heparin is a heterogenous mixture of straight-chain anionic mucopolysaccharides, called glycosaminoglycans. These chains have a high degree of sulfation, which imparts a negative charge that contributes to the anticoagulant activity through binding to AT-III. Heparin combines with AT-III in a 1:1 stoichiometric ratio and induces a conformational change in AT-III such that it binds more readily to the serine proteases in the coagulation cascade. The binding of heparin to AT-III accelerates its inactivation of factor IIa (thrombin) by 1000- to 10,000-fold and that of factors IXa, Xa, XIa, and XIIa by 10- to 100-fold.

There is a variable response to heparin therapy among individuals that may be the result of varying concentrations of AT-III or antiheparin agents such as platelet factor 4. The desired effect of heparin and the degree of anticoagulation, therefore, need to be monitored. In particular, patients with AT-III deficiencies may be quite resistant to anticoagulation. Patients who undergo prolonged therapy with heparin demonstrate decreased concentrations of AT-III with continued use. Other causes of "heparin resistance" are listed in Table 15-7.[29] Although minidose heparin therapy minimally prolongs the aPTT, increased doses of heparin produce prolongation of PT and ACT as well as aPTT by inhibiting clotting factors in both intrinsic and extrinsic coagulation pathways. Minidose therapy is accomplished through the effects of heparin on factor IXa. Because this factor is necessary for the conversion of prothrombin to thrombin, minidoses of heparin inhibit the formation of thrombin with minimal effect on thrombin itself. Therefore, if thrombin formation has already occurred, minidose heparin is not effective as an anticoagulant. Conventional-dose heparin therapy, however, because it inhibits thrombin, is an effective anticoagulant even if thrombin formation has occurred. Inactivation of thrombin prevents the conversion of fibrinogen to fibrin. Because heparin has no effect on fibrinolysis, heparin has no effect on an established thrombus except to prevent its extension. Table 15-8 presents a summary of the three levels of heparin therapy. Patients with prosthetic heart valves are converted from Coumadin therapy to standard heparin preoperatively and postoperatively because it is easily monitored and neutralized for surgery.

Regional anesthesia is often a desirable option in vascular surgical patients because of coexisting disease (see Chapter 9). Patients receiving therapeutic anticoagulation with a continuous intravenous heparin infusion producing an elevation in aPTT of 1.5 to 2 times the control are not candidates for regional anesthesia. There are at least 18 case reports of an epidural hematoma after neuraxial procedures in this setting.[30] The issue is also important for epidural catheter removal. Heparin infusions should be discontinued for 2 to 4 hours and coagulation status assessed before catheter manipulation.[30]

The use of regional anesthesia in patients receiving minidose heparin (5000 units subcutaneously twice daily) preoperatively is another consideration. By definition, blood coagulation studies are not prolonged after minidose heparin (see Table 15-8), but the potential for epidural hematoma formation does exist.[31] Problems arise because the blood concentration of heparin after subcutaneous administration is highly variable and may be therapeutic within 2 hours after administration.[32] Epidural and intraspinal hematomas have been reported with regional anesthetic techniques performed in patients receiving minidose heparin, but more than 9000 patients received this therapy without complications.[30,33,34] An evaluation of coagulation status is warranted before performing a regional anesthetic technique in debilitated patients, with coexisting coagulopathy, and with longer (more than 5 days) therapy.[30] A subset of patients may develop thrombocytopenia with prolonged minidose heparin therapy.[35]

Heparin is used intraoperatively because of its immediate onset of action as a means of preventing intravascular clot formation while vessels are clamped. Commonly, small intravenous doses such as 5000 to 8000 units are administered as an intravenous bolus before the vessels are clamped. A "top-off" dose is usually administered subsequently every hour while the vessels remain clamped. Because of patients' variable response to heparin, it is prudent to measure the response to heparin with an ACT. A baseline ACT should be determined prior to the administration of heparin. For the dose of heparin used in vascular surgery (70 to 100 units/kg), the ACT becomes prolonged to 250 to 300 seconds. Patients with AT-III

TABLE 15-7

Causes of Heparin Resistance

Ongoing active coagulation
Antithrombin III (AT-III) deficiency, congenital or acquired
Previous heparin therapy
Drug interaction as with oral contraceptives
Presence of other medical syndromes such as hypereosinophilia or coronary artery disease
Advanced age
Drug error in dose, route of administration, or product (not a true cause of heparin resistance but must always be considered)

Adapted from Ellison N, Jobes DR, Schwartz AJ: Heparin therapy during cardiac surgery. In Ellison N, Jobes DR (eds): *Effective hemostasis in cardiac surgery*, Philadelphia, 1988, WB Saunders, 1.

TABLE 15-8

Three Levels of Heparin Therapy

Dosage Level	Goal	Purpose
Minidose	Coagulation studies not prolonged	Prevention of deep venous thrombosis
Conventional dose	Prolongation of aPTT 2.0 to 2.5 times the baseline	Anticoagulation; prevention of thrombus formation
Maxidose	Total hemostatic paralysis	Institution of cardiopulmonary bypass

aPTT, activated partial thromboplastin time.

deficiency, including those who have been receiving heparin therapy for an extended period of time preoperatively, demonstrate heparin resistance, defined as lack of prolongation of the ACT for a given dose of heparin (see Table 15-7). These patients require higher doses of heparin. If the AT-III deficiency is severe, they may require administration of FFP to restore their levels of AT-III.

Controversy exists over the use of epidural or intrathecal techniques in patients who will be intraoperatively anticoagulated. The risk of intraspinal (epidural or intrathecal) bleeding exists.[36] Although a study involving large numbers of patients has shown that symptomatic hematomas are a rare complication, the risk/benefit ratio must be carefully considered.[37] Intraoperative anticoagulation with heparin after regional anesthesia is generally acceptable during vascular surgery with the following cautions recommended by Liu and Mulroy[30]:

1. Avoid the technique in patients with other coagulopathies.
2. Delay heparin administration for 1 hour after needle placement.
3. Remove catheter 1 hour before any subsequent heparin administration or 2 to 4 hours after the last heparin dose.
4. Monitor the patient's neurologic status postoperatively to provide early detection of motor blockade and consider use of a minimal concentration of local anesthetic to enhance the detection of a spinal hematoma.
5. Use clinical judgment for proceeding with surgery after a bloody or difficult neuraxial needle placement, although there are no data to support mandatory cancellation.

If good surgical hemostasis has been achieved after the vascular reconstruction is completed, heparin may not need to be neutralized. However, if bleeding persists without a surgical cause for bleeding, heparin is neutralized with a protamine dose of 1 mg per 100 units of heparin activity remaining. The ACT is again measured after neutralization with protamine in order to identify any residual heparin effect. For patients who are at risk for thrombotic events postoperatively, low-dose heparin may be continued until the patient can ambulate.

Rarely, patients demonstrate a recurrence of heparin effect after complete heparin neutralization with protamine. This phenomenon, which is termed *heparin rebound*, is usually seen several hours after surgery. Heparin rebound is identified by an increasing ACT that had returned to normal after protamine administration and is treated by administration of additional protamine.

HIT is a rare complication of heparin therapy and is characterized by a new onset of thrombocytopenia (usually in the range of 50,000 to 100,000 platelets/mm³), resistance to heparin, and thrombosis.[38] HIT has been associated with intravenous and subcutaneous administration of heparin as well as with prn heparin flush.[39] The mechanism of action is probably immunologic; heparin acts as a haptene for the development of an antibody that induces platelet activation.[38] Although the incidence of HIT is very low, it carries a high morbidity and mortality. The successful management of patients undergoing cardiovascular surgery has been described using iloprost and other antiplatelet agents to allow the safe administration of heparin.[40]

Low-Molecular-Weight Heparin and Heparinoids

In contrast to standard heparin, which is a heterogenous mixture of variable molecular weight compounds (depending on the numbers of attached polysaccharide chains), LMWH contains only low-molecular-weight compounds of heparin. LMWH is derived from standard heparin by a depolymerization process, yielding compounds with relatively more anti-Xa activity than anti-IIa activity as compared with standard heparin. These low-molecular-weight compounds are cleared from the circulation more slowly than higher molecular weight compounds. The half-life of LMWH is thus three to four times that of standard heparin, producing significant anti-Xa activity that persists 12 hours after injection.[41] The plasma half-life of LMWH increases in patients with renal failure because of the predominant renal clearance. Protamine is not fully effective in neutralizing the anti-Xa effects of LMWH because protamine binding to LMWH is reduced.[41] Several products are available, and it is important to recognize their use in vascular surgical patients because of the issues concerning regional anesthesia.

Spinal hematoma has been associated with regional anesthesia in patients receiving LMWH. It is therefore important to weigh the risks versus benefits of performing a neuraxial block on an individual basis.[41] Previously published recommendations for patients receiving LMWH by Horlocker and Wedel were updated in a consensus statement published by the American Society of Regional Anesthesia (ASRA) and Pain Medicine as follows[41,42]:

1. Monitoring of anti-Xa level is not recommended. The anti-Xa level is not predictive of the risk of bleeding and is, therefore, not helpful in the management of patients undergoing neuraxial blocks.
2. Antiplatelet or oral anticoagulant medications administered in combination with LMWH may increase the risk of spinal hematoma. Concomitant administration of medications affecting hemostasis, such as antiplatelet drugs, standard heparin, or dextran, represents an additional risk of hemorrhagic complications perioperatively, including spinal hematoma. Education of the entire patient care team is necessary to avoid potentiation of the anticoagulant effects.
3. Presence of blood during needle and catheter placement does not necessitate postponement of surgery. However, initiation of LMWH therapy in this setting should be delayed for 24 hours postoperatively. Traumatic needle or catheter placement may signify an increased risk of spinal hematoma, and it is recommended that this consideration be discussed with the surgeon.
4. Preoperative LMWH
   a. Patients on preoperative LMHW can be assumed to have altered coagulation. In these patients, needle placement should occur at least 10 to 12 hours after the LMWH dose.
   b. Patients receiving higher (treatment) doses of LMWH, such as enoxaparin 1 mg/kg every 12 hours, dalteparin 120 U/kg every 12 hours, dalteparin 200 U/kg daily, or tinzaparin 175 U/kg daily, will require delays of at least 24 hours to assure normal hemostasis at the time of needle insertion.

c. Neuraxial techniques should be avoided in patients administered a dose of LMWH 2 hours preoperatively (general surgery patients), because needle placement would occur during peak anticoagulant activity.

5. Postoperative LMWH. Patients with postoperative initiation of LMWH thromboprophylaxis may safely undergo single-injection and continuous catheter techniques. Management is based on total daily dose, timing of the first postoperative dose, and dosing schedule.

   a. Twice-daily dosing. This dosing regimen may be associated with an increased risk of spinal hematoma. The first dose of LMWH should be administered no earlier than 24 hours postoperatively, regardless of the anesthesia technique, and only in the presence of adequate (surgical) hemostasis. Indwelling catheters should be removed prior to initiation of LMWH thromboprophylaxis. If a continuous technique is selected, the epidural catheter may be left indwelling overnight and removed the following day, with the first dose of LMWH administered 2 hours after catheter removal.

   b. Single daily dosing. This dosing regimen approximates the European application. The first postoperative LMWH dose should be administered 6 to 8 hours postoperatively. The second postoperative dose should occur no sooner than 24 hours after the first dose. Indwelling neuraxial catheters may be safely maintained. However, the catheter should be removed a minimum of 10 to 12 hours after the last dose of LMWH. Subsequent LMWH dosing should occur a minimum of 2 hours after catheter removal.

Heparinoids, such as danaparoid, are mixtures of low-molecular-weight sulfated glycosaminoglycurans that are devoid of heparin or heparin fragments. Danaparoid has a much longer half-life and relatively more anti-Xa versus anti-IIa activity than LMWH. As with LMWHs, the anti-Xa activity is only partially neutralized by protamine and requires direct monitoring of anti-Xa activity or drug levels for assessing clinical effect. Vascular surgical patients who develop HIT in response to prophylactic treatment with heparin or LMWH to prevent venous thrombosis or arterial occlusion preferentially receive a heparinoid such as danaparoid for anticoagulation.

Coumadin

Coumadin is an indirect anticoagulant that interferes with the action of vitamin K in the synthesis of factors II, VII, IX, and X. The hemostatic defect produced by Coumadin is similar to vitamin K deficiency. For elective surgery, patients receiving Coumadin may be converted to heparin and then have their Coumadin discontinued. Heparin can then be discontinued just prior to surgery. This question of discontinuing anticoagulation preoperatively, however, is controversial. The advent of cardiac surgery has proved that patients can undergo surgery while their hemostatic system is totally paralyzed. Except for surgery involving the eye, central nervous system, and large raw surfaces (eg, liver bed), most authorities agree that anticoagulation can be maintained intraoperatively. The preoperative management of patients taking Coumadin is similar to that in the previous discussion on management of patients with vitamin K deficiency. Similarly, the laboratory findings show a prolonged

PT with a normal aPTT. Regional anesthesia techniques are avoided in patients with abnormal coagulation profiles. Published recommendations by Enneking and Benzon for patients who require chronic anticoagulation with Coumadin (warfarin) therapy have been updated as follows[42,43]:

1. Caution should be used when performing neuraxial techniques in patients recently discontinued from chronic warfarin therapy. The anticoagulant therapy must be stopped (ideally 4 to 5 days prior to the planned procedure) and the PT (international normalized ratio [INR]) measured prior to initiation of neuraxial block. Early after discontinuation of warfarin therapy, the PT and the INR reflect predominantly factor VII levels, and in spite of acceptable factor VII levels, factor II and X levels may not be adequate for normal hemostasis. Adequate levels of II, VII, IX, and X may not be present until the PT or INR is within normal limits.

2. The concurrent use of medications that affect other components of the clotting mechanisms may increase the risk of bleeding complications for patients receiving oral anticoagulants and do so without influencing the PT and INR. These medications include aspirin and other NSAIDs, ticlopidine, and clopidogrel, unfractionated heparin, and LMWH.

3. For patients receiving an initial dose of warfarin before surgery, the PT and INR should be checked prior to neuraxial block if the first dose was given more than 24 hours earlier or a second dose of anticoagulant has been administered.

4. Patients receiving low-dose warfarin therapy during epidural analgesia should have their PT and INR monitored on a daily basis and checked before catheter removal, if initial doses of warfarin are administered more than 36 hours preoperatively. Initial studies evaluating the safety of epidural analgesia in association with oral anticoagulation utilized mean daily doses of approximately 5 mg of warfarin. Higher dose warfarin may require more intensive monitoring of the coagulation status.

5. As thromboprophylaxis with warfarin is initiated, neuraxial catheters should be removed when the INR is less than 1.5. This value was derived from studies correlating hemostasis with clotting factor activity levels greater than 40%.

6. Neurologic testing of sensory and motor function should be performed routinely during epidural analgesia for patients receiving warfarin therapy. The type of analgesic solution should be tailored to minimize the degree of sensory and motor block. These checks should be continued after catheter removal for at least 24 hours and longer if the INR was greater than 1.5 at the time of catheter removal.

7. An INR greater than 3 should prompt the physician to withhold or reduce the warfarin dose in patients with indwelling epidural catheters. The authors can make no definitive recommendations for removal of neuraxial catheters in patients with therapeutic levels of anticoagulation during neuraxial catheter infusion.

8. Reduced doses of warfarin should be given to patients who are likely to have an enhanced response to the drug.

Platelet Inhibitors

A number of medications that interfere with platelet function are prescribed for patients with vascular disease. These include aspirin and NSAIDs, thienopyridine derivatives (ticlopidine and clopidogrel), direct thrombin inhibitors such as hirudin, and platelet glycoprotein IIb/IIIa antagonists (abciximab, epti-fibatide, tirofiban).[42] Aspirin interferes with platelet function by inhibiting cyclooxygenase, which is involved in the conversion of arachidonic acid to prostaglandin cyclic endoperoxides and thromboxane A_2. Because thromboxane A_2 is involved in platelet aggregation and vasoconstriction, interfering with its production decreases platelet aggregation and prolongs bleeding time. This inhibition is irreversible and persists for the life of the platelet, approximately 10 days. Therefore, it would be optimal for patients taking aspirin to discontinue the drug 2 weeks before elective vascular surgery, especially if major blood loss is anticipated.

Dipyridamole also interferes with platelet function and is often prescribed for patients with vascular disease because of its synergistic effects with aspirin. Dipyridamole's mechanism of action differs from that of aspirin in that intracellular cyclic adenosine monophosphate (cAMP) inhibits the platelet aggregation caused by ADP. Dipyridamole is a phosphodiesterase inhibitor, causing an increase in cAMP, resulting in decreased platelet aggregation and an increase in platelet survival time. The drug is used as an adjunct to anticoagulants in the prevention of thromboembolic events and in long-term therapy of chronic angina pectoris. Ticlopidine causes selective inhibition of adenosine phosphate–mediated platelet activation by irreversibly binding to platelets.

The use of regional anesthetic techniques in patients receiving platelet inhibitors is debatable but does not appear to be associated with an increased risk of spinal hematoma provided that these medications are not combined with other medications that interfere with coagulation. It is important to recognize that a hemostatic defect is present but that there is no evidence to suggest that regional anesthesia should be avoided in these patients. The ASRA consensus statements regarding this issue are as follows[42]:

1. There is no wholly accepted test, including the bleeding time, which will guide antiplatelet therapy. Careful preoperative assessment of the patient to identify alterations of health that might contribute to bleeding is crucial. These conditions include a history of easy bruisability/excessive bleeding, female gender, and increased age.
2. NSAIDs appear to represent no added significant risk for the development of spinal hematoma in patients having epidural or spinal anesthesia. The use of NSAIDs alone does not create a level of risk that will interfere with the performance of neuraxial blocks.
3. At this time, there do not seem to be specific concerns as to the timing of single-shot or catheter techniques in relation to the dosing of NSAIDs, postoperative monitoring, or the timing of neuraxial catheter removal.
4. The actual risk of spinal hematoma with ticlopidine and clopidogrel and the glycoprotein IIb/IIIa antagonists is unknown. Consensus management is based on labeling precautions and the surgical, interventional cardiology/radiology experience.
   a. Based on labeling and surgical reviews, the suggested time interval between discontinuation of thienopyridine therapy and neuraxial blockade is 14 days for ticlopidine and 7 days for clopidogrel.

b. Platelet glycoprotein IIb/IIIa inhibitors exert a profound effect on platelet aggregation. Following administration, the time to normal platelet aggregation is 24 to 48 hours for abciximab and 4 to 8 hours for eptifibatide and tirofiban. Neuraxial techniques should be avoided until platelet function has recovered. Glycoprotein IIb/IIIa antagonists are contraindicated within 4 weeks of surgery. Should one be administered in the postoperative period (following a neuraxial technique), the patient should be carefully monitored neurologically.

5. The concurrent use of other medications affecting clotting mechanisms, such as oral anticoagulants, unfractionated heparin, and LMWH, may increase the risk of bleeding complications. Cyclooxygenase-2 inhibitors have minimal effect on platelet function and should be considered in patients who require anti-inflammatory therapy in the presence of anticoagulation.

Herbal Therapy

An increasing number of patients who are ingesting herbal medicines may present for vascular surgery. Adverse effects such as increased bleeding and drug interactions may be a cause for concern. Available information in the literature suggests a discontinuation of all herbal medicines 2 weeks before surgery.[44] The ASRA consensus statements regarding this issue are as follows[42]:

1. The use of herbal medications alone does not create a level of risk that will interfere with the performance of neuraxial blocks. Mandatory discontinuation of these medications, or cancellation of surgery in patients in whom these medications have been continued, is not supported by available data.
2. Data on the combination of herbal therapy with other forms of anticoagulation are lacking. However, the concurrent use of other medications affecting clotting mechanisms, such as oral anticoagulants or heparin, may increase the risk of bleeding complications in these patients.
3. There is no wholly accepted test to assess adequacy of hemostasis in the patient reporting preoperative herbal medications.
4. At this time, there do not seem to be specific concerns as to the timing of neuraxial block in relation to the dosing of herbal therapy, postoperative monitoring, or the timing of neuraxial catheter removal.

Thrombolytic Therapy

Thrombolytic therapy involves the activation of fibrinolysis in order to lyse a clot. In the realm of vascular disease, thrombolytic therapy may be administered for an acute vascular occlusion, such as peripheral artery thrombosis, pulmonary embolism, deep vein thrombosis, and occluded arteriovenous dialysis cannula. This therapy is also effective for acute myocardial infarction and stroke. If emergency surgery is required after the administration of thrombolytic therapy, it is important to recognize the derangements in hemostasis that have been induced. Drugs that may be used as thrombolytics include tPA, streptokinase, and urokinase. They promote fibrinolysis through the activation of plasminogen to plasmin, which is a serine protease that can degrade fibrin, fibrinogen, and coagulation factors V, VIII, and XII (Figure 15-3).

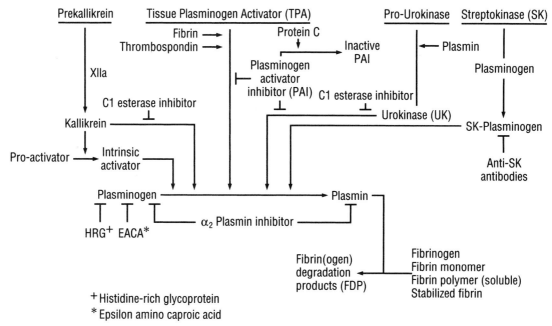

FIGURE 15-3 Biochemical pathways involved in the fibrinolytic system. (From Lucas FV, Miller ML: *Cleve Clin J Med* 55:531, 1988.)

Plasmin is inhibited by α_2-antiplasmin, α_2-macroglobulin, AT-III, and α_1-antitrypsin. These inhibitors are depleted when systemic activation of plasminogen leads to excessive amounts of circulating plasmin. tPA is selective in that it activates only fibrin-bound plasmin, whereas streptokinase and urokinase activate both fibrin-bound plasmin and freely circulating plasmin. This difference results in a more systemic fibrinolysis with streptokinase and urokinase as opposed to tPA, but tPA can also produce systemic fibrinolysis during prolonged use or in large doses.

Preoperative bleeding may occur at sites of vascular access. Intramuscular injections should be avoided. Extreme care should be taken in the institution of new sites of vascular access. Sites that are accessible to manual compression should preferably be chosen for arterial and large-bore venous access. If uncontrollable bleeding does occur, administration of FFP or cryoprecipitate may be indicated in addition to packed red cells. Therapy with an inhibitor of fibrinolysis such as EACA may also be considered. Previously published statements by Rosenquist and Brown regarding anesthetic management of patients receiving fibrinolytic or thrombolytic medications have been updated as follows[42,45]:

1. Advances in fibrinolytic/thrombolytic therapy have been associated with an increased use of these drugs, which will require further increases in vigilance. Ideally, the patient should be queried prior to the thrombolytic therapy for a recent history of lumbar puncture, spinal or epidural anesthesia, or epidural steroid injection to allow appropriate monitoring. Guidelines detailing original contraindications for thrombolytic drugs suggest avoidance of these drugs for 10 days following puncture of noncompressible vessels.
2. Preoperative evaluation should determine whether fibrinolytic or thrombolytic drugs have been used preoperatively or have the likelihood of being used intraoperatively or postoperatively. Patients receiving fibrinolytic and thrombolytic drugs should be cautioned against receiving spinal or epidural anesthetics except in highly unusual circumstances. Data are not available to clearly outline the length of time neuraxial puncture should be avoided after discontinuation of these drugs.
3. In those patients who have received neuraxial blocks at or near the time of fibrinolytic and thrombolytic therapy, neurologic monitoring should be continued for an appropriate interval. It may be that the interval of monitoring should not be more than 2 hours between neurologic checks. Furthermore, if neuraxial blocks have been combined with fibrinolytic and thrombolytic therapy and ongoing epidural catheter infusion, the infusion should be limited to drugs minimizing sensory and motor block to facilitate assessment of neurologic function.
4. There is no definitive recommendation for removal of neuraxial catheters in patients who unexpectedly receive fibrinolytic and thrombolytic therapy during a neuraxial catheter infusion. The measurement of fibrinogen level (one of the last clotting factors to recover) may be helpful in making a decision about catheter removal or maintenance.

Pentoxifylline

Pentoxifylline is a synthetic xanthine derivative used for symptomatic treatment of claudication in patients with peripheral vascular disease. Pentoxifylline's principal effect is an increase in the flexibility of red blood cells, allowing improvement in blood flow in the microcirculation, resulting in better tissue oxygenation. There are associated decreases in blood viscosity and in total systemic vascular resistance.

Pentoxifylline also has an inhibitory effect on platelet aggregation.[46] Levels of intracellular cAMP are increased by the enhanced release and synthesis of prostacyclin as well as through phosphodiesterase inhibition, which occurs with the administration of pentoxifylline.

Fibrinolytic activity is increased and fibrinogen levels are reduced with the use of pentoxifylline. This reduction in fibrinogen level is reversible and has not been reported to cause an increased risk of bleeding. The enhanced fibrinolysis is thought to occur from increased levels of plasminogen activator as well as from decreased antiplasmin activity.

Procoagulant Therapy

Protamine

Protamine sulfate is a cationic protein that is extracted from the sperm or mature testes of salmon. Its only therapeutic role is to neutralize heparin. Because of its strongly basic property, protamine binds to the acidic heparin to form a stable salt. Protamine has a rapid onset of action, and dosage depends on the amount of heparin in the circulation. Doses of 1 to 1.3 mg of protamine per 100 U heparin administered are recommended. Because serum levels decrease rapidly after an intravenous injection of heparin, the amount of protamine required for neutralization also decreases with time. Various methods have been described to determine the dose of protamine necessary for adequate heparin neutralization, including the ACT, dose-response curves, and protamine titration. It is most important, however, to monitor the adequacy of neutralization when a dose of protamine has been administered. Probably the most common, simplest, and most practical clinical method in determining adequate protamine dose involves an estimation of an initial dose based on the amount of heparin administered, elapsed time since administration, and the ACT. After the initial dose of protamine is administered, a repeated measure of the ACT is obtained, and further protamine therapy is guided by the results of the ACT.

Protamine also has weak anticoagulant properties by affecting the function of thrombin. These in vitro anticoagulant effects, however, are not clinically important, as rather large doses of protamine have been administered with minimal effects on coagulation.[47]

Adverse effects of protamine range from mild systemic hypotension, which is mostly a result of systemic vasodilation through an anaphylactic or anaphylactoid reaction, to catastrophic pulmonary vasoconstriction with severe, protracted hypotension. It is important to identify patients at risk for serious reactions to protamine; these may include diabetic patients taking insulin, patients with prior exposure to intravenous protamine, patients with cross-reacting antigens (fish allergy, history of vasectomy), and patients with a previous history of catastrophic pulmonary vasoconstriction after protamine administration.

Lysine Analogs

EACA and tranexamic acid are synthetic lysine analogs that interfere with the conversion of plasminogen to plasmin by binding to the lysine binding sites of plasminogen. This blocks the binding of tPA to plasminogen that causes the release of plasmin. These drugs are most effective for reducing operative bleeding when administered prophylactically and have been extensively studied for use during cardiac surgery. Published studies that examine the role of lysine analogs during vascular surgery are sparse. Patients treated with tranexamic acid

undergoing thoracic aortic surgery had less bleeding and fewer transfusions than patients treated with placebo in a randomized, double-blind placebo-controlled study without an increase in perioperative thrombotic complications.[48] Use of tranexamic acid in patients undergoing carotid endarterectomy at the time of coronary artery bypass grafting does not appear to increase the incidence of myocardial ischemia–related complications.[49] EACA is effective in reducing blood loss during posterior spinal fusion and reduces the risk of rebleeding before cerebral vascular surgery in patients with subarachnoid hemorrhage.[50,51]

Aprotinin

Aprotinin is a naturally occurring nonspecific serine protease inhibitor that suppresses plasmin activation and has a beneficial effect on platelet function. This drug has also been extensively studied during cardiac surgery but is more expensive and more likely to cause an allergic reaction because it is a naturally occurring substance obtained from bovine lung. The drug prolongs the result of a celite-activated ACT but does not affect kaolin-activated ACT. Studies that examine the use of aprotinin during vascular surgery are sparse despite numerous studies demonstrating decreases in blood loss and transfusion requirements during cardiac surgery. Low-dose aprotinin significantly decreases blood product transfusion requirements during thoracic aortic surgery requiring deep hypothermic circulatory arrest and does not appear to be associated with renal or myocardial dysfunction.[52]

Desmopressin

Desmopressin (DDAVP) releases vWF and plasminogen activator from endothelial cells and factor VIII from the liver. DDAVP is, therefore, useful for treatment of hemophiliacs with decreased vWF or factor VIII. The drug has been shown to reduce blood loss and yield higher levels of vWF and factor VIII during cardiac surgery.[53] The drug also has a beneficial effect on platelet function in cardiac surgical patients.[54] Mild platelet dysfunction and moderate thrombocytopenia commonly occur during vascular surgery.[55] Thrombocytopenia occurs during aortic vascular surgery because of platelet consumption in the surgical wound and the aortic prosthesis and because of the dilutional effects of hypervolemia. Although use of DDAVP might be considered in this setting, a randomized, prospective, double-blind study demonstrated no benefit in terms of blood loss, incidence of blood transfusion, or decreased bleeding time.[55]

Intraoperative Blood Loss and Replacement

More than 50% of all transfusions of packed red blood cells occur in the perioperative setting, and major vascular surgery has the potential for significant blood loss. In addition, patients undergoing vascular surgery tend to have concomitant disease states that may dictate maintenance of a higher level of hemoglobin, thus lowering the transfusion trigger for red blood cell administration. These disease states include peripheral vascular disease, cerebrovascular disease, coronary artery disease, and impaired pulmonary and myocardial function. Although healthy individuals may tolerate hemoglobin levels of 7 g/dL or lower, patients undergoing vascular surgery are not likely to tolerate even higher levels before they have exhausted their ability to compensate for the anemia. Therefore, acceptable hemoglobin levels must be individually determined for each patient, taking into account their ability to compensate, the degree of further blood loss expected, and the etiology of the anemia. Furthermore, as the hemoglobin level decreases, special attention should be given to minimizing the conditions that impair oxygen delivery to the tissues. This includes avoiding alkalosis, hypothermia, and myocardial depressants, which may lead to an impairment of cardiac output. Postoperatively, conditions such as shivering and hyperthermia, which increase oxygen requirements, should be avoided.

For each individual patient and circumstance, the anesthesiologist must weigh the benefit of the transfusion against the risks. The risks are mainly associated with transmission of disease and transfusion reactions. The human hepatitis viruses are the most frequently transmitted infections. Donor screening with specific and nonspecific tests has reduced the incidence of hepatitis infection and HIV infection, but the incidence is not zero (Table 15-9).[56,57] The advent of HIV screening actually coincided with decreased incidences of blood transfusion and number of units transfused among elderly patients undergoing carotid endarterectomy in a large retrospective study involving 1114 patients.[58] Cytomegalovirus transmission can also occur but is usually asymptomatic in immunocompetent patients.[59] Bacterial infection of blood components can also cause transfusion-transmitted infection and may exceed the risk from viral infection (Table 15-10).[60] Transfusion reactions occur in varying degrees. The most common reaction, consisting of fever, chills, and urticaria, occurs in 1 in 100 transfusions. Hemolytic transfusion reactions can be eliminated with compatibility testing but occur on the order of 1 in 6000 and are invariably due to a clerical error.[61]

Endovascular repair of abdominal aortic aneurysms is a newer technique that offers many advantages over an open procedure.[62] Although blood loss from leaky valves and the delivery systems is usually less than during open repair, trauma from femoral dissection and passage of the large delivery device may lead to vessel perforation and massive hemorrhage.[63,64]

Transfusion of homologous blood can often be avoided if blood conservation measures are taken. These include (1) preoperative collection and storage of autologous blood concomitant with iron supplementation, (2) the use of intraoperative blood salvage techniques,[65] and (3) intraoperative hemodilution. Except for intraoperative blood salvage, these techniques require that a certain degree of anemia be induced, which can be minimized in the preoperative technique by prescribing iron

TABLE 15-9

Viral Infectious Risks of Blood Transfusions

Infection	Incidence Rate among Repeat Donors per 100,000 Person-Years (95% confidence intervals)
Hepatitis B	10.43 (7.99-13.37)
Hepatitis C	3.25 (2.36-4.36)
HIV	2.92 (2.26-3.70)
Human T cell	1.59 (1.12-2.19)

HIV, human immunodeficiency virus.
From Glynn SA, Kleinman SH, Schreiber GB, et al: *JAMA* 284:238, 2000

TABLE 15-10

Bacterial Infectious Risk of Blood Transfusions

Infection	Incidence Rate of Transmission* (95% confidence intervals)	Incidence of Fatal Reactions* (95% confidence intervals)
Red blood cells	0.21 (0.03-0.40)	0.13 (0-0.27)
Single-donor platelets	9.98 (5.4-14.9)	2.22 (0.04-4.4)
Pooled platelets	10.64 (4.4-16.9)	1.94 (0-4.62)

*Events per million units distributed.
From Kuehnert MJ, Roth VR, Haley NR, et al: *Transfusion* 41:1493, 2001.

supplementation. Anemia that may be well tolerated by young, healthy patients may not be tolerated in vascular patients with concomitant disease who are not able to compensate for even mild degrees of anemia before their reserve is exhausted.

Intraoperative fluid and blood losses begin with the surgical incision. As tissues become exposed, losses occur from evaporation and by a shift of extracellular fluid to the "third-space" compartment as a result of the tissue trauma that occurs during surgery. The degree and rate of these losses depend on the extent of the incision and surgical exposure needed for the particular operation.

During aortoiliac surgery, operative bleeding is usually the result of venous injury because of the close anatomic relationship between the aorta and iliac arteries and the major veins. In addition to the inferior vena cava, these include the left renal, left gonadal, lumbar, and iliac veins.[66,67] During infrainguinal arterial surgery, major intraoperative blood loss is usually not a common problem, but it may become a problem in the recovery room. Postoperative bleeding is usually due to leaking anastomoses, an inadequately ligated branch of a vein graft, laceration of a vein wall with use of an in situ technique, inadequate reversal of heparin anticoagulation, or a preexisting defect in coagulation.[66]

As blood loss ensues, there are resultant decreases in intravascular volume, red blood cells, clotting factors, and platelets. After replacement with clear fluids and red blood cells has begun, the coagulation defect of dilutional thrombocytopenia may become apparent. Because this becomes important at counts of less than 50,000 to 100,000 platelets/mm^3, platelet transfusion becomes necessary.[68,69] Dilution of coagulation factors is usually not a problem until large quantities of replacement blood have been administered.

Operative bleeding is more common during aortoiliac surgery than infrainguinal arterial reconstruction, in which postoperative bleeding most commonly occurs. Bleeding from major venous systems is usually the source during aortoiliac surgery. Particular attention is given to the area at the level of the aortic bifurcation where the posterior lateral surface of the aorta and the iliac artery are tightly adherent to the inferior vena cava and right iliac vein.[66] Any major venous bleeding is initially controlled with application of gentle finger pressure at the site. An aortic aneurysm may rarely erode into the inferior vena cava, producing a fistula, which may not always be initially apparent.[66,70] Consequently, massive venous bleeding occurs in the aneurysmal sac during its resection while the aorta is cross-clamped. Arterial bleeding can occur during posterior aortic dissection or during resection of the aneurysm from the lumbar or inferior mesenteric arteries.[66,67]

Large disruptions in vascular integrity such as those described obviously require surgical ligation for adequate hemostasis to be achieved. Before bleeding is controlled, however, large amounts of blood loss may ensue, resulting in the defects in coagulation associated with massive blood transfusions.

Postoperative Bleeding and Reoperation

Patients undergoing vascular surgery are at risk for massive and sudden blood loss at vascular anastomoses or sutured arteriotomy sites. Postoperative bleeding may be occult for bleeding sites that are contained by surrounding tissue or when surrounding tissue can accommodate blood loss. Bleeding becomes apparent with a continued need for blood and fluid replacement, as dictated by the patient's hemodynamics, urine output, laboratory studies, and ongoing blood loss. Retroperitoneal hemorrhage after aortic surgery can produce a distended and tense flank. The cause of the bleeding is usually leaking anastomoses, inadequately ligated vessels, or unrecognized laceration of major vessels during dissection.

Postoperative bleeding after carotid surgery is detected more easily because the neck cannot accommodate significant bleeding without producing symptoms that are readily apparent, such as neck swelling, hoarseness, and difficulty breathing. Airway compromise in this situation becomes life threatening and is not easily corrected because altered anatomy makes intubation and airway management difficult, if not impossible. This situation is best managed with local anesthesia because general anesthesia may lead to complete loss of airway patency in the setting of difficult intubation. O'Sullivan et al described six patients who developed neck hematomas after carotid artery surgery, all of whom experienced immediate airway obstruction with induction of anesthesia and were difficult to intubate.[71] Airway obstruction occurred in six of seven patients described by Kunkel et al who were also difficult to intubate.[72] Two sustained perioperative myocardial infarctions, one had respiratory failure, and one died. Awake intubation or a local anesthetic technique is thus strongly advised for surgical neck exploration of a postoperative carotid hematoma. Figure 15-4 presents a

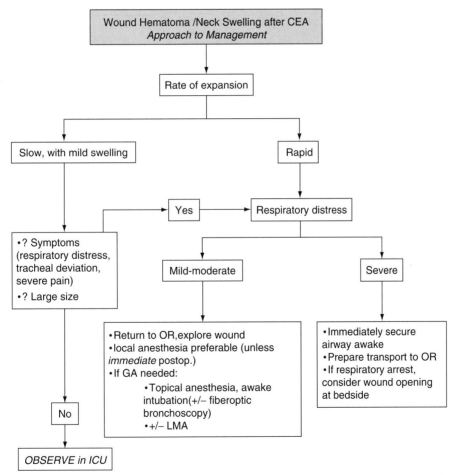

FIGURE 15-4 A suggested approach to the management of wound hematomas accompanied by neck swelling after carotid endarterectomy *(CEA)*. Mild swelling with minimal symptoms may be managed conservatively with observation in an intensive care unit *(ICU)*. The presence of respiratory symptoms or a rapid increase in neck diameter requires immediate reexploration in the operating room *(OR)* and securing of the airway while the patient is awake. Neck swelling immediately (<1 hour) after surgery may produce less glottic edema because of the short duration of bleeding, but cautious assessment of the airway is still advised before proceeding with general anesthesia *(GA)* for reexploration. Opening of the wound at the bedside is probably only appropriate for acute respiratory arrest. *LMA,* laryngeal mask airway. (From O'Connor CJ, Tuman KJ: Vascular surgery. In Troianos CA (ed): *Anesthesia for the cardiac patient,* St. Louis, 2002, Mosby.)

suggested approach to the management of wound hematomas with neck swelling after carotid endarterectomy (see Chapter 10).

Immediate reoperation is indicated for excessive postoperative bleeding. Blood volume is replaced as rapidly as possible before induction of anesthesia unless blood loss is massive or far exceeds the ability to replace the loss. As the amount of blood replacement increases, the patient's own blood begins to take on characteristics of bank blood, with low levels of 2, 3-diphosphoglycerate and low activities of factors V and VIII, as well as dilutional thrombocytopenia. While the surgeon is attempting to achieve surgical hemostasis, the anesthesiologist must continually evaluate the patient's hemostatic profile in order to recognize any defects that must also be addressed. Continued monitoring of the ACT, platelet count, fibrinogen level, PT, and aPTT should be carried out as long as active bleeding persists. These studies aid in the identification of any nonsurgical cause for bleeding, such as heparin rebound, as well as guide therapy for correction of the hemostatic defect.

Acknowledgement: The authors gratefully acknowledge Norig Ellison, MD for his contribution to this chapter in the first edition of Vascular Anesthesia.

REFERENCES

1. Ellison N: Diagnosis and management of bleeding disorders, *Anesthesiology* 47:171, 1977.
2. Fischback DP, Fogdall RP: *Coagulation: the essentials*, Baltimore, 1981, Williams & Wilkins.
3. Ellison N: Coagulation evaluation and management. In Ream AK, Fogdall RP (eds): *Acute cardiovascular management*, Philadelphia, 1982, JB Lippincott, 773.
4. Salzman EW: Hemorrhagic disorders. In *ACS manual of preoperative and postoperative care*, Philadelphia, 1983, WB Saunders, 153.
5. Ellison N, Silberstein LE: Hemostasis in the perioperative period. In Stoelting RK, Barash PG, Gallagher TJ (eds): *Advances in anesthesia*, vol 3, Chicago, 1986, Year Book Medical Publishers, 67.
6. Strauss R, Wehler M, Mehler K, et al: Thrombocytopenia in patients in the medical intensive care unit: bleeding prevalence, transfusion requirements, and outcome, *Crit Care Med* 30:1765, 2002.
7. Stoelting RK, Dierdorf SF, McCammon RL: Disorders of coagulation. In *Anesthesia and co-existing disease*, New York, 1988, Churchill Livingstone, 575.
8. Fabris F, Luzzatto G, Soini B, et al: Risk factors for thrombosis in patients with immune-mediated heparin-induced thrombocytopenia, *J Intern Med* 252:149, 2002.
9. Kaebnick H, Towne JB: Hypercoagulable states and vascular thromboses. In Ernst CB, Stanley JC (eds): *Current therapy in vascular surgery*, Toronto, 1987, BC Decker, 235.
10. Comp PC: Hereditary disorders predisposing to thrombosis. In Coller BS (ed): *Progress in hemostasis and thrombosis*, vol 8, Orlando, Fla, 1986, Grune & Stratton, 71.
11. Aoki N, Moroi M, Sakata Y, et al: Abnormal plasminogen: a hereditary molecular abnormality found in a patient with recurrent thrombosis, *J Clin Invest* 61:1186, 1978.
12. Carrell N, Gabriel DA, Blatt PM, et al: Hereditary dysfibrinogenemia in a patient with thrombotic disease, *Blood* 62:439, 1983.
13. Mueh JR, Herbst KD, Rapaport SI: Thrombosis in patients with the lupus anticoagulant, *Ann Intern Med* 92:156, 1980.
14. Atik M: Venous thrombosis. In Moore WS (ed): *Vascular surgery, a comprehensive review*, Orlando, Fla, 1986, Grune & Stratton, 1043.
15. Rosenberg RD: Actions and interactions of antithrombin and heparin, *N Engl J Med* 292:146, 1975.
16. Sas G, Blasko G, Banhegyi D, et al: Abnormal antithrombin III (antithrombin III "Budapest") as a cause of familial thrombophilia, *Thromb Diath Haemorrh* 32:105, 1974.
17. Seligsohn U, Berger A, Abend M, et al: Homozygous protein C deficiency manifested by massive venous thrombosis in the newborn, *N Engl J Med* 310:559, 1984.
18. Rick ME: Protein C and protein S, vitamin K–dependent inhibitors of blood coagulation, *JAMA* 263:701, 1990.
19. Gonzalez R, Alberca I, Sala N, Vincente V: Protein C deficiency—response to danazol and DDAVP, *Thromb Haemost* 53:320, 1985.
20. Coller B, Owen J, Jesty J, et al: Deficiency of plasma protein S, protein C, or antithrombin III and arterial thrombosis, *Arteriosclerosis* 7:456, 1987.
21. Schafer AI: The hypercoagulable states, *Ann Intern Med* 102:814, 1965.
22. Naeye RL: Thrombotic state after a hemorrhagic diathesis, a possible complication of therapy with epsilon aminocaproic acid, *Blood* 19:694, 1962.
23. Hirsh J, Cade JF, Gallus AS: Anticoagulants in pregnancy: a review of indications and complications, *Am Heart J* 83:301, 1972.
24. Ellison N, Ominsky AJ: Clinical considerations for the anesthesiologist whose patient is on anticoagulant therapy, *Anesthesiology* 39:328, 1973.
25. Eckhardt WF, Iaconetti J, Kwon JS, et al: Inadvertent carotid artery cannulation during pulmonary artery catheter insertion, *J Cardiothorac Vasc Anesth* 10:283, 1996.
26. Troianos CA, Jobes DR, Ellison N: Ultrasound-guided cannulation of the internal jugular vein. A prospective, randomized study, *Anesth Analg* 72:823, 1991.
27. Bridenbaugh PO, Greene NM: Spinal neural blockage. In Cousins MJ, Bridenbaugh PO (eds): *Neuronal blockage in clinical anesthesia and management of pain*, Philadelphia, 1988, JB Lippincott, 244.
28. Odoom JA, Sih IL: Epidural analgesia and anticoagulant therapy. Experience with one thousand cases of continuous epidurals, *Anesthesia* 38:254, 1983.
29. Ellison N, Jobes DR, Schwartz AJ: Heparin therapy during cardiac surgery. In Ellison N, Jobes DR (eds): *Effective hemostasis in cardiac surgery*, Philadelphia, 1988, WB Saunders, 1.
30. Liu SS, Mulroy MF: Neuraxial anesthesia and analgesia in the presence of standard heparin, *Reg Anesth Pain Med* 23(Suppl 2):157, 1998.
31. Parnass SM, Rothenberg DM, Fisher RI, Ivankovich AD: Spinal anesthesia and minidose heparin, *JAMA* 263:1496, 1990.
32. Gallus AS, Hirsh J, Tuttle RJ, et al: Small subcutaneous doses of heparin in prevention of venous thrombosis, *N Engl J Med* 288:545, 1973.
33. Vandermeulen EP, Van Aken H, Vermylen J: Anticoagulants and spinal-epidural anesthesia, *Anesth Analg* 79:1165, 1994.
34. Greaves JD: Serious spinal cord injury due to haematomyelia caused by spinal anaesthesia in a patient treated with low-dose heparin, *Anaesthesia* 46:613, 1997.
35. Hirsh J, Raschke R, Warkentin TE, et al: Heparin: mechanism of action, pharmacokinetics, dosing considerations, monitoring, efficacy, and safety, *Chest* 108(4 Suppl):258S, 1995.
36. Owens FL, Kasten GW, Hessel EA: Spinal subarachnoid hematoma after lumbar puncture and heparinization. A case report, review of the literature, and discussion of anesthetic implications, *Anesth Analg* 65:1201, 1986.
37. Rao TLK, El-Etr AA: Anticoagulation following placement of epidural and subarachnoid catheters: an evaluation of neurologic sequelae, *Anesthesiology* 55:618, 1981.
38. Kappa JR, Addonizio VP Jr: Heparin-induced thrombocytopenia: diagnosis and management. In Ellison N, Jobes DR (eds): *Effective hemostasis in cardiac surgery*, Philadelphia, 1988, WB Saunders, 123.
39. Kappa JR, Fisher CA, Berkowitz HB, et al: Heparin-induced platelet activation in sixteen surgical patients: diagnosis and management, *J Vasc Surg* 5:101, 1987.
40. Kappa JR, Fisher CA, Todd B, et al: Intraoperative management of patients with heparin-induced thrombocytopenia, *Ann Thorac Surg* 49:714, 1990.
41. Horlocker TT, Wedel DJ: Neuraxial block and low-molecular-weight heparin: balancing perioperative analgesia and thromboprophylaxis, *Reg Anesth Pain Med* 23(Suppl 2):164, 1998.
42. Horlocker TT, Wedel DJ, Benzon H, et al: Regional anesthesia in the anticoagulated patient: defining the risks, *Reg Anesth Pain Med* 28:172, 2003.
43. Enneking FK, Benzon H: Oral anticoagulants and regional anesthesia: a perspective, *Reg Anesth Pain Med* 23(Suppl 2):140, 1998.
44. Hodges PJ, Kam PC: The perioperative implications of herbal medicines, *Anaesthesia* 57:889, 2002.
45. Rosenquist RW, Brown DL: Neuraxial bleeding: fibrinolytics/thrombolytics, *Reg Anesth Pain Med* 23(Suppl 2):152, 1998.
46. Ward A, Clissold SP: Pentoxifylline. A review of its pharmacodynamic and pharmacokinetic properties, and its therapeutic efficacy, *Drug* 34:50, 1987.
47. Ellison N, Ominsky AJ, Wollman H: Is protamine a clinically important anticoagulant? *Anesthesiology* 35:621, 1971.
48. Casati V, Sandrelli L, Speziali G, et al: Hemostatic effects of tranexamic acid in elective thoracic aortic surgery: a prospective, randomized, double-blind, placebo-controlled study, *J Thorac Cardiovasc Surg* 123:1084, 2002.

49. Ruel MA, Wang F, Bourke ME, et al: Is tranexamic acid safe in patients undergoing coronary endarterectomy? *Ann Thorac Surg* 71:1508, 2001.

50. Florentino-Pineda I, Blakemore LC, Thompson GH, et al: The effect of epsilon-aminocaproic acid on perioperative blood loss in patients with idiopathic scoliosis undergoing posterior spinal fusion: a preliminary prospective study, *Spine* 26:1147, 2001.

51. Leipzig TJ, Redelman K, Horner TG: Reducing the risk of rebleeding before early aneurysm surgery: a possible role for antifibrinolytic therapy, *J Neurosurg* 86:220, 1997.

52. Seigne PW, Shorten GD, Johnson RG, Coumunale ME: The effects of aprotinin on blood product transfusion associated with thoracic aortic surgery requiring deep hypothermic circulatory arrest, *J Cardiothorac Vasc Anesth* 14:676, 2000.

53. Salzman EW, Weinstein MJ, Weintraub RM, et al: Treatment with desmopressin acetate to reduce blood loss after cardiac surgery. A double-blind randomized trail, *N Engl J Med* 314:1402, 1986.

54. Mongan PD, Hosking MP: The role of desmopressin acetate in patients undergoing coronary artery bypass surgery. A controlled clinical trial with thromboelastographic risk stratification, *Anesthesiology* 77:38, 1992.

55. Clagett GP, Valentine RJ, Myers SI et al: Does desmopressin improve hemostasis and reduce blood loss from aortic surgery? A randomized, double-blind study, *J Vasc Surg* 22:223, 1995.

56. Dodd R: Current viral risks of blood and blood products, *Ann Med* 32:469, 2000.

57. Glynn SA, Kleinman SH, Schreiber GB, et al: Trends in incidence and prevalence of major transfusion-transmissible viral infections in US blood donors, 1991 to 1996. Retrovirus Epidemiology Donor Study (REDS), *JAMA* 284:238, 2000.

58. Waggoner JR 3rd, Wass CT, Polis TZ, et al: The effect of changing transfusion practice on rates of perioperative stroke and myocardial infarction in patients undergoing carotid endarterectomy: a retrospective analysis of 1114 Mayo Clinic patients. Mayo Perioperative Outcomes Group, *Mayo Clin Proc* 76:376, 2001.

59. Ellison N: A commentary on three NIH Consensus Development Conferences on Transfusion Medicine, *Anesth Clin North Am* 8:609, 1990.

60. Kuehnert MJ, Roth VR, Haley NR, et al: Transfusion-transmitted bacterial infection in the United States, 1998 through 2000, *Transfusion* 41:1493, 2001.

61. Myhre BA, Bove JR, Schmidt PJ: Wrong blood—a needless cause of surgical deaths, *Anesth Analg* 60:777, 1981.

62. Kahn RA, Moskowitz DM: Endovascular aortic repair, *J Cardiothorac Vasc Anesth* 16:218, 2002.

63. Zarins CK, White RA, Schwarten D, et al: AneuRx stent graft versus open surgical repair of abdominal aortic aneurysms: multicenter prospective clinical trial, *J Vasc Surg* 29:292, 1999.

64. Sutton DC, Rother A: Endoluminal abdominal aortic aneurysm repair complicated by intracardiac guidewire placement and massive transfusion, *Anesth Analg* 91:89, 2000.

65. Patra P, Chaillou P, Bizouarn P: Intraoperative autotransfusion for repair of unruptured aneurysms of the infrarenal abdominal aorta. A multicenter study of 203 patients. Association Universitaire de Recherche en Chirurgie (AURC), *J Cardiovasc Surg* 41:407, 2000.

66. Lalka SG, Bernard VM: Noninfectious complications in vascular surgery. In Moore W (ed): *Vascular surgery: a comprehensive review*, Orlando, Fla, 1986, Grune & Stratton, 959.

67. Downs A: Problems in resection of aorto-iliac and femoral aneurysms. In Bernhard VM, Towne JB (eds): *Complications in vascular surgery*, Orlando, Fla, 1980, Grune & Stratton, 68.

68. Sheldon GF, Lim RC Jr, Blaisdell FW: The use of fresh blood in the treatment of critically ill patients, *J Trauma* 15:670, 1975.

69. Miller RD, Robbins TO, Tong MJ: Coagulation defects associated with massive transfusions, *Ann Surg* 174:794, 1971.

70. Bernhard VM: Aortocaval fistulas. In Haemovici H (ed): *Vascular emergencies*, New York, 1982, Appleton-Century-Crofts, 353.

71. O'Sullivan JC, Wells DG, Wells GR: Difficult airway management with neck swelling after carotid endarterectomy, *Anaesth Intensive Care* 14:460, 1986.

72. Kunkel JM, Gomez ER, Spebar MJ, et al: Wound hematomas after carotid endarterectomy, *Am J Surg* 148:844, 1986.

73. Barrer MJ, Ellison N: Platelet function, *Anesthesiology* 46:202, 1977.

74. Neerhout RC: Evaluation and management of surgical patients with complicating hematologic conditions, *Pediatr Clin North Am* 16: 681, 1969.

75. Lucas FV, Miller ML: The fibrinolytic system, *Cleve Clin J Med* 55: 531, 1988.

Complications of Vascular Surgery 16

Dimitri Arnaudov, MD
Maxim Benbassat, MD
Gligor Gucev, MD
Philip D. Lumb, MB, BS, FCCM

Complications of Monitoring

Most operations on peripheral vessels for relatively healthy individuals are performed with standard monitoring according to American Society of Anesthesiologists (ASA) requirements.[1] The practicing anesthesiologist has to be aware of not only the available noninvasive monitors but also their associated complications. Automatic noninvasive blood pressure monitoring is usually a minor and innocent procedure, but several cases of pain, petechiae and ecchymoses, skin damage, limb edema, venous stasis and thrombophlebitis, peripheral neuropathy, and even compartment syndrome have been reported.[2-9] Multiple uses of blood pressure cuffs predispose to bacterial colonization. For long surgical procedures, when frequent blood pressure readings are necessary, it is prudent to change the cuff position periodically or select an alternative strategy.

Other noninvasive monitors such as pulse oximetry, neuromuscular stimulators, electrocardiography, and temperature probes are also associated with hazards. Pulse oximetry has been associated with corneal abrasions, burns, pressure and ischemic injuries, and electric shock.[10-18] Nerve stimulators can be a source of burns, pressure injuries, and pain.[19,20] Even the simple act of noninvasive temperature monitoring is reported to be the cause of burns, bleeding, local damage, and bacterial colonization.[21-25] The new technologies and disposable probes have reduced incidents of this type. Contemporary capnographs expose the patient for vascular anesthesia to some unexpected harm. The mainstream capnograph has a probe, which is heavy and heated. Pressure damage and burns could result from its inappropriate use.[26] Sidestream capnographs aspirate gas samples from the circuit at a continuous rate of more than 150 mL/min. Patients undergoing low-flow anesthesia could be hypoventilated because of progressive loss of gas volume from the anesthesia system to the capnograph. The sample stream can be scavenged or returned to the breathing circuit to prevent circuit leakage (see Chapter 8).

Complications of Transesophageal Echocardiography

The use of transesophageal echocardiography (TEE) during surgery was first described in 1980, and it has become an accepted monitor in cardiovascular surgery. The most important applications for intraoperative TEE are estimating ventricular function, assessing valvular function, demonstrating the presence of residual air, and detecting other cardiac abnormalities. TEE is considered relatively safe and noninvasive. Serious complications (eg, esophageal injury or bleeding, vocal cord paralysis, arrhythmias, hypotension, seizures, cardiac arrest) occur in less than 3% of TEE examinations.[27]

Insertion and manipulation of the TEE probe may cause lip injuries or oropharyngeal, esophageal, or gastric trauma resulting in functional or structural disruption of the upper gastrointestinal tract.[28-34] Hoarseness and recurrent laryngeal nerve palsy are also complications of TEE.[35] The close relation of the TEE probe to the heart explains the incidents of arrhythmia sometimes seen in lightly anesthetized patients.[36,37] There are also reports of systemic bacteremia and sepsis.[38,39] Inadvertent endotracheal insertion of the TEE probe is uncommon in the operating room, in part because endotracheal intubation precedes placement of the TEE probe. Some other unusual complications have been reported such as cases of airway obstruction, especially in infants; spleen rupture; compression of aberrant arteries with resultant end-organ ischemia; and even carcinoid crisis induced by pressure of the TEE probe.[40,41] Increased operator skill has reduced the incidence of TEE-associated complications. Recognizing the contraindications to TEE placement also reduces complications.[42]

Complications of Invasive Monitoring

INTRA-ARTERIAL CATHETERS. Arterial cannulation was introduced in the early 1970s and described in detail by a number of authors.[43-48] Since then, this method has become a routine way to monitor vascular patients. Placement of an intra-arterial catheter allows the clinician to (1) continuously and accurately monitor arterial pressure, (2) sample arterial blood avoiding multiple arterial punctures, and (3) determine cardiac output and blood volume using various dilutional techniques. Many arteries are suitable for placement of an arterial catheter. In vascular surgery, the patients present an additional challenge for anesthesiologists performing the arterial catheter placement. These patients already have peripheral vascular disease and altered peripheral perfusion. Many of them are undergoing numerous surgical interventions with compromised arteries. It is even more difficult to find a suitable artery for cannulation in patients with previously amputated extremities or artificial arterial grafts. Usually the procedure is easily accomplished at the bedside using percutaneous methods such as the Seldinger technique to cannulate the radial, brachial, axillary, femoral, dorsalis pedis, or superficial temporal artery. The radial artery is the most frequently used site for arterial catheter placement.

Despite an initial large number of studies about complications of arterial cannulation, the technique is widely practiced.[44,45] The complications of indwelling arterial catheters are well defined in textbooks and numerous reports about them are published.[46] The major complications of arterial cannulation are ischemia and necrosis secondary to either thrombosis or embolism. The longer the catheter is in place, the greater the incidence of thrombosis. Indwelling arterial catheters in small arteries present for more than 48 hours clearly increase the risk of thrombosis.[47] Although no clear-cut guidelines exist, clinicians should attempt to use the smallest gauge catheter compatible with transcutaneous placement by direct puncture. A 20-gauge catheter is appropriate for use in the adult radial artery. Multiple punctures of the radial artery, long-lasting hypotension, hypercoagulation, and vascular occlusive disorders predispose to thrombosis and ischemic changes of the radial artery.[46,48-50] Other potential complications include embolism, hemorrhage, ischemia, arteriovenous fistula, and pseudoaneurysm formation.[51-55]

Prevention of complications from arterial cannulation requires atraumatic and meticulously aseptic technique. Emboli of various types can be avoided by flushing the arterial system in short pulses with carefully "debubbled" solutions. The connections of the entire tubing system have to be tight to avoid accidental disconnection and rapid exsanguination of the patient.

The Allen test deserves special attention. This was originally described by Allen in 1929 for diagnosis of thromboangiitis obliterans.[46,56] The original test and its more recent modifications (direct compression, Doppler or plethysmography) are not good predictors of the likelihood of developing ischemic complications of the hand. Nevertheless, use of the test, especially in patients with peripheral vascular disease, is innocuous, rapid, and simple to perform and can be recommended. Documentation of rapid capillary refill is appropriate in patients for whom invasive cannulation is planned.[57]

Evidence of distal ischemia in an extremity with proximal arterial cannulation mandates immediate removal of the catheter with simultaneous aspiration in an attempt to remove any arterial thrombus that is present. Sympathetic blockade may be beneficial for the affected limb if ischemia persists. Although distal gangrene is the most feared complication, the most common is percutaneous sloughing or necrosis at the site of cannulation. The presence of the catheter in the lumen of the artery can cause intimal thickening and accumulation of platelet aggregates. It can cause blockage of the small perforators coming off the main artery at acute angles. The intimal thickening and disruption of the arterial wall can lead to pseudoaneurysm formation after decannulation. A recognized technique during arterial decannulation is to aspirate on the catheter and try to clear as much thrombus as possible.[58]

CENTRAL VENOUS CATHETERS. Access to the central venous system is indicated when peripheral veins are not available or when indications for central venous catheters (CVCs) are present. Intermittent or continuous monitoring of central venous pressure (CVP) is necessary for many vascular patients. When vasoactive drugs are indicated, the drips are preferentially infused through a central catheter. Pulmonary artery balloon flotation catheters are placed through single- or multiple-lumen introducers, some of which possess high-flow features. Often the patients' central veins are cannulated with a high-flow introducer used as a large-bore CVP catheter, which, when indicated, is available for pulmonary artery catheterization. The

widespread use of CVP creates a risk for complications of various types (Table 16-1).

Unrecognized puncture of the arterial system (carotid, subclavian) followed by cannulation with a large-bore introducer may lead to significant complications including hemorrhage and hemothorax, damage of the recurrent laryngeal nerve, and cerebrovascular accident. Perforation of the carotid artery with subsequent needle passage into the trachea can cause a temporary tracheal-carotid fistula.[59] Overly vigorous use of a scalpel to enlarge the skin entry site prior to passage of the vessel dilator and introducer sheath has been noted to cause damage to the adjacent external jugular vein and carotid artery.[59-62]

Another serious complication of central venous cannulation is embolism caused by fragments of catheters or introduction devices (guide wires). These complications have to be recognized because they cause arrhythmias, vascular damage, thrombosis, and embolism. Foreign bodies should be removed as quickly and completely as possible using interventional radiology

---

TABLE 16-1

Complications of Percutaneous Central Venous Catheters

Access	Adverse Effect
Internal jugular vein	Needle injury to or cannulation of the carotid artery with consequent ischemic brain infarction.
	Brain infarction caused by carotid embolism or venous thrombosis extending to intracranial venous sinuses.
	Needle injury to the vagus nerve, phrenic nerve, cervical sympathetic chain, stellate ganglion, and cervical plexus.
	Injury to transverse processes of the cervical vertebrae with consequent reactions and infections of periosteum and bone.
Subclavian Vein	Injury to brachial plexus.
	Injury to the clavicle or first-rib periosteum.
Internal jugular and subclavian vein	Needle injury to or cannulation of the adjacent arteries.
	Venous air embolism.
	Injury to vertebral artery with possible brainstem ischemic damage.
	Injury of lymphatic ducts, lymphorrhagia, chylomediastinum, and chylothorax.
	Puncture of a pleural dome alone.
	Puncture of a pleural dome and lung apex.
	Catheter misplacement in pleural cavity and consequent deposition of fluids and blood infusates in the pleural space.
	Pneumothorax.
	Hemothorax and/or soft tissue and mediastinal hematoma.
All cannulation techniques and locations (external jugular, basilic, femoral veins)	Inadvertent arterial puncture only or subsequent cannulation of the artery.
	Detour of the catheter tip into a branch vein.
	Venous perforation or erosion from the catheter tip.
	Malposition of the central venous pressure catheter.
	Clot and fibrinous sleeve formation.
	Thrombosis of the vein and thromboembolism.
	Catheter-related infections.
	Catheter shredding and foreign body embolus.
	Loss of the guide wire and its embolization.
	External bleeding from catheter skin site.

Modified from Grenrik A: *Textbook of critical care*, ed 4, Philadelphia, 2000, WB Saunders.

methods.[63-65] Finally, disconnection of the central catheter with resultant risk of air entrainment has to be kept in mind. All connections have to be firmly tightened to prevent disconnection and exsanguinations.[66] During long surgical procedures, the cannulation site is often covered and remains unseen by the anesthesiologist. Silent and unrecognized bleeding through the high-flow central catheter could lead to disastrous results. The use of extension tubes with Luer-Lok system connections offers additional safety features.

Patients with implanted vena cava filters (VCFs) for prevention of pulmonary embolism are at lifelong risk for numerous complications. There are many case reports about guide wire entrapment with or without displacement of the VCF.[67,68] The usual reason is lack of awareness about the presence of the filter. The use of a J-shaped guide wire and its deep insertion are other reasons for this complication. The engagement of a guide wire or CVP catheter in a VCF is preventable if the anesthesiologist is aware of the presence of the filter. The access and depth of insertion have to be carefully chosen. Use of straight guide wires is recommended. In case of entrapment, excessive traction on the guide wire should be avoided (the VCF might be dislodged), and an interventional angiography consultation should be obtained.

PULMONARY ARTERY CATHETERS. Since their introduction into clinical practice a quarter of a century ago, pulmonary artery catheters (PACs) have been the subject of much scrutiny. Despite several investigations, studying everything from survival to multiple organ failure and duration of hospital stay, no conclusive evidence has shown the use of PACs to be specifically beneficial. Nevertheless, balloon-tipped catheters continue to be broadly used in operating rooms worldwide.[69] The major argument of the opponents of PAC is the various complications arising from their use, some of them fatal. All complications related to CVC might occur during PAC placement. For the balloon catheter itself there are specific adverse effects (Table 16-2).[70]

Atrial and ventricular arrhythmias are often seen during insertion of PACs. The occurrence of arrhythmias is higher in patients with preexisting cardiac disease, shock, hypoxemia, electrolyte abnormalities, acidosis, and prolonged catheterization time.[71] PAC insertion–induced arrhythmias are caused by stimulation of the endocardium or in some cases the distention of the pulmonary artery from the inflated balloon. Arrhythmias are the primary complication of the catheterization procedure. Minor arrhythmias, such as premature atrial and ventricular contractions, occur commonly with catheter insertion but usually resolve spontaneously after the catheter is advanced through the right ventricle and exits the pulmonary artery outflow tract. Premature ventricular contractions and short runs of ventricular tachycardia are often seen during the passage of the catheter into the pulmonary artery.

Right bundle-branch block (RBBB) is a described complication but is not seen often. It has to be considered as a risk in patients with previous existing left bundle branch block (LBBB) related to the possible trauma from the catheter on the right bundle of Hiss and resultant complete heart block (CHB). In a study of 47 critically ill patients who underwent a total of 82 pulmonary artery catheterizations, there were no episodes of CHB related to the pulmonary artery catheterization procedure in the

TABLE 16-2

Incidence of Adverse Effects with PACs

Complication	Reported Incidence (%)
Central venous access	
Arterial puncture	1.1–13
Bleeding at cutdown site (children)	5.3
Postoperative neuropathy	0.3–1.1
Pneumothorax	0.3–4.5
Air embolism	0.5
Catheterization	
Minor arrhythmias*	4.7–68.9
Severe arrhythmias (ventricular tachycardia or fibrillation)*	0.3–62.7
Right bundle-branch block*	0.1–4.3
Complete heart block (in patients with prior LBBB)*	0–8.5
Catheter residence	
Pulmonary artery rupture*	0.1–1.5
Positive catheter tip cultures	1.4–34.8
Catheter-related sepsis	0.7–11.4
Thrombophlebitis	6.5
Venous thrombosis	0.5–66.7
Pulmonary infarction*	0.1–5.6
Mural thrombus*	28–61
Valvular or endocardial vegetations or endocarditis*	2.2–100
Deaths (attributed to PA catheter)*	0.02–1.5

*Complications thought to be more common (or exclusively associated) with pulmonary artery catheterization than with central venous catheterization.
LBBB, left bundle-branch block; PA, pulmonary artery.
From Practice guidelines for pulmonary artery catheterization. A report by the American Society of Anesthesiologists Task Force on Pulmonary Artery Catheterization, *Anesthesiology* 78:380, 1993.

patients with either old LBBB or indeterminate-aged LBBB. There were two episodes of CHB in patients with new LBBB. The authors concluded that the incidence of CHB complicating pulmonary artery catheterization with balloon-tipped, flow-directed catheters in critically ill patients with old or indeterminate-aged LBBB is extremely low. Therefore, they do not recommend the routine placement of a temporary transvenous pacemaker in all patients with LBBB prior to pulmonary artery catheterization.[72] Instead, a transcutaneous pacemaker and a temporary transvenous pacing wire or pacing PAC should be readily available to treat complete atrioventricular block. It should be recognized that initiation of pacing with a specially adapted PAC may be difficult if the catheter has not been advanced into the pulmonary artery, thereby aligning the pacing port correctly in the right ventricle. The onset of the block may be delayed and become manifest after induction of anesthesia. For example, incomplete RBBB following PAC insertion has been reported to progress to complete RBBB and bradycardia following induction of anesthesia. Thus, the anesthesiologist must be prepared to treat this complication whenever it arises.[73]

Some of the mechanical complications from pulmonary catheters, such as erosions and perforation of vessels, cause increased mortality.[74] Catastrophic bleeding with bronchial obstruction and lung collapse result after perforation of a branch of the pulmonary artery. The clinical picture includes arterial blood flow from the endotracheal tube, high peak inspiratory pressures during mechanical ventilation; hemodynamic deterioration, and rapid desaturation. Treatment involves isolation of the healthy lung (usually by the means of a double-lumen tube), ventilation with 100% oxygen, and treatment of hemorrhagic shock. Positive end-expiratory pressure (PEEP) has been suggested in order to tamponade the affected lung. Immediately after the diagnosis is made, a cardiothoracic surgical team should be involved and equipment for cardiopulmonary bypass has to be available.[75,76] Some authors believe that in the absence of high-risk factors, such as pulmonary hypertension and systemic anticoagulation, pulmonary artery rupture from a PAC can be successfully treated by withdrawal of the catheter and supportive care.[77]

To prevent pulmonary artery rupture, the anesthesiologist has to recognize promptly distal catheter migration and occlusion of the pulmonary artery (spontaneous [auto] "wedge"). It is important to recognize that balloon occlusion of the pulmonary artery should be limited in duration. In order to avoid traumatic damage to the pulmonary artery secondary to overinsertion and/or balloon-induced rupture, the catheter should always be advanced into the pulmonary artery with the balloon fully inflated (1.5 mL of gas). The catheter should be withdrawn until balloon occlusion occurs with 1.25 to 1.5 mL of gas; smaller volumes indicate overinsertion into the pulmonary artery. During balloon inflation, continuous observation of the pulmonary artery waveform is mandatory. A catheter should never be advanced to the pulmonary artery occlusion pressure (PAOP) position by injection of a specific volume of gas; rather, gradual injection and waveform observation are required. During placement excessive force should never be required to overcome obstruction to passage. If resistance is encountered, the operator should reassess the cannulation and placement.

Another serious complication of PACs is coiling and knotting in the right heart cavities. Arrhythmias and blockage caused by the knotted catheter are reported. The knot itself may damage the cardiac structures.[78,79] The interventional radiology team has to be consulted in order to unknot the catheter.[80] Knot formation is unlikely if the operator recognizes the depth of insertion at the tricuspid valve and inserts the catheter no more than 15 cm before noting the characteristic pulmonary artery waveform.

Infection is the most frequent complication of PAC placement. The grades of infection range from simple colonization of the catheter site to systemic bacteremia and sepsis. Routes of infection could be breaks in the monitoring tubing, migrated bacteria and fungi along the catheter tract, and hematogenous seeding from circulating microbes.[81-83] Scrupulous attention to sterile technique during catheter insertion must be ensured. Anesthesiologists often underestimate the threat of catheter contamination because it is not immediately apparent. The patients later develop spiking fevers and become septic. This may be a delayed complication of inappropriate insertion technique. There are no recent prospective studies about the incidence of any type of infection and comparison of the cultures taken from the catheter, its sheath, and the blood cultures. Coagulase-negative staphylococci, *Staphylococcus aureus*, aerobic gram-negative bacilli, and *Candida albicans* most commonly cause catheter-related bloodstream infections. After appropriate cultures of blood and catheter samples are obtained, empirical intravenous antimicrobial therapy should be initiated on the basis of clinical signs, the severity of the patient's acute illness, underlying disease, and the potential pathogen(s) involved. In most cases of bacteremia and fungemia, the PAC and its introducer should be removed. It is not clear whether patients with positive results of catheter cultures (but with negative blood culture results) and no other obvious site of infection need to be treated with antibiotics.[84]

The postoperative management of vascular surgical patients should include steps to discover and treat monitoring complications. Physical examination should assess for presence of burns, corneal and skin abrasions, neurologic impairment, hematomas, ischemia of the extremities, and the presence of bilateral breath sounds. A chest film should be obtained after CVC and must be evaluated for the presence of pneumothorax, hemothorax, mediastinal hematoma, and misplacement of the catheter. The tip of the CVC should not be within the pericardial silhouette on chest radiographs. This finding demands an immediate correction. It is important to note that a portion of the superior vena cava lies within the pericardium. Any patient with a CVC in place who develops unexplained hypotension, dyspnea, or chest tightness has to be evaluated for cardiac tamponade.[85] Catheters inserted through the left subclavian vein or left internal jugular vein should not lie with the tip perpendicular to the sidewall of the superior vena cava because this position is suspected of increasing the likelihood of erosion through the vessel wall. The tip of a PAC should be positioned within two fingerbreadths of the sternal border to lessen the risk of pulmonary infarction and pulmonary artery rupture.

If a pneumothorax, hemothorax, or hydrothorax is noted on chest radiograph and respiratory or hemodynamic function is compromised, placement of a chest tube and connection to a water seal apparatus with suction of 20 cm of water is indicated. A small asymptomatic pneumothorax in extubated patients without respiratory compromise can be observed. However, if there is respiratory distress or if positive-pressure ventilation is planned, chest tube placement is necessary. Hydrothorax or hemothorax noted after fluid or blood infusion through an indwelling CVC is a cause for immediate concern. The catheter should be removed or repositioned until blood can be aspirated freely. In the case of a repositioned catheter, it should not be reused until its position is confirmed by repeated chest radiography. The volume of blood lost from the chest tube in a patient with hemothorax should be monitored, and bleeding greater than 200 mL/hr must be thoroughly evaluated.

Use of real-time ultrasound or Doppler ultrasound guidance for placement of internal jugular and subclavian CVCs in adult patients increases the probability of successful catheter placement and reduces the risk of complications and the need for multiple catheter placement attempts[86,87] (see Chapter 8).

Complications of the Surgical Procedure
Stroke following Carotid Artery Endarterectomy

Since the pioneer days in the early 1950s when Fisher described the syndrome of neurologic symptoms caused by narrowing, thrombosis, and embolism of the carotid sinus and Carrea, Eastcott, and DeBakey performed the first surgeries, the fate of the carotid artery endarterectomy has been significantly influenced by the incidence of perioperative complications.[88-91] After reports of complication rates as high as 10% to 20% in the 1970s, concerns were expressed about the benefits of the endarterectomy.[92-94] It is evident that the morbidity and mortality of carotid endarterectomy associated with cardiovascular and other complications have declined, but the success of the surgery is most realistically determined by the magnitude of any neurologic complications. In order to address the issues of selection of patients, risk factors, complication rate, and overall benefits, several well-controlled, randomized outcome studies were designed. The scope of current practice is shaped by the results of these studies (see Chapter 10).

The North American Symptomatic Carotid Endarterectomy Trial (NASCET) was started in 1987 in 50 centers.[95] Inclusion criteria were transient monocular blindness, hemispheric transient ischemic attack, or a nondisabling stroke on the side of the angiographically verified 30% to 99% stenosis of the carotid artery. Patients were stratified as having severe stenosis (>70%) and moderate stenosis with less than 70% decrease in the luminal diameter. Patients were randomly assigned to either a surgical or a medical treatment group. Surgeons accepted in the study had to demonstrate a less than 6% perioperative stroke and death rate over a 2-year period. The first results were published in 1991, when the trial for the severe stenosis group was stopped.[95] Carotid artery endarterectomy showed an absolute reduction in ipsilateral stroke rate of 17% and was recommended for all patients with severe stenosis. The arm of the study exploring the moderate stenosis group was continued and the results demonstrated that among patients with stenosis of 50% to 69%, the 5-year rate of any ipsilateral stroke was 15.7% among patients treated surgically and 22.2% among those treated medically ($P = 0.045$).[96] To prevent one ipsilateral stroke during the 5-year period, 15 patients would have to be treated with carotid endarterectomy. Among patients with less than 50% stenosis, the stroke rate in the surgical group was 14.9% and the medically treated group had a stroke rate of 18.7%, $P = 0.16$. Among the patients with severe stenosis who underwent endarterectomy, the 30-day rate of death or disabling ipsilateral stroke persisting at 90 days was 2.1%; this rate increased to only 6.7% at 8 years. Benefit was greatest among men, patients with recent stroke, and patients with hemispheric symptoms. Patients with stenosis less than 50% had no benefit from surgery.

For 1415 symptomatic patients, the NASCET study demonstrated an overall rate of perioperative stroke and death of 6.5%.[97] At 30 days the rate of disabling stroke was 1.8% and nondisabling stroke 3.7%. By 90 days of follow-up, the disabling stroke rate was only 0.9% and nondisabling stroke rate 4.5%. The European Carotid Surgery Trial (ECST) has reported results with comparable perioperative stroke rates.[98,99] In 1745 patients at 30 days the disabling stroke rate was 2.5% and the nondisabling stroke rate was 3.5%.

Without surgical treatment, the incidence of stroke for patients with transient ischemic attacks (TIAs) related to severe carotid stenotic lesions is 12% to 13% for the first year after onset of symptoms. The risk of stroke cumulates to approximately 30% to 35% at the end of 5 years. Stroke rates are higher if TIAs have a hemispheric distribution, recent onset, or

increasing frequency. Increased stroke rates are also observed with high-grade stenosis.[100] Patients who have had a stroke continue to be at risk for subsequent strokes at the rate of 5% to 9% per year, with approximately 25% to 45% of patients having another stroke within 5 years of the original event.[101,102]

The risk of stroke in patients with asymptomatic carotid artery stenosis is relatively modest compared with the risk of stroke in symptomatic patients. The risk/benefit ratio for these procedures is more sensitive to surgical excellence and comorbidity factors. The Asymptomatic Carotid Atherosclerosis Study (ACAS) examined 1662 patients with ultrasound-verified stenosis of greater than 60% at 39 centers in North America between 1987 and 1993.[103] In the surgical group, 2.3% of the patients suffered a stroke or death. The projected risk of ipsilateral stroke or perioperative stroke or death at the 5-year interval was 5.1%, including the risk of stroke with arteriography. Only 0.4% of the patients in the medical group suffered stroke or death in the initial period, but their projected risk of stroke or death at 5 years was 11% ($P = 0.004$, 95% confidence interval). The benefit associated with surgery was realized within the first year, and 89% of patients survived long enough to achieve that benefit with the mean age at entry of 67 years. The study was terminated after 2.7 years of median follow-up demonstrating significant advantage of surgical treatment.

Analysis of the risk /benefit ratio of carotid endarterectomy must include mention of prevalence of coexisting coronary artery disease (CAD). The appropriate management of patients with carotid artery disease and symptomatic or asymptomatic CAD has been addressed in several studies. Moore et al, in their statement on "Guidelines for carotid endarterectomy: a multidisciplinary consensus statement from the ad hoc committee, American Heart Association," reviewed 56 reports on the topic.[104] The options include operating on the carotid lesion first, with an increased risk of morbidity and mortality from myocardial infarction; operating on the coronary lesion first, with an increased risk of perioperative stroke; operating on both lesions during the same period of anesthesia; or operating on the coronary arteries alone. The results of the meta-analysis demonstrated that the perioperative stroke rate was similar if carotid and coronary artery surgeries were combined or if carotid surgery preceded coronary artery bypass grafting (CABG). If CABG was done first, the frequency of stroke was significantly greater. If carotid endarterectomy was done first, the frequency of myocardial infarction ($P = 0.01$) and that of death ($P = 0.02$) were greater. These findings are summarized in Table 16-3.

As there is no consensus on the preferred approach for management of patients with combined coronary and carotid artery disease, a well-designed prospective randomized trial is necessary. Carotid angioplasty and stenting is also being evaluated as an alternative to carotid endarterectomy. The patients treated with this method have an incidence of stroke similar to that of endarterectomy patients.[105,106]

The pathogenesis of perioperative stroke in patients undergoing endarterectomy is mostly due to thromboembolism, brain hypoperfusion during the time of carotid clamp placement, and reperfusion injury. Thromboembolism is the most frequent cause of perioperative stroke and usually occurs in the first 24

TABLE 16-3

Incidences of Complications with Three Surgical Options for Combined Disease

Option	CVA	Myocardial Infarction	Death
Simultaneous	0.0617	0.0467	0.056
Staged carotid-CABG	0.053	0.1147*	0.0938*
Staged CABG-carotid	0.1003*	0.0247	0.0358

*$P<0.05$
CABG, coronary artery bypass grafting: CVA, cerebrovascular accident.

hours and especially in the first 6 postoperative hours. It is a result of either debris entering the cerebral circulation from the site of surgery or complete thrombosis of the internal carotid artery. Both phenomena are caused by manipulation of the artery and are worsened by increased coagulability. The typical clinical picture is that of a stroke that develops in the recovery room. Presence of a new neurologic deficit requires prompt diagnosis and treatment. In this situation, most authorities recommend urgent surgical exploration or cerebral angiography followed immediately by corrective surgery.[107-110]

Strokes are thought to be thromboembolic if the infarction occurred in the territory of distribution of a main arterial trunk or its branches. The majority of perioperative strokes in the NASCET study were ipsilateral, two thirds of them occurring after the endarterectomy.[97] In the Findlay and Marchak series of 700 patients, 3.4% had a perioperative stroke.[111] Of the 13 patients who had major hemispheric symptoms, two thirds were due to thrombotic and embolic phenomena, one third had proven or possible cross-clamp ischemia, and one patient had an intracerebral hemorrhage. Radak et al reported 41 strokes in a series of 2250 carotid endarterectomies.[112] Thrombotic occlusions were found in 22% of patients who had intraoperative or immediate postoperative strokes compared with 61% of patients who had delayed-onset strokes. The patients from the delayed-onset group also had better outcomes after reoperation. The epidemiologic data are consistent with earlier observations by Imparato and Koslow and their coworkers.[113,114]

Hemodynamic Instability following Carotid Endarterectomy

Hemodynamic instability frequently follows carotid endarterectomy and may play a role in the development of neurologic, surgical, and medical complications. Several studies have observed the incidence of this phenomenon. Bove et al reported hypertension in 19% and hypotension in 28% of the patients.[115] Postoperative neurologic complications affected 9% of this group, compared with 0% complications in the normotensive group. Englund and Dean reported complications in 37% of the patients with diastolic blood pressure higher than 100 mmHg and 6% of the patients with decrease of the mean arterial pressure of 40 mmHg or more.[116] Towne and Bernhard examined 253 postendarterectomy patients with 3.4% neurologic deficit in the normotensive group and 10.2% neurologic deficit in patients whose systolic arterial pressure was greater than 200 mmHg.[117] In some cases it may be difficult to determine whether the hypertension is caused by postoperative hemodynamic instability or stroke following the operation.[118]

Relative to degree of stenosis, the blood flow in the distal areas is proportionally decreased, creating a chronic hypoperfusion state. Arteriolar-capillary beds distal to stenosis are dilated to ensure adequate blood flow. This chronic vasodilation results in loss of vascular autoregulation. Following revascularization, this vasculature is fragile and exposed to breakthrough perfusion pressure. Patients who have had previous neurologic deficits may have areas with altered arteriolar and capillary permeability. The profound increase in cerebral blood flow may cause edema and hemorrhagic infarction. Hyperperfusion syndrome occurs in patients with high-grade stenosis and longstanding hypoperfusion. Cerebral blood flow studies in six patients with postoperative unilateral headache revealed increases of cerebral blood flow from 43 ± 16 mL/100 g/min before surgery to 83 ± 39 mL/100 g/min postoperatively.[119]

The carotid sinus reflex plays an important role in perioperative hemodynamic instability following carotid endarterectomy. Arterial mechanoreceptors are located in the media and adventitia of the common carotid artery near its bifurcation. The mechanoreceptors are sensitive to both pulse pressure and heart rate. The receptors have a threshold pressure below which they are inactive. The threshold may be reset by chronic hypertension. In normotensive patients it is approximately 65 to 70 mmHg. With increases in the arterial pressure activity from the receptors, increases to the systolic maximum reached about 180 mmHg. Impulses are conducted by the carotid sinus nerve and glossopharyngeal nerve to the nucleus tractus solitarius (NTS). The efferent path starts at the NTS via the tractus bulbospinalis and reaches preganglionic adrenergic neurons, resulting in lower sympathetic tone and increased vagal tone through vagal nuclei activation.[120] Seagard et al described two different types of carotid baroreceptors.[121] Type I carotid baroreceptors, mainly large myelinated A fibers, are characterized by a sudden onset of discharge at relatively high frequency at pressure threshold. Type II carotid baroreceptors, mainly small A fibers and nonmyelinated C fibers, demonstrate a spontaneous subthreshold discharge with a slower rate of firing than those of type I. Thus, type I baroreceptors may be involved in rapid adjustment of systemic blood pressure, whereas type II baroreceptors may play a longer lasting role to maintain the baseline level of pressure.

Hypotension following endarterectomy may result from increased activity of the carotid sinus reflex. Angell-James and Lumley measured the activity of the carotid sinus nerve (CSN) in patients undergoing carotid surgery.[122] The activity of the CSN correlated with changes in arterial pressure. In three hypotensive patients after the carotid procedure, CSN activity was greater than preoperatively. In two patients with postoperative hypertension, postoperative CSN activity was lower than preoperatively.

A prospective study exploring the effects of CSN blockade on the perioperative hemodynamics after endarterectomy was done by Gottlieb et al.[123] The patients were randomly assigned to receive either bupivacaine or placebo injection into the carotid sinus during surgery. The patients receiving bupivacaine block had a significantly higher incidence of postoperative hypertension. Mehta et al compared the nerve-sparing surgical technique and the nerve-ablating technique for endarterectomy.[124] Patients who underwent nerve ablation had a significantly ($P < 0.005$) increased postoperative blood pressure and required more frequent intravenous antihypertensive medication (24%) compared with patients having nerve sparing (6%). Although the carotid sinus reflex is one of the key factors in the development of hemodynamic instability following carotid endarterectomy, the etiology appears to be multifactorial. Preoperative hypertension was found to be the single most important determinant for the development of postoperative hypertension by Towne and Bernhard.[117] Increased concentrations of renin were found in the jugular veins of patients developing hypertension.[125] Archie related hypertension to inadequate collateral circulation, and Ahn et al correlated hypertension with elevated cranial norepinephrine levels.[126,127] Management of hemodynamic instability following carotid endarterectomy is important to prevent new neurologic deficits or extension of existing ones. Aggressive treatment of perioperative hypertension and control of systolic arterial pressure under 180 mmHg are the most important objectives.[128]

Spinal Cord Injury following Major Vascular Surgery

Spinal cord damage following major vascular surgery is an unpredictable, devastating complication of multifactorial origin (see Chapter 11).[129-187] Possible causative factors include interruption of the greater radicular artery (Adamkiewicz's artery), prolonged aortic occlusion, perioperative hypotension, atheromatous embolization, and interruption of the internal iliac artery circulation.[129-135] Significant predictors of postoperative paraplegia or paraparesis in a study by Svensson et al of 1509 patients undergoing thoracoabdominal aortic operations were total aortic clamp time, extent of aorta repaired, aortic rupture, patient's age, proximal aortic aneurysm, and history of renal dysfunction.[136] As stated by Rosenthal, however, no factor could be cited as a sole cause of cord ischemia, and neurologic deficit after aortic operations "remains a tragically unpredictable and random event."[165]

The occurrence rate of spinal cord injury varies widely with the anatomic region involved, the acuity of the procedure, and the operative technique employed (open versus endovascular). Following unruptured abdominal aortic aneurysm (AAA) repair, major neurologic deficit is a rare event with a reported incidence of less than 0.25%.[137,138] In an editorial in 1993, Szilagyi reported that the approximate incidence of paraplegia after AAA was 1 in 400 and after aortoiliac reconstruction for occlusive disease was 1 in 5000.[139] In patients with ruptured AAA, the rate is reported to be slightly higher at 1.9%.[138] In a study by Keen, paraplegia following repair of aortic coarctation occurred in only 0.3% of a total of 5492 operations performed.[140] The highest incidence of spinal cord ischemia has been associated with operations involving thoracic and thoracoabdominal aortic aneurysms (TAA and TAAA), and it occurs postoperatively in 5% to 21% of these procedures.[136,145,154-159] Alternatively, experience indicates that the overall risk of cord ischemia has decreased to the 5% to 8% range.[141,142,146,147,149,150] These rather consistent results have been achieved with a variety of surgical and adjunctive methods designed to minimize spinal cord ischemia, which are reviewed in Chapter 11 and elsewhere.[151] Some studies are even showing significantly lower rates (0% to 2.7%) of neurologic deficit after TAAA

repair with use of multimodality perioperative monitoring and therapeutic protocols.[148,152,171] In a meta-analytic study concerning surgical management of acute traumatic dissection of TAA, Von Oppell et al observed an overall paraplegia rate of 9.9% in 1492 patients.[169] Simple aortic cross-clamping was associated with an incidence of neurologic deficit of 19.2% of 443 cases.

It is possible that endovascular treatment of thoracic aortic aneurysms may reduce perioperative complications, especially in debilitated patients who otherwise would be deemed poor candidates for surgery. Advantages of this approach include no need for aortic cross-clamping, avoidance of general anesthesia, and no large abdominal incisions in this high-risk population[153] (see Chapter 7). However, spinal cord ischemia after endovascular repair of thoracic aortic aneurysm has also been noted. Gravereaux et al described postoperative neurologic deficit in 3 of 53 patients (5.7%) undergoing endovascular exclusion of their TAA, with irreversible paralysis occurring in 2 patients.[153] Greenberg et al reported spinal cord ischemia in 12% of a series of 23 patients after endograft repair of TAA.[160] Following the same procedure performed in 108 patients in the study by Mitchell and colleagues, 4 patients (3.7%) sustained paraplegia.[161] Possible risk factors for neurologic deficit in this particular type of operation include long-segment thoracic aortic exclusion and concomitant or previous abdominal or thoracic aortic replacement. Both these circumstances may compromise collateral circulation to the spinal cord and result in early neurologic deficit.[153] Postoperative hypotension, on the other hand, has been blamed for causing delayed-onset spinal cord ischemia in both surgical and endovascular TAA repair.[160,162,164,176-178]

The etiology of spinal cord ischemia after major vascular surgery on the aorta is probably multifactorial, but the fundamental cause is always an alteration in blood supply to the spinal cord.[165] There are two anatomically distinct arterial systems supplying the cord: intrinsic and extrinsic.[131,134,166] The intrinsic network consists of three longitudinal arteries: one anterior and two posterior spinal arteries. The extrinsic blood supply is composed of segmental medullary feeder arteries that supply the anterior and posterior spinal arteries.[165] The anterior spinal artery extends the full length of the spinal cord, but it is narrow and sometimes discontinuous. There is also a relative lack of an intramedullary collateral circulation between the anterior and posterior spinal arteries. The wide spacing of the radicular arteries leaves "watershed" areas along the course of the anterior spinal artery, increasing the risk of infarction after loss of a single radicular artery.[152,166] The anterior spinal artery is, therefore, the major source of perfusion to the anterior portion of the thoracic cord, and interruption of the largest of its segmental radicular arteries (the artery of Adamkiewicz) has been implicated as the principal cause of spinal cord ischemia.[131] The greater radicular artery (Adamkiewicz's artery) arises between T9 and T12 in 75% of cases, between L1 and L3 in 10% of cases, and between T5 and T8 in 15% of cases.[138,168]. The key to prevention of spinal cord injury during AAA repair has been to avoid interruption of the blood flow from the Adamkiewicz's artery. Controversy exists as to whether the greater radicular artery is of such critical importance or whether neurologic injury is more likely when the normal collateral supply to the spinal cord has been compromised.[167] According to Szilagyi, the greater radicular artery may be "harmlessly occluded much more frequently than it is occluded with serious consequences."[139] He explained this observation with ample pelvic collateral flow, which prevents damaging ischemia to the spinal cord. The lower lumbar arteries that anastomose with the intrinsic network may significantly contribute to the blood supply of the terminal spinal cord.[134] In general, when the greater radicular artery is open and of normal size, the pelvic blood supply is of minor importance. When the greater radicular artery is severed, however, the pelvic blood supply becomes critically important.[165]

Two patterns of spinal cord injury are recognized: early onset and delayed paraplegia. The former type appears to be related to intraoperative surgical events, such as length and level of aortic cross-clamping, and failure to identify and reestablish critical collateral blood supply to the cord. There seems to be a consensus in the literature about a close correlation of increasing cross-clamp time and ischemic cord injury.[136,142,143,146,149,157,172] The exact safety limits of the ischemic time are unknown, but it is generally regarded as 20 to 30 minutes under normothermic condition.[138,173] Grabitz et al nevertheless pointed out that it is impossible to predict what aortic clamping time can be tolerated in a particular patient because the exact vascular anatomy, including collateral vessels that provide the spinal cord with blood, is unknown at this time.[147] This may explain why paraplegia can occur only after 30 minutes of cross-clamping in some patients and may not be present even after 60 minutes in others.

The pathogenesis of delayed paraplegia is controversial. It has been reported to occur from 1 to 21 days after surgery.[170] Ischemic spinal cord injuries are thought to be the result of complex interactions among several factors: perfusion and oxygen delivery, local metabolic rate and oxygen demand, reperfusion injury, and failure to maintain microcirculatory flow.[179] Most authors believe that delayed deficit is associated with postoperative hypotension.[160,162,164,175-178] Cambria et al have observed that hypotensive episodes, particularly during hemodialysis, precipitate paraplegia in some patients even weeks after clearly normal postoperative lower extremity neurologic function. Although in most cases a precipitating event cannot be identified, the authors recommended vigorous treatment of perioperative hypotension from any cause in order to prevent delayed neurologic deficit.[155,175] Crawford et al found that causes associated with low-flow states were myocardial infarction, multiple organ system failure, esophageal bleeding, and cardiorespiratory failure.[170] Other possible causes for delayed paraplegia include spinal cord swelling and postoperative neuronal damage resulting from an intraoperative subclinical ischemic insult.[144,163,170,174]

Strategies to prevent spinal cord injury during high-risk TAA repair have been described. In general, these are (1) surgical measures designed to minimize ischemia by maintaining cord blood supply and (2) neuroprotective adjuncts intended to reduce the spinal cord metabolism and oxygen demand. Spinal cord ischemia may be ameliorated surgically by complete intercostal reimplantation, cerebrospinal fluid drainage, distal aortic perfusion, and maintenance of proximal hypertension during cross-clamping.[145,156,177,188-190] Neuroprotective strategies in clinical use include systemic and local hypothermia, high-dose barbiturates, naloxone, papaverine, and avoidance of hyperglycemia.[142,155,180,181,183-187] Reperfusion injury is minimized by the use of mannitol, steroids, and calcium channel blockers.[182] No method has been universally effective in prevention of paraplegia. However, a multimodal strategy that combines a number of these approaches appears to be effective in diminishing cord injury after TAA repair.[148,155] Hollier et al retrospectively reviewed 150 consecutive patients undergoing thoracoabdominal aortic replacement from 1980 to 1991.[148] They found that adherence to a multimodal protocol reduced the risk for spinal cord dysfunction from 6 of 108 (6%) in the pre-protocol group to 0 of 42 in the protocol group (0%). Maintenance of hemodynamic stability in the perioperative period is also of great importance. It is hoped that careful follow-up of patients who have had aortic cross-clamping with neurologic examination and prompt institution of measures for spinal cord protection upon signs of neurologic deficit will decrease the incidence of spinal cord ischemia (see Chapter 11).[187-198]

Acute Renal Failure

Renal dysfunction following major vascular procedures remains a frequent problem today despite better understanding of perioperative fluid management and implementation of various renal prophylactic protective strategies (see Chapter 14). Postoperative acute renal failure (ARF) ranges from 1% to 13% in elective AAA surgery.[199-204] The incidence is significantly higher in ruptured AAA, reaching 24%, with a resultant mortality rate ranging from 43% to 66% in patients requiring renal replacement therapy.[198,205,206] Renal impairment after TAAA repair was reported to be between 3% and 54%.[147,155,200,207-210] The wide range in the postoperative ARF incidence may be explained by the differences in the diagnostic criteria for renal failure adopted in individual series. Some authors define kidney dysfunction as more than a 25% increase of serum creatinine above baseline level. Other studies use the presence of full-blown renal failure requiring dialysis as the inclusion criterion in their analysis. In a study involving 1220 patients undergoing acute or elective TAAA operation, LeMaire et al defined renal impairment as an elevation of the serum creatinine level greater than 3 mg/dL and renal failure as a need for postoperative hemodialysis.[202] The authors found the incidence of renal impairment to be 25% in the acute group versus 9% in the elective cases. Postoperative renal failure occurred in 10% of the emergencies and in 6% of the elective repairs. The rate of ARF was substantially lower than that reported in other acute series, which the authors attributed to their adherence to a strict definition of renal failure.

ARF continues to cause significant morbidity and mortality in the immediate postoperative period despite improved surgical techniques and advances in applied critical care management strategies. In addition, the mortality rate of patients requiring dialysis has not decreased significantly over the last 50 years.[201,211,212] In a prospective study of 43,642 patients undergoing cardiac surgery, the mortality rate for patients who needed dialysis was 63.7%, compared with 4.3% for patients without ARF.[213] In another prospective study of 475 consecutive patients undergoing TAAA surgery, death occurred most frequently in patients with postoperative ARF requiring hemodialysis (22 patients, 56%) followed by patients with ARF not requiring dialysis (31 patients, 38%).[199] Mortality was lower in patients with no renal failure (50 patients, 14%). Morbidity was also significantly higher in the ARF group. Pulmonary complications (68% vs. 33%), neurologic complications (68% vs. 15%), and digestive complications (19% vs. 5%) occurred more frequently in patients with kidney dysfunction.

In addition to being an important marker for severe morbidity, ARF has been shown to be a significant independent risk factor for mortality.[214-245] A review by Chertow et al of 42,773 patients who underwent CABG or valvular heart surgery found a 63.7% mortality rate in the group requiring renal replacement therapy versus only 4.3% in patients with no renal failure.[216] Collins et al examined more than 13,000 vascular operations performed at 123 Veterans Affairs hospitals and identified several preoperative factors that are independently associated with 30-day mortality for patients undergoing aortic surgery.[192] For AAA, the independent predictors of 30-day postoperative mortality included, among others, a creatinine level higher than 1.2 mg/dL. In the study by Safi et al on 243 patients undergoing TAAA, the univariate odds ratio of death, given ARF, was 6.7.[200] Patients with chronic renal dysfunction undergoing carotid artery surgery may experience a significant increase in the perioperative stroke rate compared with those with normal renal function.[240] They are also at higher risk for increased perioperative and long-term mortality.[239] These data emphasize the significance of renal insufficiency as a marker of poor outcome in patients after vascular surgery. Association of ARF with other organ injury is also of critical importance in determining patients' outcome. Presence of multiorgan failure carries a notoriously high mortality rate that approaches 100% when more than three organs fail simultaneously.[203,212]

Despite a wide variety of etiologic factors causing kidney dysfunction, a common pathophysiologic mechanism for perioperative ARF is ischemic injury to the nephron with subsequent reperfusion injury. A major factor here is the acute disturbance of the renal circulation by temporary interruption of the arterial blood supply and/or systemic hypotension. The risk is especially high in aortic surgery requiring suprarenal cross-clamp. Breckwoldt et al compared two groups of patients for elective AAA repair: patients who underwent infrarenal cross-clamping alone and those who underwent suprarenal cross-clamping alone or combined with infrarenal cross-clamping.[217] Transient renal insufficiency was more frequent in the suprarenal group than in the infrarenal group (28% vs. 10%), although mortality and dialysis rates were similar. In another study, postoperative renal injury was observed in 28.6% of the patients with unilateral and in 50% in the group requiring bilateral suprarenal aortic cross-clamp.[218] Kidney dysfunction was found in 8.4% of the infrarenal aortic clamp group. Again, no patient required hemodialysis.

Cross-clamping the aorta decreases renal perfusion depending on the level of clamp placement. Thoracic aorta cross-clamping diminishes renal blood flow by 85% to 94%, causing direct ischemia to the kidneys. It would seem intuitively that infrarenal cross-clamping should not influence renal perfusion drastically, but major effects on kidney hemodynamics and glomerular filtration rate do occur. In a study of 12 patients in

whom other hemodynamic variables, including heart rate, pulmonary artery occluded pressure (PAOP), cardiac output, and mean arterial pressure were unchanged, the application of an infrarenal abdominal aortic cross-clamp decreased renal blood flow by 38% during the period of clamping.[222] One hour after unclamping, renal blood flow had recovered to only 54% of baseline. Renal vascular resistance increased 75% in these patients with application of the cross-clamp. Besides location, the duration of aortic cross-clamping seems to be an important pathogenic factor in the development of acute renal injury. Wahlberg et al retrospectively reviewed 60 patients who underwent infrarenal aortic reconstruction with temporary suprarenal clamping.[244] The authors found that postoperative renal failure was unusual after temporary suprarenal aortic clamping of less than 25 minutes duration, and even slightly elevated blood urea nitrogen or creatinine levels were the exception. The risk for transient renal insufficiency was only doubled when the aorta was clamped for 25 to 50 minutes. However, the incidence of ARF increased 10-fold when clamping time exceeded 50 minutes. Accordingly, it was concluded that aortic clamping above the renal arteries for up to 50 minutes should be regarded as safe and well tolerated (see Chapter 11).

Another important factor causing ischemic injury is thromboembolism to the renal arteries. Causes include surgical manipulation with dislodgment of embolic material from an atheromatous aorta, aortic cross-clamping and unclamping, possible embolism of cardiac origin, trauma, and renal artery dissection.[200,203] Interestingly, when infra- or juxtarenal aortic control is either not possible or considered high risk for embolic complications because of the presence of calcified aortic plaques around the renal artery ostia, supraceliac cross-clamping was shown to be a safe and valuable alternative for achieving proximal control in abdominal aortic reconstruction.[219]

The cornerstone of renal protection in aortic surgery is maintenance of adequate cardiac output to ensure optimal renal perfusion before, during, and after aortic cross-clamping. Adequate preload with either crystalloid or colloid solutions should be given to maintain left ventricular filling pressure at normal or slightly supranormal levels, especially prior to removal of the aortic cross-clamp in order to maximize cardiac output.[241-243] A significant number of pharmacologic agents are available for prevention and treatment of ARF, but definitive evidence supporting specific therapy is lacking.[244-262] Although loop diuretics, mannitol, and dopamine are frequently employed to minimize perioperative kidney injury, their use is based more on individually perceived advantages and empirical clinical practices than on uniformly reproducible results from randomized, clinical trials. Other drugs with theoretical beneficial effects, such as atrial natriuretic peptide analogs, adenosine blockers, and calcium antagonists, need further investigation to justify recommendation for their routine use. A relatively new, highly selective dopamine type 1 agonist, fenoldopam mesylate, may offer renal protection in high-risk patients following major vascular interventions. It has been approved by the Food and Drug Administration for the management of hypertensive emergencies. However, fenoldopam may cause significant increases in renal blood flow, glomerular filtration rate, and natriuresis without adversely affecting the systemic blood pressure.[257] Its renal protective effect has been demonstrated in patients after cardiopulmonary bypass and in dogs during a 90-minute period of infrarenal aortic cross-clamping.[257,258] Gilbert et al used a fenoldopam infusion in 22 patients for elective repairs of AAAs.[259] They found a relatively rapid return of renal blood flow to baseline values in these patients despite profound decreases during aortic cross-clamping. The study was not blinded, and there was no control group. Once again, although the results from trials are promising, further large-scale clinical trials are necessary to investigate how fenoldopam compares with traditional (and cheaper) therapies in its ability to offer renal protection. In conclusion, ensuring adequate intravascular fluid volume remains the only approach to preventing and managing acute renal dysfunction that can be considered relatively effective and safe.[245]

Since its introduction in 1991 by Parodi et al, endovascular infrarenal aortic aneurysm repair has become a valuable alternative to open surgery in selected patients.[214] Because it is intuitively less invasive, this approach could be ideal for patients in whom the standard open procedure might cause increased perioperative morbidity and mortality. The few studies comparing endovascular aneurysm management with open surgery were unable to show significant differences in overall survival rates. However, most investigators agree that there is less blood loss, reduced need for blood replacement, and decreased length of stay in the intensive care unit (ICU) with endovascular procedures.[194-196] Teufelsbauer et al concluded that the presence of renal or pulmonary dysfunction, especially in geriatric patients or those in ASA class IV, is a clear indication for selecting endoluminal repair.[197] Others found that the major morbidities following open surgery included cardiac, respiratory, and renal complications as opposed to predominantly local wound complications following endovascular procedures.[215] Nevertheless, the long-term outcome of endoluminal repair of AAA remains uncertain, and this method has not been accepted yet as standard treatment of AAA.[197]

Infrequently, ARF may result from rhabdomyolysis as a complication from reperfusion following extended periods of limb ischemia or prolonged surgery on young patients in hyperlordotic position.[220] The released myoglobin, which is then freely filtered by the glomerulus into the renal tubules, can precipitate and cause mechanical obstruction. In addition, myoglobin can have a direct toxic effect on the tubular cell. To prevent renal injury, the goal is to maximize urine flow through intravenous crystalloid infusion, diuretic treatment, and alkalinization of the urine with sodium bicarbonate.[221] There are few published reports of rhabdomyolysis following major vascular surgery. The general impression would be that perioperative rhabdomyolysis is a rare event. Surprisingly, one study found a relatively high incidence of lumbar and lower limb rhabdomyolysis among 224 patients who underwent abdominal aortic surgery.[220] Postoperative rhabdomyolysis was diagnosed in 20 (9%) patients. In these patients, 9 (4%) experienced low back pain of unusual severity and had a large increase in creatine kinase (more than 1750 IU/L) with typical findings at tomodensitometry or muscle biopsy confirming lumbar muscle rhabdomyolysis. ARF requiring hemodialysis was recorded in three cases. The remaining 11 patients had lower limb muscle rhabdomyolysis not associated with postoperative renal failure. The authors cautioned that this syndrome should be suspected in patients operated in the hyperlordotic position who experience severe lumbar postoperative pain and great increases in creatine kinase activity.

Contrast medium–induced nephropathy (CMN) is believed to be the third leading cause of ARF in hospitalized patients.[223] It may occur after any radiographic procedure in connection with the administration of intravascular iodine-based contrast media and is usually nonoliguric in nature and of short duration (resolves within 1 to 2 weeks).[224] There seems to be a consensus in the literature that CMN is rare in patients with normal renal function, with the incidence rate ranging from 1% to 12% in general unselected series.[223,225,229] However, the occurrence may be much higher in patients with certain risk factors, reaching up to 40% to 50%.[226,227] In a large randomized trial involving 1196 patients undergoing coronary angiography, Rudnick et al found that 50% of the group with diabetic nephropathy developed contrast medium–induced renal dysfunction.[230] Fifteen percent of these patients needed dialysis. In addition, patients who develop renal failure after contrast dye administration have increased mortality.[225] In one study involving patients who received intravenous contrast dye, the mortality rate was 34% in the ARF group but only 7% in those who did not have renal injury. After adjusting for comorbid factors, renal failure was associated with an odds ratio of dying of 5.5.[234]

The underlying pathophysiologic mechanisms of contrast material toxicity to the kidneys may include direct tubular toxicity and hemodynamic effects.[228] Interestingly, radiocontrast agents appear to induce a biphasic hemodynamic response, with an initial brief period of vasodilation followed by a variable period of renal vasoconstriction and possible subsequent medullary ischemia.[231] The type and the tonicity of the contrast medium may play a major etiologic role as well. Reports have shown that the later introduction of low-osmolar contrast medium may halve the risk of renal failure compared with the previously used high-osmolar contrast medium.[229,230] Data from trials with the newly developed nonionic, iso-osmolar dimers have demonstrated even less nephrotoxicity than with low-osmolar agents.[233] Risk factors shown to augment the incidence of CMN are preexisting renal insufficiency and diabetic nephropathy.[228] In some studies, patients with diabetes mellitus but no kidney dysfunction were not found to be at risk for CMN.[232] Other conditions such as dehydration, congestive heart failure (CHF), and older age may also increase the occurrence rate. Another important factor that correlates directly with the risk of CMN is the total volume of radiocontrast medium administered. In a randomized prospective trial, Cigarroa et al found that only 2% of the group who received a limited contrast material volume developed CMN versus 26% of those in whom the limit was exceeded.[235] Other studies have confirmed that volume of contrast material is an independent risk factor for CMN.[230] Certain drugs, such as aminoglycosides, nonsteroidal anti-inflammatory drugs, and cyclosporin, are well known for their potential to cause chemical renal injury, and their administration together with iodinated contrast media significantly enhances the nephrotoxic effect of the latter.[226]

Fortunately, unlike most forms of hospital-acquired renal failure, CMN may be preventable. Several prophylactic approaches have been proposed. The most important measure remains volume expansion. If there is no contraindication to oral administration, free fluid intake should be encouraged. Otherwise, an intravenous infusion of normal or half-normal saline has to be instituted. Good hydration, designed to maintain a high urine flow rate, is a key issue.[237] Infusion of NaCl 0.9% 12 hours before and after contrast agents significantly ($P = 0.05$) reduced the incidence of contrast agent–induced ARF compared with the use of hydration plus mannitol or furosemide.[238] Diuretics and dopamine have been suggested as agents that could prevent renal injury, but studies have failed to prove their efficacy so far.[250] According to some reports, diuretics may actually contribute to the renal injury, especially if their use causes negative fluid balance.[238] Similarly, renal-dose dopamine was shown to increase the incidence rate of contrast nephropathy among patients with diabetes.[227] Thus, routine administration of diuretics and dopamine for prophylaxis of CMN cannot be recommended.[228,251] The D_1-receptor agonist fenoldopam may be of benefit to high-risk patients who need intravascular contrast injection. A number of studies have demonstrated encouraging results.[252,253] Madyoon et al evaluated the ability of fenoldopam to prevent radiocontrast nephropathy in 46 high-risk patients undergoing interventional angiographic procedures.[248] The incidence of radiocontrast nephropathy, defined as an increase in serum creatinine of 25% or more at 48 hours after the procedure, was 13% in the group treated with fenoldopam compared to 38% of the control group. Thus, the use of fenoldopam in high-risk patients appears to minimize the likelihood of radiocontrast nephropathy. Nevertheless, more large-scale, multicenter, randomized, controlled trials are needed to confirm these observations.[247] Tepel et al demonstrated that oral acetylcysteine can also reduce the incidence rate of contrast nephropathy: from 21% in the placebo group to 2% in the acetylcysteine-treated patients, which suggests that free radical formation may play a role in the pathogenesis of CMN.[249] Efforts should be made to minimize the volume of radiocontrast material given, particularly in high-risk patients. An effective step in this direction is the employment of carbon dioxide as the initial contrast medium in azotemic patients, supplemented with iodinated agents only when necessary. Because carbon dioxide is rapidly dissolved in blood and transported to the lungs for excretion, it has been demonstrated to be a safe contrast medium with few complications and no reported nephrotoxicity.[236]

In the postoperative period, management of oliguria or suspected ARF involves maintenance of appropriate cardiovascular performance to remove prerenal causes of oliguria before progression to acute tubular necrosis occurs. Following aortic surgery, hypovolemia may result from bleeding, third-space fluid loss, or inappropriate diuresis secondary to the effects of hypothermia, mannitol, or other diuretics. Hypothermia may cause diuresis by precipitating renal tubular dysfunction, insulin resistance with hyperglycemia and osmotic diuresis, and increased vascular permeability.[254] Determination of cardiac output (CO) and pulmonary artery occlusion pressure (PAOP) is useful in differentiating CHF from hypovolemia as the prerenal cause of oliguria. Inotropic support, diuretics, and preload and afterload reduction may be indicated in the treatment of the low-output state in the patient with CHF. Hypovolemia as a cause of decreased renal perfusion is treated by volume infusion titrated to PAOP and CO. In vascular surgi-

cal patients without a PAC, a fluid challenge is indicated following the exclusion of CHF by physical examination. However, because of the high incidence of CAD in vascular surgical patients of all types, if a fluid challenge does not rapidly increase urine output, a PAC should be placed to aid in management decisions.[255]

The most common form of ARF in the ICU setting is nonoliguric renal failure with urine flows greater than 15 mL/hr. Early diagnosis of ARF is important so that fluid therapy may be tailored appropriately and treatment regimens adjusted, such as by modifying the dosage of nephrotoxic antibiotics. A creatinine clearance derived from a 2-hour urine collection can provide quantification of renal function in patients with nonoliguric renal failure.[256] In oliguric ARF, management of fluid balance and azotemia necessitates some form of renal replacement therapy.[260]

In a review article, Petroni and Cohen presented a comprehensive overview of the most commonly available renal replacement therapy techniques.[246] These include standard or conventional intermittent hemodialysis (CIHD), peritoneal dialysis (PD), and continuous renal replacement therapy (CRRT). CIHD is the most commonly used therapy for ARF in the United States.[261] Possible drawbacks are hemodynamic instability with renal hypoperfusion and worsening of the ischemic injury, electrolyte imbalance, and need for heparinization, which can cause bleeding after major vascular surgery. PD, although simpler to perform than CIHD, is not considered a suitable therapy for ARF in most surgical patients. It is contraindicated in patients who have recently undergone a celiotomy or surgery with a retroperitoneal approach to the abdominal aorta. In addition, it carries risks of infection and protein loss. The third modality, CRRT, is performed by uninterrupted, extracorporeal solute and/or fluid removal. This procedure is facilitated by connecting a hemofilter with a semipermeable membrane to the patient's circulation by an arterial or venous catheter, or both. To prevent clotting of the hemofilter, citrate instead of heparin may be used because citrate can be utilized as both a buffer and an anticoagulant.[260]

When CRRT is used primarily for achieving fluid balance the mode is called hemofiltration. When solute clearance and uremic control are the goals, the method is defined as hemodialysis. Of course, both therapy modes can be employed simultaneously, which is referred to as hemodiafiltration.[246] In the continuous arteriovenous renal replacement therapy mode, blood is removed from the body by an arterial catheter and returned to the circulation through a venous catheter. The driving force for hemofiltration in this process depends solely on the patient's arterial blood pressure. The second method utilizes venous access alone and is known as continuous venovenous hemofiltration. Because the hydrostatic pressure in this case is not sufficient, an external pump provides the pressure gradient needed for hemofiltration. Both methods can be used to control uremia as well as fluid and electrolyte balance.[262] Thus, CRRT may offer a safer way to treat perioperative ARF following major procedures by overcoming some of the disadvantages of CIHD and PD including adverse hemodynamic changes and the risk of infection. However, no randomized clinical trials have shown CRRT to improve patients' survival when compared with CIHD.[246]

Other Complications

Cranial Nerve Injury during Carotid Endarterectomy

Perioperative complications of carotid endarterectomy include stroke, myocardial infarction, and death, and postoperative complications are cranial nerve injuries, wound hematoma, hypertension, hypotension, hyperperfusion syndrome, intracerebral hemorrhage, seizures, and recurrent stenosis. Of these, cranial nerve injuries and recurrent stenoses are the only ones not directly related to early postoperative care of patients with carotid endarterectomy.[263] The prevalence of peripheral cranial nerve injuries varies between 12% and 69%. The variability of these data depends on the retrospective or prospective character of the study and the sensitivity of the diagnostic techniques applied.[264]

In a number of prospective studies, cranial nerve injuries were found to be a common complication after carotid endarterectomy. Accessory, vagal, facial, hypoglossal, and recurrent laryngeal nerves in the order of their rate of damage have been reported. In a prospective study by Schauber et al of 183 carotid endarterectomy patients, 26 (14.2%) nerve injuries were identified in 21 patients. There were 14 recurrent laryngeal, 8 hypoglossal, 2 marginal mandibular, and 2 greater auricular nerve dysfunctions.[265] Ballotta et al found, in a prospective study of 89 repeated carotid endarterectomies, 25 cranial and/or cervical nerve injuries identified in 19 patients (21%).[266] They included 8 hypoglossal nerves (9%), 11 vagal nerves or branches (12%) (6 recurrent laryngeal nerves [7%], 3 superior laryngeal nerves [3%], and 2 complex vagal nerves [2%]), 3 marginal mandibular nerves (3%), 2 greater auricular nerves (2%), and 1 glossopharyngeal nerve (1%).

A number of factors related to the operation, such as general anesthesia and surgical technique and the surgeon's experience, might influence the incidence of such injuries. Repeated endarterectomy is associated with a higher incidence of cranial and/or cervical nerve injuries.[267] Most of the injuries are due to mechanical factors resulting from retractor trauma, electrocautery, hematoma formation, and direct damage from clamps and ligatures. Although frequent, cranial nerve injuries are usually transient and without residual deficit. The anesthesiologist has to recognize such complications in the early postoperative period on the basis of typical clinical signs. A damaged recurrent laryngeal nerve occurs with prolonged postoperative hoarseness, hypoglossal nerve damage arises with an ipsilateral deviation of the tongue, weakness of the trapezius muscle follows accessory nerve lesion (inability to lift the shoulder), a diaphragm elevated on the affected side is typical of phrenic nerve injury, and drop of the ipsilateral corner of the mouth hints at a marginal mandibular nerve damage. Postoperatively, if symptoms of possible cranial nerve abnormalities occur, involved patients should have a thorough head and neck evaluation in order to identify possible lesions and institute further treatment to improve their quality of life.[268]

Carotid Sinus Dysfunction and Loss of Carotid Body Chemoreceptor Function

Hemodynamic instability during carotid endarterectomy and in the early postoperative period is well known even though its mechanisms are not well understood. Both hypertension and hypotension are seen. Dangerous bradycardia can also be associated. Severe hemodynamic volatility also follows bilateral carotid body tumor resection as part of the baroreflex failure syndrome.[269] The latter appears to be caused by surgical damage to the carotid sinus (bulb) innervation. The sinus nerve of Hering, a branch of the glossopharyngeal nerve, is part of a reflex arc including the brainstem. Surgical damage to it interrupts the negative feedback system, resulting in rapid swings of the arterial blood pressure. Infiltration of the carotid bifurcation may correct this hemodynamic volatility. Conflicting data from other studies regarding the exact etiology of carotid endarterectomy and circulatory instability address other factors, such as previous hypertension, hypovolemia, or endogenous hypercatecholaminemia. Carotid sinus dysfunction, regardless of its etiology, is a serious problem during and after carotid surgery that increases surgical morbidity and mortality.[270] There is inconsistency concerning the risk of hemodynamic lability during bilateral endarterectomy with a short interval between procedures.[271]

Postoperative hypoxemia has been repeatedly discussed. The loss of carotid body chemoreceptor function is the anticipated cause. The use of a higher fraction of inspired oxygen and avoidance of high doses of respiratory depressants (opioids) are wise practice.

Repair of Coarctation of the Aorta

Coarctation of the aorta typically arises with severe hypertension resistant to medical management (see Chapter 11). Surgical correction leads to normalization of the blood pressure in most patients. Hypertension often recurs during long-term follow-up. The reported prevalence of late hypertension depends on the diagnostic criteria used and on the duration of follow-up, ranging from 30% to 75%. Paradoxical hypertension is a major reason for postoperative mortality and morbidity. It causes CAD followed by sudden death, heart failure, cerebrovascular accidents, and ruptured aortic aneurysm. The cause of late hypertension is unknown, but several theories have been proposed, including decreased aortic compliance, abnormal baroreceptor function, and neuroendocrine activation.[272] Increased renin production causes shunting of blood from mesenteric arteries and may result in mesenteric arteritis. Mesenteric arteritis typically arises on the third postoperative day and is characterized by abdominal pain and tenderness, vomiting, ileus, fever, melena, and leukocytosis. A combination of α- and β-blocking agents (labetalol) or pure arterial dilators (hydralazine) is used to manage the postcoarctectomy hypertension syndrome.

Aortic Repair

An interruption of the aortic circulation at any level for a certain time causes hypoperfusion of all organs beneath the cross-clamp (see Chapter 11). The occurrence of gastrointestinal, hepatopancreatic, and biliary ischemia after aortic repair for aneurysmal or occlusive disease is a devastating complication with a high mortality rate. It occurs more frequently after ruptured AAA repair. The causes of intestinal ischemia (ischemic colitis, IC) are ligation, prosthetic occlusion, and embolization of the inferior mesenteric artery in conjunction with insufficient collateral circulation of the colon, hypotension, or reperfusion injury.[273] The severity of ischemia in IC defines the extent of intestinal damage, varying from mucosal to transmural. The average incidence of IC is about 7%. Depending on the criteria used, retrospective reviews report incidences ranging from 3% to 30%, with mortality rates varying from 0% to 100%.[274] In a retrospective study of 4957 patients who underwent surgery of the abdominal aorta for infrarenal AAA, Longo et al reported 58 (1.2%) with subsequent IC.[275] The most frequent symptom noticed was bloody diarrhea. The diagnosis was made most frequently by colonoscopy. The mean time to diagnosis of IC was 5.5 days after aortic surgery (range 1 to 21 days). Aneurysmal rupture or perioperative hypotension was present in 35 of 49 patients. The overall mortality reported was 54%, but it was 89% if bowel resection for bowel infarction was required.

Other signs of IC include left-sided abdominal pain, tenderness, fever, leukocytosis and thrombocytopenia, and worsening diarrhea. All indicate progression of the intestinal ischemia and mandate reoperation. Colonoscopy under these circumstances must be performed cautiously.[276] The decision to continue with conservative treatment or go back to surgery depends on the dynamics of the clinical picture and repeated colonoscopies. Colonic and gastric tonometry has been used to try to ensure earlier detection of ischemia.[277,278] Conservative treatment of intestinal ischemia includes fluid management, bowel rest and decompression, and broad-spectrum antibiotics.

Other complications of interrupted perfusion have also been reported. Mehta et al described numerous adverse sequelae after hypogastric artery interruption, particularly bilateral, during standard open aortic aneurysm repair with considerable morbidity including buttock necrosis, severe lower extremity neurologic deficits, IC, impotence, and gluteal claudication.[279] Lower extremity ischemia with variable severity has been reported after TAAA or AAAA repair. In a review of 1601 aortic reconstructions, Kuhan and Raptis reported distal limb ischemia in 23 cases, 1.9%.[280] Surgery for aneurysmal disease was performed in 71% of the cases and in 29% for occlusive disease. Of those patients, 13.6% underwent an early amputation and a further 20.5% underwent a delayed amputation. Ernst, in his review of AAA, reported distal thromboembolism in 3% as an early complication.[281] The degree of ischemic insult varies from the subjective feeling of a cool and insensitive foot through claudication to necrosis mandating amputation.

The exact cause of limb ischemia is unknown, but most incidents result from embolization of atheroma or mural thrombus originating from morbidly changed arteries. Emboli from any prosthetic graft or thrombosis of distal small vessels, prolonged hypotension, and blood hypercoagulability are also possible etiologies. Other causes of distal ischemia include kinking of prosthetic grafts and the presence of intimal dissection. New techniques of endovascular abdominal aneurysm repair surgery are not free of complications. In a study involving 57 patients undergoing endovascular abdominal aortic surgery, Parent et al reported an incidence of 10.4% endograft limb dysfunction from which 3 patients developed endograft thrombosis and 4 developed graft stenosis.[282] Hypercoagulability, inadequate heparinization, and distal occlusive disease predispose to the development of distal thrombosis.

Abdominal compartment syndrome following ruptured AAA was described in four patients by Fietsam et al.[283] All four patients received more than 25 L of fluids for resuscitation and developed a typical clinical picture of increased intraabdominal pressure (IAP) with increased CVP, high peak inspiratory pressure, increased arterial carbon dioxide pressure ($PaCO_2$), decreased PaO_2, and decreased urinary output. The authors concluded that reopening the abdomen or delayed closure improves the oxygenation and oliguria. Platell et al, in a study of 42 patients who underwent abdominal aortic surgery, tried to use IAP as a valuable indication for relaparotomy in order to improve hemodynamically unstable and oliguric patients.[284] They failed to prove a causal relationship between IAP and patients' deterioration.

After Roizen et al, who reported five cases of anaphylactoid reaction after vascular graft placement, no more cases of hypersensitivity to the grafting material are available in the medical literature. This observation raises the question whether allergic reactions are a significant complication with the variety of graft materials currently available.[285]

Unusual Complications of Vascular Surgery

Sexual dysfunction is a well-known consequence of aortic surgery but has also been associated with varicose vein surgery. The published incidence averages 36% to 83%.[286,287] The clinical picture includes malfunction of erection and ejaculation. The cause is surgical disruption of the genital autonomic nerves and/or hypogastric or pudendal arteries. Sparing surgical techniques are the main way to reduce, but not completely prevent, sexual dysfunction following vascular surgery.

Urologic complications, including damage to the ureter and the urinary bladder, are unusual but occasionally reported in the literature. In most vascular surgical series, direct ureteral injury occurs in less than 1% of cases, and ureteral obstruction occurs in 2% to 14% of aortoiliac reconstructions.[288] Those injuries vary from partial ureteral damage to full transection or obstruction, with development of urinary leakage or hydronephrosis. The resulting urinary sepsis and ARF substantially increase the morbidity and mortality for vascular patients. Early recognition of these complications and appropriate treatment (eg, surgical, stent placement) are the key for successful outcome.

Kahn et al described fracture of the tibia in two female patients from 18 cases undergoing distal peroneal bypass using a lateral approach with fibula resection.[289] The patients were suffering from osteoporosis. The authors concluded that tibia fracture is a possible complication of this approach, especially in elderly women with osteoporosis.

Surgery for thoracic outlet syndrome using either the supraclavicular or transaxillary approach presents risk for various severe complications including damage to or thrombosis of the axillary artery, vein injuries or thrombosis, transient or definitive paralysis of the brachial plexus, long thoracic or phrenic nerves, hemothorax, and chylothorax.[290,291]

Bleeding

Intraoperative bleeding may complicate any vascular surgical procedure, but it is a significant perioperative consideration during aortic surgery, bypass procedures for portal hypertension, limb transplantation, and traumatic injury to the great vessels. Most of the hemorrhage occurs because of imperfect surgical technique or derangements of the coagulation cascade.

Blood loss during some procedures may be expressed in multiples of estimated blood volume and requires complete reconstitution of the patient's blood. In a multicenter prospective study of 666 patients with nonruptured AAA, Johnston reported a 4.8% incidence of intraoperative bleeding, from which 2.3% of patients had postoperative bleeding requiring transfusion or surgical treatment; and in 1.4% of the patients large volumes of blood were transfused and/or the use of a cell saver was necessary.[292]

Substantial bleeding accompanies surgery for acute aortic dissection. For thoracic and thoracoabdominal lesions the estimated blood loss (EBL) is 400 to 800 mL. Nonruptured abdominal aneurysm has an average EBL of 500 mL. During thoracoabdominal aortic repair, ongoing back bleeding from distal vessels during cross-clamping results in blood loss of 5 to 7 L. Use of a cell saver is highly recommended for those patients to return part of the lost blood.[293]

Bleeding is considered a complication if surgical treatment or transfusion of more than two units of blood is required.[294] Major postoperative bleeding in vascular surgery is infrequent. Massive intracavitary (thoracic, abdominal) bleeding usually arises as hemorrhagic shock and mandates aggressive resuscitation and surgical intervention. Those patients usually have bad outcomes because of rapid exsanguination.

Postoperative hemorrhage may arise as an expanding hematoma or wound bleeding after superficial procedures or as unexplained hemodynamic instability in the case of occult bleeding. Skin edge bleeding may be controlled by direct compression, cauterization, or nylon sutures. Small-wound hematomas may be observed. Large hematomas should be evacuated in the operating room.[295] Neck hematomas after carotid endarterectomy are life threatening because of rapid airway obstruction. After the surgeon is notified, the patient must be taken emergently back to the operating room and a controlled intubation attempted. In case of failed intubations, the surgical incision may need to be reopened to relieve pressure and resultant tracheal compression and/or deviation.

When bleeding arises as unexplained hypotension, other causes of hemodynamic instability must be excluded or treated. In clinical practice, situations are often complicated by combination of several disease states, making the correct treatment choice difficult. This problem remains unsolved even using all available means for volume assessment. Monitoring the vital signs, repeated hematocrit tests, evaluating the preload (CVP, PAOP) and CO, and diuresis have to be carried out. For some patients, low CO and increasing filling pressures suggest concurrent cardiac dysfunction and need for inotropes or/and vasodilators. If preload is decreased, occult bleeding and hypovolemia of other causes have to be differentiated. Presumably, measuring circulating blood volume by new monitors using indocyanine green or lithium would detect the downward volume trend well before extreme hemodynamic decompensation. Crystalloids, colloids, and packed red blood cells are used to correct hypovolemia, third-space fluid loss, brisk diuresis related to osmotic agents (hyperglycemia, mannitol), hypothermia, and diuretics.

The coagulation and fibrinolytic systems are activated during and after major vascular surgery. Excessive and continuous bleeding with oozing from the operative wound, bloody discharge from the drains, and increased need for hemotransfusion are all signs of coagulopathy. Causes of coagulopathy in the postoperative period include hypothermia, hemodilution, disseminated intravascular coagulation, and residual heparin and protamine effects. After obtaining a full coagulation profile (prothrombin time, partial thromboplastin time, platelet count, fibrinogen, fibrinogen-degraded products, and activated coagulation time), component therapy, fresh frozen plasma, cryoprecipitate, and/or platelets should be used. Residual heparinization (prolonged partial thromboplastin time and activated coagulation time) should be reversed with protamine. Aprotinin or ε-aminocaproic acid is used by some surgical teams for patients undergoing major or recurrent surgery intraoperatively and continued for 24 hours in order to reduce EBL and postoperative bleeding (see Chapter 15).

REFERENCES

1. Standards of the American Society of Anesthesiologists: Standards for basic anesthetic monitoring (approved by House of Delegates on October 21, 1986 and last amended on October 21, 1998), http://www.asahq.org/Standards/02.html#gen1.
2. Saul L, Smith J, Mook W: The safety of automatic versus manual blood pressure cuffs for patients receiving thrombolytic therapy, *Am J Crit Care* 7:192, 1998.
3. Pedley CF, Bloomfield RL, Colflesh MJ, et al: Blood pressure monitor–induced petechiae and ecchymoses, *Am J Hypertens* 7:1031, 1994.
4. Baetz MD, Pylypchuk G, Baetz M: A complication of ambulatory blood pressure monitoring, *Ann Intern Med* 121:468, 1994 (letter; comment).
5. Bickler PE, Schapera A, Bainton CR: Acute radial nerve injury from use of an automatic blood pressure monitor, *Anesthesiology* 73:186, 1990.
6. Lin CC, Jawan B, de Villa MV, et al: Blood pressure cuff compression injury of the radial nerve, *J Clin Anesth* 13:306, 2001.
7. Yamada M, Tsuda K, Nagai S, et al: A case of crush syndrome resulting from continuous compression of the upper arm by automatically cycled blood pressure cuff, *Masui Jpn J Anesthesiol* 46:119, 1997.
8. Sutin KM, Longaker MT, Wahlander S, et al: Acute biceps compartment syndrome associated with the use of a noninvasive blood pressure monitor, *Anesth Analg* 83:1345, 1996.
9. Vidal P, Sykes PJ, O'Shaughnessy M, Craddock K: Compartment syndrome after use of an automatic arterial pressure monitoring device, *Br J Anaesth* 72:738, 1994.
10. Ball DR: A pulse oximetry probe hazard, *Anesth Analg* 80:1251, 1995.
11. Radu A, Zellweger M, Grosjean P, Monnier P: Pulse oximeter as a cause of skin burn during photodynamic therapy, *Endoscopy* 31:831, 1999.
12. Kohjiro M, Koga K, Komori M, et al: A case report of a burn produced by the probe of a pulse oximeter, *Masui Jpn J Anesthesiol* 41:1991, 1992.
13. Shellock FG, Slimp GL: Severe burn of the finger caused by using a pulse oximeter during MR imaging. *AJR* 153:1105, 1989 (letter).
14. Pandey CK, Rani A, Srivastava K, et al: Thermal injury with pulse oximeter probe in hypothermic patient. Pulse oximeter probe burn in hypothermia, *Can J Anaesth* 46:908, 1999.
15. Wille J, Braams R, van Haren WH, van der Werken C: Pulse oximeter–induced digital injury: frequency rate and possible causative factors, *Crit Care Med* 28:3555, 2000.
16. Rubin MM, Ford HC, Sadoff RS: Digital injury from a pulse oximeter probe, *J Oral Maxillofac Surg* 49:301, 1991.
17. Clark M, Lavies NG: Sensory loss of the distal phalanx caused by a pulse oximeter probe, *Anaesthesia* 52:508, 1997.
18. Wakeling HG: Diathermy frequency shock from faulty pulse oximeter probe, *Anaesthesia* 50:749, 1995.
19. Myyra R, Dalpra M, Globerson J: Electrical erythema? *Anesthesiology* 69:440, 1988.
20. Dorsch JA, Dorsch SE: *Neuromuscular transmission monitoring in understanding anesthesia equipment*, Baltimore, 1999, Williams & Wilkins, 866.
21. Hall SC, Stevenson GW, Suresh S: Burn associated with temperature monitoring during magnetic resonance imaging, *Anesthesiology* 76:152, 1992.

22. Lau JV, Renart I, Buchon A, Gimeno V: Massive epistaxis as a rare complication in the immediate postoperative period following heart surgery, *Rev Esp Anestesiol Reanim* 43:117, 1996.

23. Siersema PD, van Buuren HR, van Blankenstein M: Anal blood loss: remember the thermometer! *Ned Tijdschr Geneeskd* 140:233, 1996.

24. Doring B, Inoue K, Reichelt W: Bronchial obstruction caused by incorrect positioning of a temperature probe, *Anaesthesist* 38:631, 1989.

25. Livornese LL Jr, Dias S, Samel C, et al: Hospital-acquired infection with vancomycin-resistant *Enterococcus faecium* transmitted by electronic thermometers, *Ann Intern Med* 117:112, 1992.

26. Huffman LM, Riddle RT: Mass spectrometer and/or capnograph use during low-flow, closed circuit anesthesia administration, *Anesthesiology* 66:439, 1987.

27. Practice guidelines for perioperative transesophageal echocardiography. A report by the American Society of Anesthesiologists and the Society of Cardiovascular Anesthesiologists Task Force on Transesophageal Echocardiography, *Anesthesiology* 84:986, 1996.

28. Kallmeyer IJ, Collard CD, Fox JA, et al: The safety of intraoperative transesophageal echocardiography: a case series of 7200 cardiac surgical patients, *Anesth Analg* 92:1126, 2001.

29. Rousou JA, Tighe DA, Garb JL, et al: Risk of dysphagia after transesophageal echocardiography during cardiac operations, *Ann Thorac Surg* 69:486, 2000.

30. Yamamoto H, Fujimura N, Namiki A: Swelling of the tongue after intraoperative monitoring by transesophageal echocardiography, *Masui Jpn J Anesthesiol* 50:1250, 2001.

31. Brinkman WT, Shanewise JS, Clements SD, Mansour KA: Transesophageal echocardiography: not an innocuous procedure, *Ann Thorac Surg* 72:1725, 2001.

32. Massey SR, Pitsis A, Mehta D, Callaway M: Oesophageal perforation following perioperative transoesophageal echocardiography, *Br J Anaesth* 84:643, 2000.

33. Spahn DR, Schmid S, Carrel T, et al: Hypopharynx perforation by a transesophageal echocardiography probe, *Anesthesiology* 82:581, 1995.

34. De Vries AJ, van der Maaten JM, Laurens RR: Mallory-Weiss tear following cardiac surgery: transoesophageal echoprobe or nasogastric tube? *Br J Anaesth* 84:646, 2000.

35. Kawahito S, Kitahata H, Kimura H, et al: Recurrent laryngeal nerve palsy after cardiovascular surgery: relationship to the placement of a transesophageal echocardiographic probe, *J Cardiothorac Vasc Anesth* 13:528, 1999.

36. Berkompas DC, Saeian K: Atrial fibrillation complicating transesophageal echocardiography, *Chest* 103:1929, 1993 (letter).

37. Suriani RJ, Tzou N: Bradycardia during transesophageal echocardiographic probe manipulation, *J Cardiothorac Vasc Anesth* 9:347, 1995.

38. Mentec H, Vignon P, Terre S, et al: Frequency of bacteremia associated with transesophageal echocardiography in intensive care unit patients: a prospective study of 139 patients, *Crit Care Med* 23:1194, 1995.

39. Nikutta P, Mantey-Stiers F, Becht I, et al: Risk of bacteremia induced by transesophageal echocardiography: analysis of 100 consecutive procedures, *J Am Soc Echocardiogr* 5:168, 1992.

40. Olenchock SA Jr, Lukaszczyk JJ, Reed J 3rd, Theman TE: Splenic injury after intraoperative transesophageal echocardiography, *Ann Thorac Surg* 72:2141, 2001.

41. Janssen M, Salm EF, Breburda CS, et al: Carcinoid crisis during transesophageal echocardiography, *Intensive Care Med* 26:254, 2000.

42. Bensky AS, O'Brien JJ, Hammon JW: Transesophageal echo probe compression of an aberrant right subclavian artery, *J Am Soc Echocardiogr* 8:964, 1995.

43. Bedford RF: Long-term radial artery cannulation: effects on subsequent vessel function, *Crit Care Med* 6:64, 1978.

44. Bedford RF: Radial arterial function following percutaneous cannulation with 18- and 20-gauge catheters, *Anesthesiology* 47:37, 1977.

45. Slogoff S, Keats AS, Arlund C: On the safety of radial artery cannulation, *Anesthesiology* 59:42, 1983.

46. *Advanced cardiac life support.* Dallas, 1997, American Heart Association, 13-3.

47. Bedford RF, Wollman H: Complications of percutaneous radial-artery cannulation: an objective prospective study in man, *Anesthesiology* 38:228, 1973.

48. Martin C, Saux P, Papazian L, Gouin F: Long-term arterial cannulation in ICU patients using the radial artery or dorsalis pedis artery, *Chest* 119:901, 2001.

49. Martin C, Crama P, Courjaret P, et al: Le cathétérisme prolongé de l'artère radiale: evaluation prospective du risque thrombogène et infectieux, *Ann Fr Anesth Reanim* 3:435, 1984.

50. Rehfeldt KH, Sanders MS: Digital gangrene after radial artery catheterization in a patient with thrombocytosis, *Anesth Analg* 90:45, 2000.

51. Clark VL, Kruse JA: Arterial catheterization, *Crit Care Clin* 8:687, 1992.

52. Edwards DP, Clarke MD, Barker P: Acute presentation of bilateral radial artery pseudoaneurysms following arterial cannulation, *Eur J Vasc Endovasc Surg* 17:456, 1999.

53. Lermi A, Cunha BA: *Pseudomonas aeruginosa* arterial line infection, *Am J Infect Control* 26:538, 1998.

54. Qvist J, Peterfreund RA, Perlmutter GS: Transient compartment syndrome of the forearm after attempted radial artery cannulation, *Anesth Analg* 83:183, 1996.

55. Lee KL, Miller JG, Laitung G: Hand ischaemia following radial artery cannulation, *J Hand Surg [Br]* 20:493, 1995.

56. Ryan JF, Raines J, Dalton BC, Mathieu A: Arterial dynamics of radial artery cannulation, *Anesth Analg* 52:1017, 1973.

57. Yao FS, Artusio JF: *Anesthesiology problem-oriented patient management*, Philadelphia, 1998, Lippincott Williams & Wilkins, 146.

58. Grenvik A: *Textbook of critical care*, Philadelphia, 2000, WB Saunders, 61.

59. Morton PG: Arterial puncture during central venous catheter insertion, *Crit Care Med* 27:878, 1999.

60. Marymount JH 3rd, Vender JS, Szokol JW, Murphy GS: Arterial or venous cannulation: no transducer needed, *Crit Care Med* 28:2676, 2000.

61. Rigg, A, Huges P, Lopez A, et al: Right phrenic nerve palsy as a complication of indwelling central venous catheters, *Thorax* 52:831, 1997.

62. Marino P: *The ICU book*, Baltimore, 1998, Williams & Wilkins, 64.

63. Schummer W, Schummer C, Gaser E, Bartunek R: Loss of the guide wire: mishap or blunder? *Br J Anaesth* 88:144, 2002.

64. Michaelis G, Biscoping J: Clinical significance and effects of foreign body embolism during the use of central venous catheters, *Anasthesiol Intensivmed Notfallmed Schmerzther* 35:137, 2000.

65. Hehir DJ, Cross KS, Kirkham R, et al: Foreign body complications of central venous catheterisation in critically ill patients, *Ir J Med Sci* 161:49, 1992.

66. Savage M, Ludher J, Brydon M, Donellan R: Central venous line disconnections with associated blood loss, *J Qual Clin Pract* 18:213, 1998.

67. Streib EW, Wagner JW: Complications of vascular access procedures in patients with vena cava filters, *J Trauma* 49:553, 2000.

68. Kaufman JA, Thomas JW, Geller SC, et al: Guide-wire entrapment by inferior vena caval filters: in vitro evaluation, *Radiology* 198:71, 1996.

69. Ivanov RI, Allen J, Sandham JD, et al: Pulmonary artery catheterization: a narrative and systematic critique of randomized controlled trials and recommendations for the future, *New Horiz* 5:268, 1997.

70. Practice guidelines for pulmonary artery catheterization. A report by the American Society of Anesthesiologists Task Force on Pulmonary Artery Catheterization, *Anesthesiology* 78:380, 1993.

71. Darovic GO: *Hemodynamic monitoring: invasive and noninvasive clinical application*, Philadelphia, 1995, WB Saunders, 313.

72. Morris D, Mulvihill D, Lew WY: Risk of developing complete heart block during bedside pulmonary artery catheterization in patients with left bundle-branch block, *Arch Intern Med* 147:2005, 1987.

73. Miller R: *Anesthesia*, Philadelphia, 2000, WB Saunders, 1162.

74. Sirivella S, Gielchinsky I, Parsonnet V: Management of catheter-induced pulmonary artery perforation: a rare complication in cardiovascular operations, *Ann Thorac Surg* 72:2056, 2001.

75. Liu C, Webb CC: Pulmonary artery rupture: serious complication associated with pulmonary artery catheters, *Int J Trauma Nurs* 6:19, 2000.

76. Brahim JJ, Cheung D, Jessurun JA, et al: Rounded mass in the middle lobe after Swan-Ganz catheterization, *Chest* 121:261, 2002.

77. Stancofski ED, Sardi A, Conaway GL: Successful outcome in Swan-Ganz catheter–induced rupture of pulmonary artery, *Am Surg* 64:1062, 1998.

78. Kainuma M, Yamada M, Miyake T: Pulmonary artery catheter passing between the chordae tendineae of the tricuspid valve, *Anesthesiology* 83:1130, 1995.

79. Arnaout S, Diab K, Al-Kutoubi A, Jamaleddine G: Rupture of the chordae of the tricuspid valve after knotting of the pulmonary artery catheter, *Chest* 120:1742, 2001.

80. Ismail KM, Deckmyn TJ, Vandermeersch E, et al: Nonsurgical extraction of intracardiac double-knotted pulmonary artery catheter, *J Clin Anesth* 10:160, 1998.

81. Sherertz RJ, Heard SO, Raad II: Diagnosis of triple-lumen catheter infection: comparison of roll plate, sonication, and flushing methodologies, *J Clin Microbiol* 35:641, 1997.

82. Sitges-Serra A: Strategies for prevention of catheter-related bloodstream infections, *Support Care Cancer* 7:391, 1999.

83. Sitges-Serra A, Girvent M: Catheter-related bloodstream infections, 23:589, 1999.

84. Mermel LA, Farr BM, Sherertz RJ, et al: Infectious Diseases Society of America, American College of Critical Care Medicine, Society for Healthcare Epidemiology of America. Guidelines for the management of intravascular catheter-related infections, *J Intravenous Nurs* 24:180, 2001.

85. Collier PE, Blocker SH, Graff DM, et al: Cardiac tamponade from central venous catheters, *Am J Surg* 176:212, 1998.

86. Randolph AG, Cook DJ, Gonzales CA, et al: Ultrasound guidance for placement of central venous catheters: a meta-analysis of literature, *Crit Care Med* 24:2053, 1996.

87. Longnecker DE, Tinker JH, Morgan GE Jr: *Principles and practice of anesthesiology*, St. Louis, 1999, Mosby, chap 41.

88. Fisher M: Occlusion of the internal carotid artery, *Arch Neurol Psychiatry* 65:346, 1951.

89. Carrea R, Molins M, Murphy G: Surgical treatment of spontaneous thrombosis of the internal carotid artery in the neck: carotid-carotideal anastomosis: report of a case, *Acta Neurol Latinoam* 1:71, 1955.

90. Eastcott HH, Pickering GW, Rob CG: Reconstruction of internal carotid artery in a patient with intermittent attacks of hemiplegia, *Lancet* 267:994, 1954.

91. DeBakey ME: Successful carotid endarterectomy for cerebrovascular insufficiency: nineteen-year follow-up, *JAMA* 233:1083, 1975.

92. Easton JD, Sherman DG: Stroke and mortality rate in carotid endarterectomy: 228 consecutive operations, *Stroke* 8:565, 1977.

93. Warlow CP: Carotid endarterectomy: does it work? *Stroke* 15:1068, 1984.

94. Barnett HJM, Plum F, Walton JN: Carotid endarterectomy—an expression of concern, *Stroke* 15:941, 1984.

95. North American Symptomatic Carotid Endarterectomy Trial (NASCET): Beneficial effect of carotid endarterectomy in symptomatic patients with high-grade carotid stenosis, *N Engl J Med* 325:445, 1991.

96. Barnett HJM, Taylor DW, Eliasziw M, et al, for the North American Symptomatic Carotid Endarterectomy Trial Collaborators: Benefit of carotid endarterectomy in patients with symptomatic moderate or severe stenosis, *N Engl J Med* 339:1415, 1998.

97. Ferguson GG, Eliasziw M, Barr HWK, et al, for the NASCET Collaborators: The North American Symptomatic Carotid Endarterectomy Trial. Surgical results in 1415 patients, *Stroke* 30:1751, 1999.

98. European Carotid Surgery Trialists' Collaborative Group: MRC European Carotid Surgery Trial: interim results for symptomatic patients with severe (70-99 percent) or with mild (0-29 percent) carotid stenosis, *Lancet* 337:1235, 1991.

99. European Carotid Trialists' Collaborative Group: Endarterectomy for moderate symptomatic carotid stenosis: interim results from the MRC European Carotid Surgery Trial, *Lancet* 347:1591, 1996.

100. Dennis M, Bamford J, Sandercock P, Warlow C: Prognosis of transient ischemic attacks in the Oxfordshire Community Stroke Project, *Stroke* 21:848, 1990.

101. Sacco RL, Wolf PA, Kannel WB, McNamara PM: Survival and recurrence following stroke: the Framingham study, *Stroke* 13:290, 1982.

102. Wiebers DO, Whisnant JP, O'Fallon WM: Reversible ischemic neurologic deficit (RIND) in a community: Rochester, Minnesota, 1955-1974, *Neurology* 32:459, 1982.

103. Executive Committee for the Asymptomatic Carotid Atherosclerosis Study: Endarterectomy for asymptomatic carotid artery stenosis. *JAMA* 273:1421, 1995.

104. Moore WS, Barnett HJ, Beebe HG, et al: Guidelines for carotid endarterectomy: a multidisciplinary consensus statement from the Ad Hoc Committee, American Heart Association, *Circulation* 91:566, 1995.

105. Brown MM, Pereira AC, McCabe DJH, for the CAVATAS Investigators: Carotid and Vertebral Artery Transluminal Angioplasty Study (CAVATAS): 3 year outcome data. *Cerebrovasc Dis* 9(Suppl 1):66, 1999.

106. Bettmann MA, Katzen BT, Whisnant J, et al: Carotid stenting and angioplasty: a statement for healthcare professionals from the Councils on Cardiovascular Radiology, Stroke, Cardio-Thoracic and Vascular Surgery, Epidemiology, and Prevention, and Clinical Cardiology, American Heart Association, *Stroke* 29:336, 1998.

107. Rosenthal D, Zeichner WD, Lamis PA, Stanton PE Jr: Neurologic deficit after carotid endarterectomy: pathogenesis and management, *Surgery* 94:776, 1983.

108. Rockman CB, Jacobowitz GR, Lamparello PJ, et al: Immediate reexploration for the perioperative neurologic event after carotid endarterectomy: is it worthwhile? *J Vasc Surg* 32:1062, 2000.

109. Krul J, van Gijn J, Ackerstaff R, et al: Site and pathogenesis of infarcts associated with carotid endarterectomy, *Stroke* 20:324, 1989.

110. Taylor CL, Selman WR, Grubb RL Jr, Ratcheson RA: Ischemic complications of carotid endarterectomy. In Loftus CM, Kresowik TF (eds): *Carotid artery surgery*, New York, 2000, Thieme Medical Publishers, 471.

111. Findlay JM, Marchak BE: Reoperation for acute hemispheric stroke after carotid endarterectomy: is there any value? *Neurosurgery* 50:486, 2002.

112. Radak D, Popovic AD, Radiceivic S, et al: Immediate reoperation for perioperative stroke after 2250 carotid endarterectomies: differences between intraoperative and early postoperative stroke, *J Vasc Surg* 30:245, 1999.

113. Imparato A, Riles T, Lamperello P, Ramirez S: The management of TIA and acute stroke after carotid endarterectomy. In Bernhard V, Towne J (eds): *Complications in vascular surgery*, Orlando, Fla, 1985, Grune & Stratton, 728-731.

114. Koslow A, Picotta J, Ouriel K, et al: Re-exploration for thrombosis in carotid endarterectomy, *Circulation* 80:73, 1989.

115. Bove EL, Fry WJ, Gross WS, Stanley JC: Hypotension and hypertension as consequences of baroreceptor dysfunction following carotid endarterectomy, *Surgery* 85:633, 1979.

116. Englund R, Dean RH: Blood pressure aberrations associated with carotid endarterectomy, *Ann Vasc Surg* 1:304, 1986.

117. Towne JB, Bernhard VM: The relationship of postoperative hypertension to complications following carotid endarterectomy, *Surgery* 88:575, 1980.

118. Hertzer N: Nonstroke complications of carotid endarterectomy. In Bernhard V, Towne J (eds): *Complications in vascular surgery*, Orlando, Fla, 1985, Grune & Stratton, 741-746.

119. Sundt TM Jr, Sharbrough FW, Piepgras DG, et al: Correlation of cerebral blood flow and electroencephalographic changes during carotid endarterectomy: with results of surgery and hemodynamics of cerebral ischemia, *Mayo Clin Proc* 56:533, 1981.

120. Reitan J: Control of the systematic circulation. In Scurr C, Feldman S (eds): *Scientific foundation of anesthesia*, Chicago, 1982, Year Book Medical Publishers, 133-134.

121. Seagard JL, Hopp FA, Drummond HA, Van Wynsberghe DM: Selective contribution of two types of carotid sinus baroreceptors to the control of blood pressure, *Circ Res* 72:1011, 1993.

122. Angell-James JE, Lumley JSP: The effects of carotid endarterectomy on the mechanical properties of the carotid sinus and carotid sinus nerve activity in atherosclerotic patients, *Br J Surg* 61:805, 1974.

123. Gottlieb A, Satariano-Jaudem P, Schoenwald P, et al: The effects of carotid sinus nerve blockade on hemodynamic stability after CEA, *J Cardiothorac Vasc Anesth* 11:67, 1997.

124. Mehta M, Rahmani O, Dietzek A, et al: Eversion technique increases the risk for post-carotid endarterectomy hypertension, *J Vasc Surg* 34:839, 2001.

125. Smith B: Hypertension following carotid endarterectomy: the role of cerebral renin production, *J Vasc Surg* 1:623, 1984.

126. Archie J: The relationship of early hypertension following carotid endarterectomy to intraoperative cerebral ischemia, *Ann Vasc Surg* 2:108, 1988.

127. Ahn S, Marcus D, Moore W: Postcarotid endarterectomy hypertension: association with elevated cranial norepinephrine, *J Vasc Surg* 7:351, 1989.

128. Cafferata HT, Merchant RF, DePalma RG: Avoidance of postcarotid endarterectomy hypertension, *Ann Surg* 196:465, 1982.

129. Zuber WF, Gaspar MR, Rothschild PD: The anterior spinal artery syndrome—a complication of abdominal surgery: report of five cases and review of the literature, *Am J Surg* 172:909, 1970.

130. Ferguson LR, Bergan JJ, Conn J Jr, Yao JST: Spinal ischemia following abdominal aortic surgery, *Ann Surg* 181:2677, 1975.

131. Picone AL, Green RM, Ricotta JR, et al: Spinal cord ischemia following operations on the abdominal aorta, *J Vasc Surg* 3:94, 1986.

132. Iliopoulos JI, Howanitz PE, Pierce GE, et al: The critical hypogastric circulation, *Am J Surg* 154:671, 1987.

133. Dimakakos P, Arapoglou B, Katsenis K, et al: Ischemia of the spinal cord following elective operative procedures of the infrarenal aorta, *J Cardiovasc Surg (Torino)* 37:243, 1996.

134. Gloviczki P, Cross SA, Stanson AW, et al: Ischemic injury to the spinal cord or lumbosacral plexus after aorto-iliac reconstruction, *Am J Surg* 162:131, 1991.

135. Senapati A, Browse NL: Gluteal necrosis and paraplegia following postoperative bilateral internal iliac artery occlusion, *J Cardiovasc Surg (Torino)* 31:194, 1990.

136. Svensson LG, Crawford ES, Hess KR, et al: Experience with 1509 patients undergoing thoracoabdominal aortic operations, *J Vasc Surg* 17:357, 1993.

137. Szilagyi DE, Hageman JH, Smith RF, Illiott JP: Spinal cord damage in surgery of the abdominal aorta, *Surgery* 83:38, 1978.

138. Elliot J, Szilagyi D, Hageman J, et al: Spinal cord ischemia secondary to surgery of the abdominal aorta. In Bernhard V, Towne J (eds): *Complications in vascular surgery*, Orlando, Fla, 1985, Grune & Stratton, 291-306.
139. Szilagyi DE: A second look at the etiology of spinal cord damage in surgery of the abdominal aorta, *J Vasc Surg* 17:1111, 1993.
140. Keen G: Spinal cord damage and operations for coarctations of the aorta: etiology, practice, and prospects, *Thorax* 42:11, 1987.
141. Acher CW, Wynn MM, Hoch JR, Kranner PW: Cardiac function is a risk factor for paralysis in thoracoabdominal aortic replacement, *J Vasc Surg* 27:821, 1998.
142. Svensson LG, Hess KR, D'Agostino RS, et al: Reduction of neurologic injury after high-risk thoracoabdominal aortic operation, *Ann Thorac Surg* 66:132, 1998.
143. Katz NM, Blackstone EH, Kirklin JW, Karg RB: Incremental risk factors for spinal cord injury following operation for acute traumatic transection, *J Thorac Cardiovasc Surg* 81:669, 1981.
144. Hill A, Kalman P, Johnston K, Vosu H: Reversal of delayed-onset paraplegia after thoracic aortic surgery with cerebrospinal fluid drainage, *J Vasc Surg* 20:315, 1994.
145. Ross SD, Kron IL, Parrino PE, et al: Preservation of intercostal arteries during thoracoabdominal aortic aneurysm surgery: a retrospective study, *J Thorac Cardiovasc Surg* 118:17, 1999.
146. Cambria R, Davison JK, Zannetti S, et al: Thoracoabdominal aneurysm repair: perspectives over a decade with the clamp-and-sew technique, *Ann Surg* 226:294, 1997.
147. Grabitz K, Sandmann W, Stuhmeirer K, et al: The risk of ischemic spinal cord injury in patients undergoing graft replacement for thoracoabdominal aortic aneurysms, *J Vasc Surg* 23:230, 1996.
148. Hollier L, Money SR, Naslund TC, et al: Risk of spinal cord dysfunction in patients undergoing thoracoabdominal aortic replacement, *Am J Surg* 164:210, 1992.
149. Coselli JS, LeMaire SA, Miller CC 3rd, et al: Mortality and paraplegia after thoracoabdominal aortic aneurysm repair: a risk factor analysis, *Ann Thorac Surg* 69:409, 2000.
150. Safi HJ, Campbell MP, Muller CC, et al: Cerebral spinal fluid drainage and distal aortic perfusion decrease the incidence of neurological deficit: the results of 343 descending and thoracoabdominal aortic aneurysm repairs, *Eur J Vasc Endovasc Surg* 14:118, 1997.
151. Cambria RP, Giglia J: Prevention of spinal cord ischemic complications after thoracoabdominal aortic surgery, *Eur J Vasc Endovasc Surg* 15:96, 1998.
152. Jacobs MJ, de Mol BA, Elenbaas T, et al: Spinal cord blood supply in patients with thoracoabdominal aortic aneurysms, *J Vasc Surg* 35:30, 2002.
153. Gravereaux EC, Faries PL, Burks JA, et al: Risk of spinal cord ischemia after endograft repair of thoracic aortic aneurysms, *J Vasc Surg* 34:997, 2001.
154. Cox GS, O'Hara PJ, Hertzer NR, et al: Thoracoabdominal aneurysm repair: a representative experience, *J Vasc Surg* 15:780, 1992.
155. Cambria RP, Davison JK, Carter C, et al: Epidural cooling for spinal cord protection during thoracoabdominal aneurysm repair: a five year experience, *J Vasc Surg* 31:1093, 2000.
156. Safi HJ, Miller CC, Carr C, et al: Importance of intercostal artery reattachment during thoracoabdominal aortic aneurysm repair, *J Vasc Surg* 27:58. 1998.
157. Coselli JS, LeMarie SA, Schmittling ZC, Koksoy C: Cerebrospinal fluid drainage in thoracoabdominal aortic surgery, *Semin Vasc Surg* 13:308, 2000.
158. Webb TH, Williams GM: Thoracoabdominal aneurysm repair, *Cardiovasc Surg* 7:573, 1999.
159. Livesay JJ, Cooley DA, Ventemiglia RA, et al: Surgical experience in descending thoracic aneurysmectomy with and without adjuncts to avoid ischemia, *Ann Thorac Surg* 39:37, 1985.
160. Greenberg R, Resch T, Nyman U, et al: Endovascular repair of descending thoracic aortic aneurysms: an early experience with intermediate-term follow-up, *J Vasc Surg* 31:147, 2000.
161. Mitchell RS, Miller DC, Dake DC: Stent graft repair of thoracic aortic aneurysms, *Semin Vasc Surg* 10:257, 1997.
162. Kasirajan K, Dolmatch B, Ouriel K, Clair D: Delayed onset of ascending paralysis after thoracic aortic stent graft deployment, *J Vasc Surg* 31:196, 2000.
163. Safi HJ, Miller CC, Azizzadeh A, Iliopoulos DC: Observations on delayed neurologic deficit after thoracoabdominal aortic aneurysm repair, *J Vasc Surg* 26:616, 1997.
164. Azizzadeh A, Huynh TT, Miller CC, Safi HJ: Reversal of twice delayed neurologic deficits with cerebrospinal fluid drainage after thoracoabdom-inal aneurysm repair: a case report and plea for a national database collection, *J Vasc Surg* 31:592, 2000.
165. Rosenthal D: Spinal cord ischemia after abdominal aortic operation: is it preventable? *J Vasc Surg* 30:391, 1999.
166. Defraigne JO, Otto B, Sakalihasan N, Limet R: Spinal ischemia after surgery for abdominal infrarenal aortic aneurysm: diagnosis with nuclear magnetic resonance, *Acta Chir Belg* 97:250, 1997.
167. Cunningham J, Laschinger J, Spencer F: Monitoring of somatosensory evoked potentials during surgical procedures on the thoracoabdominal aorta, *J Thorac Cardiovasc Surg* 94:275, 1987.
168. Lazorthes G: Arterial vascularization of the spinal cord. Recent studies of the anastomotic substitution pathways, *J Neurosurg* 35:253, 1971.
169. Von Oppell UO, Dunne TT, De Groot MK et al: Traumatic aortic rupture: twenty-year meta-analysis of mortality and risk of paraplegia, *Ann Thoracic Surg* 58:585, 1994.
170. Crawford E, Mizrahi E, Hess K, et al: The impact of distal aortic perfusion and somatosensory evoked potentials monitoring on prevention of paraplegia after aortic aneurysm operation, *J Thorac Cardiovasc Surg* 95:357, 1988.
171. Coselli JS, LeMaire SA, Koksoy C, et al: Cerebrospinal fluid drainage reduces paraplegia after thoracoabdominal aortic aneurysm repair: results of a randomized clinical trial. *J Vasc Surg* 35:631, 2002.
172. Svenson LG: New and future approaches for spinal cord protection, *Semin Thorac Cardiovasc Surg* 9:206, 1997.
173. Youngberg J: Anesthetic consideration for major vascular surgery. *1999 Annual Refresher Course Lectures*. American Society of Anesthesiology 256:1, 1999.
174. Rokkas CK, Kouchoukos NT: Profound hypothermia for spinal cord protection in operations on the descending thoracic and thoracoabdominal aorta, *Semin Thorac Cardiovasc Surg* 10:57, 1998.
175. Cambria RP, Davison JK, Zannetti S, et al: Clinical experience with epidural cooling for spinal cord protection during thoracic and thoracoabdominal aneurysm repair, *J Vasc Surg* 25:234, 1997.
176. Chuter TA, Gordon RC, Reilly LM, et al: An endovascular system for thoracoabdominal aortic aneurysm repair, *J Endovasc Ther* 8:25, 2001.
177. Teisenhausen K, Amann W, Koch G, et al: Cerebrospinal fluid drainage to reverse paraplegia after endovascular thoracic aortic aneurysm repair, *J Endovasc Ther* 7:132, 2000.
178. Brock MV, Redmond JM, Ischiwa S, et al: Clinical markers in cerebrospinal fluid for determining neurologic deficits after thoracoabdominal aortic aneurysm repairs, *Ann Thorac Surg* 64:999, 1997.
179. Svensson LG, Crawford ES, Sun J: Ischemia, reperfusion, and no-reflow phenomenon. In Svensson LG, Crawford ES (eds): *Cardiovascular and vascular disease of the aorta*, Philadelphia, 1997, WB Saunders, 194.
180. Acher CW, Wynn MM, Hoch JR, et al: Combined use of cerebral spinal fluid drainage and naloxone reduces the risk of paraplegia in thoracoabdominal aneurysm repair, *J Vasc Surg* 19:236, 1994.
181. Kouchoukos NT, Daily BB, Rokkas CK, et al: Hypothermic bypass and circulatory arrest for operations on the descending thoracic and thoracoabdominal aorta, *Ann Thorac Surg* 60:67, 1995.
182. Fowl RJ, Patterson RB, Gewirtz RJ, Anderson DK: Protection against spinal cord injury using a new 21-aminosteroid, *J Surg Res* 48:597, 1990.
183. Acher CW, Wynn MM, Archibald J: Naloxone and spinal fluid drainage as adjuncts in the surgical treatment of thoracoabdominal and thoracic aneurysms, *Surgery* 108:755, 1990.
184. Rokkas C, Sundaresan S, Shuman TA, et al: Profound systemic hypothermia protects the spinal cord in a primate model of spinal cord ischemia, *J Thorac Cardiovasc Surg* 106:1024, 1993.
185. Salzano R, Ellison LH, Altonji PF, et al: Regional deep hypothermia of the spinal cord protects against ischemic injury during thoracic aortic cross-clamping, *Ann Thorac Surg* 57(1):65, 1994.
186. Davison J, Cambria R, Vierra D, et al: Epidural cooling for regional spinal cord hypothermia during thoracoabdominal aneurysm repair, *J Vasc Surg* 20:304, 1994.
187. Quayumi AK, Janusz MT, Jamieson WE, Lyster DM: Pharmacologic interventions for the prevention of spinal cord injury caused by aortic cross-clamping, *J Thorac Cardiovasc Surg* 104:256, 1992.
188. Safi HJ, Bartoli S, Hess KR, et al: Neurologic deficit in patients at high risk with thoracoabdominal aortic aneurysms: the role of cerebrospinal fluid drainage and distal aortic perfusion, *J Vasc Surg* 20:434, 1994.
189. Safi HJ, Hess KR, Randel M, et al: Cerebrospinal fluid drainage and distal aortic perfusion: reducing neurologic complications in repair of thoracoabdominal aortic aneurysm types I and II, *J Vasc Surg* 23:223, 1996.

190. Jacobs MJHM, Meylaerts SA, de Haan P, et al: Strategies to prevent neurologic deficit based on motor-evoked potentials in type I and II thoracoabdominal aortic aneurysm repair, *J Vasc Surg* 29:48, 1999.

191. Hamilton G: In Branchereau A, Jacobs M (eds): *Complications in vascular and endovascular surgery*, Armonk, NY, 2001, Futura, 95-105.

192. Collins TC, Johnson M, Daley J, et al: Preoperative risk factors for 30-day mortality after elective surgery for vascular disease in Department of Veterans Affairs hospitals: is race important? *J Vasc Surg* 34:634, 2001.

193. Cruz CP, Drouilhet JC, Southern FN, et al: Abdominal aortic aneurysm repair, *Vasc Surg* 35:335, 2001.

194. Moore WS, Kashyap VS, Vescera CL, et al: Abdominal aortic aneurysm: a 6-yr comparison to endovascular versus transabdominal repair, *Ann Surg* 230:298, 1999.

195. Quinones-Baldrich WJ, Garner C, Caswell D, et al: Endovascular, transperitoneal, and retroperitoneal abdominal aortic aneurysm repair: results and costs, *J Vasc Surg* 30:59, 1999.

196. Sicard GA, Rubin BG, Sanchez LA, et al: Endoluminal graft repair for abdominal aortic aneurysms in high-risk patients and octogenarians: is it better than open repair? *Ann Surg* 234:427, 2001.

197. Teufelsbauer H, Prusa AM, Wolff K, et al: Endovascular stent grafting versus open surgical operation in patients with infrarenal aortic aneurysms: a propensity score–adjusted analysis, *Circulation* 106:782, 2002.

198. Joseph AY, Fisher JB, Toedter LJ, et al: Ruptured abdominal aortic aneurysm and quality of life, *Vasc Endovasc Surg* 36:65, 2002.

199. Godet G, Fleron MH, Vicaut E, et al: Risk factors for acute postoperative renal failure in thoracic or thoracoabdominal aortic surgery: a prospective study, *Anesth Analg* 85:1227, 1997.

200. Safi HJ, Harlin SA, Miller CC, et al: Predictive factors for acute renal failure in thoracic and thoracoabdominal aortic aneurysm surgery, *J Vasc Surg* 24:338, 1996.

201. Thadhani R, Pascual M, Bonventre JV: Acute renal failure, *N Engl J Med* 334:1448, 1996.

202. LeMaire SA, Rice DC, Schmittling ZC, Coselli JS: Emergency surgery for thoracoabdominal aortic aneurysms with acute presentation, *J Vasc Surg* 35:1171, 2002.

203. Hansen KJ, Deitch JS: Renal complications. In Rutherford RB (ed): *Vascular surgery*, Philadelphia, 2000, WB Saunders, 655-664.

204. Roberts KW, Lumb PD: Complications of vascular surgery. In Kaplan JA (ed): *Vascular anesthesia*, New York, 1991, Churchill Livingstone, 643-644.

205. Fielding JL, Black J, Ashton F, et al: Ruptured aortic aneurysms: postoperative complications and their aetiology, *Br J Surg* 71:487, 1984.

206. Gordon AC, Pryn S, Collin J: Outcome of patients who required renal support after surgery for ruptured abdominal aortic aneurysm, *Br J Surg* 81:836, 1994.

207. Coselli J: Thoracoabdominal aortic aneurysms: experience with 372 patients, *J Card Surg* 9:638, 1994.

208. Mauney M, Tribble C, Cope J, et al: Is clamp and sew still viable for thoracic aortic resection? *Ann Surg* 223:534, 1996.

209. Mastroroberto P, Chello M: Emergency thoracoabdominal aortic aneurysm repair: clinical outcome, *J Thorac Cardiovasc Surg* 118:477, 1999.

210. Velazquez O, Bavaria J, Pochettino A, Carpenter J: Emergency repair of thoracoabdominal aortic aneurysms with immediate presentation, *J Vasc Surg* 30:996, 1999.

211. Schepens MA, Defauw JJ, Hamerlinjnck MP, Vermeulen FE: Risk assessment of acute renal failure after thoracoabdominal aortic aneurysm surgery, *Ann Surg* 219:400, 1994.

212. Star RA: Treatment of acute renal failure, *Kidney Int* 54:1817, 1998.

213. Chertow GM, Lazarus JM, Christiansen CL, et al: Preoperative renal risk stratification, *Circulation* 95:878, 1997.

214. Parodi JC, Palmaz JC, Barone HD: Transfemoral intraluminal graft implantation for abdominal aortic aneurysms, *Ann Vasc Surg* 5:491, 1991.

215. Arko FR, Lee WA, Hill BB, et al: Aneurysm-related death: primary endpoint analysis for comparison of open and endovascular repair, *J Vasc Surg* 36:297, 2002.

216. Chertow GM, Levy EM, Hammermeister KE, et al: Independent association between acute renal failure and mortality following cardiac surgery, *Am J Med* 104:343, 1998.

217. Breckwoldt WL, Mackey WC, Belkin M, O'Donnell TF Jr: The effect of suprarenal cross-clamping on abdominal aortic aneurysm repair, *Arch Surg* 127:520, 1992.

218. Sasaki T, Ohsawa S, Ogawa M, et al: Postoperative renal function after an abdominal aortic aneurysm repair requiring a suprarenal aortic cross-clamp, *Surg Today* 30:33, 2000.

219. Nypaver TJ, Shepard AD, Reddy DJ, et al: Supraceliac aortic cross-clamping: determinants of outcome in elective abdominal aortic reconstruction, *J Vasc Surg* 17:868, 1993.

220. Bertrand M, Godet G, Fleron MH, et al: Lumbar muscle rhabdomyolysis after abdominal aortic surgery, *Anesth Analg* 85:11, 1997.

221. Eneas JF, Schoenfeld BY, Humphreys MH: The effect of infusion of mannitol–sodium bicarbonate on the clinical course of myoglobinuria, *Arch Intern Med* 139:801, 1979.

222. Gamulin Z, Forster A, Morel D, et al: Effects of infrarenal aortic cross-clamping on renal hemodynamics in humans, *Anesthesiology* 61:394, 1984.

223. Hou SH, Bushinsky DA, Wish JB, et al: Hospital-acquired renal insufficiency: a prospective study, *Am J Med* 74:243, 1983.

224. Schner RW, Gottschalk CW (eds): *Diseases of the kidney*, ed 5, Boston, 1993, Little, Brown.

225. Nash K, Hafeez A, Abrinko P, Hou S: Hospital-acquired renal insufficiency, *J Am Soc Nephrol* 7:1376, 1996 (abstract).

226. Thomsen HS: Nephrotoxicity. In Thomsen HS, Muller RN, Mattrey RF (eds): *Trends in contrast media*, Berlin, 1999, Springer-Verlag, 105.

227. Weisberg LS, Kurnik PB, Kurnik BRC: Risk of radiocontrast nephropathy in patients with and without diabetes mellitus, *Kidney Int* 45:259, 1994.

228. Waybill MM, Waybill PN: Contrast media–induced nephrotoxicity: identification of patients at risk and algorithms for prevention, *J Vasc Interv Radiol* 12:3, 2001.

229. Morcos SK, Thomsen HS, Webb JAW: Contrast-media-induced nephrotoxicity: consensus report. Contrast Media Safety Committee of the European Society of Urogenital Radiology, *Eur Radiol* 9:1602, 1999.

230. Rudnick MR, Goldfarb S, Wexler L, et al: Nephrotoxicity of ionic and nonionic contrast media in 1196 patients: a randomized trial, *Kidney Int* 47:254, 1995.

231. Barrett BJ: Contrast nephrotoxicity, *J Am Soc Nephrol* 5:125, 1994.

232. Sterner G, Nyman U, Valdes T: Low risk of contrast-medium-induced nephropathy with modern angiographic technique, *J Intern Med* 250:429, 2001.

233. Chalmers N, Jackson RW: Comparison of iodixanol and iohexol in renal impairment, *Br J Radiol* 72:701, 1999.

234. Levy EM, Viscoli CM, Horwitz RI: The effect of acute renal failure on mortality, A cohort analysis, *JAMA* 275:1489, 1996.

235. Cigarroa RG, Lange RA, Williams RH, Hillis LD: Dosing of contrast material to prevent contrast nephropathy in patients with renal disease, *Am J Med* 86:649, 1989.

236. Hawkins IF, Caridi JG: Carbon dioxide (CO_2) digital subtraction angiography: 26-years experience at the University of Florida, *Eur Radiol* 8:391, 1998.

237. Solomon R: Contrast-medium-induced acute renal failure, *Kidney Int* 53:230, 1998.

238. Solomon R, Werner C, Mann D, et al: Effects of saline, mannitol, and furosemide on acute decreases in renal function induced by radiocontrast agents, *N Engl J Med* 331:1416, 1994.

239. Ayerdi J, Sampson LN, Deshmukh N, et al: Carotid endarterectomy in patients with renal insufficiency: should selection criteria be different in patients with renal insufficiency? *Vasc Surg* 35:429, 2001.

240. Hamdan A, Pomposelli FB, Gibbons GW, et al: Renal insufficiency and altered postoperative risk in carotid endarterectomy, *J Vasc Surg* 29:1006, 1999.

241. Bush H, Huse J, Johnson W, et al: Prevention of renal insufficiency after abdominal aortic aneurysm resection by optimal volume loading, *Arch Surg* 116:1517, 1981.

242. Norris EJ, Frank SM: Anesthesia for vascular surgery. In Miller R (ed): *Anesthesia*, ed 5, New York, 2000, Churchill Livingstone, 1166.

243. Ellis SE, Roizen MF, Mantha S, et al: Anesthesia for vascular surgery. In Barash P, Cullen B, Stoelting R (eds): *Clinical anesthesia*, ed 4, Philadelphia, 2001, JB Lippincott, 1078-1079.

244. Wahlberg E, DiMuzio PJ, Stoney RJ: Aortic clamping during elective operations for infrarenal disease: the influence of clamping time on renal function, *J Vasc Surg* 36:13, July 2002.

245. Dishart MK, Kellum JA: An evaluation of pharmacological strategies for the prevention and treatment of acute renal failure, *Drugs* 59:79, 2000.

246. Petroni KC, Cohen NH: Continuous renal replacement therapy: anesthetic implications, *Anesth Analg* 94:1288, 2002.

247. Chu VL, Cheng JW: Fenoldopam in the prevention of contrast media–induced acute renal failure, *Ann Pharmacother* 35:1278, 2001.

248. Madyoon H, Croushore L, Weaver D, Mathur V: Use of fenoldopam to prevent radiocontrast nephropathy in high-risk patients, *Cathet Cardiovasc Interv* 53:341, 2001.

249. Tepel M, van der Giet M, Schwarzfeld C, et al: Prevention of radiographic-contrast-agent-induced reductions in renal function by acetylcysteine, *N Engl J Med* 343:180, 2000.

250. Stevens MA, McCullough PA, Tobin KJ, et al: A prospective randomized trial of prevention measures in patients at high risk for contrast nephropathy: results of the PRINCE study, *J Am Coll Cardiol* 33:403, 1999.

251. Weisberg LS, Kurnik PB, Kurnik BRC: Dopamine and renal blood flow in radiocontrast-induced nephropathy in humans, *Ren Fail* 15:61, 1993.

252. Tumlin JA, Wang A, Murray PT, Mathur VS: Fenoldopam mesylate blocks reductions in renal plasma flow after radiocontrast dye infusion: a pilot trial in the prevention of contrast nephropathy, *Am Heart J* 143:894, 2002.

253. Hunter DW, Chamsuddin A, Bjarnason H, Kowalik K: Preventing contrast-induced nephropathy with fenoldopam, *Tech Vasc Interv Radiol* 4:53, 2001.

254. Reuler J: Hypothermia: pathophysiology, clinical settings, and management, *Ann Intern Med* 89:519, 1979.

255. Hertzer N, Beven E, Young J, et al: Coronary artery disease in peripheral vascular patients: a classification of 1000 coronary angiograms and results of surgical management, *Ann Surg* 199:223, 1984.

256. Sladen R, Endo E, Harrison T: Two-hour versus 24-hour creatinine clearance in critically ill patients, *Anesthesiology* 67:1013, 1987.

257. Halpenny M, Lakshmi S, O'Donnell A, et al: Fenoldopam: renal and splanchnic effects in patients undergoing coronary artery bypass grafting. *Anaesthesia* 56:953, 2001.

258. Halpenny M, Markos F, Snow HM, et al: The effects of fenoldopam on renal blood flow and tubular function during aortic cross-clamping in anaesthetized dogs, *Eur J Anaesthesiol* 17:491, 2000.

259. Gilbert TB, Hasnain JU, Flinn WR, et al: Fenoldopam infusion associated with preserving renal function after aortic cross-clamping for aneurysm repair, *J Cardiovasc Pharmacol Ther* 6:31, 2001.

260. Druml W: Metabolic aspects of continuous renal replacement therapies, *Kidney Int* 56: S56, 1999.

261. Alkhunaizi AM, Schrier RW: Management of acute renal failure: new perspectives, *Am J Kidney Dis* 28: 315, 1996.

262. Garcia J, Pagini E: Acute renal failure: etiology, diagnosis and therapy. In Estafanous F (ed): *Anesthesia and the heart patient*, Boston, 1989, Butterworth, 317-324.

263. Biller J, Feinberg WM, Castaldo JE, et al: Guidelines for carotid endarterectomy: a statement for healthcare professionals from a special writing group of the Stroke Council, American Heart Association, *Circulation* 97:501, 1998.

264. Branchereau A, Jacobs M: *Complications in vascular surgery. Part I*, Armonk, NY, 2001, Futura, 141.

265. Schauber MD, Fontenelle LJ, Solomon JW, Hanson TL: Cranial/cervical nerve dysfunction after carotid endarterectomy, *J Vasc Surg* 25:481, 1997.

266. Ballotta E, Da Giau G, Renon L, et al: Cranial and cervical nerve injuries after carotid endarterectomy: a prospective study, *Stroke* 30:1162, 1999.

267. Bartolucci R, D'Andrea V, Leo E, De Antoni E: Cranial and neck nerve injuries following carotid endarterectomy intervention. Review of the literature, *Chir Ital* 53:73, 2001.

268. Maniglia AJ, Han DP: Cranial nerve injuries following carotid endarterectomy: an analysis of 336 procedures, *Head Neck* 13:121, 1991.

269. De Toma G, Nicolanti V, Plocco M, et al: Baroreflex failure syndrome after bilateral excision of carotid body tumors: an underestimated problem, *J Vasc Surg* 31:806, 2000.

270. Qureshi AI, Luft AR, Sharma M, et al: Frequency and determinants of postprocedural hemodynamic instability after carotid angioplasty and stenting, *Stroke* 30:2086, 1999.

271. Rutherford R: *Postoperative management and complications following carotid endarterectomy in vascular surgery*, Philadelphia, 2000, WB Saunders, 1884.

272. Jenkins NP, Ward C: Coarctation of the aorta: natural history and outcome after surgical treatment, *QJM* 92:365, 1999.

273. Farkas JC, Calvo-Verjat N, Laurian C, et al: Acute colorectal ischemia after aortic surgery: pathophysiology and prognostic criteria, *Ann Vasc Surg* 6:111, 1992.

274. Dadian N, Ohki T, Veith FJ, et al: Overt colon ischemia after endovascular aneurysm repair: the importance of microembolization as an etiology, *J Vasc Surg* 34:986, 2001.

275. Longo WE, Lee TC, Barnett MG, et al: Ischemic colitis complicating abdominal aortic-aneurysm surgery in the U.S. veteran, *J Surg Res* 60:351, 1996.

276. Ernst C: *Colon ischemia following aortic reconstruction in vascular surgery*, Philadelphia, 2000, WB Saunders, 1542.

277. Bannister J, Wildsmith T: *Anaesthesia for vascular surgery*, London, 2000, Arnold, 196.

278. Kuttila K, Perttila J, Vanttinen E, Niinikoski J: Tonometric assessment of sigmoid perfusion during aortobifemoral reconstruction for arteriosclerosis, *Eur J Surg* 160:491, 1994.

279. Mehta M, Veith FJ, Ohki T, et al: Unilateral and bilateral hypogastric artery interruption during aortoiliac aneurysm repair in 154 patients: a relatively innocuous procedure, *J Vasc Surg* 33(2 Suppl):S27, 2001.

280. Kuhan G, Raptis S: 'Trash foot' following operations involving the abdominal aorta, *Aust NZ J Surg* 67:21, 1997.

281. Ernst C: Current concepts: Abdominal aortic aneurysm, *N Engl J Med* 328:1167, 1993.

282. Parent FN 3rd, Godziachvili V, Meier GH 3rd, et al: Endograft limb occlusion and stenosis after ANCURE endovascular abdominal aneurysm repair, *J Vasc Surg* 35:686, 2002.

283. Fietsam R Jr, Villalba M, Glover JL, Clark K: Intra-abdominal compartment syndrome as a complication of ruptured abdominal aortic aneurysm repair, *Am Surg* 55:396, 1989.

284. Platell CF, Hall J, Clarke G, Lawrence-Brown M: Intra-abdominal pressure and renal function after surgery to the abdominal aorta, *Aust NZ J Surg* 60:213, 1990.

285. Roizen MF, Rodgers GM, Valone FH, et al: Anaphylactoid reactions to vascular graft material presenting with vasodilation and subsequent disseminated intravascular coagulation, *Anesthesiology* 71:331, 1989.

286. Lee ES, Kor DJ, Kuskowski MA, Santilli SM: Incidence of erectile dysfunction after open abdominal aortic aneurysm repair, *Ann Vasc Surg* 14:13, 2000.

287. Nevelsteen A, Beyens G, Duchateau J, Suy R: Aorto-femoral reconstruction and sexual function: a prospective study, *Eur J Vasc Surg* 4:247, 1990.

288. York JW, Money SR: Prevention and management of ureteral injuries during aortic surgery, *Semin Vasc Surg* 14:266, 2001.

289. Kahn MB, Profeta B, Hume E, et al: Tibia fracture after fibula resection for distal peroneal bypass, *J Vasc Surg* 34:979, 2001.

290. Melliere D, Becquemin JP, Erienne G, et al: Severe injuries resulting from operations for thoracic outlet syndrome: can they be avoided? *J Cardiovasc Surg (Torino)* 32:599, 1991.

291. Jonathan DB, Peter AG: *Vascular and endovascular surgery*, Philadelphia, 1998, WB Saunders, 241.

292. Johnston KW: Multicenter prospective study of nonruptured abdominal aortic aneurysm. Part II. Variables predicting morbidity and mortality, *J Vasc Surg* 9:437, 1989.

293. Jaffe R, Samuels S: *Anesthesiologist 's manual of surgical procedures*, Philadelphia, 1999, Lippincott Williams & Wilkins, 273.

294. Ahn SS, Rutherford RB, Johnston KW, et al: Reporting standards for infrarenal endovascular abdominal aortic aneurysm repair. Ad Hoc Committee for Standardized Reporting Practices in Vascular Surgery of the Society for Vascular Surgery/International Society for Cardiovascular Surgery, *J Vasc Surg* 25:405, 1997.

295. Fowl R, Hurst J: Postoperative care of the vascular surgical patient. In Yeager MP, Glass DD (eds): *Anesthesiology& vascular surgery: perioperative management of the vascular surgical patient*, Norwalk, Conn, 1990, Appleton & Lange, 275.

Postoperative Cardiovascular Low-Output Syndrome and Sepsis

17

Madhav Swaminathan, MBBS, MD
Robert N. Sladen, MBCHB, MRCP (UK), FRCPC
Mark Stafford Smith, MD, CM, FRCPC

AMONG the many clinical issues confronting the anesthesiologist in the postoperative period, low cardiac output syndrome and sepsis are two of the most serious. Patients undergoing vascular surgery are elderly, often have coronary artery disease, and sustain significant perioperative fluid shifts, putting them at risk for low-output states. Systemic inflammation, sepsis, and organ dysfunction are common consequences of vascular surgery that continue to challenge the perioperative physician. As the understanding of the process of organ dysfunction grows, new information with regard to genetic variability, cellular pathophysiology, and molecular mechanisms may enhance diagnostic and therapeutic options in the future.

In this chapter, the authors discuss the pathophysiology of postoperative low cardiac output syndrome and sepsis, systemic responses to these complications, and a logical approach to their hemodynamic management.

Low Cardiac Output Syndrome

Definition

Low cardiac output syndrome refers to a clinical state in which the heart is unable to meet the perfusion requirements of metabolizing tissues in the body or can do so only from an increased filling pressure. The low cardiac output syndrome may be seen as a part of a larger pathophysiologic state known as *circulatory failure* (Figure 17-1), in which some component of the circulation, namely the heart, blood vessels, blood volume, or oxygen content of the arterial blood, is responsible for failure to meet the perfusion demands of the body. Integral to the definition of low cardiac output syndrome is the concept that it is a syndrome and, therefore, a constellation of clinical signs resulting from failure of tissue perfusion. The hypoperfusion reduces the supply of oxygen and substrates to tissues and leads to cellular injury. The cells respond by producing inflammatory mediators that cause changes in the microvasculature, further exacerbating cellular injury. The consequent clinical picture of reduced perfusion and systemic organ responses constitutes the low cardiac output syndrome.

From the clinician's point of view, hypoperfusion states are also referred to as shock. Shock describes the clinical state consequent to inadequate perfusion of vital capillary beds. *Low-output shock* is the term used when there is a primary decrease in cardiac output with compensatory vasoconstriction (cardiogenic, hypovolemic shock). Perfusion is maintained to the coronary and cerebral circulations (relatively independent of

α-adrenergic vasoconstriction) at the expense of splanchnic and renal blood flow.

High-output shock is the term used when there is a primary decrease in systemic vascular resistance with compensatory increases in cardiac output (septic, anaphylactic shock). High output is a misnomer because considerable myocardial depression exists in sepsis and patients become hypotensive because cardiac output cannot increase sufficiently to compensate for the low systemic vascular resistance. A better term is *distributive shock* because there is excessive flow to the periphery and inadequate flow to the splanchnic, renal, and pulmonary beds. Therefore, although representing extreme ends of cardiac output, both low cardiac output syndrome and sepsis characterize the diverse pathophysiology of circulatory failure in the postoperative period.

Etiology and Classification

Shock was classified into four broad categories by Blalock in 1934—hematologic, neurologic, vasogenic, and cardiogenic. Over the years, multiple classifications based on etiology or treatment categories have evolved. However, classification according to the etiology of precipitating cause is more useful for identification and treatment of the underlying abnormality (Table 17-1; see Figure 17-1). Hypovolemic shock results from excessive blood or fluid loss, causing a decrease in circulating blood volume and, therefore, preload. Myocardial function is typically preserved in the early stages of hypovolemia. Cardiogenic shock occurs when the cardiac pump mechanism fails to generate adequate cardiac output. This type of shock may be precipitated by myocardial infarction or stunning or preexisting cardiomyopathy. Cardiogenic shock may also be simply classified according to etiology as precardiac (eg, tamponade), intracardiac (eg, myocardial infarction, cardiomyopathy), or postcardiac (eg, pulmonary embolism). Postoperative low cardiac output in vascular surgical patients is usually a result of either hypovolemia (related to surgical bleeding, coagulopathy, or inadequate fluid resuscitation) or myocardial dysfunction (related to myocardial ischemia or infarction). In critically ill patients, circulatory failure may result from excessive vasodilation caused by sepsis. Although individual conditions may precipitate shock by affecting any component of circulation, namely the heart, blood vessels, blood volume, or oxygen content of blood, significant overlap may occur and ultimately result in the progressive involvement of all components. In this chapter, low cardiac output syndrome implies hypovolemic (hemorrhagic) or cardiogenic shock as the primary etiology.

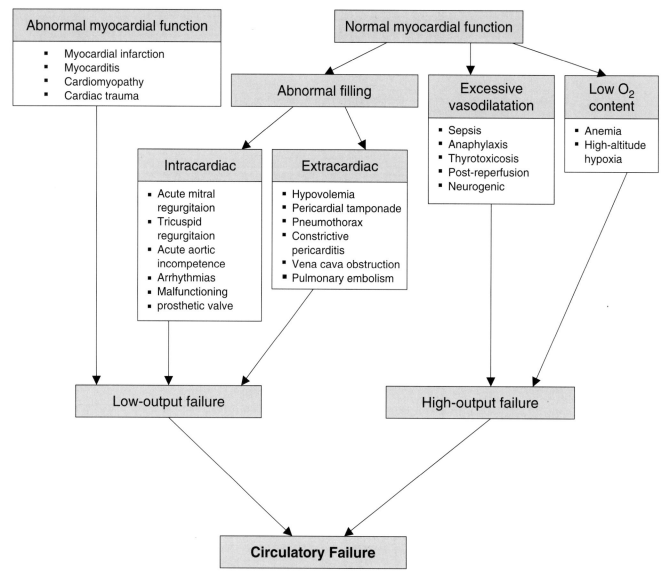

FIGURE 17-1 Classification of circulatory failure based on precipitating cause.

Pathophysiology of Low Cardiac Output Syndrome

Inadequate tissue perfusion in low cardiac output syndrome stems from an inability of the heart to pump adequate amounts of blood. The inefficient delivery of oxygen and substrate to the tissues prompts adaptive responses by cellular metabolic processes. As a consequence of oxygen deprivation, the cells turn to anaerobic mechanisms to produce energy for cellular functions. Anaerobic metabolism is not efficient in generating adenine triphosphate (ATP) and also results in the production of lactic acid. The accumulation of lactate and other vasodilator and myocardial depressant substances further worsens the hypotension, low cardiac output, and shock state and, if left untreated, results in death.

TISSUE OXYGEN IMBALANCE. Central to the concept of oxygen delivery is the fact that oxygen is not stored in the body and, therefore, the delivery of oxygen is rate limiting for cellular oxidative mechanisms. An imbalance in oxygen supply and demand may result from a reduced supply in the presence of normal demand (eg, hypovolemic or cardiogenic shock) or inadequate supply when faced with increased demand as may occur in hypermetabolic states, such as thyrotoxicosis. Oxygen imbalance (termed *dysoxia*) also occurs in sepsis because of a combination of decreased supply (regional perfusion failure) and metabolic shutdown of cellular oxidative processes (Figure 17-2).

Arterial Oxygen Content. Oxygen is present in the blood in two forms, bound to hemoglobin and dissolved in plasma. Almost all the oxygen in the blood is transported by hemoglobin, while a small amount is dissolved in plasma. Arterial oxygen content (CaO_2) is determined by the concentration of hemoglobin in the blood (g/dL), the percentage of arterial hemoglobin saturated with oxygen (SaO_2), and the volume of oxygen dissolved in plasma (mL). When fully saturated, 1 g of hemoglobin combines with 1.34 mL of oxygen. The dissolved content is determined by arterial oxygen tension and the blood

TABLE 17-1

Classification of Circulatory Failure

Abnormalities of the heart
  Abnormal myocardial function (cardiogenic shock)
    Myocardial infarction
    Cardiomyopathies
    Myocarditis
    Cardiac trauma
    Postischemic myocardial stunning
    Pharmacologic myocardial depressants
  Normal myocardial function. Abnormal filling
    Intracardiac
      Acute mitral regurgitation
      Tricuspid regurgitation
      Acute aortic incompetence
      Arrhythmias
      Malfunctioning prosthetic valve
    Extracardiac
      Pericardial tamponade
      Pneumothorax
      Constrictive pericarditis
      Vena cava obstruction
      Pulmonary embolism
Abnormalities of blood volume (hypovolemic shock)
  Depletion of blood (hemorrhagic)
    Trauma
    Surgical blood loss
    Gastrointestinal bleeding
    Retroperitoneal blood loss
  Depletion of fluid (nonhemorrhagic)
    Dehydration
    Hyperemesis
    Diarrhea
    Third-space fluid loss—thermal injury, anaphylaxis (anaphylactic shock)
Abnormalities of blood vessels
  Excessive vasodilatation
    Sepsis (septic shock)
    Reperfusion injury (after liver transplantation)
    Anaphylaxis
    Thyrotoxicosis
    Drug induced—nitroprusside
    Neurogenic (spinal shock)
    Arteriovenous shunts
  Vascular injury
    Aortic dissection
Abnormalities of oxygen content of circulating blood
  Anemia
  High-altitude hypoxia

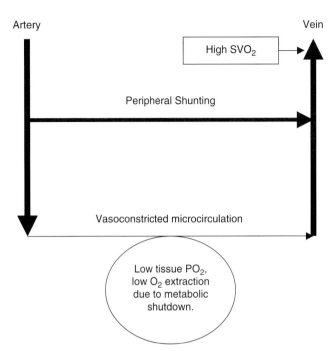

FIGURE 17-2 Mechanism of tissue hypoxia in shock. Shutdown of microcirculation in peripheral tissues results in arteriovenous shunting of blood through larger vessels. This leads to higher mixed venous oxygen saturation (SVO_2). Further tissue hypoxia occurs because of shutdown of cellular oxidative metabolic processes.

solubility coefficient for oxygen (0.003 mL/dL). This may be expressed as:

$$Ca_{O_2} \text{ (mL/dL)} = \text{(Hb g/dL) (Sa}_{O_2}\text{) (1.34 mL/g)} \quad (1)$$
$$+ \text{(Pa}_{O_2}\text{ mmHg) (0.003 mL/dL)}$$

where Hb = hemoglobin, Sa_{O_2} = percentage of hemoglobin saturated with oxygen, and Pa_{O_2} = arterial oxygen tension.

In a hypothetical example, if hemoglobin is 15 g/dL, Pa_{O_2} is 95 mmHg (i.e., normal arterial blood at sea level), and Hb is 100% saturated, the Ca_{O_2} can be calculated as:

$$Ca_{O_2} \text{ (mL/dL)} = \text{(15 g/dL) (100\%) (1.34 mL/g)} \quad (2)$$
$$+ \text{(95 mmHg) (0.003 mL/dL)}$$
$$= 20.1 \text{ mL/dL} + 0.3 \text{ mL/dL}$$
$$= 20.4 \text{ mL oxygen/dL blood}$$

It can be seen from the equation that the concentration and oxygen saturation of hemoglobin are the major determinants of Ca_{O_2}. In a postoperative vascular patient, the effect of anemia and hypoxia on oxygen content can be illustrated with the same equation. Therefore, if Hb = 9 g/dL, $\%Sa_{O_2}$ = 95%, and Pa_{O_2} = 85 mmHg, the Ca_{O_2} may be calculated as:

$$Ca_{O_2} \text{ (mL/dL)} = \text{(9 g/dL) (95\%) (1.34 mL/g)} \quad (3)$$
$$+ \text{(85 mmHg) (0.003 mL/dL)}$$
$$= 11.5 \text{ mL/dL} + 0.3 \text{ mL/dL}$$
$$= 11.8 \text{ mL/dL}$$

Thus, oxygen content has been nearly halved with figures considered "normal." The efficient delivery of oxygen-poor blood, therefore, assumes greater significance.

Oxygen delivery. Oxygen delivery to the tissues (Do_2) is the product of the oxygen content of the blood (Ca_{O_2}) and the volume of oxygen delivered per unit time (i.e., cardiac output). Therefore:

$$Do_2 = (Ca_{O_2}) \times (CO) \quad (4)$$

where Do_2 = oxygen delivery in mL/min, Ca_{O_2} = arterial blood oxygen content in mL O_2/L blood, and CO = cardiac output in L/min.

In a hypothetical example, if the normal Ca_{O_2} is 200 mL O_2/L blood (see equation 2) and cardiac output is 5 L/min, then:

$$Do_2 \text{ (mL/min)} = \text{(20 mL/dL)} \times \text{(5 L/min)} \quad (5)$$
$$= 1000 \text{ mL/min}$$

Oxygen Consumption. The tissue oxygen consumption ($\dot{V}O_2$) may be calculated using the Fick principle:

$$\dot{V}O_2 = \text{oxygen delivery (}DO_2\text{)} - \text{oxygen return}$$

Oxygen return from the tissues may be calculated by measuring mixed venous oxygen content (Cvo_2), which is normally 150 mL O_2/L blood (ie, 15 mL O_2/dL blood). In the preceding example (equation 5), mixed venous oxygen return would be $150 \times 5 = 750$ mL/min. Therefore, $\dot{V}O_2$ can be calculated as the difference between arterial oxygen delivery and venous oxygen return, or:

$$1000 \text{ mL/min} - 750 \text{ mL/min} = 250 \text{ mL/min}$$

Therefore, 75% of oxygen carried normally remains in venous blood. This is not a valid assumption for any tissue because Svo_2 applies to the blood (venous effluent). Oxygen extraction is represented by the arteriovenous oxygen content difference ($AVDO_2$). Mixed venous (ie, pulmonary artery) $AVDO_2$ represents averaged oxygen extraction for the body (normally 5 mL oxygen per 100 mL blood) but provides little information regarding regional organ perfusion and extraction. Organs may have high blood flow with relatively low extraction (ie, kidney, which receives 25% of CO but has $AVDO_2$ of only 3 mL/100mL blood) or low flow with high extraction (ie, myocardium that receives only 250 mL/min but has $AVDO_2$ of 11 mL/100 mL blood). The most desaturated blood in the body is in the coronary sinus ($Scso_2 = 50\%$, which represents a Pvo_2 of about 25 mmHg). A Pvo_2 of 22 mmHg is the lowest pressure that generates tissue diffusion of oxygen, so the coronaries have no further reserve in terms of oxygen extraction—if myocardial oxygen demand increases, coronary blood flow must

increase or ischemia results. However, because of a lack of sustainable oxygen stores in the body, cells turn to anaerobic metabolism for energy production. The heart is usually the first to suffer, mainly owing to a combination of its already maximal extraction and low reserve. Anaerobic metabolism results in the accumulation of lactate and, consequently, lactic acidosis.

LACTIC ACIDOSIS. The accumulation of lactate resulting from inadequate tissue perfusion results in type A lactic acidosis characterized by a low tissue Po_2. This type is distinct from the lactate accumulation in aerobic disorders, known as type B lactic acidosis, in which the Po_2 is usually normal. Cellular metabolic processes rely on oxidative pathways to ensure maximal efficiency in ATP generation. For each mole of glucose metabolized to carbon dioxide and water, anaerobic phosphorylation reactions generate four moles of ATP. In contrast, aerobic phosphorylation reactions generate a net yield of 32 moles of ATP. Therefore, oxidative metabolism is far more efficient at generating ATP than anaerobic metabolism. The main pathway for oxidative phosphorylation of ADP to ATP is the tricarboxylic acid (TCA) cycle (Figure 17-3). Metabolic pathways involving the β-oxidation of fatty acids and glycolysis produce a common product, acetyl coenzyme A (acetyl CoA), which enters the TCA cycle to produce ATP. However, the lack of oxygen shuts down the TCA cycle, resulting in the accumulation of acetyl CoA. The high levels of acetyl CoA inhibit pyruvate dehydrogenase, resulting in the accumulation of pyruvate. Because pyruvate can no longer enter the TCA cycle owing to inhibition of pyruvate dehydrogenase, it is reduced to lactate by an alternative pathway that generates small amounts of ATP through anaerobic glycolysis. Therefore, although energy is produced by

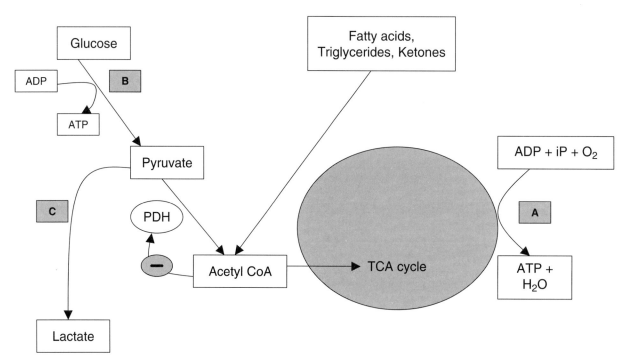

FIGURE 17-3 The accumulation of lactic acid in shock. When oxygen is unavailable at site A, acetyl coenzyme A (Acetyl CoA) accumulates in the tricarboxylic acid (TCA) cycle. Acetyl CoA inhibits pyruvate dehydrogenase (PDH), leading to accumulation of pyruvate. The excess pyruvate is converted to lactate (step C) in a process that allows the metabolism of glucose to continue to produce marginal amounts of ATP (site B). ADP, adenosine monophosphate; ATP, adenosine triphosphate; CoA, coenzyme A; iP, inorganic phosphate; PDH, pyruvate dehydrogenase; TCA, tricarboxylic acid cycle.

anaerobic metabolism, it leads to the accumulation of lactate in the blood. Lactic acidosis has major effects on most organ systems, especially the heart.[1] The decrease in cardiac output seen in acidosis is especially marked when the pH decreases below 7.20 (Figure 17-4).[2] The decrease in cardiac output further jeopardizes oxygen delivery to the tissues, resulting in a vicious cycle of increased acidosis and myocardial depression, which, if left unchecked, leads to multiple organ failure and death.

MICROCIRCULATORY CHANGES. The redistribution of cardiac output is the body's first and most important adaptive mechanism in low-output states. In an effort to maintain blood flow to important organs, such as the brain and heart, cardiac output is redirected away from other organs that are not considered a priority for survival. The microcirculation—arterioles, capillary bed, venules, and metarterioles—is the final common pathway that delivers the cardiac output and oxygen to tissues. In the presence of microcirculatory dysfunction, oxygen delivery to and metabolite clearance from tissues are impaired despite adequate hemodynamic function. Shock may also be simply defined as inadequate perfusion of the microcirculation.

Blood flow through any organ is determined by the difference between the arterial and venous pressures of vessels supplying the organ and the resistance of its vascular bed. Therefore:

$$\text{Blood flow} = \frac{(\text{mean arterial pressure} - \text{mean venous pressure})}{\text{vascular resistance}}$$

This formula is the physiologic application of Ohm's law of electrical theory, which states that current (blood flow) is directly proportional to the voltage (pressure gradient) and inversely proportional to resistance (vascular resistance).

Although vascular resistance plays an important role in controlling blood flow, other factors that influence resistance must also be highlighted. The relationship of various factors that affect blood flow through a vessel is illustrated by *Poiseuille's* equation:

$$\text{Fluid flow} = \frac{\pi \ (\text{pressure difference}) \ (\text{radius})^4}{8 \ (\text{vessel length}) \ (\text{fluid viscosity})}$$

It is apparent that the radius of the vessel is the major influence on blood flow. Smaller arteries and veins have important systemic and local regulatory mechanisms for control of vessel radius and, therefore, vascular resistance.

Vascular resistance is determined by two factors, neural control of vessel tone and local vasoactive substances released in response to stress. Neural control of vessel tone is mediated mainly by sympathetic vasoconstrictor-vasodilator fibers acting on muscular arteries that supply blood to the microcirculation. These fibers are found in arteries and veins throughout the body but not in capillaries. Sympathetic vasoconstrictor fibers cause vasoconstriction by increasing norepinephrine at nerve endings, which then acts on α_1-adrenergic receptors in vascular smooth muscle.[3] Local vasoactive substances released by tissues in response to oxygen deprivation include lactic acid, prostaglandins, histamine, nitric oxide (NO), and other vasoactive peptides. These substances are responsible for dilating or constricting capillaries in an attempt to maintain or augment blood flow through important areas within the microcirculation. Capillary flow is, therefore, dynamic and shifts from capillary bed to capillary bed and from capillary to capillary within each bed.

In low-output states, the initial response is mediated by the sympathoadrenal system, which results in intense arteriolar and venular constriction, especially in "low-priority" organs such as the abdominal viscera, so that blood flow may be redirected to the heart and brain. Sympathetically mediated vasoconstriction decreases blood flow to the microcirculation. The ensuing tissue hypoxia leads to the accumulation of lactic acid, endothelial injury, and production of other vasodilator substances. In the late stages of most forms of shock, there is a generalized failure of the vascular smooth muscle to constrict efficiently, resulting in vasodilatory shock.[4] Proposed mechanisms for this

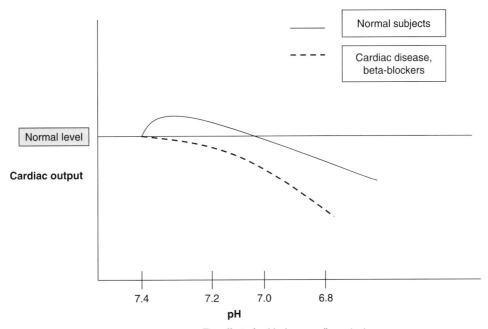

FIGURE 17-4 The effect of acidosis on cardiac output.

vasodilation include activation of ATP-sensitive potassium channels in vascular smooth muscle plasma membrane, activation of the inducible form of nitric oxide synthase, and vasopressin deficiency.[5-9] After a critical duration of shock, small precapillary arterioles are the first to lose their vascular tone. However, venular constriction persists, leading to obstruction to outflow. This increases capillary hydrostatic pressure, resulting in the leakage of intravascular fluid into the extravascular space. Interstitial edema increases, pushing cells farther away from their nutrient supply, worsening cellular hypoxia and acidosis. It also leads to the stagnation of blood flow within the capillary bed, which triggers intravascular coagulation (see later).

Cardiac Function and Low-Output Failure

Cardiac output is determined by the stroke volume and heart rate. The performance of the heart as a pump is dependent on the coupling of myocardial mechanics and vascular tone. In low-output syndrome, cardiac performance declines because of disturbances in both ventricular mechanics and vascular tone. Simplistic as the relationship may seem, there is a complex interplay of various factors that ultimately determine the ability of the heart to generate adequate stroke volume.

The stroke volume is determined by three factors: (1) left ventricular end-diastolic volume, or preload; (2) myocardial contractility; and (3) myocardial systolic wall tension (afterload), which is generated by impedance to ventricular outflow. The heart rate determines the cardiac output at any given stroke volume.

PRELOAD. The main determinants of preload are as follows:

Circulating blood volume. A decrease in circulating blood volume (because of postoperative blood loss or inadequate fluid resuscitation) results in decreased venous return to the heart with a consequent decrease in ventricular performance.

Distribution of blood volume. Although the total blood volume may be adequate, a maldistribution of this volume results in inadequate preload. Maldistribution of blood volume may be due to high intrathoracic pressures (that impede venous return), high pericardial pressures (eg, pericardial tamponade, which reduces diastolic volume), and altered venous tone (that occurs during hypovolemia to augment venous return).

Atrial contraction. Atrial systole plays an important role in ventricular diastolic filling. Patients with stiffer ventricles (hypertrophy) rely more on the atrial contraction to overcome elevated diastolic pressures for preload. Normally, atrial contraction contributes about 25% to cardiac output. In conditions with decreased ventricular compliance such as aortic stenosis or hypertrophic obstructive cardiomyopathy, its contribution may be as much as 40%. Thus, arrhythmias such as junctional rhythm or atrial fibrillation, which cause loss of the atrial kick, lead to rapid decompensation.

Myocardial muscle tension is directly dependent on muscle fiber length, which is a function of the end-diastolic volume (or preload). This classic length-tension association was described by separate investigators nearly 100 years ago and is known as the Frank-Starling relationship. However, because myocardial muscle length is impractical to measure in a clinical situation, the length-tension relationship is described by the end-diastolic pressure (assumed to be linearly related to fiber length) and the stroke volume. Hemodynamic correlates of ventricular performance are derived from central venous pressure, pulmonary artery occlusion pressure, and left atrial pressure. Unfortunately, the assumption that the left ventricular end-diastolic pressure is linearly related to the end-diastolic volume throughout the full range of values is incorrect. As illustrated in Figure 17-5, gradual increases in left ventricular end-diastolic volume are

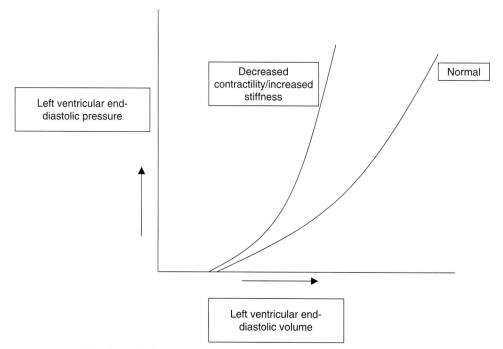

FIGURE 17-5 The relationship between left ventricular end-diastolic pressure and end-diastolic volume. In patients with poor myocardial contractility, the end-diastolic pressure is higher for a given end-diastolic volume than in those with normal cardiac function.

accompanied by disproportionately large increases in end-diastolic pressure. Therefore, an increase in pulmonary artery occlusion pressure in a stiff ventricle reflects the increasing stiffness of the ventricle rather than an increase in preload per se. On the other hand, the thin-walled right ventricle is more compliant, ensuring that right ventricular end-diastolic pressures adapt more efficiently to changes in end-diastolic volume. Therefore, right ventricular filling pressures do not change significantly with increasing right ventricular end-diastolic volumes. Thus, central venous pressure is a poor marker of right ventricular filling and an even poorer marker of left ventricular preload.

Transesophageal echocardiography enables the direct measurement of end-diastolic volumes and is being increasingly used to assess the postoperative patient. However, it is an expensive diagnostic tool that requires considerable expertise to obtain images and interpret them. The patient also needs to be sedated, which limits its usefulness as a continuous monitor of ventricular function (see Chapter 8).

CONTRACTILITY. At a given preload, ventricular performance is mainly determined by the state of myocardial contractility. Normal subjects respond to increasing preload with gradually increasing stroke volumes (Figure 17-6). However, the Frank-Starling curve is shifted to the left when contractility increases, such as with the administration of inotropic drugs. In this situation, the stroke volume is greater for any given preload. When myocardial contractility is decreased, for example, with myocardial ischemia, the same preload results in a reduced stroke volume. During myocardial ischemia, left ventricular compliance is markedly reduced, resulting in disproportionately greater increases in end-diastolic pressure for increases in left ventricular end-diastolic volume (see Figure 17-5).

Many factors influence myocardial contractility, including sympathetic activity, exogenous and endogenous catecholamines, myocardial depressants (drugs, toxins, hypoxia, lactic acid), and loss of functioning myocardium (myocardial infarction, ischemia). The postoperative vascular surgical patient is at high risk for perioperative myocardial ischemia and the residual effects of interventions, such as aortic cross-clamping, that result in a significant period of myocardial "stunning."[10] A high index of suspicion for myocardial ischemia is warranted when these patients deteriorate into a low cardiac output state despite apparently adequate intravascular volume replacement.

Because a direct measurement of ventricular contractility is impractical, indirect measures (such as pulmonary artery pressure) are used to indicate the contractile state. Echocardiographic indexes such as left ventricular ejection time, pre–ejection period, end-systolic stress, and velocity of fiber shortening, have also been shown to be preload-insensitive indicators of contractile function.[11]

Traditionally, myocardial contractility has received attention during the systolic period of the cardiac cycle. However, diastole is an active period of the cardiac cycle and abnormalities of myocardial contractile function during diastole are important determinants of global ventricular performance. The ability of the heart to fill at any given filling pressure is termed *diastolic compliance* or *lusitropy*. The energy-consuming lusitropic state enables the ventricle to accelerate its diastolic relaxation, thereby permitting it to fill at any level of diastolic pressure. Therefore, in an energy-starved environment that may occur with hypovolemic shock or myocardial ischemia, lusitropy is the first to decrease, resulting in decreased diastolic compliance (ie, ventricular stiffness) and consequent diastolic dysfunction.[12,13] Myocardial contractility is, therefore, important to both the diastolic and systolic phases of the cardiac cycle.

AFTERLOAD. The afterload may be defined as the net load against which myocardial muscle fibers must contract during systole. The afterload on the heart is determined by the size of the heart and the aortic pressure.

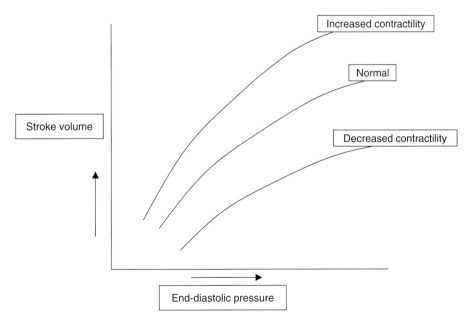

FIGURE 17-6 The relationship between left ventricular stroke volume and end-diastolic pressure. In patients with poor myocardial contractility, there is little increase in stroke volume on increasing preload in the "flat" portion of the curve. Increasing contractility with inotropic therapy shifts the curve upward and toward the left, optimizing the preload and increasing stroke volume.

Heart size. The internal radius of the left ventricle is an important component of afterload (or myocardial wall tension) according to Laplace's law:

$$\text{Wall tension} = \frac{(P)\,(r)}{2(T)}$$

where P = pressure generated by the myocardium during systole, r = internal radius of the left ventricle, and T = ventricular wall thickness.

The effect of afterload on heart size can be illustrated in patients with abnormal heart size. The Laplace relationship implies that afterload is increased by an increase in intramyocardial systolic pressure (P), an increase in the internal radius (r), and a decrease in wall thickness (T). Conditions that impose a pressure load (ie, aortic stenosis) result in *parallel* sarcomere replication, which increases wall thickness at the expense of the intracavitary radius (concentric hypertrophy)—that is, compensates for the increase in P. Conditions that impose a volume load (ie, mitral regurgitation) result in *series* sarcomere replication, which increases intracavitary radius (eccentric hypertrophy) and afterload, making pharmacologic afterload reduction through vasodilation beneficial.

Aortic pressure. The aortic pressure is principally influenced by peripheral vascular resistance, physical characteristics of the arterial tree (arteriosclerosis, arteriovenous shunting, coarctation), and the volume of blood within it at onset of systole.

When the afterload increases, the preload also increases to maintain cardiac output. However, when the limit of preload reserve is reached, the ventricular performance becomes exquisitely sensitive to the effects of afterload. In low cardiac output states related to myocardial dysfunction (or cardiogenic shock), stroke volumes are low owing to a combination of decreased myocardial contractility and intense vasoconstriction (high afterload). The limited ability of the myocardium to increase contractility and an already maximal preload reserve make the stroke volume dependent on the afterload conditions. This pathophysiology is the basis for afterload reduction therapy in advanced cardiac failure.[14,15]

HEART RATE. An increase in heart rate is the simplest mechanism by which an individual can increase cardiac output for a given stroke volume. The increase in heart rate also results in an increase in myocardial contractility (inotropy) and an improvement in diastolic relaxation (lusitropy). This force-frequency relationship is also known as the *Bowditch effect* or *treppe or staircase phenomenon.*[16,17] The Bowditch effect appears to be more apparent as an advantage in the normally functioning heart. However, a sudden decrease in heart rate that occurs with a compensatory pause can result in "recuperation" and consequent increase in contractile strength, a phenomenon termed the *Woodworth effect* or *reverse staircase phenomenon.*[18,19] It must also be kept in mind that an increase in heart rate occurs at the expense of diastolic time, a period on which coronary perfusion is dependent. Therefore, in patients with myocardial ischemia or fixed coronary artery stenosis, an increase in heart rate not only increases myocardial oxygen demand but also decreases oxygen supply by reducing the time available for coronary perfusion.

Neurohormonal Responses to Low Cardiac Output

SYMPATHOADRENAL ACTIVATION. The sympathoadrenal response to reduced arterial blood pressure and circulating blood volume restores blood pressure by augmenting myocardial contractility and increasing peripheral vasoconstriction. The resulting renal vasoconstriction also activates the renin-angiotensin-aldosterone axis.

Sympathoadrenal activation in response to hypoperfusion occurs as a result of reduced firing of baroreceptors situated in the great arteries and atria. Inhibition of sympathetic tone is reduced, leading to increased release of epinephrine from the adrenal medulla and norepinephrine from sympathetic nerve endings (from spinal segments T1 to L2, the thoracolumbar sympathetic outflow tract). Further activation of sympathetic tone by aortic and carotid chemoreceptors occurs in response to hypoxia and acidosis. Increased endogenous circulating catecholamine levels lead to several effects on the heart, blood vessels, and metabolic systems through the activation of different adrenergic receptor subtypes (Table 17-2).[20] There is an increase in myocardial contractility mediated by β_1-adrenergic receptors, while α_1-receptors mediate vasoconstriction and, therefore, redistribution of blood to the cardiocerebral circulation. In addition, venous reservoirs in the pulmonary, hepatic, splanchnic, and cutaneous circulation are mobilized to augment circulating blood volume. In the initial stages of low cardiac output syndrome, sympathetic stimulation of the heart occurs because of increased circulating and intramyocardial levels of norepinephrine. As cardiac function deteriorates, baroreceptor desensitization and β-adrenergic receptor downregulation occur to leave the heart functionally denervated.[21] This denervation stimulates further sympathetic activation that worsens the existing myocardial dysfunction.

The sympathetic system also mediates its actions in low cardiac output syndrome through direct effects on the kidneys. The rich sympathetic innervation of renal cortical vessels ensures a brisk renal response to hypovolemia. Blood flow within the kidneys is preferentially redistributed to the juxtamedullary nephrons, enhancing the kidneys' ability to concentrate urine.

Metabolic effects of sympathetic activation improve energy substrate availability during reduced tissue perfusion. Glycogen stores in the liver are mobilized to produce glucose (glycogenolysis), and lipolysis results in the increased availability of free fatty acids. Both glucose and fatty acids are essential substrates for cellular metabolic processes that produce energy in the form of ATP.

RENIN-ANGIOTENSIN-ALDOSTERONE ACTIVATION. The activation of the renin-angiotensin-aldosterone axis constitutes one of the most important compensatory mechanisms and underlines the role of the kidneys in circulatory homeostasis (Figure 17-7). The kidneys begin to secrete renin within a few hours of cardiac decompensation. Renin secretion in the kidneys is controlled by (1) afferent arteriolar constriction, (2) macula densa sodium-sensitive receptors, and (3) negative feedback from elevated angiotensin II levels.

Renin enzymatically cleaves angiotensinogen, a glycoprotein produced in the liver, into angiotensin I, which is then converted to angiotensin II (an octapeptide) by the angiotensin-converting enzyme (ACE). Angiotensin II exerts profound effects on the circulatory system, including arterial vasoconstriction and aldosterone release from the adrenal cortex. Angiotensin II

TABLE 17-2

Adrenergic Receptors

Subtypes	alpha-Adrenergic Receptors		beta-Adrenergic Receptors		
	alpha₁	alpha₂	beta₁	beta₂	beta₃
Agonists	Epi, NE		Isoproterenol, Epi, NE		
Agonist potency	Epi ≥ NE		Iso > NE ≥ Epi	Iso > Epi >> NE	Iso ≥ NE >> Epi
Representative selective agonists	Phenylephrine, methoxamine	Clonidine, α-methyl NE	Denopamine	Terbutaline, clenbuterol	BRL 37344, oxprenolol
Antagonists	Phentolamine, phenoxybenzamine		Propranolol, nadolol, timolol, oxprenolol		—
Representative selective antagonists	Prazosin, terazosin	Yohimbine, rauwolscine	Metoprolol, atenolol	ICI 118551	—
Second messenger	Phosphatidyl inositol turnover, ↑intracellular Ca²⁺	↓Cyclic AMP, ↓or↑ Ca²⁺ influx, Na⁺/H⁺ exchange	↑ Cyclic AMP	↑ Cyclic AMP	↑ Cyclic AMP
Representative responses	Vasoconstriction, intestinal relaxation, uterine contraction, pupillary dilation	↓ NE (presynaptic), platelet aggregation, vasoconstriction, ↓ insulin secretion	↑ Heart rate, ↑contractility, ↑lipolysis, ↑ renin secretion	Smooth muscle relaxation, ↑ glycogenolysis in skeletal muscle, ↑ NE (presynaptic)	↑ Brown fat thermogenesis, ↑ lipolysis
Desensitization	Yes	Yes	Yes (+)	Yes (++)	No

Epi, epinephrine; Iso, isoproterenol; NE, norepinephrine.
From Young JB, Landsberg L: Catecholamines and the adrenal medulla. In Wilson JD, Foster DW, Kronenberg HM, Reed Larsen P (eds): *Williams Textbook of Endocrinology,* ed 9, Philadelphia, 1998, WB Saunders, 684.

increases mesangial cell contraction, leading to a greater glomerular surface area for filtration, increased release of norepinephrine from nerve endings, myocyte hypertrophy, and fibroblast growth. Aldosterone promotes reabsorption of sodium and excretion of potassium by the distal tubules and collecting ducts. Angiotensin II and aldosterone together increase arterial pressure and augment intravascular volume. However, sustained vasoconstriction may worsen kidney function, and elevation in blood volume may be deleterious in cardiogenic shock states. This highlights the observation made often in the clinical setting that although compensatory

mechanisms may compensate for hypovolemia, with increasing stresses, these responses rapidly decompensate unless corrective measures are taken.

HYPOTHALAMIC-PITUITARY ACTIVATION. Osmoreceptors in the hypothalamus are activated in response to a change in plasma osmolality to induce secretion of arginine vasopressin (AVP), a nonapeptide that is stored in the posterior pituitary.[22] The secretion of AVP is also triggered by hypovolemia (through venous stretch receptors), decreased vasomotor tone (arterial baroreceptors), and several neuropeptides (acetylcholine, angiotensin II, histamine, and bradykinin).[23-25] The principal action of AVP

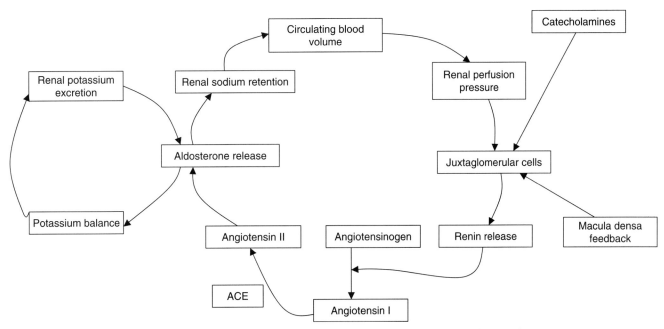

FIGURE 17-7 The renin-angiotensin system in circulatory homeostasis. ACE, angiotensin-converting enzyme.

is to promote water reabsorption through the renal collecting duct epithelium by acting on specific V2 receptors.[26] The normal physiologic range of AVP for antidiuresis (V2 receptor effect) is 1 to 5 pg/mL. Plasma AVP increases to 30 to 100 pg/mL in hypotension, at which levels it stimulates the V1 vascular receptors to augment vasoconstriction and contributes to increased systemic vascular resistance.[27] During end-stage shock, sustained baroreceptor stimulation results in depletion of AVP stores in the posterior pituitary, and plasma AVP may be as low as 3 ng/mL. Low-dose infusions (1 to 6 U/hr) restore plasma AVP to appropriate levels for V1 stimulation. The vasoconstrictive effect of AVP is used therapeutically for the treatment of refractory vasodilation after cardiopulmonary bypass,[28] sepsis,[29] and historically for esophageal varices.[30]

NATRIURETIC PEPTIDES. Natriuretic peptides play an important role in cardiovascular homeostasis. The family of natriuretic peptides includes four main peptides—atrial natriuretic peptide (ANP), B-type or brain natriuretic peptide (BNP), C-type natriuretic peptide (CNP), and urodilatin.[31,32] ANP is secreted by specialized atrial cells and BNP is secreted by ventricular myocytes, both in response to increased intracardiac filling pressures.[31,33,34] In contrast, CNP is produced in the brain and vascular endothelium, and urodilatin is the C-terminal peptide fragment of the ANP prohormone that is produced in the kidneys.[35] The principal actions of ANP and BNP are natriuresis, diuresis, and vasodilation. In addition, BNP and CNP have prominent antifibrotic effects on cardiac myocytes, and CNP also has a positive lusitropic and a negative inotropic effect.[36-38] In the early stages of cardiogenic shock or acute heart failure, these peptides are secreted in response to elevated intracardiac pressures and counter the actions of endogenous vasoconstrictors. In contrast to those in cardiogenic shock, natriuretic peptide levels are low in hemorrhagic shock (low intracardiac pressures). With progression of heart failure, the natriuretic effect seems to be blunted.[33] Several studies have also shown elevated BNP to be a strong predictor of adverse outcome after myocardial infarction and heart failure.[39-41] Natriuretic peptides have important regulatory actions on the circulatory and renal systems. They also have complex control mechanisms governing their synthesis and actions. As researchers further elucidate their roles in critical illness, it is conceivable that these molecules will be utilized for the diagnosis and treatment of various cardiovascular diseases.

Renal Function and Low Cardiac Output Syndrome

Vascular surgery is often complicated by postoperative renal dysfunction.[42,43] Depending on the degree of damage, renal dysfunction may either remain subclinical or evolve into renal failure requiring some form of replacement therapy. Evidence supports a multifactorial basis for perioperative renal injury including (1) acute tubular necrosis (ischemic or nephrotoxic), (2) vascular injury (thrombosis or embolism, arterial or venous), (3) acute or chronic renal failure, and (4) inflammatory syndromes.

A primary response of the kidneys during the low-output states is to conserve body fluid. This renal response is a result of a reduced perception of circulating volume and is designed to conserve sodium and water. There are two parts of the renal response, an afferent limb that senses the inadequacy of circu-

lating volume and an efferent limb that activates retention of sodium and water (see Chapter 14).

THE AFFERENT LIMB. Changes in intravascular volume are sensed by mechanoreceptors in the atria and ventricles. Changes in arterial pressure are sensed by baroreceptors in the aortic arch and carotid sinuses. Their usual function in normovolemic states is to inhibit the sympathetic outflow and stimulate parasympathetic control of circulation.[44-46] However, in cardiogenic shock, despite high filling pressures, these mechanoreceptors exhibit a blunted response and, in concert with reduced arterial pressure, decrease the inhibitory influence on the sympathetic system. As a result, there is an increase in sympathetic activity, leading to activation of the efferent limb of the renal response.[47] In hypovolemic conditions, the renal response is activated by reduced arterial baroreceptor control over the sympathetic system. Therefore, in both hypovolemia and cardiogenic shock, there is a reduced perception of circulating volume leading to the renal sympathetic response.

THE EFFERENT LIMB. The effect of perceived volume depletion is an activation of neurohormonal systems that primarily affect glomerular hemodynamics. There is an increase in renal vascular resistance, a decrease in glomerular filtration rate, and an increase in the filtration fraction. The degree of efferent arteriolar constriction exceeds afferent arteriolar resistance, causing the increase in filtration fraction. The increase in efferent arteriolar resistance is mediated by angiotensin II.[48] This mechanism conserves glomerular filtration rate in the initial stages of low cardiac output syndrome despite reduced renal blood flow. However, during the later stages of low cardiac output syndrome, angiotensin II also constricts the afferent arteriole, resulting in marked reductions in filtration fraction and glomerular filtration rate (see Acute Renal Failure). The use of ACE inhibitors may accelerate renal dysfunction by eliminating the angiotensin II–mediated mechanism of conserving the glomerular filtration rate. The changes in glomerular hemodynamics prompt an increase in reabsorption of sodium and water in the proximal and distal tubules. These changes are due to physical factors brought about by an increase in the filtration fraction and by the actions of angiotensin II on epithelial transport, which serve to amplify the increase in sodium and water reabsorption.

ACUTE RENAL FAILURE. Acute renal failure (ARF) is an important cause of in-hospital mortality. Despite the use of dialysis, the mortality of perioperative ARF remains about 60%. ARF in low cardiac output syndrome usually results from a combination of reduced renal perfusion and tubular injury secondary to obstruction by cellular debris (Figure 17-8), leading to a condition termed *acute tubular necrosis*.[49] The renovascular theory of ARF suggests that an increase in afferent arteriolar constriction accompanied by a decrease in efferent arteriolar dilatation in the presence of reduced renal blood flow leads to a net decrease in glomerular plasma flow and hydrostatic pressure. The tubular theory of ARF suggests that cellular debris physically obstructs renal tubules, leading to an increase in intraluminal pressure and "back-leak" of fluid across the damaged epithelium. Altered glomerular capillary permeability is yet another theory of ARF. In low cardiac output syndrome, a combination of vascular and tubular factors may be responsible for the development of ARF. Even if adequate renal blood flow is restored, medullary renal

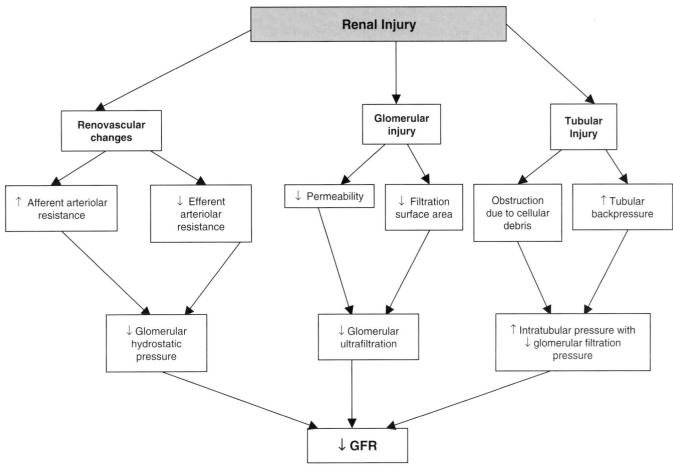

FIGURE 17-8 The pathophysiology of reduced glomerular filtration rate (GFR) in acute renal failure. (From Anderson RJ, Schrier RW: Acute renal failure. In Braunwald E, Isselbacher KJ, Petersdorf RG, et al [eds]: *Harrison's Principles of Internal Medicine,* ed 11, New York, 1987, McGraw-Hill, 1149.)

congestion and intrarenal vasoconstriction persist for several hours, leading to renal dysfunction that extends well into the postoperative period.[50] Vascular surgery patients may be at further "renal risk" because of contrast agents frequently used in the operating room to visualize graft flow or facilitate endovascular stent deployment, and vessel wall plaque detachment resulting in atheroembolic renal injury.[51,52] A combination of preexisting cardiac disease, intraoperative blood loss, use of nephrotoxic agents, and myocardial stunning owing to aortic clamping places the vascular surgical patient at high risk for sustaining acute perioperative renal injury (see Chapter 16).

Other Organ Systems in Low Cardiac Output Syndrome

As with the kidneys, other organs are equipped with autoregulatory systems that provide reserves during low-output states. The brain is also protected by these autoregulatory mechanisms that maintain cerebral perfusion until the mean arterial pressure drops below 50 mmHg. During sepsis-related circulatory failure, inflammatory mediators may be responsible for neuronal damage despite adequate cerebral perfusion. Acute lung injury may occur because of a combination of increased pulmonary capillary permeability, inflammatory exudates, alveolar collapse, and cellular aggregates in the microcirculation. These changes result in widespread shunting of blood through nonventilated areas, impaired gas exchange, severe hypoxemia, and, ultimately, the high-mortality condition termed the *acute respiratory distress syndrome.* The liver and gut also suffer ischemic consequences of low cardiac output syndrome. Gut barrier integrity is compromised, leading to translocation of gut bacteria into the bloodstream. Hepatocellular damage from hypoperfusion is reflected by an increase in serum transaminases and a decrease in synthesis of clotting factors. Sustained hypoperfusion to all organs results in exhaustion of reserve mechanisms and the consequent development of multiorgan failure.

The responses of the hematologic and inflammatory systems are important in the pathophysiology of low cardiac output syndrome and in many respects are similar to the response seen in sepsis syndromes. In fact, much of the current understanding of the inflammatory response in shock has evolved from studies in sepsis. However, low perfusion states result in cellular hypoxia that subsequently triggers the inflammatory response.

Differential Diagnosis of Low-Output Syndrome

The most common causes of postoperative low-output syndrome are hypovolemia and cardiogenic shock. It is imperative to differentiate hypovolemic from cardiogenic shock because the management differs in several fundamental ways. However, both conditions may exist simultaneously. Hypovolemia and hypotension may result in myocardial ischemia in the susceptible patient. Alternatively, excessive bleeding and consequent hypovolemia may complicate cardiogenic shock related to myocardial depression. The physician caring for the patient with low cardiac output syndrome must have a careful, complete history of perioperative events to diagnose accurately the type of shock encountered during the postoperative course.

Frequently, preoperative factors exist that place the vascular patient at risk for postoperative hypovolemia or cardiogenic shock. For instance, a history of excessive gastrointestinal fluid losses (eg, extended period without fluid intake) or hemorrhage (eg, during invasive vascular procedures) may cause the patient to be hypovolemic at the start of surgery. Similarly, a history of coronary artery disease or cardiomyopathy increases the likelihood of cardiac complications. Intraoperative factors must also be taken into account. Inadequate hemostasis, hypothermia, and prolonged aortic occlusion may also contribute to shock states in the postoperative period. Hypothermia in the operating room may cause platelet dysfunction and vasoconstriction leading to increased bleeding and hypotension during postoperative rewarming. An algorithm for the approach to the patient with postoperative circulatory failure is presented in Figure 17-9.

The diagnosis of the type of shock is supported by hemodynamic measurements made by pulmonary artery catheter, transesophageal echocardiography, and by monitoring temperature, acid-base status, urine output, electrocardiogram, chest radiograms, and blood loss. The typical hemodynamic profiles of hypovolemic and cardiogenic shock are outlined in Table 17-3.

TABLE 17-3

Typical Hemodynamic Profiles in Hypovolemic and Cardiogenic Shock

Parameter	Normal Range	Hypovolemic	Cardiogenic
HR, beats/min	60-120	>120	>120
CI, L/min/m^2	2.2-4.0	<2.2	<2.2
SI, mL/beat/m^2	30-50	<30	<30
PAOP, mmHg	6-12	<4	>18
SVRI, dyne sec cm^{-5}/m^2	1500-3000	>3000	>3000
Svo$_2$, %	70-80	<55	<55

HR, heart rate, CI, cardiac index, SI, stroke index, PAOP, pulmonary artery occlusion pressure, SVR, systemic vascular resistance, Svo$_2$, mixed venous oxygen saturation.

Management of Low-output Syndrome

Regardless of etiology, the management of low cardiac output syndrome must follow a logical sequence based on accurate clinical and hemodynamic data (Table 17-4).

STABILIZE HEART RHYTHM AND RATE. Cardiac arrhythmias are common in the perioperative period in vascular surgical patients. Arrhythmias may be secondary to hypovolemia, myocardial ischemia, or metabolic derangements and may be refractory to therapy until the underlying disorder is corrected. One of the cardinal manifestations of postoperative low cardiac output syndrome is tachycardia. Tachyarrhythmias often reflect the severity of the underlying hemodynamic derangement. Bradycardia and bradyarrhythmias more commonly reflect underlying conduction system disease or drug effects.

Tachyarrhythmias. Sinus tachycardia in the postoperative patient may be due to pain, myocardial ischemia, hypoxemia, or hypercarbia. These underlying conditions must be aggressively

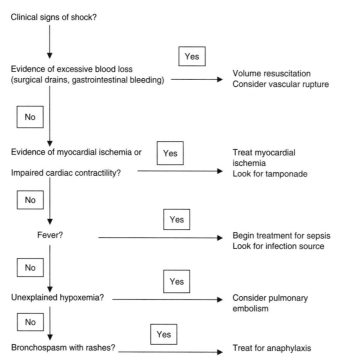

FIGURE 17-9 Algorithm for an approach to the patient with postoperative circulatory failure. (Modified from: Kline JA: Shock. In Marx JA [ed]: *Rosen's Emergency Medicine: Concepts and Clinical Practice*, ed 5, Philadelphia, 2002, Mosby, 40.)

TABLE 17-4

Principles of Hemodynamic Management of the Low Cardiac Output Syndrome

1. Stabilize heart rhythm and rate
   a. Treat tachycardia and bradycardia
   b. Treat supraventricular and ventricular arrhythmias
2. Optimize preload
   a. Increase deficient preload (hypovolemic [hemorrhagic] shock)
      Blood transfusion, blood products, colloid, crystalloid
   b. Decrease excessive preload [cardiogenic shock]
      Diuretics, venodilators (nitroglycerin), inotropic support
3. Enhance contractility
   a. Normalize pH and electrolyte milieu
      Control ventilation, correct acid-base and electrolyte imbalance
   b. Select appropriate inotropic agent
      Dopamine, epinephrine, norepinephrine
4. Normalize systemic vascular resistance (SVR)
   a. Reduce excessive afterload
      i. Vasodilator therapy
         Nitroprusside, nitroglycerin
      ii. Inodilator therapy
          Dobutamine, amrinone
   b. Restore inadequate SVR
      Phenylephrine, norepinephrine

treated. Resolution of tachycardia is a reliable indicator of clinical improvement. Tachycardia with a heart rate greater than 160 beats/min is usually due to supraventricular tachycardia including atrial fibrillation, atrial flutter, and paroxysmal supraventricular tachycardia.

Atrial fibrillation is commonly seen in elderly patients in the postoperative period.[53,54] The most important factor in the etiology of supraventricular arrhythmias is high circulating endogenous catecholamines, which is an integral component of low cardiac output syndrome. Factors that increase catecholamines include pain, acidosis, hypoxemia, and hypercarbia.

Patients with chronic atrial fibrillation often have some form of underlying valvular disease. The valvular disorder combined

with the lack of an atrial kick reduces cardiac reserve, and, consequently, these patients are more vulnerable to the development of low cardiac output syndrome.

Bradyarrhythmias. Bradycardia in the setting of low cardiac output syndrome is an ominous sign that requires aggressive management. Postoperative bradycardia may be due to intrinsic sinus node dysfunction, therapy with β-adrenergic blockers, hypothermia, inferior wall myocardial infarction, or digitalis toxicity. Initial treatment may be attempted with anticholinergic agents. Although these drugs may suffice for the treatment of transient bradycardia, electrical pacing is the safest and most reliable method of treating potentially life-threatening bradycardias. A transvenous pacemaker can usually be placed by the right internal jugular approach without difficulty and capture achieved by monitoring the P wave on an electrocardiogram attached to the pacing wire, with or without the help of fluoroscopy. Instead of isolated transvenous pacing leads, a pulmonary artery catheter with pacing capability may also be used.[55] External pacing may also be used if access for transvenous pacing is difficult or impossible.[56]

Ventricular arrhythmias. One of the most important features of myocardial ischemia is the onset of increasing ventricular irritability. In cardiogenic shock, recurrent ventricular arrhythmias may become increasingly refractory to therapy and are often the cause of death.[57] The approach to treatment of ventricular arrhythmias is summarized in Table 17-5.

OPTIMIZE PRELOAD.

Identify optimal preload. Optimal preload describes the filling pressures necessary to ensure effective cardiac function in a prevailing situation of myocardial contractility and afterload. In hypovolemic shock, filling pressures are low and myocardial contractility is usually normal. In this situation, optimal preload is achieved when cardiac function is enhanced to restore organ perfusion defined by a cardiac index greater than 2.2 L/min/m^2, mixed venous oxygen saturation of greater than 65%, stable arterial blood pressure, and urine output greater than 1 mL/kg/hr. Patients with cardiogenic shock have high filling

TABLE 17-5

Treatment of Ventricular Arrhythmias: Therapeutic Modalities

Modality	Administration	Remarks
DC cardioversion	Use synchronous mode for VT, asynchronous for VF; 100-400 J	First-line, emergency treatment for VT, VF
Amiodarone	300 mg IV bolus. 150 mg can be repeated once	First-tier treatment for VF, pulseless VT
Lidocaine	IV loading dose 1.0-1.5 mg/kg over 30-60 sec	First-line therapy for ventricular ectopy; rapid bolus may cause hypotension
	Maintenance infusion 1-4 mg/min	
	Therapeutic level 2-6 μg/mL	
Procainamide	IV loading dose 10-15 mg/kg *slowly* over 60 min	May provide control of arrhythmias refractory to lidocaine
	Maintenance infusion 1-4 mg/min	Not recommended in refractory VF
	Therapeutic range 4-8 μg/mL	
Bretylium	IV loading dose 5-10 mg/kg over 10-20 min	May cause transient hypertension followed by quite marked hypotension catecholamine depletion
	Maintenance 1-2 mg/min	
Magnesium	IV 2 mL of 25% solution over 10-20 min (= 0.5 g, or 9.6 mEq of Mg^{2+})	Use early in resistant arrhythmias
Sotalol	80 mg orally twice daily up to 240-320 mg per day	Recommended for stable VT; IV formulation not FDA approved in the United States; QTc must be monitored during treatment

Note: Ventricular arrhythmias may remain refractory to cardioversion or pharmacologic therapy until abnormal pH, blood gases, potassium, and magnesium are corrected.
DC, direct current; FDA, Food and Drug Administration; IV, intravenous; QTc, corrected QT interval; VF, ventricular fibrillation; VT, ventricular tachycardia.

pressures, reduced myocardial contractility, and high afterload. Optimal preload in this situation is achieved when cardiac function is enhanced to achieve similar endpoints but with reduced pulmonary congestion and edema. This condition usually involves decreasing filling pressures, enhancing myocardial contractility and decreasing afterload.

An essential step in the management of low cardiac output syndrome, therefore, involves either restoring deficient preload or decreasing excessive preload.

Restore deficient preload. The most fundamental management principle in hypovolemic shock is restoring deficient preload. Adequate preload is achieved by administering intravenous fluid in a series of challenges. The adequacy of fluid resuscitation is indicated by improvement in hemodynamic parameters. Fluid replenishment should be continued until target hemodynamic indexes are achieved or until no further improvement in cardiac output occurs (the flat part of the Starling curve); further fluid administration results in pulmonary congestion. Steps must then be taken to improve myocardial contractility with appropriate inotropic therapy.

The choice of fluid is important; although the risks of blood transfusion are well known, hypovolemia in the setting of excessive surgical blood loss is likely to require transfusion of blood or blood components. Blood product transfusion should be guided by hematocrit and coagulation parameters. Although no target hematocrit has been defined as a trigger for transfusion, studies indicate that excessive hemodilution (eg, less than 20%) may be associated with higher morbidity in cardiac surgical patients.[58,59]

The crystalloid versus colloid controversy is so far unresolved. The advantages of colloids (ie, 25% or 5% human albumin, 5% purified plasma derivative, 6% hetastarch, 10% pentastarch) include the rapid expansion of intravascular volume, an osmotic effect drawing extravascular fluid into the plasma space, and reduced risk of disease transmission with heat-treated blood derivatives.[60] However, the disadvantages of colloids are that these solutions do not rehydrate depleted extracellular volume and may worsen dilutional coagulopathy through effects on platelets.

Crystalloids (eg, 0.9% saline, lactated Ringer's solution) are relatively cheap and associated with low probability of adverse reaction. Their main disadvantage is that, relative to colloid, larger amounts of fluid are required to resuscitate from hemorrhagic shock for an equivalent increase in preload. Large amounts of normal saline can also cause hyperchloremic metabolic acidosis.

Reduce excessive preload. Low cardiac output syndrome caused by reduced myocardial contractility (cardiogenic shock) is defined by high filling pressures (flattening of the Frank-Starling curve). Any further increase in preload results in pulmonary congestion, edema, atelectasis, and increased intrapulmonary shunting with resultant hypoxemia. High filling pressures also result in higher left ventricular end-diastolic volume, increased myocardial wall stress, and reduced subendocardial coronary perfusion. If left uncorrected, this situation may rapidly lead to progressive myocardial ischemia and myocardial failure. Excessive preload may be reduced by administering venodilators, diuretics, and inodilators.

Venodilators (eg, nitroglycerin) exert their effects predominantly by dilating the venous reservoir, thereby decreasing preload to the right ventricle. In addition, pulmonary vessels are dilated. Intravenous nitroglycerin in low doses (0.5 to 1.5 μg/kg/min) also reduces myocardial wall stress and improves coronary blood flow to ischemic subendocardial vessels. However, this may be accompanied by systemic hypotension related to arterial vasodilation and reflex tachycardia that negates the benefit of improved myocardial oxygen supply.

Loop diuretics (eg, furosemide) are helpful in reducing intravascular volume by promoting diuresis. In the setting of low cardiac output syndrome, there is reduced renal blood flow and intense intrarenal vasoconstriction. Diuretics are, therefore, most useful after intravascular volume and renal perfusion pressure have been normalized.

Inodilators (eg, milrinone) enhance myocardial contractility and decrease afterload by causing peripheral vasodilation (Table 17-6). A reduction in excessive preload is achieved by shifting the Frank-Starling curve upward and toward the left (see Figures 17-5 and 17-6). Therefore, augmented preload is optimized by enhancing myocardial contractility and improving cardiac performance.

ENHANCE CONTRACTILITY. Prior to selecting an inotropic agent, any acidosis and electrolyte imbalance must be corrected. Acidosis has a negative inotropic effect and reduces myocardial response to catecholamines. Administration of sodium bicarbonate to a pH greater than 7.25 is an important first step in managing the acidosis. Frequent monitoring of arterial blood gases and serum lactate levels is essential in order to assess the adequacy of bicarbonate therapy. Hypocalcemia may also impair myocardial contractility by reducing the amount of extracellular calcium available to facilitate cardiac contraction. Low ionized calcium levels may be seen following rapid blood transfusion with large quantities of citrated blood; citrate toxicity is particularly common in the setting of hepatic ischemia (such as during open repair of thoracic aortic aneurysms). A normal extracellular-to-intracellular potassium ratio is essential for the maintenance of resting membrane potential in excitable tissue, such as the myocardium. Serum potassium levels may be increased (ARF, muscle ischemia, blood transfusion) or decreased (hemodilution, excessive diuresis). Hypokalemia decreases the resting membrane potential and delays ventricular repolarization. Myocardial contractility is impaired, and there is an increased risk of ventricular arrhythmias. Hyperkalemia results in prolonged depolarization, prolonged PR interval and QRS duration, and increased risk of

TABLE 17-6

Inodilators

Drug	Class	β_1	β_2	α_1	DA_1	PDE I
Isoproterenol	Catecholamine	++++	+++			
Dobutamine	Catecholamine	+++	+++			
Dopamine	Catecholamine	++	++	++	+++	
Dopexamine	Catecholamine	±	++++		+	
Amrinone	Bipyridine					+++
Enoximone	Imidazole					+++
Piroximone	Imidazole					+++
Milrinone	Bipyridine					+++

β_1, β_2, α_1, adrenergic activity; DA_1, dopaminergic activity (DA_1 receptors); PDE I, phosphodiesterase III inhibition.

ventricular fibrillation or asystole. Both hypokalemia and hyperkalemia must be corrected prior to administration of inotropes. Table 17-7 describes the actions of various inotropes and vasopressors.

β-Adrenergic agents. Increase in myocardial contractility is achieved predominantly by stimulation of β_1-adrenergic receptors. However, most sympathomimetic agents have mixed β_1 and β_2 effects and may cause undesirable tachycardia and/or arrhythmias. Usually, β_1 stimulation is the dominant inotropic mechanism in cardiac muscle. However, about 20% of inotropic activity is mediated by β_2-receptors, so that the normal ratio of β_1- to β_2-receptors is 80:20. In chronic congestive heart failure (CHF), long-standing sympathetic stimulation of β_1-receptors leads to their downregulation, in direct proportion to the degree of ventricular impairment.[21] The mechanism of downregulation is thought to involve increased G_i-protein activity and is associated with a decrease in β_1-receptor density. In chronic CHF, the ratio of β_1- to β_2-receptors is decreased to about 60:40, thereby increasing the importance of β_2-receptor stimulation (Figure 17-10).[61] This suggests that in chronic CHF, nonselective β-adrenergic agents such as dobutamine, dopexamine, epinephrine, or isoproterenol induce a substantial proportion of their inotropic effect through stimulation of cardiac β_2-receptors. There is some evidence that small doses of β-blocking agents may actually enhance ventricular function in CHF and after cardiopulmonary bypass because they reduce β-receptor stimulation (ie, downregulation) and increase β-receptor density.

Peripheral action of an inotrope may be mediated by either β_2-receptors (vasodilation) or α_1-receptors (vasoconstriction). Under normal circumstances, adrenergic agents mediate their positive *inotropic* effect (increase in force of contraction) on the cardiac β_1-receptor. However, there are three other cardiac effects mediated through the β_1-receptor. Stimulation of the sinus node from β-adrenergic drug therapy results in tachycardia (positive *chronotropic* effect), increased conduction velocity through the cardiac conducting system (positive *dromotropic* effect), and decreased arrhythmia threshold (positive *bathmotropic* effect).

The dose-response relationship for each of these effects may vary from one agent to another. For example, isoproterenol is such a potent chronotropic agent that increased heart rate always precedes its inotropic effect, and tachycardia and tachyarrhythmias limit its use as an inotropic agent. In contrast, dobutamine has significantly less chronotropic effect and is, therefore, a useful inotropic agent. The effect of positive dromotropism is well illustrated by the introduction of a β_1-agonist agent in a patient with atrial fibrillation. There is frequently an increase in the ventricular rate; that is, conduction is enhanced through the atrioventricular node. β_1-Adrenergic agents increase the risk and susceptibility to both supraventricular and ventricular arrhythmias and usually

---

TABLE 17-7

Preparation, Dosage, and Actions of Inotropic and Vasopressor Agents

Drug	Preparation	Concentration	Dosage	Predominant Action	Clinical Effects
Adrenergic Agents: Catecholamines					
Dopamine	400 mg/250 mL	1600 µg/mL	1-2 µg/kg/min	Dopaminergic	Saluresis
				β_1-adrenergic	inotropy, chronotropy,
			3-10 µg/kg/min	α_1-adrenergic	vasoconstriction
			>10 µg/kg/min		
Epinephrine	2 mg/250 mL	8 µg/mL	20-200 ng/kg/min	$\beta_{1,2}$-adrenergic	Inotropy, chronotropy,
				α_1-adrenergic	vasoconstriction
Dobutamine	250 mg/250 mL	1000 µg/mL	5-25 µg/kg/min	$\beta_{1,2}$-adrenergic	Inotropy, chronotropy,
					vasodilation
Norepinephrine	4 mg/250 mL	16 µg/mL	10-100 ng/kg/min	α_1-adrenergic	Vasoconstriction
				β_1-adrenergic	Inotropy
Adrenergic Agents: Noncatecholamines					
Phenylephrine *Direct-acting agents*	20 mg/250 mL	80 µg/mL	20-80 µg/kg/min	α_1-adrenergic	Vasoconstriction
Vasopressin*	20 units/mL	1 unit/mL	20 units (bolus)	Vascular smooth muscle	
		0.2-0.4 units/min		contraction	Vasoconstriction
Nonadrenergic Agents: Phosphodiesterase Inhibitors					
Inamrinone	Ampoule	10 mg/mL	1.5-3 mg/kg (l)	PDE III inhibition	Inotropy, chronotropy,
					vasodilation
	400 mg/250 mL[†]	1600 µg/mL	5-20 µg/kg/min (m)		
Milrinone	10/20/50 mL vial	20 µg/mL	50 µg/kg (l)	PDE III inhibition	Inotropy, chronotropy,
	1 mg/mL[‡]		0.375 – 0.75 µg /kg/min (m)		vasodilation

*Non–FDA-approved indication.
[†]Must be prepared in normal saline and shielded from light.
[‡]Reconstituted in 5% dextrose.
(l), loading dose; (m), maintenance dose; PDE III, phosphodiesterase III.

Normal

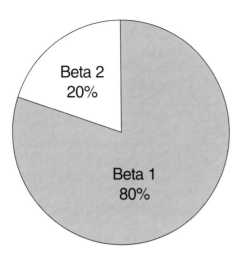

Congestive Heart Failure

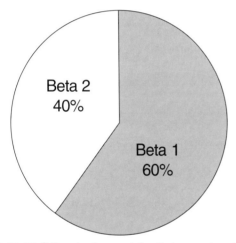

FIGURE 17-10 β-Receptor downregulation. Under normal conditions, 20% of all β-adrenergic receptors in the heart are β_2-receptors. In congestive heart failure, β_2-receptor density may increase to 40%.

exacerbate existing arrhythmias. Stimulation of cardiac β_2-receptors can also precipitate arrhythmias through reflex catecholamine release secondary to β_2-receptor–mediated peripheral vasodilation.

Inoconstriction versus inodilation. Norepinephrine, epinephrine, and dopamine (the endogenous catecholamines) have potent α_1-agonist activity. In the higher dosage range, their inotropic effect is accompanied by increasingly intense peripheral, renal, splanchnic and pulmonary vasoconstriction. This property may be useful in treating patients who have myocardial depression associated with states of low systemic vascular resistance, for example, after cardiopulmonary bypass or as a component of septic shock. However, excessive vasoconstriction ultimately leads to tissue hypoperfusion, metabolic acidosis, and organ ischemia and failure.

Dopexamine, dobutamine, and isoproterenol (the synthetic catecholamine derivatives) have potent β_2-agonist activity. Their inotropic effect is accompanied by systemic and pulmonary vasodilation. There is added advantage in the combination of decreased afterload and improved stroke volume resulting from these agents, for both the systemic and the pulmonary circulation. Limitations of these agents include hypotension from peripheral vasodilation and reflex tachycardia.

Dopamine. Dopamine is a precursor of the endogenous catecholamines (epinephrine, norepinephrine) that acts directly on dopaminergic, α- and β-adrenergic receptors and also exerts about half of its activity indirectly through the release of endogenous stores of norepinephrine from nerve terminals.[62] In cardiomyopathies or severe myocardial dysfunction, in which endogenous norepinephrine stores are depleted, dopamine is less effective as an inotrope.[63] Low-dose dopamine (less than 3 μg/kg/min) is used to selectively activate dopaminergic receptors that cause splanchnic and renal vasodilation. However, dopamine causes predominantly β_1-mediated inotropic effects at higher infusion doses (3 to 10 μg/kg/min). Animal studies have shown that dopamine may confer protection on the splanchnic vasculature against the vasoconstrictive effects of other inotropes, such as norepinephrine.[64] The preservation of dopaminergic receptor-mediated splanchnic effects, combined with β_1-receptor–mediated inotropic effects, has made dopamine a popular first-line inotropic agent. Unfortunately, the precise dose at which dopamine exerts dopaminergic versus adrenergic effects is unpredictable in any given patient. Although low-dose dopamine may increase renal artery blood flow, in clinical trials it has not been shown to improve outcomes in the setting of cardiac surgery or critical care.[65] Increasing infusion rates beyond 10 μg/kg/min promotes predominantly α_1-mediated vasoconstricting effects of dopamine.

Epinephrine. Epinephrine is a potent sympathomimetic agent that acts on β-adrenergic receptors. At low doses its β effects predominate, and at higher doses (>0.01 μg/kg/min), α_1-mediated effects are seen.[66] Its potent β effects make it a powerful inotrope capable of significantly shifting a failing myocardial performance curve upward and toward the left (see Figure 17-5). Epinephrine is used in the dosage range of 0.02 to 0.2 μg/kg/min. As with norepinephrine, its β-adrenergic effects are prominent in the lower dose range, and α-adrenergic effects predominate at higher dosages. When the inotropic action of epinephrine is combined with afterload reduction, provided by either a pure vasodilator such as sodium nitroprusside or a phosphodiesterase inhibitor such as milrinone, the enhancement of stroke volume is greater than if either agent is used alone.

Dobutamine. Dobutamine is a synthetic derivative of isoproterenol with predominantly β-adrenergic effects. It enhances cardiac performance by increasing contractility and decreasing afterload. Unlike dopamine, it does not depend on the release of norepinephrine from nerve endings, making it a useful agent in low cardiac output syndrome related to cardiomyopathy. However, its positive chronotropic effects may prove to be undesirable in the setting of myocardial ischemia. Used in the dosage range of 5 to 25 μg/kg/min, dobutamine is a potent inodilator, through β_1-receptor–mediated inotropic action and β_2-receptor–mediated arterial vasodilation. It decreases both systemic and pulmonary vascular resistance and thereby decreases left and right ventricular afterload. It also decreases preload by venodilation, which increases venous capacitance. Chronotropic and bathmotropic activities occur as a result of cardiac β_1- and β_2-receptor stimulation and reflex baroreceptor response to arterial vasodilation. However, dobutamine's propensity to cause tachycardia or tachyarrhythmias is far less than that of isoproterenol. Dobutamine has no dopaminergic activity. Increases in renal blood flow and diuresis are secondary to increased cardiac output. The most common limitations to the use of dobutamine are hypotension caused by vasodilation, which is likely to occur in hypovolemic states, and severe sepsis, tachycardia, and tachyarrhythmias.

Norepinephrine. Norepinephrine is structurally similar to epinephrine and has a profound stimulatory effect on α_1-adrenergic receptors, causing an increase in afterload of the right and left ventricles. Myocardial contractility is also increased by an effect on β_1-receptors. Norepinephrine is indicated when myocardial depression is associated with hypotension because it provides both direct inotropic action and peripheral vasoconstriction (inoconstriction). Combined administration with a phosphodiesterase inhibitor such as milrinone augments stroke volume better than either agent used alone and helps to avoid hypotension induced by phosphodiesterase inhibitors. When norepinephrine is used in low systemic vascular resistance states, care must be taken to return vascular resistance only to a low normal level. Excessive vasoconstriction leads to increased cardiac afterload and may induce acute cardiac failure, myocardial ischemia, and pulmonary edema. Peripheral vasoconstriction can induce splanchnic, renal, or peripheral ischemia and metabolic acidosis.

Isoproterenol. This powerful β-adrenergic stimulant has limited use as an inotrope. Its positive chronotropic effects predominate over its inotropic effects, reducing its utility in situations in which tachycardia is undesirable. It may be useful as a chronotrope in the treatment of sinus bradycardia or other bradyarrhythmias. However, it is rarely recommended as an inotrope or chronotrope because of its unfavorable pharmacologic profile.

Dopexamine. Dopexamine is a synthetic catecholamine that is available in Europe but is considered an investigational drug in the United States. It stimulates β_2-adrenergic and dopaminergic receptors and has a weak β_1 effect.[67] As a result, it helps restore organ flow through its vasodilating properties. However, human trials with dopexamine have not shown that it improves outcome in patients undergoing major abdominal surgery or in the setting of sepsis.[68-70] Its place in the pharmacopoeia of catecholamines awaits further clinical experience.

Phosphodiesterase inhibitors. Cyclic adenosine monophosphate (cAMP) controls intracellular calcium concentration, cardiac muscle contractility, and smooth muscle relaxation. The levels of cAMP may be increased by β-adrenergic stimulation or by preventing its breakdown by the enzyme phosphodiesterase III (PDE III). A major advantage of phosphodiesterase inhibitors is that their mechanism of action is independent of β-receptors and they are, therefore, effective in the presence of β-adrenergic blocking drugs or β-receptor downregulation. With the widespread use of β-adrenergic blocking drugs, the "postreceptor" action of PDE III inhibitors assumes great significance with regard to inotropy. Myocardial efficiency and oxygen bal-

ance are improved by decreased afterload and preload and a positive lusitropic effect on wall stress. Inamrinone and milrinone belong to a class of bipyridine derivatives that selectively inhibit PDE III. Both drugs have significant vasodilator effects with marked reductions in systemic and pulmonary vascular resistance. The combination of afterload reduction with mild chronotropic effect makes these drugs ideal inotropes for low cardiac output syndrome related to cardiomyopathy or myocardial ischemia. However, their significant vasodilatory effects may result in hypotension necessitating the use of vasopressors such as norepinephrine or vasopressin.[71] Another advantage of PDE III inhibitors is that they can be combined with other β-adrenergic agonists to produce a synergistic inotropic effect.

Inamrinone is particularly useful in the treatment of right ventricular failure associated with pulmonary hypertension; in fact, its ability to decrease pulmonary vascular resistance and right ventricular afterload may be superior to that of dobutamine and less likely to be associated with tachycardia. Inamrinone has a short redistribution half-life of 1 to 2 minutes and a long elimination half-life of 2 to 6 hours. As about 40% of the drug is excreted unchanged in urine, careful dose titration is required in patients with renal insufficiency. Its long-term use is also associated with thrombocytopenia (an effect attributed to its principal metabolite, *N*-acetylamrinone).[72] Although both inamrinone and milrinone also possess potential for producing cardiac rhythm disturbances owing to their effect on intracellular cAMP levels, the risk of life-threatening arrhythmias is less when compared with β-adrenergic agents.[73-76]

Milrinone has a more favorable pharmacokinetic profile and has shown promise as an inotrope in chronic heart failure.[77] However, a clinical trial has not shown any significant benefit in this population of patients compared with placebo,[78] and others have argued that similar benefits may be achieved with dobutamine at a lower cost.[79] Nonrandomized studies suggest that milrinone appears to be more stable and is associated with less development of tolerance than dobutamine.[80] Currently, milrinone enjoys popularity as a first-choice inotrope in acute and chronic heart failure seen in the postoperative period.

Thyroid hormones. The thyroid hormones thyroxine (T_4) and triiodothyronine (T_3) are important endocrine regulators of metabolism, temperature, and cardiovascular function. Critically ill patients frequently have low T_4 and T_3 despite normal circulating thyroid-stimulating hormone (TSH) levels, a condition termed euthyroid sick syndrome.[81] Most commonly, there is a reduction in peripheral conversion of T_4 to T_3, resulting in low T_3 levels. Later on in the illness, T_4 levels may also decrease, accompanied by decreased pituitary responsiveness to T_4 and T_3, resulting in low levels of TSH.[82,83] Low levels of T_3 have been shown in patients with low cardiac output syndrome following cardiac surgery.[84] T_3 has been investigated as a possible inotropic agent or adjunct to other inotropes for weaning from bypass. However, although some investigators have shown that intravenous T_3 improves postoperative left ventricular function after cardiac surgery, others have not been able to confirm these findings.[85-87]

NORMALIZE SYSTEMIC VASCULAR RESISTANCE
Reduce excessive afterload. An ischemic or severely dysfunctional left ventricle is critically dependent on afterload reduction in order to increase efficacy of myocardial contraction.

Reducing afterload with vasodilators increases stroke volume for a given preload. This issue is particularly important for the patient with myocardial depression and elevated systemic vascular resistance.

Sodium Nitroprusside. Sodium nitroprusside has a direct, potent vasodilator action on vascular smooth muscle with a very rapid onset and offset of action. The goal of vasodilator therapy is to increase cardiac output by decreasing systemic vascular resistance. A sudden drop in blood pressure in response to a low dose of sodium nitroprusside may indicate undertreated hypovolemia; in this case, afterload reduction should be continued after fluid challenges to restore preload. Sodium nitroprusside also decreases aortic diastolic pressure and coronary perfusion pressure and promotes intracoronary steal by shunting blood away from ischemic myocardium. Myocardial ischemia may, therefore, occur because of a combination of coronary steal and reflex tachycardia. Hypoxemia may also result from inhibition of the hypoxic pulmonary vasoconstrictor response.

Nitroglycerin. Nitroglycerin is primarily a venodilator and is useful in reducing preload. However, nitroglycerin also decreases afterload by reducing myocardial wall stress and by a direct vasodilating effect on arteries at higher doses. Because its venodilator effects predominate, nitroglycerin seldom causes an increase in cardiac output, and if preload reduction is excessive, cardiac output decreases. The beneficial effects of nitroglycerin on myocardial oxygen balance make it a useful adjunct in the therapy of low cardiac output syndrome in postoperative vascular surgical patients who have demonstrated ischemic heart disease.

Calcium Channel Blockers. Calcium channel blockers (CCBs) have vasodilatory effects on the coronary, pulmonary, and systemic circulations. Specific CCBs may have little or no significant negative inotropic and negative chronotropic action. They have been used to reduce afterload and improve systolic function in patients with CHF.[88] However, depression of ventricular contractility along with excessive vasodilation, hypotension, and reflex tachycardia may preclude their use in the setting of low cardiac output syndrome in the postoperative period.

Inodilator Therapy (see Table 17-6). When inotropic activity is combined with afterload reduction in a single agent, hemodynamic management is potentially simplified. Inodilators decrease not only systemic and pulmonary vascular resistance but also heart size, wall stress, and cardiac work, making them attractive agents in the therapy of cardiogenic shock.[89,90] Isoproterenol is associated with undesirable tachycardia that limits its use in states of myocardial ischemia. Dopamine exhibits vasodilator activity in the low-dose range only (probably less than 5 μg/kg/min); above this range, its α_1-adrenergic action causes increasing vasoconstriction. Dobutamine, milrinone, and inamrinone are currently available inotropic agents that also have the advantage of simultaneous afterload reduction (inodilation).

Restore inadequate systemic vascular resistance (vasopressor therapy). Systemic vascular resistance may be abnormally low because of autonomic neuropathy (diabetes, chronic renal failure), arteriovenous shunts (liver failure), sepsis, or drugs (long-acting vasodilators, such as ACE inhibitors, calcium blockers).

Excessive vasodilation may result in low aortic diastolic pressure and reduced coronary perfusion pressure. However, vasopressors must be carefully titrated to achieve the most effective balance between perfusion and flow. Excessive vasoconstriction may induce splanchnic, renal, and peripheral ischemia, exacerbate cellular hypoxia, and increase myocardial wall stress, resulting in a vicious circle of cardiac decompensation and pulmonary edema.

Vasopressor agents should, therefore, be used only when all efforts to restore blood pressure by the use of aggressive fluid administration and inotropic support have failed and the calculated systemic vascular resistance is abnormally low. Vasopressors may complement the use of inodilators by counteracting their excessive vasodilating effects. In this situation, they may allow the titration of the inodilator to produce an optimal inotropic response without excessive afterload reduction.

Phenylephrine and norepinephrine stimulate α_1-adrenergic receptors to produce vasoconstrictor effects. Both agents are useful when selective vasoconstriction is required without an increase in heart rate. Another vasopressor agent that has gained popularity is vasopressin. It has been successfully used to manage hypotension in the setting of sepsis, vasodilatory shock seen after cardiac surgery, and as an adjunct to milrinone therapy.[71,91-93] Vasopressin is discussed in greater detail in the section dealing with sepsis.

MECHANICAL SUPPORT. When interventions to optimize cardiovascular function fail to correct a low cardiac output state, the prognosis is generally poor. However, if myocardial function is temporarily reduced (eg, because of myocardial ischemia), cardiac assist devices may be used to augment tissue perfusion and assist the heart as a short-term solution. These devices are discontinued when there is return of cardiac function amenable to pharmacologic control or when there is no further improvement despite maximal support.

Intra-aortic balloon pump. The intra-aortic balloon pump (IABP) is used for circulatory support in patients with left ventricular dysfunction or cardiogenic shock to minimize extension of myocardial infarction and treat refractory myocardial ischemia. The IABP consists of a nonocclusive balloon that is placed percutaneously in the descending aorta. The balloon inflates during diastole (providing diastolic pressure augmentation, thereby increasing coronary perfusion pressure) and deflates during systole (providing afterload reduction during left ventricular ejection) in a process known as *counterpulsation*. This increases cardiac output and coronary and cerebral perfusion and decreases left ventricular work. Maximal benefits of counterpulsation are achieved in patients with moderate left ventricular failure related to acute reversible ischemia. Hemodynamic support with the IABP improves outcome when used for temporary hemodynamic control in acute cardiogenic shock.[94] Effective counterpulsation generally results in decreased heart rate and left ventricular end-diastolic and pulmonary capillary wedge pressures and increased cardiac output. These effects also allow more effective pharmacologic control of hemodynamics. Secondary benefits are also seen with an increase in peripheral perfusion and a reduction in tissue acidosis. However, the benefits of IABP must be weighed against possible complications, and these devices are rarely used in vascular surgery patients because of their intrinsic vascular disease. The use of IABP may be associated with limb ischemia, thrombus formation around an inactive balloon, detachment of atheromatous aortic lesions, occlusion of renal artery ostia, and balloon rupture.

Ventricular assist devices. Cardiogenic shock that does not respond to either pharmacologic measures or IABP support may require more aggressive support in the form of ventricular assist devices (VADs). These devices have been approved in the United States for two indications—temporary support of potentially reversible cardiac dysfunction secondary to postcardiotomy or postinfarction cardiogenic shock and as a "bridge" to transplantation in irreversible myocardial dysfunction. VADs are used most frequently after cardiac surgery or when heart transplant candidates demonstrate acute deterioration of cardiac function. They are not commonly used following major vascular surgery because patients presenting with severe aortic disease are frequently not suitable as heart transplant candidates. However, successful combined VAD placement with aortic aneurysm repair has been reported.[95]

Newer Perspectives in Management of Low Cardiac Output Syndrome

PHARMACOGENOMICS. Many anesthesiologists are familiar with variability in clinical response to drugs in the perioperative setting.[96-99] The increasing burden of diagnostic and therapeutic facts can make the complexities of genomics seem overwhelming for the practicing anesthesiologist. The basic facts, however, remain simple: genes are composed of coded strands of DNA, which produce messenger RNA (mRNA), which encodes proteins that are responsible for specific cellular actions. Small genetic differences between individuals known as polymorphisms may result in subtle changes in the amount or functional properties of proteins. Depending on the functional importance of the proteins, these subtle differences may have profound effects on outcome from disease (eg, tumor necrosis factor α polymorphism and outcome in sepsis[100]). The complex relationship among environmental factors, mRNA protein products, and genetic variability is just beginning to be understood. These factors may combine in several ways to increase susceptibility to disease and modify its responsiveness to therapy.

Pharmacogenomics is defined as the use of genetic screening to determine how a patient will respond to a specific pharmacologic therapy. Whereas pharmacogenomics implies a more general study of gene variations in response to small molecules, *pharmacogenetics* refers to the effect of inheritance or polymorphisms on individual variations in response to specific drugs. To explain this variation, pharmacogenetics has mainly focused on the influence of genetic heterogeneity among (1) enzymes involved in drug biotransformation (pharmacokinetics) and (2) allele-specific variations among drug receptors that contribute to drug response (pharmacodynamics). Drug biotransformation takes place in two phases—phase I reactions, in which mainly the cytochrome family of enzymes add or expose a functional group in the molecule that serves as a site for conjugation reactions, and phase II reactions, in which the molecule is conjugated with another to enhance its elimination. Pharmacogenetic variability in cytochrome enzymes has been identified to classify some individuals as "poor metabolizers."

The important implication for anesthesiologists is that some patients may possess polymorphisms of cytochrome genes that express themselves as poor metabolizer phenotypes. These patients may exhibit inefficient metabolism of several drugs, including β-adrenergic blockers (especially metoprolol), anesthetics (such as propofol), warfarin, and opiates—all of which are highly dependent on hepatic metabolism for termination of effect. Similarly, variability in adrenergic receptor subtypes has been identified, which places individuals at risk for the development of heart failure once cardiac injury has occurred. Some of this variability may also explain why there is a wide range in cardiovascular response to many vasoactive drugs used in critically ill patients, making standardized therapeutic decisions difficult. It is conceivable that genomic studies may be able to identify individuals at risk before they undergo major vascular surgery, which would make it easier for the critical care physician to tailor therapy for better outcomes.

GENE THERAPY. Gene therapy involves the introduction of foreign DNA into native host cells to treat a disorder through synthesis of a missing or defective gene product, usually a protein. The process involves transferring DNA directly to target cells with vectors, a process termed *transfection*. Transfection may be achieved by viral vectors, such as adenovirus, adeno-associated virus, and retrovirus, or nonviral vectors, such as liposomes. Current gene therapy trials have met with limited success because of concerns of host infection and unfavorable inflammatory and immunogenic responses to viral vectors.[101-103] Nonviral vectors have shown promise in eliminating some of these concerns.[104] Gene therapy for vascular diseases involves delivery of recombinant DNA to local tissue sites in the vasculature by specially designed intravascular catheters.[105,106] To increase new blood vessel formation (angiogenesis) at target sites, the intramyocardial application of vectors encoding growth factors, such as vascular endothelial growth factor and fibroblast growth factor, has shown clinical promise. Studies have shown improvement in new vessel formation and amelioration of ischemia related to increased expression of growth factor proteins in a host that previously showed inadequate gene expression.[107-110] Because low cardiac output syndrome can be essentially described as a defect in perfusion, the application of gene therapy for increasing angiogenesis in underperfused areas of the vasculature may seem like an attractive option. However, this new area of therapeutics must be adopted with caution, as it is also accompanied by several concerns: enhanced immunogenicity in an already compromised host, increased vascular permeability in an "inflamed" environment, and ethical concerns regarding societal concepts of gene therapy.

Sepsis

Sepsis is the most common cause of death in noncardiac critical care units and the tenth most common cause of death overall.[111] In 2000, sepsis was responsible for 31,613 deaths in the United States, representing an increase of 1.8% from the previous year.[111] The cost of caring for septic patients is estimated to be between $5 billion and $10 billion per year in the United States, with a mortality rate estimated between 20% and 50%.[112-115] Despite predictions of a decreasing trend in infection-related complications in surgical patients, the incidence of sepsis in a rapidly aging and increasingly morbid surgical population is on the rise.[116]

Vascular surgical patients are frequently at risk for postoperative sepsis because of a number of factors, including the inflammatory response to surgery and the presence of prosthetic grafts within the vasculature.[117,118] The syndrome that occurs in response to an infection or shock in the critically ill patient represents the systemic inflammatory response mediated by cellular and chemical messengers. The host homeostatic defense mechanisms are overwhelmed by the activated inflammatory response. If this insult persists, host defenses are unable to respond sufficiently and the patient deteriorates into progressive shock, cellular injury, multiorgan failure, or death.

Definitions

One problem that plagued researchers and data analysts in the past was the lack of a unifying definition of sepsis and related disease states.[119-125] In 1992, the American College of Chest Physicians and the Society of Critical Care Medicine evolved a consensus statement to define sepsis and its sequelae clearly as a continuum (Table 17-8).[126] The onset of systemic inflammatory response syndrome (SIRS) according to the definition describes the systemic inflammatory response to a variety of insults, infectious or noninfectious (eg, trauma). This description is an important contribution of the consensus statement. The definition of SIRS identifies insults unrelated to infection, which lead to systemic inflammation as separate entities. When SIRS is accompanied by infection, it is termed *sepsis*. Severe sepsis describes the progression of sepsis to include organ dysfunction, hypotension, and hypoperfusion. When hypotension and perfusion abnormalities seen with sepsis persist despite adequate fluid resuscitation, septic shock ensues. Ultimately, sustained abnormalities seen in septic shock culminate in the development of multiorgan dysfunction syndrome (MODS), defined as "the presence of altered organ function in an acutely ill patient such that homeostasis cannot be maintained without intervention."[126]

TABLE 17-8

Definitions of Systemic Inflammatory Response Syndrome, Sepsis, Septic Shock, and Multiple Organ Dysfunction Syndrome

Systemic inflammatory response syndrome (SIRS): At least two of the following conditions in response to a variety of clinical insults:
(1) Oral temperature of $>38^{\circ}C$ or $<36^{\circ}C$
(2) Respiratory rate of >20 breaths/min or $Paco_2$ of <32 mmHg
(3) Heart rate of >90 beats /min
(4) Leukocyte count of $>12,000/mm^3$ or $<4000/mm^3$ or $>10\%$ immature (band) forms

Sepsis: The presence of two or more SIRS criteria in response to an infection

Severe sepsis: Sepsis with one or more signs of organ dysfunction, hypoperfusion, or hypotension, such as:
(1) Metabolic acidosis,
(2) Acute alteration in mental status, or
(3) Oliguria

Septic shock: Sepsis with hypotension that is unresponsive to fluid resuscitation plus organ dysfunction or perfusion abnormalities as listed above from severe sepsis. Patients may be receiving inotropes or vasopressors and, therefore, not hypotensive but still in septic shock.

Multiple organ dysfunction syndrome (MODS): Dysfunction of more than one organ, requiring intervention to maintain homeostasis

---

Despite the progress made in characterizing sepsis and related diseases, the consensus definition also has its problems. It is now known that MODS may result from both direct organ injury and secondary consequences of sepsis; however, the consensus statement does not recognize MODS with a noninfectious etiology.[127] Controversy also exists regarding the association between SIRS as a precise definition and severity of illness.[114,128] There is also concern that including noninfectious causes of SIRS has reduced incentive for the clinician to search for treatable infectious sources.[129] Although these definitions have helped to focus research efforts, the increasing trend of mortality related to sepsis has prompted pleas to reevaluate this area.[130]

Pathophysiology of Sepsis

The progression from SIRS to MODS usually involves an infecting pathogen. However, SIRS represents the body's systemic inflammatory response to a variety of insults that may not necessarily include infection. In fact, there appears to be no difference in outcome between culture-positive and culture-negative septic patients.[131] Nevertheless, the presence of infection is central to the concept of sepsis. The following subsections discuss the pathophysiology of sepsis from initiation of infection by microorganisms to the coordinated host response leading to unregulated mediators of inflammation culminating in MODS.

THE MICROBIOLOGY OF SEPSIS. The increasing incidence of septicemia (the official term used for calculation of national statistics in the United States) has been attributed to (1) increase in number of immunocompromised hosts, (2) more frequent use of invasive procedures and devices, (3) greater ability to diagnose septicemia, (4) increase in antibiotic-resistant pathogens, and (5) a rapidly aging population in need of health care.[114,132] A variety of microorganisms may produce sepsis. Gram-negative rods are responsible for about 50% of all cases of sepsis, and only half of these are associated with positive blood culture.[133] More than 50% of gram-negative bacteremias are complicated by septic shock, compared with 5% to 10% for gram-positive or fungal infections.[134] However, studies have highlighted the increasing prevalence of gram-positive bacteria as a cause of sepsis.[135-137] The increase in gram-positive septicemia has been attributed to (1) empirical antibiotic regimens designed primarily against gram-negative microbes that have selected out resistant gram-positive pathogens, (2) more frequent use of long-term intravascular devices, (3) increase in the use of prosthetic devices, and (4) antibiotic resistance among gram-positive organisms, such as methicillin-resistant *Staphylococcus aureus* and vancomycin-resistant enterococci.

Gram-negative sepsis. Gram-negative bacteria are normal commensals in the human gastrointestinal tract. Infection usually begins as a local infection of the gastrointestinal or urinary tract and, in the presence of predisposing factors, invades the bloodstream to produce septicemia (Table 17-9). The most common organism responsible for sepsis is *Escherichia coli*, followed by *Klebsiella, Enterobacter, Serratia,* and *Pseudomonas*. *Klebsiella* and *Pseudomonas* are the most virulent, and *Pseudomonas* and *Enterobacter* are increasingly becoming resistant to antimicrobial agents. Gram-negative sepsis is initiated by endotoxin, a lipopolysaccharide (LPS) component of the outer cell wall of bacteria. In 1989, Suffredini et al demon-

TABLE 17-9

Predisposing Factors for the Development of Gram-Negative Sepsis

Extremes of age
Diabetes
Renal insufficiency
Chronic immunosuppression
    Acquired immunodeficiency syndrome
    Chemotherapy
    After solid organ transplantation
Instrumentation
    Endotracheal intubation
    Intravascular catheter
    Urinary catheter
    Vascular surgical prostheses
Surgery
    Gastrointestinal procedure
    Genitourinary procedure
    Obstetric procedure
Trauma

---

strated that injection of purified endotoxin produced sepsis-like symptoms in healthy human volunteers.[138] The sepsis-like symptoms are actually due to various chemical mediators of the inflammatory cascade, such as cytokines that are elaborated by LPS-responsive cells (macrophages, endothelial cells, neutrophils). Similar signs and symptoms of sepsis are also seen with the direct administration of cytokines, such as tumor necrosis factor α (TNF-α), in the absence of endotoxemia.[139] Therefore, the sequence of events is postulated to be liberation of LPS endotoxin by gram-negative bacteria, interaction between LPS and macrophages (and other LPS-responsive cells), and the release of cytokines into the bloodstream, with subsequent signs and symptoms of sepsis.

Gram-positive sepsis. Gram-positive bacteria are found on the skin, wounds, and catheter sites, accounting for the association of gram-positive sepsis with intravascular devices, surgical prostheses, and postoperative wounds.[135] In contrast to gram-negative sepsis, in which endotoxin is a central pathogenic feature, gram-positive bacteria depend on the interaction of their cell wall polymers with host defenses and the production of powerful exotoxins (eg, botulin) for their effects. Gram-positive cell wall polymers, lipoteichoic acid and peptidoglycan, are capable of binding to several host cell surface receptors, such as CD14, and activating the inflammatory and complement cascades. Host defenses against these bacteria (eg, C-reactive protein) target these lipoteichoic moieties on the bacterial cell wall, enabling more efficient elimination from the body.[140,141] Exotoxins, on the other hand, lead to massive T-cell activation and release of cytokines, resulting in cellular injury and MODS.[142]

It is now becoming clear that gram-negative and gram-positive bacteria have distinct pathophysiologic mechanisms, necessitating different and appropriate therapeutic strategies. Ongoing research trials will, in the future, enable even more rapid pathogen identification and institution of specific therapy.

ENDOTOXEMIA AND SEPSIS. Endotoxin is released by gram-negative bacteria in the gut and then translocates into the bloodstream following disruption of gut mucosal defenses.[143,144]

A breakdown of the gut mucosal barrier is thought to be due to intestinal ischemia secondary to diversion of blood flow from the splanchnic bed to cardiocerebral circulation. This provides the opportunity for translocation of endotoxin from the gut to the bloodstream through mesenteric lymphatics.[143,145,146] Defective gut mucosal perfusion by gastric tonometry has been reported in infrarenal aortic aneurysm surgery.[147] Gut ischemia has also been shown to be more severe with open repair of abdominal aortic aneurysms compared with endovascular repair.[148] Both studies imply impaired visceral perfusion during aortic occlusion. In addition, gut ischemia and portal endotoxemia are seen more often with the intraperitoneal approach to abdominal aortic aneurysm surgery, possibly because of increased gut handling.[149]

Although a large number of virulence factors have been identified, LPS (the active component of endotoxin) bears the strongest association with toxicity. LPS exerts its toxic effects by binding to specific cell membrane receptors (CD14, leukocyte integrins) and soluble proteins (soluble CD14).[150-152] These receptors and soluble proteins enable the expression of cytokines TNF-α and interleukin-1β (IL-1β) from macrophages and interleukin-4 from B lymphocytes and increase the phagocytic ability of polymorphonuclear leukocytes (PMNs).[153-155] The intracellular events that translate LPS induction to enhanced cytokine transcription by mRNA are mediated by second messengers, principally nuclear factor κB (NF-κB).[156] The activation of cellular and humoral components of the inflammatory response thus represents the central pathophysiologic feature of gram-negative sepsis. Endotoxin was thought to depress myocardial function directly, but studies show that this effect is secondary to myocardial cytokines acting through NO and cyclic guanosine monophosphate (cGMP).[157,158] Although serum levels of endotoxin have shown an inconsistent relationship with morbidity, antiendotoxin antibodies have shown correlation with adverse outcomes.[159-162] Because endotoxin appears to be responsible for most of the effects of gram-negative sepsis, trials with antiendotoxin agents or LPS antagonists have received much attention. However, initial trials with first-generation LPS antagonists have not yielded encouraging results.[163,164] As new knowledge of the molecular mechanisms of LPS action emerge, LPS antagonists will undoubtedly be further refined to yield more effective therapeutic options.

The Immune Response to Sepsis

It is generally believed that the hypotension, coagulopathy, and organ dysfunction that accompany sepsis are due to the activation of the immune system resulting from pathogenic organisms or tissue injury seen in low cardiac output syndrome. Over the last decade, research efforts have been focused toward identifying new inflammatory molecules, cytokines, and other cellular messengers responsible for cell injury. The large number of mediators, second messengers, regulators, and modulators within the immune system ensure that specific pathways are activated to counter a specific challenge. Other redundant pathways are suppressed. New knowledge has provided opportunities for understanding immunomodulation and developing new therapeutic strategies to achieve better outcomes for critically ill postoperative patients. Two essential components of the immune response can be broadly categorized: (1) activation of inflammation and (2) release of mediators of inflammation.

ACTIVATION OF INFLAMMATION. The first step in the immune response is the recognition of cellular injury, microbial cell wall components, or antigen-antibody complexes. There are two main pathways of immune activation that are independent of immunoglobulins, the lipopolysaccharide pathway and the complement pathway.

Lipopolysaccharide pathway. As discussed earlier, gramnegative bacteria possess endotoxin, an LPS component of the outer cell wall. LPS interacts with monocytes and other cellular components of the inflammatory cascade through the CD14 receptor. This essential interaction is mediated by the lipopolysaccharide binding protein (LBP) and leads to macrophage activation and release of cytokines, prostaglandin E_2 (PGE_2) and NO.[165-167] This pathway is also regulated because LPS-mediated cytokine release is also controlled by interferon-γ (IFN-γ) and interleukin-10 (IL-10), and LPS itself can suppress IL-2 production.[168]

Complement pathway. The complement system normally functions as an efficient defense system against pathogenic organisms.[169] Complement activation results in the release of inflammatory molecules, opsonization of microbes, induction of host cell lysis, and activation of the coagulation system. Sustained intravascular complement activation, occurring during prolonged hypoperfusion and shock, sets up an inflammatory response that amplifies tissue damage and organ dysfunction. The classic pathway of complement activation is initiated by the binding of component C1 to antigen-antibody complexes; the alternative pathway is activated by particulate polysaccharides, fungi, bacteria, and viruses. The final common pathway results in a "membrane attack complex," a supramolecular organization of about 20 proteins, and the release of soluble proinflammatory mediators C3a and C5a. C3a enables phagocytosis of foreign particles and clearance of immune complexes.[170] C5a induces PMN activation, cell migration, adherence, and aggregation.[171] It also increases pulmonary vascular resistance, enhances vascular permeability, decreases systemic vascular resistance, and induces leukopenia.[171-173] More important, C5a induces monocytes to enhance production of TNF-α, which produces the characteristic hemorrhagic necrosis seen in sepsis.[170] Appropriately, these activated complement molecules are called anaphylatoxins. The membrane attack complex incorporates itself into the lipid membrane and forms transmembrane channels that activate membrane-bound phospholipases, causing lethal disruption.

MEDIATORS OF INFLAMMATION. The principal mediators of inflammation are the cytokines. This large family of interleukins, growth factors, and necrosis factors (eg, TNF-α) initiate the response, maintain a proinflammatory state, and mount an anti-inflammatory response. Other important inflammatory mediators are the eicosanoids, platelet-activating factors (PAFs), and free oxygen radicals.

The initiators—TNF-α and interleukin-1. The first cytokine released by monocytes and macrophages in response to LPS induction is TNF-α.[166] It plays a central role in the induction of both pro- and anti-inflammatory cytokines, thus regulating its own actions. Among other agents that regulate the production or release of TNF-α are drugs that increase cAMP, such as phosphodiesterase inhibitors (amrinone, milrinone) and β-agonists.[174,175] The other central cytokine initiator is IL-1,

TABLE 17-10

Range of Actions of Tumor Necrosis Factor-α and Interleukin-1

Sepsis-like syndrome in animal models
Repression of endothelial proliferation
Stimulation of interleukin-1β secretion
Pulmonary neutrophil sequestration
Inhibition of lipoprotein lipase activity
Procoagulant effect
Antifibrinolytic effect
Natriuresis
Hyperglycemia
Increased vascular permeability
Increased hypothalamic thermostat—fever

which is produced by almost any nucleated cell. Along with TNF-α, IL-1 has multiple actions on various organ systems (Table 17-10).[176-185]

The proinflammatory cytokines. The principal proinflammatory cytokines are IL-6, IL-8, and IL-12. These interleukins are produced by a variety of cells, including monocytes, macrophages, endothelial cells, and fibroblasts.[186-189] The most significant actions of IL-6 involve the induction and mediation of the acute phase reaction in the liver.[188,190] The generation of acute phase proteins results in pyrexia and increased corticosteroid production.[186] IL-8 functions as a significant mediator in chemotaxis and transendothelial migration of neutrophils.[187,191]

The anti-inflammatory cytokines. The anti-inflammatory cytokines are important regulators of cytokine actions. They help modulate and tailor the immune response at target sites in order to achieve maximum efficiency. The principal cytokines in this category are IL-4, IL-10, IL-13, and transforming growth factor-β (TGF-β). Most of these interleukins and TGF-β can suppress the production of initiators IL-1 and TNF-α. Apart from interleukins, soluble receptors also play an important anti-inflammatory role. These proteins are IL-1 receptor antagonist (IL-1ra) and soluble TNF receptor. By suppressing the initiators, anti-inflammatory cytokines exert a significant effect as they limit the intensity of the inflammatory cascade at the beginning. In addition, they exert regulatory effects at multiple levels to suppress production of other proinflammatory cytokines. Because IL-1 is known to have potent proinflammatory actions, antagonists such as IL-1ra have been investigated as potential therapeutic strategies against the inflammatory surge that occurs in sepsis. However, a multicenter phase III trial did not show encouraging results with this anti-inflammatory agent.[192]

Eicosanoids. Eicosanoids are a family of polyunsaturated 20-carbon fatty acids synthesized from arachidonic acid. Cyclooxygenase cleaves arachidonic acid to form endoperoxides, which are precursors of prostaglandins. In platelets, endoperoxides yield thromboxane (TxA_2), which promotes vasoconstriction and platelet aggregation. In capillary endothelial cells, endoperoxides yield prostacyclin (PGI_2), which inhibits platelet aggregation, promotes vasodilation, and maintains capillary perfusion. Normally, there is a finely tuned balance between these two systems. During sepsis, increased levels of PAF and proinflammatory cytokines, endothelial damage, and tissue hypoxia interact to increase eicosanoid production in tissues.[193] With platelet activation and damage in shock, especially with hemorrhage, a massive release of thromboxane overwhelms prostacyclin, triggers microthrombi and vasoconstriction, and exacerbates tissue ischemia.[194]

In granulocytes, the enzyme lipoxygenase converts arachidonic acid to leukotrienes. The leukotrienes contribute to the characteristic pathophysiologic changes of shock, especially in the lung. These changes include vasoconstriction, microthrombi formation, increased vascular permeability, and the release of myocardial depressant factors, lysosomal hydrolases, and proteolytic agents. Increased capillary permeability leads to interstitial edema, which further compromises the microcirculation. A vicious cycle of tissue ischemia and cellular dysfunction, leading to further leukotriene release, is set up.

Specific thromboxane receptor inhibitors, leukotriene antagonists, and prostacyclin releasers (difibropeptides) enhance survival in animals subjected to experimental hemorrhagic shock but have not proved as promising in models of sepsis.[193,195-197] Nonspecific prostaglandin inhibitors, such as ibuprofen, although having shown a mortality benefit in animals, have not improved survival in human trials.[198,199] Vasodilator prostaglandins exert a renal protective effect in shock; as a consequence, patients receiving nonsteroidal anti-inflammatory drugs are more susceptible to ARF during a hemodynamic insult.[200]

Platelet-activating factors. PAFs belong to a heterogenous family of acetylated phosphoglycerides whose role in the pathophysiology of shock is becoming increasingly apparent. PAFs are generated from cell membrane lipids in a variety of cells, including platelets, neutrophils, macrophages, and endothelial cells, all of which possess specific membrane receptors for PAFs. PAFs enhance TNF-α production by macrophages and increase IL-1β production by monocytes.[201,202] PAFs may also alter endothelial cell structure, causing increased intercellular gaps and increased vascular permeability seen in sepsis.[203] In animal models, PAFs have been shown to contribute to a number of features of sepsis similar to those seen in humans.[204] However, human trials of PAF antagonists in sepsis have not shown a significant benefit in survival with their use (see Chapter 1).[205,206]

Disseminated Intravascular Coagulation

Disseminated intravascular coagulation (DIC) is a recognized complication of sepsis and is also cited as the cause of coagulation abnormalities seen after major aortic surgery.[207,208] As a consequence of maldistribution of blood flow that occurs in sepsis, there is blood stasis within tissues accompanied by hypoxia and acidosis. The cellular hypoxia also occurs in other forms of shock and forms the basis of ensuing microvascular thrombosis and DIC seen in most forms of circulatory failure, including sepsis. Endothelial injury resulting from cellular hypoxia not only acts as a stimulus for contact activation of factor XII (Hageman factor) and the intrinsic pathway of coagulation, but also activates fibrinolysis by plasmin and the kinin system. The extrinsic pathway of coagulation is also activated through procoagulants, which are activated by the release of thromboplastins from injured tissues, platelets, and leukocytes. Active fibrinolysis causes the liberation of large amounts of fibrin degradation products, which in turn inhibit fibrin polymerization. Fibrin deposition may occur in both intra- and

extravascular spaces and is also triggered directly by hypoxia.[209] The extensive fibrin deposition that occurs in DIC has inflammatory effects as well.[210] Fibrin encapsulates bacteria, and fibrinolysis may trigger the release of endotoxin. DIC is especially likely to occur in situations in which shock is associated with hemorrhage and hematoma, in which hemostasis and fibrinolysis can trigger further consumption of platelets and coagulation factors.

Microvascular thrombosis from DIC leads to end-organ ischemia and infarction and may hasten the onset of MODS. However, the role of DIC as a cause of MODS or simply as a marker of severe tissue perfusion abnormalities is still disputed. Certainly, the consumption of hemostatic factors by DIC can significantly influence the severity of bleeding from surgical wounds and trauma.

Laboratory findings of DIC typically include prolongation of all coagulation tests and a rapidly falling platelet count (in fact, a normal stable platelet count would make the diagnosis of DIC unlikely). Fibrinogen levels are typically preserved until later in the course of DIC, when stores of fibrinogen in the liver are depleted. Coexisting fibrinolysis is reflected by increasing levels of fibrin degradation products, in particular the D-dimer. Although replacement of blood products and treatment with low-dose heparin infusion with or without antifibrinolytic agents (i.e., ε-aminocaproic acid) address the immediate problems caused by DIC, only correction of the underlying acidosis and hypoxemia by improving tissue perfusion can address the cause of DIC (see Chaper 15).

Renal Function in Sepsis

ARF occurs in about 5% of all hospitalizations and 30% of critical care admissions and is associated with 35% to 75% mortality.[211,212] Vascular surgical patients are frequently at risk for postoperative renal dysfunction because of a combination of factors, such as advanced age, preexisting renal insufficiency, atheroembolic injury, and intraoperative renal ischemia. This places them in a precarious position if sepsis complicates the clinical picture. Two of the reasons why ARF carries a higher mortality rate are the associated illnesses and the lack of adaptive responses required to blunt the effects of increasing azotemia.

The ARF seen with sepsis and septic shock fits in with the vascular theory of ARF (see earlier). Rather than intrarenal injury, there is an impairment of intrarenal vasomotor control, a condition termed *vasomotor nephropathy*. Sepsis is the most extreme example of a vasomotor nephropathy, in which progressive renal dysfunction is associated with intense intrarenal vasoconstriction despite systemic vasodilation. Loss of autoregulation of renal blood flow is the principal abnormality in the vasomotor nephropathy seen with severe sepsis. This prerenal etiology is characterized by oliguria and low urinary sodium excretion, consistent with elevated plasma renin activity.[213] Later during the course of sepsis, direct tubular injury may also occur, adding to the vasomotor nephropathy.

In sepsis, hypovolemia and hypotension evoke systemic vasoconstrictor responses that lead to renal dysfunction.[214] Endotoxin, along with the various vasoactive compounds it activates (endothelin, TxA_2, prostaglandin F_2, and leukotrienes), induces afferent arteriolar constriction, mesangial contraction, and direct tubular injury.[214] Renal blood flow may also be reduced by a combination of endotoxin-mediated endothelial injury and microvascular thrombosis. Endothelial injury is associated with a loss of local vasodilators, such as prostacyclin and NO, which increases intrarenal vasoconstriction.[215] The net effect is decreased renal blood flow, glomerular filtration rate, sodium excretion, and urine output. Although endotoxin induces a general decrease in vascular responsiveness to vasoconstrictors, therapy with norepinephrine and vasopressin helps normalize arterial pressure, renal blood flow, and autoregulation.[8,29,216-218] Other causes of ARF in sepsis are intrarenal hypoxic injury, nephrotoxic antibiotics, infectious interstitial nephritis, and immunologically mediated glomerular injury (see Chapter 14).[219-221]

Therapeutic Strategies

Traditional therapy of sepsis has centered on antimicrobial agents, consistent with the acceptance of an infectious etiology. However, over the last decade, new knowledge has emerged highlighting the contribution of noninfectious etiologies, inflammatory mechanisms, and genetic predisposition to the pathophysiologic features seen in sepsis and MODS. Accordingly, new therapeutic strategies have also emerged, attempting to target the disease at a molecular level. However, in the critical care unit, treatment of the septic patient mainly involves antimicrobials, hemodynamic support, and prevention of progression of sepsis to MODS.

ANTIMICROBIALS. Surgical patients are at a higher risk of nosocomial infections than other hospitalized patients.[116] Many vascular surgical patients are smokers and may have other comorbidities, such as diabetes, obesity, or end-stage renal disease, or may have been in the hospital for a prolonged period—all risk factors for the development of surgical site infection.[222] Whenever postoperative sepsis is suspected, cultures of blood and appropriate body fluids should be sent for analysis. In addition, other noninfectious conditions that mimic sepsis such as myocardial infarction, acute pancreatitis, and acute blood loss should be ruled out before starting antimicrobial therapy. Antimicrobial agents may be selected on the basis of the microbes likely to be found in the organ identified as the possible source of infection. For example, sepsis related to intravascular devices is likely to be due to gram-positive cocci, and pulmonary infections are likely to isolate gram-negative rods.

The distribution of pathogens isolated from operative wound sites has not changed much during the last decade. *S. aureus*, coagulase-negative staphylococci, enterococcus, and *E. coli* are still the most frequently isolated pathogens.[223] The dose of antibiotics should be based on the likely pathogen rather than the nature and severity of organ dysfunction. After the infectious source has been identified, the antimicrobial regimen should not be altered to treat febrile episodes or worsening appearance of chest radiographs. In appropriate doses, antibiotics effectively control in vivo microbial activity. Increasing the recommended antibiotic dosage or duration does not increase the antimicrobial effect and may adversely affect the functioning of other organs in a critically ill patient. Additional antibiotic coverage is usually unnecessary and is unlikely to result in a more rapid improvement.

It is important to recognize that critically ill patients may have renal and/or hepatic impairment that must be taken into account in the selection and dosage of the appropriate antibiotics. In patients with hepatic dysfunction, a renally eliminated antibiotic is preferable, whereas in renal dysfunction, an agent with hepatic elimination is preferred. It may also be important to adjust the timing of drug administration because some antibiotics have time-dependent kinetics rather than concentration-dependent kinetics.[224-226] Antibiotic failure is usually a rare cause of persistent fever or worsening of symptoms. More often, it is related to poor antibiotic selection, inadequate dosage, incorrect spectrum, or suprainfection. Antibiotics may also encourage the release of endotoxin as a consequence of bacterial cell lysis.[227] Because bactericidal agents have a greater potential for endotoxin release than bacteriostatic antibiotics, the choice of agent, if other factors are equal, should favor the latter.[228] Early institution, appropriate selection, and adequate coverage of antimicrobial agents are vital to ensure the successful treatment of the septicemic patient.

HEMODYNAMIC SUPPORT. The goal of hemodynamic support in septic patients is to restore effective tissue perfusion. In sepsis, regional and local blood flows are impaired, making it difficult to define the goals of hemodynamic therapy. Organ perfusion is impaired despite an elevated cardiac output and low systemic vascular resistance. However, because most organs are dependent on perfusion pressure for adequate blood flow, the first task is to normalize the mean arterial pressure and restore the perfusion pressure. Hemodynamic support, therefore, centers on appropriate inotrope and vasopressor therapy.

Hemodynamically unstable septic patients who do not respond to fluid resuscitation should have a trial of vasopressor therapy.[229] Although the goal of vasopressor therapy is to normalize arterial pressure, it is important to understand that normal pressure does not equal normal flow. However, because autoregulation of blood flow is impaired in most organs below a mean arterial pressure of 50 mmHg, normalization of systemic blood pressure is a reasonable first step in restoring perfusion.[229] The ultimate effect of the vasopressor depends on the balance between direct vasoconstrictive effects and indirect increase in blood flow related to an increase in the perfusion pressure. Simultaneous assessment of organ perfusion is, therefore, essential to monitor the adequacy of vasopressor therapy. The effect on splanchnic perfusion is an important consideration when selecting a vasopressor. Adequate perfusion of the splanchnic vasculature helps maintain gut mucosal integrity, which is considered to be an important protective feature in the pathogenesis of sepsis. Vasopressors differ in their actions on the splanchnic circulation, and this effect may well be the deciding factor when selecting the appropriate agent.

Dopamine It is common practice to use dopamine in conjunction with norepinephrine in sepsis. Although dopamine ameliorates the splanchnic or renal vasoconstriction associated with norepinephrine in controlled conditions, this finding has not been confirmed in the setting of sepsis.[64,230-233] Some studies have shown an increase in gut mucosal perfusion attributable to dopamine, whereas others have reported the opposite.[234-237] The effects of dopamine on the splanchnic circulation remain controversial.

Epinephrine. Epinephrine is usually added to the hemodynamic support regimen as a last resort. It increases mean arterial pressure and cardiac output but decreases gut perfusion and increases lactate levels.[238-240] However, it is a useful agent for hemodynamic support in patients who are unresponsive to other therapeutic strategies.

Norepinephrine. Norepinephrine is the vasopressor of choice in septic patients who cannot maintain an adequate mean arterial pressure. This potent vasoconstrictor was initially reserved for the most critically ill patients who did not respond to any other measures. However, studies have shown that norepinephrine can predictably raise the mean arterial pressure and, therefore, the perfusion pressure to vital organs without causing direct vasoconstrictive organ damage in septic patients.[241-244] Norepinephrine has also been shown to be superior to dopamine in reversing the hypotension seen with hyperdynamic septic shock.[245] The beneficial effects of norepinephrine seem to stem from its ability to increase the mean arterial pressure in an environment of high cardiac output, low systemic resistance, and hyperdynamic septic shock. These effects override any local vasoconstrictive detrimental effects. Several studies have shown that the addition of norepinephrine to nonresponsive hypotensive septic patients significantly improves the renal filtration function, as seen by an increase in urine flow and creatinine clearance.[241,242,244,245] The norepinephrine-mediated rise in perfusion pressure results in an increase in regional blood flow, as evidenced by a significant reduction in plasma lactate levels.[245] Splanchnic perfusion is increased by norepinephrine, provided the cardiac index is maintained, if necessary, by the addition of other agents, such as dopamine or dobutamine.[239,246] Norepinephrine has shown significant beneficial effects in septic patients as a result of its generalized vasoconstrictive properties and should be used early in septic patients when hemodynamic support is required for maintaining adequate perfusion.

Vasopressin. Vasopressin, an endogenous nonapeptide secreted from the posterior pituitary, is also a potent vasopressor used for hemodynamic support in sepsis. In the early stages of sepsis or vasodilatory shock, plasma levels of vasopressin are elevated as a response to increased baroreceptor firing.[247] As shock progresses and the hypotension is sustained, endogenous vasopressin levels decline; this decrease is thought to occur as a consequence of a number of factors, including excessive baroreceptor firing, high norepinephrine levels, and autonomic insufficiency.[9,91,248] In the setting of sepsis, vasopressin infusion therapy increases the mean arterial pressure as a result of its vasoconstrictive effects on vessels in the skin and skeletal muscle. More important, it increases vascular responsiveness to norepinephrine and other vasopressors.[249,250] Septic patients also demonstrate heightened sensitivity to the pressor effects of vasopressin.[8] Several trials have shown a beneficial effect of vasopressin in various forms of vasodilatory shock, when other pressors, including norepinephrine, failed to elicit an adequate response.[29,92,93,251,252] However, vasopressin may also cause mesenteric vasoconstriction, an undesirable effect in shock states. This effect is dose dependent and not seen during low-dose therapy. A therapeutic trial of low-dose vasopressin is warranted for patients in shock who do not respond to norepinephrine. Further prospective, randomized trials are needed to determine whether vasopressin has a role in improving outcomes in septic shock.

RENAL PROTECTION. The most important deleterious consequence of sustained sepsis or SIRS is progression to MODS. The pathophysiology of renal dysfunction in sepsis has already been outlined. In patients with septic shock, the incidence of ARF may approach 51% and the requirement for dialysis within 24 hours of onset of sepsis increases the relative risk of death by twofold.[253, 254] Preservation of renal function, therefore, assumes significant importance in the management of sepsis.

Interventions for renal protection are commonly attempted in the critically ill patient. Unfortunately, in this setting increases in urine output are often confused with improvement in global renal function. There are no drugs currently available that have demonstrated renal protective properties.[255] Among the drugs evaluated for renal protection, the most common are diuretics, low-dose dopamine, and CCBs.

The use of loop diuretics in ARF has been evaluated in several studies. Although these agents may increase urine output, loop diuretics have not been shown to benefit renal function, prevent ARF, or improve outcome in patients undergoing major vascular or cardiac surgery.[256,257] There is no supportive rationale for the use of loop diuretics for the prevention of ARF in septic patients. Mannitol, an osmotic diuretic, has also been evaluated for renoprotection in vascular and renal transplant surgery.[258,259] The hypothesized mechanisms for the renoprotective effects of mannitol include osmotic reduction of tubular obstruction, prostaglandin-mediated increase in renal blood flow, and free radical scavenging. However, few studies have researched the use of mannitol in septic patients. Accordingly, apart from renal transplantation, there is no recommended rationale for the use of mannitol in the prevention or treatment of ARF.

Low-dose dopamine is commonly used in the intensive care unit. Unfortunately, the renoprotective potential of dopamine is based more on theoretical considerations than clinical evidence. Low-dose dopamine (also known as renal-dose dopamine—1 to 3 µg/kg/min) is used to avoid α- and β-adrenergic receptor–mediated cardiovascular effects and promote a dopaminergic receptor–mediated increase in renal blood flow. Dopamine is also thought to prevent norepinephrine-mediated vasoconstriction in renal and splanchnic vessels. Although these observations are relevant in controlled, experimental ARF in animal models, extrapolation to critically ill human subjects has not been successful. Dopamine has been shown to increase urine output in critically ill, oliguric patients in the intensive care unit, but randomized trials have not shown a benefit with dopamine with regard to the prevention of postoperative ARF or improvement in outcome in patients with ARF.[260-263] It is important to consider that dopamine may result in undesirable cardiovascular effects in patients at risk for myocardial ischemia and is, therefore, not without risk. Current recommendations support the use of dopamine for hemodynamic therapy, in which it may result in a renal benefit because of improved hemodynamics, but caution against its use solely for renal protection.[229,264] Fenoldopam, an antihypertensive agent with selective dopaminergic properties without adrenergic effects, has been considered for renal protection, but no rigorous clinical trials have been performed to evaluate the role of this agent in the setting of sepsis.

The rationale for the use of CCB agents for renal protection stems from the important role played by calcium in renal homeostasis. The potential renoprotective effects of CCBs are attributed to three possible mechanisms: (1) the ability of these drugs to increase renal blood flow by inhibiting voltage-dependent, calcium-channel–mediated vasoconstriction; (2) a direct cytoprotective effect related to their antioxidant or free radical–scavenging action; and (3) blockade of the cascade of calcium-dependent cell death, therefore reducing or preventing ischemia-reperfusion injury.[265,266] Evidence for the renoprotective role of CCBs came from the reduced incidence of renal dysfunction in the long-term follow-up of hypertensive patients treated with CCBs or β-blockers.[267,268] In the acute perioperative setting, some benefit has been observed with felodipine and nifedipine in aortic surgery.[269-271] Although these agents may prove to be beneficial for renal protection in patients undergoing major surgery, their use in sepsis may be limited by their vasodilatory actions.

Evolving Concepts in Sepsis

Over the past decade, an overwhelming amount of information has been derived from both basic science and clinical critical care research on the molecular basis of sepsis and its clinical correlates. Accordingly, new therapeutic targets have been identified, mainly aimed at the immune and coagulation systems. New knowledge in gene expression of cellular messengers has also led to the possibility of genetic profiling of susceptible patients in order to better target therapy.

GENETIC VARIABILITY AND SUSCEPTIBILITY TO SEPSIS. In an observational study in 1988, Sorensen and colleagues suggested that genetic influences were the strongest determinants of susceptibility to infection.[272] Since this article was published, other studies have also shown that genetic variability is strongly associated with outcome for a number of infections. A key prognostic factor of the severity of sepsis is the balance between the host pro- and anti-inflammatory responses. Genetic polymorphisms may confer protection by increasing the ability to mount a more effective anti-inflammatory response. On the other hand, genetic variability may also increase susceptibility to infection by reducing the efficiency of the anti-inflammatory response. Therefore, all genes encoding proteins involved in the inflammatory cascade are candidate genes that determine the interindividual susceptibility to sepsis.

A key proinflammatory molecule that initiates the inflammatory cascade is TNF-α. This molecule has received special attention because genetic variants that modulate TNF-α activity may play an important role in determining the clinical response to sepsis, and anti-TNF-α agents may be potentially useful as therapeutic tools in sepsis. Genetic polymorphisms may account for up to 60% of the observed interindividual variability in TNF-α production.[273] Polymorphisms of the TNF-α promoter gene are associated with greater susceptibility to infection and poorer outcome after surgical sepsis.[274,275] Although animal studies have shown that anti-TNF-α antibodies promote survival after septic shock, phase III trials in human septic patients have not been as consistent despite the enrollment of more than 10,000 patients.[276,277] A small subset of severely septic patients with elevated TNF-α levels may, however, benefit from anti-TNF-α therapy.

Genetic variability of genes encoding the production of the potent anti-inflammatory cytokine IL-1ra is also known to be associated with differences in outcome after an infectious challenge. This has been demonstrated in genetically deficient mice and suggested in human observational studies.[278,279] Polymorphisms of other cytokine genes (IL-1 and IL-6) and noncytokine genes (nitric oxide synthase, heat shock protein, and PAF) have also been suggested as potential factors in the immune response to sepsis.[280]

GENE THERAPY. There is evidence that a number of single-gene inherited disorders may benefit from the addition of a missing or defective gene or silencing of an overexpressive gene. Because sepsis has a multifactorial etiology, clinical trials with single-gene therapies are unlikely to be dramatically successful. However, gene therapy even for a defective single polymorphism may improve clinical outcome by reducing the severity of the disease process. Gene therapy for sepsis has centered on this premise. Both viral and nonviral vector–based gene therapies modulating the immune response have been shown to be beneficial in animal models of sepsis and endotoxemia.[281-284] Extrapolation from animal models to relevant human populations is unfortunately complicated. Because sepsis is multifactorial and involves multiple redundant pathways, modulating a single pathway is unlikely to alter the outcome of sepsis in a major way. The beneficial effects of gene therapy seen in animals cannot be simply extrapolated to humans. In contrast to animal models, in which gene therapy is initiated before the septic insult, critically ill patients already have an ongoing septic process. However, preoperative therapy for vascular surgery patients may be possible because a potential insult is anticipated. The degree and duration of gene expression required to sustain a therapeutic effect are, as yet, unknown. Finally, vectors for gene therapy used in animal models cannot be administered to humans in comparable doses. For the time being, the potential for gene therapy to alter the severity of sepsis, and therefore the outcome, remains only a promising idea.

NITRIC OXIDE. Since NO was identified as the primary constituent of endothelium-derived relaxing factor, studies have shown this important molecule to be the principal regulator of vasomotor tone.[285,286] A brief overview of NO production is shown in Figure 17-11. The production of NO is catalyzed by nitric oxide synthase (NOS), which exists in three isoforms—two constitutive and one inducible (or iNOS). It has been demonstrated that iNOS is the primary source of NO generation, which is largely responsible for the hypotension and vasodilation associated with septic shock.[286-288] Patients with sepsis demonstrate elevated levels of nitrite and nitrate, consistent with the hypothesis that NO is responsible for the vasodilation and decreased sensitivity to vasopressors seen in these patients.[286,289-291] NO has been reported to play important physiologic roles and may function as a platelet inhibitor, intracellular bactericidal agent, neurotransmitter, and inhibitor of mitogenesis in vascular smooth muscle and cause myocardial depression seen in sepsis.[285,286,288,292] Some of these effects, such as platelet inhibition, vasodilation, and cytokine induction, represent beneficial host defense mechanisms against the harmful effects of the septic process. It is the unregulated excessive production of NO that may be counterproductive in septic shock.

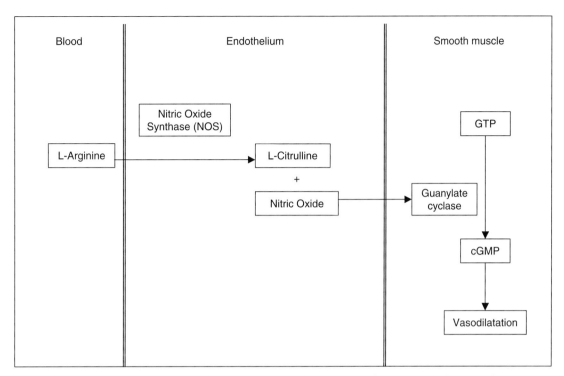

FIGURE 17-11 Formation of nitric oxide and mechanism of vasodilatation. cGMP, cyclic guanylate monophosphate; GTP, guanylate triphosphate.

The important role of NO in the pathophysiology of sepsis makes it an attractive therapeutic target. Competitive inhibitors of iNOS have received attention as potential therapeutic targets, including N^G-monomethyl-L-arginine (L-NMA), N^G-nitro-L-arginine (L-NNA), and N^G-nitro-L-arginine methyl ester (L-NAME). In animal studies, L-NMA was associated with increased mean arterial pressure, systemic vascular resistance, and pulmonary vascular resistance with reduced cardiac output and cardiac index.[293-295] However, outcome results from NO inhibition in these animal studies are equivocal.[295,296] Human trials of NO inhibitors, such as L-NAME, have not demonstrated benefit. Principal among the undesirable effects have been a decrease in cardiac index and increase in pulmonary vascular resistance that may be deleterious for tissue perfusion.[297-300] Although successful in increasing mean arterial pressure, NOS inhibitors do not seem to have a major impact on the inflammatory cascade and the progress of sepsis.

ENDOGENOUS OPIOIDS. The endogenous opioid peptides, endorphins and enkephalins, are present in the hypothalamus, endocrine glands, and gastrointestinal tract. This family of 10 to 15 neuropeptides has morphine-like analgesic actions, behavioral effects, and regulatory functions on the neuroendocrine system. Initial animal and human experiments with the opioid antagonist naloxone in the treatment of shock suggested that endogenous opioids are beneficial in reducing pain and arterial pressure, counteracting vasoconstrictive mechanisms.[301,302] However, the use of opioid antagonists in the treatment of shock has produced inconsistent results.[303-307] These differences in results have been attributed to variability in dose, timing, and method of administration of naloxone combined with the variability in age, gender, disease type, and treatment of shock patients.[308] The mechanism of action of naloxone in improving hemodynamics in critically ill patients is speculative.[309,310] Naloxone may be beneficial in certain cases of septic shock when other resuscitative measures such as fluid therapy and vasopressors fail. However, it remains a temporary therapeutic measure and must be viewed as an adjunct to the management of critically ill patients.

CORTICOSTEROIDS. The use of corticosteroids in sepsis remains a controversial issue. Steroids exert their anti-inflammatory effect by inhibiting the second messenger NF-κB, an activator of cytokines; increasing the synthesis of lipocortin 1, a phospholipase 2 inhibitor; inhibiting the induction of cyclooxygenase-2; and preventing the release of adhesion molecules, all of which are important mediators of the various steps of the inflammatory process.[311-313] In addition to anti-inflammatory actions, steroids increase hepatic synthesis of glucagon, glucose, and protein; supplement endogenous steroid levels; inhibit downregulation of α-adrenergic receptors and increase receptor density, restoring catecholamine sensitivity; and improve cardiac performance by inhibiting β-endorphin production.[313-316] However, long-term treatment with steroids is not without complications. The development of superinfection related to immunosuppression, hyperglycemia, gastrointestinal bleeding, psychosis, and arrhythmias may limit their usefulness in the setting of sepsis.[314]

Two large studies have demonstrated no mortality benefit and greater infection rates with the use of steroids in the treatment of sepsis.[317,318] However, more recent investigation in this area has generated renewed interest. Bollaert and colleagues reported a beneficial effect of supraphysiologic doses of hydrocortisone on hemodynamics and mortality in an elegant prospective, placebo-controlled trial.[319] Although reporting no difference in mortality, Briegel et al found that hydrocortisone significantly reduced time to cessation of vasopressor support compared with placebo.[320] These studies suggest that short-term high-dose steroids may be harmful, but moderate doses, administered over a longer period of time, may have beneficial effects. Long-term treatment with steroids may supplement endogenous hormone levels and restore the balance among intracellular second messengers (such as NF-κB).

IMMUNOMODULATION. Evidence suggests that a hyperinflammatory response is central to the pathophysiology of sepsis. Clinical studies demonstrate elevated levels of proinflammatory mediators (TNF-α, IL-1) in all septic patients. Animal studies confirm that exogenous administration of these mediators faithfully mimicked most of the signs of sepsis. Inhibition of these mediators and other anti-inflammatory strategies to limit inflammation have, therefore, become attractive therapeutic targets for study. In general, although animal models have shown promising results in this line of investigation, clinical trials have yet to demonstrate useful therapeutic interventions.

Proinflammatory cytokine inhibitors IL-1ra (IL-1 receptor antagonist), sTNFr (soluble TNF receptor), and TNFMAb (TNF monoclonal antibody, afelimomab) have been tested in human subjects with sepsis. Despite enrolling more than 8600 patients, 16 human trials have not demonstrated any significant benefit with the use of any of these inhibitors. Although individual agents have not shown a benefit, combination therapy may hold more promise.[321] When these trials are examined together, there is a modest trend toward improvement in mortality with mediator-specific therapy.[322,323]

The success of anti-inflammatory therapy in other diseases characterized by immune-mediated injury (eg, Crohn's disease, rheumatoid arthritis) is in contrast to the failure of these agents in sepsis.[324-327] The consistent failure of clinical sepsis trials to replicate the successes of animal models questions the validity of immunomodulation as a viable approach to therapy.

ANTICOAGULATION. The immune and coagulation systems are intimately related, leading to the characteristic hemostatic derangements seen in sepsis. The coagulation system has been evaluated as a therapeutic target in the treatment of sepsis. Much attention has been paid to the relationship between thrombin and activated protein C. Thrombin plays a central role in the balance between a procoagulant state (related to fibrin generation) and an anticoagulation state. Once formed, thrombin leads to generation of activated protein C (APC), which inactivates factors V and VIII, thereby blocking thrombin generation (Figure 17-12). This APC-based intrinsic inhibitory feedback mechanism ensures that thrombin generation does not result in unregulated coagulation.[328] Factors that reduce the levels of APC, therefore, critically shift the balance toward a pathologic procoagulant state.

Activated protein C inhibits thrombin generation, promotes fibrinolysis, and has been shown to exert anti-inflammatory effects through inhibition of release of proinflammatory mediators and prevention of leukocyte adhesion.[329-336] Studies also suggest that APC may protect endothelial function and reduce apoptosis by altering gene expression of modulators of inflammatory molecules (see Chapter 15).[336,337]

The activation of protein C depends on endothelial cell membrane integrity and endothelial receptor function. In sepsis and allied inflammatory states, the loss of endothelial integrity,

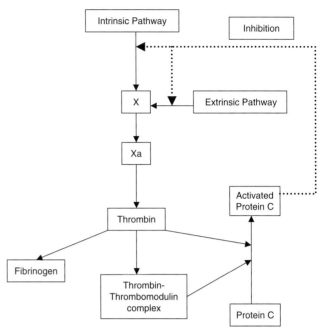

FIGURE 17-12 Generation of activated protein C and mechanism of inhibition of the coagulation cascade.

widespread thrombin generation, and sustained fibrinolysis combine to consume existing protein C and reduce further activation leading to low plasma APC levels. Low levels of APC are consistently seen in septic patients and have been strongly associated with MODS and mortality.[332,338,339] Protein C deficiency seems to develop early in the course of sepsis and has been suggested as a valuable prognostic indicator.[340-342] This scenario laid the foundation for a possible role for APC as a therapeutic agent in sepsis.[343] After the generation of the human recombinant form of APC (also known as activated drotrecogin α) and demonstration of its efficacy in animal sepsis models, the drug was evaluated in the Recombinant Human Activated Protein C Worldwide Evaluation in Severe Sepsis (PROWESS) trial.[344] This trial enrolled 1690 septic patients and found that APC reduced the relative risk of death at 28 days by 19.4%.[344] Although this trial is the first to show a significant mortality benefit in sepsis, there was also an increased risk for serious bleeding in the study group. Current recommendations limit the use of APC to patients who meet the criteria for the PROWESS trial and do not support its use in patients at risk for severe bleeding. The apparent success with APC as a therapeutic agent is attributed to more than just its antithrombotic effect. The beneficial effects of APC on fibrinolysis, immunomodulation, endothelial integrity, and apoptotic injury seem to combine favorably in the setting of sepsis.

Summary

Patients undergoing vascular surgery are at high risk for postoperative complications, including low cardiac output states and sepsis. Clinical management of both these conditions is dependent on the understanding of the basic pathophysiologic processes involved. Timely institution of a logical sequence of interventions aimed at optimizing hemodynamic status and correcting underlying abnormalities is central to current therapeutic strategies. For the future, there is hope that ongoing research will identify new targets for more specific interventions, particularly in the therapy of sepsis. New insights into the role of genetics in the pathophysiology of disease and the variability in response to therapy may provide new tools to individualize treatment to achieve improved clinical outcomes.

REFERENCES

1. Kamel KS, Mazer CD: Effect of $NaHCO_3$ on cardiac energy metabolism and contractile function during hypoxemia, *Crit Care Med* 29:344, 2001.
2. Steenbergen C, Deleeuw G, Rich T, Williamson JR: Effects of acidosis and ischemia on contractility and intracellular pH of rat heart, *Circ Res* 41:849, 1977.
3. Schlant RC, Sonnenblick EH, Katz AM: Normal physiology of the cardiovascular system. In Alexander RW, Schlant RC, Fuster V (eds): *Hurst's the heart*, ed 9, New York, 1998, McGraw-Hill, 81.
4. Landry DW, Oliver JA: The pathogenesis of vasodilatory shock, *N Engl J Med* 345:588, 2001.
5. Jackson WF: Ion channels and vascular tone, *Hypertension* 35:173, 2000.
6. Quayle JM, Nelson MT, Standen NB: ATP-sensitive and inwardly rectifying potassium channels in smooth muscle, *Physiol Rev* 77:1165, 1997.
7. Thiemermann C, Szabo C, Mitchell JA, Vane JR: Vascular hyporeactivity to vasoconstrictor agents and hemodynamic decompensation in hemorrhagic shock is mediated by nitric oxide, *Proc Natl Acad Sci USA* 90:267, 1993.
8. Landry DW, Levin HR, Gallant EM, et al: Vasopressin pressor hypersensitivity in vasodilatory septic shock, *Crit Care Med* 25:1279, 1997.
9. Landry DW, Levin HR, Gallant EM, et al: Vasopressin deficiency contributes to the vasodilation of septic shock, *Circulation* 95:1122, 1997.
10. Cuypers PW, Gardien M, Buth J, et al: Cardiac response and complications during endovascular repair of abdominal aortic aneurysms: a concurrent comparison with open surgery, *J Vasc Surg* 33:353, 2001.
11. Skiles JA, Griffin BP: Transesophageal echocardiographic (TEE) evaluation of ventricular function, *Cardiol Clin* 18:681, 2000.
12. Munt B, Jue J, Gin K, et al: Diastolic filling in human severe sepsis: an echocardiographic study, *Crit Care Med* 26:1829, 1998.
13. Bonow RO, Udelson JE: Left ventricular diastolic dysfunction as a cause of congestive heart failure. Mechanisms and management, *Ann Intern Med* 117:502, 1992.
14. McGhie AI, Golstein RA: Pathogenesis and management of acute heart failure and cardiogenic shock: role of inotropic therapy, *Chest* 102:626S, 1992.
15. Chatterjee K, Parmley WW: Vasodilator therapy for acute myocardial infarction and chronic congestive heart failure, *J Am Coll Cardiol* 1:133, 1983.
16. Sonnenblick EH, Morrow AG, Williams JF Jr: Effects of heart rate on the dynamics of force development in the intact human ventricle, *Circulation* 33:945, 1966.
17. Freeman GL, Little WC, O'Rourke RA: Influence of heart rate on left ventricular performance in conscious dogs, *Circ Res* 61:455, 1987.
18. Woodworth RS: Maximal contraction, staircase contraction, refractory period, and compensatory pause of the heart, *Am J Physiol* 8:213, 1902.
19. Hajdu S: Mechanism of the Woodworth staircase phenomenon in heart and skeletal muscle, *Am J Physiol* 216:206, 1969.
20. Young JB, Landsberg L: Catecholamines and the adrenal medulla. In Wilson JD, Foster DW, Kronenberg HM, Reed Larsen P (eds): *Williams textbook of endocrinology*, ed 9, Philadelphia, 1998, WB Saunders, 684.
21. Bristow MR, Ginsburg R, Minobe W, et al: Decreased catecholamine sensitivity and beta-adrenergic-receptor density in failing human hearts, *N Engl J Med* 307:205, 1982.
22. McKinley MJ, Denton DA, Coghlan JP, et al: Cerebral osmoregulation of renal sodium excretion—a response analogous to thirst and vasopressin release, *Can J Physiol Pharmacol* 65:1724, 1987.
23. Share L: Role of vasopressin in cardiovascular regulation, *Physiol Rev* 68:1248, 1988.
24. Budzikowski AS, Paczwa P, Szczepanska-Sadowska E: Central V1 AVP receptors are involved in cardiovascular adaptation to hypovolemia in WKY but not in SHR, *Am J Physiol* 271:H1057, 1996.
25. Grindstaff RR, Cunningham JT: Cardiovascular regulation of vasopressin neurons in the supraoptic nucleus, *Exp Neurol* 171:219, 2001.
26. Kjaer A, Hesse B: Heart failure and neuroendocrine activation: diagnostic, prognostic and therapeutic perspectives, *Clin Physiol* 21:661, 2001.
27. Bichet DG: Vasopressin receptors in health and disease, *Kidney Int* 49:1706, 1996.

28. Mets B, Michler RE, Delphin ED, et al: Refractory vasodilation after cardiopulmonary bypass for heart transplantation in recipients on combined amiodarone and angiotensin-converting enzyme inhibitor therapy: a role for vasopressin administration, *J Cardiothorac Vasc Anesth* 12:326, 1998.
29. Malay MB, Ashton RC Jr, Landry DW, Townsend RN: Low-dose vasopressin in the treatment of vasodilatory septic shock, *J Trauma* 47:699, 1999.
30. Gimson AE, Westaby D, Hegarty J, et al: A randomized trial of vasopressin and vasopressin plus nitroglycerin in the control of acute variceal hemorrhage, *Hepatology* 6:410, 1986.
31. Ogawa K, Ito T, Hashimoto H, et al: Plasma atrial natriuretic factor in congestive heart failure, *Lancet* 1:106, 1986.
32. Nakaoka H, Imataka K, Amano M, et al: Plasma levels of atrial natriuretic factor in patients with congestive heart failure, *N Engl J Med* 313:892, 1985.
33. Cody RJ, Atlas SA, Laragh JH, et al: Atrial natriuretic factor in normal subjects and heart failure patients. Plasma levels and renal, hormonal, and hemodynamic responses to peptide infusion, *J Clin Invest* 78:1362, 1986.
34. Raine AE, Erne P, Burgisser E, et al: Atrial natriuretic peptide and atrial pressure in patients with congestive heart failure, *N Engl J Med* 315:533, 1986.
35. Kone BC: Molecular biology of natriuretic peptides and nitric oxide synthases, *Cardiovasc Res* 51:429, 2001.
36. Tamura N, Ogawa Y, Chusho H, et al: Cardiac fibrosis in mice lacking brain natriuretic peptide, *Proc Natl Acad Sci USA* 97:4239, 2000.
37. Komatsu Y, Itoh H, Suga S, et al: Regulation of endothelial production of C-type natriuretic peptide in coculture with vascular smooth muscle cells. Role of the vascular natriuretic peptide system in vascular growth inhibition, *Circ Res* 78:606, 1996.
38. Brusq JM, Mayoux E, Guigui L, Kirilovsky J: Effects of C-type natriuretic peptide on rat cardiac contractility, *Br J Pharmacol* 128:206, 1999.
39. Richards AM, Nicholls MG, Yandle TG, et al: Plasma N-terminal probrain natriuretic peptide and adrenomedullin: new neurohormonal predictors of left ventricular function and prognosis after myocardial infarction, *Circulation* 97:1921, 1998.
40. Richards AM, Doughty R, Nicholls MG, et al: Neurohumoral prediction of benefit from carvedilol in ischemic left ventricular dysfunction. Australia-New Zealand Heart Failure Group, *Circulation* 99:786, 1999.
41. Tsutamoto T, Wada A, Maeda K, et al: Attenuation of compensation of endogenous cardiac natriuretic peptide system in chronic heart failure: prognostic role of plasma brain natriuretic peptide concentration in patients with chronic symptomatic left ventricular dysfunction, *Circulation* 96:509, 1997.
42. Godet G, Fleron MH, Vicaut E, et al: Risk factors for acute postoperative renal failure in thoracic or thoracoabdominal aortic surgery: a prospective study, *Anesth Analg* 85:1227, 1997.
43. Huynh TT, Miller CC 3rd, Estrera AL, et al: Determinants of hospital length of stay after thoracoabdominal aortic aneurysm repair, *J Vasc Surg* 35:648, 2002.
44. Linden RJ: Atrial reflexes and renal function, *Am J Cardiol* 44:879, 1979.
45. Quail AW, Woods RL, Korner PI: Cardiac and arterial baroreceptor influences in release of vasopressin and renin during hemorrhage, *Am J Physiol* 252:H1120, 1987.
46. Myers BD, Peterson C, Molina C, et al: Role of cardiac atria in the human renal response to changing plasma volume, *Am J Physiol* 254:F562, 1988.
47. Taneyama C, Goto H, Goto K, et al: Attenuation of arterial baroreceptor reflex response to acute hypovolemia during induced hypotension, *Anesthesiology* 73:433, 1990.
48. Levens NR, Peach MJ, Carey RM: Role of the intrarenal renin-angiotensin system in the control of renal function, *Circ Res* 48:157, 1981.
49. Anderson RJ, Schrier RW: Acute renal failure. In Braunwald E, Isselbacher KJ, Petersdorf RG, et al (eds): *Harrison's principles of internal medicine*, ed 11, New York, 1987, McGraw-Hill, 1149.
50. Hilberman M, Derby GC, Spencer RJ, Stinson EB: Sequential pathophysiological changes characterizing the progression from renal dysfunction to acute renal failure following cardiac operation, *J Thorac Cardiovasc Surg* 79:838, 1980.
51. Carpenter JP, Fairman RM, Barker CF, et al: Endovascular AAA repair in patients with renal insufficiency: strategies for reducing adverse renal events, *Cardiovasc Surg* 9:559, 2001.
52. Modi KS, Rao VK: Atheroembolic renal disease, *J Am Soc Nephrol* 12:1781, 2001.
53. Valentine RJ, Rosen SF, Cigarroa JE, et al: The clinical course of new-onset atrial fibrillation after elective aortic operations, *J Am Coll Surg* 193:499, 2001.
54. Mathew JP, Parks R, Savino JS, et al: Atrial fibrillation following coronary artery bypass graft surgery: predictors, outcomes, and resource

utilization. MultiCenter Study of Perioperative Ischemia Research Group, *JAMA* 276:300, 1996.

55. Simoons ML, Demey HE, Bossaert LL, et al: The Paceport catheter: a new pacemaker system introduced through a Swan-Ganz catheter, *Cathet Cardiovasc Diagn* 15:66, 1988.

56. Zoll PM, Zoll RH, Falk RH, et al: External noninvasive temporary cardiac pacing: clinical trials, *Circulation* 71:937, 1985.

57. Al-Khatib SM, Granger CB, Huang Y, et al: Sustained ventricular arrhythmias among patients with acute coronary syndromes with no ST-segment elevation: incidence, predictors, and outcomes, *Circulation* 106:309, 2002.

58. DeFoe GR, Ross CS, Olmstead EM, et al: Lowest hematocrit on bypass and adverse outcomes associated with coronary artery bypass grafting. Northern New England Cardiovascular Disease Study Group, *Ann Thorac Surg* 71:769, 2001.

59. Fang WC, Helm RE, Krieger KH, et al: Impact of minimum hematocrit during cardiopulmonary bypass on mortality in patients undergoing coronary artery surgery, *Circulation* 96:II-194-9, 1997.

60. Hankeln K, Radel C, Beez M, et al: Comparison of hydroxyethyl starch and lactated Ringer's solution on hemodynamics and oxygen transport of critically ill patients in prospective crossover studies, *Crit Care Med* 17:133, 1989.

61. Brodde OE, Schuler S, Kretsch R, et al: Regional distribution of beta-adrenoceptors in the human heart: coexistence of functional beta 1- and beta 2-adrenoceptors in both atria and ventricles in severe congestive cardiomyopathy, *J Cardiovasc Pharmacol* 8:1235, 1986.

62. Goldberg LI: The dopamine vascular receptor, *Biochem Pharmacol* 24:651, 1975.

63. Anderson FL, Port JD, Reid BB, et al: Effect of therapeutic dopamine administration on myocardial catecholamine and neuropeptide Y concentrations in the failing ventricles of patients with idiopathic dilated cardiomyopathy, *J Cardiovasc Pharmacol* 20:800, 1992.

64. Schaer GL, Fink MP, Parrillo JE: Norepinephrine alone versus norepinephrine plus low-dose dopamine: enhanced renal blood flow with combination pressor therapy, *Crit Care Med* 13:492, 1985.

65. Marik PE: Low-dose dopamine: a systematic review, *Intensive Care Med* 28:877, 2002.

66. Freyschuss U, Hjemdahl P, Juhlin-Dannfelt A, Linde B: Cardiovascular and metabolic responses to low-dose adrenaline infusion: an invasive study in humans, *Clin Sci (Lond)* 70:199, 1986.

67. Baumann G, Felix SB, Filcek SA: Usefulness of dopexamine hydrochloride versus dobutamine in chronic congestive heart failure and effects on hemodynamics and urine output, *Am J Cardiol* 65:748, 1990.

68. Takala J, Meier-Hellmann A, Eddleston J, et al: Effect of dopexamine on outcome after major abdominal surgery: a prospective, randomized, controlled multicenter study. European Multicenter Study Group on Dopexamine in Major Abdominal Surgery, *Crit Care Med* 28:3417, 2000.

69. Smithies M, Yee TH, Jackson L, et al: Protecting the gut and the liver in the critically ill: effects of dopexamine, *Crit Care Med* 22:789, 1994.

70. Colardyn FC, Vandenbogaerde JF, Vogelaers DP, Verbeke JH: Use of dopexamine hydrochloride in patients with septic shock, *Crit Care Med* 17:999, 1989.

71. Gold JA, Cullinane S, Chen J, et al: Vasopressin as an alternative to norepinephrine in the treatment of milrinone-induced hypotension, *Crit Care Med* 28:249, 2000.

72. Ross MP, Allen-Webb EM, Pappas JB, McGough EC: Amrinone-associated thrombocytopenia: pharmacokinetic analysis, *Clin Pharmacol Ther* 53:661, 1993.

73. Goldstein RA, Gray EL, Dougherty AH, Naccarelli GV: Electrophysiologic effects of amrinone, *Am J Cardiol* 56:25B, 1985.

74. Davidenko JM, Antzelevitch C: The effects of milrinone on conduction, reflection, and automaticity in canine Purkinje fibers, *Circulation* 69:1026, 1984.

75. Anderson JL, Askins JC, Gilbert EM, et al: Occurrence of ventricular arrhythmias in patients receiving acute and chronic infusions of milrinone, *Am Heart J* 111:466, 1986.

76. Naccarelli GV, Goldstein RA: Electrophysiology of phosphodiesterase inhibitors, *Am J Cardiol* 63:35A, 1989.

77. Milfred-LaForest SK, Shubert J, Mendoza B, et al: Tolerability of extended duration intravenous milrinone in patients hospitalized for advanced heart failure and the usefulness of uptitration of oral angiotensin-converting enzyme inhibitors, *Am J Cardiol* 84:894, 1999.

78. Cuffe MS, Califf RM, Adams KF Jr, et al: Short-term intravenous milrinone for acute exacerbation of chronic heart failure: a randomized controlled trial, *JAMA* 287:1541, 2002.

79. Yamani MH, Haji SA, Starling RC, et al: Comparison of dobutamine-based and milrinone-based therapy for advanced decompensated congestive heart failure: hemodynamic efficacy, clinical outcome, and economic impact, *Am Heart J* 142:998, 2001.

80. Mehra MR, Ventura HO, Kapoor C, et al: Safety and clinical utility of long-term intravenous milrinone in advanced heart failure, *Am J Cardiol* 80:61, 1997.

81. Wartofsky L, Burman KD: Alterations in thyroid function in patients with systemic illness: the "euthyroid sick syndrome," *Endocr Rev* 3:164, 1982.

82. Docter R, Krenning EP, de Jong M, Hennemann G: The sick euthyroid syndrome: changes in thyroid hormone serum parameters and hormone metabolism, *Clin Endocrinol (Oxf)* 39:499, 1993.

83. Wehmann RE, Gregerman RI, Burns WH, et al: Suppression of thyrotropin in the low-thyroxine state of severe nonthyroidal illness, *N Engl J Med* 312:546, 1985.

84. Reinhardt W, Mocker V, Jockenhovel F, et al: Influence of coronary artery bypass surgery on thyroid hormone parameters, *Horm Res* 47:1, 1997.

85. Bettendorf M, Schmidt KG, Grulich-Henn J, et al: Tri-iodothyronine treatment in children after cardiac surgery: a double-blind, randomised, placebo-controlled study, *Lancet* 356:529, 2000.

86. Mullis-Jansson SL, Argenziano M, Corwin S, et al: A randomized double-blind study of the effect of triiodothyronine on cardiac function and morbidity after coronary bypass surgery, *J Thorac Cardiovasc Surg* 117:1128, 1999.

87. Bennett-Guerrero E, Jimenez JL, White WD, et al: Cardiovascular effects of intravenous triiodothyronine in patients undergoing coronary artery bypass graft surgery. A randomized, double-blind, placebo-controlled trial. Duke T3 study group, *JAMA* 275:687, 1996.

88. Gattis W, O'Connor CM: Calcium antagonists in the treatment of heart failure. Re-evaluation of therapeutic strategies, *Drugs* 59:17, 2000.

89. Cargnelli G, Piovan D, Bova S, et al: Present and future trends in research and clinical applications of inodilators, *J Cardiovasc Pharmacol* 14:S124, 1989.

90. Dei Cas L, Metra M, Visioli O: Clinical pharmacology of inodilators, *J Cardiovasc Pharmacol* 14:S60, 1989.

91. Reid IA: Role of vasopressin deficiency in the vasodilation of septic shock, *Circulation* 95:1108, 1997.

92. Argenziano M, Chen JM, Choudhri AF, et al: Management of vasodilatory shock after cardiac surgery: identification of predisposing factors and use of a novel pressor agent, *J Thorac Cardiovasc Surg* 116:973, 1998.

93. Rosenzweig EB, Starc TJ, Chen JM, et al: Intravenous arginine-vasopressin in children with vasodilatory shock after cardiac surgery, *Circulation* 100:II182, 1999.

94. Hollenberg SM, Kavinsky CJ, Parrillo JE: Cardiogenic shock, *Ann Intern Med* 131:47, 1999.

95. Pasic M, Hummel M, Hetzer R: Combined aortic surgery and implantation of a left ventricular assist device, *N Engl J Med* 346:711, 2002.

96. Court MH, Duan SX, von Moltke LL, et al: Interindividual variability in acetaminophen glucuronidation by human liver microsomes: identification of relevant acetaminophen UDP-glucuronosyltransferase isoforms, *J Pharmacol Exp Ther* 299:998, 2001.

97. Court MH, Duan SX, Hesse LM, et al: Cytochrome P-450 2B6 is responsible for interindividual variability of propofol hydroxylation by human liver microsomes, *Anesthesiology* 94:110, 2001.

98. Dundee JW, Hassard TH, McGowan WA, Henshaw J: The 'induction' dose of thiopentone. A method of study and preliminary illustrative results, *Anaesthesia* 37:1176, 1982.

99. Christensen JH, Andreasen F: Individual variation in response to thiopental, *Acta Anaesthesiol Scand* 22:303, 1978.

100. Stuber F, Petersen M, Bokelmann F, Schade U: A genomic polymorphism within the tumor necrosis factor locus influences plasma tumor necrosis factor-alpha concentrations and outcome of patients with severe sepsis, *Crit Care Med* 24:381, 1996.

101. Murohara T, Horowitz JR, Silver M, et al: Vascular endothelial growth factor/vascular permeability factor enhances vascular permeability via nitric oxide and prostacyclin, *Circulation* 97:99, 1998.

102. Floege J, Kriz W, Schulze M, et al: Basic fibroblast growth factor augments podocyte injury and induces glomerulosclerosis in rats with experimental membranous nephropathy, *J Clin Invest* 96:2809, 1995.

103. Baumgartner I, Pieczek A, Manor O, et al: Constitutive expression of phVEGF165 after intramuscular gene transfer promotes collateral vessel development in patients with critical limb ischemia, *Circulation* 97:1114, 1998.

104. Nabel EG, Gordon D, Yang ZY, et al: Gene transfer in vivo with DNA-liposome complexes: lack of autoimmunity and gonadal localization, *Hum Gene Ther* 3:649, 1992.

105. Willard JE, Landau C, Glamann DB, et al: Genetic modification of the vessel wall. Comparison of surgical and catheter-based techniques for delivery of recombinant adenovirus, *Circulation* 89:2190, 1994.

106. Nabel EG, Plautz G, Nabel GJ: Site-specific gene expression in vivo by direct gene transfer into the arterial wall, *Science* 249:1285, 1990.

107. Nabel EG, Yang ZY, Plautz G, et al: Recombinant fibroblast growth factor-1 promotes intimal hyperplasia and angiogenesis in arteries in vivo, *Nature* 362:844, 1993.

108. Schumacher B, Pecher P, von Specht BU, Stegmann T: Induction of neoangiogenesis in ischemic myocardium by human growth factors: first clinical results of a new treatment of coronary heart disease, *Circulation* 97:645, 1998.

109. Schumacher B, Stegmann T, Pecher P: The stimulation of neoangiogenesis in the ischemic human heart by the growth factor FGF: first clinical results, *J Cardiovasc Surg (Torino)* 39:783, 1998.

110. Rosengart TK, Budenbender KT, Duenas M, et al: Therapeutic angiogenesis: a comparative study of the angiogenic potential of acidic fibroblast growth factor and heparin, *J Vasc Surg* 26:302, 1997.

111. Minino AM, Smith BL: *Deaths: preliminary data for 2000*, National vital statistics reports, vol 49, no 12, Hyattsville, Md, 2001, National Center for Health Statistics.

112. Parrillo JE: Pathogenetic mechanisms of septic shock, *N Engl J Med* 328:1471, 1993.

113. Pinner RW, Teutsch SM, Simonsen L, et al: Trends in infectious diseases mortality in the United States, *JAMA* 275:189, 1996.

114. Rangel-Frausto MS: The epidemiology of bacterial sepsis, *Infect Dis Clin North Am* 13:299, 1999.

115. Sharkey R, Mulloy E, O'Neill G, et al: Toxic shock syndrome following influenza A infection, *Intensive Care Med* 25:335, 1999.

116. Mangram AJ, Horan TC, Pearson ML, et al: Guideline for prevention of surgical site infection, 1999. Centers for Disease Control and Prevention (CDC) Hospital Infection Control Practices Advisory Committee, *Am J Infect Control* 27:97, 1999.

117. Welborn MB, Oldenburg HS, Hess PJ, et al: The relationship between visceral ischemia, proinflammatory cytokines, and organ injury in patients undergoing thoracoabdominal aortic aneurysm repair, *Crit Care Med* 28:3191, 2000.

118. Giordanengo F, Cugnasca M, Giorgetti PL, Miani S: Prosthetic infection in vascular surgery, *Minerva Chir* 46:251, 1991.

119. Silverman H: Equivocal definitions of sepsis and septic shock, *Crit Care Med* 18:1048, 1990.

120. Bone RC: Let's agree on terminology: definitions of sepsis, *Crit Care Med* 19:973, 1991.

121. Sprung CL: Definitions of sepsis—have we reached a consensus? *Crit Care Med* 19:849, 1991.

122. Bone RC, Sprung CL, Sibbald WJ: Definitions for sepsis and organ failure, *Crit Care Med* 20:724, 1992.

123. Young GB, Bolton CF, Austin TW: Definitions for sepsis and organ failure, *Crit Care Med* 21:808, 1993.

124. Hayden WR: Sepsis and organ failure definitions and guidelines, *Crit Care Med* 21:1612, 1993.

125. Lowry SF: Sepsis and its complications: clinical definitions and therapeutic prospects, *Crit Care Med* 22:S1, 1994.

126. American College of Chest Physicians/Society of Critical Care Medicine Consensus Conference: Definitions for sepsis and organ failure and guidelines for the use of innovative therapies in sepsis, *Crit Care Med* 20:864, 1992.

127. Piper RD, Sibbald WJ: Multiple organ dysfunction syndrome: the relevance of persistent infection and inflammation. In Fein AM, Abraham AD, Balk RA et al (eds): *Sepsis and multiorgan failure*, Baltimore, 1997, Lippincott, Williams & Wilkins, 189.

128. Salvo I, de Cian W, Musicco M, et al: The Italian SEPSIS study: preliminary results on the incidence and evolution of SIRS, sepsis, severe sepsis and septic shock, *Intensive Care Med* 21(Suppl 2):S244, 1995.

129. Vincent JL: Dear SIRS, I'm sorry to say that I don't like you, *Crit Care Med* 25:372, 1997.

130. Abraham E, Matthay MA, Dinarello CA, et al: Consensus conference definitions for sepsis, septic shock, acute lung injury, and acute respiratory distress syndrome: time for a reevaluation, *Crit Care Med* 28:232, 2000.

131. Perl TM, Dvorak L, Hwang T, Wenzel RP: Long-term survival and function after suspected gram-negative sepsis, *JAMA* 274:338, 1995.

132. Centers for Disease Control: Increase in national hospital discharge survey rates for septicemia—United States, 1979-1987, *MMWR Morb Mortal Wkly Rep* 39:31,1990.

133. Wenzel RP: The mortality of hospital-acquired bloodstream infections: need for a new vital statistic? *Int J Epidemiol* 17:225, 1988.

134. Parrillo JE, Parker MM, Natanson C, et al: Septic shock in humans. Advances in the understanding of pathogenesis, cardiovascular dysfunction, and therapy, *Ann Intern Med* 113:227, 1990.

135. Bone RC: Gram-positive organisms and sepsis, *Arch Intern Med* 154:26, 1994.

136. Cockerill FR 3rd, Hughes JG, Vetter EA, et al: Analysis of 281,797 consecutive blood cultures performed over an eight-year period: trends in microorganisms isolated and the value of anaerobic culture of blood, *Clin Infect Dis* 24:403, 1997.

137. Valles J, Leon C, Alvarez-Lerma F: Nosocomial bacteremia in critically ill patients: a multicenter study evaluating epidemiology and prognosis. Spanish Collaborative Group for Infections in Intensive Care Units of Sociedad Espanola de Medicina Intensiva y Unidades Coronarias (SEMIUC), *Clin Infect Dis* 24:387, 1997.

138. Suffredini AF, Fromm RE, Parker MM, et al: The cardiovascular response of normal humans to the administration of endotoxin, *N Engl J Med* 321:280, 1989.

139. Michie HR, Spriggs DR, Manogue KR, et al: Tumor necrosis factor and endotoxin induce similar metabolic responses in human beings, *Surgery* 104:280, 1988.

140. Polotsky VY, Fischer W, Ezekowitz RA, Joiner KA: Interactions of human mannose-binding protein with lipoteichoic acids, *Infect Immun* 64:380, 1996.

141. Dunne DW, Resnick D, Greenberg J, et al: The type I macrophage scavenger receptor binds to gram-positive bacteria and recognizes lipoteichoic acid, *Proc Natl Acad Sci USA* 91:1863, 1994.

142. Herman A, Kappler JW, Marrack P, Pullen AM: Superantigens: mechanism of T-cell stimulation and role in immune responses, *Annu Rev Immunol* 9:745, 1991.

143. Moore FA, Moore EE, Poggetti R, et al: Gut bacterial translocation via the portal vein: a clinical perspective with major torso trauma, *J Trauma* 31:629, 1991.

144. Deitch EA, Winterton J, Li M, Berg R: The gut as a portal of entry for bacteremia. Role of protein malnutrition, *Ann Surg* 205:681,1987.

145. Magnotti LJ, Upperman JS, Xu DZ, et al: Gut-derived mesenteric lymph but not portal blood increases endothelial cell permeability and promotes lung injury after hemorrhagic shock, *Ann Surg* 228:518, 1998.

146. Sambol JT, Xu DZ, Adams CA, et al: Mesenteric lymph duct ligation provides long-term protection against hemorrhagic shock–induced lung injury, *Shock* 14:416, 2000.

147. Nakatsuka M: Assessment of gut mucosal perfusion and colonic tissue blood flow during abdominal aortic surgery with gastric tonometry and laser Doppler flowmetry, *Vasc Endovasc Surg* 36:193, 2002.

148. Elmarasy NM, Soong CV, Walker SR, et al: Sigmoid ischemia and the inflammatory response following endovascular abdominal aortic aneurysm repair, *J Endovasc Ther* 7:21, 2000.

149. Lau LL, Halliday MI, Lee B, et al: Intestinal manipulation during elective aortic aneurysm surgery leads to portal endotoxaemia and mucosal barrier dysfunction, *Eur J Vasc Endovasc Surg* 19:619, 2000.

150. Morrison DC, Kirikae T, Kirikae F, et al: The receptor(s) for endotoxin on mammalian cells, *Prog Clin Biol Res* 388:3, 1994.

151. Tobias PS, Soldau K, Gegner JA, et al: Lipopolysaccharide binding protein–mediated complexation of lipopolysaccharide with soluble CD14, *J Biol Chem* 270:10482, 1995.

152. Anderson DC, Springer TA: Leukocyte adhesion deficiency: an inherited defect in the Mac-1, LFA-1, and p150,95 glycoproteins, *Annu Rev Med* 38:175, 1987.

153. Wright SD, Ramos RA, Tobias PS, et al: CD14, a receptor for complexes of lipopolysaccharide (LPS) and LPS binding protein, *Science* 249:1431, 1990.

154. Hu H, Moller G: Lipopolysaccharide-stimulated events in B cell activation, *Scand J Immunol* 40:221,1994.

155. Wilson ME, Jones DP, Munkenbeck P, Morrison DC: Serum-dependent and -independent effects of bacterial lipopolysaccharides on human neutrophil oxidative capacity in vitro, *J Reticuloendothel Soc* 31:43, 1982.

156. Muller JM, Ziegler-Heitbrock HW, Baeuerle PA: Nuclear factor kappa B, a mediator of lipopolysaccharide effects, *Immunobiology* 187:233, 1993.

157. Evans HG, Lewis MJ, Shah AM: Interleukin-1 beta modulates myocardial contraction via dexamethasone sensitive production of nitric oxide, *Cardiovasc Res* 27:1486, 1993.

158. Finkel MS, Oddis CV, Jacob TD, et al: Negative inotropic effects of cytokines on the heart mediated by nitric oxide, *Science* 257:387, 1992.

159. Bennett-Guerrero E, Ayuso L, Hamilton-Davies C, et al: Relationship of preoperative antiendotoxin core antibodies and adverse outcomes following cardiac surgery, *JAMA* 277:646, 1997.

160. Stafford-Smith M, Phillips-Bute B, McCreath B, et al: Relationship of preoperative antiendotoxin core antibodies and acute renal injury following cardiac surgery, *Anesthesiology* 95:A 404, 2001 (abstract).

161. Parsons PE, Worthen GS, Moore EE, et al: The association of circulating endotoxin with the development of the adult respiratory distress syndrome, *Am Rev Respir Dis* 140:294, 1989.

162. Goldie AS, Fearon KC, Ross JA, et al: Natural cytokine antagonists and endogenous antiendotoxin core antibodies in sepsis syndrome. The Sepsis Intervention Group, *JAMA* 274:172, 1995.

163. Warren HS, Amato SF, Fitting C, et al: Assessment of ability of murine and human anti-lipid A monoclonal antibodies to bind and neutralize lipopolysaccharide, *J Exp Med* 177:89, 1993.

164. McCutchan JA, Wolf JL, Ziegler EJ, Braude AI: Ineffectiveness of single-dose human antiserum to core glycolipid (*E. coli* J5) for prophylaxis of bacteremic, gram-negative infections in patients with prolonged neutropenia, *Schweiz Med Wochenschr Suppl* 14:40, 1983.

165. Harbrecht BG, Wang SC, Simmons RL, Billiar TR: Cyclic GMP and guanylate cyclase mediate lipopolysaccharide-induced Kupffer cell tumor necrosis factor-alpha synthesis, *J Leukoc Biol* 57:297, 1995.

166. Salgado A, Boveda JL, Monasterio J, et al: Inflammatory mediators and their influence on haemostasis, *Haemostasis* 24:132, 1994.

167. Cebon J, Layton JE, Maher D, Morstyn G: Endogenous haemopoietic growth factors in neutropenia and infection, *Br J Haematol* 86:265, 1994.

168. Gough DB, Jordan A, Mannick JA, Rodrick MI: Impaired cell-mediated immunity in experimental abdominal sepsis and the effect of interleukin 2, *Arch Surg* 127:859, 1992.

169. Damerau B: Biological activities of complement-derived peptides, *Rev Physiol Biochem Pharmacol* 108:151, 1987.

170. Deitch EA, Mancini MC: Complement receptors in shock and transplantation, *Arch Surg* 128:1222, 1993.

171. Bone RC: The pathogenesis of sepsis, *Ann Intern Med* 115:457, 1991.

172. Donnelly TJ, Meade P, Jagels M, et al: Cytokine, complement, and endotoxin profiles associated with the development of the adult respiratory distress syndrome after severe injury, *Crit Care Med* 22:768, 1994.

173. Dofferhoff AS, de Jong HJ, Bom VJ, et al: Complement activation and the production of inflammatory mediators during the treatment of severe sepsis in humans, *Scand J Infect Dis* 24:197, 1992.

174. Giroir BP: Mediators of septic shock: new approaches for interrupting the endogenous inflammatory cascade, *Crit Care Med* 21:780, 1993.

175. Severn A, Rapson NT, Hunter CA, Liew FY: Regulation of tumor necrosis factor production by adrenaline and beta-adrenergic agonists, *J Immunol* 148:3441, 1992.

176. van der Poll T, Buller HR, ten Cate H, et al: Activation of coagulation after administration of tumor necrosis factor to normal subjects, *N Engl J Med* 322:1622, 1990.

177. Okusawa S, Gelfand JA, Ikejima T, et al: Interleukin 1 induces a shock-like state in rabbits. Synergism with tumor necrosis factor and the effect of cyclooxygenase inhibition, *J Clin Invest* 81:1162, 1988.

178. van der Poll T, van Deventer SJ, Hack CE, et al: Effects on leukocytes after injection of tumor necrosis factor into healthy humans, *Blood* 79:693, 1992.

179. Dinarello CA, Cannon JG, Wolff SM, et al: Tumor necrosis factor (cachectin) is an endogenous pyrogen and induces production of interleukin 1, *J Exp Med* 163:1433, 1986.

180. Strieter RM, Koch AE, Antony VB, et al: The immunopathology of chemotactic cytokines: the role of interleukin-8 and monocyte chemoattractant protein-1, *J Lab Clin Med* 123:183, 1994.

181. Graham RM, Strahan ME, Norman KW, et al: Platelet and plasma platelet-activating factor in sepsis and myocardial infarction, *J Lipid Mediat Cell Signal* 9:167, 1994.

182. Nakagami H, Cui TX, Iwai M, et al: Tumor necrosis factor-alpha inhibits growth factor–mediated cell proliferation through SHP-1 activation in endothelial cells, *Arterioscler Thromb Vasc Biol* 22:238, 2002.

183. Calkins CM, Heimbach JK, Bensard DD, et al: TNF receptor I mediates chemokine production and neutrophil accumulation in the lung following systemic lipopolysaccharide, *J Surg Res* 101:232, 2001.

184. Beutler B, Cerami A: The biology of cachectin/TNF—a primary mediator of the host response, *Annu Rev Immunol* 7:625, 1989.

185. Meulders Q, He CJ, Adida C, et al: Tumor necrosis factor alpha increases antifibrinolytic activity of cultured human mesangial cells, *Kidney Int* 42:327, 1992.

186. Bellomo R: The cytokine network in the critically ill, *Anaesth Intensive Care* 20:288, 1992.

187. Van Zee KJ, DeForge LE, Fischer E, et al: IL-8 in septic shock, endotoxemia, and after IL-1 administration, *J Immunol* 146:3478, 1991.

188. Green RM, Whiting JF, Rosenbluth AB, et al: Interleukin-6 inhibits hepatocyte taurocholate uptake and sodium-potassium-adenosinetriphosphatase activity, *Am J Physiol* 267:G1094, 1994.

189. Ertel W, Krombach F, Kremer JP, et al: Mechanisms of cytokine cascade activation in patients with sepsis: normal cytokine transcription despite reduced CD14 receptor expression, *Surgery* 114:243, 1993.

190. Buck C, Bundschu J, Gallati H, et al: Interleukin-6: a sensitive parameter for the early diagnosis of neonatal bacterial infection, *Pediatrics* 93:54, 1994.

191. Solomkin JS, Bass RC, Bjornson HS, et al: Alterations of neutrophil responses to tumor necrosis factor alpha and interleukin-8 following human endotoxemia, *Infect Immun* 62:943, 1994.

192. Opal SM, Fisher CJ Jr, Dhainaut JF, et al: Confirmatory interleukin-1 receptor antagonist trial in severe sepsis: a phase III, randomized, double-blind, placebo-controlled, multicenter trial. The Interleukin-1 Receptor Antagonist Sepsis Investigator Group, *Crit Care Med* 25:1115, 1997.

193. Quinn JV, Slotman GJ: Platelet-activating factor and arachidonic acid metabolites mediate tumor necrosis factor and eicosanoid kinetics and cardiopulmonary dysfunction during bacteremic shock, *Crit Care Med* 27:2485, 1999.

194. Alemayehu A, Sawmiller D, Chou BS, Chou CC: Intestinal prostacyclin and thromboxane production in irreversible hemorrhagic shock, *Circ Shock* 23:119, 1987.

195. Bitterman H, Yanagisawa A, Lefer AM: Beneficial actions of thromboxane receptor antagonism in hemorrhagic shock, *Circ Shock* 20:1, 1986.

196. Bitterman H, Smith BA, Lefer AM: Beneficial actions of antagonism of peptide leukotrienes in hemorrhagic shock, *Circ Shock* 24:159, 1988.

197. Fletcher JR, Short BL, Casey LC, et al: Thromboxane inhibition in gram-negative sepsis fails to improve survival, *Adv Prostaglandin Thromboxane Leukot Res* 12:117, 1983.

198. Bernard GR, Wheeler AP, Russell JA, et al: The effects of ibuprofen on the physiology and survival of patients with sepsis. The Ibuprofen in Sepsis Study Group, *N Engl J Med* 336:912, 1997.

199. Fletcher JR, Ramwell PW: Modification, by aspirin and indomethacin, of the haemodynamic and prostaglandin releasing effects of *E. coli* endotoxin in the dog, *Br J Pharmacol* 61:175, 1977.

200. Dunn M: The role of arachidonic acid metabolites in renal homeostasis. Non-steroidal anti-inflammatory drugs renal function and biochemical, histological and clinical effects and drug interactions, *Drugs* 33:56, 1987.

201. Maier RV, Hahnel GB, Fletcher JR: Platelet-activating factor augments tumor necrosis factor and procoagulant activity, *J Surg Res* 52:258, 1992.

202. Poubelle PE, Gingras D, Demers C, et al: Platelet-activating factor (PAF-acether) enhances the concomitant production of tumour necrosis factor-alpha and interleukin-1 by subsets of human monocytes, *Immunology* 72:181, 1991.

203. Bussolino F, Camussi G, Aglietta M, et al: Human endothelial cells are target for platelet-activating factor. I. Platelet-activating factor induces changes in cytoskeleton structures, *J Immunol* 139:2439, 1987.

204. Mathiak G, Szewczyk D, Abdullah F, et al: Platelet-activating factor (PAF) in experimental and clinical sepsis, *Shock* 7:391, 1997.

205. Dhainaut JF, Tenaillon A, Le Tulzo Y, et al: Platelet-activating factor receptor antagonist BN 52021 in the treatment of severe sepsis: a randomized, double-blind, placebo-controlled, multicenter clinical trial. BN 52021 Sepsis Study Group, *Crit Care Med* 22:1720, 1994.

206. Froon AM, Greve JW, Buurman WA, et al: Treatment with the platelet-activating factor antagonist TCV-309 in patients with severe systemic inflammatory response syndrome: a prospective, multi-center, double-blind, randomized phase II trial, *Shock* 5:313, 1996.

207. ten Cate H: Pathophysiology of disseminated intravascular coagulation in sepsis, *Crit Care Med* 28:S9, 2000.

208. Anagnostopoulos PV, Shepard AD, Pipinos II, et al: Hemostatic alterations associated with supraceliac aortic cross-clamping, *J Vasc Surg* 35:100, 2002.

209. Abraham E: Coagulation abnormalities in acute lung injury and sepsis, *Am J Respir Cell Mol Biol* 22:401, 2000.

210. Tapper H, Herwald H: Modulation of hemostatic mechanisms in bacterial infectious diseases, *Blood* 96:2329, 2000.

211. Hou SH, Bushinsky DA, Wish JB, et al: Hospital-acquired renal insufficiency: a prospective study, *Am J Med* 74:243, 1983.

212. Neveu H, Kleinknecht D, Brivet F, et al: Prognostic factors in acute renal failure due to sepsis. Results of a prospective multicentre study. The French Study Group on Acute Renal Failure, *Nephrol Dial Transplant* 11:293, 1996.

213. Cumming AD, Driedger AA, McDonald JW, et al: Vasoactive hormones in the renal response to systemic sepsis, *Am J Kidney Dis* 11:23, 1988.

214. Badr KF: Sepsis-associated renal vasoconstriction: potential targets for future therapy, *Am J Kidney Dis* 20:207, 1992.

215. Wardle EN: Acute renal failure and multiorgan failure, *Nephron* 66:380, 1994.

216. Pastor CM: Vascular hyporesponsiveness of the renal circulation during endotoxemia in anesthetized pigs, *Crit Care Med* 27:2735, 1999.

217. Tsuneyoshi I, Yamada H, Kakihana Y, et al: Hemodynamic and metabolic effects of low-dose vasopressin infusions in vasodilatory septic shock, *Crit Care Med* 29:487, 2001.

218. Hesselvik JF, Brodin B: Low dose norepinephrine in patients with septic shock and oliguria: effects on afterload, urine flow, and oxygen transport, *Crit Care Med* 17:179, 1989.

219. Kaloyanides GJ: Antibiotic-related nephrotoxicity, *Nephrol Dial Transplant* 9:130, 1994.

220. Cameron JS: Immunologically mediated interstitial nephritis: primary and secondary, *Adv Nephrol Necker Hosp* 18:207, 1989.

221. Montseny JJ, Meyrier A, Kleinknecht D, Callard P: The current spectrum of infectious glomerulonephritis. Experience with 76 patients and review of the literature, *Medicine (Baltimore)* 74:63, 1995.

222. Nagachinta T, Stephens M, Reitz B, Polk BF: Risk factors for surgical-wound infection following cardiac surgery, *J Infect Dis* 156:967, 1987.

223. National Nosocomial Infections Surveillance (NNIS) report, data summary from October 1986–April 1996, issued May 1996. A report from the National Nosocomial Infections Surveillance (NNIS) system, *Am J Infect Control* 24:380, 1996.

224. Tschida SJ, Vance-Bryan K, Zaske DE: Anti-infective agents and hepatic disease, *Med Clin North Am* 79:895, 1995.

225. Cunha BA, Friedman PE: Antibiotic dosing in patients with renal insufficiency or receiving dialysis, *Heart Lung* 17:612, 1988.

226. Maderazo EG: Antibiotic dosing in renal failure, *Med Clin North Am* 79:919, 1995.

227. Eng RH, Smith SM, Fan-Havard P, Ogbara T: Effect of antibiotics on endotoxin release from gram-negative bacteria, *Diagn Microbiol Infect Dis* 16:185, 1993.

228. Bucklin SE, Fujihara Y, Leeson MC, Morrison DC: Differential antibiotic-induced release of endotoxin from gram-negative bacteria, *Eur J Clin Microbiol Infect Dis* 13:S43, 1994.

229. Practice parameters for hemodynamic support of sepsis in adult patients in sepsis. Task Force of the American College of Critical Care Medicine, Society of Critical Care Medicine. *Crit Care Med* 27:639, 1999.

230. Richer M, Robert S, Lebel M: Renal hemodynamics during norepinephrine and low-dose dopamine infusions in man, *Crit Care Med* 24:1150, 1996.

231. Strigle TR, Petrinec D: The effect of renal range dopamine and norepinephrine infusions on the renal vasculature, *Am Surg* 56:494, 1990.

232. Lherm T, Troche G, Rossignol M, et al: Renal effects of low-dose dopamine in patients with sepsis syndrome or septic shock treated with catecholamines, *Intensive Care Med* 22:213, 1996.

233. Juste RN, Panikkar K, Soni N: The effects of low-dose dopamine infusions on haemodynamic and renal parameters in patients with septic shock requiring treatment with noradrenaline, *Intensive Care Med* 24:564, 1998.

234. Meier-Hellmann A, Bredle DL, Specht M, et al: The effects of low-dose dopamine on splanchnic blood flow and oxygen uptake in patients with septic shock, *Intensive Care Med* 23:31, 1997.

235. Ruokonen E, Takala J, Kari A, et al: Regional blood flow and oxygen transport in septic shock, *Crit Care Med* 21:1296, 1993.

236. Marik PE, Mohedin M: The contrasting effects of dopamine and norepinephrine on systemic and splanchnic oxygen utilization in hyperdynamic sepsis, *JAMA* 272:1354, 1994.

237. Neviere R, Mathieu D, Chagnon JL, et al: The contrasting effects of dobutamine and dopamine on gastric mucosal perfusion in septic patients, *Am J Respir Crit Care Med* 154:1684, 1996.

238. Levy B, Bollaert PE, Charpentier C, et al: Comparison of norepinephrine and dobutamine to epinephrine for hemodynamics, lactate metabolism, and gastric tonometric variables in septic shock: a prospective, randomized study, *Intensive Care Med* 23:282, 1997.

239. Meier-Hellmann A, Reinhart K, Bredle DL, et al: Epinephrine impairs splanchnic perfusion in septic shock, *Crit Care Med* 25:399, 1997.

240. Day NP, Phu NH, Bethell DP, et al: The effects of dopamine and adrenaline infusions on acid-base balance and systemic haemodynamics in severe infection, *Lancet* 348:219, 1996.

241. Martin C, Saux P, Eon B, et al: Septic shock: a goal-directed therapy using volume loading, dobutamine and/or norepinephrine, *Acta Anaesthesiol Scand* 34:413, 1990.

242. Desjars P, Pinaud M, Potel G, et al: A reappraisal of norepinephrine therapy in human septic shock, *Crit Care Med* 15:134, 1987.

243. Meadows D, Edwards JD, Wilkins RG, Nightingale P: Reversal of intractable septic shock with norepinephrine therapy, *Crit Care Med* 16:663, 1988.

244. Redl-Wenzl EM, Armbruster C, Edelmann G, et al: The effects of norepinephrine on hemodynamics and renal function in severe septic shock states, *Intensive Care Med* 19:151, 1993.

245. Martin C, Papazian L, Perrin G, et al: Norepinephrine or dopamine for the treatment of hyperdynamic septic shock? *Chest* 103:1826, 1993.

246. Reinelt H, Radermacher P, Fischer G, et al: Effects of a dobutamine-induced increase in splanchnic blood flow on hepatic metabolic activity in patients with septic shock, *Anesthesiology* 86:818, 1997.

247. Wilson MF, Brackett DJ, Tompkins P, et al: Elevated plasma vasopressin concentrations during endotoxin and *E. coli* shock, *Adv Shock Res* 6:15, 1981.

248. Day TA, Randle JC, Renaud LP: Opposing alpha- and beta-adrenergic mechanisms mediate dose-dependent actions of noradrenaline on supraoptic vasopressin neurones in vivo, *Brain Res* 358:171, 1985.

249. Karmazyn M, Manku MS, Horrobin DF: Changes of vascular reactivity induced by low vasopressin concentrations: interactions with cortisol and lithium and possible involvement of prostaglandins, *Endocrinology* 102:1230, 1978.

250. Medina P, Noguera I, Aldasoro M, et al: Enhancement by vasopressin of adrenergic responses in human mesenteric arteries, *Am J Physiol* 272:H1087, 1997.

251. Argenziano M, Choudhri AF, Oz MC, et al: A prospective randomized trial of arginine vasopressin in the treatment of vasodilatory shock after left ventricular assist device placement, *Circulation* 96:II-286, 1997.

252. Argenziano M, Chen JM, Cullinane S, et al: Arginine vasopressin in the management of vasodilatory hypotension after cardiac transplantation, *J Heart Lung Transplant* 18:814, 1999.

253. Rangel-Frausto MS, Pittet D, Costigan M, et al: The natural history of the systemic inflammatory response syndrome (SIRS). A prospective study, *JAMA* 273:117, 1995.

254. Pittet D, Thievent B, Wenzel RP, et al: Bedside prediction of mortality from bacteremic sepsis. A dynamic analysis of ICU patients, *Am J Respir Crit Care Med* 153:684, 1996.

255. Hsu CY, Chertow GM: Chronic renal confusion: insufficiency, failure, dysfunction, or disease, *Am J Kidney Dis* 36:415, 2000.

256. Lassnigg A, Donner E, Grubhofer G, et al: Lack of renoprotective effects of dopamine and furosemide during cardiac surgery, *J Am Soc Nephrol* 11:97, 2000.

257. Shilliday IR, Quinn KJ, Allison ME: Loop diuretics in the management of acute renal failure: a prospective, double-blind, placebo-controlled, randomized study, *Nephrol Dial Transplant* 12:2592, 1997.

258. van Valenberg PL, Hoitsma AJ, Tiggeler RG, et al: Mannitol as an indispensable constituent of an intraoperative hydration protocol for the prevention of acute renal failure after renal cadaveric transplantation, *Transplantation* 44:784, 1987.

259. Conger JD: Interventions in clinical acute renal failure: what are the data? *Am J Kidney Dis* 26:565, 1995.

260. Flancbaum L, Choban PS, Dasta JF: Quantitative effects of low-dose dopamine on urine output in oliguric surgical intensive care unit patients, *Crit Care Med* 22:61, 1994.

261. Pass LJ, Eberhart RC, Brown JC, et al: The effect of mannitol and dopamine on the renal response to thoracic aortic cross-clamping, *J Thorac Cardiovasc Surg* 95:608, 1988.

262. Paul MD, Mazer CD, Byrick RJ, et al: Influence of mannitol and dopamine on renal function during elective infrarenal aortic clamping in man, *Am J Nephrol* 6:427, 1986.

263. Parks RW, Diamond T, McCrory DC, et al: Prospective study of postoperative renal function in obstructive jaundice and the effect of perioperative dopamine, *Br J Surg* 81:437, 1994.

264. Denton MD, Chertow GM, Brady HR: "Renal-dose" dopamine for the treatment of acute renal failure: scientific rationale, experimental studies and clinical trials, *Kidney Int* 50:4, 1996.

265. Thalen PG, Nordlander MI, Sohtell ME, Svensson LE: Attenuation of renal ischaemic injury by felodipine, *Naunyn Schmiedebergs Arch Pharmacol* 343:411, 1991.

266. Greif F, Anais D, Frei L, et al: Blocking the calcium cascade in experimental acute renal failure, *Isr J Med Sci* 26:301, 1990.

267. Bakris GL, Mangrum A, Copley JB, et al: Effect of calcium channel or beta-blockade on the progression of diabetic nephropathy in African Americans, *Hypertension* 29:744, 1997.

268. Madsen JK, Zachariae H, Pedersen EB: Effects of the calcium antagonist felodipine on renal haemodynamics, tubular sodium handling, and blood pressure in cyclosporin-treated dermatological patients, *Nephrol Dial Transplant* 12:480, 1997.

269. de Lasson L, Hansen HE, Juhl B, et al: Effect of felodipine on renal function and vasoactive hormones in infrarenal aortic surgery, *Br J Anaesth* 79:719, 1997.

270. Bergman AS, Odar-Cederlof I, Westman L: Renal and hemodynamic effects of diltiazem after elective major vascular surgery—a potential renoprotective agent? *Ren Fail* 17:155, 1995.

271. Antonucci F, Calo L, Rizzolo M, et al: Nifedipine can preserve renal function in patients undergoing aortic surgery with infrarenal cross-clamping, *Nephron* 74:668, 1996.

272. Sorensen TI, Nielsen GG, Andersen PK, Teasdale TW: Genetic and environmental influences on premature death in adult adoptees, *N Engl J Med* 318:727, 1988.

273. Westendorp RG, Langermans JA, Huizinga TW, et al: Genetic influence on cytokine production and fatal meningococcal disease, *Lancet* 349:170, 1997.

274. Mira JP, Cariou A, Grall F, et al: Association of TNF2, a TNF-alpha promoter polymorphism, with septic shock susceptibility and mortality: a multicenter study, *JAMA* 282:561, 1999.

275. Tang GJ, Huang SL, Yien HW, et al: Tumor necrosis factor gene polymorphism and septic shock in surgical infection, *Crit Care Med* 28:2733, 2000.

276. Tracey KJ, Cerami A: Tumor necrosis factor: a pleiotropic cytokine and therapeutic target, *Annu Rev Med* 45:491, 1994.

277. Reinhart K, Karzai W: Anti-tumor necrosis factor therapy in sepsis: update on clinical trials and lessons learned, *Crit Care Med* 29:S121, 2001.

278. Fang XM, Schroder S, Hoeft A, Stuber F: Comparison of two polymorphisms of the interleukin-1 gene family: interleukin-1 receptor antagonist polymorphism contributes to susceptibility to severe sepsis, *Crit Care Med* 27:1330, 1999.

279. Hirsch E, Irikura VM, Paul SM, Hirsh D: Functions of interleukin 1 receptor antagonist in gene knockout and overproducing mice, *Proc Natl Acad Sci USA* 93:11008, 1996.

280. Stuber F: Impact of genomic variation on inflammatory processes and sepsis. In Eichacker PQ, Pugin J (eds): *Evolving concepts in sepsis and septic shock*, Boston, 2001, Kluwer Academic Publishers, 81.

281. Kolls J, Peppel K, Silva M, Beutler B: Prolonged and effective blockade of tumor necrosis factor activity through adenovirus-mediated gene transfer, *Proc Natl Acad Sci USA* 91:215, 1994.

282. Chen GH, Reddy RC, Newstead MW, et al: Intrapulmonary TNF gene therapy reverses sepsis-induced suppression of lung antibacterial host defense, *J Immunol* 165:6496, 2000.

283. Oberholzer C, Oberholzer A, Bahjat FR, et al: Targeted adenovirus-induced expression of IL-10 decreases thymic apoptosis and improves survival in murine sepsis, *Proc Natl Acad Sci USA* 98:11503, 2001.

284. Minter RM, Ferry MA, Murday ME, et al: Adenoviral delivery of human and viral IL-10 in murine sepsis, *J Immunol* 167:1053, 2001.

285. Furchgott RF: Studies on relaxation of rabbit aorta by sodium nitrite: the basis for the proposal that the acid-activatable inhibitory factor from retractor penis is inorganic nitrite and the endothelium-derived relaxing factor is nitric oxide. In Vanhoutte PM (ed): *Vasodilatation: vascular smooth muscle, peptides, and endothelium*, New York, 1988, Raven Press, 401.

286. Cobb JP, Danner RL: Nitric oxide and septic shock, *JAMA* 275:1192, 1996.

287. From the bench to the bedside: the future of sepsis research. Executive summary of an American College of Chest Physicians, National Institute of Allergy and Infectious Disease, and National Heart, Lung, and Blood Institute Workshop, *Chest* 111:744, 1997.

288. Natanson C, Hoffman WD, Suffredini AF, et al: Selected treatment strategies for septic shock based on proposed mechanisms of pathogenesis, *Ann Intern Med* 120:771, 1994.

289. Moncada S, Higgs A: The L-arginine-nitric oxide pathway, *N Engl J Med* 329:2002, 1993.

290. Loscalzo J: Nitric oxide and vascular disease, *N Engl J Med* 333:251, 1995.

291. Lowenstein CJ, Dinerman JL, Snyder SH: Nitric oxide: a physiologic messenger, *Ann Intern Med* 120:227, 1994.

292. Murad F: The 1996 Albert Lasker Medical Research Awards. Signal transduction using nitric oxide and cyclic guanosine monophosphate, *JAMA* 276:1189, 1996.

293. Kilbourn RG, Gross SS, Jubran A, et al: NG-methyl-L-arginine inhibits tumor necrosis factor-induced hypotension: implications for the involvement of nitric oxide, *Proc Natl Acad Sci USA* 87:3629, 1990.

294. Freeman BD, Zeni F, Banks SM, et al: Response of the septic vasculature to prolonged vasopressor therapy with N(omega)-monomethyl-L-arginine and epinephrine in canines, *Crit Care Med* 26:877, 1998.

295. Strand OA, Leone AM, Giercksky KE, et al: N(G)-monomethyl-L-arginine improves survival in a pig model of abdominal sepsis, *Crit Care Med* 26:1490, 1998.

296. Cobb JP, Natanson C, Hoffman WD, et al: N omega-amino-L-arginine, an inhibitor of nitric oxide synthase, raises vascular resistance but increases mortality rates in awake canines challenged with endotoxin, *J Exp Med* 176:1175, 1992.

297. Petros A, Lamb G, Leone A, et al: Effects of a nitric oxide synthase inhibitor in humans with septic shock, *Cardiovasc Res* 28:34, 1994.

298. Avontuur JA, Biewenga M, Buijk SL, et al: Pulmonary hypertension and reduced cardiac output during inhibition of nitric oxide synthesis in human septic shock, *Shock* 9:451, 1998.

299. Avontuur JA, Tutein Nolthenius RP, van Bodegom JW, Bruining HA: Prolonged inhibition of nitric oxide synthesis in severe septic shock: a clinical study, *Crit Care Med* 26:660, 1998.

300. Avontuur JA, Tutein Nolthenius RP, Buijk SL, et al: Effect of L-NAME, an inhibitor of nitric oxide synthesis, on cardiopulmonary function in human septic shock, *Chest* 113:1640, 1998.

301. Holaday JW, Faden AI: Naloxone reversal of endotoxin hypotension suggests role of endorphins in shock, *Nature* 275:450, 1978.

302. Faden AI, Holaday JW: Opiate antagonists: a role in the treatment of hypovolemic shock, *Science* 205:317, 1979.

303. Peters WP, Johnson MW, Friedman PA, Mitch WE: Pressor effect of naloxone in septic shock, *Lancet* 1:529, 1981.

304. Hughes GS Jr: Naloxone and methylprednisolone sodium succinate enhance sympathomedullary discharge in patients with septic shock, *Life Sci* 35:2319, 1984.

305. Groeger JS, Carlon GC, Howland WS: Naloxone in septic shock, *Crit Care Med* 11:650, 1983.

306. DeMaria A, Carven DE, Heffernan JJ, et al: Naloxone versus placebo in treatment of septic shock, *Lancet* 1:1363, 1985.

307. Roberts DE, Dobson KE, Hall KW, Light RB: Effects of prolonged naloxone infusion in septic shock, *Lancet* 2:699, 1988.

308. Boeuf B, Gauvin F, Guerguerian AM, et al: Therapy of shock with naloxone: a meta-analysis, *Crit Care Med* 26:1910, 1998.

309. Boyd JL, 3rd, Stanford GG, Chernow B: The pharmacotherapy of septic shock, *Crit Care Clin* 5:133, 1989.

310. Shenep JL: Septic shock, *Adv Pediatr Infect Dis* 12:209, 1996.

311. Auphan N, DiDonato JA, Rosette C, et al: Immunosuppression by glucocorticoids: inhibition of NF-kappa B activity through induction of I kappa B synthesis, *Science* 270:286, 1995.

312. Chi EY, Henderson WR, Klebanoff SJ: Phospholipase A2–induced rat mast cell secretion. Role of arachidonic acid metabolites, *Lab Invest* 47:579, 1982.

313. Carlet J: From mega to more reasonable doses of corticosteroids: a decade to recreate hope, *Crit Care Med* 27:672, 1999.

314. Melby JC: Drug spotlight program: systemic corticosteroid therapy: pharmacology and endocrinologic considerations, *Ann Intern Med* 81:505, 1974.

315. Vale W, Spiess J, Rivier C, Rivier J: Characterization of a 41-residue ovine hypothalamic peptide that stimulates secretion of corticotropin and beta-endorphin, *Science* 213:1394, 1981.

316. Barnes PJ: Beta-adrenergic receptors and their regulation, *Am J Respir Crit Care Med* 152:838, 1995.

317. Effect of high-dose glucocorticoid therapy on mortality in patients with clinical signs of systemic sepsis. The Veterans Administration Systemic Sepsis Cooperative Study Group, *N Engl J Med* 317:659, 1987.

318. Bone RC, Fisher CJ Jr, Clemmer TP, et al: A controlled clinical trial of high-dose methylprednisolone in the treatment of severe sepsis and septic shock, *N Engl J Med* 317:653, 1987.

319. Bollaert PE, Charpentier C, Levy B, et al: Reversal of late septic shock with supraphysiologic doses of hydrocortisone, *Crit Care Med* 26:645, 1998.

320. Briegel J, Forst H, Haller M, et al: Stress doses of hydrocortisone reverse hyperdynamic septic shock: a prospective, randomized, double-blind, single-center study, *Crit Care Med* 27:723, 1999.

321. Remick DG, Call DR, Ebong SJ, et al: Combination immunotherapy with soluble tumor necrosis factor receptors plus interleukin 1 receptor antagonist decreases sepsis mortality, *Crit Care Med* 29:473, 2001.

322. Zeni F, Freeman B, Natanson C: Anti-inflammatory therapies to treat sepsis and septic shock: a reassessment, *Crit Care Med* 25:1095, 1997.

323. Natanson C, Esposito CJ, Banks SM: The sirens' songs of confirmatory sepsis trials: selection bias and sampling error, *Crit Care Med* 26:1927, 1998.

324. van Deventer SJ, Elson CO, Fedorak RN: Multiple doses of intravenous interleukin 10 in steroid-refractory Crohn's disease. Crohn's Disease Study Group, *Gastroenterology* 113:383, 1997.

325. Taylor PC, Williams RO, Maini RN: Anti-TNF alpha therapy in rheumatoid arthritis—current and future directions, *Curr Dir Autoimmun* 2:83, 2000.

326. Ulfgren AK, Andersson U, Engstrom M, et al: Systemic anti-tumor necrosis factor alpha therapy in rheumatoid arthritis downregulates synovial tumor necrosis factor alpha synthesis, *Arthritis Rheum* 43:2391, 2000.

327. Maini RN, Taylor PC: Anti-cytokine therapy for rheumatoid arthritis, *Annu Rev Med* 51:207, 2000.

328. Esmon C: The protein C pathway, *Crit Care Med* 28:S44, 2000.

329. Hanson SR, Griffin JH, Harker LA, et al: Antithrombotic effects of thrombin-induced activation of endogenous protein C in primates, *J Clin Invest* 92:2003, 1993.

330. Araki H, Nishi K, Ishihara N, Okajima K: Inhibitory effects of activated protein C and heparin on thrombotic arterial occlusion in rat mesenteric arteries, *Thromb Res* 62:209, 1991.

331. Gruber A, Griffin JH, Harker LA, Hanson SR: Inhibition of platelet-dependent thrombus formation by human activated protein C in a primate model, *Blood* 73:639, 1989.

332. Hesselvik JF, Malm J, Dahlback B, Blomback M: Protein C, protein S and C4b-binding protein in severe infection and septic shock, *Thromb Haemost* 65:126, 1991.

333. Bajzar L, Manuel R, Nesheim ME: Purification and characterization of TAFI, a thrombin-activable fibrinolysis inhibitor, *J Biol Chem* 270:14477, 1995.

334. Grey S, Hau H, Salem HH, Hancock WW: Selective effects of protein C on activation of human monocytes by lipopolysaccharide, interferon-gamma, or PMA: modulation of effects on CD11b and CD14 but not CD25 or CD54 induction, *Transplant Proc* 25:2913, 1993.

335. Grey ST, Tsuchida A, Hau H, et al: Selective inhibitory effects of the anticoagulant activated protein C on the responses of human mononuclear phagocytes to LPS, IFN-gamma, or phorbol ester, *J Immunol* 153:3664, 1994.

336. Murakami K, Okajima K, Uchiba M, et al: Activated protein C attenuates endotoxin-induced pulmonary vascular injury by inhibiting activated leukocytes in rats, *Blood* 87:642, 1996.

337. Joyce DE, Gelbert L, Ciaccia A, et al: Gene expression profile of antithrombotic protein c defines new mechanisms modulating inflammation and apoptosis, *J Biol Chem* 276:11199, 2001.

338. Roman J, Velasco F, Fernandez F, et al: Protein C, protein S and C4b-binding protein in neonatal severe infection and septic shock, *J Perinat Med* 20:111, 1992.

339. Fourrier F, Chopin C, Goudemand J, et al: Septic shock, multiple organ failure, and disseminated intravascular coagulation. Compared patterns of antithrombin III, protein C, and protein S deficiencies, *Chest* 101:816, 1992.

340. Lorente JA, Garcia-Frade LJ, Landin L, et al: Time course of hemostatic abnormalities in sepsis and its relation to outcome, *Chest* 103:1536, 1993.

341. Kidokoro A, Iba T, Fukunaga M, Yagi Y: Alterations in coagulation and fibrinolysis during sepsis, *Shock* 5:223, 1996.

342. Mesters RM, Helterbrand J, Utterback BG, et al: Prognostic value of protein C concentrations in neutropenic patients at high risk of severe septic complications, *Crit Care Med* 28:2209, 2000.

343. Kanji S, Devlin JW, Piekos KA, Racine E: Recombinant human activated protein C, drotrecogin alfa (activated): a novel therapy for severe sepsis, *Pharmacotherapy* 21:1389, 2001.

344. Bernard GR, Vincent JL, Laterre PF, et al: Efficacy and safety of recombinant human activated protein C for severe sepsis, *N Engl J Med* 344:699, 2001.

Respiratory Complications and Management

18

Christine A. Doyle, MD
Ronald G. Pearl, MD, PhD

G IVEN the diversity of patients and procedures related to vascular surgery, it is not surprising that vascular surgical procedures vary greatly in their postoperative respiratory complications and management. Many patients can be extubated in the operating room upon completion of surgery. However, others require mechanical ventilatory support for a period ranging from hours to days. Even in previously healthy patients, the risk of postoperative pulmonary complications after upper abdominal procedures is 20% to 30%.

Risk Factors

Pulmonary Disease

CHRONIC OBSTRUCTIVE PULMONARY DISEASE. The patient with underlying lung disease is at increased risk for pulmonary complications and the need for prolonged postoperative ventilation. Patients with chronic obstructive pulmonary disease (COPD) have an expiratory flow limitation with resulting end-expiratory hyperinflation. The total lung capacity, functional residual capacity (FRC), and residual volume are all increased. Positive-pressure mechanical ventilation may cause or worsen this dynamic hyperinflation (intrinsic positive end-expiratory pressure [PEEP]). End-expiratory hyperinflation may occur even when end-expiratory airway pressure returns to zero. Most authors agree that the end-inflation hold pressure (plateau pressure) should be less than 35 cmH$_2$O in order to prevent lung parenchymal strain.[1] Some patients may have exaggerated hypoxic vasoconstriction, polycythemia, or undiagnosed cor pulmonale.[2] Use of nitrous oxide may further expand bullae in the lung and increase the risk of pneumothorax.

ASTHMA. Patients with asthma are at greatly increased risk for bronchospasm during induction of anesthesia, surgery, emergence, and recovery. Increased airway resistance can cause severe difficulties with ventilation, even leading to death. The major physiologic consequences are hypoxemia, hypercarbia, barotrauma, and increased work of breathing. Both physicians and patients frequently fail to appreciate the severity of asthma. As with COPD, air trapping may occur. Because barotrauma is related to the dynamic hyperinflation of alveolar units, a ventilator strategy utilizing lower volumes and pressures is suggested.[3] Expiratory time must be increased to minimize the hyperinflation. This hyperinflation can cause significant hemodynamic effects (see the section on PEEP).

RESTRICTIVE LUNG DISEASE. Restrictive lung disease causes proportional decreases in all lung volumes; airway resistance is unchanged. The decrease in FRC causes a decrease in compli-ance. At any given lung volume, transpulmonary pressure is abnormally high. Thus, the airway pressures required for adequate tidal volume (V$_T$) are significantly increased. Both physiologic deadspace and shunt are increased, and both the partial pressure of oxygen in arterial blood (Pao$_2$) and carbon dioxide (Paco$_2$) (assuming compensatory hyperventilation) are decreased. The increased ventilation/perfusion (V/Q) mismatch is the predominant cause of hypoxia, and relative hyperventilation is thought to be the cause of the hypocarbia. Arterial pH is generally normal at rest, but hyperventilation with exertion may induce a significant respiratory alkalosis. Respiratory function is always worse with exertion, and rapid shallow breathing is typical even at rest.[4]

SMOKING. Smoking causes two physiologic changes: decreased mucociliary function and increased carboxyhemoglobin. Mucociliary function takes approximately 2 weeks to return to normal after smoking cessation and may cause significantly increased secretions, which can last for several days. Carboxyhemoglobin levels return to normal within 24 hours.[5]

Cardiac Disease

Many patients undergoing vascular surgery have underlying cardiac disease, which increases the risk of intraoperative and postoperative events. Mechanical ventilation may be beneficial by decreasing both systemic and myocardial oxygen demands.

MYOCARDIAL ISCHEMIA OR INFARCTION. The most significant risk factors for overall morbidity and mortality are cardiac ischemia and infarction within the first postoperative week and are believed to be related to the exaggerated sympathetic response.[6] Underlying ischemic cardiomyopathy is the most important risk factor for cardiac morbidity and mortality.

HEART FAILURE. Heart failure (or congestive heart failure) is the common endpoint of most cardiac diseases. No matter what the cause, the heart is unable to pump enough blood for basic metabolic needs. There are approximately 500,000 new cases of heart failure per year in the United States, and 6% to 10% of all patients older than 65 years have some degree of heart failure.[7] The preoperative ejection fraction (EF) is a significant predictor of operative risk; an EF less than 40% increases risk eightfold. These patients may benefit from preoperative optimization of preload (diuretics) and afterload (vasodilators) as well as intraoperative inotropes. Postoperative development of pulmonary edema may necessitate prolonged mechanical ventilation.

ARRHYTHMIAS. The variety of possible arrhythmias can lead to many different problems in the perioperative period. The use of implanted devices (pacemakers or automatic implantable cardioverter-defibrillators) may require specialized management.

Atrial arrhythmias (fibrillation and flutter) are present in 1% of patients older than 60 years and 5% to 10% of those older than 75 years. Associated risk factors include coronary artery disease, COPD, hypertension, and cardiomyopathy. Rapid heart rates may produce coronary insufficiency. Furthermore, the risk of stroke is increased approximately fivefold with atrial fibrillation.[8] Patients are chronically anticoagulated because of the risk of mural thrombus and embolization; they are generally not candidates for regional anesthesia unless their coagulation status is normalized.

Atrioventricular (AV) heart block is generally an acquired disease, most often related to prior cardiac ischemia. Although first-degree block is relatively inconsequential, second- and third-degree blocks indicate significant cardiac risk. Type II second-degree AV block is generally associated with a bundle-branch pattern related to a block below the bundle of His. The PR interval is constant, and the dropped beats are due to intermittent block of the *other* bundle branch. The greatest risk is progression to third-degree block. Third-degree block (complete heart block) is associated with one of two possibilities: asystole or a junctional escape rhythm. The treatment remains emergent pacemaker implantation.[9,10]

More and more patients now have implanted devices to regulate the electrical activity of the heart. Pacemakers and implantable cardiac defibrillators are inserted in approximately 200,000 and 60,000 patients per year, respectively. The most recent guidelines from the American College of Cardiology and the American Heart Association recommend device interrogation both before and after planned surgical procedures. Rate-responsive pacemaker modes and cardioversion modes should be disabled immediately before surgery.[11]

Emergency Surgery

The patient who requires urgent or emergent surgery is likely to have many of these comorbidities. Unfortunately, a complete history may be unobtainable. The physiologic changes associated with vascular disease and these other problems are likely to be greater in the patient presenting for emergency surgery (e.g., wider blood pressure swings, more third spacing). Risk of aspiration is significantly higher. Transfusion requirements are also higher. These patients are more likely to require postoperative ventilation and have other complications.

Preventative Measures

Most preventative measures center around optimizing preoperative status. Complete understanding of the preoperative comorbidities and their physiology is critical (see Chapter 6). Bronchodilators, diuresis, antiarrhythmics, and so on must be optimized. Smoking cessation is beneficial. Intraoperative and postoperative continuation of these treatment modalities is also important.

Physiologic Changes Associated with Surgery

Vascular surgery encompasses procedures in nearly every part of the body. Each anatomic location has particular associated issues.[12]

Carotid endarterectomy is the second most commonly performed procedure in the United States. Most patients should be awake and extubated at the end of the case to allow neurologic evaluation. Blood pressure may be labile and can contribute to postoperative bleeding.

Thoracic vascular procedures include aortic aneurysms and dissections. Other vessels may also require operative repair. These cases are associated with a variety of pulmonary issues in each phase of the procedure (preoperatively, intraoperatively, postoperatively). Preoperative considerations have been previously discussed (Chapters 5 and 6). Intraoperatively, there is generally a need for one-lung ventilation if full cardiopulmonary bypass is not used. Postoperatively, the incision (thoracotomy or sternotomy) is a source of significant pain, and most patients splint significantly. Pain and splinting contribute to a decrease in V_T, which may not be offset by an increase in respiratory rate. Most patients require mechanical ventilation for a period ranging from hours to days.

Abdominal vascular surgery, whether for aneurysms or occlusive disease, is generally associated with an extensive midline or paramedian incision. Even with a retroperitoneal approach, there is significant pain, which extends into the upper abdomen, contributing to decreased V_T. There may be extensive third-space losses, which may preclude early extubation. A small percentage of patients require mechanical ventilation for more than 24 hours. Postoperative epidural use may facilitate early extubation, ambulation, and maximal pulmonary function.

Peripheral vascular surgery includes procedures on both arteries and veins. Most arterial procedures involve a form of infrainguinal bypass (e.g., femoral-femoral, femoral-distal). Venous procedures involve both the arms and legs. Patients may have poor exercise tolerance and a relatively sedentary lifestyle, contributing to a preoperative decrease in pulmonary function. Epidural pain management may facilitate early ambulation and maximize pulmonary function after surgery.

Physiologic Changes Associated with Anesthesia

Whether the patient is asleep or awake, lung volumes decrease with supine positioning and V/Q mismatch increases. Supine positioning decreases FRC as much as 10% to 15%. General anesthesia decreases FRC by an additional 5% to 10% within 10 minutes of the commencement of anesthesia. PEEP or continuous positive airway pressure (CPAP) may reverse this decrease in the FRC, but the effects do not continue after extubation. This decrease in FRC persists up to 2 weeks after surgery. FRC decreases even with regional techniques.

Anesthesia and surgery decrease vital capacity (VC) by 25% to 50% and 1 to 2 weeks are required for VC to return to normal. Expiratory reserve volume can decrease by up to 60% for upper abdominal procedures and 25% for lower abdominal procedures. V_T decreases 20% within 24 hours of surgery and does not return to normal for 1 to 2 weeks.[13-15]

Need for Prolonged Postoperative Ventilation

Patients may need mechanical ventilation for a variety of reasons, which can be considered in two broad categories: physiologic and surgical. Increased work of breathing, acidosis (metabolic and/or respiratory), and inadequate oxygenation are the most common indications for intubation and mechanical ventilation. Less often, hemodynamic compromise is also an indication. There are additional indications that are specific to the postoperative patient, including the need for sedation to protect a vascular repair and anticipated fluid shifts that may produce pulmonary edema. Concerns about the potential need for reoperation may also be appropriate indications for short-term postoperative mechanical ventilation.

Fast-Tracking

The term *fast tracking* generally refers to the planned early extubation of the postoperative patient. Although the term and approach are used most commonly in reference to cardiac surgery patients, the concept applies to other surgeries.

The fast-track patient is usually extubated within hours after completion of surgery, if not in the operating room. Changes in anesthetic techniques (lower total doses of anesthetic agents, particularly of opioids, and the use of shorter acting agents) as well as postoperative management (less sedation and a willingness to extubate at night) are required for successful early extubation. Close attention to pain management is critical, and regional techniques can be helpful (see Chapter 19). Advantages of fast-tracking include the ability to assess neurologic status, earlier ambulation (decreased risk of deep venous thrombosis, pneumonia), patients' satisfaction, and shorter stay in the intensive care unit (ICU). The risks include precipitation of complications including the need for reintubation.[16-19]

A variety of studies in the cardiac population have identified factors associated with "prolonged" postoperative ventilation—ventilation for 4 or more days—which include female gender, increasing age, low body mass index (perhaps related to malnutrition or cachexia), preexisting renal failure, coronary artery disease, COPD, prior stroke, preoperative ventilation, intra-aortic balloon pump, or use of pressors or inotropes.[20]

Regional Anesthesia

Most vascular procedures are amenable to regional anesthesia, either as the primary anesthetic technique or as an adjunct (see Chapter 9). Use of such techniques can facilitate the rapid extubation of patients in addition to promoting early ambulation and minimizing postoperative complications (e.g., pneumonia).

Goals of Mechanical Ventilation

Oxygenation

Postoperative ventilation of the vascular surgery patient initially uses an increased fraction of inspired oxygen (F_IO_2) (50% to 100%) to compensate for altered ventilation-perfusion matching. The F_IO_2 can usually be decreased below 0.5 within the first few hours. Pulse oximetry, rather than arterial blood gases, can be used to monitor the decreasing F_IO_2.

Prolonged use of a high F_IO_2 (greater than 70% to 80%) can produce pulmonary oxygen toxicity, partly by providing a source for free radical formation, particularly in patients who have been hypotensive or septic. It is currently impossible to distinguish between the toxic effects of a high F_IO_2 and other mediators of lung injury. Absorption atelectasis at high F_IO_2 (over 0.95) is also of concern, particularly in the patient who already has a loss of FRC.

Minute Ventilation

Whether using a volume preset mode or a pressure preset mode, there must be a minute ventilation goal for each patient. This goal must take into account the patient's underlying diseases. For most patients the goal should be normocapnia and normal pH. There are two components that determine the minute ventilation: V_T and rate. Cookbook ventilator settings, such as a V_T of 10 mL/kg and a rate of 10, may be inadequate and lead to acidemia or alkalemia, depending upon the patient. A typical minute ventilation (V_E) is 5 L/min in the normal patient. Patients with COPD typically require 8 to 12 L/min; acute respiratory distress syndrome (ARDS) or sepsis can increase this demand to 15 to 20 L/min.

DETERMINING RESPIRATORY RATE. Optimal respiratory rate is affected by both restrictive and obstructive lung disease. In the normal patient an initial ventilator rate of 8 to 12 breaths per minute is appropriate, and the V_T and rate should be titrated to the arterial blood gases or end-tidal carbon dioxide pressure ($P_{ET}CO_2$). Although hypocapnia is frequently induced in the ventilated patient, it may also be seen in patients with early asthma or acute lung injury.[21] Restrictive lung disease requires a higher rate to compensate for the smaller V_T; obstructive lung disease may require a low rate to allow for prolonged exhalation and prevent hyperinflation.

DETERMINING TIDAL VOLUME. In the otherwise normal patient, an initial V_T of 8 to 10 mL/kg is appropriate. However, this can lead to hyperinflation and damage of *normal* lung units in some patients. In general, patients with restrictive disease require smaller volumes; those with obstructive disease require normal volumes. In patients with acute lung injury, the aerated and recruitable lung is much smaller than normal so that when a "normal" V_T is used, the airway pressure in those units is much higher. Plateau pressures over 35 cmH_2O should be avoided, as the normal lung is maximally distended at this pressure.

Role of peak pressure limits. In volume modes, there is generally a peak pressure pop-off valve; the full V_T is *not* delivered if the peak inspiratory pressure (PIP) exceeds the set pop-off pressure. This limit can help to prevent barotrauma. Although pressure is generally the measured variable, as with hemodynamics, the real variable is the end-expiratory *volume*, which causes alveolar overdistention.

DETERMINING PEAK INSPIRATORY PRESSURE. When using pressure modes, the goal is to set a pressure that generates the desired V_T. Compliance is measured as the change in lung volume per unit change in applied pressure and is the reciprocal of elastance. Given a fixed end-inspiratory pressure, variations in compliance can cause wide variations in the delivered V_T. Compliance changes are a particular problem in the patient with a rapidly changing clinical course.

A major difference between pressure and volume modes is the inspiratory flow pattern. During pressure control modes, inspiratory pressure is constant and maximal flow occurs during the initial portion of the inspiratory cycle. During volume control modes, inspiratory flow is constant and maximal pressure occurs at the end of the respiratory cycle (when a constant flow pattern is used).

Endotracheal tube compensation. The endotracheal tube (ETT) is the narrowest component of the connection between patient and ventilator. Hence, the ETT acts as a large flow-dependent resistor; every form of ventilatory assist has to counterbalance this mechanical effect.

The flow pattern changes from laminar to turbulent as the flow rate is increased. The critical flow rates (at which flow becomes turbulent) range up to about 400 mL/sec in an adult ETT of 9 mm internal diameter. Typical inspiratory flow rate on a ventilator is 60,000 mL/sec. Thus, at the flow rates and respiratory frequencies usually occurring during assisted spontaneous breathing, the flow is predominantly turbulent, explaining the curvilinear pressure-flow relationship.[22]

Compensation for the resistance of the ETT can be provided by pressure support. Some ventilators have an automatic tube compensation specifically designed to offset this tube resistance.

Positive End-Expiratory Pressure

PEEP can be applied in any of the modes of ventilation. It provides a constant supra-atmospheric pressure throughout exhalation and can improve oxygenation by recruiting and stenting open alveolar units. CPAP is the provision of supra-atmospheric pressure throughout the entire respiratory cycle in the spontaneously breathing patient.

The recruitment of alveoli with PEEP decreases intrapulmonary shunting, thus V/Q matching is improved. PEEP may improve oxygenation by redistributing intra-alveolar edema, although PEEP does *not* drive fluid out of the alveoli. PEEP also increases FRC toward normal.

PEEP can decrease cardiac output, predominantly by decreasing venous return. Pulmonary vascular resistance may also increase. Cardiac contractility and rate are generally not affected. These effects are particularly exaggerated during hypovolemia. PEEP can also affect hemodynamic measurements, including pulmonary artery occlusion pressure.

PEEP can be extrinsic (set on the ventilator) or intrinsic (generated within the lungs); intrinsic PEEP (PEEPi, auto-PEEP) is more likely with short expiratory times and in patients with underlying lung disease, particularly COPD. Although it is intrinsic to the patient, it causes the same pulmonary and cardiovascular effects as PEEP. The adverse hemodynamic effects of PEEP are increased in patients with (overly) compliant lungs, such as patients with emphysema. Clinical evidence of auto-PEEP includes breath stacking. Although most often seen in patients with chronic airflow obstruction, it may also be seen in those with an increased V_T or an inadequate expiratory time.

Optimal PEEP is typically determined by oxygenation, but lung mechanics are the best (but more difficult) determinant. The most beneficial effects of PEEP occur when it is titrated to maximize lung compliance and alveolar recruitment. Plotting pressure versus lung volume during positive-pressure ventilation produces a sigmoidal curve. The lower inflection point defines an area of maximum compliance change; above this point most alveoli remain open. Setting a PEEP above this value serves to keep these alveoli recruited, and shear stress caused by cyclic collapse and reopening of the alveolar units is minimized. An upper inflection point defines an area of minimum compliance change, where alveoli are maximally inflated without overdistention. The risk of barotrauma or volutrauma is significantly increased at this point. Figure 18-1 demonstrates a typical pressure-volume curve.[23-26]

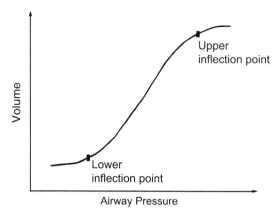

FIGURE 18-1 Static pressure-volume curve (positive end-expiratory pressure inflection points). The lower inflection point of this static pressure-volume curve represents the pressure below which alveoli collapse. The upper inflection point represents the pressure above which alveoli become overdistended.

Modes of Ventilation

All modern ventilators are positive-pressure ventilators. A supra-atmospheric pressure is generated, which creates a gradient that pushes air into the lungs. No matter what mode is used, there are several variables that may be set; the modes are generally divided into two groups depending on whether the volume or the peak pressure is preset. The most common of these modes are discussed in the following sections. Other variables may include the respiratory frequency, the inspiratory time, and the inspiratory flow pattern.

In addition, all modern ventilators contain at least one microprocessor that facilitates control and trending. It is the microprocessor capabilities that have made many of the modern modes possible. Each manufacturer has a (proprietary) set of algorithms that determine triggering timing, triggering sensitivity, flow characteristics, and so on.[27-30]

Many of these algorithms are designed to make ventilators function more like the native pulmonary system. The use of linear models to describe the function of organ systems is limited at best. Although such linear systems involve gross oversimplifications, they can be useful in understanding the mechanical properties of the respiratory system.

Whether the volume or pressure is set, the goal is to achieve a certain minute volume within a given pressure limit. Boyle's law defines the relationship between pressure and volume of a confined gas: $V \times P = $ constant. In this case, the constant is defined by the elastance and resistance of the lung (and is not necessarily constant over time). Elastance is the term used to describe the tendency of the lungs and chest wall to collapse. Compliance is the inverse of elastance and is calculated by dividing the V_T by the difference between the plateau pressure and PEEP. Typical compliance is 80 to 100 mL/cmH_2O; it is reduced to 40 to 60 mL/cmH_2O in the postoperative patient and may be as low as 20 mL/cmH_2O in the patient with respiratory disease. Resistance is the limitation in flow imposed by the ETT and the large airways. It is calculated by dividing the difference between the peak and plateau pressures by the flow.

No matter what mode is selected, three things must be set: breath initiation, limiting target, and breath cessation.

The obvious dichotomy is the limiting target, either a set volume or a set pressure. Breath initiation can be pressure (spontaneous) or time (mechanical) driven, or a combination; breath cessation can be determined by pressure, volume, time, or flow (Table 18-1).

Volume Modes

CONTROLLED MECHANICAL VENTILATION. Controlled mechanical ventilation (CMV) is the simplest of the modes. It is used on most anesthesia machines and some transport ventilators. Rate and V_T are set. The inspiratory flow or inspiratory/expiratory (I/E) ratio is also preset. The machine delivers the set volume at the set rate; the patient is unable to breathe at any other time. Thus, it requires significant sedation in awake patients. Figure 18-2 shows the pressure-time loops for the volume modes.

ASSIST-CONTROL VENTILATION. Assist control (AC) is a patient-triggered mode with a controlled backup ventilation mode. Both a rate and V_T are set. Breaths are delivered when either (1) the patient triggers the ventilator by attempting to inspire or (2) the machine does not sense a breath within the preselected time period. If the patient's respiratory drive is sufficient, all breaths may be triggered spontaneously. Each breath delivered has the set V_T. If the patient inhales during the exhalation phase, a second breath is delivered; breath stacking can easily occur. Approximately one third of the work of breathing may be done by the patient during AC ventilation.

INTERMITTENT MANDATORY VENTILATION. Intermittent mandatory ventilation (IMV) is a mode that allows both spontaneous ventilation and volume-preset assisted ventilation. By synchronizing the machine-triggered breaths with the spontaneous breaths, the delivery of a second (machine-driven) breath during exhalation is prevented, thus synchronized IMV or SIMV. The triggering mechanism is much like that of a sensing pacemaker. Although algorithms vary, the microprocessor sets a refractory period after each breath, the duration of which is determined by the set rate. After that period, the machine is in a "sensitive" period, and if the patient does not spontaneously trigger a breath, the machine triggers a breath.

MANDATORY MINUTE VENTILATION. Originally described by Hewlett et al in 1977 as a weaning mode, mandatory minute ventilation (MMV) guarantees a preselected minute volume.[31]

A. Controlled Mechanical Ventilation (CMV)

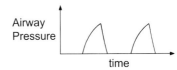

B. Assist-Control Ventilation (AC)

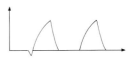

C. Intermittent Mandatory Ventilation (IMV) with PEEP

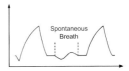

D. Mandatory Minute Ventilation (MMV) with PEEP

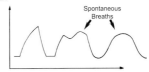

FIGURE 18-2 Volume-mode pressure-time loops. **A,** Controlled mechanical ventilation. Note that each breath appears identical. **B,** Assist-control ventilation. The first breath is spontaneously triggered (note the downward initial inflection). **C,** Intermittent mandatory ventilation with positive end-expiratory pressure. The first breath is spontaneously triggered and assisted, the second is spontaneous, and the third is controlled. **D,** Mandatory minute ventilation. The first breath is machine driven, the second occurs as the patient begins to start spontaneous breathing, and the last is fully spontaneous ventilation.

If the patient spontaneously generates the minute volume, the machine does not initiate a breath. Various algorithms are used to determine how often the patient breathes and the V_T. Trend data can be reviewed to determine what percentage of time the patient is being mechanically ventilated. This mode can be useful in weaning. However, the patient can become quite fatigued

---

TABLE 18-1

Modes of Ventilation

Mode	Breath Initiation	Limiting Target	Breath Cessation	Comments
CMV	Mechanical timer		Time	
AC	Mechanical timer and spontaneous flow trigger or spontaneous pressure trigger	Volume	Volume or time or pressure pop-off	I/E set
SIMV	Synchronized mechanical timer and spontaneous flow trigger or spontaneous pressure trigger		Volume or time or pressure pop-off	
MMV	Mechanical timer and/or spontaneous flow trigger or spontaneous pressure trigger		Volume or time	
PC	Mechanical timer	Pressure	Time	Inspiratory time is set
PS	Spontaneous flow trigger or spontaneous pressure trigger		Flow	Typically 25% of maximal flow will stop PS
CPAP	Spontaneous		None (continuous)	

AC, assist control; CMV, controlled mechanical ventilation; CPAP, continuous positive airway pressure; I/E, inspiratory/expiratory ratio; MMV, mandatory minute ventilation; PC, pressure control; PS, pressure support; SIMV, synchronized intermittent mandatory ventilation.

if the spontaneous V_T falls and the spontaneous respiratory rate increases to maintain V_E.

Pressure Modes

PRESSURE CONTROL. Pressure control (PC) uses a set PIP as well as a set rate and inspiratory time to determine the delivered V_T. Delivered volume is dependent on lung compliance and can be quite variable if the compliance is rapidly changing. Although it has long been the preferred mode for neonates, it has been more difficult to use in adults because of the variable V_T. PC minimizes the PIP for a given V_T, and the inspiratory flow pattern may be beneficial in preventing barotrauma. Figure 18-3 shows the pressure-time loops for the pressure modes.

PRESSURE SUPPORT. Pressure support (PS) may be used independently or in conjunction with the volume modes. It is a mode that can optimize muscle work, encouraging reconditioning and preventing atrophy, yet avoiding fatigue of the respiratory muscles.

PS uses a flow trigger. The patient's inspiratory effort triggers an increase in the airway pressure, which persists until the preset support condition is met. The breath lasts as long as the patient continues to inspire; exhalation occurs when inspiratory flow drops below a certain amount (either a percentage of maximum flow or a fixed L/min). Setting a higher pressure support

level increases the augmented V_T. A variety of mechanisms are used to determine the initial rapid flow rate of the ventilator to achieve the PS value, including pressure slope control (Viasys Healthcare, Palm Springs, CA), inspiratory rise time control (Siemens Elema AB, Solna, Sweden), or percentage inspiratory time control (Drägerwerk, Lübeck, Germany). The delivered V_T during PS is determined by the patient's spontaneous inspiratory time and the resistance and compliance of the patient's respiratory system.

CONTINUOUS POSITIVE AIRWAY PRESSURE. CPAP sets a continuous (both inspiratory and expiratory) positive airway pressure that may be generated by a variety of expiratory pressure valves or demand flow valves. These valves create a preselected resistance on the expiratory limb of the ventilator circuit. Airflow is adjusted to maintain this set pressure. CPAP is typically set between 5 to 10 cmH$_2$O and is rarely over 15 to 18 cmH$_2$O. It is typically used as a weaning method and can also be used noninvasively.

AIRWAY PRESSURE RELEASE VENTILATION. Airway pressure release ventilation (APRV) involves the intermittent *decrease* in airway pressure from the preselected CPAP. This mode was developed to minimize barotrauma caused by high PIPs. It can be used in spontaneously breathing patients. Increasing the baseline airway pressure improves oxygenation, and the timed release facilitates carbon dioxide removal.

APRV requires a continuous flow generator (Down's flow or similar) and a low-flow threshold pressure valve on the expiratory limb. The valve solenoid opens at preset intervals, abruptly dropping the airway pressure. The amount of CPAP required to support this mode is 1.5 to 2 times that required in IMV.

Noninvasive Modes

Noninvasive modes of ventilatory support provide no control of the airway. Thus, they are not indicated for patients who are unable to control their airway spontaneously. Patients must be able to coordinate spontaneous breathing with an external source of positive pressure and be able to keep their mouth closed if a nasal mask is used.

CONTINUOUS POSITIVE AIRWAY PRESSURE. CPAP by either nasal or full face mask improves oxygenation by recruiting atelectatic alveoli, which increases FRC above the closing volume. It also improves pulmonary compliance and reduces the work of breathing. In addition, in patients with PEEPi, the pressure gradient between the alveoli and the mouth at end-expiration is reduced, thus minimizing the work required to initiate airflow during inspiration. An obstructive component, such as that found in sleep apnea, is also minimized.

In the patient with congestive heart failure, the reduction in venous return caused by CPAP may decrease pulmonary edema and improve cardiac function by unloading the failing left ventricle and decreasing the ventricular transmural pressure.[32]

BILEVEL POSITIVE AIRWAY PRESSURE. Bilevel positive airway pressure (BiPAP) involves the use of differential positive airway pressure augmentation. Inspiratory (iPAP) and expiratory (ePAP) pressures are set, typically with the iPAP 5 to 10 cmH$_2$O above the ePAP. Both inspiratory and expiratory lung volumes are augmented. FRC is increased as with CPAP; the work of breathing is decreased, as the inspiratory muscles do not need to generate as much of a negative pleural pressure. This mode

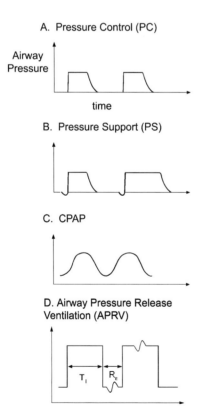

FIGURE 18-3 Pressure-mode pressure-time loops. **A,** Pressure control. Note that each breath is identical. **B,** Pressure support (PS). Note the variation in duration of the breath. The duration of the inspiratory effort determines the tidal volume. **C,** Continuous positive airway pressure (CPAP) with PS. The sinusoidal appearance is typical of spontaneous ventilation. **D,** Airway pressure release ventilation. The patient may breathe spontaneously at either pressure. The relatively high CPAP is maintained for time T$_I$ (equivalent to the inspiratory time) and released for time R$_E$ (the release expiratory time).

can be useful in the patient with an exacerbation of COPD or acute cardiogenic pulmonary edema.[32]

Several machines can provide BiPAP, including most modern ventilators (using PS for the iPAP and CPAP for the ePAP). For freestanding systems the oxygen is bled into the main inspiratory line and cannot provide F_IO_2 over 0.4. The patient who has a high oxygen requirement may need to receive BiPAP from a ventilator.

BiPAP also has a role in the immediate postextubation period, particularly in the patient with underlying COPD. Nearly 25% of all patients who are intubated for more than 48 hours have some level of respiratory distress, and of these patients up to two thirds require reintubation.[33] The studies that have looked at BiPAP in patients with COPD exacerbations have shown a decreased need for mechanical ventilation, a decreased duration of mechanical ventilation, as well as a decreased risk of reintubation after extubation.[34-36] This advantage, however, is less distinct in patients without chronic lung disease.[33]

Weaning and Extubation

There are no objective criteria for determining when to start weaning. Several indices may be used to determine whether the patient is ready for extubation. Despite such tools, physicians do not accurately predict whether mechanical ventilation can be successfully discontinued. As many as 50% of patients who self-extubate do not need reintubation.[37]

Most important, the original reason for ventilation must be resolved. It is important to prepare the patient psychologically, before surgery if possible, for the process. It is unwise to impose additional cardiac stress in patients with ischemic cardiac disease. Mental status must be such that the patient is able to participate in the process and protect the airway if extubated.[23,38-42]

Weaning Parameters

A variety of physiologic indices are available to predict the ability to extubate. They use different objective measurements and have different definitions of success or failure. In general, most agree that success is a patient who is extubated for at least 24 hours. The failure criteria include a variety of measured and observed values (Table 18-2).

Although there is controversy about the "best" weaning method, most would agree that weaning trials should be performed regularly (each day) until the patient is extubated. There is extensive literature about standardized trial protocols, including earlier extubation in these patients.[37,38,41,43] These protocols usually use preliminary measurements to determine whether the patient is ready to attempt a trial (maximal inspiratory force [MIF], maximal V_T) and then commence a spontaneous breathing trial that lasts until the patient is extubated or becomes fatigued. Figure 18-4 shows a sample weaning parameters form (Table 18-3).

Changes upon Cessation of Positive Pressure

Because positive pressure and PEEP do contribute to the redistribution of intra-alveolar edema, removal of these may lead to an apparent increase in pulmonary edema. The removal of positive pressure may increase venous return, contributing to pulmonary edema. Lung volume decreases as well.

Respiratory Complications

In general, complications of mechanical ventilation fall into three major groups: (1) mechanical, (2) psychological, and (3) medical. The mechanical complications include problems associated with intubation and extubation, problems with the ETT, or problems in operation of the ventilator. The psychological complications are varied but include dependence. The medical complications can be significant and are discussed in greater detail.

Pulmonary Edema

Pulmonary edema is a frequently seen postoperative complication. It is considered to be more common in those with underlying coronary artery disease; there are neurogenic causes as well. The clinical manifestations of *postoperative* pulmonary edema are not well defined.

Arieff examined more than 8000 major inpatient operations and found an overall incidence of pulmonary edema of 7.6%; approximately two thirds of these patients had a comorbidity (acute myocardial infarction, acute renal failure, acute gastrointestinal bleed, stroke, pneumonia, pulmonary embolus, or hyponatremia).[44]

Contributing to this problem is difficulty in assessing third-space losses despite a variety of objective assessments. Patients

TABLE 18-2
Weaning Criteria—Predictors of Failure

Objective criteria	$Paco_2 \geq 50$ mmHg OR Increase in $Paco_2 \geq 8$ mmHg $pH \leq 7.33$ OR Decrease in $pH \geq 0.07$ $Pao_2 \leq 60$ mmHg ($Fio_2 \geq 0.5$)
Subjective criteria	Diaphoresis Increasing respiratory effort (excessive work of breathing) Tachycardia Arrhythmias Hypotension Poor nutritional status, including magnesium and phosphate deficiencies

Fio_2, fraction of inspired oxygen; $Paco_2$, partial pressure of carbon dioxide in arterial blood.

TABLE 18-3
Weaning Criteria—Predictors of Success

	Value
Minute ventilation (L/min)	$\leq 10-15$
Tidal volume (mL)	≥ 325
Tidal volume/weight (mL/kg)	$\geq 4-5$
Vital capacity (mL/kg)	$\geq 10-15$
Respiratory frequency (breaths/min)	$\leq 25-38$
Frequency/tidal volume ratio (breaths/min/L) "rapid/shallow" index	≤ 105
Maximum inspiratory pressure (cmH$_2$O)	$\leq -30-15$
Dynamic compliance (mL/cmH$_2$O)	≥ 22
Static compliance (mL/cmH$_2$O)	≥ 33
Pao_2/Pao_2 ratio	≥ 0.35

Pao_2, partial pressure of oxygen in arterial blood.

| Addressograph Stamp - Patient Name, Medical Record Number | **WEANING ASSESSMENT CONSULTATION** |

Date:_____   Time:_____   Unit:_____   Days Post-Intubation:_____

Diagnosis:_____   Airway size/diameter:_____   Original Intubation Indication:_____

Screen #1: GENERAL / SUBJECTIVE OVERVIEW:

1. Hemodynamic stability	❏Unstable	❏Stable with vasopressors	❏Stable
2. Fluid balance	❏Fluid (+) _____L	❏Fluid (−) _____L	❏Euvolemic
3. Metabolic demand factors	❏Febrile	❏Afebrile	❏Other_____
4. Chest x-ray	❏Diffuse infiltrates	❏Focal infiltrates	❏Clear
5. Sedation/Analgesia	❏IV sed._____	❏IV analgesia_____	❏PRN_____
6. Spontaneous respiratory pattern	❏Absent	❏Asynchronous	❏Normal
7. Cough reflex	❏Absent	❏Weak with suction	❏Strong
8. Secretion characteristics	❏Thick	❏Thin	❏Quantity_____
9. Neuro status/responsiveness	❏Unresponsive	❏Somnolent	❏Alert & oriented

Screen #2: OXYGENATION / VENTILATION CRITERIA:

1. PaO_2/FiO_2:_____ (>200)   2. FiO_2____ (<.60)   3. PEEP____ (<10)

Comparative RSBI

ABG: _____ Date:_____ Time:____   Current PS_____ RR/V_T ____/____ RSBI_____ V_E_____

Vent settings:_____   PS 5 cm H_2O RR/V_T ____/____ RSBI_____ V_E_____

ASSESSMENT / SCREENING RECOMMENDATIONS:

❏ **Patient meets criteria for Spontaneous Breathing Trial (SBT)**   ❏ **Patient does not meet criteria for SBT**

Physician Contact (Time)_____

SPONTANEOUS BREATHING TRIAL (SBT)   *Performed on PSV @_____cm H_2O*

Start Time:_____   Stop Time:_____   Duration:_____

RSBI_____   RSBI_____

V_E_____ V_E_____   Post Trial ABG: _____

Respiratory Muscle Strength:

Maximum inspiratory force: ❏ Pre-Trial   ❏ Post-Trial   ❏ Not Assessed

---

SBT OUTCOME / RECOMMENDATIONS:

❏ **Patient Passed SBT**   ❏ **Patient failed SBT**

Recommendation / Comments:_____

Respiratory Care Services   Performed and Reported by: _____

White - Medical Records   **Canary** - Respiratory Care Services

FIGURE 18-4 Sample weaning parameters form.

with preexisting left ventricular dysfunction or renal failure may develop pulmonary edema with smaller changes in intravascular volume. There is a poor correlation of the chest radiograph with physiologic status. Some authors feel that a pulmonary artery catheter is necessary to distinguish between cardiogenic and low-pressure pulmonary edema in postoperative patients.[45]

Pleural Effusion

The most common cause of pleural effusion in the United States is congestive heart failure, with an estimated annual incidence of 500,000. Coronary artery bypass surgery is sixth, with an estimated incidence of 60,000.[46]

Most postoperative effusions are transudative, related to a relative imbalance between hydrostatic and oncotic pressures. As with pulmonary edema, intraoperative and postoperative fluid administration may contribute to the development of the problem. Initial management should focus on fluid restriction and diuresis if the patient has stable hemodynamics and renal function.

Pleural effusions are frequently seen after cardiac surgery. Nearly half of all patients who undergo coronary artery bypass grafting develop pleural effusion, generally on the left side after internal mammary artery dissection. Most of these resolve spontaneously.[47] The frequency of effusions after other types of surgery is poorly defined.

Pneumonia

Ventilator-associated pneumonia (VAP) is the second most common nosocomial infection (after urinary tract infections) in hospitalized patients; it is the most common infection in the ICU. Frequency ranges from approximately 25% to 50% of all ventilated patients. It is the greatest single influence on length of stay in the ICU, length of stay in the hospital, and number of ventilator days.[48,49]

There are many risk factors for VAP. Among the most significant are emergent intubation (and reintubation), aspiration, mechanical ventilation lasting more than 72 hours, major surgery, COPD, and frequent changes of ventilator circuits (<48 hours). Patients who require reintubation have a 47% rate of VAP, compared with 10% in those who do not.[48] In addition, antibiotics add to the risk of all pneumonias, particularly for resistant organisms such as *Pseudomonas aeruginosa*.

Perhaps the greatest obstacle is the lack of consistent diagnosis of VAP. The Centers for Disease Control has separate parameters, as does the American Thoracic Society.[50,51] An International Conference Consensus Panel was formed in 2001 to discuss strategies for diagnosis and treatment (Table 18-4).[52]

There has been interest in minimizing aspiration of oral and upper airway secretions that may contribute to VAP. Pooling of secretions on the ETT cuff has been documented, and a specially designed ETT, with a subglottic suction port, has been used. One study showed a difference in incidence of 4.1% versus 17.9%, which was not statistically significant, although the calculated incidence based upon episodes per 1000 ventilator days was.[53]

Ventilator-Induced Lung Injury

Lung injury may be caused or extended by the process of mechanical ventilation. Ventilator-induced lung injury is perhaps better described as volutrauma rather than barotrauma.

TABLE 18-4

Definition of Ventilator-Associated Pneumonia

CDC (A)[50]	Rales or dullness on examination
	AND any of the following:
	    Purulent or changed sputum
	    Positive blood cultures
	    Pathogen in a sputum specimen obtained by transtracheal aspirate, bronchial brushing, or biopsy

CDC (B)	Chest x-ray with new or progressive infiltrate or consolidation or cavitation or effusion
	AND any of the following:
	    Purulent or changed sputum
	    Positive blood cultures
	    Pathogen in a sputum specimen obtained by transtracheal aspirate, bronchial brushing, or biopsy
	    Isolation of virus or vital antigen in respiratory secretions
	    Diagnostic antibody titers (acute IgM or convalescent IgG)
	    Histopathologic evidence of pneumonia

ATS (1995)[51]
"Severe" hospital acquired pneumonia
	Admission to the intensive care unit
	Respiratory failure, defined as the need for mechanical ventilation or the need for >35% oxygen to maintain an arterial oxygen saturation >90%
	Rapid radiographic progression, multilobar pneumonia, or cavitation of a lung infiltrate
	Evidence of severe sepsis with hypotension and/or end-organ dysfunction:
	    Shock (systolic blood pressure < 90 mmHg or diastolic blood pressure < 60 mmHg)
	    Requirement for vasopressors for more than 4 hr
	    Urine output < 20 mL/hr or total urine output < 80 mL in 4 hr (unless another explanation is available)
	    Acute renal failure requiring dialysis

Consensus Group[52]	New, persistent pulmonary infiltrates not otherwise explained on chest x-ray
	AND At least two of the following:
	    T > 38.0°C
	    WBC > 10,000 cells/mL
	    Purulent respiratory secretions

ATSD, American Thoracic Society; CDC, Centers for Disease Control; IgM, immunoglobulin M; T, temperature; WBC, white blood count.

Injury from alveolar overdistention may be seen even with relatively low PIPs. Normal lung is maximally distended when the transpulmonary pressure (expiratory airway pressure less the pleural pressure) is 30 to 35 cmH$_2$O. This transpulmonary pressure is the equivalent of the plateau pressure (Pplat).[54] Incidence of barotrauma is higher in groups of patients with Pplat greater than 35 cmH$_2$O, especially if compliance is less than 30 mL/cmH$_2$O.[55]

Computed tomography of the lungs in ARDS typically reveals heterogeneous intraparenchymal disease. Approximately one third of the lung is unaerated, one third is poorly aerated, and one third is normally aerated. The last subset is most susceptible to alveolar overdistention, as it is the most compliant. Localized overdistention can be prevented not only by decreasing V$_T$ and PIPs but also by measures that decrease overall compliance or increase the pleural pressure (such as strapping the thorax).[56,57]

Acute Respiratory Distress Syndrome

ARDS is a spectrum of disease with local and systemic manifestations, defined by four criteria: acute onset (24 to 48 hours after the precipitant), disturbances in oxygenation ($Pao_2/F_iO_2 <$ 200), bilateral diffuse infiltrates on chest radiograph, and absence of left-sided heart failure.[58,59]

ARDS can be classified by clinical phases or by pathophysiology. The clinical phases begin with the acute injury, followed by a latent period lasting hours to days. This phase is followed by acute respiratory failure, lasting days to a week. The final clinical phase is severe physiologic abnormalities. The pathologic phases are characterized by an initial exudative picture, followed by fibroproliferation (organization), and ending with fibrosis, scarring, and cyst formation.[25]

Unfortunately, the acute and latent clinical phases are often not appreciated until the acute respiratory failure phase has commenced. In addition, the varied and "staggered" clinical response may make the phases indistinguishable, and not all cases of ARDS progress in a stepwise fashion. Furthermore, the rapidity of transition from one phase to another may preclude any reasonable treatment time frame.

The distinct clinical and pathophysiologic phases would seem to imply focused treatment for different phases. This understanding has fostered ongoing clinical trials. In 1994 the ARDS network (ARDSnet) was formed with the goal of carrying out multicenter trials to develop effective therapy for ARDS. The initial project was determining a unified "best" ventilation strategy. Therapeutic goals were redefined to emphasize protection of the lung from excessive stretch; pH and pCO_2 became secondary goals. Ventilation with a lower volume (6 mL/kg ideal body weight) and lower plateau pressures (<30 cmH$_2$O) was demonstrated to decrease mortality as well as ventilator time (Table 18-5).[60] Ongoing studies include evaluation of fluids and use of pulmonary artery catheters (the Fluids and Catheters Treatment Trial [FACTT]) and the use of steroids in *late* (over 1 week) ARDS (the Late Steroid Rescue Study [LaSRS]).

Miscellaneous

Double-Lung Ventilation

Thoracotomy typically requires selective lung ventilation, most often using a double-lumen endotracheal tube (DLT). Although common in the operating room, the use of a DLT in the ICU may be precipitated by a difficult (operative) intubation or anticipated difficulty in replacing the DLT with a standard ETT. It may also be mandated by a variety of clinical situations, most often bronchopleural fistula and less commonly selective airway protection, unilateral lung disease, and severe bilateral lung disease. Despite the use of the DLT, one-lung or split-lung ventilation in the ICU is not common.

Both synchronous and asynchronous split ventilation of the two lungs have been described. Synchronous ventilation can be achieved by "slaving" two ventilators together, using an external control device, or manually setting the rate and relying on accurate internal timing devices. This synchrony can be alternating so that

TABLE 18-5

ARDSnet Ventilator Settings

Variable	Traditional Volumes	Lower Volumes
Ventilator mode	Volume assist control	
Initial tidal volume (mL/kg predicted body weight)	12	6
Plateau pressure (cmH$_2$O)	≤ 50	≤ 30
Ventilator rate setting to achieve a pH goal of 7.30 to 8.45 (breath/min)	6-35	
I/E ratio	1:1 – 1:3	
Oxygenation goal	Pao$_2$ 55-80mmHg or Sao$_2$ 88-95	
Allowable combinations of Fio2 and PEEP		0.3 and 5
		0.4 and 5
		0.4 and 8
		0.5 and 8
		0.5 and 10
		0.6 and 10
		0.7 and 10
		0.7 and 12
		0.7 and 14
		0.8 and 14
		0.9 and 14
		0.9 and 16
		0.9 and 18
		and 18
		and 20
		1.0 and 22
		1.0 and 24
Weaning	By pressure support; required by protocol when Fio2 ≤ 0.4	

Fio$_2$, fraction of inspired oxygen; I/E, inspiratory/expiratory ratio; Pao$_2$, partial pressure of oxygen in arterial blood; PEEP, positive end-expiratory pressure; Sao$_2$, oxygen saturation. Adapted from Acute Respiratory Distress Syndrome Network: *N Engl J Med* 342:1301, 2000.

one lung is in full inhalation while the other is in full exhalation. Alternatively, a single ventilator can be used with two circuits with a variety of devices to provide different flow and PEEP in each limb. Asynchronous ventilation occurs when two ventilators are used without any attempt to match respiratory rates.[61]

REFERENCES

1. Burns D, West TA, Hawkins K, et al: Immediate effects of positive end-expiratory pressure and low and high tidal volume ventilation upon gas exchange and compliance in patients with acute lung injury, *J Trauma* 51:1177 2001.
2. West JB: *Pulmonary pathophysiology, the essentials*, ed 5, Philadelphia, 1995, Lippincott Williams & Wilkins, 49.
3. National Institute of Health, National Heart, Lung and Blood Institute: *Expert panel report 2: guidelines for the diagnosis and management of asthma*, NIH Publication No. 97-4051, Bethesda, Md, 1997, US Department of Health and Human Services.
4. West JB: *Pulmonary pathophysiology, the essentials*, ed 5, Philadelphia, 1995, Lippincott Williams & Wilkins, 77.
5. West JB: *Pulmonary pathophysiology, the essentials*, ed 5, Philadelphia, 1995, Lippincott Williams & Wilkins, 115.
6. Mangano DT, Layug EL, Wallace A, et al: Effect of atenolol on mortality and cardiovascular morbidity after noncardiac surgery, *N Engl J Med* 335:1713, 1996.
7. Hunt SA, Baker DW, Chin MH, et al: A report of the American College of Cardiology/American Heart Association Task Force on Practice Guidelines (Committee to Revise the 1995 Guidelines for the Evaluation and

Management of Heart Failure), http://www.acc.org/clinical/guidelines/failure/hf_index.htm, accessed July 21, 2002.

8. Lin HJ, Wolf PA, Kelly-Hayes M, et al: Stroke severity in atrial fibrillation. The Framingham study, *Stroke* 27:1760, 1996.
9. Marriott HJL: *Practical electrocardiography*, ed 7, Baltimore, 1983, Williams & Wilkins, 322.
10. Gregoratos G, Cheitlin MD, Cinill A, et al: ACC/AHA guidelines for implantation of cardiac pacemakers and antiarrhythmia devices: a report of the American College of Cardiology/American Heart Association Task force on Practice Guidelines, *J Am Coll Cardiol* 31:1175, 1998.
11. Eagle KA, Berger PB, Calkins H, et al: ACC/AHA guideline update for perioperative cardiovascular evaluation for noncardiac surgery, http://www.acc.org/clinical/guidelines/perio/update/periupdate_index.htm, accessed July 2, 2002.
12. Fann JI, Mitchell RS, Peterson KL, Haddow GR: Vascular surgery. In Jaffe RA, Samuels SI (eds): *Anesthesiologist's manual of surgical procedures*, ed 2, Philadelphia, 1999, Lippincott Williams & Wilkins, 263.
13. Stock MC: Respiratory function in anesthesia. In Barash PG, Cullen BG, Stoelting RK (eds): *Clinical anesthesia*, ed 3, Philadelphia, 1997, Lippincott-Raven, 747.
14. Eisenkraft JB, Cohen E, Neustein SM: Anesthesia for thoracic surgery. In Barash PG, Cullen BG, Stoelting RK (eds): *Clinical anesthesia*, ed 3, Philadelphia, 1997, Lippincott-Raven, 769.
15. Ferguson MK: Preoperative assessment of pulmonary risk, *Chest* 115:58S, 1999.
16. Meade MO, Guyatt G, Butler R, et al: Trials comparing early vs late extubation following cardiovascular surgery, *Chest* 120(6 Suppl):445S, 2001.
17. Silbert BS, Santamaria JD, O'Brien JL, et al: Early extubation following coronary artery bypass surgery: a prospective randomized controlled trial, *Chest* 113:1481, 1998.
18. Doering LV, Esmailian F, Laks H: Perioperative predictors of ICU and hospital costs in coronary artery bypass graft surgery, *Chest* 118:736, 2000.
19. Wilmore DW, Kehlet H: Management of patients in fast-track surgery, *Br Med J* 322:473, 2001.
20. Branca P, McGaw P, Light RW, et al: Factors associated with prolonged mechanical ventilation following coronary artery bypass surgery, *Chest* 119:537, 2001.
21. Laffey JG, Kavanaugh BP: Hypocapnia, *N Engl J Med* 347:43, 2002.
22. Guttmann J, Haberthur C, Mols G: Automatic tube compensation, *Respir Care Clin North Am* 7:475, 2001.
23. Irwin RS, Hubmayr RD: Mechanical ventilation: weaning. In Irwin RS, Cerra FB, Rippe JM (eds): *Intensive care medicine*, ed 4, Philadelphia, 1999, Lippincott-Raven, 742.
24. Amato MBP, Barbas CSV, Meeiros DM, et al: Effect of a protective-ventilation strategy on mortality in the acute respiratory distress syndrome, *N Engl J Med* 338:347, 1998.
25. Weinacker AB, Vaszar LT: Acute respiratory distress syndrome: physiology and new management strategies, *Annu Rev Med* 52:221, 2001.
26. Ward NS, Lin DY, Nelson DL, et al: Successful determination of lower inflection point and maximal compliance in a population of patients with acute respiratory distress syndrome, *Crit Care Med* 30:963, 2002.
27. Banner MJ, Lampotang S, Blanch PB, Kirby RR: Mechanical ventilation. In Civetta JM, Taylor RW, Kirby RR (eds): *Critical care*, ed 3, Philadelphia, 1997, Lippincott Williams & Wilkins, 715.
28. Fitzgerald J: *Auto flow: 20 questions–20 answers*, Lübeck, Dräger Medizintechnik GmbH (undated).
29. *Evita 4 Intensive Care Ventilator, operating instructions software 4.n*, Lübeck, 2001, Dräger Medizintechnik GmbH.
30. *Servo Ventilator 300/300A operating manual 8.0/9.0*, Solna, Sweden, 1999.
31. Hewlett AM, Platt AS, Terry VG: Mandatory minute volume. A new concept in weaning from mechanical ventilation, *Anaesthesia* 32:163, 1977.
32. Kosowsky JM, Storrow AB, Carleton SC: Continuous and bilevel positive airway pressure in the treatment of acute cardiogenic pulmonary edema, *Am J Emerg Med* 18:91, 2000.
33. Keenan SP, Powers C, McCormack DG, Block G: Noninvasive positive-pressure ventilation for postextubation respiratory distress, *JAMA* 287:3238, 2002.
34. Brochard L, Mancebo J, Wysocki M, et al: Noninvasive ventilation for acute exacerbations of chronic obstructive pulmonary disease, *N Engl J Med* 333:817, 1995.

35. Kramer N, Meyer TJ, Meharg J, et al: Randomized, prospective trial of noninvasive-positive pressure-ventilation in acute respiratory failure, *Am J Respir Crit Care Med* 151:1799, 1995.
36. Girault C, Daudenthun I, Chevron V, et al: Noninvasive ventilation as a systemic extubation and weaning technique in acute-on-chronic respiratory failure, *Am J Respir Crit Care Med* 160:86, 1999.
37. Ely EW, Baker AM, Dunagan DP, et al: Effect on the duration of mechanical ventilation of identifying patients capable of breathing spontaneously, *N Engl J Med* 335:1864, 1996.
38. MacIntyre NR, Cook DJ, Ely EW Jr, et al: Evidence-based guidelines for weaning and discontinuing ventilatory support. A collective task force facilitated by the American College of Chest Physicians, the American Association for Respiratory Care; and the American College of Critical Care Medicine, *Chest* 120(6 Suppl):375S, 2001.
39. Dupont H, LePort Y, Paugam-Burtz C, et al Reintubation after planned extubation in surgical ICU patients: a case control study, *Intensive Care Med* 27:1875, 2001.
40. Keenan SP: Weaning protocols: here to stay, *Lancet* 359:186, 2002.
41. Khamiees M, Raju P, DeGirolamo A, et al: Predictors of extubation outcome in patients who have successfully completed a spontaneous breathing trial, *Chest* 120:1262, 2001.
42. Hess D: Ventilator modes used in weaning, *Chest* 120(6 Suppl):474S, 2001.
43. Marelich GP, Murin S, Battistella F, et al: Protocol weaning of mechanical ventilation in medical and surgical patients by respiratory care practitioners and nurses: effect on weaning time and incidence of ventilator-associated pneumonia, *Chest* 118:459, 2000.
44. Arieff AI: Fatal postoperative pulmonary edema. Pathogenesis and literature review, *Chest* 115:1371, 1999.
45. Fischer JE, Fegelman E, Johannigman J: Surgical complications. In Schwartz SI, Shires GT, Spencer FC, et al (eds): *Principles of surgery*, ed 7, New York, 1999, McGraw-Hill, 455.
46. Light RW: Pleural effusion, *N Engl J Med* 346:1971, 2002.
47. Sadikot RT, Rogers JT, Cheng D, et al: Pleural fluid characteristics of patients with symptomatic pleural effusion after coronary artery bypass graft surgery, *Arch Intern Med* 160:2665, 2000.
48. Brown DL, Hungness ES, Campbell RS, et al: Ventilator-associated pneumonia in the surgical intensive care unit, *J Trauma* 51:1207, 2001.
49. Fowler RA, Flavin KE, Barr J, et al: Variability in antibiotic prescribing patterns and outcomes in patients with clinically suspected ventilator-associated pneumonia, *Chest* 123:835, 2003.
50. CDC definitions for nosocomial infections, 1988, *Am Rev Respir Dis* 139:1058, 1989.
51. American Thoracic Society: Hospital-acquired pneumonia in adults: diagnosis, assessment of severity, initial antimicrobial therapy, and preventative strategies, *Am J Respir Care Crit Med* 153:1711, 1995.
52. Rello J, Paiva JA, Baraibar J, et al: International conference for the development of consensus on the diagnosis and treatment of ventilator-associated pneumonia, *Chest* 120:955, 2001.
53. Smulders K, van der Hoeven H, Weers-Pothoff I, Vandenbroucke-Grauls C: A randomized clinical trial of intermittent subglottic secretion drainage in patients receiving mechanical ventilation, *Chest* 121:858, 2002.
54. Tobin MJ: Advances in mechanical ventilation, *N Engl J Med* 344:1986, 2001.
55. Broussarsar M, Thierry G, Jaber S, et al: Relationship between ventilatory settings and barotrauma in the acute respiratory distress syndrome, *Intensive Care Med* 28:406, 2002.
56. Burns D, West TA, Hawkins K, et al: Immediate effects of positive end-expiratory pressure and low and high tidal volume ventilation upon gas exchange and compliance in patients with acute lung injury, *J Trauma* 51:1177, 2001.
57. Hess DR, Kacmarek RM: Determining appropriate physiologic goals. In *Essentials of mechanical ventilation*, New York, 1996, McGraw-Hill, 59.
58. Murray JF, Matthay MA, Luce JM, Flick MR: An expanded definition of the ARDS, *Am Rev Respir Dis* 138:720, 1988.
59. Bernard GR, Artigas A, Brigham KL, et al: The American-European Consensus Conference on ARDS: definitions, mechanisms, relevant outcomes, and clinical trial coordination, *Intensive Care Med* 20:225, 1994.
60. Acute Respiratory Distress Syndrome Network: Ventilation with lower tidal volumes as compared with traditional tidal volumes for acute lung injury and the acute respiratory distress syndrome, *N Engl J Med* 342:1301, 2000.
61. Tuxen D: Independent lung ventilation. In Tobin MJ (ed): *Principles and practice of mechanical ventilation*, New York, 1994, McGraw-Hill, 571.

Pain Management after Vascular Surgery

Peter F. Dunn, MD

Shihab U. Ahmed, MB, BS, MPH

Kevin C. Dennehy, MB, BCh, FFARCSI

19

"For all the happiness man can gain is not in pleasure but in rest from pain" are powerful words penned by the 17th century poet Sir John Dryden that still ring true today. Providing relief from pain is a natural extension of the basic tenet "do no harm" and has been a goal of health care providers since antiquity.[1] However, as a profession, physicians have not been effective at relieving patients of the pain associated with surgery, trauma, and medical disease and this may cause harm. Advances in the understanding of pain mechanisms, new and improved analgesia therapies, increased public desire for better pain relief, and enhanced physician awareness of the need for adequate pain relief have produced guidelines aimed at improving postoperative pain therapy.[2-4] The adequate treatment of postoperative pain goes beyond the humanitarian aspect of relieving obvious suffering and discomfort. Studies have shown that adequate perioperative analgesia not only has immediate physiologic benefits but also results in long-term reductions in morbidity and mortality.[5] Effective treatment of postoperative pain results in faster recovery and shorter hospital stays, which are important considerations in the current health care environment.[6]

Preemptive analgesia, the administration of analgesics before tissue damage, is an old concept for which there is renewed enthusiasm. In the early 1900s, Crile used preoperative blocks to mitigate central nervous system (CNS) changes and postoperative pain brought about through noxious surgical stimuli.[7] More recently, Mendell, Woolf, and others have described the relationship between peripheral and CNS sensitization related to noxious stimuli.[8-10] Preemptive analgesia may attenuate sensitization of nociceptive pathways and the subsequent development of neuropathic pain.[11,12]

Although the experimental evidence is convincing, many studies have questioned the true clinical benefit of preemptive analgesia.[13-15] Kissin identified five potential problems to explain the apparent disparity between the success in the laboratory and the clinical realm.[7] First, the terminology, definition, and concept of preemptive analgesia are not uniform. He pointed out that the noxious stimuli leading to central hyperexcitability may be initiated not only during the surgery but also during the secondary inflammatory stage in the early postoperative period. The design of many studies may not take this into account, and, thus, absence of outcomes from preincisional versus postincisional therapy (unwittingly defined as pre- vs. post-noxious stimuli) may miss the true preemptive benefit that both therapies have on this secondary stage of noxious stimuli. In addition, it may be that postoperative pain at rest and incisional pain evoked by movement are transmitted by different fibers and/or receptors.[16,17] Furthermore, the timing of the therapeutic

regimen in relationship to the noxious stimuli for a preemptive effect is unknown.[13,18] Second, the antinociceptive blockade may not be complete. Incomplete blockade of afferent signals may be a reason some studies have failed to demonstrate preemptive effects.[19,20] Third, many studies incorporate potentially effective preemptive regimens, such as systemic opioids or nitrous oxide, in their control groups.[21,22] The true effect of specific preemptive regimens compared with such groups may appear less beneficial. Fourth, noxious stimuli during surgery are not controlled and are difficult to quantitate. Often, the stimulus may not be noxious enough to induce pathologic pain, for which preemptive analgesia may be effective. Finally, the outcome measures of most studies, namely pain intensity and opioid consumption, may not be reliable. The true clinical benefit of preemptive analgesia to date remains unproved.

The optimum regimen for perioperative analgesia is unknown. Some studies have advocated the use of epidural anesthesia and analgesia (EAA) for vascular patients. Decreased time of intubation, time in the intensive care unit (ICU), number of pulmonary and myocardial complications, and improved coagulation status have been attributed to using EAA.[23-25] In other studies, myocardial outcomes in high-risk patients scheduled for abdominal aortic reconstruction were no different for patients randomly assigned to either epidural or intravenous opioid analgesia regimens.[26,27] Bois et al evaluated the difference in postoperative myocardial ischemia after aortic surgery for patients randomly assigned to either thoracic epidural analgesia (bupivacaine and fentanyl) or intravenous patient-controlled analgesia (morphine).[27] Although there was better pain control in the epidural group, there was no difference in the incidence of postoperative myocardial ischemia between the two analgesia regimens. Low statistical power of analysis related to small numbers of patients, difficulty in defining high-risk patients, and overall poor study designs have been mentioned by the critics of these and other studies in discussing why no benefit of the use of epidural analgesia was found.[28]

A large meta-analysis of randomized controlled studies found a significant reduction in postoperative myocardial infarction (MI) in patients receiving postoperative thoracic epidural analgesia compared with systemic analgesic techniques.[24] A randomized, multi-institutional study compared four groups of anesthetic and postoperative analgesic regimens on outcome for patients having elective abdominal aortic aneurysm repair.[29] Thoracic epidural anesthesia combined with a light general anesthesia (GA) followed by either intravenous or epidural patient-controlled analgesia (PCA) offered no major advantage compared with GA followed by either analgesia regimen. Epidural analgesia was associated with shorter times to extubation but offered no benefit in time to discharge from the ICU, advancement to diet, time to ambulation, or pain scores. More recently, pain and fatigue scores were lower and global outcome measures were improved in patients after colonic surgery who received epidural analgesia compared with those who were treated with intravenous PCA.[30] The primary outcome measure of functional exercise capacity and secondary outcome of health-related quality of life were attributed to the better analgesia associated with the epidural regimen, and the benefit extended to the 6-week follow-up period. Further study is needed to clarify the true benefit to the patients and to justify the cost differential associated with epidural analgesia regimens[31] (Table 19-1).

A significant portion of the vascular surgery population is elderly. The cultural, psychological, and physiologic differences of elderly patients must be understood to treat their postoperative pain effectively. Elderly patients often have the misconception that pain is a normal and expected part of the aging process, and they may be stoic in reporting their symptoms. Effective pain assessment may also be difficult because of cognitive impairment associated with delirium and dementia. Auditory and visual impairments make assessment techniques, such as the visual analog scale, difficult to utilize. Alterations in cardiovascular, pulmonary, hepatic, and renal systems may affect the delivery, side effects, and clearance of the pain medications, respectively. Although the aging process per se does not alter the pain threshold or tolerance, elderly patients are more sensitive to the analgesic effects of opiate drugs and their side effects.[32] Alternative therapies may be used in combination with opiates to limit the dose-dependent side effects of the opiates.

Postoperative pain management for vascular surgery patients remains a challenge because of significant comorbid disease. For instance, peripheral polyneuropathy related to diabetes mellitus, central neuropathy associated with a previous stroke, or limb amputation because of peripheral vascular disease may all result in chronic pain syndromes. Patients with such chronic pain syndromes are often treated with a multifaceted therapeutic regimen that needs to be considered when planning their postoperative analgesia. In these circumstances,

TABLE 19-1

Physiologic Sequelae and Outcome Measures after Surgery

Cardiovascular stress and morbidity
Intraoperative blood loss
Autonomic hyperactivity
Neuroendocrine stress response
Catabolism
Increased metabolic rate
Hypercoagulability and thromboembolism
Pulmonary dysfunction and morbidity
Fluid retention
Immune system dysfunction
Postoperative ileus
Length of hospitalization and health care costs
Chronic pain syndromes
Mortality

early consultation and involvement of the acute-chronic pain service may help optimize the patient's perioperative care.

Mechanism of Pain

Pain is a protective measure that forces clinicians to avoid further injury to the area experiencing the pain. When surgery is performed on a patient under anesthesia, pain is an unwelcome result. Tissue injury causes release of potent mediators of inflammation and pain. If pain is not treated, changes occur at the spinal cord level that potentiate pain. Postoperative pain results in discomfort of the patient, prolonged recovery, and increased risk of pulmonary and cardiac morbidity. The goal, therefore, is to attenuate the sensation of pain.

Initial Injury

Cutaneous receptors that respond preferentially and in a graded fashion to noxious stimuli are termed *nociceptors*. Nociceptors transduce mechanical, heat, cold, and chemical noxious stimuli to electrical signals that are then transmitted to the CNS. The threshold at which a nociceptor responds to stimulation is, in general, lower than the psychophysical pain threshold so that low levels of stimulation that activate the nociceptor may not be interpreted as pain.[33] It is likely that both spatial and temporal summation of nociceptor input at central levels is necessary for the appreciation of pain.

The type of initial stimulus is also important. A mechanical stimulus that evokes the same response in a C-fiber nociceptor as a heat stimulus evokes less pain than the heat stimulus. This difference may be due to recruitment of more nociceptors by the heat stimulus being distributed over a greater area or to the mechanical stimulus, but not the heat stimulus, causing coactivation of mechanical receptors resulting in suppression of pain through a "gate control" mechanism.[34] The initial stimulus that is interpreted as painful is followed by continued stimulation of the nociceptor. Subsequent stimulation is based on continued direct effects and the effects of locally released chemicals on nociceptors. These inflammatory mediators include bradykinin, prostaglandins, leukotrienes, serotonin, histamine, substance P, thromboxanes, platelet-activating factor, protons, and free radicals. Some mediators directly stimulate and others sensitize the nociceptor.[35] Sensitization of nociceptors is characterized by a lowering of the stimulus threshold to which they respond, an increased response to suprathreshold stimuli, and ongoing spontaneous activity.

Subsequent Pain

It is believed that injury to afferent axons results in changes in ion channel proteins causing a hyperexcitable membrane. Injury causes a local increase in the concentration of Na^+ channels.[36] The increase in the concentration of Na^+ channels in the axon correlates with the occurrence of peak ectopic discharge following neuroma formation, and this discharge may be reduced by sodium channel blockers. Potassium conductance also plays a role in the electrophysiology of injured nerve fibers. Potassium channel blockers have been shown to increase intracellular K^+ and increase the firing rate of myelinated sensory neurons following injury.[37] Regenerating nerve fibers have been observed to have increased concentrations of endoneurial potassium.[38]

Injury to sensory neurons causes changes in the amount of neuroactive agents present in the dorsal root ganglia (DRG). Substance P and calcitonin gene–related peptide (CGRP) immunoreactivity both decrease in the DRG. Vasoactive intestinal peptide (VIP) and galanin both increase in the DRG.[39,40] Certain populations of cells increase their expression of nitric oxide in response to injury.[41] The functional significance of these changes in neuropeptides is not obvious. In the periphery, substance P and CGRP cause capillaries to be leaky and vasodilated, respectively, with CGRP facilitating the actions of substance P both in the periphery and in the CNS.[42,43] In contrast to these excitatory effects, galanin inhibits the effects of substance P and CGRP in the periphery and CNS.[44] VIP is considered to be a neurotrophic factor by stimulating glycogenolysis, increasing glucose utilization, and increasing blood flow after nerve injury.[39]

Comorbid Processes

Diabetes mellitus is a common disorder in patients with vascular disease, and neuropathy is a common complication of diabetes. Pain and other abnormal sensations have been described in all types of diabetic neuropathy, but the precise etiology of these altered sensations in human diabetic neuropathy is unclear. Simple changes in glucose levels do not appear to be solely responsible; however, hyperglycemia has been shown to suppress the antinociceptive effects of opioids.[45] The peripheral nervous system has been studied more extensively than the CNS. Pathologic changes include atrophy of axons and degeneration followed by regeneration of clusters of nerve fibers with resulting changes in nerve structure, sensory neurotransmitters, and electrophysiology.

Nerve structure studies have shown myelin splitting in the spinal roots of long-term diabetic rats, which is more notable in the DRG than in the ventral roots.[46] Axonal atrophy is thought to arise from impaired transport and uptake of cytoskeletal proteins by the sensory cell bodies in the DRG.[47] Although reduced levels of substance P and CGRP along with reduced retrograde transport of neuronal growth factor (NGF) have been demonstrated, it is not known whether this contributes to the pain associated with diabetic neuropathy.[48,49] Motor and sensory nerve conduction velocities have been shown to be reduced within weeks of the onset of chemically induced diabetes.[50] Treating the hyperglycemia with insulin allows the conduction velocities to return toward normal. Alternatively, inhibitors of aldose reductase can prevent or reverse nerve conduction deficits in diabetic rodents without altering plasma insulin or glucose levels.[51] Schwann cell–derived neurotrophic factor (CNTF) is reduced in the sciatic nerve of both diabetic and galactose-fed rats. CNTF treatment prevents sensory, but not motor, nerve conduction velocity reductions.[52,53]

Patients with diabetes may be receiving various methods of pain control prior to vascular surgery. Good glycemic control has been shown to help prevent the progression of peripheral neuropathy.[54] Tricyclic antidepressants are effective in the relief of painful neuropathy in patients with both normal and depressed mood.[55] Selective serotonin reuptake inhibitors have been shown to relieve sensory symptoms.[56] Anticonvulsants and antiarrhythmics such as carbamazepine and mexiletine have been shown to help control painful diabetic neuropa-

thy.[57,58] A prolonged course of aldose reductase inhibitors has shown efficacy against both the development of spontaneous pain and loss of sensory function.[59] The topical application of capsaicin has been shown to improve the pain of diabetic neuropathy, possibly through depletion of substance P from sensory nerve terminals.[60] The severe pain of diabetic neuropathy has also been shown to be amenable to treatment with a spinal cord stimulator.[61]

Amputation

The sensation of the intact limb being present after amputation is referred to as "phantom limb." If pain is present in the limb at the time of amputation, the same pain is commonly experienced after amputation and is referred to as "phantom limb pain."[62] It has been reported that there is less phantom limb pain if there is a pain-free interval between the pain and the amputation.[63] This observation led to a study by Bach et al that suggested that continuous epidural block for 3 days prior to amputation decreased the incidence of phantom limb pain to a greater extent than did epidural anesthesia initiated at the time of surgery.[64] Criticisms of this study include a small sample size (25), investigators not "blinded" to therapy, unequal numbers of patients with diabetes in each group, and the fact that, although the epidural group had less pain at 6 months, there was no statistical difference between the groups at 1 week and at 1 year.[64] The results of this study have not been repeated, and the findings have not been extrapolated to universal practice.

Preemptive Analgesia

Analgesic techniques employed prior to a painful stimulus may result in less pain and analgesia requirement than if the technique is employed after the painful stimulus. In addition to controlling physiologic pain, preemptive analgesia reduces the development of pathologic pain by preventing central sensitization caused by the initial incisional injury and potentiated by subsequent inflammatory injury. Therefore, for preemptive analgesia to be effective, the analgesic technique must be employed prior to incision, during surgery, and during the initial postoperative period.[65] Evidence of the effectiveness of preemptive analgesia is present in animal studies, but the results of clinical studies are less uniform and depend on the methodology chosen to demonstrate the preemptive effect.[7]

A number of potential problems have been identified in the clinical studies. The absence of sufficient afferent blockade allows nociceptive input to the CNS and negates any preemptive analgesic effect. Moller et al demonstrated that only an extensive epidural block from T4 to S5 prevents the cortisol response to lower abdominal surgery.[19] Shir et al observed that preemptive analgesia occurred in patients undergoing radical prostatectomy under epidural analgesia alone but not in those having general or combined general and epidural anesthesia because the effectiveness of the epidural was guaranteed only in the patients who were awake.[66] A balanced analgesic regimen does not provide a preemptive effect.[20]

Results of studies in which a partial preemptive effect was inadvertently administered to patients in the control group are difficult to interpret. Opioids used during induction and maintenance of anesthesia, as well as those provided at emergence, all have a preemptive effect. It is, therefore, difficult in clinical studies to maintain a difference between groups with regard to the level of nociceptive input into the CNS. Surgery that is not associated with enough nociceptive input does not generate central sensitization regardless of the method of analgesia. Preemptive analgesia can therefore be demonstrated only when surgery is painful enough to induce both physiologic and pathologic pain.

Systemic Therapy—Opioids

Patient-Controlled Analgesia

Opioid analgesics are one of the most effective classes of analgesic medications for moderate-to-severe pain. Pain management after surgery, especially during the initial postoperative period, requires parenteral opioid administration for rapid and effective pain control. In the immediate postoperative period, oral routes are often not tolerated because of nausea and impaired bowel motility. Postoperative pain is poorly controlled with intermittent administration of intramuscular (IM) analgesics.[67] Intravenous (IV) PCA was introduced in 1970 as an alternative to intermittent subcutaneous (SC) and IM injection of opioid for postoperative pain control.[68] PCA refers to a process of delivering analgesic medications in which patients can determine when and how much medication they receive regardless of the route and the drug. Review has supported superior analgesia with the use of intravenous PCA after major surgery.[69]

The rationale for the use of PCA as the preferred mode of delivery of opioids is supported by studies on opioid pharmacology. There is considerable interindividual and intraindividual variability in the response after opioid administration. Opioid requirements after surgery may vary 10-fold depending on the heterogeneity of the population (interindividual variability).[70] An individual patient's analgesic requirement may increase with greater periods of stimulation, such as during ambulation, physical therapy, and dressing changes, whereas the same patient's analgesic requirement may decrease during periods of minimal stimulation, such as bed rest (intraindividual variability).

The relationship between opioid dose and analgesia is not a linear one but rather a sigmoidal relationship (Figure 19-1).[71] After surgery, the serum opioid level needs to reach a minimum level before the onset of analgesia becomes clinically manifest (analgesic threshold). As the serum opioid level increases above the analgesic threshold, small increases may provide excellent analgesia. The minimum effective analgesic concentration (MEAC) indicates the serum concentration of opioid that correlates with effective clinical analgesia. Serum opioid levels above the MEAC result in a high incidence of side effects, such as nausea, vomiting, sedation, and respiratory depression. In postoperative patients, MEAC changes constantly because of intra- and interindividual variability. Effective postoperative analgesia may be accomplished by maintaining opioid levels at the MEAC during rest and allowing supplemental dosing during periods of increased stimulation. A decrease in serum concentration of opioid below the MEAC can quickly lead to significant pain, and a small increase of serum level from the analgesic threshold can lead to effective analgesia. The challenge is how to achieve this goal.

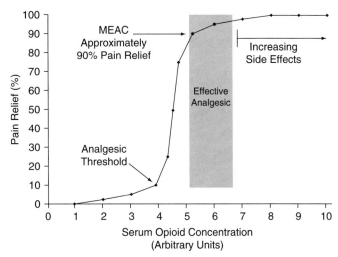

FIGURE 19-1 The steep sigmoidal dose-response curve for opioid analgesics. The minimum effective analgesic concentration (MEAC) is the lowest serum opioid concentration at which the patient obtains effective analgesia. Increasing the serum opioid concentration above MEAC does not significantly improve analgesia but does increase the incidence of unwanted side effects. The analgesic threshold is the serum concentration at which a small increase in serum concentration greatly increases the quality of analgesia. (Adapted from Etches RC: *Surg Clin North Am* 79:297, 1999.)

Because of the interindividual variability, an arbitrary dose given as IM, SC, or IV boluses may be below or above the MEAC for a given individual. Intermittent dosing, regardless of the route, may result in highly variable plasma opioid concentrations (Figure 19-2). Initial peak concentrations much higher than the MEAC may lead to side effects, and prolonged trough

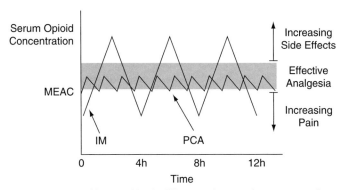

FIGURE 19-2 Pharmacokinetic differences between intravenous patient-controlled analgesia (PCA) and 4-hourly intramuscular injections. With the injections, patients may experience periods of excessive pain and side effects, especially sedation. In contrast, prompt administration of small doses by way of intravenous PCA allows the patient to reestablish analgesia quickly, with less risk of increasing the serum opioid concentration to the levels associated with increasing side effects. MEAC, minimum effective analgesic concentration. (Adapted from Ferrante FM: Patient-controlled analgesia: a conceptual framework for analgesic administration. In Ferrante FM, VadeBoncouer TR [eds]: *Postoperative Pain Management*, New York, 1993, Churchill Livingstone, 269.)

levels below the MEAC may result in periods of inadequate analgesia. Studies have demonstrated that when parenteral analgesia is administered every 3 to 4 hours, an adequate serum analgesic concentration is achieved only 35% of the time.[72] The continuous infusion of opioids may also provide inadequate analgesia despite its ability to reach a steady-state serum level. This inadequacy occurs because the intraindividual variability requires the adjustment of the serum level at the times of stimulation, such as during ambulation or physical therapy. If the continuous infusion achieves a steady-state level of analgesia during ambulation, the level may be too high during inactivity and cause unacceptable side effects.

Intravenous PCA allows the administration at the patient's demand of small doses of the drug with or without a low-dose background infusion. This technique adjusts for intra- and interpatient variations in response to therapy. PCA allows patients to maintain a sense of control in their care. This control may be particularly important in patients with anxious or neurotic personalities, who may need higher serum opioid concentrations to achieve adequate analgesia.[73] Pain threshold or pain tolerance and coping skills may vary from individual to individual. Pain has both physical and emotional components, and giving the patient the control to choose when and how much medication to use can improve the patient's overall satisfaction.

The PCA device is an infusion pump that delivers a preset bolus dose when the patient triggers the device by pressing a button (demand dose). The demand dose can be repeated at a specified time interval. The time interval between the demand doses (lockout time) is the period of inactivation. Thus, in spite of the frequency with which a patient presses the demand dose button, actual drug delivery occurs only at the end of the lockout time. This helps prevent overdosing the drug. Although most patients use the demand bolus one to three times per hour, because of intra- and interindividual variability, the lockout interval should be between 6 to 10 minutes. This setting gives the patient the flexibility to give a bolus preemptively before any activity such as ambulation. The PCA pump can also be programmed to deliver a continuous infusion of medication (basal infusion) in addition to the demand doses. A total dose per unit time is also programmed after taking into consideration both the demand dose and the basal infusion. The unit has a mechanical lock to reduce the risk of tampering and a software lock that prevents reprogramming by unauthorized personnel. PCA devices also keep an electronic event log that tracks the pump activity, such as the number and timing of total attempts by the patient, including successful ones.

When possible, patients should be educated about PCA during the preoperative visit. Patients who are informed about PCA for the first time in the immediate postoperative period have difficulty following the instructions on how to use the device and understanding the concept. It is important to explain the incident pain (pain with activity such as ambulation or physical therapy) and to use the demand dose preemptively to prevent worsening pain. Patients should be reassured of the safety mechanisms, including the lockout interval and hourly limit, to prevent an overdose. It is also important to explain to the patient that PCA usage is associated with an exceptionally low risk of addiction or dependence when there is no previous history of alcohol or substance abuse.

PCA orders should specify the opioid, its concentration, demand dose, lockout interval, basal infusion, and 1- or 4-hour limit (Table 19-2). The order should also include monitoring requirements and must specifically prohibit the administration of opioid or other CNS depressants drugs without prior discussion with the physician responsible for the PCA order.

Many opioids have been used for PCA, and most provide satisfactory analgesia. Morphine is the most commonly used opioid against which all others are compared. Hydromorphone, fentanyl, and meperidine account for almost all of the remainder. After an IV bolus administration of morphine, the onset of action is within 1 minute and the action peaks in 5 to 20 minutes. Plasma levels of morphine are poorly correlated with analgesia.[74] Morphine is metabolized primarily in the liver and is excreted through the kidney. Morphine-6-glucuronide is an active metabolite, more potent than morphine, and accumulates in severe renal insufficiency. For this reason, hydromorphone or fentanyl may be preferable to morphine in patients with renal insufficiency.

Hydromorphone is a derivative of morphine and is approximately five times more potent.[75] Because of its higher lipid solubility, hydromorphone has more rapid redistribution and elimination and shorter duration of action compared with morphine. Some suggest that hydromorphone is better tolerated and causes fewer side effects after major surgery, especially in elderly patients, when compared with morphine.[76] It has no known active metabolites in humans and is a preferred opioid for patients with severe renal insufficiency.

Fentanyl is a highly lipid-soluble synthetic opioid that is 125-fold more potent than morphine and has an onset of action within 30 seconds and peak effect within 5 to 15 minutes. Unlike the case of morphine, there seems to be a correlation between the plasma concentration of fentanyl and its effects on analgesia and ventilation. The therapeutic window for fentanyl is approximately 0.6 to 2.0 ng/mL for analgesia without clinically significant respiratory depression.[77] Fentanyl has a longer elimination half-life (185 to 219 minutes) than morphine (120 minutes) because of its larger volume of distribution secondary to its higher lipid solubility.[76] Fentanyl is metabolized in the liver and excreted in the urine and bile. Fentanyl's metabolism is minimally reduced in the presence of hepatic disease.

Meperidine is structurally similar to atropine and also unique in that it has local anesthetic properties.[78] It is more lipid soluble and has a faster onset of action than morphine, but it is one tenth as potent as morphine.[74] Meperidine has a stronger correlation between its plasma concentrations and its pharmacologic effect compared with morphine.[76] There seems to be a larger variability of MEAC of meperidine among patients, but the

TABLE 19-2

Patient-Controlled Analgesia Dosages and Lockout Intervals

Opioids	Demand Dose	Lockout Interval (min)	Basal Rate
Morphine	0.5-2.0 mg	6-10	0.5-2.0 mg/hr
Hydromorphone	0.25-1.0 mg	6-10	0.25-1.0 mg/hr
Fentanyl	10-25 μg	6-10	25-50 μg/hr
Meperidine	10-20 mg	6-15	10-20 mg/hr

concentration is consistent within each individual patient.[76] Meperidine is primarily metabolized to normeperidine in the liver and then excreted by the kidney. In patients with normal renal function, the elimination half-life of normeperidine is about 15 to 40 hours. Dosages of more than 800 mg of meperidine per day, or the presence of significant renal insufficiency, may cause normeperidine to accumulate to toxic levels.[76] Normeperidine has excitatory CNS effects including twitching, hyperreflexia, agitation, confusion, hallucinations, myoclonus, and seizures. Compared with morphine, meperidine may cause less constipation, urinary retention, and biliary tract spasm.[76]

The primary goal of the PCA technique is to maintain analgesia rather than to establish analgesia. Prior to starting PCA, it is essential to establish analgesia through administration of bolus doses in sufficient amounts. In the authors' experience, postoperative analgesia may be achieved in the vast majority of adult patients by giving 2 to 5 mg of morphine IV every 5 minutes up to a total of 10 to 20 mg. As an alternative to morphine, hydromorphone, 0.5 to 1.0 mg, can be given every 5 minutes to a total of 6 to 10 mg. Patients with a prior history of chronic opioid use may need higher loading doses of opioids because of tolerance. After the effective analgesic level is established, the patient should be able to maintain analgesia by utilizing the demand dose, keeping the serum concentration level at the MEAC. Macintyre and Jarvis retrospectively reviewed the first 24-hour morphine consumption of 1010 postsurgical adult patients.[79] They found that the age of the patient is strongly correlated with the amount of morphine consumed (average 24-hour morphine consumption in mg = 100 − age). They also noted that weight and male gender were weakly correlated with 24-hour morphine consumption. The surgical site was not found to be a predictor of morphine consumption.

Although many physicians avoid prescribing a basal rate in addition to the PCA demand dose because of the potential for an increase in side effects, including sedation and respiratory depression, the basal rate may be advantageous in certain circumstances. Low-dose infusions at night may improve sleep and reduce pain experienced after long periods of sleep when demand doses cannot be given. Basal infusions during the day, the peak time for opioid use, may reduce the need for demand dosing to maintain the MEAC and help to optimize the analgesic regimen.[80] Basal rates may be effectively used for patients who have received opioids before surgery for chronic pain. For morphine PCA, basal infusion can be adjusted between 0.5 and 1.0 mg per hour in patients with no prior history of significant opioid use. When the basal infusion is added, a higher level of vigilance is needed because of an increased risk of respiratory depression.

PCA pumps have the option to limit the total dose (demand and basal infusion) per 1 hour or every 4 hours for additional safety. For a morphine PCA, the typical limit is 10 mg per hour or 30 mg in 4 hours. It is important to keep in mind that when the demand dose and/or basal rate is changed, hourly limits may need to be adjusted accordingly to prevent a time lapse without medication. An order for supplemental bolus doses administered by the nursing staff should be included with the PCA orders. These supplemental doses may maximize the patient's participation during physical therapy and alleviate the increased pain associated with dressing changes and other procedures.

If PCA does not provide effective analgesia, a systematic assessment of the patient and the PCA pump is required. Assessment of the PCA-related problem should begin with pump malfunction, programming error, or drug preparation error. It is also important to find out whether the patient has been using the demand button properly. There may be a need for reeducation, reassurance, and encouragement. If excessive side effects occur with one drug, a change to another drug on the list (see Table 19-2) may produce a better effect.[4]

PCA is a safe way to provide effective analgesia despite some scattered reports of respiratory depression.[81,82] The reported incidence of potentially serious respiratory depression with PCA is approximately 0.5%.[71,83] Patients at increased risk for respiratory depression are elderly persons and patients with obstructive sleep apnea.[71,83] Other factors such as drug error, programming error, pump malfunction, or inappropriate PCA parameters can also cause respiratory depression. Providing inservice training to the nursing staff and standardizing the drug orders and the pump throughout the hospital can reduce these risk factors. Physicians should keep in mind that concomitant administration of CNS depressants and a background basal infusion increases the risk of respiratory depression.

Ballantyne et al published the result of a meta-analysis in which they examined the evidence in published randomized controlled trials comparing clinical outcomes of PCA and conventional IM analgesia.[84] They compared IV PCA without background infusion with IM opioid given every 3 to 4 hours on an as-needed basis. They found significantly better analgesia with IV PCA over intermittent IM opioid injection. However, a more recent review revealed contradictory findings in a comparison of PCA with intermittent IM, IV, SC, or simple continuous infusion.[69] Some studies showed significantly better analgesia with PCA, whereas others found no difference. Some studies in which no difference among the regimens was found were performed in an ICU. In the ICU setting with a higher nurse/patient ratio, effective analgesia with intermittent injection may be achieved without delay. Some studies have found no difference in analgesia through PCA or IV bolus by the nursing staff while the patient was in the ICU, but significantly better analgesia was obtained from PCA on the regular floor after their transfer from the ICU. Ballantyne et al also found "considerable evidence" of higher satisfaction of patients with PCA compared with intermittent IM opioid.[84] Studies on the effects of PCA on pulmonary function are contradictory. Some studies show that PCA regimens offer no improvement in pulmonary function and oxygenation compared with intermittent IM injection, whereas other studies have found significant improvement in forced vital capacity and peak expiratory flow rate.[85-87]

In summary, PCA is not a "one-size-fits-all" modality or "set and forget" therapy for postoperative pain control. The optimal postoperative pain relief depends on continued assessment of pain intensity and the monitoring of the side effects of the medication. The assessment should be followed by appropriate adjustments of the bolus dose, lockout intervals, and the basal infusion. PCA is an effective and safe way to provide analgesia to postsurgical patients. It provides safe, efficient analgesia with minimal sedation and improved pulmonary function with minimal side effects. Optimal drug dosage can be achieved with the ability to alter doses to match the changing demands of the patients. PCA allows individualization of therapy. The lag time for nursing response is eliminated. This decreased dependence on the nursing staff allows greater spontaneous activity of the patient. Acceptance by both nursing staff and patients is high.[85]

The duration of parenteral opioid therapy during the postoperative period depends on the extent of the surgical incision, opioid-induced side effects, and the patient's ability to tolerate oral intake. When the patient starts to tolerate oral intake, transition to oral opioids should be considered. The transition to oral opioids should start with a short-acting opioid for breakthrough pain. This replaces the patient-activated PCA demand dose or nurse-administered parenteral bolus dose per patient's request. If there was no previous history of adverse reaction to a given opioid, any short-acting opioid can be administered by the oral route for postoperative pain. Immediate-release morphine, oxycodone, and hydromorphone are appropriate in most cases. The initial starting doses are 5 to 15 mg of morphine sulfate, 2.5 to 5 mg of oxycodone, or 1 to 2 mg of hydromorphone. For elderly patients with a prior history of opioid sensitivity, a so-called weaker opioid such as propoxyphene and hydrocodone can be chosen for the transition to the oral pain medication. The dose can be repeated in 3- to 4-hour intervals.

During the transition from the parenteral to the oral route, it is important to assess the efficacy of the prescribed dose frequently to avoid inadequate analgesia. The oral doses should be increased gradually if analgesia is not sufficient. When a combination of opioid and acetaminophen is used for breakthrough pain, the recommended total daily dose of acetaminophen (4 g in patients with normal liver function) should not be exceeded. When applicable, addition of a nonsteroidal anti-inflammatory drug (NSAID) may reduce the dose of opioid medication required.[88,89] The newer NSAIDs (cyclooxygenase II inhibitors) may be useful adjuncts to opioids in relieving postoperative pain. Patients taking chronic opioids should receive their usual daily dose of opioid medication as soon as they are able to tolerate oral medications. Patients treated for chronic pain should follow up with their pain physician after they are discharged from the hospital to review their analgesic regimen.

Opioids may result in clinically significant side effects, such as respiratory depression, nausea and vomiting, ileus and constipation, urinary retention, and pruritus. Other medications have been used to limit the opioid-related side effects. Aspirin, NSAIDS, and cyclooxygenase II inhibitors may act synergistically with opioids and have been shown to reduce the amount of opioid needed for the treatment of postoperative pain.[88,90] In vascular patients with significant comorbid disease, the use of NSAIDs for postoperative analgesia may have a limited role. NSAIDs are associated with potentially significant renal effects.[4,91] A systematic review of the literature suggests that for patients with normal preoperative renal function, NSAIDs cause a clinically unimportant transient reduction in renal function.[92] For patients with baseline renal insufficiency or in whom perioperative renal injury may be a concern, such as patients undergoing suprarenal aortic cross-clamping or receiving a perioperative IV contrast agent, the use of NSAIDs may not be prudent. NSAIDs, especially IV or IM ketorolac, may also cause significant gastrointestinal effects.[93,94] Finally, vascular patients may be at risk for thrombocytopenia related to consumption in the perioperative period. In such patients, the inhibition of platelet function associated with the NSAIDs may be undesirable. α_2-Agonists, anticonvulsants, calcium channel blockers, nitrates, and many other categories of drugs have also been used as postoperative analgesics.[95-98] It remains for future study to evaluate what role these drugs will have in postoperative analgesia regimens and in reducing opioid-related side effects.

Side effects related to opioids may be reduced by switching to another opioid, changing the route of opioid administration, or using specific therapies to treat the side effects. No specific opioid is associated with a lower incidence of nausea and vomiting compared with another.[99] Anecdotal evidence of treating postoperative nausea and vomiting by switching opioids needs to be evaluated in crossover studies.[4,99] Thus, nausea and vomiting may best be treated with antiemetics. Lack of extrapyramidal side effects and lower incidence of sedation make ondansetron and other antiserotonergic agents attractive first-line choices over antidopaminergic drugs.[100,101] Ileus and constipation may be lower with parenteral than enteral opioids.[90] Pruritus may be high with neuraxial opioids. Switching to other routes and/or to other opioids associated with low levels of histamine release may be an effective method of treating the pruritus. Ondansetron has also been reported to be effective therapy for pruritus associated with intrathecal morphine.[102]

Regional Anesthesia and Analgesia
Epidural

Multiple physiologic sequelae that can influence outcome occur after major surgery (see Table 19-1). The ability to attenuate these sequelae is in the best interests of the patient. Pain relief, specifically regional analgesia, has shown considerable benefit in this regard. Although brachial plexus and lower extremity blocks have their application in patients with vascular disease, EAA has been more studied and is more widely practiced for major vascular surgery. An interesting and highly critiqued study by Yeager et al demonstrated significant benefits for EAA over GA and IV analgesia in patients considered to be "high risk" undergoing major vascular, thoracic, and upper abdominal surgery.[6] The benefits included lower mortality, lower incidences of major infections and cardiovascular problems, shorter time to extubation, and reduced hospital costs. Unfortunately, the groups included a mixture of surgical procedures and management of the epidural was not controlled[6] (see Chapter 9).

EAA was also found to be superior to GA and IV analgesia in a study by Tuman et al.[25] Patients were randomly assigned to receive epidural anesthesia–GA followed by EAA versus GA followed by IV PCA for major vascular surgery. There was no difference in mortality but the incidence of congestive heart failure, MI, and infection was less in the epidural group. The new finding was a dramatic reduction in vascular graft occlusion favoring the epidural anesthesia group (2.5% versus 22.5%). Thromboelastograph findings indicated that the GA group became hypercoagulable whereas the EAA group did not. Christopherson et al demonstrated similar results in patients having infrainguinal revascularization randomly assigned to EAA versus GA.[103] The incidence of early graft occlusion was 4% in the EAA group and 22% in the GA group.

They determined that the fibrinolytic system was inhibited in the GA group but not in the EAA group, thus promoting formation of clot. Epidural anesthesia has been demonstrated to reduce length of stay after endoluminal abdominal aortic aneurysm repair (2.5 versus 3.2 days in the epidural and GA groups, respectively) and need for admission to the ICU (0 versus 11%, respectively.[104]

Other studies have not found EAA to provide a significant improvement in outcome. Baron et al compared EAA-GA with GA for intraoperative management of anesthesia during major vascular surgery and reported no difference in outcome.[26] Of note, there was significant crossover in this trial with patients from both groups receiving postoperative epidural analgesia. Norris et al compared epidural anesthesia and GA with GA alone intraoperatively followed by epidural or IV PCA postoperatively for patients having major vascular surgery.[29] They found that all outcome data were similar among the four groups except for a shorter time to extubation in the epidural PCA groups. Nevertheless, there was no difference among the four groups in time to discharge from the ICU. Neither the intraoperative nor the postoperative anesthetic and analgesic techniques influenced outcome in this study.[29] In a retrospective analysis, Schunn et al found that the choice of anesthetic (epidural versus general) did not influence the rate of early infrainguinal graft thrombosis (14% versus 9.4%, respectively).[105] Bode et al prospectively studied 423 patients randomly assigned to receive GA, epidural anesthesia, or spinal anesthesia.[106] Monitoring was with arterial and pulmonary artery catheters in an intensive care setting for 48 to 72 hours postoperatively. There was a nonsignificant trend for fewer postoperative cardiac events in the GA group with the incidence of MI being 3.6%, 5.2%, and 4.7% and the incidence of death being 2.9%, 2.9%, and 3.4% in the GA, spinal anesthesia, and epidural anesthesia groups, respectively.[106]

The role of regional anesthesia in reducing the incidence of pulmonary dysfunction, blood loss, thromboembolism, immune dysfunction, and gastrointestinal dysmotility has not been studied well in patients undergoing vascular surgery. There is evidence that EAA provides beneficial effects for these outcomes following nonvascular surgery, and it has been studied in other situations.[107,108] It is, therefore, for these perceived beneficial effects on outcome that postoperative pain following major and peripheral vascular surgery is commonly treated with epidural analgesia. The use of anticoagulation is common in the perioperative period. Recommendations regarding the use of regional anesthesia in the anticoagulated patient are listed in the Appendix.

Intrathecal Opioids

The discovery of opioid receptors in the spinal cord, together with the evidence of inhibitory effects of morphine on nociceptive impulses, prompted a great deal of focus on the role of the spinal cord in nociception in the mid-1970s. In 1976 Yaksh and Rudy reported that small doses of intrathecal morphine produced prolonged, naloxone-reversible, analgesia in rats.[109] In 1979, Wang et al reported the first use of intrathecal opioid injection for analgesia in a group of cancer patients.[110] They conducted a double-blind, placebo-controlled, crossover study in eight patients. The subjects received 0.5 to 1.0 mg of intrathecal morphine. Six patients obtained 12 to 24 hours of complete pain relief without sedation, respiratory depression, or neuromuscular deficit. The first report of intrathecal opioid therapy for postoperative pain relief was in a group of patients undergoing herniorrhaphies in 1981.[111]

Opioid receptors have been found in high concentration in the marginal layer and substantia gelatinosa of the dorsal horn of the spinal cord.[112] When introduced into the subarachnoid space, opioids bind with receptors located in both pre- and postsynaptic sites. At the presynaptic terminal, opioids inhibit the release of excitatory neurotransmitters including substance P, CGRP, and neurokinin A.[113] Opioids cause hyperpolarization of the postsynaptic neuron by G protein–mediated opening of potassium channels.[113]

Several pharmacologic variables influence the intensity, onset, duration, and spread of intrathecal opioids. These variables include lipid solubility, degree of ionization, and receptor affinity. Lipid solubility plays an important role in determining the onset, the extent of the spread, and the duration of analgesia.[114,115] Highly lipid-soluble opioids, such as sufentanil, have a more rapid analgesic onset than water-soluble agents such as morphine. Sufentanil, when injected into the subarachnoid space, is rapidly transferred from the cerebrospinal fluid (CSF) to the spinal cord and is quickly transferred from the tissues into the vascular space for redistribution and elimination.[116] More ionized hydrophilic drugs such as morphine and, to a lesser extent, hydromorphone remain in the CSF for a longer period of time, resulting in a longer duration of action. Also, because of their relative lipid insolubility, morphine and hydromorphone have greater cephalad migration through the rostral flow of CSF. Although there is a greater extent of analgesia, the cephalad migration of the drug to the brain produces nausea, sedation, and respiratory depression. The difference in receptor affinity for various opioids plays a relatively minor role in pharmacokinetics when the medications are administered intrathecally.

Since the first reported administration of intrathecal opioids for analgesia, there have been many studies showing the efficacy of intrathecal opioids after abdominal, orthopedic, thoracic, and vascular procedures.[117-119] The major advantage of intrathecal opioid administration for postoperative analgesia is the relative absence of sympathetic or motor block that is commonly encountered with the spinal administration of local anesthetics. These features of intrathecal opioid administration may facilitate early ambulation of postoperative patients without significant risk of orthostatic hypotension or motor weakness. Gwirtz et al prospectively evaluated nearly 6000 patients who received intrathecal opioid therapy for pain relief after major abdominal, thoracic, vascular, and orthopedic procedures.[117] Patients received 0.65 to 0.8 mg of morphine for abdominal aortic aneurysm and 0.4 to 0.5 mg for hip and knee surgery. Doses were reduced by 0.1 mg for patients older than 65 years or debilitated patients and were increased by 0.1 mg for extremely tall patients. The majority of patients (74%) received 25 μg of fentanyl along with morphine. On a scale of 1 to 10 (1 indicating complete dissatisfaction and 10 indicating complete satisfaction with analgesia), the study found a mean satisfaction score of 8.51. Although the incidence of respiratory depression ($PaCO_2$ >50 mmHg and/or respiratory rate <8 breaths/min) was 3%, there was no case of life-threatening respiratory depression. They concluded that a single injection of intrathecal opioids provides excellent analgesia after major surgery for the initial 24-hour postoperative period.

The common side effects of intrathecal opioid administration are pruritus, nausea, urinary retention, somnolence, and respiratory depression.[117,120] Respiratory depression after intrathecal administration is an insidious process occurring over a period of 8 to 20 hours or occasionally longer. Morphine, through cephalad migration, can reach the brainstem respiratory center and cause delayed respiratory depression. Mild depression of CO_2 responsiveness can occur after only 0.2 mg of intrathecal morphine, but clinically significant respiratory compromise is a rare event, ranging from 0.1 and 0.4%.[118,121] Earlier reports of high rates of delayed respiratory depression were related to the large dose (2 to 15 mg) of injected morphine.[122,123] Currently, the recommended dose for a single intrathecal morphine injection is 0.2 to 0.8 mg.[117] A single intrathecal bolus of lipophilic opioids has not been associated with delayed respiratory depression.[120]

Pruritus is the most common side effect of intrathecal opioid administration.[117] It usually involves the face, neck, and upper thorax, although generalized pruritus can occur, especially when morphine is used. The possible etiologies include: release of histamine, especially in the tissue near the peripheral nerve endings, and interaction of opioids with the trigeminal nucleus at the medulla.[124] Most cases can be easily managed with the use of diphenhydramine, although IV naloxone may be needed in severe cases.[117] Ten milligrams of IV propofol has also been shown to provide rapid relief of pruritus caused by spinal opioid administration.[125] Nausea may result either from cephalad spread of the opioid through the CSF or from systemic absorption and delivery to the vomiting center located in the medulla. It may be treated with conventional antiemetic therapy.[117] Administration of 4 mg of IV ondansetron given prior to the placement of intrathecal opioid reduced the incidence of nausea, vomiting, and pruritus.[126] Urinary retention after the administration of spinal opioids does occur and may be due to inhibition of sacral parasympathetic outflow with relaxation of the detrusor muscle and sphincter spasm.[127] Intravenous naloxone and urocholine may be helpful in relieving symptoms in some patients.[127]

Intrathecal opioids provide excellent postoperative analgesia during the first 24 hours after major surgical procedures. Although delayed respiratory depression from intrathecal opioids is a concern, it is rare, usually develops progressively, and is generally preceded by nausea, vomiting, and increased somnolence.[114,128,129] Administration of concomitant opioid therapy or other CNS depressants can increase the risk and should be done cautiously. A written protocol and nursing education should guide continuous assessment of patients. A physician should be available around the clock to assess pain and side effects from the medications.

Cervical Plexus Block

Tangkanakul et al conducted a systematic review of trials comparing regional versus GA for carotid endarterectomy[130] (see Chapter 10). There were too few events in the randomized trials to determine whether there were important differences between regional and GA in risks of death, stroke, or MI. There was a significant reduction in the incidence of local hemorrhage and shunt insertion in the regional group. Nonrandomized studies

suggested a potential benefit of regional anesthesia, but these studies are likely to be biased. The most common regional techniques for carotid endarterectomy are superficial cervical plexus block, deep cervical plexus block, and a combination of both. Deep cervical plexus block is associated with potentially serious complications, such as diaphragmatic dysfunction, epidural or subarachnoid injection, or vertebral artery injection.[131] In a randomized study comparing superficial and deep cervical plexus block, Stoneham et al found that the patients with superficial block had higher analgesia requirements in the first 24 hours after surgery.[132] Other studies have found no difference in postoperative analgesia requirements between patients treated with superficial versus combined superficial and deep blocks.[131] Given the lack of superiority and greater risk associated with deep cervical plexus block, superficial cervical plexus blocks alone may be used as the regional technique for carotid endarterectomies.

Acute Pain Service

A team approach is necessary for safe and effective implementation of an individualized analgesia regimen for each vascular surgery patient. Acute pain service teams, comprising physicians with expertise in pain management, pharmacists, clinical nurse specialists and/or physician assistants, and administrative personnel, may provide daily pain management for the patients. The team may also provide educational support for the nurses and other hospital staff who provide daily care of the patients so that modern techniques, such as PCA and epidural-intrathecal regimens, may be safely used.[133] The guidelines established in 1992 by the U.S. Department of Health and Human Services stated that institutions must provide resources to provide the best and most modern pain relief appropriate to their patients.[2] In addition, quality assurance procedures should be used to assure that the following pain management practices are being carried out: patients are informed that effective pain relief is an important part of their treatment; clear documentation of pain assessment and management is provided; there are institution-defined levels for pain intensity and relief that elicit review of current pain therapy, modifications in treatment, and its efficacy; and there is an internal review of the effectiveness of the program. The acute pain service should be established to meet these guidelines. In addition, the establishment of institutional protocols may be beneficial in helping to manage the analgesia techniques.[134] A review of current hospital practice in the United States found that fewer than half of the hospitals surveyed had acute pain management programs, but an additional 13% were planning to implement such programs.[135] Through education of patients and nursing and hospital staff, implementation of acute pain service teams, and establishing institutional guidelines and protocols for pain management, effective, safe, and individualized pain therapy can be provided to vascular surgical patients.[136]

Appendix

Recommendations of the Second Consensus Conference of the American Society of Regional Anesthesia and Pain Medicine on Regional Anesthesia and the Anticoagulated Patient. Available on line at the American Society of Regional Anesthesia web site.

1. Thrombolytic and fibrinolytic therapy—Avoid spinal or epidural anesthesia except in unusual circumstances. Avoid these drugs within 10 days of puncture of noncompressible blood vessels. Data regarding the safety of neuraxial catheter removal while receiving therapy are not available.

2. Prophylactic subcutaneous heparin—Neuraxial techniques are not contraindicated. The risk of neuraxial bleeding may be reduced by delaying the dose of heparin until after the performance of the block and may be increased in the debilitated patient or during prolonged treatment. Patients receiving heparin for longer than 4 days should have a platelet count prior to performance of a block.

3. Therapeutic intraoperative anticoagulation with heparin— Avoid neuraxial techniques in patients with other coagulopathies. Delay heparin administration by 1 hour after block. Remove the catheter 1 hour before or 2 to 4 hours after subsequent heparin doses. No data to support mandatory canceling of the case in the setting of a bloody or difficult neuraxial procedure.

4. Prolonged therapeutic anticoagulation with heparin—Avoid neuraxial blocks in this setting as risk of neuraxial bleeding appears to be increased particularly when associated with concurrent administration of antiplatelet medications, low-molecular-weight heparin (LMWH), and oral anticoagulants. Discontinue therapy 2 to 4 hours prior to neuraxial catheter removal and monitor coagulation status.

5. LMWH—Neuraxial techniques should occur 12 hours after a prophylactic dose of LMWH and 24 hours after therapeutic dosing. There is no utility to monitoring the anti-Xa level as it is not predictive of the risk of bleeding. Concomitant administration of antiplatelet drugs, oral anticoagulants, standard heparin, or dextran increases the risk of perioperative hemorrhagic complications. Traumatic needle or catheter placement should warrant a 24-hour delay of postoperative LMWH therapy.
   a) Twice-daily dosing of LMWH—The first dose should be administered 24 hours postoperatively after removal of indwelling catheters and at least 2 hours after removal of catheter.
   b) Single daily dosing of LMWH—The first dose should be administered 8 hours postoperatively with the second dose 24 hours after the first. Indwelling catheters may be safely maintained. Catheters should be removed 12 hours after a dose of LMWH and subsequent dosing should occur at least 2 hours after catheter removal.

6. Oral anticoagulants—These should be stopped 4 to 5 days prior to neuraxial technique and prothrombin time/international normalized ratio (PT/INR) measured. Caution is urged if other medications that affect clotting mechanisms are being used, such as LMWH, aspirin, heparin, antiplatelet agents, and NSAIDs. Neuraxial catheters should be removed when the INR is less than 1.5. Clinical judgment should govern removal or maintenance of neuraxial catheters in the setting of therapeutic INR.

7. Antiplatelet agents—There is no accepted test that will guide antiplatelet therapy. The use of NSAIDs alone does not represent increased risk. Recommended time intervals between discontinuation of medication and neuraxial block are 14 days for ticlopidine, 7 days for clopidogrel, 2 days for abciximab, and 8 hours for eptifibatide and tirofiban. COX-2 inhibitors have minimal effect on platelet function and should be considered in patients who require anti-inflammatory therapy in the presence of anticoagulation.

8. Herbal therapy—The use of herbal medications does not preclude the performance of neuraxial anesthesia. The combination of herbal therapy with other antithrombotic agents may increase the risk of bleeding complications but data are lacking.

9. New anticoagulants—Fondaparinux, a synthetic pentasaccharide, was approved by the FDA in 2001 for deep venous thrombosis (DVT) prophylaxis for hip fracture and hip and knee replacement surgery. It works by inhibiting factor Xa. The FDA issued a black box warning against the performance of spinal anesthesia or puncture while on this medication due to spinal hematoma development and paralysis.

REFERENCES

1. Todd EM: Pain: historical perspectives. In Wall PD, Melzack R (eds): *Textbook of pain*, New York, 1999, Churchill Livingstone, 1.
2. Carr DB: *Acute pain management in infants, children, and adolescents: operative and medical procedures*, AHCPR publication No. 92-0032, Rockville, Md, 1992, Agency for Health Care Policy and Research, Public Health Service, U.S. Department of Health and Human Services.
3. Practice guidelines for acute pain management in the perioperative setting. A report by the American Society of Anesthesiologists Task Force on Pain Management, Acute Pain Section, *Anesthesiology* 82:1071, 1995.
4. Max MB: Principles of analgesic use in the treatment of acute pain and cancer pain. Glenview, Ill, 1999, American Pain Society.
5. Ballantyne JC, Carr DB, deFerranti S, et al:. The comparative effects of postoperative analgesic therapies on pulmonary outcome: cumulative meta-analyses of randomized, controlled trials, *Anesth Analg* 86:598, 1998.
6. Yeager MP, Glass DD, Neff RK, Brinck-Johnsen T: Epidural anesthesia and analgesia in high-risk surgical patients, *Anesthesiology* 66:729, 1987.
7. Kissin I: Preemptive analgesia. Why its effect is not always obvious, *Anesthesiology* 84:1015, 1996.
8. Woolf CJ, Salter MW: Neuronal plasticity: increasing the gain in pain, *Science* 288:1765, 2000.
9. Woolf CJ: Evidence for a central component of post-injury pain hypersensitivity, *Nature* 306:686, 1983.
10. Mendell LM: Physiological properties of unmyelinated fiber projection to the spinal cord, *Exp Neurol* 16:316, 1966.
11. Pedersen JL, Crawford ME, Dahl JB, et al:. Effect of preemptive nerve block on inflammation and hyperalgesia after human thermal injury, *Anesthesiology* 84:1020, 1996.
12. Yashpal K, Katz J, Coderre TJ: Effects of preemptive or postinjury intrathecal local anesthesia on persistent nociceptive responses in rats. Confounding influences of peripheral inflammation and the general anesthetic regimen, *Anesthesiology* 84:1119, 1996.
13. Fletcher D, Kayser V, Guilbaud G: Influence of timing of administration on the analgesic effect of bupivacaine infiltration in carrageenin-injected rats, *Anesthesiology* 84:1129, 1996.
14. Dahl JB, Hansen BL, Hjortso NC, et al:. Influence of timing on the effect of continuous extradural analgesia with bupivacaine and morphine after major abdominal surgery, *Br J Anaesth* 69:4, 1992.
15. Nikolajsen L, Ilkjaer S, Christensen JH, et al: Randomised trial of epidural bupivacaine and morphine in prevention of stump and phantom pain in lower-limb amputation, *Lancet* 350:1353, 1997.
16. Kawamata M, Watanabe H, Nishikawa K, et al:. Different mechanisms of development and maintenance of experimental incision–induced hyperalgesia in human skin, *Anesthesiology* 97:550, 2002.
17. Brennan TJ: Frontiers in translational research: the etiology of incisional and postoperative pain, *Anesthesiology* 97:535, 2002.
18. Abdi S, Lee DH, Park SK, Chung JM: Lack of pre-emptive analgesic effects of local anaesthetics on neuropathic pain, *Br J Anaesth* 85:620, 2000.
19. Moller W, Rem J, Brandt R, Kehlet H: Effect of posttraumatic epidural analgesia on the cortisol and hyperglycaemic response to surgery, *Acta Anaesthesiol Scand* 26:56, 1982.

20. Rockemann MG, Seeling W, Bischof C, et al:. Prophylactic use of epidural mepivacaine/morphine, systemic diclofenac, and metamizole reduces postoperative morphine consumption after major abdominal surgery, *Anesthesiology* 84:1027, 1996.

21. Goto T, Marota JJ, Crosby G: Nitrous oxide induces preemptive analgesia in the rat that is antagonized by halothane, *Anesthesiology* 80:409, 1994.

22. O'Connor TC, Abram SE: Inhibition of nociception-induced spinal sensitization by anesthetic agents, *Anesthesiology* 82:259, 1995.

23. Major CP Jr, Greer MS, Russell WL, Roe SM: Postoperative pulmonary complications and morbidity after abdominal aneurysmectomy: a comparison of postoperative epidural versus parenteral opioid analgesia, *Am Surg* 62:45, 1996.

24. Beattie WS, Badner NH, Choi P: Epidural analgesia reduces postoperative myocardial infarction: a meta-analysis, *Anesth Analg* 93:853, 2001.

25. Tuman KJ, McCarthy RJ, March RJ, et al:. Effects of epidural anesthesia and analgesia on coagulation and outcome after major vascular surgery, *Anesth Analg* 73:696, 1991.

26. Baron JF, Bertrand M, Barre E, et al:. Combined epidural and general anesthesia versus general anesthesia for abdominal aortic surgery, *Anesthesiology* 75:611, 1991.

27. Bois S, Couture P, Boudreault D, et al:. Epidural analgesia and intravenous patient-controlled analgesia result in similar rates of postoperative myocardial ischemia after aortic surgery, *Anesth Analg* 85:1233, 1997.

28. de Leon-Casasola OA, Lema MJ: Epidural analgesia and intravenous patient-controlled analgesia result in similar rates of myocardial ischemia after aortic surgery. *Anesth Analg* 87:745, 1998.

29. Norris EJ, Beattie C, Perler BA, et al:. Double-masked randomized trial comparing alternate combinations of intraoperative anesthesia and postoperative analgesia in abdominal aortic surgery, *Anesthesiology* 95:1054, 2001.

30. Carli F, Mayo N, Klubien K, et al:. Epidural analgesia enhances functional exercise capacity and health-related quality of life after colonic surgery: results of a randomized trial, *Anesthesiology* 97:540, 2002.

31. Ammar AD: Postoperative epidural analgesia following abdominal aortic surgery: do the benefits justify the costs? *Ann Vasc Surg* 12:359, 1998.

32. Kaiko RF, Wallenstein SL, Rogers AG, et al:. Narcotics in the elderly, *Med Clin North Am* 66:1079, 1982.

33. Van Hees J, Gybels J: C-nociceptor activity in human nerve during painful and non-painful skin stimulation, *J Neurol Neurosurg Psychiatry* 44:600, 1981.

34. Melzack R, Wall PD: Pain mechanisms: a new theory, *Science* 150:971, 1965.

35. Raja SN, Meyer RA, Campbell JN: Transduction properties of the sensory afferent fibers. In Yaksh TL, Lynch CI, Zapol WM, (eds): *Anesthesia: biologic foundations*, Philadelphia, 1998, Lippincott-Raven, 515.

36. Devor M, Govrin-Lippmann R, Angelides K: Na$^+$ channel immunolocalization in peripheral mammalian axons and changes following nerve injury and neuroma formation, *J Neurosci* 13:1976, 1993.

37. Kajander KC, Bennett GJ: Onset of a painful peripheral neuropathy in rat: a partial and differential deafferentation and spontaneous discharge in A$_{beta}$ and A$_{delta}$ primary afferent neurons, *J Neurophysiol* 68:734, 1992.

38. Low PA: Endoneurial potassium is increased and enhances spontaneous activity in regenerating mammalian nerve fibers—implications for neuropathic positive symptoms, *Muscle Nerve* 8:27, 1985.

39. Nielsch U, Keen P: Reciprocal regulation of tachykinin- and vasoactive intestinal peptide-gene expression in rat sensory neurones following cut and crush injury, *Brain Res* 481:25, 1989.

40. Zhang X, Ju G, Elde R, Hokfelt T: Effect of peripheral nerve cut on neuropeptides in dorsal root ganglia and the spinal cord of monkey with special reference to galanin, *J Neurocytol* 22:342, 1993.

41. Verge VM, Xu Z, Xu XJ, et al:. Marked increase in nitric oxide synthase mRNA in rat dorsal root ganglia after peripheral axotomy: in situ hybridization and functional studies, *Proc Natl Acad Sci USA* 89:11617, 1992.

42. Lembeck F, Holzer P: Substance P as neurogenic mediator of antidromic vasodilation and neurogenic plasma extravasation, *Naunyn Schmiedebergs Arch Pharmacol* 310:175, 1979.

43. Brain SD, Williams TJ, Tippins JR, et al:. Calcitonin gene–related peptide is a potent vasodilator, *Nature* 313:54, 1985.

44. Wiesenfeld-Hallin Z, Bartfai T, Hokfelt T: Galanin in sensory neurons in the spinal cord, *Front Neuroendocrinol* 13:319, 1992.

45. Raz I, Hasdai D, Seltzer Z, Melmed RN: Effect of hyperglycemia on pain perception and on efficacy of morphine analgesia in rats, *Diabetes* 37:1253, 1988.

46. Tamura E, Parry GJ: Severe radicular pathology in rats with longstanding diabetes *J Neurol Sci* 127:29, 1994.

47. Mohiuddin L, Fernyhough P, Tomlinson DR: Reduced levels of mRNA encoding endoskeletal and growth-associated proteins in sensory ganglia in experimental diabetes, *Diabetes* 44:25, 1995.

48. Diemel LT, Stevens EJ, Willars GB, Tomlinson DR: Depletion of substance P and calcitonin gene–related peptide in sciatic nerve of rats with experimental diabetes; effects of insulin and aldose reductase inhibition, *Neurosci Lett* 137:253, 1992.

49. Lindsay RM, Harmar AJ: Nerve growth factor regulates expression of neuropeptide genes in adult sensory neurons, *Nature* 337:362, 1989.

50. Moore SA, Peterson RG, Felten DL, O'Connor BL: A quantitative comparison of motor and sensory conduction velocities in short- and long-term streptozotocin- and alloxan-diabetic rats, *J Neurol Sci* 48:133, 1980.

51. Tomlinson DR: Aldose reductase inhibitors and the complications of diabetes mellitus, *Diabet Med* 10:214, 1993.

52. Calcutt NA, Muir D, Powell HC, Mizisin AP: Reduced ciliary neuronotrophic factor-like activity in nerves from diabetic or galactose-fed rats, *Brain Res* 575:320, 1992.

53. Mizisin A, Bache M, DiStefano P, et al:. Effects of BDNF or CNTF treatment on galactose neuropathy, *Soc Neurosci Abstr* 21:1535, 1995.

54. The effect of intensive treatment of diabetes on the development and progression of long-term complications in insulin-dependent diabetes mellitus. The Diabetes Control and Complications Trial Research Group, *N Engl J Med* 329:977, 1993.

55. Max MB, Culnane M, Schafer SC, et al:. Amitriptyline relieves diabetic neuropathy pain in patients with normal or depressed mood, *Neurology* 37:589, 1987.

56. Sindrup SH, Bjerre U, Dejgaard A, et al:. The selective serotonin reuptake inhibitor citalopram relieves the symptoms of diabetic neuropathy, *Clin Pharmacol Ther* 52:547, 1992.

57. Rull JA, Quibrera R, Gonzalez-Millan H, et al:. Symptomatic treatment of peripheral diabetic neuropathy with carbamazepine (Tegretol): double-blind crossover trial, *Diabetologia* 5:215, 1969.

58. Dejgard A, Petersen P, Kastrup J: Mexiletine for treatment of chronic painful diabetic neuropathy, *Lancet* 1:9, 1988.

59. Goto Y, Hotta N, Shigeta Y, et al:. Effects of an aldose reductase inhibitor, epalrestat, on diabetic neuropathy. Clinical benefit and indication for the drug assessed from the results of a placebo-controlled double-blind study, *Biomed Pharmacother* 49:269, 1995.

60. Treatment of painful diabetic neuropathy with topical capsaicin. A multicenter, double-blind, vehicle-controlled study. The Capsaicin Study Group, *Arch Intern Med* 151:2225, 1991.

61. Tesfaye S, Watt J, Benbow SJ, et al: Electrical spinal cord stimulation for painful diabetic peripheral neuropathy, *Lancet* 348:1698, 1996.

62. Jensen TS, Krebs B, Nielsen J, Rasmussen P: Immediate and long-term phantom limb pain in amputees: incidence, clinical characteristics and relationship to pre-amputation limb pain, *Pain* 21:267, 1985.

63. Katz J, Melzack R: Pain 'memories' in phantom limbs: review and clinical observations, *Pain* 43:319, 1990.

64. Bach S, Noreng MF, Tjellden NU: Phantom limb pain in amputees during the first 12 months following limb amputation, after preoperative lumbar epidural blockade, *Pain* 33:297, 1988.

65. Kissin I: Preemptive analgesia, *Anesthesiology* 93:1138, 2000.

66. Shir Y, Raja SN, Frank SM: The effect of epidural versus general anesthesia on postoperative pain and analgesic requirements in patients undergoing radical prostatectomy, *Anesthesiology* 80:49, 1994.

67. Ferrante FM, Covino BG: Patient-controlled analgesia: a historical perspective. In Ferrante FM, Ostheimer GW, Covino BG (eds): *Patient-controlled analgesia*, Boston, 1990, Blackwell Scientific, 3.

68. Forrest WH Jr, Smethurst PW, Kienitz ME: Self-administration of intravenous analgesics, *Anesthesiology* 33:363, 1970.

69. Macintyre PE: Safety and efficacy of patient-controlled analgesia, *Br J Anaesth* 87:36, 2001.

70. Austin KL, Stapleton JV, Mather LE: Relationship between blood meperidine concentrations and analgesic response: a preliminary report, *Anesthesiology* 53:460, 1980.

71. Etches RC: Patient-controlled analgesia, *Surg Clin North Am* 79:297, 1999.

72. Austin KL, Stapleton JV, Mather LE: Multiple intramuscular injections: a major source of variability in analgesic response to meperidine, *Pain* 8:47, 1980.

73. Lim AT, Edis G, Kranz H, et al: Postoperative pain control: contribution of psychological factors and transcutaneous electrical stimulation, *Pain* 17:179, 1983.

74. Stoelting RK: Opioid agonists and antagonists. In *Pharmacology and physiology in anesthetic practice*, ed 3, Philadelphia, 1998, Lippincott Williams & Wilkins, 77.

75. Drover DR, Angst MS, Valle M, et al: Input characteristics and bioavailability after administration of immediate and a new extended-release formulation of hydromorphone in healthy volunteers, *Anesthesiology* 97:827, 2002.

76. Austrup ML, Korean G: Analgesic agents for the postoperative period. Opioids, *Surg Clin North Am* 79:253, 1999.

77. Peng PW, Sandler AN: A review of the use of fentanyl analgesia in the management of acute pain in adults, *Anesthesiology* 90:576, 1999.

78. Sandler AN: Clinical pharmacology and applications of spinal opioids. In Bowdle TA, Horita A, Kharasch ED (eds): *The pharmacologic basis of anesthesiology*, New York, 1994, Churchill Livingstone, 149.

79. Macintyre PE, Jarvis DA: Age is the best predictor of postoperative morphine requirements, *Pain* 64:357, 1996.

80. Burns JW, Hodsman NB, McLintock TT, et al: The influence of patient characteristics on the requirements for postoperative analgesia. A reassessment using patient-controlled analgesia, *Anaesthesia* 44:2, 1989.

81. Hammonds WD, Hord AH: Additional comments regarding an anesthesiology-based postoperative pain service, *Anesthesiology* 69:139, 1988.

82. White PF: Mishaps with patient-controlled analgesia, *Anesthesiology* 66:81, 1987.

83. Etches RC: Respiratory depression associated with patient-controlled analgesia: a review of eight cases, *Can J Anaesth* 41:125, 1994.

84. Ballantyne JC, Carr DB, Chalmers TC, et al: Postoperative patient-controlled analgesia: meta-analyses of initial randomized control trials, *J Clin Anesth* 5:182, 1993.

85. Wheatley RG, Somerville ID, Sapsford DJ, Jones JG: Postoperative hypoxaemia: comparison of extradural, IM and patient-controlled opioid analgesia, *Br J Anaesth* 64:267, 1990.

86. Boldt J, Thaler E, Lehmann A, et al: Pain management in cardiac surgery patients: comparison between standard therapy and patient-controlled analgesia regimen, *J Cardiothorac Vasc Anesth* 12:654, 1998.

87. Gust R, Pecher S, Gust A, et al: Effect of patient-controlled analgesia on pulmonary complications after coronary artery bypass grafting, *Crit Care Med* 27:2218, 1999.

88. Williams JT: The painless synergism of aspirin and opium, *Nature* 390:557, 1997.

89. Reuben SS, Connelly NR, Steinberg R: Ketorolac as an adjunct to patient-controlled morphine in postoperative spine surgery patients, *Reg Anesth* 22:343, 1997.

90. Barratt SM: Advances in acute pain management, *Int Anesthesiol Clin* 35:27, 1997.

91. Clive DM, Stoff JS: Renal syndromes associated with nonsteroidal anti-inflammatory drugs, *N Engl J Med* 310:563, 1984.

92. Lee A, Cooper MC, Craig JC, et al: Effects of nonsteroidal anti-inflammatory drugs on postoperative renal function in normal adults, *Cochrane Database Syst Rev* CD002765, 2001.

93. Buchman AL, Schwartz MR: Colonic ulceration associated with the systemic use of nonsteroidal anti-inflammatory medication, *J Clin Gastroenterol* 22:224, 1996.

94. Wolfe PA, Polhamus CD, Kubik C, et al: Giant duodenal ulcers associated with the postoperative use of ketorolac: report of three cases, *Am J Gastroenterol* 89:1110, 1994.

95. Park J, Forrest J, Kolesar R, et al: Oral clonidine reduces postoperative PCA morphine requirements, *Can J Anaesth* 43:900, 1996.

96. Dirks J, Petersen KL, Rowbotham MC, Dahl JB: Gabapentin suppresses cutaneous hyperalgesia following heat-capsaicin sensitization, *Anesthesiology* 97:102, 2002.

97. Choe H, Kim JS, Ko SH, et al: Epidural verapamil reduces analgesic consumption after lower abdominal surgery, *Anesth Analg* 86:786, 1998.

98. Lauretti GR, Oliveira AP, Rodrigues AM, Paccola CA: The effect of transdermal nitroglycerin on spinal S(+)-ketamine antinociception following orthopedic surgery, *J Clin Anesth* 13:576, 2001.

99. Woodhouse A, Mather LE: Nausea and vomiting in the postoperative patient-controlled analgesia environment, *Anaesthesia* 52:770, 1997.

100. Desilva PH, Darvish AH, McDonald SM, et al: The efficacy of prophylactic ondansetron, droperidol, perphenazine, and metoclopramide in the prevention of nausea and vomiting after major gynecologic surgery, *Anesth Analg* 81:139, 1995.

101. Paech MJ, Pavy TJ, Evans SF: Single-dose prophylaxis for postoperative nausea and vomiting after major abdominal surgery: ondansetron versus droperidol, *Anaesth Intensive Care* 23:548, 1995.

102. Arai L, Stayer S, Schwartz R, Dorsey A: The use of ondansetron to treat pruritus associated with intrathecal morphine in two paediatric patients, *Paediatr Anaesth* 6:337, 1996.

103. Christopherson R, Beattie C, Frank SM, et al: Perioperative morbidity in patients randomized to epidural or general anesthesia for lower extremity vascular surgery. Perioperative Ischemia Randomized Anesthesia Trial Study Group, *Anesthesiology* 79:422, 1993.

104. Cao P, Zannetti S, Parlani G, et al: Epidural anesthesia reduces length of hospitalization after endoluminal abdominal aortic aneurysm repair, *J Vasc Surg* 30:651, 1999.

105. Schunn CD, Hertzer NR, O'Hara PJ, et al: Epidural versus general anesthesia: does anesthetic management influence early infrainguinal graft thrombosis? *Ann Vasc Surg* 12:65, 1998.

106. Bode RH Jr, Lewis KP, Zarich SW, et al: Cardiac outcome after peripheral vascular surgery. Comparison of general and regional anesthesia, *Anesthesiology* 84:3, 1996.

107. Rodgers A, Walker N, Schug S, et al: Reduction of postoperative mortality and morbidity with epidural or spinal anaesthesia: results from overview of randomised trials, *BMJ* 321:1493, 2000.

108. Grass J: The role of epidural anesthesia and analgesia in postoperative outcome, *Anesthesiol Clin North Am* 18:407, 2000.

109. Yaksh TL, Rudy TA: Analgesia mediated by a direct spinal action of narcotics, *Science* 192:1357, 1976.

110. Wang JK, Nauss LA, Thomas JE: Pain relief by intrathecally applied morphine in man, *Anesthesiology* 50:149, 1979.

111. Katz J, Nelson W: Intrathecal morphine for postoperative pain relief, *Reg Anesth* 6:1, 1981.

112. Gouarderes C, Cros J, Quirion R: Autoradiographic localization of mu, delta and kappa opioid receptor binding sites in rat and guinea pig spinal cord, *Neuropeptides* 6:331, 1985.

113. Dickenson AH: Mechanisms of the analgesic actions of opiates and opioids, *Br Med Bull* 47:690, 1991.

114. Cousins MJ, Mather LE: Intrathecal and epidural administration of opioids, *Anesthesiology* 61:276, 1984.

115. Gourlay GK, Cherry DA, Plummer JL, et al: The influence of drug polarity on the absorption of opioid drugs into CSF and subsequent cephalad migration following lumbar epidural administration: application to morphine and pethidine, *Pain* 31:297, 1987.

116. Sabbe MB, Grafe MR, Mjanger E, et al: Spinal delivery of sufentanil, alfentanil, and morphine in dogs. Physiologic and toxicologic investigations, *Anesthesiology* 81:899, 1994.

117. Gwirtz KH, Young JV, Byers RS, et al: The safety and efficacy of intrathecal opioid analgesia for acute postoperative pain: seven years' experience with 5969 surgical patients at Indiana University Hospital, *Anesth Analg* 88:599, 1999.

118. Holmstrom B, Laugaland K, Rawal N, Hallberg S: Combined spinal epidural block versus spinal and epidural block for orthopaedic surgery, *Can J Anaesth* 40:601, 1993.

119. Davis I: Intrathecal morphine in aortic aneurysm surgery, *Anaesthesia* 42:491, 1987.

120. Etches RC, Sandler AN, Daley MD: Respiratory depression and spinal opioids, *Can J Anaesth* 36:165, 1989.

121. Kafer ER, Brown JT, Scott D, et al: Biphasic depression of ventilatory responses to CO_2 following epidural morphine, *Anesthesiology* 58:418, 1983.

122. Davies GK, Tolhurst-Cleaver CL, James TL: Respiratory depression after intrathecal narcotics, *Anaesthesia* 35:1080, 1980.

123. Glynn CJ, Mather LE, Cousins MJ, et al: Spinal narcotics and respiratory depression, *Lancet* 2:356, 1979.

124. Ballantyne JC, Loach AB, Carr DB: Itching after epidural and spinal opiates, *Pain* 33:149, 1988.

125. Borgeat A, Wilder-Smith OH, Saiah M, Rifat K: Subhypnotic doses of propofol relieve pruritus induced by epidural and intrathecal morphine, *Anesthesiology* 76:510, 1992.

126. Yeh HM, Chen LK, Lin CJ, et al: Prophylactic intravenous ondansetron reduces the incidence of intrathecal morphine–induced pruritus in patients undergoing cesarean delivery, *Anesth Analg* 91:172, 2000.

127. Rawal N, Mollefors K, Axelsson K, et al: An experimental study of urodynamic effects of epidural morphine and of naloxone reversal, *Anesth Analg* 62:641, 1983.

128. Bromage PR, Camporesi EM, Durant PA, Nielsen CH: Nonrespiratory side effects of epidural morphine, *Anesth Analg* 61:490, 1982.

129. Rawal N, Schott U, Dahlstrom B, et al: Influence of naloxone infusion on analgesia and respiratory depression following epidural morphine, *Anesthesiology* 64:194, 1986.

130. Tangkanakul C, Counsell CE, Warlow CP: Local versus general anaesthesia in carotid endarterectomy: a systematic review of the evidence, *Eur J Vasc Endovasc Surg* 13:491, 1997.

131. Pandit JJ, Bree S, Dillon P, et al: A comparison of superficial versus combined (superficial and deep) cervical plexus block for carotid endarterectomy: a prospective, randomized study, *Anesth Analg* 91:781, 2000.

132. Stoneham MD, Doyle AR, Knighton JD, et al: Prospective, randomized comparison of deep or superficial cervical plexus block for carotid endarterectomy surgery, *Anesthesiology* 89:907, 1998.

133. Frenette L: The acute pain service, *Crit Care Clin* 15:143, 1999.

134. Rawal N, Allvin R: Epidural and intrathecal opioids for postoperative pain management in Europe—a 17-nation questionnaire study of selected hospitals. Euro Pain Study Group on Acute Pain, *Acta Anaesthesiol Scand* 40:1119, 1996.

135. Warfield CA, Kahn CH: Acute pain management. Programs in U.S. hospitals and experiences and attitudes among U.S. adults, *Anesthesiology* 83:1090, 1995.

136. Ferrante FM: Patient-controlled analgesia: a conceptual framework for analgesic administration. In Ferrante FM, VadeBoncouer TR (eds): *Postoperative pain management*, New York, 1993, Churchill Livingstone, 269.

Ethical Decisions/End-of-Life Care in Patients with Vascular Disease

20

Gail A. Van Norman, MD

Anesthesiology and Medical Ethics

The field of biomedical ethics is rich with important contributions from anesthesiologists. The hallmark legal decision in 1914 regarding informed consent in the United States, *Schloendorff v Society of New York Hospital*, involved anesthesia care.[1] Anesthesiologists were key in the development of mechanical ventilation during the polio epidemics of the 1940s and 1950s and were among the first to recognize the ethical challenges this technology posed.[2] A declaration by Pope Pius XII about the morality of refusing or discontinuing life-sustaining care was delivered during the International Congress of Anesthesiologists in 1957, paving the way for the later broader social debate on limiting or ending life-sustaining therapies.[3] John S. McDonald attributed the mid-20th century change in the Catholic church's stance regarding labor analgesia to the influence of the Pope's "personal friend" John J. Bonica, chairman of the Department of Anesthesiology at the University of Washington.[4] After horrific revelations regarding human experimentation in Nazi Germany, descriptions of similarly disturbing abuses by medical researchers in the United States were published in the *New England Journal of Medicine* by Henry Beecher, the first professor and chair of the Harvard Medical School Department of Anesthesiology. His work was directly responsible for the development of institutional review boards to protect human subjects from abuses by physician researchers. The Ad Hoc Committee of the Harvard Medical School, also led by Dr. Beecher, developed the concept of brain death to answer the ethical challenges of limiting invasive medical care, distributing limited intensive care unit resources, and obtaining vital organs for transplantation.[5,6]

The leadership of anesthesiologists in many of the most problematic ethical challenges of 20th century medicine is not coincidental. Anesthesiologists are and have been a vital part of health care teams in the operating room, pain clinic, emergency department, and intensive care unit, providing invasive care to patients when they are most vulnerable and when ethical decision making is most critical.

The Health Care "Team"

The tenacious but false image of anesthesiology practice as one that is confined to the operating room, together with gross misconceptions that anesthesiologists are subordinate to the moral and legal authority of surgeons or other physicians, leads many anesthesiologists to believe mistakenly that they have lesser ethical obligations in care of patients.

The increasing complexity of medical practice demands that patients' care involve the efforts of physicians of different disciplines as well as skilled nursing professionals, technologists, and therapists. The health care "team" has evolved from a hierarchy, in which one physician assumed a "command" position, to that of team consensus and integration, in which many health care givers share duties. Many physicians who are accustomed to the hierarchical approach have difficulty adjusting to one in which majority opinion, deference to other experts, and unanimity or consensus may be more appropriate than autocratic rule. The operating room and intensive care unit are especially rich in examples of patients' care requiring multidisciplinary cooperation, conflict, and compromise.

Many anesthesiologists find false comfort in the misconception that a "captain of the ship doctrine" relieves them of ethical obligations to the patient. The captain of the ship doctrine, however, is a concept that is not only baseless both medically and ethically, but also no longer widely accepted legally. Although the courts have in the past sometimes relied on parallels in maritime law to assign medical, legal, and moral authority to the surgeon as the captain of the ship, they now recognize that the scope and complexity of medical practice are such that no single provider has complete knowledge and control over a patient's care. Most states have discarded the captain of the ship doctrine and hold nurses, nurse anesthetists, anesthesiologists, radiologists, radiology technologists, and surgeons separately accountable for medical and ethical mischief that occurs in the operating room.[7] Anesthesiologists, therefore, have special ethical and legal duties toward patients, based on their specialized knowledge, scope of practice, and individual skills.

The Changing Physician-Patient Relationship

Principles of medical ethics can be best understood in light of changes in the historical doctor-patient relationship and developments in Western philosophy. For much of history, physicians were unable to alter the outcome of disease significantly. Medical ethical principles derived from the writings of Hippocrates and others emphasized maintaining the exclusivity and authority of the medical profession, promoting the moral integrity of physicians, and protecting the physician-patient relationship through vows of confidentiality and compassion.[8] In the 1700s and 1800s a scientific approach to the treatment of disease developed, with increasing knowledge of anatomy, circulation, and genetics, the development of the germ theory of disease, and medical advances such as the development of vaccines. The physician could sometimes change the natural course of illness, and with that power came the authority that accompanies specialized knowledge.

During the 1900s, the wealth of Western governments increased, and they could respond to growing social concerns about the sick and underprivileged. Strategies to provide health care to poor and elderly people included government programs, such as nationalization of health care in some Western countries and government-financed programs such as Medicare and Medicaid in the United States.

The wealth of physicians also increased. Many joined the upper classes, separated culturally and economically from the patients whom they served. Meanwhile, widespread immigration from Africa, the Middle East, and Asia brought to the United States and Europe more diverse and fundamentally different cultural and religious beliefs. The relative homogeneity of Western culture was transformed; not only were physicians less likely to identify personally with their patients, they were less likely to share even common religious or moral values.[9]

In the wake of World War II, revelations about the role of physicians in experimentation, torture, and executions involving human prisoners in Nazi Germany shook the image of physicians as humanitarians. Despite renewed commitment of physicians to the humanitarian vows of medical practice in the Helsinki Declaration, revelations about continued abuses in clinical research in the United States during the 1960s further eroded the professional image of physicians and the trust of patients.[5]

The rights-based social movement toward self-determination of the 1950s and 1960s also affected the physician-patient relationship. The civil rights movement was paralleled in medicine by concerns about the rights of patients with psychiatric illnesses, such as abuses of civil commitment rules and the rights of patients to refuse treatment. These issues quickly found their way into mainstream medical practice as advances in medical technology made it possible to prolong dying, seemingly indefinitely. Patients and their families questioned whether the prolongation of life at almost any cost was desirable or even moral, then sought and secured religious, constitutional, and legal support to refuse even life-sustaining therapies when such therapies were in conflict with their personal values. The very foundation of the professional "ethic" of medicine was shaken to the core: preservation of life was no longer always the epitome of "doing good," and allowing patients to die without costly and sometimes seemingly cruel interventions no longer appeared to violate the rule *primum non nocere*. It is no coincidence that the discipline of bioethics coalesced in the 1970s in the midst of these social and technological changes.

Today, the physician-patient relationship bears little resemblance to that of the past. Many of the prevalent conceptions of the moral obligations of health professionals and society to meet the needs of the sick have been challenged or even overturned. An educated and demanding public expects both readily available and high-quality health care despite the increasing cost of medical therapies. A looming crisis in health care costs and delivery presents physicians with new ethical dilemmas about whom to serve: the interests of an individual patient, the interests of the managed care system that pays their fees, or the best interests of society as a whole. Physicians and patients alike have increasingly turned to the courts to resolve issues when the goals and values of patients and physicians conflict, when medical care does not meet expectations or results in injury to the patient, and when efforts to contain rising health care costs result in restriction of health care resources.

Anesthesiologists find themselves in conflict with patients over medical decision making, surrogate decision makers, end-of-life care, do-not-resuscitate orders, physician-assisted suicide, and many other issues. Conflicts also occur with insurers, managed care organizations, and government-sponsored health care over allocation of health care dollars and efforts to dictate health care techniques and technologies. To help the anesthesiologist navigate the complex and often emotional ethical issues in care of patients, it is valuable to review basic concepts in medical ethics and how they are applied in patients' care issues.

Biomedical Ethical Principles

A simplified way to consider modern moral reasoning in medicine is to divide ethical approaches into two broad categories: the ethics of rules and the ethics of consequences.

The ethics of rules, or *deontological* ethics, states that there are features of actions other than their consequences that determine whether they are right or wrong. This moral theory can be traced to its religious roots in Judeo-Christian culture and was formulated in the writings of Immanuel Kant in the 1700s. In Kantian philosophy, the rules governing an action must be capable of being universalized; that is, the principle on which one acts should be one that people consistently desire *everyone* to act upon. Further, an act is morally right *only* if the actor is motivated by "good will." In deontological ethics, the intentions of the actor and the principles under which he or she acts determine the morality of the action. There is no direct relationship between the morality of an act and its actual consequences. Kantians recognize that despite best efforts, uncontrollable things sometimes happen, which are not the moral responsibility of the actor. The ends, in other words, *never* justify the means. Moreover, in Kantian philosophy, the value of the individual is paramount: individuals and groups cannot be sacrificed for the collective self-interest. Deontologists are criticized when "morally right" actions, according to this definition, have negative or even unacceptable results.[8,10]

An example of deontological reasoning is the well-known ethical principle of "double effect." A physician administers increasing doses of narcotics to relieve the pain and suffering of a patient with terminal cancer. Eventually, the physician faces the possibility that the dose of narcotic required to relieve pain will cause respiratory depression and death. Is intentionally administering a potentially fatal dose of narcotic to a patient for the purpose of relieving pain ethical? Intentional killing of another person is considered by most of society to be morally unacceptable and legally prosecutable. Kantians would argue that even if the patient dies, the act is morally good, but *only* if the physician is acting on a principle of doing good—relieving suffering—and *only* if the physician does not actually intend to kill the patient. The so-called double effect of the physician's action, the patient's death, is irrelevant.[8,10,11]

In the ethics of consequences, or *consequentialism*, the morality of an action is determined by the balance of good and bad consequences that result from it. There is no intrinsic right or wrong value to actions. The right action in any circumstance is that which produces the best result, presumably as judged by some disinterested third party. The most prominent consequentialist theory is called *utilitarianism*. It asserts that there is only *one* ethical principle, that of utility, which states that people ought always to produce the best balance of maximum positive results and minimum negative results. Consequentialists are criticized about definitions of which results are "positive" and "negative." Should positive value be assigned only to the things that all reasonable persons would want or to the things valued by individuals?[8,10]

Consequentialist reasoning is applied, for example, in the debate about whether permanently comatose patients should be used as donors of vital organs. Deontologists argue that universalized rules against killing strictly prohibit such actions and that no living individual should be sacrificed for another because each has intrinsic and equal value. Some consequentialists argue that it is morally acceptable because by using the vital organs of such patients physicians benefit thousands of other patients, eliminate expenses associated with medically supporting permanently comatose patients, and decrease expensive medical care to patients who require medical support until a brain-dead donor can be found. Other consequentialists argue that it is morally unacceptable because it would cause mistrust of doctors, it may produce an unacceptable devaluation of certain types of lives, it would lead to discrimination against the handicapped and vulnerable in society, and it would result in a net decrease in the rates of organ donation because of adverse public perceptions.

Deontological and consequentialist theories are both applied to varying degrees in discussions of medical ethical principles. As a society that values individualism and affords high protection to the rights of individuals, people tend to turn to deontological arguments and Kantian philosophy when ethical questions arise that weigh the authority of the physician against the goals and values of the patient. When there is an attempt to resolve broad-based, societal issues such as the allocation of increasingly limited economic and technological resources, consequentialist arguments, are often used. Some of the toughest ethical questions in medicine arise when the rights and the desires of individual patients run counter to societal policies and deontological principles clash with consequentialist principles. Such issues are common in the intensive care unit and managed care settings and in the management of poor or elderly patients whose care is subsidized by government funding.

Four basic principles of medical ethics are generally invoked when ethical issues in medicine arise and are referred to in this chapter: respect for patients' autonomy, beneficence (doing good), nonmaleficence (avoiding harm), and justice.

Respect for Patients' Autonomy

The principle of respect for patients' autonomy is the idea that autonomous patients have the right to determine what should be done to them medically. The principle has roots in Western philosophy, which places primary importance on individualism, personal freedoms, and limitations of social government. Legal principles protect individual freedoms, such as the right to privacy, the right to defense of self and property, and guarantees

of noninterference, and impose limitations generally only when there is a perceived overriding benefit to society or one person's actions endanger others. "Autonomy" refers to the ability to make independent decisions that are "free from both controlling influences by others and from personal limitations that prevent meaningful choice, such as inadequate understanding."[10] The principle of respect for patients' autonomy demands that physicians give the patient's values and goals in medical care primary consideration. Further, the principle of respect for patients' autonomy requires that physicians do their utmost to *promote* patients' autonomy and correct reversible conditions that might interfere with it, such as patients' lack of knowledge or temporary impediments related to illness or medication. The classic example of respect for patients' autonomy occurs during the informed consent process, when the physician educates the patient about the risks, benefits, and alternatives to a proposed treatment and then respects the patient's decision.

Beneficence

The principle of beneficence requires doctors to strive to contribute to the positive welfare of patients. It demands more than simply avoiding harming patients; it requires that active and positive steps toward helping them are taken. The principle of beneficence has evolved from the simple goal of prolonging life to that of producing benefits *that are meaningful and beneficial in the eyes of the individual patient.*[10] Treatments that prolong life, for example, may not represent a benefit to a patient who perceives such interventions as producing overriding harms such as physical or psychological suffering, economic impoverishment, or social isolation. An example of this concept of beneficence is employed when a physician respects the wishes of a Jehovah's Witness patient not to undergo a lifesaving blood transfusion because in the patient's eyes it would produce a spiritual harm that is much greater than loss of life.

Nonmaleficence

Nonmaleficence is the principle of avoiding harm to patients found in the Hippocratic oath, "I will use treatment to help the sick according to my ability and judgment, but I will never use it to injure or wrong them."[11] The concept of nonmaleficence is most controversial in end-of-life issues, such as the differences between killing and letting die, intending and foreseeing harmful outcomes, and withholding and withdrawing life-sustaining treatments. It is also prominent in issues involving medical research, in which the researcher has moral obligations to protect the safety and health of human subjects and to minimize the suffering and maltreatment of animals. The principle of nonmaleficence includes harms that are not merely physical but economic, spiritual, and social in nature.[10,11]

Justice

The principle of justice considers that which is fair, equitable, and appropriate. Justice implies entitlement, and the term *injustice* implies a wrongful act or omission that unfairly distributes burdens or denies someone something to which they have a right.[10] The principle of justice is invoked in discussing allocation of health care resources. There are many ways in which such resources might be distributed that meet different definitions of fairness: distribution might be equal or proportional to need, effort, actual contribution, or merit, for example. Debates about Medicare allocations thus include questions of whether the program should cover all health care for patients older than 65 (equal distribution) or should cover health care for such patients only if they cannot otherwise afford it (distribution proportional to need).

Both deontological and consequentialist influences can be seen in the four basic principles. Respect for patients' autonomy and the principle of nonmaleficence are derived from deontological principles that respect individualism, demand that physicians act out of good will, assign intrinsic value to life, and do not allow sacrifice of one person for another. The principle of beneficence has deontological roots in the maxim to act with good will, as well as consequentialist implications. Because it is not always possible to produce benefits or eliminate harms without incurring some risk or cost, the utilitarian concept of determining the value of an act by the balance of benefits and harms it produces often comes into play in the principles of beneficence and nonmaleficence. The principle of justice involves the deontological concepts of good will and the intrinsic value of life but is also utilitarian when it weighs costs and benefits to produce the most good for the greatest number of people.

Ethical Problems and Vascular Surgical Patients

The vascular surgical patient may present with a broad variety of disorders, including cerebrovascular disease, diseases of the aorta, peripheral vascular disease, and coronary artery disease. Vascular diseases can occur at any age but are most often associated with middle age and beyond, are a leading cause of morbidity and disability in elderly people, and present a high monetary cost to society. The highest incidence of peripheral arterial disease is in the sixth and seventh decades of life. Aortic disease becomes more prevalent in both women and men older than 50. Stroke increases in incidence with age, is the third leading cause of death in the United States, and is the leading cause of long-term disability, costing $30 billion to $40 billion dollars per year. It is estimated that by the year 2020, cardiovascular diseases will become the leading global cause of total disease burden, defined as the years subtracted from a healthy life by disability or death.[12]

Patients with vascular disease are, therefore, more likely to be confronted with the social and economic problems of aging. They face conflicts over autonomy and choice, competence to make medical decisions, surrogate decision making, refusal of or limitations to medical treatments, allocation of limited medical resources, and end-of-life issues such as withdrawing or withholding care and assisted suicide. The ethical principles guiding the care of vascular surgical patients are not different from those concerning the care of others, but many ethical challenges are common in this population of patients.

Informed Consent

Until recently, American physicians resisted providing information to patients in order to gain and hold professional stature and were professionally encouraged to be "authoritative, manipulative, and even deceitful" with patients.[13] Today, the principle of respect for patients' autonomy requires that physi-

cians respect medical decisions made by competent patients, irrespective of their age. Further, physicians have the duty to *promote* the ability of patients to make reasoned medical choices by providing all truthful, accurate, and relevant information. Patients also have the right to refuse medical therapy, even if their decision is at odds with what the physician feels would be in the patient's best interests. This principle is supported in the United States by constitutional guarantees of privacy and noninterference. The legal doctrine embodying respect for patients' autonomy is that of informed consent.

One of the earliest legal cases in the United States establishing the rights of patients to consent to and to refuse therapy occurred in 1914. In the case of *Schloendorff v Society of New York Hospital*, a woman agreed to undergo anesthesia for a gynecologic examination but refused surgery. Surgery was nevertheless performed while she was unconscious. During the operation she sustained a brachial plexus injury and later required the amputation of several fingers. Justice Cardozo ruled for the plaintiff in his now famous pronouncement that "every human being of adult years and sound mind has the right to determine what shall be done to his own body," a decision that is cited to this day in cases involving informed consent.[1]

Several elements are essential to the informed consent process. Consent must be voluntary and given by a person with the functional capacity to make medical decisions.[10] Coercive pressures that interfere with voluntariness as well as concerns about competence frequently arise in the care of elderly patients.

Coercive social and economic pressures common to older patients may interfere with their ability to make truly voluntary decisions. Fear of dependence or of becoming a social, economic, or emotional burden to family members may pressure geriatric patients to undertake medically onerous therapies they would otherwise refuse. Economic pressures may play a significant role in the decisions of patients with limited monetary resources to forgo otherwise beneficial therapies. Although these pressures can affect any population of patients, elderly patients are especially likely to face these pressures while simultaneously confronting medical problems that involve difficult treatment decisions.

COMPETENCE. Competence, or the functional capacity to make medical decisions, requires that patients be capable of understanding the need to make a decision, be able to receive and understand information relevant to the decision, and have the ability to express a decision that considers the information presented to them. It should be noted that the term "competence" is a legal term applied to all adults older than 18 years who have not been adjudged incompetent. Medical authorities use the terms "competence" and "capacity" almost interchangeably to refer to a set of abilities necessary to engage in the informed consent process, regardless of age. Decision-making capacity can be adversely affected by conditions common in vascular patients, such as dementia, cerebrovascular disease, depression, and medication. The presence of such medical diagnoses, however, is not de facto evidence of incompetence; the courts have recognized that even patients suffering from some types of dementia may still possess the capacity to give informed consent.[14] Physical barriers to communication that are more common in elderly patients, such as aphasia and hearing loss, can give the false impression of impaired capacity, even though no such impairment exists.[15] Determining whether a patient has the capacity to make health care decisions is challenging in the setting of anesthesia and surgery, when health care providers are often strangers to the patient and when time and resources for making complex determinations about competence can be limited.

Despite extensive study, physicians poorly understand patients' decision making, and both paternalism and prejudice plague physicians' behavior in the informed consent process. When physicians refer patients for evaluation of competence to make medical decisions, it is most often because the patient has refused the physician's advice.[16] One study found that physicians do not adequately inform patients about basic medical decisions more than 80% of the time and inform them about complex medical decisions less than 1% of the time (Figure 20-1).[17] Studies have also shown that physicians regularly ascribe a lower quality of life to impaired and handicapped patients than do the patients themselves. They are incorrect about patients' preferences regarding life-extending therapies more than half of the time and underestimate older patients' desire for life-extending therapy more than 30% of the time (Figure 20-2).[18] Surveys of physicians and other health care workers indicate that they are also likely to *act* on personal prejudices regarding handicapped or impaired patients.[19]

Assumptions about a patient's ability to make medical decisions that are based on age or diagnostic categories are not consistent with ethical medical care. Capacity is also not based on the perceived quality of the decision a patient makes but on whether the patient has the abilities necessary for making a reasoned decision.[10,14,20] When determining whether a patient is capable of making a medical decision, the anesthesiologist should focus on the functional capacity of the patient and ask the following questions: (1) Can the patient communicate a decision? (2) Can the patient receive and understand information that is relevant to the required decision? (3) Can the patient understand the potential consequences of the decision, including risks and benefits? (4) Can the patient make a decision, express it, and disclose his or her values and desires with regard to the medical advice being given? A patient who is capable of each of these actions is competent to make medical decisions, even if the decisions made appear to be bad decisions in the eyes of the physician.[14,16,20,21]

Competence is a relative and task-dependent quality; competence in one activity does not ensure or even imply competence in another, and incompetence in some tasks is not proof of incompetence in others.[14] An elderly patient may have problems remembering specific names and dates, for example, and yet thoroughly understand the ramifications of undergoing a leg amputation. Capacity to make decisions can also change in

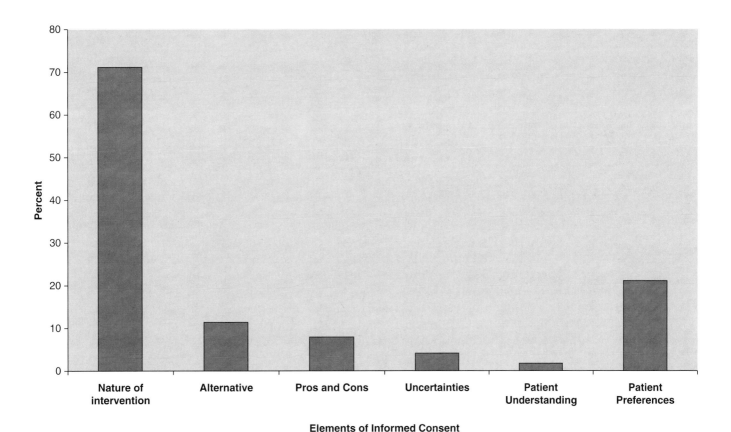

Elements of Informed Consent

FIGURE 20-1 How often are essential elements of informed consent included in consent discussions with patients? Essential elements in the informed consent process are missing from consent discussions more than 80% of the time. In more than 3000 consent discussions, pros and cons of therapy and uncertainties and risks were discussed less than 10% of the time, patients' understanding was evaluated 1.5% of the time, and patients' preferences were elicited only 21% of the time. (Adapted from Braddock C, Edwards K, Hasenberg N, et al: *JAMA* 282:2313, 1999.)

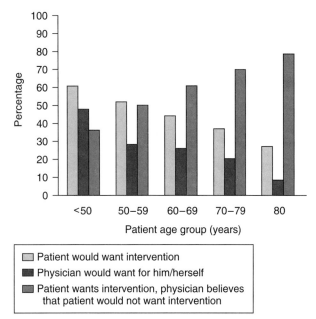

FIGURE 20-2 Disparity of patients' preferences and physician's perceptions of patients' preferences. A higher percentage of patients would want life-sustaining interventions than their physicians would want for themselves if they were in the same situation. The disparity between patients' desire for interventions and their physician's belief about whether they would want interventions increases with patients' age. (Adapted from Hamel M, Teno J, Goldman L, et al: *Ann Intern Med* 130:116, 1999.)

response to environmental factors, such as time of day, familiarity of surroundings, the presence of distractions, and response to medications.[22,23] It is the ethical duty of the anesthesiologist to promote competence and maximize patients' capacity to make their own medical decisions whenever possible and not simply rely on surrogate decision makers. It may be obvious during a preoperative conversation with a patient that the patient is or is not capable of carrying out the preceding tasks. When a patient's capacity is unclear, however, consultation with an expert may be necessary to determine the patient's competence or to overcome physical barriers to communication.

When conditions that interfere with medical decision making can be remedied, it is the physician's ethical duty to do so to promote autonomy in making a decision. Examples include language difficulties that might be remedied by an interpreter, confusion as the result of medication that can reasonably be withheld, and lack of adequate knowledge, which can be corrected by discussion and education. In such cases, elective surgery should be postponed until the patient can participate in medical decision making.[15,22]

In many cases, however, impairments to competence are not temporary, or surgery is urgent and must take place in a time frame that does not permit restoration of competence. When a patient is impaired by an irreversible condition affecting competence, such as irreversible changes in cognition and/or consciousness, the anesthesiologist may have to rely on a proxy decision maker.

DISCLOSURE AND TRUTH TELLING. Disclosing medical information to patients includes both presentation of facts and applica-

tion of bias. How much factual information must or should be disclosed to patients in the informed consent process, and is it ethical to try to influence patients' decisions?

Courts in the United States have cited three standards for the factual content in medical information. The oldest is the "professional standard" in which the physician tells the patient only the facts that other physicians of the same specialty would tell them. This standard sets the stage for systematic secrecy and manipulation among professional colleagues and is not considered adequate by U.S. courts. The courts are evenly divided between a "reasonable person" standard, in which the physician must disclose any information a so-called reasonable person would want to know, and a "subjective standard," in which the physician has a duty to disclose any additional information the individual patient is likely to consider important. In general, informed consent standards require that physicians discuss the proposed therapy, the common risks (because they occur frequently), the serious risks (because the consequences are severe), and alternatives to the proposed therapy, including the option of no therapy.[10]

Physicians sometimes cite a doctrine of "therapeutic privilege" to justify incomplete disclosure or nondisclosure of relevant facts to obtain informed consent. Therapeutic privilege is the assertion that some medical information is so inherently stressful to patients that disclosing it might cause the patient psychological or physical harm.[8,10] Many anesthesiologists cite this as an argument for not talking about the risk of death to patients about to undergo anesthetics, for example. Studies emphatically do *not* support the contention that disclosing stressful information has significant adverse effects on patients who are about to undergo anesthetic care.[24] One possibility is that therapeutic privilege is cited primarily by anesthesiologists who find the process of discussing medical information with patients uncomfortable and stressful *to themselves*. It is ethically acceptable to forgo or limit disclosure of medical information to patients who request it, but such decisions are not ethically or legally within the physician's unilateral discretion.

Physician bias is present in all medical decision making. The physician-patient relationship is an inherently unequal one: the patient is vulnerable because of disability or illness, and the physician possesses specialized knowledge and authoritative influence over the patient. The physician has ethical duties not to exploit the inequality of the relationship and the patient's trust to accomplish his or her own ends. Thus, although physicians always include subjective bias in informed consent discussions, principles of modern medical ethics and legal precedents strictly limit the ways in which a physician can influence the behavior and decisions of autonomous patients.

Coercion, manipulation, and rational persuasion represent techniques by which physicians influence patients.[10] Coercion involves presenting an implied or overt threat of significant harm to the patient unless the patient cooperates with medical therapy. It may be hard to imagine circumstances in which anesthesiologists use threats to obtain patients' cooperation, but coercive circumstances are in fact common in anesthesia care. A patient who desires palliative surgery for vascular disease, but who does not want cardiopulmonary resuscitation, may be coerced into accepting resuscitation in the operating room if doctors or hospital policies insist on suspension of do-not-resuscitate (DNR) orders before anesthesia and surgery. Patients who are denied needed analgesics or anxiolytics prior to signing consent forms may be coerced into signing agreements they do not really understand in order to obtain relief of suffering related to pain or anxiety. Potential subjects of medical studies may feel that they will not have access to potentially lifesaving therapy unless they agree to be a "human guinea pig." To quote Eliot Freidson, "It is my impression that clients are more often bullied than informed into consent, their resistance weakened in part by their desire for the general service if not the specific procedure, in part by the oppressive setting they find themselves in, and in part by the calculated intimidation, restriction of information, and covert threats of rejection by the professional staff itself."[25] Threats capable of altering a patient's free decisions completely usurp the patient's autonomy and are unethical in almost all circumstances. One notable exception might be cases in which a patient's behavior poses a direct danger to medical staff or other persons.

Manipulating medical information includes lying, omitting important facts, or making misleading exaggerations in order to influence patients' decisions. Manipulation alters patients' understanding of a situation in order to motivate them to do what the physicians want. It literally causes the patient to believe something that is false, is therefore inconsistent with autonomous choice, and is unethical.[10]

On the other hand, patients expect physicians to have opinions about medical therapies because of their specialized knowledge and experience. Rational persuasion is influence that is noncontrolling. It neither compels the patient to do what the physician desires (as in coercion) nor deliberately misrepresents the implications of the choice (as in manipulation). In presenting anesthetic choices, for example, it is legitimate and ethical for anesthesiologists to offer an opinion and sound reasoning about how to proceed as long as they do not support it with false or misleading information.

Proxy Decision Making

Frequently, the need to make critical medical decisions arises at times when disease has rendered the patient unconscious or too ill to formulate or express his or her wishes. Legal decisions in the United States recognize the legal and moral authority of surrogate decision makers when patients are unable to express their wishes directly. In 1976, the matter of Karen Ann Quinlan established the rights of unconscious patients to have their previously expressed wishes regarding health care implemented through appropriate surrogate decision makers, even if the medical decision involved potentially life-sustaining therapy. Karen Ann Quinlan was a young woman who suffered a respiratory arrest of uncertain etiology and subsequently became ventilator dependent. Doctors refused to discontinue ventilator therapy at the request of her family. The New Jersey State Supreme Court rendered a decision that Karen was a living person who possessed the right to have her wishes regarding health care implemented by a surrogate decision maker, in this case her father. Subsequent legal decisions in the cases of Clair Convoy and Nancy Cruzan allowed surrogate decision makers to discontinue nutrition and hydration that was life sustaining. In the case of Helen Wanglie, the courts supported a surrogate's decision to *continue* life-sustaining therapy over the objections of physicians because it was what a patient would have wanted. Most states now have laws allowing patients' wishes regarding medical care to be implemented through durable powers of attorney (DPAs), living wills, and proxy decision makers.[5]

Three assumptions are involved in proxy decision making: (1) that decisions made by a competent patient can be implemented by proxy if the patient is unable to express them at the time that treatment is needed, (2) that the proxy will make the same decision the patient would make if the patient could express it (the proxy will "don the mantle" of the patient), and (3) that in the absence of proxies, doctors might act less out of interest for the patient than out of fear of litigation.

Family members are the most common proxy decision makers for incompetent patients. It is assumed that family members have the patient's best interests at heart, are most likely to have discussed decisions with the patient when the patient was capable of expressing wishes, and, by virtue of sharing a common cultural background, are most likely to know what the patient would decide. Studies clearly demonstrate, however, that family members often have *not* discussed issues and values surrounding the use of life-sustaining treatments with loved ones and that family proxy decision makers often come no closer than chance alone to predicting what a family member would want (Figure 20-3).[26-28] In some cases, family members may have conflicts of interest that cause them to make decisions that are not in the best interests of the patient at all. It has also been shown that physicians themselves are incorrect in predicting resuscitation preferences in more than half of their patients.[18] Proxy decision making is, therefore, a poor substitute for patients' decision making, and should thus be utilized *only* when a patient cannot participate in medical decision making and cannot be restored to competence in a time frame during which the medical therapy is meaningful.

Mechanisms for proxy decision making can include advanced directives or living wills, DPAs, legal guardians, and legally designated hierarchies. Advanced directives and living wills are documents in which competent patients state their wishes regarding future health care decisions, to be used when the patients are not able to express their decisions. DPAs are

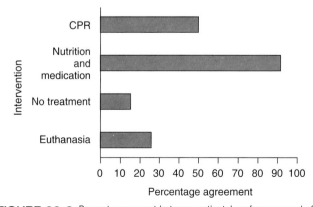

FIGURE 20-3 Percent agreement between patients' preferences and offspring requests. Offspring requests regarding medical intervention for a parent agreed with parents' requests 50% of the time, except in the requests for nutrition and hydration, where concordance was more than 90%. (Adapted from Sonnenblick M, Friedlander Y, Steinberg A: *J Am Geriatr Soc* 41:599, 1993.)

documents in which patients designate a specific person to make medical decisions for them if they later become incompetent. Legal guardians are persons appointed by a court as surrogate medical decision makers, often when incompetent patients either have never been competent or have not provided a designated DPA for health care decisions when they were competent. Finally, most states designate a hierarchy of family members who can act as surrogate health care decision makers (Table 20-1).

In the United States, the Patient Self-Determination Act of 1990 requires any hospital receiving federal health care funding to supply every patient upon admission with information regarding advanced directives.[29] Thus, many vascular surgery patients present to the operating room or intensive care unit with advanced directives or designated proxy decision makers. The anesthesiologist should review any advanced directives, discuss any potential conflicts with planned anesthesia care, and identify persons who will be the patient's designated surrogate decision makers should questions arise in the operating room. Intensive care physicians have ethical and legal obligations to engage competent patients actively in any discussions about advanced directives, limitations of medical care, and surrogate decision making and not to bypass the patient in favor of family members or other surrogates. Because the medical condition of any patient can change rapidly and unexpectedly, advanced directives should be clarified as early as possible in the vascular patient's hospital course, even if life-threatening events are not expected to happen.

End-of-Life Issues and Informed Refusal of Medical Therapy

Informed consent is meaningless if physicians do not also accept the concept of "informed refusal." Without the right to refuse therapy, patients do not consent but simply acquiesce to the will of the physician. Anesthesiologists face issues of withdrawing or withholding care and supportive care of the dying patients in their roles as intensivists, palliative pain management experts, and in the operating room when they provide anesthesia for terminally ill patients having palliative surgery or for patients who have DNR orders.

Today, over 80% of the deaths in the United States occur in health care facilities, and the majority of deaths in the intensive care unit (ICU) happen after a decision has been reached to withhold treatment.[30] Patients and doctors alike recognize that aggressive medical interventions may not be appropriate or desired in the presence of advancing disease. Termination or refusal of specific therapies, however, does not imply termination of other medical care. In the words of Albert Jonsen, "when the goals of curing are exhausted, the goals of caring must be reinforced."[11] What are these goals of caring? According to a 1996 review of the literature published by the American Medical Association, issues of foremost importance to patients at the end of life are control over the timing and location of death; management of symptoms such as pain, dyspnea, and depression; financial management of medical care, and maintenance of therapeutic options, including physician-assisted suicide.[31]

REFUSING, WITHDRAWING, AND WITHHOLDING CARE. Despite the fact that legal decisions have firmly established that both oral and written decisions by patients to withhold or forgo life-sustaining therapy are legally binding, studies show that physicians have persistently ignored patients' self-determination in the institution of medical therapies at the end of life. The Study to Understand Prognoses and Preferences for Outcomes and Risks of Treatments (SUPPORT) demonstrated that more than a third of patients who died in hospitals spent at the least the last 10 days of their life in intensive care, comatose, or on a ventilator against their wishes. Many of these patients spent their entire life savings on their end-of-life care. Even more discouraging was the finding that aggressive programs to change physicians' behavior and decision making through patients' advocacy and physician education had no effect.[32,33]

Physicians' resistance to respecting patients' decisions to forgo resuscitation and/or life-sustaining care has been based on false assumptions that the legal authority of patients' decisions and advanced directives is relatively limited. They also express discomfort with ethical distinctions, such as the differences between affirmative acts and omissions and extraordinary versus ordinary care.

Legal precedents have firmly established the rights of patients and their surrogates to decide to forgo virtually any medical therapy, even when it could be lifesaving. In 1983, two physicians in California were charged with murder and conspiracy to commit murder for terminating life support in accordance with family wishes for a patient who was left deeply comatose after a postoperative stroke. A California Court of Appeals ruled that there was no duty to continue treatment if "further treatment would be of no reasonable benefit to the patient" and that cessation of heroic life support measures did not constitute an "affirmative act" but simply omission of further treatment.[34] Legal decisions in the cases of Karen Ann Quinlan, Claire Convoy, and Nancy Cruzan all support the right to forgo life-sustaining medical therapy.[5]

The courts have punished physicians who ignore the wishes of patients or their surrogate decision makers to terminate life-sustaining care by awarding economic damages for the costs of continued health care and punitive damages for pain, suffering, and mental anguish of the patients' survivors. In *Osgood v Genesys Regional Medical Center*, for example, the court awarded $16 million to a patient and her family after life support was initiated despite contrary instructions from the patient's legal surrogate.[35]

Ethicists argue that withdrawing and withholding care does not violate the rules against killing patients because there is a difference between killing and letting die and between acts of commission, such as lethal injection, and acts of omission, such

---

TABLE 20-1

Hierarchy for Surrogate Decision Making

Patient, if competent
Appointed guardian
Person holding durable power of attorney (DPA)
Patient's spouse
Patient's children older than 18 years, if unanimous
Patient's parents, if unanimous
Adult siblings, if unanimous

as withdrawal of a ventilator. These distinctions are often both confused and confusing to physicians, and many ethicists now endorse a "principle of proportionality."[11] In this principle, treatment is "mandatory" to the extent that it is likely to confer greater benefits than burdens to the patient. The benefits and burdens are measured not solely by medical outcome and preservation of life but also by the patient's perceptions of the medical, social, and psychological benefits and burdens. The principle of proportionality is thus inextricably linked to the patient's understanding and choices regarding end-of-life care. The dying patient may reasonably decide to forgo therapies that physicians traditionally think of as extraordinary, such as ventilator support and cardiopulmonary resuscitation (CPR), yet seek other interventions that seem even more invasive, such as surgery to relieve ischemic limb pain. Pursuing invasive care while forgoing resuscitative care can be entirely consistent with a patient's end-of-life goals and is completely compatible with ethical medical care.

Should anesthesiologists be involved in withdrawal of life support from dying patients? There are two common scenarios in which the anesthesiologist may face this possibility—in the intensive care unit and in the operating room during a "non–heart-beating" cadaveric organ donation. Withdrawal of life-sustaining therapy is a complex and solemn undertaking that requires special physician knowledge, experience, and training. Competence in the care of patients forgoing life-supportive therapy includes the ability to support and counsel patients and families, understanding of and respect for a patient's autonomy and religious and cultural beliefs, knowledge about the physiology and pharmacology of end-of-life care, knowledge about the prevention and treatment of suffering, ability to meet the nonphysical needs of patients, ability to work in complex health care teams, ability to communicate, and empathy.[36] Anyone undertaking the care of a patient from whom life-sustaining therapy is to be withdrawn must also have intimate familiarity with the ethical and legal issues involved.

The principle of nonmaleficence can easily be violated by those who are unfamiliar with complex legal, medical, and social aspects of withdrawal of care. Without adequate expertise, physicians may fail to treat suffering appropriately or adequately, may mishandle important social and psychological issues concerning the patient and family, and may cause undue suffering of the family and loved ones. Accordingly, the specialties of internal medicine, family medicine, and intensive care medicine have each designated core curricula that include specific training in end-of-life care, terminal weaning of ventilator support, palliative care, and the legal and ethical dimensions of decisions and procedures during withdrawal of life-sustaining therapy.[37–39] The Joint Commission on Accreditation of Healthcare Organizations has also published standards for the palliative care of dying patients and withdrawal of life support.[40] As yet, anesthesiology residency and the anesthesiology subspecialty critical care medicine do not outline or require competence in end-of-life issues or withdrawal of life-sustaining therapy.[41] Therefore, it cannot be assumed that most anesthesiologists have either adequate education or adequate experience to provide this care. For this reason, only anesthesiologists who have specialty training and/or significant practice experience should ever be involved with

withdrawing life-sustaining care, whether it be in an ICU patient, or a patient undergoing non–heart-beating cadaveric organ donation.

The actual process of withdrawal of life-sustaining therapy should take into account an understanding of the patient's physiology, level of dependence on the therapy to be withdrawn, level of consciousness, preferences regarding analgesia and sedation, and preferences regarding level of family involvement. Once the decision is made to withdraw life-sustaining therapy, all of the patient's treatment orders should be reviewed and rewritten according to the redirection of treatment goals. Therapies that promote the patient's comfort should be continued, and those promoting physiologic homeostasis or treating the underlying disease process might all be withdrawn.[29] In keeping with the principle of proportionality, any treatment that the patient considers more burdensome than beneficial should be stopped (Table 20–2).

Three interventions are worthy of special consideration: fluid and nutritional therapy, the administration of potentially lethal doses of sedatives and/or narcotics for the purpose of relieving pain or anxiety, and the administration of neuromuscular blocking agents. The withdrawal of fluids and nutrition in the dying patient is controversial, even though it is definitely permissible under American law.[5] The medical and palliative benefits of fluids and nutrition may in many cases be outweighed by the burdens. Adverse effects of nutrition and hydration include fluid overload, diarrhea and abdominal cramping, complications and discomfort presented by placing and maintaining intravenous or enteral access, and prolongation of the dying process through hemodynamic homeostasis. Critically ill patients often experience decreased appetite or even nausea and may not experience "starvation" as a form of suffering. Dehydration can be associated with analgesic and anesthetic effects mediated through ketone production and endogenous opioid release. On the other hand, feeding and hydration of the dying patient may hold important value for family members as well as members of the health care team, as acts of nurturing. In all cases, symptomatic suffering of the patient is to be avoided, and families should be allowed to participate in nurturing activities to comfort the patient.[29]

Pain, dyspnea, and depression are symptoms of suffering, which are altogether too common at the end of life. Is it ethical to take the risk that medications used to alleviate suffering, such as sedatives and analgesics, may as a side effect hasten death? Medical, legal, and religious authorities accept the principle of double effect discussed earlier in this chapter, although it confuses many physicians. Whereas it is entirely ethical to administer medications with the intention of relieving suffering, even if they happen to hasten death, it is not ethical to administer the same agents *for the purpose* of hastening death. It is not ethically justifiable, for example, to administer narcotics to stop respiration in an unconscious patient, who is not aware and therefore cannot have symptoms of suffering.[10,29]

Neuromuscular blocking agents have no anesthetic, analgesic, or sedative properties; have no place in the palliative care of the patient from whom life-sustaining care is being withdrawn; and should not be initiated if withdrawal of mechanical ventilation is planned. When withdrawal of mechanical ventilation is anticipated in a patient who is receiving neuromuscular

TABLE 20-2

Steps in Withdrawing Life-Sustaining Therapy

Actions/Therapy to Initiate or Continue	Actions/Therapy to Discontinue

Review and rewrite medical orders to reflect the new goals of therapy.
Continue or initiate therapies that might increase patients' comfort. Consider:
  Antipyretics
  Antiemetics
  Antipruritics
  Prophylaxis against GI bleeding
  Anticonvulsants
  Herpes zoster treatment
  Antisialagogues to control secretions
Treat patients' suffering. Consider modifying or initiating
  Analgesics
  Anxiolytics
Continue nurturing forms of care, provided the balance of burdens and
    benefits is toward patients' comfort.
  Bathing
  Less frequent dressing changes
  Mouth care
	Discontinue medications/therapies designed to support physiologic homeostasis
	    or treat the underlying disease process. Consider:
	  Ventilatory support/artificial airway
	  Intra-aortic balloon pump support
	  Left ventricular assist devices
	  Pacemakers
	  Dialysis
	  Cerebrospinal fluid drainage
	  Antibiotics, antifungals, antivirals
	  Vasopressors and antiarrhythmics
	  Chronic endocrine therapies
	  Transfusions
	  Supplemental oxygen
	  Muscle relaxants
	Consider deactivating automatic implantable defibrillators, to avoid shock to
	    patient during the dying process.
	Discontinue prophylactic therapy that may be more uncomfortable than the condition
	    it is prophylactic against:
	  Subcutaneous heparin for deep venous thrombosis prophylaxis
	Other routine procedures and treatments to discontinue:
	  Routine phlebotomy
	  Routine radiographic studies, such as chest x-ray study
	  Wound débridements
	  Dressing changes beyond those needed to provide cleanliness and comfort
	  Endotracheal suctioning, unless it adds to patient's comfort
	Consider whether IV fluids and nutrition contribute to patient's or family's comfort
	    or should be withdrawn

Adapted from Lowenstein E (ed): *Medical Ethics. International Anesthesiology Clinics*, vol 39, no 3, Philadelphia, 2001, Lippincott Williams & Wilkins.

blocking agents, the agents should be stopped in all but very exceptional circumstances. Paralyzing the patient so that the family sees no movement is not ethically or medically justifiable and, even worse, might mask signs of distress that would alert the medical team to treat suffering, such as pain or anxiety.[29,42]

PHYSICIAN-ASSISTED SUICIDE AND EUTHANASIA. Physician-assisted suicide and euthanasia are distinct from withdrawing and withholding treatment in that both involve actions whose *primary intention* is to cause death. In the case of physician-assisted suicide, the physician provides either medication or prescriptions that the patient must self-administer, which are intended to cause death. Assisted suicide requires the participation of a patient who is competent to make medical decisions and who is autonomous. Euthanasia involves the direct administration by the physician of drugs to hasten death.[10]

To date, euthanasia is legal in only one Western country, The Netherlands, where it was legalized in 2002. In Australia, legalized euthanasia was overturned 9 months after a law permitting it passed, and an Oregon state physician-assisted suicide law is currently under federal challenge. Supporters of physician-assisted suicide argue that respect for patients' autonomy and privacy requires that the circumstances, timing, and location of death should, as far as possible, be the choice of the patient. Fears of inadequate control of suffering at the end of life are cited as a compelling reason for the availability of assisted suicide. Opponents of assisted suicide argue that, far from returning death to the privacy and control of the patient, it

"medicalizes" death and overly idealizes the morality of physicians and their relationships with patients. Many ethicists agree that there are certainly individual circumstances in which patients' suffering cannot be controlled and in which assisted suicide would be ethical and even kind. But most have reservations about public policies that sanction assisted suicide, citing fears that the option will be abused and that poor, elderly, and otherwise vulnerable members of society might choose or experience financial or social pressure to choose suicide instead of palliative care.

There is evidence to support fears that the assisted suicide option can be abused, can unfairly burden vulnerable populations, and may even be used to disguise acts of euthanasia in communities in which it is legalized. Carlos Gomez studied assisted suicide in The Netherlands in the early 1990s. At that time, although technically illegal, assisted suicide would not be investigated or prosecuted in The Netherlands if certain conditions were met: the request came from a conscious patient, the desire to die was enduring and repeated over time, and no reasonable alternative to end suffering could be offered. Gomez described cases that violated the conditions, including that of an infant who was euthanized and that of a critically injured motorist who was unconscious when the physician elected to administer a lethal injection of potassium chloride. In others, alternatives to lethal injection were available.[43] Later review of the Netherlands experience confirmed that euthanasia without a patient's request accounted for 0.7% of all deaths and that 23% of physicians admitted to performing euthanasia without a patient's request.[44] An Australian study found that more than one third of surgeons surveyed admitted to administering drugs to hasten death, often without a patient's request to do so.[45] Finally, a report describing the first year's experience of legal physician-assisted suicide in the state of Oregon demonstrated that patients who committed assisted suicide were elderly and more likely than controls to be divorced or never married.[46] This suggests that patients who committed suicide were more likely than controls to lack family and social supports. The authors made no inquiry into the social circumstances or economic status at the time of suicide, and the authors' conclusion that neither played a significant role in the patients' decisions does not seem supportable.

Perhaps the most powerful reason cited for opposing physician-assisted suicide is that it could provide a disincentive to physicians and the health care system to seek other solutions to health, social, and economic problems common in the elderly by providing a simpler and less expensive solution.

Do-Not-Resuscitate Orders in the Operating Room

Patients who have DNR orders sometimes present to the operating room for anesthesia and surgery. In the SUPPORT database, which contained 4301 seriously ill patients, 745 underwent surgery, of whom 57 had a DNR order. The surgical procedures performed included vascular access procedures, tracheotomies, liver transplantation, and coronary artery bypass grafting.[47]

Surveys have shown that a majority of anesthesiologists do not understand their ethical and legal obligations regarding DNR orders in the anesthetized patient. In one study, 59% of anesthesiologists assumed that DNR orders are automatically suspended during anesthesia and surgery.[29] This assumption is contrary to practice guidelines established by the American Society of Anesthesiologists (Table 20–3), the American College of Surgeons, and guidelines of the Joint Commission on Accreditation of Healthcare Organizations.[48–50]

Anesthesiologists cite several reasons to support automatic suspension of DNR orders in the anesthetized patient. In contrast to in-hospital cardiac arrest, cardiac arrest in the operating room carries a favorable prognosis, with a mortality of only 8%.[51] This outcome appears to occur because arrests in the operating room are witnessed events that are often due to reversible causes such as hemorrhage or drug effects and because resuscitation is instituted within seconds.

Although many anesthesiologists feel it may be appropriate to allow a patient to die as a result of a terminal disease, many also feel it is inappropriate for patients to prevent them from treating an arrest that has resulted from something the anesthesiologist has done. But complications are a known risk of modern medical practice, are not always or even usually attributable to one action or cause, and are not necessarily the result of negligence. A "moral line" probably cannot be drawn around interventions used to treat complications of the patient's illness and complications of treatments of the illness because they both originate in the process that caused the patient to seek medical attention.[52] Truog and Waisel noted that the DNR patient is often someone who is vulnerable to these kinds of complications and that DNR orders are often written with such events in mind and specifically to spare the patient from an aggressive and technological response.[29]

Some anesthesiologists invoke a popular, but misguided, statement that "anesthesia is merely ongoing resuscitation" to propose that it is impossible to distinguish resuscitation in the operating room from otherwise routine anesthetic care. This approach gives the unfortunate impression that patients need constant rescue from their anesthesiologist and that dangers related to cardiac arrest are even greater in the operating room than they are on the ward, when in fact the opposite is true. Although many anesthetic interventions are also common to

---

TABLE 20-3

Summary of Guidelines for the Anesthesia Care of Patients with Do-Not-Resuscitate Orders

I. Communication among all involved parties is key; relevant aspects of communication must be documented.

II. Policies automatically suspending DNR orders or other advanced directives prior to procedures involving anesthesia may not address a patient's rights in a responsible and ethical manner. Such policies should be reviewed and revised.

III. Because anesthetic care may involve therapies that might be regarded as resuscitation in other circumstances, directives limiting care should be reviewed prior to procedures with the patient or their appropriate surrogate. The status of those directives should be clarified or modified, based on patient's preference.

IV. Any clarifications or modifications should be documented in the medical record.

V. Plans for postoperative care should indicate if and when the original advanced directives will be reinstated. Consideration should be given as to whether providing the patient with a time- or event-limited postoperative trial of therapy can help the patient or surrogate evaluate whether continued therapy is consistent with the patient's goals.

VI. Exceptions, if any, to injunctions against therapy in the case of complications of anesthesia and surgery should be discussed and documented

VII. Concurrence among the primary physician, surgeon, and anesthesiologist is desirable; other members of the health care team should, if feasible, be included in the process.

VIII. If conflicts arise, the following resolutions are suggested:
   A. If the patient's wishes conflict with the anesthesiologist's moral views, the anesthesiologist should, if possible, withdraw from care in a timely fashion.
   B. If the patient's or surgeon's limitations of intervention are in conflict with generally accepted standards of care, ethical practice, or institutional policies, the anesthesiologist should voice such concerns and present them to the appropriate institutional body.
   C. If these alternatives are not feasible in a time frame to prevent morbidity or suffering, care should proceed with reasonable adherence to the patient's directives.

IX. The anesthesiology service should establish liaisons with surgical and nursing services to present these guidelines.

X. Modification of these guidelines may be appropriate under certain circumstances and in emergency situations.

Adapted from the *Ethical Guidelines for the Anesthesia Care of Patients with Do-Not-Resuscitate Orders or Other Directives that Limit Treatment*, American Society of Anesthesiologists, October 2001.

cardiopulmonary resuscitation, they can usually be clearly distinguished from it: would an intensivist say patients are being "resuscitated" simply because they are on a ventilator?

The objections of anesthesiologists do have merit but are not powerful enough to override the imperative requiring physicians to respect patients' autonomy. It is one thing to propose that a pneumonectomy or a thoracic vascular procedure requires the use of an endotracheal tube and that a patient who wants the surgery must agree to intubation; the procedure literally cannot be done without it. It is a very different thing to insist that the use of CPR is an integral part of most surgeries when in fact it is rarely employed in the general operating room and then only to treat an uncommon complication that the physician is actively trying to avoid. When a physician threatens to withhold anesthesia or surgery until the patient consents to another, distinct intervention, such as CPR, which is not absolutely necessary for the surgery itself, he or she is engaging in coercion. In the words of Walker, "Surgery may provide palliative treatment for otherwise untreatable disease. Suspension of DNR orders in the perioperative period places patients in the unfair position of having to weigh the benefits of palliative treatment against the risks of unwanted resuscitation."[53]

Early in the patients' rights movement, court decisions focused on defining the rights of patients to refuse or limit medical care and protecting physicians who subsequently cooperated with the patient's decision to do so. Despite those legal protections, however, studies show that physicians have placed little systematic priority on patients' own decisions with regard to end-of-life care and resuscitation. The SUPPORT study found that fewer than half of the treating physicians even knew when their patients did not want resuscitation.[32]

Because education has failed to effect widespread changes in physician behaviors with regard to patients' decision making, the legal system is stepping in to apply pressure. Legal scholars in the United States have proposed creating a tort of "wrongful living" (to distinguish it from cases of "wrongful life," which arise over neonatal conception, delivery, and health issues) to award damages to a patient whose right to refuse medical treatment has been violated through an unconsented resuscitation. Advocates of the wrongful living cause of action, such as Tricia Hackleman, argue that physicians' disrespect for patients' decision making is common and a new cause of action is the only way to force physicians to respect patients' rights.[54]

Legal decisions now penalize doctors who resuscitate patients against their wishes. Unwanted resuscitation now carries with it both the real risk of litigation against the physician for economic and punitive damages and potential criminal charges of battery. In *Anderson v St. Francis-St. George Hospital, Inc*, in Ohio, Edward Winter sued for damages when he suffered a stroke after surviving a resuscitation he had specifically stated he did not want.[55] The court found that he had cause for an action of battery against the physicians involved. In *Klavan v Chester Crozier Medical Center* in Pennsylvania in 2001, surrogates for Marshall Klavan, MD, filed suit for ignoring known and explicit directives from him to not to perform CPR or use a ventilator or intravenous devices. Resuscitation left him in a persistent vegetative state, and damages are anticipated to run to millions of dollars.[56]

How should the anesthesiologist manage the vascular patient presenting for surgery with a DNR order? The patient's primary physician or surgeon may have some knowledge of resuscitation issues in the operating room, but the anesthesiologist who will be responsible for CPR in the operating room is best qualified to discuss these risks and benefits with the patients and/or their surrogate decision makers. The approach to the patient with a DNR order involves the following steps: (1) determining what the patient's goals are; (2) establishing what exactly is meant by "resuscitation"; (3) educating the patient about the risks of resuscitation; (4) documenting the agreements reached with the patient about interventions commonly associated with resuscitation, such as intubation and ventilation, chest compressions, cardioversion and DC countershock, and the administration of vasoactive drugs; and (5) establishing agreement among care providers in the operating room about the nature of resuscitation efforts, if any, to be undertaken.[29,48]

Many patients have elected to forgo CPR because of fears that resuscitation will lead to poor outcome or because they believe CPR will be futile. Education and reassurance about the favorable prognosis of operating room resuscitation may convince some patients to rescind their DNR orders for the perioperative period. Patients also commonly fear that events in the operating room may leave them dependent on burdensome therapies, such as a ventilator or artificial nutrition. Some patients may accept resuscitation in the operating room if it is agreed that such therapy will be discontinued after an agreed-to period of time in accordance with their wishes when meaningful recovery is not anticipated. Many patients may agree to resuscitative therapies that they do not feel are invasive, such as the administration of medications.

It is not always possible to accommodate a patient's demands to limit interventions and still provide nonnegligent care. A patient's desire to have thoracic aortic aneurysm surgery under general anesthesia without endotracheal intubation seems beyond the limits of competent care, for example. The duty to respect the patient's autonomy does not require the anesthesiologist to provide care that is negligent, and there may be times when a reasonable agreement with the patient cannot be reached and the surgery and anesthesia cannot be done.

Operating room care requires the intense cooperation of many health care providers, each with ethical duties to the patient, and it is important that any resuscitation agreements between the patient and the anesthesiologist be made apparent to the other members of the team. This prevents disagreements about resuscitation from arising during a critical event, when interventions must be carried out or forgone quickly. It also permits "conscientious objectors" to the agreements to withdraw from the health care team.

Finally, DNR orders should never be construed as a "do-not-care" mandate. A patient's decision to limit one medical intervention does not imply limitations of others. The use of invasive hemodynamic monitoring, for example, may be necessary to ensure optimal anesthetic management of a patient with a DNR order and to avoid critical situations in which the DNR status of the patient becomes pivotal.

Allocation of Scarce Resources: Extrinsic and Intrinsic Rationing

Health care expenditures consume an increasing percentage of the nation's resources: total national health care expenditures in the United States increased from $143 per capita and 5% of the gross domestic product (GDP) in 1960 to $4358 per capita and 14% of the GDP in 1999. Critical care expenditures account for 1% of the annual U.S. GDP, and end-of-life care consumes 10% to 12% of all health care costs and 27% of all Medicare expenditures[57,58] (Figure 20-4).

Private insurers pay one third of all health care expenses in the United States, public funding pays for another third, and individual out-of-pocket payments account for only about 15%.[59] The third-party payer system complicates equitable distribution of health care spending by disconnecting patients and providers from the direct cost of treatment, thus facilitating patients' and providers' overconsumption. Demand for service remains high while perception about cost is unrealistic. In the words of Papper, "This simultaneous desire for new inventions and unwillingness to pay for them is analogous . . . to a decision that not only is everyone entitled to personal vehicular transportation, but that the vehicle purchased should always be a Cadillac."[60] Cost savings introduced by managed care systems and restraints on development and deployment of new technology will not provide sufficient reductions to corral rising health care expenditures driven at least in part by an aging cohort of demanding health care consumers.[57] Controlling costs will ultimately rest on some form of rationing of health care resources.

The debate on health care rationing is couched in terms implying futurity—the idea that rationing is something yet to happen. But in fact physicians, including anesthesiologists, engage right now in both *explicit* rationing and *implicit* rationing, which has important ethical implications for patients' care.[61]

Explicit rationing is the practice of limiting health care resource utilization by formal, enforceable rules that are known or knowable by all. Such rules might be based on the availability of service or dollars or on preset criteria related to the expected outcomes of treatment. Explicit rationing of dollars occurs when an insurer excludes specific services or providers or limits payments according to contract. In organ transplantation centers, explicit rationing of service occurs through policies that establish the criteria by which patients are determined eligible for service and how they are prioritized in the transplant queue. Many examples of explicit rationing can be found in anesthesia practice. An anesthesiologist who requires cash payment prior to providing anesthesia services for elective cosmetic surgery, for example, is effectively rationing the service according to ability to pay. An anesthesiologist's decision to not transfuse a hemorrhaging patient because the patient has exceeded an amount predetermined by policy effectively rations blood bank resources in equal portions to all, based at least in part on criteria related to patients' outcome. Explicit rationing has the advantage of openness, accountability, and the ability to establish patients' expectations prospectively. It tends to minimize potential provider bias through preset rules. But it has the disadvantage of inflexibility. Once the rules are established, individual exceptions are difficult to make without charges that the system is unfairly biased when it serves someone who would not normally qualify or excludes someone who would otherwise be treated—even if there is a reasonable rationable for doing so.

Implicit rationing, on the other hand, encompasses limitations that are imposed as a result of ad hoc decisions by practitioners, informal criteria, or conditions that indirectly affect the eligibility of a patient for services but are never openly identified as such. Implicit rationing occurs on a societal level, where the poor and underinsured receive fewer services, for example. It also occurs at the physician-patient level; the decision not to offer renal dialysis to an 85-year-old patient who has suffered a devastating stroke and acute renal failure after vascular surgery is implicit rationing based on perceived probability of reasonable outcomes. A decision to proceed directly to amputation in an immobile, severely demented patient with an ischemic foot, rather than undertake a series of revascularization attempts, is one of implicit rationing. Implicit rationing is covert, potentially arbitrary, and presents accountability problems; when decisions are questioned, it is hard to determine who is accountable and to whom to appeal. Physician bias about patients' motivation, capability, and quality of life may play an unfair role in rationing decisions. Decisions could come to be based on patient-related criteria that society tends to consider unfair, such as age, race, sex, handicaps, intellectual ability, and employment status. However, implicit rationing has the advantage of flexibility; because rules are not set, medical decisions can take into account individual case characteristics that might influence the appropriateness of therapy and therefore maximize individual outcomes.

Is implicit rationing unethical? Implicit rationing and its effects are hard to examine precisely because it is covert. But studies have clearly shown that implicit rationing on the societal level affects large numbers of patients in a discriminatory way. It is clear that poor and uninsured patients in the United States not only receive fewer services but also have significantly poorer health as a result.[62,63] Subpopulations most likely to be affected are those who are underemployed, work part time, or work for companies in which health care is not an employee benefit. Women and minorities are disproportionately represented among the uninsured.[64,65] In a society that

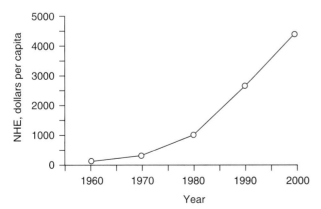

FIGURE 20-4 National health expenditures (NHE) per capita. (Adapted from Osborne and Patterson[57] and Cowen et al.[59])

values justice and is beginning to assert that health is a "right," this outcome is clearly undesirable. Intrinsic rationing strategies that knowingly allow unjustifiable inequities are unethical.

On a physician-patient level, studies of intrinsic rationing are inconsistent. Age does not appear to play a consistent or significant role in hemodialysis treatment decisions or in timing of coronary surgery in Canadian referral centers, for example; and race does not appear to have a significant effect on ICU care adjusted for severity of illness.[66-68] Lung cancer treatments do appear to differ according to age, but one explanation might be that older patients actually tend to *choose* less aggressive therapy than younger patients do, a possibility consistent with free choice of the patient and not necessarily physician rationing.[69] On the other hand, studies have also shown that physicians and other health care providers admit to negative bias in resuscitation decisions for patients who are perceived to be severely handicapped.[19] When intrinsic rationing decisions are based on patient-related criteria such as individual prognostic indicators and patients' goals, they may actually be more consistent with ethical care than extrinsic criteria that do not fairly consider individual variations in the patient's condition.

Until a national consensus is reached about how health resource allocation should be prioritized, physicians have an ethical duty in individual interactions with patients to be the patient's trustworthy advocate regardless of what combination of extrinsic and intrinsic rationing pressures come into play.[70] In medical decision making, the physician should press for the safest care that carries the most reasonable probability of a positive health outcome. Frequently, this recommendation may involve forgoing care that is futile or has a low probability of meeting the patient's goals. But it may conversely involve pressing for meaningful and beneficial care that is expensive and/or runs contrary to a third-party payer's stated intention to pay. Morreim reminds physicians of how central their duty is to advocate meaningfully, vigorously, and, most of all, sincerely: "As the physician pleads his patient's case while others allot or deny benefits, the physician can tell the patient that 'they', not he, are rationing care. He maintains unsullied his unequivocal loyalty to the patient. But at a terrible price. He is no longer practicing medicine."[71]

Ethical Issues in Research

Human Subjects Research

The fundamental ethical relationship between patients and physicians is based on a premise that the doctor will at all times put the interests of the patient first. This covenant may be broken when medical research is introduced into the relationship. As Katz stated, "Investigators who appear before patient-subjects as physicians in white coats create confusion. Patients come to hospitals with the trusting expectations that their doctor will care for them. They will view an invitation to participate in research as a professional recommendation that is intended to serve their individual interests."[72] Human research subjects are asked to put aside or at least deemphasize their own interests and share a goal with the researcher to serve the interests of some future, hypothetical group of patients. They become, in the words of Miller, "tokens to be acted upon for ends that they may but do not necessarily share."[29] Prime

examples of such objectification of patients include research in healthy humans in which there are no potential beneficial medical results for the subject and phase I cancer trials in terminally ill patients in which the goal is to examine the toxicity of the treatment and not to produce cure, remission, or even palliation.

The clinical researcher faces personal conflicts of interest when academic or corporate career opportunities and advancement, professional prestige, and/or financial incentives are a part of the research milieu.[73,74] A researcher who accepts stock options in a company for which he or she is conducting a phase I product trial, for example, raises serious concerns about his or her objectivity in performing and analyzing the results of the experiment and ability or desire to protect the patients upon whom the research is conducted. Achieving an ethical balance among the needs of the research subject, the interests of a hypothetical group of future patients, and the physician's own conflicts of interest is beyond the abilities of most individuals. This is the primary reason why human subjects research is more closely scrutinized and controlled than any other area of medicine.

Historically, regulation of research in human subjects was formulated following World War II, when the Nuremberg Code and the Helsinki Declaration* codified ethical obligations of physicians to perform useful and relevant human experiments and to protect the subjects of those experiments (Table 20-4). Surprisingly, researchers in the United States were slow to draw parallels between Nazi research and American experiments being conducted at the time of the Doctor's Trial, some of which were cited by the Nuremberg defendants as being analogous to their own. In the words of David Rothman, "the prevailing view was that [the Nuremberg medical defendants] were Nazis first and last; by definition nothing they did, and no code drawn up in response to them was relevant to the United States."[9] This view was aided in part by an American press that gave minor attention to the Doctor's Trial and its results and even extolled the nobility of prisoners, students, and army conscripts who endured the sometimes gruesome treatment of American researchers[75] (Table 20-5). Medical researchers were far from ignorant of the strict standards set by the Nuremberg Code and Helsinki Declaration, however. In 1959, Renee Fox described her observations of human experimentation on a medical ward, and reported that researchers were sometimes troubled by their "inability" to apply the standards enunciated at the Nuremberg Medical Trial.[76]

In 1966, Henry Beecher published an analysis of mainstream medical experiments in which serious ethical violations were apparent.[77] In 1974, the National Research Act was introduced, establishing the National Commission for the Protection of Human Subjects of Biomedical and Behavioral Research, out of which the modern institutional review board (IRB) was born.[5]

Three guiding principles are set forth in the ethical conduct of human subjects research: (1) respect for persons, including respect for autonomy and the obligation to protect subjects with limited autonomy; (2) beneficence, which is the obligation to minimize risks to subjects, maximize benefits, and ensure that

---

*The Helsinki Declaration was most recently amended in the year 2000; the current declaration can be obtained through the World Medical Association.

TABLE 20-4

Summary of the Nuremberg Code

I. The voluntary consent of the human subject is essential.
   a. Subjects should have legal capacity to give consent.
   b. Subjects should be so situated as to exercise free power of choice.
   c. Subjects should have sufficient knowledge to make an understanding and enlightened decision, including the nature, duration, and purpose of the experiment, the experimental methods, the conveniences and hazards to be expected, and the possible effects on his health or person.
   d. The duty for assuring the quality of consent rests with each individual who initiates, directs, or engages in the experiment, and cannot be delegated to others.
II. The experiment should offer possible fruitful results for the good of society that are unprocurable by any other means. It should not be random or unnecessary.
III. The experiment should be based on animal experiments, knowledge of the disease, or other problems under study, so that the anticipated results will justify the experiment.
IV. All unnecessary physical and mental suffering and injury is to be avoided.
V. No experiment should be done where there is a reason to believe that death or disability injury will occur, except when the experimental physicians are also the subjects.
VI. The risks should never exceed the humanitarian importance of the problem to be solved by the experiment.
VII. Adequate preparations and facilities must be provided to prevent even the remote possibility of injury, disability, or death.
VIII. The experiment should be conducted only by scientifically qualified persons.
IX. The subjects must be able to end the experiment at any time.
X. The investigator must terminate the experiment if he has reason to believe that continuation of the experiment will result in injury, disability, or death of the subject.

Adapted from Jonsen A, Veatch R, Walters L: *The Source Book for Bioethics: A Documentary History*, Washington DC, 1998, Georgetown University Press.

research design is scientifically sound; and (3) justice, which is the obligation to treat each person with regard to what is morally right and to ensure a fair distribution of benefits and burdens. Ethical principles involved in research can conflict when the rights and freedoms of individual subjects are pitted against potential benefits to humankind and society.

Respect for autonomy and informed consent in research carry the obligation to disclose accurate and balanced information and the duty to protect the confidentiality of the subjects. Research subjects should be informed of the procedures to be performed, the risks and benefits (including the possibility of no benefit to the individual), the possibility of commercializa-tion of the research findings, and the presence or perceived presence of any potential conflict of interest on the part of researchers, their institutions, or their sponsors. Subjects or their surrogates must possess the capacity to understand the information provided and to weigh risks and benefits. It should be noted that the Nuremberg Code and the original Helsinki Declaration *exluded* nontherapeutic experimentation on persons who are unable to provide consent themselves.[5]

Consent must be given without coercion. Subjects must be free to refuse to participate or to end participation at any time without penalty. One form of coercion of particular concern in human subjects research is that of "situational coercion," in

TABLE 20-5

Some Notorious Experiments Conducted on Human Subjects During the 20th Century by American Investigators

Year; Location	Experiment	Comments
1906; Manila	To investigate the effect of cholera on inmates	13 fatalities attributed to mistaken substitution of a bottle of bubonic plague for cholera.
1918-1922; California	To investigate the effects of transplanted testicles from executed convicts to "senile and devitalized men"—later goat testicles were used	Unknown outcomes.
1934; Denver	Trial of a tuberculosis "vaccine"	2 inmates: one became very ill. Both survived and were granted clemency.
1940s; Illinois	To investigate treatment and "cure" of malaria	400 prisoners; morbidity included raging fever, nausea, loss of consciousness, relapses.
1949; New York	To investigate human blood "cleansing" of cancer cells	1 subject, connected by rubber tubing vein-to-vein with a child dying of cancer, to see if the prisoner's circulation would "cleanse" her of cancer cells.
1950s: Ohio	To investigate "the natural killing-off processes of the human body"	Over 100 prisoners injected with live cancer cells—inmates told they faced no danger; any cancer they contracted would "spread slowly and could be removed surgically."
1960s; Oklahoma, Arkansas, Alabama	To investigate for a commercial pharmaceutical company effects of drugs and blood plasma products	Deaths from adverse drug effects; some prisoners received the wrong blood type; up to 30 inmates per month contracted hepatitis B.
1970s; New York	Cancer study	22 senile patients injected with live cancer cells.
1960s and 1970s; Tuskegee, Alabama	Placebo-controlled trial of treatment of syphilis	Rural black male subjects: outcomes of death, tertiary syphilis.

Adapted from Hornblum A: *Br Med J* 315:1437, 1997.[75]

which the subject may feel they are not truly free to refuse because of their particular circumstances. Examples of subjects in whom situational coercion may be a problem include prisoners, whose terms and experiences of incarceration might be affected by their decisions regarding participation in research, and hospitalized patients, who might feel that their hospital care could be compromised if they refuse to participate.[78]

Questions often arise about whether monetary or other reimbursement of human subjects is ethical. Inducements to participate are probably ethical if they do not undermine the freedom to refuse under reasonable circumstances. Significant monetary reimbursement could have detrimental effects on both the ethical balance and the scientific quality of the research. Individuals might choose to endure suffering to which others in less desperate circumstances would not subject themselves. Subjects might also conceal factors that would otherwise make them ineligible for participation, thus compromising the research results and subjecting themselves to increased risks.[10]

Obligations of beneficence require that researchers maximize benefits for their subjects and future beneficiaries of the results as well as minimize harms, including psychological, physical, legal, social, and economic harms. The scientific design of the research must address a question of sufficient value to justify the risk posed to participants, the research must follow the approved protocol, and findings should be reported accurately and promptly. The principle of nonmaleficence requires researchers to terminate research immediately if it is judged to be harmful to the participant.[10,79,80]

In the field of anesthesiology, special concern is devoted to research into the prevention or treatment of unpleasant symptoms, such as pain and nausea. The principle of nonmaleficence generally limits research protocols involving pain to studies that compare different treatments that have known efficacy, rather than placebo-controlled trials. Even when both experimental arms utilize interventions that are known to have efficacy, "escape" analgesia or antiemetics must be provided upon the patient's request.[29]

Another important question arises when physicians perform procedures on patients that are new or with which the physician has little or no experience. This is particularly common in surgical and anesthesia specialties, which are technologically oriented and in which practitioners are frequently developing and learning new techniques. When does practice innovation become experimentation? Jones suggests that a new procedure is a clinical innovation, and not experimentation, if it is not contraindicated, does not depart from scientific theory, carries no substantive risk, would be considered a viable option under similar circumstances by other competent physicians, and offers some therapeutic advantage. As always, protection of the patient and honest disclosure are paramount; informed consent for conventional treatment concentrates on what is known, whereas discussion of experimental or innovative treatment must concentrate on what is *not* known.[81]

Finally, the concept of justice addresses the protection of individuals and groups who are subject to research but who may not benefit directly from it. The risks and benefits of the research should be fairly distributed among all possible subject populations. The Helsinki Declaration underlined the principle that concern for the individual research subject must always

prevail over the interests of society.[5] Worthy intentions do not justify violating a research subject's civil rights.

Ethics of Animal Research

Although public concerns about unregulated animal experimentation date back to the antivivisection movement in England of the 1800s, the animal rights movement did not gain a foothold in the United States until recently. The U.S. animal welfare debate followed in the wake of the civil rights movement and paralleled increasing awareness of the human impact on the environment and other animal species. The first federal law concerning the laboratory use of animals, the Laboratory Animal Welfare Act, was enacted in 1966 and was amended in 1970 to become the Animal Welfare Act (AWA). In response to public pressure, the Health Research Extension Act of 1985, and amendments to the AWA, required the establishment of institutional animal care and use committees (IACUCs). These committees are required to oversee conditions of laboratory animals; to review and approve animal research protocols; to educate and train investigators in ethical issues and aspects of animal handling, anesthesia, analgesia, and euthanasia; and to act as a liaison with the community.[82]

The debate between researchers and animal rights activists has been political, emotional, and divisive; has been characterized by intransigence and shrill rhetoric; and at times has involved acts of vandalism and even violence. Researchers have resisted the concept that animal experimentation could be subject to any moral reservations and have asserted that the therapeutic advancements in medicine are utterly dependent on continued animal research. Many animal welfare activists have insisted on the moral equivalence of animal research to experiments on humans and have accused researchers of being blind to or, even worse, actually unmoved by the suffering of their animal subjects. Opponents of animal research propose that many, if not most, animal experiments either do not provide new knowledge of sufficient significance to warrant the animal suffering and death involved or else are poorly designed and of questionable application in humans.

Neither side tells the complete tale. Benefits that have been reaped from animal experimentation are myriad, including advances in anesthesia, cardiovascular and orthopedic surgery, treatments of diabetes and hemophilia, vaccines, antimicrobial agents, cancer chemotherapy, treatment of trauma and shock, and many, many others.[83] But it is not entirely sensible to assert that medical science would have come to a halt without animal experimentation. In the words of Harold Hewitt, himself an animal researcher, "it underrates the ingenuity of researchers to assert that medical progress would have been seriously impeded had animal experiments been illegal, although a different strategy would have been required. It is the skill of the scientist to find a way round the intellectual, technical and ethical limitations to investigation. No one complains, surely that we have been denied the benefit of potential advances by prohibiting experiments on unsuspecting patients, criminals, or idiots."[84] Researchers themselves have started to question the quality and validity of many animal experiments. In one review of animal experiments, the authors found that studies were fraught with problems of poor design, were statistically underpowered, were possibly subject to publication bias, and were not regularly subjected to cross-species or meta-analysis to determine whether or not results were actually applicable in humans.[85]

Most ethicists have broadened their perspective to include the possibility that animals have sufficient awareness to possess some moral status, but how much is still debated. The growing consensus is that many, if not all, animals are capable of feelings of pleasure, pain, discomfort, and fear and thus can experience enjoyment and suffering. The treatment of animals, therefore, has moral connotations that the use of inanimate objects simply does not. An act that causes an animal to suffer because of pain, fear, sickness, or poor standards of care constitutes a moral harm that is to be avoided, mitigated, and weighed against the benefits it produces.[86] Even without postulating a "moral status" for animals, traditional ethics maintains that cruelty to animals is illicit—animals should be protected from cruelty, not because they have rights but because he who is cruel to animals is more likely to be cruel to humans.[87]

Researchers have moral obligations to provide clean and humane living conditions and appropriate veterinary care for their animal subjects. They should use animals only when absolutely necessary and minimize any suffering incurred by the research. Duplicative or mediocre research that causes the deaths of many animals should not be allowed. As physician R. Burns urged in 1989, "As physicians, researchers, and educators, we must take a long-overdue objective look at how and why we use animals in research and education. A great deal of animal-based research adds very little to our understanding in the diagnosis and treatment of our patients."[88]

When Ethical Issues Transcend the Doctor-Patient Relationship: The Ethics Consultation Service and Institutional Review Boards

Education can help anesthesiologists recognize ethical conflicts but may not be sufficient to enable them to define, articulate, and resolve issues in an authoritative way. Anesthesiologists may find that they need help with evaluating ethical issues in a structured and disciplined way, aid in communication with involved parties, and mediation of conflicts. Researchers benefit from a dispassionate review of the scientific rationale, protocol, and methods of protecting both human and animal subjects from risk or frank abuse. Expertise in ethical issues is usually available through two common avenues in medical practice: the ethics committee or consultation service and IRBs.

Clinical Ethics Committees and Consultations

Dr. Karen Teel proposed the concept of ethics committees to provide a forum for patients, physicians, theologians, attorneys, and social workers to "review the individual circumstances of ethical dilemma and . . . [provide] assistance and safeguards for patients and their medical caretakers."[89] Her review was noted and incorporated by Chief Justice Hughes in his decision regarding Karen Ann Quinlan in 1976, and ethics committees and consultation services have been encouraged by the courts to resolve conflicts about care of patients without sacrificing patients' privacy through the public exposure of a legal proceeding.[5] Such committees find themselves used most to resolve conflicts among physicians, patients, and families, but

they can and often do provide valuable education, both in answering questions about clinical situations and in providing formal continuing medical education in ethics to health care providers and institutions. Ethics committees are involved in creating and defending institutional and practice policies, such as policies about discontinuing life support, managing patients with unusual religious beliefs, and informed consent. Ethics experts can help anesthesiologists and intensivists in decision making that involves the allocation of scarce resources, such as policies and practices defining patients' eligibility for vital organ transplantation. Finally, clinical ethics committees can be a valuable resource and ally when patients' interests conflict with the interests of institutions and third-party payers. This aspect may become increasingly important, as there is evidence that doctors perceive that managed care regulations sometimes prevent them from behaving in an ethical manner and have the potential to put patients' care in conflict with the professional and financial interests of the physician.[90,91]

The constitution of ethics committees varies, usually involving representation from health care providers specifically educated in medical ethics and experienced in resolving clinical conflicts as well as interested clinicians and nurses, social workers, theologians, attorneys, and patients or other lay members. It is widely acknowledged that a specialized knowledge of ethics and certain interpersonal skills are "core competences" to providing ethics consultation.[92,93] The Society for Bioethics Consultation Task Force on Standards for Bioethics Consultation stated that ethics consultants should have knowledge in multiple areas, including moral reasoning, bioethical concepts, relevant codes of ethics, institutional policies, relevant law, and others, as well as skills in ethical assessment, resolution of conflict, and interpersonal communication. The same task force, however, recommended *against* certification of individuals or groups providing ethics consultation because certification carries the risk of displacing patients and their physicians as primary decision makers, could undermine diversity, might institutionalize a particular moral perspective and exclude others, would require the creation of a new certification bureaucracy, and would be difficult to implement as there is no experience in evaluating ethics consultants' competence.[93]

Do ethics consultations "work"? Clinical ethics consultation is a young process and relatively few outcome data exist. Nevertheless, several conclusions can be drawn from recent studies. Physicians have found such consultations sufficiently useful that most—in one study up to 90%—state that they would seek another under appropriate circumstances.[94] Many patients and families also find ethics consultation helpful, and only a small percentage find it detrimental.[95] In addition, proactive ethics consultation in ICU patients has led to a statistically significant increase in the frequency and documentation of communications, increases in the number of decisions to forgo life-sustaining intervention and reductions in length of ICU stay.[96]

Early hospital ethics committees served mostly as a means of ensuring that the physician's choice of clinical options entailed the least legal risk.[92] More recently, ethics consultation has come to be seen as a service of facilitation, not authoritarian decision making.[93,97] Modern ethics committees can be helpful in conflict resolution and education but should not supplant the decision-making relationship between the primary physician and the patient and family. Furthermore, regulatory functions, such as investigating physician competence issues, are more appropriately handled by the assigned regulatory or disciplinary process in a given institution and are not the appropriate purview of a modern ethics committee.

Institutional Review Boards

After the revelations of the Doctor's Trial at Nuremberg and Henry Beecher's exposure of U.S. medical research abuses, federal legislative steps culminated in the National Research Act of 1974 requiring every institution receiving federal funding to establish a committee to review research protocols involving human subjects.[5] The National Commission for the Protection of Human Subjects of Biomedical and Behavioral Research issued recommendations for the principles that should govern human subjects research, known as the Belmont Report, in 1978, laying the groundwork for the modern IRB.[79] Researchers responded negatively to the imposition of oversight into the research process. As one congressional witness stated, "I would urge you with all the strength I can muster to leave this subject to conscionable people in the profession who are struggling to advance medicine."[80]

The mandated responsibility of the IRB is to ensure that all ethical issues have been fully addressed in the protection of human subjects of biomedical and behavioral research. The IRB is charged with reviewing all research protocols involving human subjects, weighing any and all ethical issues raised, assessing potential benefits against risks, assuring that appropriate recruitment and consent procedures are used, and at least annually reviewing the progress of each project. As of April 2003, federal law requires strict measures to protect patients' privacy, and IRBs are required within the review process to implement privacy protection for patients who are research subjects.[98]

Because IRBs are allied with institutions and not projects, they function independently of one another. Without common oversight, there is concern that the quality of review carried out by IRBs is highly variable, may overlook important aspects of projects that should be reviewed, and may be subject to institutional bias. There is further worry that some IRBs abdicate their responsibilities to carry out independent reviews in cases of multi-institutional research, thus weakening the review process.[74,80]

IRBs commonly place special emphasis on consent and recruitment procedures, but concerned voices have begun to ask whether IRBs adequately review issues such as (1) whether the research is of sufficient significance to warrant even a small risk to human subjects, (2) whether the investigator has thoroughly and honestly analyzed and presented background data to support contentions that the protocol is safe, (3) whether the research design is scientifically sound, and (4) whether the investigators is qualified to carry on the research.[74,80] Such important issues were underscored by the death of a normal volunteer subject of research studying pulmonary reflexes in asthma and another death during a phase I gene therapy trial.[99] One IRB chair reported that over a 1-year period, of 260 projects submitted for review, 31 were exempted from review, 71 were allowed expedited review because of minimal risk, and 158 underwent full review. Conditional or full approval was awarded to 126 (79%), discussion was tabled in 19, and only 13 were dispproved (8%).[74] A low rate of disapproval may indicate that a high percentage of studies have exemplary design, but it might also suggest insufficiently critical review. Additional attention may be warranted in reviewing both financial (salary and stock options) and nonfinancial (career advancement, peer recognition, publications) conflicts of interest in the research process.[73,74]

It is common for medical researchers to view the IRB as an obstacle on the road to medical advances. Particularly in light of historical and current problems protecting the autonomy and safety of research subjects, however, IRBs continue to fulfill a vital role in ethical oversight of medical investigation.

Recognizing the Physician's Moral Integrity— Conscientious Objection in Medicine

The practice of medicine is fundamentally a moral enterprise because it is guided by physicians' obligations to patients rather than themselves and because medical decision making is or should be based on ethical values and professional standards. Physicians, in other words, should not act as mere technicians, performing services on demand. Nor should physicians be guided only by their personal values, irrespective of content, but by the values and goals of medicine.

The anesthesia care of patients can involve moral controversy, disagreement, and ethical uncertainty. How should the physician respond when accepted ethical standards of care conflict with his or her own personal values? What if, for example, the anesthesiologist cannot agree to forgo resuscitation in the event of a cardiac arrest in the operating room? Or if withdrawal or withholding of nutrition and hydration runs counter to the physician's concept of ethical care?

Both medical ethicists and medical professional societies have long recognized conscientious objection in medical care. The British Medical Association, the American Thoracic Society, and the Hastings Center, for example, all provide statements recognizing the physician's right to withdraw from situations in which ethical considerations in care of patients run counter to the personal values of the physician.[100] Conscientious objection has limitations, however. Whereas acceptance of the moral objections of individual physicians to certain contentious issues such as abortion and physician-assisted suicide seems reasonable, moral objection to established standards, such as informed consent, is not. If the practice of medicine were characterized by complete value neutrality—the idea that medicine holds *no* moral or ethical values—physicians would be unable to uphold *any* ethical standards because no standards would prevail over others. Ethical decisions would be left up to the individual physician's conscience.

Conscientious objection is more likely to be supportable if the objection can be accommodated without compromising patients' rights and interest. When physicians' values conflict with established ethical standards of care, for example, they should withdraw from the care of the patient and remand care to a colleague whose beliefs do not conflict with established professional standards. The American Society of

Anesthesiologists specifically recognizes conscientious withdrawal from care in the case of patients with DNR orders or other directives that limit treatment.[48] Moral objections of physicians are also likely to have more weight if they involve conceptions the physician holds for himself or herself as an ethical doctor rather than as an ethical person, as those concepts are more likely to be founded in professionally accepted standards rather than personal beliefs.

Summary

The anesthesiologist today faces many issues in the ethical care of patients, including physician-patient conflicts, research controversies, societal issues such as allocation of health care resources, and conflicts of interest with third-party payers. These issues are particularly common and problematic in the care of patients with vascular disease, who face significant health problems while at the same time presenting the physician with ethical questions in care. Knowledge about the ethical principles in medical practice and accepted professional standards in the ethical approach to patients' care and research is essential to the practice of anesthesiology, which is and must remain more than a mere provision of technical service on demand. Anesthesiologists may at times find themselves forced to withdraw conscientiously from the care of patients when the ethical values of medicine conflict with their own personal values. Expert ethics consultation is available through hospital ethics committees and IRBs to anesthesiologists who face complex ethical issues and conflicts in patients' care and research.

REFERENCES

1. *Schloendorff v Society of New York Hospital*, 311 NY 125, 127, 129; 105 NE 92, 93, 1914.
2. Hoellerich V, Maccioli G, Coursin D: Critical care and private practice: it's the right thing to do, *Am Soc Anesthesiol Newslett* 65(8), 2001.
3. Pope Pius XII, to the International Congress of Anesthesiologists, November 24, 1957, *The Pope Speaks* 4:393, 1958.
4. MacDonald J: John J. Bonica makes obstetric anesthesia an academic concern, *ASA Newslett* 61(9), 1997.
5. Jonsen A, Beatch R, Walters L: *Source book in bioethics: a documentary history*, Washington, DC, 1998, Georgetown University Press.
6. Kopp V: Henry Knowles Beecher and the development of informed consent in anesthesia research, *Anesthesiology* 90:1756, 1999.
7. Price S: The sinking of the "captain of the ship." Reexamining the vicarious liability of an operating surgeon for the negligence of assisting hospital personnel, *J Legal Med* 10:323, 1989.
8. Scott W, Vickers M, Draper H (eds): *Ethical issues in anaesthesia*, London, 1994, Butterworth-Heinemann.
9. Rothman D: *Strangers at the bedside: history of how law and bioethics transformed medical decision-making*, New York, 1991, HarperCollins.
10. Beachamp T, Childress J: *Principles of biomedical ethics*, ed 4, New York, 1994, Oxford University Press.
11. Jonsen A, Siegler M, Winslade W: *Clinical ethics*, ed 3, New York, 1992, McGraw-Hill.
12. Braunwald E, Fauci A, Kasper D, et al (eds): *Harrison's principles of internal medicine*, ed 15, New York 2001, McGraw-Hill.
13. Furrow B: Informed consent: A thorn in medicine's side? An arrow in law's quiver? *Law Med Health* Dec:268, 1984.
14. Rizzolo P: Does a demented patient lose the right to refuse surgical intervention? *NC Med J* 53, 213, 1992.
15. Braunack-Mayer A, Hersh D: An ethical voice in the silence of aphasia: judging understanding and consent in people with aphasia, *J Clin Ethics* 12:388, 2001.

16. Mebane A, Rauch H: When do physicians request competency evaluations? *Psychosomatics* 31:40, 1990.
17. Braddock C, Edwards K, Hasenberg N, et al: Informed decision making in outpatient practice: Time to get back to basics, *JAMA* 282:2313, 1999.
18. Hamel M, Teno J, Goldman L, et al: Patient age and decisions to withhold life-sustaining treatments from seriously ill, hospitalized adults, *Ann Intern Med* 130:116, 1999.
19. Madorsky J: Is the slippery slope steeper for people with disabilities? *West J Med* 166:410, 1997.
20. Culver C, Gert B: The inadequacy of incompetence, Milbank Q 68:619, 1990.
21. Carney M, Neugroschl J, Morrison S, et al: The development and piloting of a capacity assessment tool, *J Clin Ethics* 12:17, 2001.
22. Lo B: Assessing decision-making capacity, *Law Med Healthcare* 18:193, 1990.
23. Buchanan A, Brock D: *The ethics of surrogate decision making*, Cambridge, 1991, Cambridge University Press.
24. Kain Z: Perioperative information and parental anxiety; the next generation, *Anesth Analg* 88:237, 1999.
25. Friedson E: *The profession of medicine*, New York, 1970, Dodd, Mead.
26. Layde P, Beam C, Broste S, et al: Surrogates' predictions of seriously ill patients' resuscitation preferences, *Arch Fam Med* 4:503, 1995.
27. Suhl J, Simons P, Reedy T, et al: Myth of substituted judgment: surrogate decision making regarding life support is unreliable, *Arch Intern Med* 154:90, 1994.
28. Sonnenblick M, Friedlander Y, Steinberg A: Dissociation between the wishes of terminally ill parents and decision by their offspring, *J Am Geriatric Soc* 41:599, 1993.
29. Lowenstein E (ed): *Medical ethics. International anesthesiology clinics*, vol 39, no 3, Philadelphia, 2001, Lippincott Williams & Wilkins.
30. Karlawish J: Managing death and dying in the intensive care unit, *Am J Respir Crit Care Med* 155:1, 1997.
31. Council on Scientific Affairs, American Medical Association: Good care of the dying patient, *JAMA* 275:474, 1996.
32. A controlled trial to improve care for seriously ill hospitalized patients. The Study to Understand Prognoses and Preferences for Outcomes and Risks of Treatments (SUPPORT). The SUPPORT principle investigators, *JAMA* 274:1591, 1995.
33. Covinsky K, Goldman L, Cook E, et al: The impact of serious illness on patients' families. SUPPORT investigators. Study to Understand Prognoses and Preferences for Outcomes and Risks of Treatment, *JAMA* 272:1839, 1994.
34. *Barber v Superior Court*, 147 Cal App 3d 1006, 195 Cal Rptr 484, 491, 1983.
35. *Osgood v Genesys Regional Medical Center*, Mich, no 94-26731-NH, Circuit Ct for Genesee County.
36. Von Gunten C, Ferris F, Emanuel L: The patient-physician relationship. Ensuring competency in end-of-life care: communication and relational skill, *JAMA* 284:3051, 2000.
37. *Recommended curriculum guidelines for family practice residents: end-of-life care*, Leawood, Kans, 1998, American Academy of Family Physicians.
38. *Graduate education in internal medicine: a resource guide to curriculum development*, Philadelphia, 1997, American College of Physicians.
39. Guidelines for resident training in critical care medicine, *Crit Care Med* 23:1920, 1995.
40. *Comprehensive accreditation manual for hospitals*, Oakbrook Terrace, Ill, 1996, The Joint Commission on Accreditation of Healthcare Organizations.
41. *Program requirements for residency education in anesthesiology critical care medicine*, Chicago, 1995, ACGME.
42. Rushton C, Terry P: Neuromuscular blockade and ventilator withdrawal: ethical considerations. *Am J Crit Care* 4:112, 1995.
43. Gomez C: *Regulating death: euthanasia and the case of the Netherlands*, New York, 1991, Free Press.
44. Van der Maas P, van der Wal G, Haverkate I, et al: Euthanasia, physician-assisted suicide, and other medical practices involving the end of life in the Netherlands, 1990-1995, *N Engl J Med* 335:1699, 1996.
45. Douglas C, Kerridge I, Rainbird K, et al: The intention to hasten death: a survey of attitudes and practices of surgeons in Australia, *Med J Aust* 175:511, 2001.
46. Chin A, Hedberg K, Higginson G, et al: Legalized physician-assisted suicide in Oregon—the first year's experience, *N Engl J Med* 340:577, 1999.

47. Wenger N, Greengold N, Oye R, et al: Patients with DNR orders in the operating room: surgery, resuscitation, and outcomes, *J Clin Ethics* 8:250, 1997.
48. American Society of Anesthesiologists: *ASA standards, guidelines and statements* Park Ridge, Ill, 2001, ASA.
49. American College of Surgeons: Statement on advance directives by patients: do not resuscitate in the operating room, *ACS Bull* 79(9):29, 1994.
50. Joint Commission on Accreditation of Healthcare Organizations: Patient rights chapter, *Manual of the Joint Commission on Accreditation of Health Care Organizations*, Chicago, 1994, JCAHO.
51. Olsson G, Hallen B: Cardiac arrest during anaesthesia. A computer-aided study in 250, 543 anesthetics, *Acta Anaesthesiol Scand* 32:653, 1988.
52. Casarett D, Ross L: Overriding a patient's refusal of treatment after an iatrogenic complication, *N Engl J Med* 336:1908, 1997.
53. Walker R: DNR in the OR. Resuscitation as an operative risk, *JAMA* 266:2407, 1991.
54. Hackleman T: Violation of an individual's right to die: the need for a wrongful living cause of action, 64 *U Cin L Rev*, 1355, 1370-1, 1966.
55. *Anderson v St. Francis-St. George Hospital, Inc*, 77 Ohio St 3d 82, 1996.
56. Martin R: Liability for failing to follow advanced directives. Narberth, Pa, 1999, *Physician's News Digest*.
57. Osborne M, Patterson J: Ethical allocation of ICU resources: a view from the USA, *Intensive Care Med* 22:1009, 1996.
58. Emanuel E: Cost savings at end of life: what do the data show? *JAMA* 275:1907, 1996.
59. Cowen C, Lazenby A, Martin P, et al: National health expenditures, 1999, *Health Care Financ Rev* 22:77, 2001.
60. Papper E: Rationing medical care, *Semin Anesth* 10:201, 1991.
61. Mechanic D: Dilemmas and rationing health care services: the case for implicit rationing, *BMJ* 310:1655, 1995.
62. Pawlson L, Glover J, Murphy D: An overview of allocation and rationing: implications for geriatrics, *J Am Geriatr Soc* 40:628, 1992.
63. Baker D, Shapiro M, Schur C: Health insurance and access to care for symptomatic conditions, *Arch Intern Med* 160:1269, 2000.
64. Custer W, Ketsche P: *Health insurance coverage and the uninsured: 1990-1998*, Washington DC, 1999, Health Insurance Association of America.
65. Fiscella K, Franks P, Doescher M, et al: Disparities in health care by race, ethnicity, and language among the insured: findings from a national sample, *Med Care* 40:52, 2002.
66. Kee F, Patterson C, Wilson A, et al: Stewardship or clinical freedom? Variations in dialysis decision making, *Nephrol Dial Transplant* 15:1647, 2000.
67. Naylor D, Levinton C, Wheeler S, et al: Queueing for coronary surgery during severe supply-demand mismatch in a Canadian referral centre: a case study of implicit rationing, *Soc Sci Med* 37:61, 1993.
68. Phillips R, Hamel M, Teno J, et al: Patient race and decisions to withhold or withdraw life-sustaining treatments for seriously ill hospitalized adults. SUPPORT Investigators. Study to Understand Prognoses and Preferences for Outcomes and Risks of Treatments, *Am J Med* 108:14, 2000.
69. Arndt K, Coy P, Schaafsma J: Implicit rationing criteria in non–small-cell lung cancer treatment, *Br J Cancer* 73:781, 1996.
70. Zawacki B: ICU physician's ethical role in distributing scarce resources, *Crit Care Med* 13:57, 1985.
71. Morreim E: Fiscal scarcity and the inevitability of bedside budget balancing, *Arch Intern Med* 149:1012, 1989.
72. Katz J: Human experimentation and human rights, *St. Louis Univ Law J* 7, 1993.
73. Cohen JJ: Trust us to make a difference: ensuring public confidence in the integrity of clinical research, *Acad Med* 76:209, 2001.
74. Micetich K: Reflections of an IRB chair, *Camb Q Health Ethics* 3:506, 1994.
75. Hornblum A: They were cheap and available: prisoners as research subjects in twentieth century America, *Br Med J* 315:1437, 1997.
76. *Final report of the Advisory Committee on Human Radiation Experiments*, Washington, DC, 1995, Government Printing Office.
77. Beecher H: Ethics and clinical research, *N Engl J Med* 74:1354, 1966.
78. Cohn C: Medical experimentation on prisoners, *Perspect Biol Med* Spring: 357, 1978.
79. National Commission for Protection of Human Subjects of Biomedical and Behavioral Research: *The Belmont report: ethical principles and guidelines for the protection of human subjects of research*, DHEW publication No. (OS) 78-0012, Washington, DC, 1978.
80. Silverman WA: Bad science and the role of institutional review boards, *Arch Pediatr Adolesc Med* 154:1183, 2000.
81. Jones J: Ethics of rapid surgical technological advancement, *Ann Thorac Surg* 69: 676, 2000.
82. Shapiro H: Animal rights and biomedical research: no place for complacency, *Anesthesiology* 64:142, 1986.
83. Report of the American Medical Association Council on Scientific Affairs. Animals in research, *JAMA* 261:3602, 1989.
84. Hewitt H: Benefits of animal research and the doctor's responsibility, *Br Med J* 300:811, 1990.
85. Roberts I, Kwan I, Evans P, et al: Does animal experimentation inform human healthcare? Observations from a systematic review of international animal experiments on fluid resuscitation, *Br Med J* 324:474, 2002.
86. Donnelly S, Nolan K (eds): *Animals, science and medicine* Hastings Center report, special supplement, New York, 1990, Hastings Center.
87. Martin J: The rights of man and animal experimentation, *J Med Ethics* 16:160, 1990.
88. Burns R: Animals in research, *Acad Med* 62:780, 1989.
89. Teel K: The physician's dilemma: a doctor's view: what the law should be, 27 *Baylor L Rev*, 6, 8-9, 1975.
90. Johnson S: Managed care as regulation: functional ethics for a regulated environment, *J Law Med Ethics* 23:266, 1995.
91. Council on Ethical and Judicial Affairs, American Medical Association: Ethical issues in managed care, *JAMA* 273:330, 1995.
92. Waisel D, Troug R: How an anesthesiologist can use the ethics consultation service, *Anesthesiology* 87:1231, 1997.
93. Aulisio M, Arnold M, Youngner S: Health care ethics consultation: nature, goals, and competencies. A position paper from the Society for Health and Human Values–Society for Bioethics Consultation Task Force on Standards for Bioethics Consultation, *Ann Intern Med* 133:59, 2000.
94. La Puma J, Stocking CB, Darling Cm, et al: Community hospital ethics consultation: evaluation and comparison with a university hospital service, *Am J Med* 92:346, 1992.
95. Orr R, Morton K, deLeon D, et al: Evaluation of an ethics consultation service: patient and family perspective, *Am J Med* 101:135, 1996.
96. Dowdy M, Robertson C, Bander J: A study of proactive ethics consultation for critically and terminally ill patients with extended length of stay, *Crit Care Med* 26:252, 1998.
97. Spike J, Greenlaw J: Ethics consultation: high ideals or unrealistic expectations? *Ann Intern Med* 133:55, 2000.
98. Annas G: Medical privacy and medical research—judging the new federal regulations, *N Engl J Med* 346:216, 2002.
99. Savulescu J: Two deaths and two lessons: is it time to review the structure and function of research ethics committees? *J Med Ethics* 28:1, 2002.
100. Wicclair M: Conscientious objection in medicine, *Bioethics* 14:205, 2000.

Index

Note: Page numbers followed by f indicate figures; those followed by t indicate tables.